WARREN HOLLEMAN

WARREN HOLLEMAN

# Fundamentals of
# Clinical Practice, Second Edition

# Fundamentals of Clinical Practice, Second Edition

Edited by

## *Mark B. Mengel, M.D., M.P.H.*

St. Louis University
St. Louis, Missouri

## *Warren L. Holleman, Ph.D.*

Baylor College of Medicine
Houston, Texas

and

## *Scott A. Fields, M.D.*

Oregon Health Sciences University
Portland, Oregon

**Kluwer Academic / Plenum Publishers**
**New York, Boston, Dordrecht, London, Moscow**

ISBN 0-306-46692-9

© 2002 Kluwer Academic / Plenum Publishers
233 Spring Street, New York, N.Y. 10013

http://www.wkap.nl/

10   9   8   7   6   5   4   3   2   1

A C.I.P. record for this book is available from the Library of Congress

Printed in the United States of America

To those dedicated practitioners of the art who taught us that
the core of clinical practice remains the
patient–physician relationship

# Contributors

**Bruce Ambuel, Ph.D., M.S.,** Associate Professor of Family & Community Medicine, Waukesha Family Practice Residency Program, Waukesha, Wisconsin 53188

**Elisabeth D. Babcock, Ph.D.,** President/CEO, Committee to End Elder Homelessness, Boston, Massachusetts 02118

**Cyndi Jewell Baily, J.D.,** Associate General Counsel, Senior Vice-President and General Counsel, Baylor College of Medicine, Houston, Texas 77030

**Kristen Lawton Barry, Ph.D.,** Senior Associate Research Scientist, Department of Psychiatry, University of Michigan, Ann Arbor, Michigan 48108

**Alan M. Blum, M.D.,** Professor and Gerald Wallace Chair, Department of Family Medicine, College of Community Health Sciences, University of Alabama School of Medicine, Tuscaloosa, Alabama 35401

**Thomas L. Campbell, M.D.,** Professor of Family Medicine and Psychiatry, University of Rochester School of Medicine and Dentistry, Rochester, New York 14620

**William M. Chop, Jr., M.D.,** Education and Research Foundation, Waco Family Practice Residency Program, Heart of Texas Community Health Center, Waco, Texas 76707-2291

**John L. Coulehan, M.D., M.P.H.,** Professor of Preventive Medicine and Director, Institute for Medicine in Contemporary Society, SUNY at Stony Brook, Stony Brook, New York 11794-8036

**Mark R. Cullen, M.D.,** Professor of Medicine and Public Health, Program Director, Yale Occupational & Environmental Medicine Program, Yale University School of Medicine, New Haven, Connecticut 06510

**Larry Culpepper, M.D., M.P.H.,** Professor and Chairman, Department of Family Medicine, Boston University School of Medicine, Boston, Massachusetts 02118-2393

**Annette M. David, M.D., M.P.H.,** Associate Professor, Department of Physiology, Clinical Associate Professor, Department of Medicine, University of the Philippines, Philippine General Hospital Medical Center, Manila, Philippines

**Frank Verloin deGruy III, M.D., M.S.F.M.,** Woodward-Chisholm Professor and Chair, Department of Family Medicine, University of Colorado Health Sciences Center, Denver, Colorado 80220

**Larry L. Dickey, M.D., M.P.H.,** Chief, Office of Clinical Preventive Medicine, Department of Family and Community Medicine, University of California at San Francisco, San Francisco, California 94143-0900

**Diane L. Elliot, M.D.,** Professor of Medicine, Division of Health Promotion and Sports Medicine, Oregon Health Sciences University, Portland, Oregon 97201

**Ronald M. Epstein, M.D.,** Associate Professor of Family Medicine and Psychiatry, University of Rochester School of Medicine and Dentistry, Rochester, New York 14620

**Kathleen R. Farrell, D.O.,** Assistant Professor, Division of General Internal Medicine, Oregon Health Sciences University, Portland, Oregon 97201-3098

**Laura B. Frankenstein, M.D.,** Physician, St. Alexius Senior Health Center, St. Louis, Missouri 63105

**L. Kevin Hamberger, Ph.D.,** Professor of Family & Community Medicine, Racine Family Practice Center, Medical College of Wisconsin, Racine, Wisconsin 54401-0548

**Linn Goldberg, M.D.,** Professor, Internal Medicine, Oregon Health Sciences University, Portland, Oregon 97201

**Warren L. Holleman, Ph.D.,** Associate Professor and Director, Baylor/Star of Hope Family Counseling Center, Department of Family and Community Medicine, Baylor College of Medicine, Houston, Texas 77030

**James N. Hyde, M.A., M.S.,** Associate Professor, Department of Family Medicine and Community Health, Tufts University School of Medicine, Boston, Massachusetts 02111

**Ann C. Jobe, M.D., M.S.N.,** Dean and Professor of Family Medicine, Mercer University School of Medicine, Macon, Georgia 31207

**Victoria S. Kaprielian, M.D.,** Associate Clinical Professor and Director, Quality Improvement and CME, Department of Community and Family Medicine, Duke University Medical Center Durham, North Carolina 27710

**Dana E. King, M.D.,** Associate Professor of Family Medicine, Department of Family Medicine, Medical University of South Carolina, Charleston, South Carolina 29425

**Eliana C. Korin, Dipl. Psic.,** Senior Associate Faculty, Director of Behavioral Science, Department of Family Medicine and Community Health, Montefiore Medical Center, Bronx, New York 10467

**John P. Langlois, M.D.,** Associate Clinical Professor and Director, MAHEC Division of Family Medicine, Department of Family Medicine, University of North Carolina, Mountain AHEC Asheville, North Carolina 28804

**Barry S. Levy, M.D., M.P.H.,** Adjunct Professor of Community Health, Tufts University School of Medicine, Sherborn, Massachusetts 01770.

**Mark Loafman, M.D., M.P.H.,** Associate Director, Loyola-West Suburban Family Practice Residency Program, Oak Park, Illinois 60302

**Christopher J. Mansfield, MS, Ph.D.,** Associate Professor and Director, Center for Health Services Research and Development, The Brody School of Medicine, East Carolina University, Greenville, North Carolina 27858

**Larry B. Mauksch, M.Ed.,** Clinical Associate Professor, Department of Family Medicine, University of Washington Family Medicine Residency, Seattle, Washington 98105

**Susan H. McDaniel, Ph.D.,** Professor of Psychiatry and Family Medicine, and Director, Wynne Center for Family Research, University of Rochester, Rochester, New York 14620

**Monica McGoldrick, M.A., M.S.W., Ph.D. (Honorary),** Director, Multicultural Family Institute of New Jersey, Highland Park, New Jersey 08904

**Catherine P. McKegney, M.D., M.S.,** Assistant Professor, Department of Family Practice and Community Health, University of Minnesota, Minneapolis, Minnesota 55408

**James W. Mold, M.D.,** Professor of Family Medicine and Preventive Medicine, University of Oklahoma Health Sciences Center, Oklahoma City, Oklahoma 73190-1050

**William Monroe, Ph.D.,** Professor of English and Associate Dean, The Honors College, University of Houston, Houston, Texas 77204-2090

**Warren P. Newton, M.D.,** William B. Aycock Professor and Chair, Department of Family Medicine, University of North Carolina School of Medicine, Chapel Hill, North Carolina 27599-7595

**John S. Rolland, M.D.,** Clinical Professor and Co-Director, Center for Family Health, University of Chicago Pritzker School of Medicine, Chicago, Illinois 60611

**Roger A. Rosenblatt, M.D., M.P.H.,** Professor and Vice Chair, Department of Family Medicine, University of Washington, Seattle, Washington 98195-4795

**David B. Seaburn, Ph.D.,** Assistant Professor, Psychiatry and Family Medicine, University of Rochester School of Medicine and Dentistry, Rochester, New York 14620

**Sara G. Shields, M.D., M.S.,** Assistant Professor, University of Massachusetts Family Practice Residency Program, Worcester, Massachusetts 01655

**Peggy B. Smith, Ph.D.,** Professor, Departments of Psychiatry, Obstetrics and Gynecology, and Pediatrics; Director, Teen Health Clinics; Director, Baylor Population Program, Baylor College of Medicine, Houston, Texas 77030

**Eric J. Solberg,** Program Director, Clinical Cancer Genetics, M. D. Anderson Cancer Center, Houston, Texas 77030

**Howard F. Stein, Ph.D.,** Professor of Family Medicine and Preventive Medicine, University of Oklahoma Health Sciences Center, Oklahoma City, Oklahoma 73190-1050

**Elizabeth Steiner, M.D.,** Assistant Professor, Department of Family Medicine, Oregon Health Sciences University, Portland, Oregon 97201

**Jeff Susman, M.D.,** Professor and Chair, Department of Family Medicine, University of Cincinnati, Cincinnati, Ohio 45267-0582

**Marlene F. Watson, Ph.D.,** Assistant Professor and Director, Graduate Program in Couple and Family Therapy, MCP Hahnemann University, Philadelphia, Philadelphia 19102

**Kathleen A. Zoppi, Ph.D., M.P.H,** Assistant Professor and Behavioral Science Director, Department of Family Medicine, Indiana University, Indianapolis, Indiana 46202

# Preface

*Fundamentals of Clinical Practice, Second Edition*, is an introductory textbook focusing on the patient, the physician, and society from a biopsychosocial perspective. Readers will be introduced to many important areas of clinical practice that have been neglected in more disease-based textbooks, including the patient's perspective on illness, what it means to be a physician both from a historical perspective and in today's society, important skills physicians will need to practice medicine, relationships and their importance to health, values and their importance to health, and special problems that all physicians should learn how to treat. This edition should prove very useful to medical students during their first- and second-year clinical skill courses.

The second edition was born in response to suggestions of readers and faculty regarding the first edition of *Fundamentals of Clinical Practice* and its companion volume, *Introduction to Clinical Skills*. Based on a survey of users, it was clear to us that users of both of the above textbooks wanted a one-volume text that included elements of both books. New content on the physician in literature, law in medicine, and spirituality in medicine was desired. Additionally, a second edition was desperately needed owing to advances in research in these areas and thus all of the chapters have been thoroughly updated.

As in our last edition, all chapters include numerous illustrative cases and conclude with cases for discussion that we hope will be utilized by small groups of learners to further discuss these important issues. Since our textbook cannot provide all of the information a practicing physician will need, each chapter concludes with a section of recommended readings that allows students to pursue more in-depth information in these areas. Finally, in response to the recommendations of predoctoral directors, we have developed a teacher's guide to assist faculty in facilitating discussion groups and evaluating students' understanding of this material through sample test questions.

To organize this material, this text is divided into three parts, Part I on the patient, Part II on the doctor, and Part III on society. Part I, "The Patient," begins with a discussion on human health and disease followed by a chapter on the individual and family life cycle, describing developmental issues from the patient's perspective.

Part II, "The Doctor," contains three sections. The first section on the person of the physician describes the emotional and moral effects of medical school and residency, what it means to be a physician in today's society, and a historical perspective of the physician's role in society through literature. The second section describes those basic clinical skills required of all clinicians including interviewing, taking a history, performing a physical examination, using laboratory tests appropriately, making a diagnosis, instituting treatment, and keeping accurate records. More advanced skills are described in the third section including performing a clinical interview in difficult circumstances, managing chronic illness, counseling patients for behavioral change, assessing functional status, promoting health and preventing disease, and critically appraising the literature.

Part III, "Society," also contains three sections: relationships, values, and special problems. Important relationships that can affect the patient's health are described in the first section, starting with the patient–physician relationship. Important societal systems including the family, community, workplace, environment, patient's culture, and the overall healthcare system are explored in depth to show the learner how these multiple contexts shape the patient–physician relationship and the care that is delivered to patients. The second section on values covers ethics, economics, the law, and spirituality. A third section on societal problems focuses on those difficult issues that have a profound effect on our patients' health including tobacco use, substance abuse, violence, mental illness, sexually transmitted diseases, and maternal and child health problems. These topics have often been ignored within the medical school curriculum because they do not fit neatly into a disease-oriented model of care.

Our hypothesis is that by exploring these issues in more depth, medical students will be able to form more effective therapeutic relationships with their patients—by attending to issues that do not fit neatly within a disease-oriented biomedical model of care—and will be better able to understand and advise their patients on ways they can improve their health, not just cure or control a disease.

Finally, a cautionary note: Skill development takes time. While many learners will master quickly the knowledge contained in these chapters, the skills described require practice. Many students will not feel comfortable with the more complex skills until residency training. Do not be discouraged. Continue to practice, and as you practice and watch the health of your patients improve, gain satisfaction in your efforts. Just as learning the technology and science associated with a disease-based biomedical model is important, learning these clinical skills will complement that knowledge and lead to greater professional satisfaction.

Mark B. Mengel, M.D., M.P.H
*St. Louis, MO*

Warren L. Holleman, Ph.D.
*Houston, TX*

Scott A. Fields, M.D.
*Portland, OR*

# Acknowledgments

Without the aid of many people this textbook simply would not be possible. Numerous colleagues have supported this project, even to the point of being chapter authors.

Special thanks go to our students, who have stimulated us to update and improve our ideas on generalist clinical skills development and the physician–patient relationship. In particular, first- and second-year medical students have asked the "embarrassing" questions that have prompted us to conceptualize and then reconceptualize our understanding of which skills are necessary to improve health and to establish the therapeutic patient–physician relationship.

Our secretaries Marie Michaud, Christine Sargus, and Pamela Tise have performed well and tirelessly in helping us meet deadlines. Michael M. Le developed or redesigned many of the images and figures in this volume. We also thank the editorial staff at Kluwer Academic / Plenum Publishing, headed by Mariclaire Cloutier, who has been very supportive and understanding of our many foibles. They have been particularly helpful in editing our rather long-winded confusing prose into much briefer, more understandable sentences.

Lastly we thank our families, without whose support the long hours necessary—usually after work—to put together a book of this size and scope would not have been possible. Our wives Marsha Cline Holleman, Vicki Fields, and Laura Frankenstein, and our children Annie, Tom, and Sally also helped in bringing us back to reality.

# Contents

# PART I

# The Patient

The premise that the patient is the focus of the physician's efforts is so obvious that is does not warrant stating. As physicians focus on disease, however, the personhood of a patient often gets lost as an irrelevant or insignificant detail. These chapters help to reestablish the focus on the patient—not only their disease, but also their personhood—by explaining the complex nature of human health and disease and also the developmental life cycles that are important for physicians to understand when caring for patients of all ages.

## CHAPTER 1

# Human Health and Disease

*Roger A. Rosenblatt*

*An elderly woman consulted her physician because she was having dizzy spells and couldn't sleep. Her husband had recently died, and her only child lived on the other coast. The results of her physical exam were essentially normal, except for mild hypertension.*

*The physician, unsure of the diagnosis, ordered a series of tests, which included a 24-hour electrocardiogram searching for arrhythmias, an electroencephalogram, a CT scan of the head, and a variety of blood tests. When these were unrevealing, he referred her to a neurologist, who did some additional tests, again finding nothing abnormal. The neurologist referred her to an otolaryngologist, suspecting middle ear dysfunction, but more tests were not helpful. Medicare paid for about half of the charges incurred, and the patient received sheaves of bills for the balance. Six months later, her symptoms were unchanged.*

## EDUCATIONAL OBJECTIVES

1. Provide students with a picture of the social and organizational context in which modern U.S. medicine is provided
2. Give students insight into the balance between benefit and harm that results from encounters with the medical care system
3. Introduce students to epidemiology and health services research as tools to help gauge the extent to which medical care interventions are likely to benefit patients

## U.S. MEDICINE AS AN ANOMALY

The U.S. medical enterprise is an anomaly on the world stage. Put simply, the United States spends more on medical care than any other nation, yet millions of citizens lack ready access to even the most basic healthcare services. Despite an enormous investment in healthcare—over a trillion dollars annually in 1995 and growing rapidly—healthcare status as measured by such conventional measures as infant mortality or

3

longevity is only fair, lagging far behind other countries that invest much smaller shares of their national wealth in providing medical care (Rice, 1994; Schieber *et al.*, 1994).

U.S. medicine has evolved along a path quite different from that taken by other industrialized countries (Reinhardt, 1997). Although medical care occupies much of our interest and our wealth, the basic strategy for delivering medical care services has been left largely to the vagaries of chance and self-interest. Not only is the United States without an organized national health service, but it also lacks any financing mechanism to ensure that individuals can obtain needed healthcare without plunging into penury. Healthcare policy is determined primarily by groups who profit from the decisions that they make, namely, insurance and pharmaceutical companies, hospitals, physicians, and other healthcare professionals. Medical care in the United States is a "market-oriented health care system spinning out of control" (Relman, 1994).

Not only is the medical enterprise careening across the social landscape without anyone at the helm, there is also considerable question as to whether the activities on which we spend our time and money contribute to the health of either the individual patient or the society of which she is a part (McKinlay *et al.*, 1989). The woman described in Case 1-1 presents her physician with the problem of dizziness, and he deploys an impressive array of technical gadgets to try to find that part of her anatomy causing her to experience this disquieting symptom. But as is usually the case, her symptom cannot be understood simply as a mechanical failure; it is just as likely to be caused by depression following her husband's death, despair related to social isolation, or a normal consequence of an aging neurological system. The physician's traditional approach generates considerable revenues for those who survey and interpret the tests, but the woman herself does not benefit. In fact, awash in additional bills and made anxious by the cascade of tests, she has actually been harmed by her encounter with the medical care system (Fisher & Welch, 1999).

The purpose of this chapter—and this entire book—is to place the medical endeavor in a broader biological, psychological, and social context. Specifically, this chapter will:

1. Introduce readers to the determinants of health, illness, and disease, placing the role and importance of medical care within a broad social, cultural, and economic context
2. Explore the role of the physician in modern industrial/technological society and the potential benefits and harm that derive from the physician's activities
3. Encourage physicians to be parsimonious and skeptical in their approach to medical care
4. Introduce the powerful tools provided by epidemiology and health services research to determine how physicians can best do those things that are most likely to improve the well-being of individuals and society

As practitioners of the healing arts, we have the ability to assist people in confronting and addressing the inevitable health problems that are as much a part of life as breathing or walking. But we cannot discharge this trust adequately if we become passive parts of a dysfunctional machine.

## CASE 1-2

*The old black man was found crumpled beside a wall, flaccid and unconscious. When brought to the emergency room, he was awake but unable to talk or move the left side of his body. His blood pressure was elevated and he smelled of alcohol and tobacco. When the ER staff reached his ex-wife, she told them that he had lost his job as a school custodian 6 months earlier when rising Medicaid costs led to a reduction in state funding for schools. Two days later the patient had a second, more massive stroke and died after a short period on a ventilator. The resident wrote "cerebrovascular accident" in the space on the death certificate reserved for cause of death.*

## The Health of the Individual

Medicine is a reductionist endeavor; we break human beings down into organs, cells, and molecules to gain insight into and power over fundamental biological processes. But for us as complete human beings, biochemical pathways are less important than psychological states of being. Individuals search for peace and wholeness, and health is the end point of only one ingredient of that quest.

Operationalizing health, that is, coming up with a definition that lets us know whether our activities are enhancing the health of individuals, is difficult. The World Health Organization offers a lofty but essentially vacuous formula: "Health is a state of complete physical, mental, and social well-being, and not merely the absence of disease or injury." Such a state is both unobtainable and unmeasurable, although it does generate humility in pointing out both how wide of that mark we are as humans and how medicine contributes only a small part to the attainment of such an Elysian state.

A more parsimonious and more useful approach is to define health as the absence of pain and dysfunction. Although there is an element of subjectivity even in this spare yardstick, we can at least measure whether our interventions have made people more comfortable or more functional. From a practical stand-point, it is usually physical or psychological pain that leads patients to consult physicians, and it is only fair that physicians focus their efforts on the identified problems of the individuals seeking help.

The major source of our discomfort in wrestling with all of these definitions is the fact that living is also dying. Aging seems to be woven anarchically into the very process of cell division, so that the embryo sows the seeds of its ultimate dissolution. If we examine human longevity historically, it becomes evident that the total human life span has changed little across the centuries for which we have accurate records, Methuselah and his cousins notwithstanding. The triumph of science—particularly public health interventions—is that a greater proportion of the population survives the random physical and biological agents of destruction to reach their 70s and 80s. Until we repeal the seemingly inexorable limits built into cellular biology, our goal is not so much to lengthen life as to decrease suffering and premature death.

Thus, we as physicians often find ourselves pulled in different directions by the desires of our patients and our scientific formulation of the problems with which they present. Patients bring us their symptoms and their sorrows, and we turn them into diseases that we hope can be found in the pages of texts like this one. The art of medicine lies in using our scientific knowledge to address the existential needs of our patients, without lapsing into quackery on the one hand or irrelevant technological sophistication on the other. The most powerful tool for doing this is to understand that our patients are part of larger social structures that are just as important as the smaller structures of which they are composed (Adler *et al.*, 1993).

The resident was "anatomically correct" in assigning the cause of death of our second patient to a cerebrovascular accident. The terminal event occurred when a bit of eroded atherosclerotic plaque from the intimal surface of the carotid artery lost its moorings, drifted downstream, and lodged in the distribution of the middle cerebral artery. Deprived of blood flow and oxygen, part of the brain died, and the patient with it. But was it an "accident"? And was the cause of death cerebral anoxia, or was it the patient's unemployment, alcoholism, or social status? The pathologist who sliced the brain may have ignored these questions, but an accurate autopsy would encompass more than blood vessels and clotting parameters. In the following discussion we will rise above the autopsy table, searching for causation not in end points, but in antecedents.

## The Health of the Family

Humans cannot exist as solitary organisms. As Bowlby's pioneering work on human development demonstrated, infants raised in hygienic but nonnurturing settings become autistic, physically perfect but functionally flawed (Bowlby, 1983). Even more subtle deprivation can thwart normal development, as the modern epidemics of sexual abuse and the growth of the underclass demonstrate.

With rare exceptions, physicians are constantly reminded that their patients exist as parts of family units, even though families come in many shapes and sizes. Even as we hone in on the underlying pathophysiology that is the material stuff of disease, we realize that the impact of illness on the individual is mitigated or amplified by the family of which the patient is a part. The aging man whose wife dies is much more likely to join her in death than is his peer with an even worse disease but whose wife is hale and hearty (Gallagher *et al.*, 1982).

It is literally impossible to understand the patient without understanding both his family of origin and the current family structure. This may sound ludicrous when talking about something as cut-and-dried as a fractured ankle, upper respiratory infection, or metastatic breast cancer. But in each of these cases the family structure—in all of its variation—is important both in the etiology of the disease and in our ability to help the patient overcome the problem.

The patient with a broken ankle may have suffered the injury on the ski slopes, but his ability to use crutches while the injury heals depends to a certain extent on both the physical and social environments of the family. Who will do the shopping during the 6 weeks in the cast? The child with URI and repeated ear infections may have gotten them because the mother smokes or because the child spends much of the day in an overcrowded and underventilated day-care center. The patient with breast cancer is likely to have different feelings about aggressive chemotherapy—and different desires about long-term goals—depending on the health of her spouse, the desires of her children, and her own experience watching her mother die of the same disease.

The situation becomes even more graphic when the diseases themselves arise in the cauldron of the family. Certainly emotional disabilities, from garden-variety depression to exotic forms of obsessive–compulsive disorder, have at least some of their roots in the family situation. But the real challenge to the clinician is to remember—and incorporate—the family dimension into even the most mundane of presenting complaints. Although the divorce of the school custodian in Case 1-2 did not "cause" the subsequent stroke, a stable marriage might well have prevented or mitigated the physiological changes that led ultimately to the fatal event. Understanding family dynamics is just as important for the cardiologist as for the family physician—all patients come supplied with families, just as all patients come supplied with hearts. And both are needed for human beings to live, function, and thrive.

## The Health of the Social Group and the Effect of Society on Health

Individuals belong to an interlocking series of social groups, from the small circle of the nuclear family to ever-widening circles that include neighborhoods, communities, cultures, and nations. The composition of these social groups—and the person's place within them—has a profound effect on every aspect of life. In the same way that the manner in which a child is raised shapes intelligence and personality, a person's position within society affects employment, happiness, health, and longevity.

A growing body of evidence demonstrates that a person's health depends on many factors that are frequently ignored by practitioners (Evans *et al.*, 1994). We tend to look for the causes of disease in such things as genetic defects, specific pathogens, deleterious health habits, or harmful accidents. But the health of the individual is also strongly related to much more amorphous social distinctions such as social class, employment, race, and ethnicity. It is the interaction among all of these factors that raises or lowers a person's susceptibility to illness and affects the chances of recovery once illness has begun (Adler *et al.*, 1993; McEwen, 1998). Sidebar 1 is a graphic illustration that something as fundamental as infant mortality is exquisitely dependent on the parental race, independent of rural or urban residential location.

Medical care has a part to play in determining the health status of the individual and the larger society, but the part is relatively small compared with other social forces. Even the most sophisticated diagnostic and

## INFANT MORTALITY BY RACE AND RURAL/URBAN
## RESIDENTIAL STATUS, UNITED STATES, 1991–1995

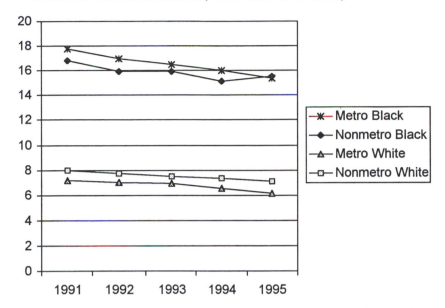

*Graph adapted from: Slifkin RT, Goldsmith LJ, Ricketts TC: Race and place: Urban–rural differences in health for racial and ethnic minorities. Working Paper No. 66, North Carolina Rural Health Research Program, Chapel Hill, NC, 2000, 7.*

therapeutic technologies are of less importance than the basic ingredients of life, such as food, shelter, clothing, and self-respect. The absence of any of these latter factors is just as devastating as most cancers. In addition, most of the medical interventions that have improved the health of populations have little to do with the traditional patient–physician relationship. Safe food and water, the development of vaccines, and the implementation of immunization programs, the use of seat belts, and efforts to curb smoking all depend on broad social programs aimed at populations, not individuals (Cluff, 1987).

Thus, it is critical to view medical care as just one way in which society attempts to improve the well-being of individuals, as well as the larger population. All too frequently, the immediacy and drama of the individual clinical encounter crowd out the prosaic but effective strategies that concentrate on improving everyone's health rather than the health of one person. This enormous concentration of resources directed at the individual diverts social investment in other interventions—education, social programs, and so forth—that have greater potential to improve the social and physical milieu. The irony is that the enormous resources that we pour into medical care tend to be taken away from services such as education or social services that ultimately have a much greater impact on whether a person lives a healthy life. The United States expends a far greater proportion of its national wealth on medical care than any other country, but this vast investment is not reflected in such a basic measure as our infant mortality rate.

We should return for a moment to our hapless patient in the emergency room, terminally ill from a stroke. Although we can and will use sophisticated imaging technologies to locate and describe the lesion in his brain, the real lesion lies in the society from which he sprung. Black men in our society have dismal health prospects, and real improvements in the health of African-Americans will require policies that address racism, employment, social status, and income distribution. Although it may seem artificial to suggest that rising Medicaid costs drain resources from the education budget, this dynamic is being played out in innumerable state legislatures as this book is being written. The physician with an interest in the health of his or her patients

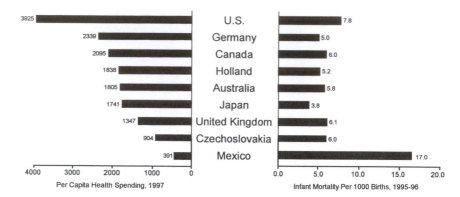

*International comparisons of health expenditures and infant mortality. Taken from an address by Larry Green, MD, at the annual meeting of the Association of Departments of Family Medicine, San Juan, Puerto Rico, 2000.*

must also become involved in broader social policies that affect the well-being of the entire population, messy and fractious as this arena always is.

# The Health of the Planet

Humanity's ultimate hubris is anointing itself as the pinnacle of creation. In this view, the world exists to further the aims of humankind, and all other species are at best subservient and at worst irrelevant to our pursuit of our own ends. The consequences of this world-view surround us: environmental degradation, wholesale destruction of species and habitat, and rampant pollution.

The root cause of many of these catastrophic effects lies in the tremendous overpopulation of the planet in the last 100 years. Medicine has played a significant part in this most devastating of biological changes (Green, 1992). Just as the industrial revolution created the technological tools to radically alter the biosphere in which we live, the emergence of modern medical interventions vastly increased effective human fertility. Declining environmental quality is now beginning to affect directly the health of individual humans, just as it has already begun to affect the quality of life for humans and many of the other species with whom we share this planet (Leaf, 1989).

What role do the medical profession and the individual physician have to play in averting this looming tragedy? The most important step is to acknowledge the problem in all of its depressing enormity and to educate ourselves and our families, colleagues, and patients about its personal and general importance at every opportunity. Denial and repression are perhaps the strongest psychodynamic mechanisms within the human mind. When confronted with a threat to global existence, the natural tendency is to consign it to some distant future date, outside our personal realm of interest or control. But the reality is that these changes have occurred relatively quickly and can be reversed just as quickly, given our technological capacity. The difficulty lies in changing two behaviors—reproduction and consumption—that are so powerful that modifying them is considerably more difficult than, say, stopping smoking.

In the clinical arena, the individual physician can have an enormous impact by giving couples the information and the techniques needed to control their own fertility. A very large proportion of pregnancies are unplanned and unwanted, disrupting and impoverishing the families involved (Gottlieb, 1995). By eliminating all unintended pregnancies in the United States, we could achieve a dramatic reduction in the overall birth rate, a reduction that if replicated worldwide could have a marked impact on the rate of population rise.

Physicians play an important role in educating children and adolescents about sexual development and fertility control. All primary care physicians—and most specialists—have the opportunity to raise the issue of family planning with their patients as part of routine health maintenance activities. And while most physicians will not perform abortions, the physician has the responsibility to make patients aware that this is a safe and legal procedure, even while trying to provide the patient with the knowledge and the tools to prevent unwanted pregnancies. If the individual clinician does not wish to provide these services because of moral or ethical reservations, he or she should support the right of other members of the profession to include termination of pregnancy in their repertoire.

The physician is sanctioned by society as a healer, and as such has the opportunity to influence the conditions that promote or undermine good health. All of our efforts at helping individual patients deal with their infirmities and diseases will be swept away unless we are part of the process that also restores and protects the health of the earth.

## CASE 1-3

*The patient, moribund on Friday, had revived by Monday. After conventional chemotherapy had failed to arrest his terminal lymphosarcoma, the attending physician had given him a shot of Krebiozin, heralding the event with a sense of drama and pageantry. Although there was no scientific evidence that Krebiozin was effective, the tumors had melted to half their original size, and the patient returned home for two glorious disease-free months. He relapsed and quickly died after the newspaper printed an AMA article stating flatly that Krebiozin was worthless.* *

# THE PHYSICIAN'S ROLE—WHAT PART DO WE PLAY?

## The Physician as Healer—Source of Our Social Legitimacy

The role of physician has multiple roots, the sturdiest of which is that of healer (McWhinney, 1998). In every prehistoric or primitive culture, selected individuals are sanctioned by their community as healers, charged with diagnosing and treating the illnesses of individuals or at times groups. Healers are expected to have acute powers of observation, extensive knowledge about the natural realm, and the ability to mediate and intervene between the causes of illness and their impacts on individuals.

In primitive and prehistoric societies, the role of healer was grafted onto and combined with that of religious leader. The mysteries of life and death were intermingled, and it was natural that the role of healer be conferred on that individual who mediated between the natural and the supernatural. Although the shaman or medicine man may have had limited empirical knowledge of disease as we understand it, he was not ineffective. By tapping into a shared communal understanding of life and its travails, he had the trust and confidence of the patient and the family (Bloom, 1965). And trust and faith can heal, whether we call this the placebo effect, the inevitable consequence of self-limited illnesses, or the use of "alternative" physical and medicinal agents that promote the restorative functions of normal physiology.

As far as we know, empiricism was first grafted onto the shamanistic role with the emergence of the Greek schools of medicine in the fourth century B.C. (Sigerist, 1960). The schools at Cos and Cnidus developed systematic approaches to the study of human anatomy, physiology, and the coherence of certain types of illness. The Greek physician may still have traveled like a minstrel from town to town, but he was judged more on his diagnostic and prognostic accuracy than on his ability to commune with the gods.

*Adapted from an article by Bruno Klapfer, *Journal of Projective Techniques*, 1957—cited in articles by Anne Harrington, *Probing the Secrets of Placebos*, Harvard Medical Alumni Bulletin, Winter 1995, 35.

The evolution of the modern role of the physician derives from both of these sources. Medicine emerged as a guild or profession during medieval times, not much more scientifically advanced than the early Greeks. The emergence of the scientific method during the fifteenth century enabled a better understanding of basic physical and biological processes. Medicine as a profession benefited enormously. But even though today's physician-technician may interpret genetic patterns and employ lasers, the social role of the physician as healer still undergirds our relationship to patients and our place in society. When we forget these foundations, we unnecessarily limit our ability not only to provide comfort, but also to promote healing (White, 1988).

Physicians in today's society still stand at the interface between the secular and the priestly. Although most patients will not have spontaneous remissions when their cancers are treated with placebos like Krebiozin, we do have the power to heal because of the patient's belief in our skill, expertise, and commitment. In our frenetic world, many problems that patients bring to the physician are expressions of disequilibrium, anxiety, or the cumulative effects of physical, psychological, and social stress (McEwen, 1998). We are most effective in restoring balance and relieving suffering when we use tools such as empathy and concern, when we listen and support rather than probe and test.

## CASE 1-4

*The child lay on the gurney, seemingly intact, but mute after having fallen off her bicycle. The pediatric emergency room physician did his best to find some remediable cause of the child's coma, but it was clear that she had a severe closed-head injury, with little chance of recovery. The pediatrician established with the parents that the child had not been wearing a bicycle helmet, trying not to blame them for the injury to their daughter. These cases bothered the pediatrician more than all of the cases of leukemia and meningitis that he saw, because they seemed to be so preventable.*

*After his shift was over, the pediatrician sat down with some of his colleagues and planned a study to determine the frequency of children's head injuries and what could be done to make helmets more available and more likely to be used. The campaign took several years, but ultimately the proportion of kids wearing helmets increased, and the number of head injuries coming to emergency rooms decreased. After this experience, the pediatrician decided to tackle another problem that brought kids into his ER, namely, gun injuries. He is still working on that one.*

## The Evolution of Public Health and Its Relationship to Medical Care

One of the great ironies of medicine is that the most effective interventions are directed at populations, while most of the resources go for the care of individuals. We have explored this concept earlier and now must grapple with how this anomaly can be addressed by the individual physician. In the country as a whole, we have done a spectacularly poor job of partitioning resources between curative and public health. Yet the individual physician can help restore the balance not only by providing the best care to each patient who walks in the door, but also by keeping in mind the *population* of patients who could benefit from the skills of the physician.

We acknowledge that most of the work that physicians will do is with individual patients, and much of the job of medical school and residency is to make physicians excel in their care of individual patients. Yet most physicians want to have an impact on the people whom they treat, and an important way to multiply one's impact is to intervene at the family, social group, or population level.

The targets of opportunity exist in virtually every segment of medicine, no matter how specialized. One can draw the inspiration to pursue these issues from one's clinical practice and special expertise, as did the pediatrician in Case 1-4. The primary care physician has limitless opportunities, based on the type of practice, from prevention of falls in the elderly to improving vaccination rates among immigrants. But a population-based perspective is by no means limited to primary care. The neurosurgeon certainly can get involved in both the prevention of head injuries by emphasizing the use of seat belts for motorists and helmets for motorcyclists and better treatment of patients with head injuries by emergency medical technicians. Oncologists can get involved in reducing the presence of carcinogens in the community or encouraging people to avoid excessive exposure to the sun. Thoracic surgeons may choose to be involved with programs designed to help parents stop smoking or to prevent kids from starting.

Public health is likely to remain weak in the United States, if only because of the relentlessly individualistic focus of our society. One way to redress this imbalance is for all physicians to incorporate the public health perspective in their work and in their lives. Not only will these efforts pay off in better health for the population, and for individual patients, but they are a potent antidote to the burnout and the cynicism that can invade the life of the busy practitioner. You may not be able to get Mrs. Smith to give up cigarettes, even though her emphysema propels her into your office every time the air pollution increases, but you may be able to help her child avoid the same dismal outcome.

For those with a particular interest in population-based medicine, the concept and practice of community-oriented primary care (COPC) may have special appeal (Tollman, 1991). The basic tenet of COPC is that the individual physician can effectively care not only for a collection of individual patients, but also for an entire defined community (Waitzkin & Hubbell, 1992). Even in the disorganized chaos of our disjointed medical care system, most physicians provide care to some group of patients that can be counted and described. For the rural physician, it may be possible to characterize all of the people living in a small town or within the catchment area of a specific rural hospital. For the urban physician, it may be a collection of neighborhoods or a particular suburb.

In all of these cases, the physician—wearing a public health hat—can find out about the prevalence of disease that afflicts this particular group of people. And knowledge confers power, because an understanding of the cause of the disease allows the physician to get involved in organized efforts to intervene. The target can be something as straightforward as making sure that the elderly have flu vaccines or as complex as trying to tackle the problem of teenage pregnancy in a rural high school. But in either case, there are sets of tools and approaches that the physician can use to multiply his or her effectiveness and combine the mantle of healer with that of physician to the community.

---

## CASE 1-5

*The stylish woman flew into the office, trailing an overloaded briefcase, an umbrella, and a few wisps of errant cigarette smoke. "My allergies are killing me," she said, almost before the physician entered the room. "That Seldane you gave me didn't do a thing; haven't you got something better?"*

*The physician glimpsed the chart: a succession of brief visits for episodic ills, all annoying, none serious. His eyes glanced at the health maintenance form he kept at the front of every chart, unsullied in this case by any entries. He noticed that he'd written "Smoking" on the problem list, but realized that was as far as he'd ever gotten.*

*"I have just the thing for you," he said. "There's a new steroid nasal inhaler that will knock out those allergy symptoms. But I don't think we'll make a lot of progress until we talk a bit about your smoking. And I also notice that you haven't had a Pap smear or a breast exam in years."*

*"Oh, doctor, be a dear and write me a prescription for the allergy puffer. I'll be sure to make an appointment to get that Pap smear."*

# FROM PREVENTION TO CURE TO PALLIATION—WHEN TO INTERVENE?

In the previous section, we confronted the dilemma faced by the physician trying to decide what portion of his energy to spend wrestling with the fundamental public health problems that cause disease and what portion to spend with individual patients who manifest these diseases. In this section, we address a different sort of priority setting: the competition between taking care of the acute episodic problems that patients bring to us and focusing our energies on preventing the appearance of disease.

The patient who breezes into the office wanting a nostrum for her nostrils—but postponing the Pap smear and avoiding any mention of her smoking—exemplifies the dilemma. Many physicians act like outfielders, i.e., the patient hits the ball, the physician fields it briskly, handles it briefly, tosses it back, and then turns to the next fungo, hoping that it won't go over the fence. The physician lives in the present, and the workday is defined by what gets past the second baseman, or the receptionist in this case.

Although every primary care physician must learn to become a good fielder, the job requires more than the ability to handle whatever ball is hit his way. Although some of the promises of the health promotion/ disease prevention approach have been overblown by individual medical disciplines and the popular press, many preventive activities make good sense. In our particular case, the physician can have more impact on the health, longevity, and well-being of this young woman by tackling the smoking issue than by writing a ream of prescriptions.

The unique asset of the primary care physician is that he has the knowledge, the leverage, and the opportunity to interweave curative and preventive medicine together. Our harried young female executive might prefer to avoid discussion of her smoking, but her allergies won't let her. And she has enough faith in her personal physician—faith distilled out of repeated visits during which her physician has solved other problems—that she can be forced to confront the more fundamental issue of smoking. This may not be the visit where she decides to quit, but evidence shows that the concerned physician, probably more than any other person in society, can encourage and sustain smoking cessation.

Our physician is also armed with an extremely powerful tool, namely, the health maintenance protocol. For every patient, there are a handful of health promotion and disease prevention activities that have been shown to be effective in detecting or preventing disease. Customized for each patient—based on his or her age, sex, racial and ethnic heritage, occupation, family history, and personal behaviors—are a set of health maintenance activities that are inexpensive and efficacious (U.S. Preventive Services Task Force, 1990).

The key to an effective health maintenance program is a program that is customized for each patient and contains only those elements that are both efficacious and cost-effective, both in the economic and in the social sense. Routine chest x-rays and electrocardiograms will occasionally reveal unexpected "pathology" in patients, but to what effect? Many of the tests that are glibly espoused by groups with a particular interest in a disease—from routine prostate-specific antigen (PSA) to mammograms at age 30—may do the individual patient more harm than good. Tests can cause harm either by exposing patients to radiation, finding conditions that either cannot or should not be treated, or simply causing unnecessary cost and anxiety. The key for the primary care physician is to focus on those conditions where early detection will make a difference to the particular patient to whom they are applied.

Fortunately, an enormous amount of superb work has been done in helping to craft such health maintenance protocols. Frame and Carlson, community physicians in upper New York state, pioneered the work in this field, and their papers inspired scores of physicians who have followed in their footsteps (Frame & Carlson, 1975a–d). Their approach, originally presented in 1975 and updated in 1986, subjects each potential test or intervention to six critical criteria (from Frame & Carlson, 1975a):

1. The condition must have a significant effect on the quality or quantity of life.
2. Acceptable methods of treatment must be available.
3. The condition must have an asymptomatic period during which detection and treatment significantly reduce morbidity or mortality.
4. Treatment in the asymptomatic phase must yield a therapeutic result superior to that obtained by delaying treatment until symptoms appear.
5. Tests that are acceptable to patients must be available at reasonable cost to detect the condition in the asymptomatic period.
6. The incidence of the condition must be sufficient to justify the cost of screening.

**13**

PRESERVING
CONTEXT WHILE
ADDRESSING THE
NEEDS OF THE
INDIVIDUAL:
MARSHALING THE
TOOLS

These six principles are enormously powerful in focusing our attention on areas where prevention works, makes sense, and is economical. This approach is not static: As our understanding of the pathophysiology and natural progression of disease expands, and as new tests are developed, the list expands and contracts. An extremely practical product of this approach has been the recommendations of the Canadian Task Force on the Periodic Health Examination and the U.S. Preventive Services Task Force. Both groups used the Frame and Carlson approach, and both forged practical age-specific guidance to the application of preventive healthcare in the context of primary care practice (Goldbloom *et al.*, 1989; U.S. Preventive Services Task Force, 1990). See Chapter 15 on Health Promotion and Disease Prevention in *Introduction to Clinical Skills: A Patient-Centered Textbook*.

One of the important ingredients of a successful health maintenance program in primary care is a medical care system that supports such an approach, both financially and organizationally. If the physician works in a community where there are too few healthcare providers, the effort of caring for individual patients crowds out attention to potentially more important public health issues. If the physician works for a hospital that expects each physician to see 25 patients a day to earn a yearly incentive bonus, the tendency will be to write the prescription and ignore the wisps of tobacco smoke. And if the insurance for the patient specifically excludes health maintenance, both the physician and the patient will have to examine the fiscal impact of tests and activities that the insurance company will not cover.

Fortunately, most employers, managed care organizations, and insurance companies have realized that carefully designed health maintenance protocols save money as well as improve the length and quality of life. To the extent that physicians see their role as caring for patients rather than for individual episodes of illness, health maintenance becomes a more sensible and rewarding activity. The adept and successful physician will blend prevention seamlessly into the more traditional practice of curative medicine.

## CASE 1-6

*Annie was referred from Port Angeles, a logging town on the Olympic peninsula, after her catastrophic GI bleed sent her into acute renal failure. By the time she arrived at University Hospital, she was in a coma, caused by the combination of profound blood loss, renal failure, and sepsis.*

*The intern struggled for days to try to restore some semblance of biochemical homeostasis. Dialysis was begun, antibiotics were given, and Annie was monitored in the ICU. One crisis followed another, as one physiological system after another in her aging body was overwhelmed by the illness.*

*The intern became obsessed with the goal of keeping Annie alive; he slept on a cot in the corridor rather than go home even on the nights he wasn't on call. He was partly goaded on by the troop of relatives who stood around Annie's bed, watching these medical heroics. They were mute, almost sullen, but present for every blood gas measurement, x-ray, or dressing change.*

*On the seventh day of her hospitalization, Annie developed disseminated intravascular coagulation and bled to death. The intern was at her bedside with the family and looked at them apologetically, feeling as if he were a complete failure. The patient's brother looked back at him, bobbed his head wearily, and said, "Thank God it's finally over; we have been hoping she would be spared this torture for days." (This case is a description of one of the author's first patients during his first rotation on the medical service during his internship year.)*

## PRESERVING CONTEXT WHILE ADDRESSING THE NEEDS OF THE INDIVIDUAL: MARSHALING THE TOOLS

When physicians sit for their board exams in the specialty they have chosen, they will have spent at least a decade mastering material relevant to the exam. From that first premed biochemistry course in college, through anatomy in medical school, to the rigors of residency, physicians are immersed in a series of educational experiences designed to make them reasonably comfortable with taking care of the problems brought to them by patients. Although the medical curriculum has its flaws, U.S. physicians are arguably the best practitioners of the science of medicine in the world.

U.S. medicine is far from perfect, however, as we have discussed in this introductory chapter. While the U.S. physician can bring more scientific firepower to bear on the physical problems of any particular patient than most physicians in other countries, it does not follow that the U.S. physician is more effective than his peers. The fault lies both in the organization of the medical care system and in the role of the physician within society.

Although the individual physician cannot remedy these imperfections alone, there is a set of tools that can multiply the effectiveness of physicians. In this section we briefly review a handful of those that can be simply and practically applied in the day-to-day practice of medicine. The three tools are the biopsychosocial perspective, population-based medicine, and clinical epidemiology. They have been touched on in different ways in the discussion thus far in this chapter, but they are so important to effective clinical medicine that it is worth revisiting them briefly in a slightly different way.

## Treat Human Beings, Not Patients

I will never forget Annie, in Case 1-6, because I never knew her when she was alive. She appeared in the ward of our tertiary care hospital, and I did what I had been trained to do: try to restore physiological equilibrium to a body that had been ravaged by disease. I couldn't talk to her—she was comatose. I didn't talk to her family, even though they surrounded me, because it never occurred to me that they would have anything of value to tell me. Had I asked, I would have learned that Annie would have rejected the vain attempt to rescue her from what turned out to be irreversible pathophysiologic processes. I was devastated by her death; her family was relieved.

Annie, unfortunately, was and is a typical hospital patient. The failure in this case was not our inability to forestall death, but the failure to ensure that the medical response was meaningful in terms of the patient's life and illness. She may have been unable to provide any detail, but her family was available and was not consulted. She came from a different culture and a different social class from the physicians who cared for her, and that was a part of the barrier between us. But the major impediment was our narrow focus on vital signs, culture reports, and lab tests. We maintained our distance from the patient to protect ourselves from the overwhelming enormity of her illness. We pursued our own goals and interests, rather than allowing her to die with dignity. Excessive medical care can cause harm for patients, their families, and society, as the accompanying figure shows.

Medicine does not exist in a vacuum, even though the actions of physicians often seem to be unconnected to the larger world. The essential tool for the physician is breadth of vision, the ability to place the patient in a context. It is not a question of injecting humanism into medicine. Rather, medicine needs to be reformulated as a scientific endeavor within the human domain (Schwartz & Wiggins, 1988). The biopsychosocial perspective is just as important to the relevance and effectiveness of the modern physician as the germ theory of disease (Engel, 1977).

## Population-Based Medicine: A Way to Set Goals for Yourself and Your Practice

Unfortunately, we do not always have the luxury of totally separating ourselves from the organizational structures that shape many aspects of the medical encounter. In the rapidly disappearing fee-for-service model of medicine, physicians have subtle (and sometimes not so subtle) incentives to schedule more visits, perform more tests, and do more procedures. Equally pernicious are those managed care systems that install physician gatekeepers, especially when physicians benefit financially from stinting on the care provided to an individual patient. When physicians benefit personally from either giving too much or too little care to their patients, a conflict of interest arises that can undermine the trust that cements the physician–patient relationship.

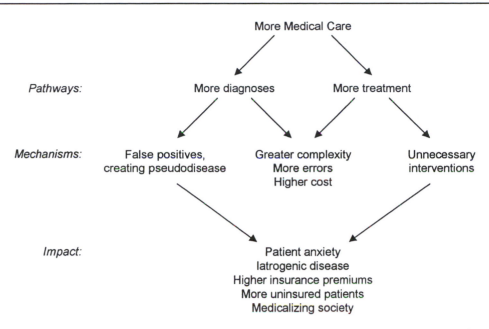

*Adapted from: Fisher ES, Welch HG. Avoiding the unintended consequences of growth in medical care. How might more be worse? JAMA 281:446–453, 1999.*

Retaining a patient-centered focus when dealing with individuals does not, however, release the physician from concern about the fiscal and social ramifications of his actions. As I discussed in my review of community-oriented patient care, the physician is in a privileged position to focus not only on the problems that patients bring to the medical visit, but also on the underlying public health issues that cause illness and suffering in the population generally. In that respect, the physician also has the responsibility to think about whether medical expenditures would have more impact if spent on other activities, from improvements in the educational system, to bolstering family planning capability, to job creation or environmental protection.

Population-based medicine is in many ways the antithesis of personal medical care. Population-based medicine deals with the denominator, an entire group of people defined by residence, race, social class, or culture; personal medical care deals usually with the individual, although at times the family unit—broadly defined—is the target of the medical intervention. Population-based medicine is a tool used to change social policies, priorities, and programs that affect large groups of people. Personal medical care is aimed at individuals, often when they are sick or in an attempt to detect or prevent illness.

Although physicians are not usually trained in the skills of population-based medicine, they need to be active participants in the arenas where these decisions are made. The relatively little attention paid to population-based medicine and public health in the United States does not mean that policies are not articulated. Rather, the healthcare system that has evolved has embedded within it the implicit value that the quality and range of medical services will be determined by patient income, employment, and social status (Reinhardt, 1997). To the extent that individual physicians do not agree with those decisions, they need to be involved in resetting these broader social goals.

## CASE 1-7

*The man sat sheepishly in the exam room, a piece of paper in his hand. "My wife sent me in for a PSA test," he explained. "You know, one of those tests that tells me if I have cancer of the prostate. She read about it in* **Good Housekeeping.***"*

*The physician tried to dissuade the man from getting the test, who was a vigorously healthy 70-year-old, had normal findings on prostate exam, and had no symptoms, but the wife's instructions prevailed. The test came back elevated, and the physician sent him on to a urologist. The patient underwent a biopsy, which was negative. He began to get annual PSA exams and had several repeat biopsies, each of which was quite painful and left the patient feeling old and weak.*

## Epidemiological Principles as a Way to Understand the Balance between Health and Illness

Most physicians understand the logic of the biopsychosocial approach to medical care, even if the rigors of daily medical practice may leave them without the time or energy to ask about family and friends. Population-based medicine is even more remote, both because physicians receive little training in its application and because it seems to exist in a realm far removed from the day-to-day practice of medicine.

Clinical epidemiology provides a tool that ties together many of the themes of this chapter, bridging the world where physicians interpret the tests of individual patients and policymakers try to make decisions about the policies that shape medical practice in this country (Fletcher *et al.*, 1982). Epidemiologists—and their partners in crime, biostatisticians—use their observations of the incidence, prevalence, and natural course of illness and medical treatment to try to extract generalizable rules about both illnesses and treatments. Clinical epidemiology harnesses those observations to the work of the individual physician.

The patient described in Case 1-7 is one you will see a thousand times, with minor variations. Is ordering a PSA logical for this 70-year-old, or would his life have been better if he had gone without? Should one get an exercise tolerance test for the middle-aged man who would like to run a marathon? Should one use expensive pills to reduce the cholesterol level in a 70-year-old woman from 230 to 190? And what does it mean when the alkaline phosphatase reading on the routine blood test is 5% above the normal range?

The individual clinician must become a professional skeptic, armed with enough knowledge of epidemiology to critically evaluate the unending stream of data spewed out by the professional and popular press. Not only are many of the nostrums, tests, and interventions urged on us expensive irritations, many of them are potentially dangerous. The patient in Case 1-7 was lucky. Had the biopsy showed a small focus of cancer, he might have ended up with a radical prostatectomy, which carries a high risk of impotence and incontinence. Those might be acceptable outcomes if the procedure were lifesaving, but we don't yet know whether prostate cancer in elderly males is even a disease, much less whether lives will be saved by surgery. This hasn't prevented an explosion in the number of radical prostatectomies, largely because physicians and patients alike are much more comfortable with action than inaction, even when evidence is lacking for efficacy.

I would argue that clinical epidemiology is a subject just as essential to the modern physician as a basic understanding of anatomy. We expect physicians to have a fairly precise idea of the locations of the main organs and the way they are interconnected, even though the ability to name all of the metacarpals generally fades as soon as the faintly prurient acronymic ditty is forgotten. By the same token, the physician should have a firm understanding of the concepts of specificity, sensitivity, prevalence, and predictive value, even if the nuances of odds ratios are something that has to be looked up. Health and illness are not pure states of being, but exist as physical, social, and epidemiological constructs. The competent physician will understand health and illness from all of these perspectives.

## CONCLUSION: THE HUMAN COMEDY— MAN AS PART OF NATURE

Although Galileo had the intellectual courage to revoke man's place at the center of the universe, he paid a heavy price for his heresy. Although we know with our minds that man is but a mote on a speck of dust lost in the immensity of space, we know with our bellies that we are the masters of creation and that the stars continue to revolve around the earth.

The central challenge of life is accepting the brevity of our individual existence. We are born into pain and shackled to mortality. We spend much of our existence looking for nostrums or diversions to blur this painful reality or deny it by invoking magical kingdoms where we will leave our corporeal bodies behind.

Medical care as an organized human activity grows out of our unwillingness to accept passively the anonymous but destructive effects of entropy and accident. Part of the allure of the medical profession is the chance to struggle against the impersonal forces of nature, to deal with our own mortality by mitigating the suffering of others. This book seeks to put this struggle into a broader context, to acknowledge the interrelationships between the individual, the society in which she is embedded, and the entire planetary community of which that society is a part. Most of medical education focuses on the powerful tools of a focused trade. But physicians are more than body mechanics, and we fail in our quest to improve the lives of individuals if we don't also direct attention to the broader social and ecological context in which they lead their lives.

Becoming an effective physician requires more than technical competence or even well-honed interpersonal skills. Although it will be a continual and often frustrating challenge, the physician has a responsibility both to herself and to the species to engage in the broader issues while also responding to the very real existential suffering of the individual.

These two activities will at times exist together and at times proceed in parallel. The goal is not ultimate success—just as with the life cycle of individuals, the art is in the process as opposed to the product. Medicine is a rewarding struggle, but a struggle nonetheless.

## CASES FOR DISCUSSION

### CASE 1

*Mrs. O'Callahan is a 48-year-old clerical worker who lives alone after a painful divorce 3 years ago. Since then she has had a succession of physical problems, including headaches, reflux, insomnia, and foot pain. She comes in to see you now because she has been having twinges of chest pain for about 2 weeks, getting worse particularly in the last 3 days. Her physical exam is unrevealing.*

1. *Your initial suspicion is that her chest pain is psychophysiologic, but you know that she has a strong history of heart disease in her family. How would you proceed with the initial workup?*
2. *Although the results of the first tests that you order are normal, the symptoms do not abate. Mrs. O'Callahan becomes more and more concerned about them and asks whether or not she should be referred to a cardiologist. Her managed care plan is structured in such a way that any referrals to outside specialists come out of your capitation (the insurance that you receive monthly for taking care of Mrs. O'Callahan). How does this affect your decision?*
3. *While you are trying to unravel the problem, you learn from another physician that he was sued by the patient because she charged that he was negligent in working up her arthritis. How does this affect your relationship with the patient and the decisions you make regarding her care?*
4. *The patient starts showing up in the emergency room without calling your office and demanding that she be admitted to the coronary care unit. You suggest that she might want to consider psychological counseling, but she rejects that suggestion angrily. What do you do now?*
5. *There is obviously no one correct answer for this problem, and part of the reason for these questions is to help the student and instructor discuss the task of dealing with difficult patients. The key concepts that the student and teacher might address include the importance of understanding the health belief model that the patient brings to the encounter and the very strong relationship between psychological distress and physical symptoms.*

### CASE 2

*Phyllis was only 15 when she came into your office, but she wanted to get pregnant. She lived in a housing project not too far from your office with her 35-year-old mother and three younger sisters. She smoked, was doing poorly in school, and fought with her mother and her mother's boyfriends. She also had bad asthma, which got worse in the spring and after she and her mother had been at war. She had been having unprotected intercourse for about 4 months and wondered why nothing had happened.*

1. *Your first inclination is to talk to Phyllis's mother, but the teenager doesn't want her mother to know that she's coming in to see you. Are you willing to continue seeing Phyllis without the mother's involvement?*
2. *On further questioning, you find that Phyllis has been suspended from school after getting into a shoving match with another girl during lunch. What responsibility do you have for following up on this?*
3. *Phyllis eventually does get pregnant and asks if you would be willing to deliver the baby. What is your response?*
4. *You are a bit worried about Phyllis's sisters, whom you haven't seen for quite a while. Is there anything you can do about their healthcare?*

## CASE 3

*Mary, a 42-year-old white woman, has been seeing you for years as her family physician. You've also been taking care of her husband Roy, a 45-year-old black Vietnam veteran with a long-term drinking problem. Mary has terrible headaches that get worse before her periods and also has been having trouble with their teenage son.*

1. *Mary comes in one day and asks you what you think of feverfew, a homeopathic headache remedy that one of her friends recommends. What is your opinion?*
2. *Although Mary has been trying to get Roy to stop drinking for years, it has been to no avail. Recently he's told her to shut up or get out. What advice can you offer Mary?*
3. *Roy has worsening hypertension, hypercholesterolemia, and a terrible family history of heart disease. Should you try to get him started on antihypertensive and lipid-lowering agents?*
4. *The teenage son has run away from home, been picked up by the police, and ends up in the youth shelter. Mary calls you in a panic. What is your response?*

## CASE 4

*You have just gone to work in a small apple-growing town in the eastern part of the state. Although many of the surrounding farm families are well-off, the town itself is decrepit. There is a large population of Hispanic migrant workers, some who still migrate and some who have settled in. There is quite a lot of racial tension between the older white families and the migrants who pick the crops, and everyone drives around with a rifle in the pickup and a handgun in the glove compartment. You are struggling to make your practice a success but also would like to do something to reduce the number of accidents and traumatic injuries from fights that keep you up nights in the emergency room.*

1. *You have a sense that the accident rate is much higher in your town than in others like it in the state but aren't sure. What can you do to find out if your appraisal is correct?*
2. *The state comes out with a program to improve emergency medical services in rural towns but requires that the money go to an elected community board. What role do you have in establishing or running such a board?*
3. *The hospital administrator is at his wit's end because the government's healthcare program for migrants doesn't pay for inpatient care. What advice do you offer him?*
4. *Juan, a 32-year-old migrant apple picker, comes in with scabies, which he got from the dirty bedding in one of the shacks provided by a local farmer. What do you prescribe for Juan, and what do you tell your county health department?*

## CASE 5

*You live in a town in the central United States where there is a large open pit mine, the main industry for that region. You notice that your patients are showing signs and symptoms of lead poisoning, which is confirmed by blood tests. The mine is financially tenuous, with old technology and marginal yields; it seems unlikely that it could afford to install appropriate pollution control equipment.*

*1. What do you tell your patients when their children show elevated levels of lead in their blood?*
*2. How do you inform the local industry?*

**Acknowledgments.** I would like to acknowledge the helpful suggestions of Theodore Phillips, John Geyman, and Robert Beaglehole.

# RECOMMENDED READINGS

Bloom SW: *The Doctor and His Patient: A Sociological Interpretation.* New York, Free Press, 1965.

> The classic—but still relevant—study of the role and function of the physician from the sociologic perspective.

Evans RG, Barer ML, Marmor TR: *Why Are Some People Healthy and Others Not? The Determinants of Health of Populations.* New York, Aldine de Gruyter, 1994.

> A comprehensive and readable analysis of the relationship between social organization and the health of the individual.

Illich I: *Medical Nemesis: The Expropriation of Health.* New York, Pantheon Books, 1976.

> This perceptive social critic details the extent to which the medicalization of ordinary life can undermine the health of both the individual and the larger society.

White KW: *The Task of Medicine: Dialogue at Wickenburg.* Menlo Park, Calif, Henry J. Kaiser Foundation, 1988.

> A modern reexploration of the biopsychosocial model of human disease.

# REFERENCES

Adler NE, Boyce WT, Chesney MA, Folkman S, Syme SL: Socioeconomic inequalities in health: No easy solution. *JAMA* 269:3140–3145, 1993.
Bloom SW: *The Doctor and His Patient: A Sociological Interpretation.* New York, The Free Press, 1965.
Bowlby J: Attachment and loss: Retrospect and prospect. *Annu Prog Child Psychiatry Child Dev*, 1983, pp 29–47.
Cluff LE: New agenda for medicine. *Am J Med* 82:803–810, 1987.
Engel GL: The need for a new medical model: A challenge for biomedicine. *Science* 196:129–136, 1977.
Evans RG, Barer ML, Marmor TR: *Why Are Some People Healthy and Others Not? The Determinants of Health of Populations.* New York, Aldine De Gruyter, 1994.
Fisher ES, Welch HG: Avoiding the unintended consequences of growth in medical care: How might more be worse? *JAMA* 281:446–453, 1999.
Fletcher RH, Fletcher SW, Wagner EH: *Clinical Epidemiology—The Essentials.* Baltimore, Williams & Wilkins Co, 1982.
Frame PS, Carlson SJ: A critical review of periodic health screening using specific screening criteria. Part 1. Selected diseases of respiratory, cardiovascular, and central nervous systems. *J Fam Pract* 2:29–36, 1975a.
Frame PS, Carlson SJ: A critical review of periodic health screening using specific screening criteria. Part 2. Selected endocrine, metabolic, and gastrointestinal diseases. *J Fam Pract* 2:123–129, 1975b.
Frame PS, Carlson SJ: A critical review of periodic health screening using specific screening criteria. Part 3. Selected diseases of the genitourinary system. *J Fam Pract* 2:189–194, 1975c.
Frame PS, Carlson SJ: A critical review of periodic health screening using specific screening criteria. Part 4. Selected miscellaneous diseases. *J Fam Pract* 2:283–289, 1975d.
Gallagher DE, Thompson LW, Peterson JA: Psychosocial factors affecting adaptation to bereavement in the elderly. *Int J Aging Hum Dev* 14(2):79–95, 1982.
Goldbloom R, Battista RN, Haggerty J: Periodic health examination, 1989 Update: 1. Introduction. *Can Med Assoc J* 141(3):205–207, 1989.
Gottlieb BR: Abortion—1995. *N Engl J Med* 332:532–533, 1995.
Green CP: The Environment and Population Growth: Decade for Action. Population Reports, Series M, No. 10. Baltimore, Johns Hopkins University Population Information Program, 1992.
Leaf A: Potential health effects of global climatic and environmental changes. *N Engl J Med* 321:1577–1583, 1989.
McEwen BS: Protective and damaging effects of stress mediators. *N Engl J Med* 338(3):171–179, 1998.
McKinlay JB, McKinlay SM, Beaglehole R: A review of the evidence concerning the impact of medical measures on recent mortality and morbidity in the United States. *Int J Health Serv* 19:181–208, 1989.
McWhinney IR: Primary care: Core values in a changing world. *Br Med J* 316:1807–1809, 1998.
Reinhardt UE: Wanted: A clearly articulated social ethic for American health care. *JAMA* 278:1446–1447, 1997.
Relman AS: The health care industry: Where is it taking us? in Lee PR, Estes CL (eds): *The Nation's Health.* Boston, Jones & Bartlett, 1994, pp 67–75.
Rice DP: Health status and national health priorities, in Lee PR, Estes CL (eds): *The Nation's Health.* Boston, Jones & Bartlett, 1994, pp 45–58.
Schieber GJ, Poullier J-P, Greenwald LM: Health system performance in OECD countries, 1980–1992. *Health Affairs* 13:100–112, 1994.

Schwartz MA, Wiggins LP: Scientific and humanistic medicine: A theory of clinical methods, in White KW (ed): *The Task of Medicine: Dialogue at Wickenburg*. Menlo Park, Calif, The Henry J. Kaiser Family Foundation, 1988, pp 137–171.

Sigerist HE: The physician's profession through the ages, in Marti-Ibanzez (ed): *Henry Sigerist on the History of Medicine*. New York, MD Publications, 1960, pp 3–15.

Tollman S: Community oriented primary care: Origins, evolution, applications. *Soc Sci Med* 32:633–642, 1991.

U.S. Preventive Services Task Force: The periodic health examination age-specific charts. *Am Fam Physician* 41:189–204, 1990.

Waitzkin H, Hubbell FA: Truth's search for power in health policy: Critical applications to community-oriented primary care and small area analysis. *Med Care Rev* 49:161–189, 1992.

White KL: *The Task of Medicine: Dialogue at Wickenburg*. Menlo Park, Calif, The Henry J. Kaiser Family Foundation, 1988.

## CHAPTER 2

# The Individual and Family Life Cycle

*Eliana C. Korin, Monica McGoldrick, and Marlene F. Watson*

*A family physician was worried about a patient, a 53-year-old woman whose blood pressure had become progressively elevated despite appropriate treatment; no cause for secondary hypertension or noticeable changes in her life were identified. Mrs. Garcia, the patient, a pleasant and energetic Latina widow, was living with her daughter and two grandchildren. One day, she brought her 18-month-old granddaughter to her physician for a routine medical visit with complaints of sleep problems. The toddler often cried or had temper tantrums at bedtime.*

*While assessing the child's development, the physician also explored the family situation. The child was the result of an unexpected though welcomed pregnancy of a a full-time working mother, who already had a 12-year-old son. When the grandmother was asked how this unexpected return to childrearing responsibilities had been for her, she confessed that in her enthusiasm to have a granddaughter, she did not anticipate the emotional and physical demands posed by an active toddler at this stage of her life. The patient's stress was exacerbated because of feelings of discomfort in renegotiating childcare arrangements with her daughter, whom she had promised to support when her husband had left home. Moreover, given the present situation, she could not pursue her plans to spend the winter holidays with siblings in her hometown.*

*At this point, the physician realized the impact of the family dynamics and life cycle issues on his patients' health. The grandmother's blood pressure and the child's sleep problems were successfully addressed as the physician promoted a dialogue between grandmother and mother focusing on the symptoms as responses to the family's adaptation to a new life-cycle stage.*

## EDUCATIONAL OBJECTIVES

1. Understand and formulate clinical problems from a life-cycle and sociocultural perspective
2. Define specific emotional issues and tasks individuals and families face as they go through the life cycle, and relate them to particular medical issues
3. Anticipate the types of clinical problems that will arise for patients as they go through the life cycle

As Case 2-1 indicates, the individual and family life-cycle perspective provides a useful framework for understanding and addressing everyday clinical problems. Over time, the family moves through various life-cycle stages, and new demands emerge requiring individual adaptation and family reorganization. When individuals and/or families resist or fail to adapt to these changes, symptoms are likely to appear. Therefore, the clinician should always ask: "In which life-cycle stage is this patient and his family? How are they dealing with life-cycle transitions?" As illustrated in Case 2-1, the unexpected birth of a child disrupted the natural cycle of life in the family, resulting in interpersonal conflicts and health problems. The symptoms—the grandmother's blood pressure and the child's sleep problems—were successfully addressed when the physician recognized the symptoms as resulting from the family's difficulty in adapting to a new life stage.

The family life cycle is an important predictor of stress, which is often greatest at transitional points when the family is moving from one developmental stage to another (Carter & McGoldrick, 1999). Medical visits tend to occur at times of transitions, such as the birth of a child, the launching of a child into adulthood, and the disability or death of a parent. An understanding of family life-cycle stages assists physicians in

- Anticipating medical problems
- Developing preventive and health promotion strategies
- Formulating hypotheses about medical problems
- Designing effective treatment strategies

To assist the student in understanding the impact of the family on the health of its members, this chapter will discuss individual development as it occurs within the family life cycle (FLC), describe the FLC stages in relation to health problems, and illustrate the application of the FLC model in medical practice. To appreciate the FLC, however, we must first understand basic patterns in the life cycle of the individual and the relationship between individual and family life cycles.

## CASE 2-2

*Mary Petlock was already pregnant with her second child when she learned that her first, David, aged 2, who had been developmentally delayed in speech and motor skills, was indeed retarded. As the physician spoke with her about David's diagnosis and prognosis, Mary began to realize that the family would be having to deal with his developmental disabilities throughout their future. She worried about how to deal with the loss of the many dreams and hopes she and her husband had for David's life, and about how the other children might have to sacrifice some of their own interests and activities and assume caretaking roles themselves. Mary also worried about how she and the rest of the family would make these adjustments.*

*The following year Mary's husband, Joseph Verdum, lost his job as a salesman for a large corporation and was unable to find another job. Because of the financial pressures of the new baby, Sam, their retarded son, David, and Joe's unemployment, the couple moved in with Mary's parents. This new living arrangement put pressure on Mary and Joe's relationship, as Mary felt more like a daughter than a mother in her parental home, subject to her mother's continual comments about how she was handling her children and her "lazy" husband. Joe, who did not feel at home with his in-laws, began staying out more, drinking at the local bar. Joe resented his wife's attention to her parents. He also resented David's disability and refused to help care for him. To help support the family, Mary took a part-time nursing job. The following year, with Joe still unemployed, Mary's mother, Anna, aged 55, was diagnosed with Alzheimer's disease.*

## THE INDIVIDUAL LIFE CYCLE IN CONTEXT

Evaluating problems in terms of both individual and family life cycles is an important part of the medical assessment. The accomplishment of certain physical, intellectual, social, spiritual, and emotional life-cycle

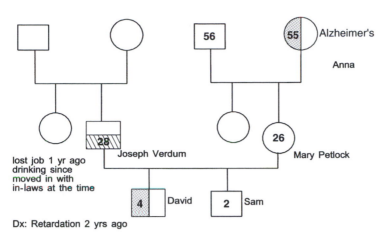

**Figure 2.1** Genogram of the Verdum/Petlock family.

tasks is part of normative development. Each person's individual life cycle intersects with the family life cycle at every point, at times causing conflict of needs. For instance, in Case 2-1, the toddler's developmental needs conflicted with the grandmother's life plans. Furthermore, when individual family members do not fit into normative expectations for development, there are repercussions on family development, as indicated in Case 2-2 (see Fig. 2.1). Similarly, a family's adaptation to its tasks will influence how individuals negotiate their individual development.

Traditional Western formulations of human development have begun with the individual as a psychological being and defined development as growth in the human capacity for autonomous functioning. In Eastern cultures the very conception of human development begins with the definition of a person as a social being and defines development as the evolution of the human capacity for empathy and connection. We present a theory of individual and family development in a social context integrating race, class, gender, and culture as central factors that structure development in fundamental ways. This theory defines maturity by our ability (1) to live in respectful relation to others and to our complex and multifaceted world, while being able (2) to control our own impulses, and (3) to think and function for ourselves, on the basis of our own values and beliefs, even if others around us do not share them. Maturity requires the ability to empathize, trust, communicate, collaborate, and respect others who are different, and to negotiate our interdependence with our environment and with our friends, partners, families, communities, and society in ways that do not exploit others.

## Developing a Self in Context

In every society, gender, class, culture, and race form a basic structure within which individuals learn what behaviors, beliefs, values, ways of expressing emotion and relating to others they will be expected to demonstrate throughout life. It is this context that carries every child from birth and childhood through adulthood to death and defines his or her legacy for the next generation. And each generation is different, as cultures evolve through time, influenced by the social, economic, and political history of their era, and making their world-view different from that of those born in other times. The gender, class, and cultural structure of any society profoundly influences the parameters of a child's evolving ability to empathize, share, negotiate, and communicate. It prescribes his or her way of thinking for self and of being emotionally connected to others. Healthy development requires establishing a solid sense of our unique selves in the context of our connections to others. Connecting to others becomes a particular challenge when they are different from us.

Because our society so quickly assigns roles and expectations based on gender, culture, class, and race, children's competences are obviously not simply milestones that they reach individually, but rather accomplishments that evolve within a complex web of racial, cultural, and familial contexts. A child's acquisition of cognitive, communicative, physical, emotional, and social skills is necessarily circumscribed by the particular social context in which he or she is raised. Thus, our evaluation of these abilities can only be meaningful if these constraints are taken into account. We urge a perspective of human development that views child development in the richness of its entire context of multigenerational family relationships as well as within its sociocultural context. The cultural, socioeconomic, racial, and gender context of the family will influence all of these developmental transitions.

A suggested schema for exploring normative individual life-cycle tasks is offered in Table 2.1 (McGoldrick & Carter, 1999). There are serious limitations to any attempt to condense the complications of life in an oversimplified framework. Obviously there is an overlap between the physical, intellectual, and social/emotional tasks, so that certain tasks could fit into each realm. Communication, for example, is a physical, intellectual, and social/emotional task of development. Table 2.1 presents a skeletal framework for assessing a person's passage through life. The phases of human development have been defined in many ways in different cultures. This outline is a rough guideline, not a statement of the true and fixed stages of life. People vary greatly in their pathways through life. The schema here is meant to be suggestive rather than definitive. Furthermore, accomplishing the individual tasks of a stage depends on resources available to individuals and families to help them develop their abilities.

During the *first stage* (0–2 years) of life, babies need to learn to communicate their needs and have some sense of trust, comfort, and relationship to their caretakers and the world around them. Their needs have to be satisfied consistently so they can develop trust for others and a sense of trustworthiness and security. They learn to coordinate their bodies and begin to explore the world. It is during this stage that empathy, the earliest emotion, begins to develop. David, the older son in Case 2-2, was obviously having trouble accomplishing the tasks of this phase. He had been delayed in speech and motor skills, which led to his being evaluated for retardation. His difficulties accomplishing the tasks required extra parental caretaking. All future life stages will be influenced by David's retardation, and extra adaptive skills will be called on from other family members throughout his life to provide him with the special supports he will need. The family will have to do more caretaking and for a longer period than with another child and deal with the lost dreams created by his disabilities for their whole lives. Children not yet born, future siblings and cousins, and even future children of these siblings will need to find the strength to deal with his limitations and offer support to him. The physician will have to help the family to adjust their expectations to David's possibilities while continuing to provide him with the necessary stimulation and support.

The *second stage*, the child's preschool years (2–4 years), is a time of great development of language and motor skills and abilities to explore and relate to the world around oneself. The child develops cognitive skills with numbers, words, and objects. Children learn to take direction, cooperate, share, trust, explore, and be aware of themselves as different from others. As early as 2½, children recognize that someone else's pain is different from their own and are able to comfort others. How discipline is handled at this phase influences the development of emotional competence, e.g., ''Look how sad you've made her'' versus ''That was naughty'' (Goleman, 1997). It is at this time that children begin to form peer relationships and to be aware of themselves as different from others. They start learning to deal with frustration and to accept limits and delay gratification, and also to obey rules. During this phase children learn where, how, and when to show aggression (Comer & Poussaint, 1992), and they need to be taught control of their anger, aggression, distress, impulses, excitement and to regulate their moods and delay gratification, and also to obey rules. This self-management, along with the continued development of empathy, is the basis of relationship skill (Goleman, 1997). By age 3 children become actively interested in defining how they are like or different from others, including skin color and hair texture (Comer & Poussaint, 1992; Matthias & French, 1996). They can start to share and be fair rather than to exclude others; they take their cues from the adults around them for how to treat others. Imagination plays an important role at this stage. Through fantasy play, and later, dramatic play, children learn to master their behavior and to deal with fears and anxieties. Physicians can be helpful to parents by highlighting the value of play and fantasy at this stage, fostering emotional and cognitive development. David in Case 2-2 reached this phase, but his developmental disabilities slowed him down increasingly with age-appropriate skills. He was behind in language and motor skills and in ability to relate to the world around him. He was slower than his peers in developing interpersonal relationships. One might predict that his younger brother, Sam, would outdistance him in developmental skills in the not too distant future. David's ongoing individual developmental difficulties will continue to create extra family life-cycle tasks for other family members in terms of extra caretaking and accommodation to his problems by his brother, who may soon

**Table 2.1**
The Individual Life Cycle in Context[a]

1. Infancy (approximately birth to age 2)
   The development of empathy and emotional attunement to others
   *Our brains are wired in a way that allows emotional learning throughout the lifespan, as long as our caretakers are reasonably well attuned to our emotions and capable of mirroring them back to us in the first 18 months of life* (Borysenko, 1996, p. 19)
   - Communicate frustration and happiness
   - Develop beginning of empathy for others
   - Talk
   - Make needs known and get them met
   - Develop coordination
   - Sit, stand, walk, run, manipulate objects, feed self
   - Recognize self as separate person
   - Trust others, primarily caretakers
   - Overcome fears of new situations
2. Early childhood (approximate ages 2 to 6)
   A growing understanding of interdependence
   *The bio-psycho-spiritual basis of the ... life cycle is wired firmly into place by the end of early childhood, conferring the gifts of empathy, relationality, interdependent perception and intuition* (Borysenko, 1996, p. 35)
   - Develop language and ability to relate and communicate
   - Learn to regulate and control emotions and impulses
   - Develop motor skills, eye–hand coordination, etc.
   - Develop control of bodily functions (bowels, urine)
   - Start to become aware of self in terms of gender and abilities
   - Start to become aware of self in relation to world around
   - Start to become aware of "otherness" in terms of gender, race, and disability
   - Learn cooperative play, ability to share
   - Learn to obey rules
   - Learn to delay gratification
   - Increase ability to develop trusting relationships
   - Start to develop peer relationships
   - Develop ability to dramatize and engage in fantasy play to master own behavior and control anxieties
3. Middle childhood (approximate ages 6 to 11 or 12)
   Moral development: including "heart logic" along with "mind logic"
   *Developing the capacity to use linear logic while retaining the inter-relational interdependent perceptual capability developed early in childhood* (Borysenko, 1996, p. 38)
   - Increase skill with language
   - Begin development of morality
   - Increase capacity for empathy
   - Increase physical coordination and motor skills
   - Develop ability to play team games
   - Learn reading, writing, and math
   - Develop knowledge about nature
   - Increase understanding of self in terms of gender, race, culture, and abilities
   - Increase understanding of self in relation to family, peers, and community
   - Develop intuition
   - Increase awareness of "otherness" in terms of gender, race, sexual orientation, culture, class, and disability
   - Increase ability to conduct peer relationships
   - Increase ability to conduct relationships with authorities
   - Develop ability to be intimate and to express anger, fear, and pain in nondestructive ways
   - Develop tolerance for difference

---

[a]Adapted from: McGoldrick M, Carter B: The self in context: The individual life cycle in systemic perspective. In Carter B, McGoldrick M (eds): *The Expanded Family Life Cycle: Individual, Family, and Social Perspectives*, ed 3. Boston, Allyn & Bacon, 1999.

*continued*

become developmentally more advanced than David. This situation will create a reversal of the expected family hierarchy, where the younger brother and any future siblings will become caretakers to the oldest, while usually it is the oldest who does more caretaking for the younger ones.

The *third developmental phase* might be said to cover the school-age years of childhood, from about age 6 to 12. At this time children typically make many developmental leaps in their cognitive skills, motor skills,

**Table 2.1**
*(Continued)[a]*

4. Pubescence (approximate ages 11–13 for girls; 12–14 for boys)
Finding one's own voice: the beginning development of authenticity
*The ability to see relationships with clarity, the uncanny tendency to recognize instances of relational injustice and cry foul, and the development of the morality of the heart ...* (Borysenko, 1996, p. 59)
- Cope with dramatic bodily changes of puberty
- Ability to assert oneself
- Increase development of emotional competence
- Develop awareness of own and others' sexuality
- Begin to learn to control one's sexual and aggressive impulses
- Recognize injustices
- Increase capacity for moral understanding
- Increase physical coordination and physical skills
- Increase ability to read, write, think conceptually and mathematically
- Increase understanding of self in terms of gender, race, culture, sexual orientation, and abilities
- Increase understanding of self in relation to peers, family, and community
- Increase ability to handle social relationships and complex social situations
- Increase ability to work collaboratively and individually

5. Adolescence (approximate ages 13 or 14–21)
Looking for an identity: continuing to voice authentic opinions and feelings in the context of societal, parental, and peer pressure to conform to age, gender, and racial stereotypes
Learning to balance caring about self and caring about others
*By this time, we can think our own thoughts, we have opinions that are separable from other people's, we can group concepts and calculate probabilities and we can stand back and reflect on ourselves* (Borysenko, 1995, p. 75)
- Continue to deal with rapid bodily changes and cultural ideals of body image
- Increase awareness and ability to deal with one's own and others' sexuality
- Learn to handle one's sexual and aggressive impulses
- Develop one's sexual identity
- Increase physical coordination and physical skills
- Increase ability to think conceptually and mathematically and learn about the world
- Increase discipline for physical and intellectual work, sleep, sex, and social relationships
- Increase understanding of self in relation to peers, family, and community
- Begin to develop a philosophy of life and a moral and spiritual identity
- Begin to develop ability to handle intimate physical and social relationships as well as increase ability to judge and handle complex social situations
- Increase ability to work collaboratively and individually
- Increase emotional competence and self-management

6. Early adulthood (approximate ages 21 to 35)
Development of the ability to engage in intense relationships committed to mutual growth, and in satisfying work. A commitment to parity for care of the family and the importance of career
*The development of a core self, a strong, yet pliable identity in which the previous development of relationality, intuition, and the logic of the heart are combined in a conscious way, bestow life's most precious gift—the ability to relate to both self and others with true intimacy* (Borysenko, 1996, p. 76)
- Increase ability to care for self and one's own needs, financially, emotionally, and spiritually
- Increase awareness and ability to deal with one's own and others' sexuality
- Increase discipline for physical and intellectual work, sleep, sex, social relationships
- Learn to focus on long-range life goals regarding work, intimate relationships, family, and community
- Develop ability to negotiate evolving relationships to one's parents, peers, children, and community, including work relationships
- Develop ability to nurture others physically and emotionally
- Develop ability to support one's children financially and emotionally
- Increase ability to tolerate delayed gratification to meet one's goals
- Evolve further one's ability to respect and advocate for those less fortunate than oneself
- Evolve ability to help onself if socially disadvantaged

[a]Adapted from: McGoldrick M, Carter B: The self in context: The individual life cycle in systemic perspective. In Carter B, McGoldrick M (eds): *The Expanded Family Life Cycle: Individual, Family, and Social Perspectives*, ed 3. Boston, Allyn & Bacon, 1999.

and emotional skills. Children expand their social world in terms of their ability to communicate and handle relationships with an increasing range of adults and children beyond their families. They learn how to conduct relationships in terms of fairness, tolerance for others who are different, conflict resolution, competition, collaboration, and intimacy. They begin to understand their identity in terms of gender, race, culture, and sexual orientation and to differentiate themselves from others. They learn to follow directions, to tolerate

**Table 2.1**
(*Continued*)[a]

27

THE INDIVIDUAL LIFE
CYCLE IN CONTEXT

7. Middle adulthood (approximate ages 35 to 50 or 55)

The emergence into authentic power. Becoming more aware of the problems of others

*Along with balancing many life tasks, there is a review of one's priorities, a striving towards balance and harmony with self and others while resisting pressure to pursue traditional gender patterns. There is greater community involvement and participation in social and political action* (Borysenko, 1996, pp. 135, 181)

- Firm up and make solid all of the tasks of early adulthood
- Nurture and support one's children and partner, including caretaking of older family members
- Deepen and solidify family friendships
- Reassess one's work satisfaction and financial adequacy and consider possibility of changing work or career to achieve greater life balance
- Involve oneself in improving community and society whether one is personally advantaged or disadvantaged
- Recognize one's accomplishments and accept one's limitations
- Accept the choices that made some dreams and goals attainable but precluded others
- Focus on mentoring the next generation
- Solidify one's philosophy of life and spirituality

8. Late middle age (approximate ages 50 or 55 to early 70s)

The beginning of the wisdom years: reclaiming the wisdom of interdependence

*An intensification of the altruism and service begun in the previous phase. Helping other, serving the community and mentoring: passing along our values and experience.... There is a need to resist our culture's dismissal of older people, especially older women.... The pendulum swings away from the active and productive principles back to the spiritual principles that value nature as well as technology, that honor cultural diversity, that foster caring for the less fortunate and that seek physical, emotional and spiritual harmony* (Borysenko, 1996, pp. 202, 219)

- Handle some declining physical and intellectual abilities
- Deal with menopause, decreasing sexual energies, and one's changing sexuality
- Come to terms with one's failure and choices with accountability but without becoming bitter
- Plan and handle work transitions and retirement
- Define one's own grandparenting and other "senior" roles in work and community
- Take steps to pass the torch and attend to one's connections and responsibilities to the next generations
- Accept one's limitations and multiple caretaking responsibilities for those above and below
- Deal with death of parents and others of older generations

9. Aging (approximate ages from 75 on)

Grief, loss, resiliency, retrospection, and growth

*This is a time to reflect and review one's life with appreciation of its successes and compassion for its failures, and with an effort to extract new levels of meaning that had previously been unappreciated* (Borysenko, 1996, p. 243)

- Respond to loss and change by using these as opportunities to reevaluate life circumstances and create new fulfilling pathways
- Remain as physically, psychologically, intellectually, and spiritually active, and as emotionally connected as possible
- Come to terms with death while focusing on what else one can still do for oneself and others
- Bring careful reflection, perspective, and balance to the task of life review
- Accept dependence on others and diminished control of one's life
- Affirm and work out one's financial, spiritual, and emotional legacy to the next generation
- Accept death of spouse and need to create a new life without a spouse
- Accept one's own life and death

[a]Adapted from: McGoldrick M, Carter B: The self in context: The individual life cycle in systemic perspective. In Carter B, McGoldrick M (eds): *The Expanded Family Life Cycle: Individual, Family, and Social Perspectives*, ed 3. Boston, Allyn & Bacon, 1999.

frustration, and to work independently and with others. Accomplishing these tasks depends both on the child's innate resources and on family and community supports to foster the child's development. If deprived of any of these resources the child may develop physical, emotional, or social symptoms. Children may develop fears, anxieties, phobias, stomach or headaches, or aggressive or withdrawn behaviors. In Case 2-2, David's brother Sam and any future siblings will have special tasks at this phase to adapt to a retarded older brother and his special needs.

Between ages 6 and 8 children develop a great passion to *belong*. They exclude others so they can fit *in*. Children of color, in particular, must be taught at this age to handle racist acts in ways that are not self-destructive (Comer & Poussaint, 1992). At this phase children learn competitiveness by comparing themselves to others, and cooperation to the degree their parents, caretakers, or teachers teach them. Otherwise competitiveness remains a problem. Sex segregation increases, greatly influenced by the fact that boys' behavior, unless checked, becomes characterized by competition, demands, and dominance. Girls have great difficulty having influence in play with boys, and thus avoid them (Maccoby, 1990). Boys tend to play more roughly in larger groups, and girls to form close friendships with one or two other girls. Goleman (1997) reports studies in which 50% of 3-year-olds have friends of the opposite sex, 20% of 5-year-olds, and virtually no 7-year-olds. Children begin to develop respect for the rights and needs of self and others. They tattle on wrongdoers and discussion about rule-breaking and commitments to rules and fairness is very important at this stage (Comer & Poussaint, 1992). How children learn life's "rules" will form the foundation of their morals. If they are continuously put down, they lose faith in themselves; if they are not admonished for selfish or unfair acts, they will grow up with a false sense of privilege. Boys especially can be physically aggressive and need to be taught fairness and to have plenty of outlets for their physical energy. Games and hobbies can mitigate social conflicts. By ages 9–12 children spend a lot of time discussing, arguing, and changing the rules of their games. Children may play adults off against each other to get what they want, because they do not yet know how to confront adults to let them know they feel neglected or ignored (Comer & Poussaint, 1992). The quality of a child's relationships with adults is more important than the gender of the adults, for both male and female children. Children between 9 and 12 are aware of unfairness and hypocrisy of adults and officials. It is important for adults to help them understand adult failings and model doing something about it so they don't feel powerless and cynical.

We might consider the *fourth developmental stage* to be pubescence, the early part of adolescence, from about age 11 to 13 for girls and age 12 to 14 or 15 for boys. Adolescence is not universal and was never particularly defined prior to the Industrial Revolution, which required a lengthier apprenticeship to learn the skills necessary for adult functioning. During this phase, young people go through puberty and begin developing the ability to function independently. At this time children are normally ambivalent, rebellious, bored, uninterested, or difficult. They are highly critical of others who don't look or act like them and they identify with a preferred group of friends who agree on dress, music, and even language. They now view morality and rules as imposed by parents and not society and experiment with new rules, valuing peer values more than those of parents.

During certain phases in development including preschool and adolescence, children seem to hold rigidly to sex-role stereotypes, even more so than their parents or teachers. It is important not to encourage this stereotyping, but instead to encourage girls to develop their own opinions, values, aspirations, and interests. It is in keeping with social norms that during the adolescent years girls often confuse identity with intimacy by defining themselves through relationships with others. Advertising and adult attitudes toward girls, which define their development in terms of their ability to attract a male, are bound to be detrimental to their mental health, leaving them lacking in self-esteem, fearing to appear smart, tall, assertive, or competent, worrying about losing their chances of finding an intimate relationship with a male. It is important to raise questions about such norms, since they put the girl into an impossible bind, i.e., you are only healthy if you define your identity not through your self but through your mate.

Children renegotiate their identity in relation to their parents as they mature; refine their physical, social, and intellectual skills; develop their spiritual and moral identity; and begin to define who they want to become as adults. Family life-cycle problems may interfere with this individual development. For example, if a mother dies leaving three adolescent daughters, the oldest may sacrifice her own individual development, e.g., forego college plans and her social development to become a caretaker for her father and sisters, out of a sense that they need her as caretaker. At the same time her short-circuiting of her individual development will be influenced by how other family members have handled earlier life-cycle dilemmas and by how they are handling this loss of the mother. Special problems may emerge for the family in Case 2-2 when David becomes an adolescent because of his retardation, since his physical development will outdistance his emotional and intellectual development. Special tasks are common, for example, in helping a retarded adolescent deal with his or her emerging sexuality and wish to connect with peers in ways that are appropriate, given the intellectual limitations.

The *fifth phase*, adolescence, goes from about 13 for girls and about 14 or 15 for boys and continues until age 21. Erikson (1968) described the development of adolescent girls as fundamentally different from that of boys, in that girls supposedly hold their identity in abeyance as they prepare to attract men by whose name they will be known and by whose status they will be defined. But after the challenges of the women's movement in the 1970s, Gilligan in her landmark study of pre- and early adolescent girls (Gilligan, 1982; Pipher, 1994) attributed the girls' loss of voice and low self-esteem to their fear of appearing too smart, assertive, or competent to attract a male. This sexist attitude is now seen as cultural, not inherent in girls' development. During this phase young people go through major bodily, emotional, sexual, and spiritual changes, evolve their sexual and gender identities, learn to relate to intimate partners, and develop the ability to function more independently. Adolescents react to social hostility and are attracted to causes. Black adolescents may succumb to despair and give up hope of a productive future. Minority adolescents may have identity problems if they are completely segregated from whites or if they live in mostly white communities. Sexual issues and information should be discussed with adolescents at home and at school, building on earlier sex education. Powerful attraction to members of the opposite sex does not mean that gender segregation disappears. Young people continue to spend a good portion of their social time with same-sex partners (Maccoby, 1990). However, the higher rates of depression in females may have their onset during adolescence, because of the difficulties of cross-sex interaction.

Adolescents are actively searching for an identity. Sexual, religious, and racial issues that seemed settled are reevaluated and subject to new understanding and revision. Similarities and differences, even within groups, cause the formation of "in and out" groups and "for and against" attitudes. The community climate regarding race and religion is important. Minority–majority ratios in school have great influence on the social atmosphere. Older teens finally understand morals and values not as impositions but as necessary for order and fairness. The media depict teens as selfish, aimless, and immoral, which can become a self-fulfilling prophecy. In a disorderly and unfair society they can stumble into drugs, alcohol, eating disorders, sexually transmitted disease, and pregnancy. Parents must try to have their influence felt to counteract that of the peer group and the larger society—an uphill struggle (Matthias & French, 1996). Teens are aware of social hypocrisy. To remain credible to teens, parents must reveal their own uncertainties, beware of double messages delivered nonverbally, speak clearly from the heart, and keep the door open for discussion now and in the future (Matthias & French, 1996).

We might think of the *sixth phase of development* as covering the decades of young adulthood (from about age 20 to the mid-30s). Of course there are great differences in the pathways at this phase based on gender or class, but in general it is the phase of generativity in terms of partnering, work, and raising children. By this time adults are expected to function without the physical or financial support of their parents. They begin not only to care for themselves but also to take on responsibilities for the care of others—both children and aging parents who need support.

Several groups encounter major developmental problems during this phase, due to social factors. By age 30, one out of every three black males is already dead, on probation, on parole, or in prison (Roberts, 1994). Many of those who are able and ready to work find themselves shut out of meaningful jobs because they lack the necessary education, technical skills, or training. Lack of stable wage earning for young black men impedes their ability to marry and creates in turn a problem for young women in this phase, who find a diminished pool of marital prospects. Taken together the massive obstacles of racism and poverty impede the forward development of young adults of color at this phase and may derail potentially productive people into the underclass, from which escape becomes harder as the life cycle continues. Gay and lesbian young adults also have difficulties at this stage because of the stigma attached to their partnering and parenting, as well as the frequent necessity to keep their true lives secret at work. These struggles created by the social system, with what should be normal developmental tasks, have implications for their smooth emotional development and well-being.

Even for those without these societal level disadvantages, this phase can be stressful. It is at this phase that adults must juggle their own jobs, their personal needs, and caretaking responsibilities. Joe Verdum, the husband in Case 2-2, obviously got off the track at this stage in his own individual life cycle in terms of his responsibility to contribute to the emotional, physical, and financial support of his wife and children. He had not dealt with his disappointment that David was retarded and was avoiding his parental responsibilities for his son. He resented his wife's attention to her parents and said she was not helping him. His irresponsibility shows that he was off the track in his own life cycle at a time in his life when it was appropriate for him to manage his own frustrations and contribute to the care of others. His individual problems increase the burden on all other family members (his wife, children, in-laws, and his family of origin) in their own life-cycle tasks.

The *seventh stage* of the life cycle might be thought of as midlife (a new stage, since in 1900 the average life span in the United States was 43 years), lasting somewhere between ages 35 and 50 or 55. Generally speaking, adults are still in good health, their children are teenagers or being launched into adulthood. This is the last opportunity for active, hands on, parenting. In addition to the usual power struggles with teenagers pushing toward launching, it is a time to shift parental gears and start treating adolescents more like the young adults they will soon be, emphasizing the wish to trust rather than constrict or punish them. It is a time for parents—unmarried, married, divorced, or remarried—to recognize the grave dangers and temptations facing today's adolescents and to resolve their own differences with partners or other adult family members enough to be able to guide their adolescents as a team, united in concern and advice. This is a time when people often do a philosophical reexamination of their lives, or even several reexaminations, and may need to "reinvent" themselves in their work and community to fit changing circumstances. There is often caretaking responsibility for older or ailing relatives, as well as for their children. It is during this phase that women go through menopause, which often allows them to concentrate their energies on new projects, having been freed up from major caretaking and deciding that it is their "turn." Symptoms might occur when the woman's individual needs do not match family and societal expectations.

It is a time when people are coming to terms with the fact that they cannot do it all. They have to let go of certain dreams and recognize their limitations to concentrate on what they can do. The family in Case 2-2 experienced individual life-cycle problems as well as family life-cycle problems at this stage, when the wife's mother, Anna, at age 55, who had been disoriented and forgetful for about a year, was diagnosed with Alzheimer's disease. Her diagnosis obviously interfered with the normative tasks of her middle-age life, in that she would lose her intellectual, physical, and emotional functioning prematurely and require caretaking herself. Her individual developmental problems will increase the burdens on the others in the family as well as her husband, her daughters, her son-in-law, and her grandchildren. Necessarily, when a person has individual developmental problems such as this, there is a double burden on the family, which loses the support of the person and now must devote energy to taking care of her.

The *eighth stage*, from about 50 or 55 to the mid-70s, might be called late middle age or early aging, a time when adults are beginning to retire, take up new interests, and still, in our times, likely to feel in good health and have the energy for major undertakings. They are by this time freed from childrearing or financial responsibilities, though they are often now helping the next generation, their grandchildren. At this stage, people have to be concerned about husbanding their financial resources and future healthcare needs. It is a time to work out increasing supports and find ways to manage decreasing physical strength and endurance. At this stage, physicians need to be alert to the emotional impact of the onset of disabling symptoms and/or chronic illness on patients' self-esteem, and its possible consequences to treatment. This is also a time of facing increasing losses of peers, older friends, and relatives. Grief and feelings of isolation often cause depression and facilitate onset of physical symptoms. Spiritual resources are important to maintain one's health and accept decline of one's abilities.

The *ninth or last stage of life*, aging and death, covers roughly the ages from 75 to 100 as people come to terms with their own mortality and that of their peer group and prepare for death. It is a time to affirm and work out one's legacy and to complete the organization of relationships with one's legatees. Any pending personal business with one's descendants and with oneself will need to be addressed. At this stage one must face decreasing ability to function and increasing dependence on others while continuing to maximize one's abilities.

Recalling Case 2-2, the special individual life-cycle problems of three members of the Verdum/Petlock family, Joseph, David, and Anna, will affect the other family members at both an individual and a family level. These issues, of course, also have extended family implications. Mary's and Joe's siblings and aunts and uncles are also affected by the problems, having to decide how much each of them could or should do to help out. The problems also have community ramifications. David's disabilities will require various community resources throughout his school-age and adult years. The community resources or lack thereof to help Joseph with his alcohol problem and to help Anna and the rest of the family with the disabilities created by Alzheimer's disease will have profound implications for this family's future negotiation of their individual and family life cycles.

## FAMILY LIFE-CYCLE STAGES

The stages of the family life cycle are by no means universal markers. In different cultures and historical eras, the demarcation of life-cycle stages will vary from current definitions in our society in terms of timing, importance, and roles expected. In our present classification (Table 2.2) of the life-cycle stages, modified from Carter and McGoldrick (1999), we try to be sensitive to differences in class and ethnicity as well as changes in society influencing family relations. What follows are descriptions of each life-cycle stage and developmental tasks illustrated by clinical vignettes.

**Table 2.2**
The Stages of the Family Life Cycle[b]

| Family life cycle stage | Emotional process of transition: key principles | Changes in family status required to proceed developmentally |
|---|---|---|
| 1. Young adulthood | Accepting emotional and financial responsibility for self | a. Differentiation of self in relation to family of origin<br>b. Development of intimate peer relationships<br>c. Establishment of self regarding work and financial independence |
| 2. Becoming a couple: partnership and marriage | Commitment to a new system | a. Formation of couple system<br>b. Realignment of relationships with extended family and friends to include partner<br>c. Balancing between individual and couple needs/identity<br>d. Deciding on parenting |
| 3. Families with young children | Accepting new members into the system | a. Adjusting marital system to make space for child(ren)<br>b. Joining in childrearing, financial, and household tasks<br>c. Realignment of relationships with extended family to include parenting, grandparenting, and other roles |
| 4. Families with adolescents | Increasing flexibility of family boundaries to accept children's independence and grandparents' frailties | a. Shifting of parent–child relationship to permit adolescent to move in and out of system<br>b. Refocus on midlife personal/conjugal and work issues<br>c. Beginning shift toward joint caring for older generation |
| 5. Midlife stage: launching children and moving on | Accepting a multitude of exits from and entries into the family system | a. Renegotiation of conjugal system as dyad<br>b. Development of adult-to-adult relationships between grown children and their parents<br>c. Realignment of relationships to include in-laws and grandchildren<br>d. Dealing with disabilities and death of parents (grandparents) |
| 6. Families in later life | Accepting the shifting of generational roles | a. Maintaining own and/or couple functioning and interests in face of physiological decline; exploration of new familial and social role options<br>b. Support for a more central role of middle generation<br>c. Making room in the system for the wisdom and experience of the elderly, supporting the older generation without overfunctioning for them<br>d. Dealing with loss of spouse, siblings, and other peers and preparation for own death. Life review and integration |

[b]Adapted from Carter B, McGoldrick M: *The Expanded Family Life Cycle: Individual Family and Social Perspectives*, ed 3. Boston, Allyn & Bacon, 1999.

## CASE 2-3

*Lucia, a 24-year-old Italian-American woman, presented to a health center experiencing headaches, stomach and chest pains, nervousness, insomnia, and fainting. Results of her physical exam and lab tests were negative. The treating physician, suspecting social and developmental factors, proceeded with symptomatic treatment and a psychosocial evaluation.*

*One year previously the patient had begun a management training program of a major company and had relocated to another city, which meant moving away from her family. When the physical symptoms became debilitating she left the training program, moved back home with her family, and took a job with a local company. Lucia's physical symptoms initially lessened but then became worse. She reported experiencing physical distress whenever she anticipated being away from home for a prolonged period with friends, especially her fiancé. Lucia's fiancé was well liked by her family, but Lucia secretly was having second thoughts about the marriage. The physician, realizing that the symptoms were anxiety-related, requested a consultation with a family therapist.*

## YOUNG ADULTHOOD

The "young adulthood" stage is defined as the period between the individual separating from the family and forming a family of his or her own. This stage varies for families depending on socioeconomic factors, cultural values, and job opportunities as well as on the health status of the individual and family members.

This phase of the life cycle includes those individuals in their 20s who have established separate dwellings from their families, are postcollege or postmilitary, and, for the most part, are financially independent. It also includes those individuals who bypassed this stage by marrying young and divorcing within a few years as well as those who are living together without formal commitment. It may also include adult children of any age who have never left home and who, along with their families, engage in the tasks associated with this phase of development. Just as physical separation from the family is not synonymous with emotional differentiation from the family, remaining in the home because of cultural values or limited economic and educational opportunities does not necessarily mean foreclosure of identity formation. In fact, Watson and Protinsky (1988) found that *enmeshment*, a family therapy term meaning overinvolvement and lack of differentiation, was positively correlated with identity achievement for African-American youths. We prefer to name this stage "young adulthood" rather than "leaving home," "unattached adult," or "in-between families" to avoid identifying differentiation and independence with disconnection and emotional distancing from the family. In many working-class families from diverse cultures, unmarried adult children are expected to live at home and contribute a portion of their earnings to the family (Strelnick & Gilpin, 1986). Increasing costs of higher education and limitations in the job market have forced middle-class children to prolong their dependence on the family, especially for housing.

Lucia's experience in Case 2-3 illustrates the conflict created by the overemphasis on male norms and reliance on white Anglo-Saxon Protestant middle-class values as the ideal for individuals and their families. Under this value system, Lucia was expected to leave home in her early 20s and to make career development her single most important goal. The failure to value intimacy and attachment along with individuation and separation seriously complicate the process of defining one's adult identity, especially for women and members of other cultures.

The key tasks (Table 2.1) for the individual at this stage of the life cycle are to become emotionally and financially responsible. To achieve these goals the individual must differentiate the self from the family of origin; develop intimate peer relationships; and establish vocational identity, work, and financial independence (Carter & McGoldrick, 1999). The essential task for the family is to support the young adult in her quest for identity and independent functioning and to accept her adoption of new values and life choices. In this phase, problems may occur because of perceived or actual expectations that the adult child will comply with familial life plans and wishes at the expense of her own. Since the expectations may not come directly from parents but indirectly from grandparents or other extended kin, or be prescribed by the community (Strelnick & Gilpin, 1986), it is necessary to think more broadly than the nuclear family when assessing the dynamics of the family.

The developmental conflict faced by the young woman in Case 2-3 also involved her relationships with her brother and grandmother. When her parents divorced and the father abandoned the family, she made an unspoken pact with her brother and mother that they would always take care of each other. Close to her ailing grandmother, Lucia often mediated conflicts between her mother and grandmother. Feelings of guilt and disloyalty to the family of origin competed with her need for autonomy and career advancement. Cultural values, family expectations, and additional stressors such as divorce and illness were important factors in this young woman's transitional conflict.

The impact of parental divorce, illness, and death can be particularly significant at this developmental phase. Although these stressors affect individual and family functioning at all phases of the life cycle, parents who lose their spouse to divorce are likely to expect increased support from their adult children at a time when their children need to invest their energies outside the family. Such a situation may place young adults in a difficult bind indeed.

Since ethnicity shapes the family life cycle at every stage (Hines *et al.*, 1999), understanding cultural patterns is critical for physicians who wish to provide effective care for young adults. For example, while the dominant culture in the United States values the young adult's autonomy and independence, many cultural groups such as Italian-Americans tend to value interdependence among family members. Thus, patients such as Lucia face special challenges in differentiating from their families. Individual developmental dilemmas are further amplified as families struggle to assimilate into mainstream American culture while maintaining core values of their cultural heritage. Lucia must negotiate some difficult compromises: "How can I succeed in the outside world and be viewed as an adult while maintaining strong ties with my family?" "How can I continue to be loyal and supportive to my family while allowing myself new life options?" A successful transition at this stage will require that Lucia, or any young adult, learn how to increase emotional distance from the family while remaining connected.

When these issues are presented clinically, the task of the physician is to frame symptoms developmentally and to normalize emotional distancing as a necessary transition while encouraging renegotiation of relationships with family as an alternative to estrangement. Young adults who cut off their parents and families do so reactively and are in fact still emotionally bound to rather than independent of the family "program" (Carter & McGoldrick, 1999). Those who learn to relate in a new way, adult to adult, will be able to maintain an ongoing and mutually respectful relationship in which each appreciates others as they are.

This is an especially challenging task for homosexual young adults and their families. In a similar case to Lucia in Case 2-3, a young woman's headaches were associated with her fear of family rejection because of her homosexuality. The experience of treating homosexual AIDS patients makes physicians painfully aware of the unfortunate consequences of these cutoffs, having witnessed the distress of patients, and sometimes families. But illness also brings opportunities for rapprochement. Family and individual counseling may hopefully facilitate healing and, eventually, reconnection between patients and their families.

Except for HIV patients and others facing chronic illness, medical visits are less frequent at this stage. Healthy young adults tend to come to physicians for work-related reasons, such as health assessment, on-the-job injuries, accidents, sports injuries, or problems related to sexuality. These encounters provide the physician an opportunity to address disease prevention and health promotion, including a review of this stage's developmental tasks. Recurrent somatic complaints are often responses to developmental and other social stressors. Young adults with chronic illness, especially men, often present with problems of compliance. Their sense of physical vulnerability is often associated with fear of losing their maleness. A focus on developmental tasks will guide the physician toward an understanding of the patient's situation.

## CASE 2-4

*Vanessa, a 28-year-old educated African-American woman, married for the first time 6 months ago, visited her physician suspecting she might be pregnant. The physician is surprised to find that Vanessa has missed her menses for 2 months without checking or sharing the possibility of a pregnancy with her husband. Despite their original plan to have children early in their marriage, Vanessa now feels ambivalent because of increasing tensions in the marriage. She reports that their relationship has been changing since they moved closer to his close-knit Jamaican family. Mark, her husband, has become less playful and affectionate, and she has become more withdrawn and intolerant. For the physician, this report reflects a contrasting scenario to earlier visits when the couple seemed happy together.*

*From Vanessa's earlier visits the physician knew the patient as an attractive, intelligent, and career-oriented woman who was completing an MBA degree when she met her husband. The patient was delighted that Mark was smart, outgoing, and responsible, proud of her achievements, and shared her goals of raising a family. They had lived together 8 months and decided to get married in response to her ailing mother's desire to attend her wedding while in good health.*

## BECOMING A COUPLE: FORMING PARTNERSHIP AND MARRIAGE

The stage of the new couple is one of the most complex and difficult transitions of the family life cycle (McGoldrick *et al.*, 1999). The two partners must renegotiate a variety of issues previously defined by each as individuals and by their respective families and cultures. They must decide on the rules that will govern their relationship and the boundary that will define them as a couple.

Recent trends, such as unmarried couples establishing households and the formation of committed homosexual partnerships, require us to explore models of partnership other than traditional marriages. The unifying element to these diverse couples is that they form a partnership with a goal of sharing a future together and deciding whether to have children.

The tasks (Table 2.2) that the new couple must successfully resolve are (1) making a commitment to the marital or partnership dyad, (2) realignment of relationships with the extended family and friends to take the partner into consideration (Carter & McGoldrick, 1999), and (3) balancing the needs of the individual with those of the couple. The ability of the partners to make a commitment to each other will be determined by the extent to which they have achieved emotional differentiation from the family of origin and established an identity of their own. Each partner should view the relationship as a means of enriching one's self, not completing one's self. The couple also needs to achieve a balance between the need for intimacy and the need for individual fulfillment. Finally, each has to grapple with expectations from parents and siblings in view of the partner's expectations. For instance, one issue facing the couple in Case 2-4 was that the husband, the only married male sibling, was dealing with his brothers' tendency to dismiss his new identity as a married man, expecting him to continue to socialize without his wife.

To support couples in their quest to establish and define a bond, the physician must assess the couple's relationship. The physician should explore each partner's desire for intimacy, the couple's decision-making

### SUPPORTING COUPLES' BONDING: QUESTIONS TO ASK COUPLES

- *"What is your idea of what a marriage/partnership should be like?"*
- *"How has this marriage, or getting together, changed or supported your plans for the future?"*
- *"In which ways do you feel you are, or are not, complementing each other?"*

process, contacts with relatives or friends, and the extended family's feelings about the marriage. Differences of education and income should also be explored to determine the balance of power between them.

Cultural differences between the partners regarding styles of socialization, family rituals, and patterns of contact with family of origin need to be identified, revised, and selectively combined in the couple's life. The complexity of marriage may not be fully appreciated by the young couple until they are faced with the challenge of deciding such issues as: how and where to celebrate the holidays; whose family traditions to follow; who does what in the household; and the degree of intimacy in the relationship.

When assessing the dynamics of the relationship, physicians should differentiate the impact of culture from race and class. For example, in another case an African-American wife's physical symptoms were caused by stress resulting from her African husband's differing views on gender roles in the marriage. Because the couple shared the same social and class backgrounds, the physician might have overlooked significant cultural differences contributing to the wife's presenting illness. Case 2-4 describes the increasing marital tension between an African-American woman and her Jamaican-Caribbean husband, which was jeopardizing her pregnancy and perhaps her health. The wife, a woman from a small and middle-class nuclear-oriented family, felt left out because of the husband's inattentiveness since the couple moved closer to his tightly knit Jamaican family. Vanessa's withdrawal and irritability reflected her disappointment that her husband's allegiance and loyalty were to his family of origin and not to her. The ambivalence she felt about the pregnancy was linked to conflict over her husband's level of commitment to the couple bond. When interviewed, Mark, the husband, was delighted about the news of the pregnancy, reaffirmed his commitment to the relationship, and criticized her ideas of a social life without family contact. He resented her distant and reserved style with his family and interpreted her request to have meals by themselves as a rejection of his family. The situation called for a compromise across personal styles, family legacies, and cultural background, along with consideration of gender differences.

Societal expectations that the man should be the major wage earner and that the woman's career is secondary in the marriage have significant implications for the health of both men and women in addition to how well the couple can jointly address the predictable crises of this stage. For instance, in Case 2-4, the patient's ambivalence about her pregnancy was related to her conflicts between motherhood obligations and the possible demands of a career. She was reluctant to discuss her conflicts with her husband, being skeptical that, as a man, he would understand her ambivalence. Like many other women, she found herself in a bind— to be a devoted mother or a successful professional—a typical dilemma at this stage, when childbearing decisions must be negotiated. Given our society's expectations for women and the lack of support for parenting, it is not surprising that an increasing number of couples and individuals are deciding to be childless.

The physician in Case 2-4 validated and normalized this patient's ambivalence, acknowledging gender differences and highlighting to the patient and her husband the social implications of childbearing for women. Their mutual expectations and frustrations regarding marriage were also examined and reframed in relation to their different cultural backgrounds. This approach promoted dialogue, understanding, and support. The husband conveyed to his wife her prerogative in making a decision about the future of this pregnancy. She decided to continue with the pregnancy, which unfortunately resulted in an early miscarriage.

Interestingly, these family and cultural differences were not a problem until the couple moved closer to the husband's family. Excessive family participation in a new couple's lives tends to undermine their relationship, whereas physical distance between family members places much more burden on the couple to define relationships by themselves (Carter & McGoldrick, 1999). In the above case, for instance, a change in the couple dynamics would be likely to occur if the wife's family became more present in their lives, bringing a balance between the two family legacies. The genogram (McGoldrick *et al.*, 1999) is a most useful clinical tool for exploring these dynamics (see Chapter 6 on the Family System). In our individual-oriented society, we often forget that marriage involves the joining of two families, not simply two individuals.

Physical closeness to family is an important factor when dealing with cases of spouse abuse, which is quite common at this life stage. Family-of-origin involvement often has a buffering effect against violence, besides providing potential support for the victim. Violence, sexual dysfunction, somatic complaints, and infertility are some common clinical problems arising at this stage of the family life cycle. Physicians aware of these tendencies will be able to detect these problems and address them in an effective and timely manner.

## CASE 2-5

*Joseph is a moderately overweight but otherwise healthy 7-year-old boy who was brought to the clinic three times in a period of 7 weeks for episodes of acute abdominal pain. Physical exam and initial ancillary tests revealed no abnormalities. The physician treated the boy for constipation and suggested dietary changes and increased physical activities to address the weight problem. Before considering further exams, he decided to explore more carefully the patient's social and family situation. This shy yet articulate and pleasant boy talked positively about school and friends but became evasive when asked about his baby brother and family subjects. Joseph's mother reported that her son was probably missing the special attention he was accustomed to receiving from his stepfather before the birth of his young brother. Most of his exclusive time with his mother or stepfather was related to homework activities. The family had also moved to a new apartment in an attractive neighborhood. He was sharing his parents' attention not only with the new baby but also with the new demands created by this move. The stepfather was very involved with house repairs and the mother seemed overwhelmed.*

## FAMILY WITH YOUNG CHILDREN

In Case 2-5, 7-year-old Joseph feels abandoned by the parents when the new baby arrives. The stress he experiences as a result of losing his parents' exclusive focus is manifested in recurrent abdominal pain. The parents face multiple demands as they expand their family and improve their life conditions. Like other couples at this stage, they struggle to meet the emotional needs of each child and their own needs as a couple and as individuals, while fulfilling work, household, and extended family demands. Needless to say, this stage of the life cycle poses a significant threat to individual, couple, and family functioning.

Children's symptoms are often indicators of family stress. Recurrent abdominal pain, along with somatic complaints in general, are problems most commonly seen by physicians working with school-age children. The pediatric literature reports that the majority of children with recurrent pain have real pain that results from the interplay of multiple factors: physiological, psychological, temperamental, and environmental (Poole *et al.*, 1995). Furthermore, they might be manifestations of stress connected to developmental and life-cycle transitions or social stressors experienced by the individual and the family.

This stage is a time for family expansion. New members are added, requiring more physical and emotional space and additional financial resources. New pursuits regarding living conditions, work status, and/or career development are explored. Even when individual and family are both progressing and basic family relationships are positive, as in the case of Joseph and his family, symptoms might occur as responses to stressful transitions.

The three main tasks (Table 2.2) of the family with young children are (1) adapting the marital system to include children; (2) sharing in childrearing, financial, and household responsibilities; and (3) realignment of familial relationships to include new roles: parents, grandparents, siblings, aunts, uncles, and so on (Carter & McGoldrick, 1999).

Another key issue at this stage of the family with young children is the formation and strengthening of the sibling system. In this phase, siblings learn how to share, build alliances, and support each other. Questions regarding sibling conflicts are commonly presented in medical visits. Sibling competition is determined not only by the availability of parents but also by how parents relate to the children.

The birth of a child requires a major realignment of family relationships. When the first child is born, adults move up a generation and assume caretaking responsibilities for the young generation. The couple's own emotional and sexual intimacy may be placed on the back burner as the couple struggles to meet the demands of parenthood. Parenting styles are defined and differences related to culture and family of origin may become pronounced with the birth of a child. Additionally, the couple or single parent may have to renegotiate boundary issues with the families of origin to accommodate the child's relationship to grandparents and other extended kin. Grandparents have to move to a less central role, supporting parents' authority. In the case of single parents, grandparents' and other family members' roles are negotiated differently, as they are most often needed for caretaking functions. Depending on cultural and class background, older children are expected to help care for younger siblings.

A crucial issue during this stage of the life cycle is the disposition of childcare responsibilities and household chores. The lack of social provision for adequate childcare in our society (McGoldrick and Carter, 2002) and the decrease of social support in general often cause children to be left without proper attention or force families, especially women, to make sacrifices to attend to family needs. In Case 2-5 Joseph's mother, a medical technician, decided to quit her job to take care of the children, while her husband continued in his career as a computer manager. Childcare is not affordable for the many two-paycheck or single-parent families with small children. When Joseph was younger, his mother, a single parent, had to rely on her own mother to take care of him to be able to work. As illustrated in Case 2-1, grandmothers are often called on to share childcare responsibilities. Financial pressures also require that the husband/father increase his hours of work, thus decreasing family contact and creating family and marital tension. In Case 2-5, as the physician realized later, the mother's statement about Joseph missing his stepfather's presence also indicated her own need for his attention.

An African proverb says that "it takes a village to raise a child," but these are times in which parents, and mothers in particular, are often left alone to take care of their families. The absence of familial or other support for the parents can lead to role strain and stress for the parents, especially the primary caretaker. Consequently, tension may develop between the couple, between parent(s) and extended family, and between parent(s) and children.

The experience of becoming a parent differs greatly for the couple, depending on each parent's gender. The socially accepted standard that mothers should be the primary caretaker for children can cause tremendous stress and anxiety among employed and career-oriented women. For those women totally involved in home life, depression, somatic complaints, or eating disorders often result. Child abuse or neglect may occur as a consequence of feelings of isolation and lack of a partner's and others' support. Research indicates that the transition to parenthood is accompanied by a general decrease in marital satisfaction and a lowering of self-esteem for women (Cowan & Cowan, 1992). Also, this phase has the highest rate of divorce (Carter & McGoldrick, 1999).

Rather than focusing only on the mother–child bond, it is important that physicians make a concerted effort to value, support, and reinforce the inclusion of fathers (McGoldrick and Carter, 2002) and other family or community members. Our clinical experiences and those of other colleagues indicate that among many Latino and African-American families (McAdoo, 1980), men are very involved with childcare even though women are primarily responsible for identifying and responding to the child's needs. Many children are not raised by their parents for cultural, socioeconomic, psychological, and legal reasons. Grandmothers as primary caretakers are a growing phenomenon (Buchanan & Lappin, 1990). In assessing and counseling families, physicians need to be aware that different family configurations tend to be stigmatized by norms dictated by the dominant culture. Moreover, childrearing practices vary enormously among cultures and social classes regarding approaches to discipline, styles of nurturance, and physical contact.

When assessing the child, her emotional, physical, cognitive, social, and neurological development must be considered in terms of family resources and responsiveness (McGoldrick and Carter, 2002). The child's temperament plays an important role in family life. Joseph's quiet, pleasant, and easygoing way had

# ASSESSING FAMILY FUNCTION:
# QUESTIONS TO ASK PARENTS OF YOUNG CHILDREN

## Couple/Individual

- *"Do you have time for yourselves as a couple?"*
- *"Do each of you find time to respond to your personal needs?"*
- *"How satisfied are you with the support and attention received from your partner and others?"*

## Parenting

- *"How did you learn to be parents?"*
- *"Are you prepared or skillful as parents?"*
- *"What are your sources of support and, if necessary, guidance?"*
- *"What are your styles of parenting?"*
- *"Do these styles conflict with your extended family, your children's school, or your physician or therapist?"*

## Child/Parent

- *"What is the 'fit' between your temperament and that of each of your children?"*
- *"How do you as parents respond to your children's special needs?"*
- *"What is it like to be a parent of children at this developmental stage?"*

facilitated the formation of the couple. The acceptance and bonding with the stepfather was facilitated by the fact that the stepfather also missed the presence of a father in own childhood.

Joseph's feelings of abandonment in Case 2-5 were exacerbated by his colicky baby brother's demands on his mother, as well as her adjustment to her new roles. As the physician could observe in their office interactions, he was missing her direct attention. This is the stage when physicians have the most frequent contact with families. Medical visits—for prenatal and child healthcare, acute illness, family planning, and so on—are very frequent. This is a stage when the physician's role can be most meaningful, as it will affect the course of life for many family members.

## CASE 2-6

*A physician was planning to discharge a 16-year-old Latina adolescent hospitalized for a severe asthmatic attack, when the nurse reported that the patient was planning to run away because of conflicts with her mother, a very religious Pentecostal believer. During the last 6 months, Rose, the patient, a college-bound straight A student, had become less interested in school and more rebellious toward her mother. She complained to the nurse of her mother's "unreasonable demands": expecting her to be responsible for household chores; babysitting for three smaller brothers; and forbidding her to visit friends. When talking to the nurse, Rose came across as a reasonable, thoughtful young woman. When interviewed with her mother, she became very angry and accused her mother of exploiting her as a servant and always taking sides with her brothers. Her mother responded by saying that she expected more from this daughter because she was the oldest. Rose's mother approached the physician privately requesting a gynecological exam to check her daughter's virginity. The young woman had already shared with the physician that she was seeing a boy from school, sometimes visiting his house, but had denied any sexual involvement.*

Adolescence calls for major changes in the family, involving a shift of the adolescent's position within the family and renegotiation of relationships at many levels: parent–child, grandparent–parent, husband–wife, and others.

This is a time of intense emotions and polarizations between family members, especially between the parents and the defiant adolescent. These conflicts typically involve a third person, such as a grandparent, a sibling, an aunt or uncle, a friend, and, frequently, a helping professional. As illustrated in Case 2-5, physicians are often pulled in as the conflict escalates and evolves into a medical event. Common medical events include exacerbation of physical symptoms, poor compliance with treatment of life-threatening illnesses, suicide attempts, drug use, and eating disorders. As in Case 2-6, the physician is often asked by the parent or child to intervene. As parents and adolescent attempt to gain control, they often enlist the support of others for their position, or in some cases, mediation of the conflict. The physician's timely involvement is often crucial to interrupt escalating conflicts that might ultimately lead to tragic outcomes. Typically, as in Case 2-6, the physician was caught in a power struggle between the adolescent and her mother, precipitated by the adolescent's budding sexuality and her demands for more autonomy and independence. In collaboration with a family therapist, the physician interviewed mother and daughter individually to identify their concerns and needs and to attempt a negotiation between them.

As the adolescent searches for autonomy and independence—a life space beyond the boundaries of the family—parental authority and control are challenged. Old rules and established values are questioned, while new ideals and mores are proposed by the adolescent, causing conflict and challenging the stability of the family. This process is less tumultuous when parents learn to be flexible enough to allow the youngster room for new experiences and autonomy, and yet know when to be firm and clear about limits in order to provide a point of reference for the experimenting adolescent. Developing flexible boundaries that allow the adolescent to move in and out, to be dependent at times of vulnerability, and to be independent to the point of taking serious risks is a stressful task for parents, especially in times of increasing violence in many communities. Parents might also feel hurt or rejected by statements such as "I don't want to be like my father or mother" or "Get out of my life," which represent the adolescent's attempts to differentiate from the family and define his or her self-identity.

The youngster's ability to differentiate from others will depend on how well she can handle intense emotions in the context of conflicting social expectations about sexual roles and norms of behavior dictated by family, community, peers, and the media (Garcia-Preto, 1999). The physical and sexual changes that take place at this stage have a dramatic effect on how adolescents see and evaluate themselves and radically alter how they are perceived by others. It is not uncommon for family members to experience confusion and fear when adolescents begin to express their sexual interests. As illustrated in Case 2-6, Mrs. Rodriguez, fearing that her daughter might be sexually active because she had a boyfriend, attempted to control her sexuality by asking the physician to check her virginity. The family's culture and religion are also significant factors in this case, as they restrict adolescent female sexuality and independence. Sometimes the adolescent's growing sexuality is ignored or rejected by parents, which may affect her self-esteem or lead her into premature rebellious and risky sexual activity. Promiscuous sexual behavior, unwanted pregnancy, and unprotected sex are possible consequences. Rose's acceptance of her mother's religious values along with her own abilities, academic aspirations, and the presence of other supports served as powerful buffers against sexual acting-out and other risky behaviors and facilitated the formation of a positive self-concept.

The process of identity formation at this stage involves the adolescent's gender and sexual identity. Considering society's bias toward heterosexuality, the physician has to be attentive to the particular needs of gay, lesbian, and bisexual adolescents, whose conflicts of identity might be expressed through somatization, repeated visits for unspecific complaints, suicidal ideation, or depressive symptoms. Ethnic minority youths also face conflicts related to their experiences of racism or other prejudice in dating, groups, schools, and work situations.

Parents usually confront the adolescent's demands for autonomy at the same time that they face their own midlife issues (Carter & McGoldrick, 1999), such as reexamining their life experiences and choices and reviewing their life plans as individuals and as a couple. Divorce or career changes are not uncommon at this period. In addition, this is a time when the family is often dealing with frail grandparents or other older relatives, a burden that usually falls on women. Parents are challenged to keep a balance between their availability to the family and to themselves, between the new and old generation's needs. Clinical problems in adult patients at this stage are frequently related to these life-cycle stressors (Table 2.2).

Some families become more vulnerable at this stage. Some parents and families are not prepared for changes and feel threatened by the adolescent's developmental needs. They become rigid and controlling and, in response, the child may often escalate rebellious behaviors. As illustrated in Case 2-6, Rose's mother, a single parent, resisted giving her oldest daughter more freedom and time outside the family because of her fear that this would weaken family ties and undermine her authority as a parent with the younger children. As a single parent who had to face many adversities, such as an abusive husband, homelessness, and poverty, she had to maintain strong control over her children and rely on her daughter's help to raise her other children successfully. Her fear of losing Rose's support, companionship, and love did not allow her to recognize and accept her daughter's needs. Like many other parents of adolescent children, she experienced her daughter's requests for autonomy as rejection.

Families that have the most difficulty letting go of their children are those that have come to rely on them for their support (Strelnick & Gilpin, 1986). In single-parent or divorced families, the oldest child often becomes an essential partner to the parent, caught in a parentified position. The adolescent's separation from the family becomes especially difficult if the parent is not able to restructure his life and build new supports. The independence of the youngest adolescent, the last to move on, can also be complicated when the marital bond is fragile and the parents avoid dealing directly with their issues. For instance, the hospitalization of a diabetic young man for ketoacidosis coincided with his discovery of his emotionally distant father's extra-marital affair and the son's concerns for his mother. A family life-cycle perspective allowed the physician to understand the importance of getting both parents involved in their son's treatment and life plans.

The adolescent's development does not depend solely on individual abilities and family competence but, to a large extent, on external factors: the economy, the availability of educational and occupational opportunities, community support, and the influence of the media, to name a few. Many families are disempowered by the intrusion of social institutions and, on occasion, well-intended professionals, which result in clashes of cultural values that undermine their authority as parents. Their disciplinary approaches are criticized or misunderstood, their cultural legacies are devalued, and determinations about their lives are made without proper family participation.

The adolescent's demands for more autonomy and independence tend to activate unresolved conflicts the parents have within themselves, with each other, and with their own parents. In this regard, questioning parents about their own adolescence will often promote understanding and healing across generations and defuse parent–child conflicts. In this case, 2 years after her own mother died, Mrs. Rodriguez, Rose's mother, was thrown out of the house by her alcoholic father when he found out she had a boyfriend. Previous experiences of loss and rejection made her especially sensitive to her daughter's need to separate from the family.

Adolescence marks a period of turmoil and conflicts but also renewal for individuals and the family. In most families, relationships are renegotiated, new life agendas are set, and families continue their developmental trajectory without major disruptions. In some families change cannot occur without a serious crisis. The role of the physician as a family mediator and life consultant is most valuable at this stage.

## CASE 2-7

*Mr. Johnson is a 55-year-old man who had worked as a regional sales manager for a large company until a massive heart attack, which resulted in a quadruple bypass 2 years ago. Previously well stabilized with diet, exercise, and medication, his recent lab results revealed a high cholesterol value, particularly the LDL component. Interviewing the patient, his physician found out that Mr. Johnson had been careless about his diet. He appeared irritable and less communicative than usual. Further inquiry focusing on possible life changes indicated that the patient was upset at his wife's increased involvement with school work and limited availability to assist in cooking and in planning family meals. Initially supportive of his wife's decision to return to graduate school, Mr. Johnson now argued constantly with his wife about her increased absence while at the same time claiming his support for her educational goals.*

## FAMILY AT MIDLIFE

At this stage the renegotiation of the marital relationship is a central task. As the parents become less involved with raising children, they can pay more attention to their own needs, assessing their satisfaction with their personal lives, considering new directions, and often revising their marital arrangement. The decision to pursue one's own needs may pose a threat to the conjugal relationship or to the partner who might expect the marriage to be center stage. The couple in Case 2-7 is an example of the partners' different expectations at this phase of their lives. Mr. Johnson's interests are now limited to the home, where he has had to adjust to a life of limited activity after many years of intense driving and traveling. In contrast, after many years of devotion to her family, raising their two daughters and adjusting to her husband's needs, Mrs. Johnson expects now to have her turn at fulfilling her own goals.

There is a tendency for men and women to be going in opposite directions psychologically at this point (McGoldrick, 1999). Men tend to become more interested in relationships and intimacy, while women's energies are more directed toward personal needs and experiences in the outside world, often resulting in marital conflicts and estrangement. When one partner is disabled or significantly older, the disparity between each spouse's needs may strain the relationship. When the marital bond has been established on principles of mutual care and respect, and companionship is valued by both partners, the couple has a better chance to renegotiate their needs despite inevitable conflicts. Fortunately, this was the case for the Johnsons once their physician facilitated a dialogue about their mutual expectations and priorities. A family life-cycle perspective helped the physician understand and address Mr. Johnson's health in the context of the couple's developmental issues. While addressing Mr. Johnson's feelings, the physician did not support his formulation for his problem—"my wife does not care"—and was able to diffuse the couple's conflicts by focusing on the developmental issues and encouraging the partners toward understanding this role reversal.

This transition has been seen negatively as a time of physical and psychological distress for women. It is at this time that women typically experience menopause, to which their reaction will depend largely on their social status and opportunities (Neugarten & Kraines, 1965). When women have more control over their lives, they are less likely to become anxious and symptomatic. Certainly, women whose only source of affirmation has been mothering are more vulnerable to depression, though they usually recover after a period of adjustment (Harbin, 1978). A significant characteristic of this stage is the great number of entries and exits of family members: children leave, but the family is enlarged by the addition of in-laws; grandparents become ill and die, while grandchildren expand the family.

The renegotiation of the parent–child relationship as the child moves into adulthood is another important task at this stage. For many families this is an easy and rewarding period, marked by the possibility of forming positive relationships with grown children and sharing their accomplishments. For others, the changing economics in our society have made launching difficult, when their adult children cannot support themselves. The youngest of the Johnsons' daughters had lived with them off and on and had been unable to find a stable job. Many middle-aged parents must provide financial or childcare support for younger families, as illustrated in Case 2-1. Problems affecting their adult children, such as marital difficulties, divorce, and unemployment, are often a major source of stress for their parents, eventually resulting in poor health and an increase in medical visits.

This group has been referred to as "the sandwich generation." They are pressed by the needs of the

## ASSESSING FAMILY FUNCTION:
## QUESTIONS TO ASK MIDDLE-AGED PATIENTS

- *"How are things with you and your family now that the children are older and more independent?"*
- *"Thinking about your life, what are the things that make you feel accomplished or happy, and what are the things you wish could be different?"*
- *"And what do you think would be your spouse's response to these questions? To your answers?"*
- *"What do you like about your marriage now? What could be different?"*
- *"How are your parents doing?" "How much does their life situation affect your own life now?"*
- *"How are other family members doing?"*

young, who may still be financially and emotionally dependent on them, and are also pressed by the needs of their aging parents, who become increasingly dependent (Asen *et al.*, 1992; McGoldrick, 1999).

Women are almost always the main caretakers in the family. The physical and emotional demands of caretaking make them more vulnerable to somatic and psychological problems. When a family member has a flareup of a chronic illness or does not respond to treatment, the physician should be alert to life-cycle issues, including burnout of the caretaker. Stress at this stage may also signal unresolved issues from earlier life-cycle stages. The physician should assess changes in the marriage, marital satisfaction, caretaking of elderly parents, the strength of the family's support system, relationships with adult children and grandchildren, unfulfilled needs and goals, and the impact of losses.

## CASE 2-8

*Mrs. Casey, a 65-year-old-woman with a past history of well-controlled non-insulin-dependent diabetes mellitus and hypertension who had been quite independent and active, was hospitalized for a stroke, a left-sided cerebrovascular accident. After that, her ability to walk and use her right hand became quite impaired. The patient was responding well to rehabilitation, but her level of activity was very restricted, requiring constant support in all activities of daily living. Mrs. Casey had five children and was living with the youngest, who was feeling overwhelmed by the prospect of being the main caregiver for her mother. Three other children had been involved, visiting their mother regularly. They appeared to be a close and well-functioning family. The physician noticed, however, some tension among the siblings. The daughters resented their brothers' passivity regarding their mother's needs. One day the patient had a fall in the hospital while trying to stand up without help, resulting in a minor injury. The physician was approached by one of the sons, whom he did not know well. The son angrily criticized him for delaying arrangements for discharge and blamed him for the incident. The physician was taken by surprise, considering his positive and close relationship with the patient and other children, who had praised him in the past for his availability to the family.*

## FAMILY AT LATER LIFE

The family in later life is faced with the painful task of accepting and adjusting to the physical decline of their older members. Adult children are required to make a shift in relational status with their aging parents and to reorganize their lives to provide them with emotional and physical support. Responses of anxiety, anger, and confusion are not uncommon, as the younger generation tries to cope with the new situation. Past unresolved family issues might emerge, amplifying these emotional reactions. Mrs. Casey's son's accusations can be interpreted as a displacement of feelings of anger and helplessness regarding her physical condition. This was exacerbated by unrecognized guilt as a result of his distancing from his family during other critical moments. The physician–patient–family relationship is especially likely to be affected when family members cannot accept the parents' decline or deal with their own conflicts and responsibilities constructively. In this case, the physician scheduled a family meeting with all of the siblings to help them identify and share their feelings and thoughts regarding their mother's condition and to foster mutual support around caregiving responsibilities.

It is distressing to witness a parent who was once active and healthy become frail and dependent. In Case 2-8, this process was especially challenging to the family, given the fact that Mrs. Casey, a vibrant woman, still held a job until the occurrence of this medical event. A proud and independent person, she avoided asking for help and tried to overcome her physical limitations, resulting in an injury. In general, most aging parents are reluctant to ask family members for support in an effort to maintain their dignity and to avoid being seen as a burden in their children's lives. However, some older adults become totally dependent on the next generation, placing excessive demands on their children. Given time constraints, financial pressures, and conflicting multiple demands on families these days, they are especially challenged to fulfill their caregiving obligations to the older generation. When parents have been independent and self-sufficient, adult children may fail to recognize a parent's needs and delay making the required shift of status in their relations with the ailing or aging parent. In these cases, the physician may have a critical role in facilitating support for the patient by taking the initiative to mobilize the children's involvement in the treatment.

Financial and caregiving demands are a major source of stress for the middle generation, at a stage when they still might be involved with childrearing responsibilities as well as facing financial pressures related to older children's education and their own life changes. Geographic distance is often an additional factor limiting availability of support and straining family relations. Women are especially burdened by becoming the sole or main caregiver for their relatives. Physicians need to be alert to the high incidence of depressive and somatic symptoms among caregivers. It is not surprising that Mrs. Casey's youngest daughter was distressed: she was trying to juggle the competing demands of being an attentive daughter, caring mother, and responsible worker. Typically, Mrs. Casey's daughters were more willing to make personal sacrifices to attend their mother's needs than were her sons, and resentment inevitably emerged. This imbalance of responsibilities is likely to be reinforced when the physician minimizes expectations for men as caregivers in their contacts with the family. The physician's role is also crucial when considering institutionalization. Besides addressing the patient's feelings of rejection and fear, the physician can help the family deal with their guilt and facilitate the decision-making process.

Awareness of ethnic and multigenerational traditions can help physicians distinguish normative patterns of caregiving from dysfunctional responses of detachment or overinvolvement (Rolland, 1994). Latino families, for instance, tend to have strong intergenerational ties and are likely to be closely involved and protective of patients. In the case of terminal illness, they might prefer to "protect" the patient from knowing the diagnosis. African-American families often share responsibility among immediate and extended family members, forming a kin network to support the needs of aging parents.

For the frail or disabled parent, the transition of status is also difficult as the parent has to grieve the loss of the competent self and adjust to the reality of a less independent and active life. In health or in sickness, the aging individual is challenged to find a dignified role in a society where old people tend to be devalued and marginalized. Many people postpone retirement for these reasons.

Grandparenthood can offer a "new lease on life" as it brings opportunities for meaningful interactions and facilitates resolution regarding one's mortality (Walsh, 1999). The acceptance of one's life and death, a major task at this stage, occurs when the individual is able to achieve a sense of integrity versus despair (Erikson, 1968).

## ASSESSING FAMILY FUNCTION:
## QUESTIONS TO ASK OLDER PATIENTS AND THEIR FAMILIES

- *How well does the patient understand his or her situation?*
- *How well does the family understand the patient's situation?*
- *Are the adult children prepared to deal with their parents' aging, disability, and increased dependence?*
- *Are they able to shift roles to respond to the new needs?*
- *What is the distribution of caregiving responsibilities among family members?*

Death and terminal illness of the older generation are particularly emotional events for adult children, as they are forced to face their own mortality and aging (Rolland, 1994). For widows and widowers, feelings of loss, disorientation, and loneliness contribute to an increase in death and suicide rates during the first year, especially for men. Advances in medical technology have extended life expectancy and allowed people to be more functional to enjoy life into older age. Physical and psychological well-being will also depend on financial security, access to health services, and social contacts.

A consultation with the family is always advised when treating older patients. Such a consultation can assess and enlist family support and ensure physician–patient–family collaboration.

## CONCLUSION

This chapter has described how the individual and family life-cycle perspective is a useful framework to address medical problems as it relates typical clinical presentations to predictable stages and specific developmental tasks. However, the life cycle should not be understood as a static concept. It needs to be examined in relation to particular life contexts with special attention to cultural differences, socioeconomic factors, and societal changes. Social stressors such as poverty and migration, and also critical events such as sickness, death, and divorce, have a major impact on the course of the individual and family life cycles.

The application of the individual and family life-cycle models in medicine has been criticized for promoting the idea of "normal" development and the traditional bias against women and different cultural

## SELF-DISCOVERY QUESTIONS

- *"Where are you in your individual life cycle development?" (see Table 2.1)*
- *"Which developmental tasks have you found most challenging?" (see Table 2.1) "Why do you think this was so?"*
- *"Which developmental tasks do you think each of your parents found most challenging?" "Why?"*
- *"What do you think will be the biggest challenge for you at your next life cycle stage?" (see Table 2.1)*
- *"What stage of the family life cycle are you at?" (see Table 2.2)*
- *"How do you assess your handling of the emotional processes in your current family life cycle phase?"*
- *"What changes in family status may be required for you to proceed to the next developmental stage?' (see Table 2.2)*
- *"How do you think you will handle the last phase of the life cycle?"*

groups (Candib, 1989). When and how families negotiate a life transition vary according to their ethnicity, class, and religion.

It is important that clinicians examine their own cultural values, especially their assumptions about "normality" and the notion of "family" in assessing individual and family development and functioning, and to avoid pathologizing patients' experiences. Finally, the physician should be aware of his or her own family experiences and life-cycle stage to evaluate how these will affect understanding and identification with each patient and family.

## CASES FOR DISCUSSION

### CASE 1

*A 50-year-old middle-class African-American professional woman, a dynamic high-school principal, came for a follow-up visit 6 months after surgery for breast cancer. The physician was struck by the patient's reaction to his good news about the surgery and lab results. This assertive and engaging woman started crying, revealing an unexpected sense of hopelessness and helplessness about her life situation, caused by marital distress after 23 years of a very happy marriage. The physician noticed that her husband, recently retired, did not come with her to the visit as he usually does.*

1. *Considering life-cycle issues and the impact of her illness, what kind of questions would you ask this patient about herself, her husband, and their relationship to understand her depression?*
2. *What hypothesis would you have regarding her depression and marital distress?*

### CASE 2

*A 17-year-old man with a history of well-controlled asthma is hospitalized for the second time in a period of 10 months. No major environmental changes explain this exacerbation of his illness. On visiting the patient in the hospital, the physician noticed that the patient seemed distraught after a family visit. This young man, usually cheerful and positive about life, broke down in tears when asked about his distress.*

1. *What information would you elicit from this patient to understand his symptoms from an individual and family life-cycle perspective?*
2. *Suppose he comes from a middle-class family whose parents are facing life transitions. What are these possible transitions and how might they be related to the patient's symptoms?*
3. *Now suppose a different situation: he is college bound and from a poor inner-city family. Considering possible issues related to differences of values, formulate some different hypotheses for the exacerbation of his illness and his emotional response. Take into consideration (a) socioeconomic factors, (b) intergenerational conflicts related to cultural clashes, and (c) issues of sexual identity.*

### CASE 3

*A 32-year-old mother brought her two children—a 6-year-old girl and a 4-year-old boy—for a routine visit. While in your office the children started to fight over a toy. The mother lost her temper and slapped the older child, scolding her for reacting to her brother's provocation. She apologized for the incident and asked for your advice.*

1. *How do you understand each child's behavior in relation to life-cycle stages and related tasks? Take into consideration gender differences.*
2. *Focusing on this family's life-cycle stage, what would you like to know about the family situation to help this mother deal with the sibling fights?*

## CASE 4

*A powerful business executive, a 56-year-old man of German descent, was hospitalized for congestive heart failure. A medical student went to check the patient and found him arguing with his wife, expressing disapproval of his only daughter's decision to marry before finishing law school. The wife, unable to calm her husband, asked the student to talk to him.*

1. *Considering life-cycle issues, what questions should the student ask the patient to understand his feelings?*
2. *Using your knowledge of family life cycle, what could be a possible script explaining the patient's reactions and the family crisis?*
3. *What would be each family member's view of the problem?*

## CASE 5

*A physician was worried about a 35-year-old diabetic patient whose blood glucose levels became increasingly higher during the past 2 months. While focusing on her social situation, the physician learned that the patient, the youngest of three daughters from a Jewish family, was considering postponing her wedding because of her 70-year-old mother's recent disability as a result of a stroke.*

1. *How do you understand this woman's dilemma, taking into consideration this family life-cycle stage?*
2. *Discuss caretaking issues in relation to gender and sibling order.*

## RECOMMENDED READINGS

Carter B, McGoldrick M: *The Expanded Facility Life Cycle: Individual, Faculty, and Social Perspectives*, ed 3. Boston, Allyn & Bacon, 1999.

> A classic text in the field of family systems that presents a well-conceptualized view of the family as it evolves through the life cycle. A must-read for medical providers interested in expanding their knowledge and skills in family work.

Rolland J: *Families, Illness and Disability: An Integrative Treatment Model*. New York, Basic Books Inc, 1994.

> A most useful text which provides a conceptual framework—a psychosocial typology and time phases of illness—which integrates chronic illness, disability, family and the individual life cycle.

Asen KE, Tomson T, Canavan B: *Family Solutions in Family Practice*. Lancaster, England, Quay Publishing, 1992.

> This readable book is a practical guide for medical practitioners on how to manage typical problems in primary care practice from a family perspective. It includes many concrete suggestions on how to interview patients, conduct family meetings, and intervene in problem situations.

McDaniel S, Campbell T, Seaburn D: *Family-Oriented Primary Care: A Manual for Medical Providers*. Berlin, Springer-Verlag, 1990.

> This excellent book is designed for physicians who want to enhance their skills in family systems medicine. The book provides a useful conceptual framework including relevant research on family systems and a practical guide to clinical practice illustrated with case examples and protocols.

Doherty WJ, Baird MP: *Family Therapy and Family Medicine: Towards the Primary Care of Families*. New York, Guilford Press, 1983.

> This pioneering book introduces a family-oriented model to medical practice applying family therapy theory and techniques. It is practical, clearly written, and still remarkably up-to-date even though it was published in the early 1980s.

## REFERENCES

Asen KE, Tomson T, Canavan B: *Family Solutions in Family Practice*. Lancaster, England, Quay Publishing, 1992.

Borysenko J: *A Woman's Book of Life: The Biology, Psychology, Spirituality of the Feminine Life Cycle*. New York, Riverhead Books, 1996.

Buchanan, B, Lappin J: Re-storying the soul of the family. *The Family Networker*, November/December, 1990, pp 46–52.

Candib L: Family life cycle theory. *Fam Syst Med* 7(4), 1989.

Carter B: Becoming parents: The family with young children, in Carter B, McGoldrick M (eds): *The Expanded Family Life Cycle: Individual, Family and Social Perspectives*, ed 3. Boston, Allyn & Bacon, 1999.

Carter B, McGoldrick M (eds): *The Expanded Family Life Cycle: Individual, Family and Social Perspectives*, ed 3. Boston, Allyn & Bacon, 1999.

Comer JP, Poussiant AF: *Raising Black Children*. New York, Penguin Books, Inc, 1992.

Cowan CP, Cowan H: *Where Partners Become Parents: The Big Life Change for Couples*. New York, Basic Books Inc, 1992.

Erikson EH: *Identity: Youth and Crisis*, ed 2. New York, WW Norton & Co, Inc, 1968.

Garcia-Preto N: *Transformation of the family system in adolescence*, in Carter B, McGoldrick M (eds): *The Expanded Family Life Cycle: Individual, Family and Social Perspectives*, ed 3. Boston, Allyn & Bacon, 1999, pp 274–286.

Gilligan C: *In a Different Voice*. Cambridge, Mass, Harvard University Press, 1982.

Goleman D: *Emotional Intelligence*. New York, Bantam Books, Inc, 1997.

Harbin E: Effects on the empty nest transition: A self-report of psychological well-being. *J Marriage Fam* 40:549–556, 1978.

Hines PM, Garcia-Preto N, McGoldrick M, Almeida R, Weltman S: Culture and the family life cycle, in Carter B, McGoldrick M (eds): *The Expanded Family Life Cycle: Individual, Family and Social Perspectives*, ed 3. Boston, Allyn & Bacon, 1999.

Maccoby EE: Gender and relationships: A developmental account. *Am Psychol* 45:513–520, 1990.

Matthias B, French MA: *Forty Ways to Raise a Non-racist Child*. New York, Harper, 1996.

McAdoo JR: The roles of black fathers in the socialization of black children, in McAdoo H (ed): *Black Families*, ed 2. Newbury Park, Calif, Sage Publications, 1980, pp 257–259.

McGoldrick M: Women and the family life cycle, in Carter B, McGoldrick M (eds): *The Changing Family Life Cycle: A Framework for Family Therapy*, ed 2. New York, Gardner Press, 1988a, pp 29–64.

McGoldrick M: Ethnicity and family life cycle, in Carter B, McGoldrick M (eds): *The Changing Family Life Cycle: A Framework for Family Therapy*, ed 2. New York, Gardner Press, 1988b, pp 69–86.

McGoldrick M: Women and the family life cycle, in Carter B, McGoldrick M (eds): *The Expanded Family Life Cycle: Individual, Family and Social Perspectives*, ed 3. Boston, Allyn & Bacon, 1999.

McGoldrick M, Carter B: The self in context: The individual life cycle in systemic perspective, in Carter B, McGoldrick M (eds): *The Expanded Family Life Cycle: Individual, Family and Social Perspectives*, ed 3. Boston, Allyn & Bacon, 1999.

McGoldrick M, Carter B: The changing family life cycle, in F. Walsh (ed): *Normal Family Processes*, ed. 3. New York, Guilford Press, 2002.

McGoldrick M, Heiman M, Carter B: The changing family life cycle, in Walsh F (ed): *Normal Family Processes*, ed 2. New York, Guilford Press, 1993, pp 405–443.

McGoldrick M, Gerson R, Shellenberger S: *Genograms: Assessment and Intervention*. New York, WW Norton & Co, Inc, 1999.

Neugarten B, Kraines RJ: Menopausal symptoms in women of various ages. *Psychosom Med* 27:256–273, 1965.

Pipher M: *Reviving Ophelia: Saving the Selves of Adolescent Girls*. New York: Ballantine Books, Inc, 1994.

Poole SR, Schmitt BD, Mauro R: Recurrent pain syndrome in children: A streamlined approach. *Contemp Pediatr* 12(1), 1995.

Roberts S: *Who We Are: A Portrait of America Based on the Latest U.S. Census*. New York Times Books, Random House, 1994.

Rolland JS: *Families, Illness and Disability: An Integrative Treatment Model*. New York, Basic Books, Inc, 1994.

Strelnick AH, Gilpin M: The family life cycle in the urban context, in Birrer R (ed): *Urban Family Medicine*. Berlin, Springer-Verlag, 1986, 27–41.

Walsh F: The families in later life: Challenges and opportunities, in Carter EA, McGoldrick M (ed): *The Expanded Family Life Cycle: Individual, Family and Social Perspectives*, ed 3. Boston, Allyn & Bacon, 1999, pp 307–326.

Watson MF, Protinsky HO: Black adolescents' identity development: Effects of perceived family structure. *Fam Relat* 37:288–292, 1988.

# PART II

# The Doctor

As with patients, the personhood of the physician often gets lost during medical education as physicians in training attempt to assimilate a vast amount of information and utilize that information for the good of their patients. These chapters will bring the personhood of the physician into focus and also help physicians in training understand the effect of that training process on their psyches and values. Understanding the physician's roles in society, through literature, will also help physicians in training understand the unique medical culture they are entering. Without such an understanding, physicians in training are at risk of losing their values and becoming less humane.

The successful physician must also develop all of the diagnostic, treatment, and technical skills that are the purview of a clinician. Interviewing a patient and taking a history, performing a physical exam, appropriately ordering laboratory tests, making a diagnosis, instituting treatment, and keeping good records and then presenting those findings to consultants are all important skills that must be learned.

Finally, more advanced skills are becoming necessary as patients demand more from their physicians. The advanced skills section describes how to interview patients in difficult circumstances, involve patients and their families in the management of chronic illness, counsel patients to change their behaviors to improve health, assess their functional status and quality of life, promote their health as well as ordering tests to screen for disease early, and then finally critically appraising new research findings, which will enable physicians to appropriately integrate new knowledge and techniques into their practice. The development of these more advanced clinical skills will enable physicians to function much more effectively in today's ever-changing clinical environment.

## CHAPTER 3

# A. The Physician

# **Becoming a Physician**

*Catherine P. McKegney*

*Helen, the ward clerk (unit secretary) on Harris 3, was legendary. She had worked at the University Hospital for somewhere between 15 and 50 years, no one knew for sure how long. The house staff figured she had the secretarial equivalent of tenure. She was intelligent and acerbic, and clearly burned-out.*

*Yia was very excited to be beginning her first rotation in the hospital on Harris 3. As her instructor had suggested, she introduced herself to the ward clerk politely and enthusiastically. Helen's response was, "I eat medical students for lunch, you know." Yia responded, "I don't think I'd taste very good," and hurried off to warn the other student on her team.*

## EDUCATIONAL OBJECTIVES

1. Understand emotions as natural and useful to physicians
2. Possess skills for managing emotions without simply suppressing them in the name of professionalism
3. Identify the varieties of uncertainty in medicine and the role that mistakes must play in learning
4. Recognize ways that medical hierarchy and privilege influence professional identity and interactions with patients and other medical professionals
5. Articulate the quandaries of boundaries between professionals and between clinicians and patients, recognizing the dialectic between the therapeutic use of joining with others and the need for asymmetry in healing and teaching relationships

## INTRODUCTION

How do we become physicians? How do we transform ourselves into those mysterious creatures? Although professional transformation can be as idiosyncratic as the initiates who begin it, there are patterns to the process. These patterns are portrayed in popular media, on television shows such as *ER* and in best-selling books like Samuel Shem's *The House of God* (Shem, 1978). Though popular culture is attending more to the stories of physician development, insights into the intricacies of how professional transformation occurs are rarely found there. Many medical educators and sociologists have written about the transformations that occur in medical trainees, but collapsing their discussions into a coherent story is very difficult.

In this chapter, I will explore the academic constructs offered by these observers within a metaphor of human development in the context of the family. This metaphor is not reality—medical students are not really children—but it illuminates the process and highlights the individuality of the trainee within the commonality of the training experience and the context of the U.S. medical system. If we decide to view the medical system as a family (McKegney, 1989), who is in and who is outside the family? Who takes what roles? What does this family look like? What does it do well? What are some of its pathologies?

Medical students are the newest members of the family. They don't know the rules and therefore depend on their teachers' guidance to avoid mistakes and to learn how learning occurs in this family. In the preclinical years, they are often confused by the political wrangling that involves their faculty and older trainees, hearing the feelings without understanding the issues. In their clinical years, medical students, like kindergartners, want to demonstrate their vast knowledge of (in this instance) basic science only to find that much of it doesn't apply in the new world of the teaching hospital. They recognize that they can learn from everyone in the hospital, from the department chairs to the orderlies, and are hurt (Silver & Glicken, 1990), like Yia in Case 3-1, by the trickle-down resentment that lands on them at the bottom of the heap.

Continuing with the family metaphor, interns are school-age children, learning as fast as they ever will, with new responsibilities, new opportunities, and new vulnerability to a system that has little time to accommodate individual talents or shortcomings. Intern mistakes have the potential to be lethal, since their orders no longer must be "cosigned." Some are overwhelmed by the independence, others become cocky, and most muddle through, learning the basic procedures of the system from the nurses, respiratory technicians (nannies and foster mothers), and senior residents (older siblings). The faculty physicians teach, but focus more on large concepts and pathophysiology than the essential basics of night-to-night management of sick patients.

Senior residents, like adolescents, vacillate between deserved confidence in their specialized knowledge and the anxiety of the impending "real world" waiting for them outside the teaching hospital at the completion of their training. On the one hand, they take on the semiparental function of supervising interns and medical students. These older sibs tend to evaluate their youngers by how well they get the chores done (care of patients) than how well they do their homework (reading or attending lectures) (Hundert *et al.*, 1996). On the other hand, they worry what they'll do when they need help "on the outside," seeing adulthood as complete independence from interference or assistance.

Fellows are a bit like adult children who still live at home at an age when most of their peers are settled and on their own. They are often the preferred consultant of their younger "siblings," who are less intimidated about asking them questions than asking the attending faculty. Like "big brother" or "big sister" home from college, the fellow is in the most temporary position of all with the shortest time left before true adulthood.

In the medical education "family" there are several generations of adults, and a variety of in-laws. The fledgling attending physicians are like new parents. They are unsure of exactly how to "raise the children," but fairly certain that they can do a better job than their predecessors. Though they require the assistance of their seniors, some of that help feels like interference, and an imposition of old ways. Compared with academic faculty, community-based physicians are less connected to their family of origin and less available to students as well. On the other hand, they are living the career goals of most medical students. Senior faculty physicians have been through the challenges of launching a few generations of trainees and have made a few runs at changing the system. They can see that not all of the new tricks are all that new, or necessarily better than the old tricks. Some have grown cynical and have stopped trying to make a difference.

Nonphysician faculty and staff in hospitals and training programs have vital roles in teaching but, like in-laws or stepparents, they are never quite counted as "real members" of the physician family. Teachers of the basic sciences and the behavioral sciences are valued and gain academic status within the university, but they are in the peculiar position of nurturing trainees who are pursuing a different discipline from their own. They seem all-powerful during the clinical years, but usually have a lower status in the hospital. Compared with physicians, they have less hierarchical power and less acknowledgment of their roles as teachers.

Like stepparents, gardeners, nannies, cooks, and maiden aunts in a huge extended household, the nurses, ward clerks, and radiology technicians do most of the work of patient care in the teaching hospital. The power of these unacknowledged teachers to help or hinder the neophyte physician in learning medicine and in performing the required "scut work" is enormous (Lassetter, 1984; Stein, 1967; Wolf, 1997). Operating room nurses make sure that medical students know how to scrub properly and the nursing assistants on the wards take the time to help house staff find essential supplies. Like most groups whose contributions are undervalued, they resent the invisibility of their contributions to patient care and teaching. They anticipate the induction of the students into the unselfconsciously privileged role of physician, at the top of the medical hierarchy, though they are currently the most vulnerable because of their dependent state. In these circumstances, they are the obvious target for retaliation, although usually more indirectly than in Case 3-1.

Deans, department chairs, and most senior faculty are like the grandparents. They sometimes usurp the active parenting role of the younger faculty and sometimes step in to balance the system in essential ways that only years of experience can guide. The grandparents know the myths of the family and the history; they have the clearest vision of the family's place in the community at large.

What are the strengths of this family? Its members are all intelligent, dedicated, energetic, and capable. Most come to their chosen work to heal the sick and assuage their patients' pain. The work is exhausting and joyful: It involves participation in the deepest human experiences and offers unparalleled opportunity for personal growth. The training process is both arduous and exhilarating. Though all members of this "family" are doing their best most of the time, the interaction patterns that are the legacy of medical education can be very painful, contributing to physician impairment and burnout. Like parents who raise their children as they themselves were raised, medical educators tend to teach as they were taught (Hundert *et al.*, 1996), perpetuating patterns of isolation, rigidity, unrealistic expectations, secret keeping, triangulation, blaming, and denial of the pain that they themselves experienced in training (see Table 3.1) (McKegney, 1989).

Growth from infancy to maturity within the medical family involves development in a number of key ways: "managing emotions" (Smith & Kleinman, 1989), "training for uncertainty" (Fox, 1989), facing

**Table 3.1**

Comparison of Common Dysfunctional Family Patterns and Similar Dynamics in the Medical Education System

| | Family system | Medical education system |
|---|---|---|
| Isolation | Insists on minimal interaction with the community | Separates trainees and physicians from the community of patients |
| | Won't let in-laws give suggestions | Discounts criticism from nonphysicians: "How could they understand?" |
| Rigidity | Continues autocratic parenting long after children are old enough to make their own choices | Maintains overextension of on-call hours despite more intensive inpatient care demands |
| Unrealistic expectations | Feeds children junk food, neglecting nutritional needs | Requires house staff to work 30-hour shifts |
| | Leaves a 10-year-old without supervision overnight | Expects students not to make mistakes even if appropriate given their level of expertise |
| Secret keeping | Avoids revealing family problems to outsiders | Hides physician impairment and student abuse |
| Triangulation | Mom talks about disappointments in dad with teenage daughter | University professor criticizes community physician to students, not face to face |
| Blaming | "You're a bad kid" | "A good intern doesn't forget that kind of thing" |
| Denial | "There's nothing wrong in our family" | "Internship wasn't that bad—all of us did one" |

mistakes, adapting to a new identity, and delineating boundaries. The remainder of this chapter will examine these themes offering clarity for students who are struggling to become physicians in the context of the medical education system.

---

### CASE 3-2

*The first semester of the first year of medical school. Gross anatomy. Six medical students to a cadaver, beginning the first day and for the next 4 months, they will skin her, and then take her apart, beginning with her back and arm, ending with her head—deconstructing her completely before they take the formaldehyde-soaked paper towels from her face.*

*The six of them talk about her as they use her irreproducible body to see, feel, and embed in their memories the intricacies of human construction. They become a team around her, talking little about the repulsion of filleting human flesh, but acknowledging their respect for her donation, as they are initiated into this new mystery of the human reality.*

*Most teams named "their" cadavers: Across the room, the young man with the cherry red muscles was called "Godzilla" because of his bulk. And everyone visited him when they had trouble finding the smaller muscles of their wizened "80-something" woman. They all speculated whether he had committed suicide with carbon monoxide because of his color. Of course, they never knew. Each team wondered about what had killed their cadaver. The team gathered around the "80-something" woman was grateful she had everything except her gallbladder; it meant they didn't have to lean over another team's shoulders too often to learn. And they named her "Madonna" after a blonde bombshell of the era, in part as a joke about how old and tiny she was, and in part as a grateful accolade.*

---

### CASE 3-3

*Sandra, a fourth-year medical student on her cardiology rotation, is the acting intern caring for a 45-year-old woman, Mrs. Jones, who had a cardiac arrest at home, was resuscitated by the EMTs after ineffective CPR by her husband, and has persistent hypoxic encephalopathy. For the one year prior to this disaster, she was the breadwinner because of her husband's disabling back pain from a work injury. He visits her constantly, traveling from their home 50 miles away. Over the second week of hospitalization, as the patient's cognitive impairment appears more permanent, Sandra notices that the couple verbally deny Mrs. Jones's limitations; all the while, Mr. Jones does so much for his wife that she is not learning the skills she needs to adapt to her disability.*

*At morning rounds, Sandra recommends a psychiatric consultation regarding the dysfunctional dynamic she sees developing between husband and wife: organizing their relationship yet again around the illness role of one of them. The attending looks askance, implying that Sandra is overly sensitive, and states that the couple's relationship will have little effect on Mrs. Jones's recovery. Much to her own shock, Sandra begins to cry, and the senior resident guides her into an empty patient room until she can pull herself together, which she does hurriedly in order to join the team as they finish rounds. Neither the resident, the attending, nor any of Sandra's fellow medical students ever mentions this incident. Sandra is left feeling that she became too involved, and worries that her display of emotion will affect her evaluation.*

---

## MANAGING EMOTIONS

One of the goals of the medical training process, it seems, is to exorcise emotional expression by the developing physician. The normal feelings evoked by close contact with another person—shyness, sexual attraction, fear, revulsion, pity—are deemed "unprofessional." When instructors see evidence of these strong feelings, they often fear that the trainee is not in control, and may not be able to do the job. The initiate is expected to panic, in a very minor way, at the beginning of the first year; after that, the student should be able to hide, if not override, intense responses. After all, a physician should keep a cool head, focus on what can be fixed, remaining warm and therapeutic all the while. Medical students, no longer "laypeople" and not yet physicians, are neither fish nor fowl; the transition from obeying normal societal taboos about what is discussed and what is touched to the full breaking of those taboos as physicians is an awkward process (Harper, 1993).

For the physician in training, this acquisition of "affective neutrality" (Smith & Kleinman, 1989) begins at the very beginning: in gross anatomy lab as in Case 3-2. The revulsion felt when facing the formaldehyde-preserved cadaver is commonplace and seldom discussed. To help the new students stay calm, the instructors are strategically matter-of-fact. The students are recognized as being in transition; they have not yet acquired the distance necessary to perform in the medical system, and they are taught by example. In striving to obey the rules of the medical family, they imitate the calm of the professors, even though they have strong reactions which this placid behavior belies. As adults, they feel fear when facing death and revulsion about urine, feces, and other excreta. Many students are left with the sense that they are the only ones who experience conflict and confusion because of the paucity of opportunities to directly address these feelings. Smith and Kleinman (1989) observed that most students would turn an emotionally charged situation into a scientific problem to be solved, ignoring the affective components, both the patient's and their own. Solving problems is vastly more comfortable than facing the reflection of one's own fear of illness in the patient's. Focusing on the details of technique or points to be learned turns the situation into an intellectual puzzle like the ones they have been playing with for their previous 16 years of education. Consciously ignoring that they are crudely cutting up what once was a human being, students also use humor, joking, as in Case 3-2, gently or disrespectfully to dissipate less acceptable feelings of disgust or anxiety (Fox, 1989).

And what about sexual feelings? Physicians have license to touch others in ways usually associated with intimate relationships. Parents with their infants and lovers with each other have this right—and physicians. Even in this day of magnetic resonance imaging and the Human Genome Project, physicians examine their patients. Patients expect it, and information absorbed through the eyes, ears, nose, and hands of the physician is still the fastest, most "cost-effective" to acquire, and most efficiently integrated. Breaking social taboos to gather information during a history and physical examination requires an adjustment (Harper, 1993). Students often express the confusion they feel as if it were only about technique: uncertainty about what the epididymis feels like, or how to move aside a woman's breast to listen to her heart. To admit to the uncontrollable intrusion of sexual feelings during this basic ritual of the profession hints somehow at unfitness for the job rather than an intact hypothalamus.

Discussion of technical details is one way of ignoring the feelings evoked by physical examinations; total avoidance is another popular way to manage this problem. House officers supervising medical students will overlook the "rectal deferred" on the physical examination form, ignoring the student's discomfort just as they ignore their own. In some circumstances, the patient's condition is a legitimate reason for delaying aspects of the examination. Most often, the students' discomfort and their supervisors' are the reasons for incomplete histories or examinations. Since the physicians' discomfort is rarely addressed explicitly, the student gets little guidance in deciding when it is truly appropriate not to do a rectal examination on a patient, and when the student needs to do the examination in order to provide good care. Avoiding the examination because of embarrassment or sexual feelings may be appropriate, but only if arrangements are made for another to complete the examination for the patient's sake.

Calm in the face of crisis is an appropriate goal for a professional who will face pain and death on a regular basis. Recognizing, naming, accepting, and honoring these feelings might better prepare students for their clinical responsibilities. As one study has shown, unrecognized feelings can interfere with the young physicians' performance of the clinical interview (Epstein *et al.*, 1998; Smith, 1986). Unfortunately, most medical students are taught to ignore their emotions, in a silent curriculum of denial. By the time they finish medical school, most students will exclaim excitedly about the latest "great case," but will be unable to feel

## COPING WITH FEELINGS

*When you feel feelings, find someone whom you can tell. Do this especially when it seems the feelings are silly or inappropriate. Remember to use feeling words. Confusion is more of a thinking process than a feeling one. Feeling words include mad, sad, bad, glad, scared, lonely, turned on, hurt. Find someone you can trust to support you, a professional counselor, your advisor, a minister, or your sibling, and who can keep confidences.*

the fear of vulnerability, disability, and loneliness that produced Sandra's tears in Case 3-3. The silence that greeted those tears taught her to suppress them the next time.

Though medical students are intentionally trained to suppress emotional expression, they are also expected to learn how to remain warm and compassionate with patients and their families. This empathy with patients is stated as a value by teachers, but students are left to find it within themselves rather than being guided to balance their level headedness with compassion. In expressing compassion, students and house staff are expected to draw on precisely those sensitivities that they silently discarded during gross anatomy and their uncomfortable clinical encounters. The chasm between social self and professional self is too deep for some, and they settle into a cool, distant style. This is familiar as the classic style of the university-based consultant who often knows only parts of his patients' lives, those bits that are relevant to his specialty. Since medical students spend most of their time with university-based physicians, this "expert" style is the professional style they often incorporate as their own.

As Renee Fox documented during the 1960s (Fox, 1989), the humanist movement within medicine articulated the value of the warmer, more collaborative physician that the patient advocacy movement also emphasized. When medical students and residents attempt to build a collaborative bridge with their social skills, they can find themselves awash in feelings: patients', families', and their own. They relied on "analytic transformation" and denial to cope during their own initiations, and so have no personal experience on which to draw while caring for their patients. Awkwardly and ineffectively, they resort to reassuring patients and families with intellectual explanations. Or they assume that patients and families will remain so "emotional" and irrational that explanations will be useless. Instructing students in "patient education" may provide skills, but without attention to the emotional scars and habits of denial that remain from training, the skills will be difficult to incorporate into patient encounters. For example, if we follow Sandra in Case 3-3 into her residency, we find that she feels confused about discussing increasing activities after an MI with a patient and his wife. She knows what the equivalences are between activity achieved in cardiac rehab and the effort needed for home activities. She knows that most couples have questions that they rarely ask about sexual activities after a heart attack. In seminar sessions, she practiced eliciting and answering precisely these questions. Still, she hesitates. Her supervisor comments on her hesitation and she feels ashamed, and gets teary again. After delicate questioning, she remembers the story of her crying on rounds in medical school. When her supervisor agrees with her assessment of the Jones's marital style, and congratulates her for her courage in bringing up the subject, she feels enormous relief. After that she is eager to help her current patient and his wife with their questions, both spoken and silent.

## CASE 3-4

*James is enjoying his fourth-year rotation on infectious disease (ID) consult service. The attending, Dr. Janacek, is approachable, smart, and a good teacher. The consults are interesting; James was worried that all he'd see would be patients with AIDS, but there have been some "interesting cases" in people with intact immune systems. The most recent was a consult from the ENT service about a woman with a persistent sinusitis who was HIV negative and had no risk factors. On rounds, the ID team all commented on how the initial outpatient choice of antibiotics made sense, but that when the woman was admitted 2 days before, the ENT service had missed the boat in their choice of parenteral antibiotic coverage. James was honored to be asked to write the consult note in the patient's chart. He worked very hard to display the ID team's thought processes that led to their recommendation of a change in medications.*

*When Dr. Janacek reviewed the note, she obviously was not pleased. She felt that James had insulted the ENT service in the way he presented the ID team's recommendations. James was confused. He thought that he had accurately described the deliberations of the team. He hadn't realized the importance of editing the condescension that the team had expressed in their discussions.*

## TRAINING FOR UNCERTAINTY

Renee Fox observed what she called "training for uncertainty" in the medical schools of the 1950s. She defined this as "the flow of medical school experiences that successively and cumulatively taught students to perceive medical uncertainty." They were taught to accept uncertainty as the fate of the physician; without the imaging procedures available today, often only pathologists had the ultimate answers, after doing the autopsy. With acknowledgment of the role of uncertainty in clinical decision-making, physicians developed "shared, patterned ways of coping with its meaning and consequences as well as its de facto existence" (Fox, 1989). She also described training for "detached concern" where some empathy is maintained, but an emotional distance allows effective clinical decision-making. Both of these tasks continue to be important for medical trainees to accomplish, but the training in these areas is hampered by a ballooning body of facts to be memorized. The rapid availability of more information than ever contributes to more precise diagnoses (before autopsy), although these diagnoses are still based on probabilities, not absolute certainty. The United States's infatuation with technologically derived "facts" obscures this reality, even while medical educators recognize the importance of inculcating problem-solving processes rather than teaching facts (Novak *et al.*, 1999).

Patients used to spend a significant length of time in hospitals. They were diagnosed, treated, and got better or died in hospitals, in full view of medical students and residents. Extended stays had some disadvantages for patients and contributed to the high cost of medical care, but with shortening lengths of stay, medical trainees rarely see the entire process of diagnosis, treatment, and healing in continuity. These disjointed experiences obscure the evolving nature of diagnosis, the use of therapeutic trial as a diagnostic modality, and the iterative hypothesis testing that occurs with patients with complex diagnostic dilemmas. Because they do not follow cases closely for extended periods, each hypothesis seems like a conclusion, a certainty. On the next admission, or outpatient visit, the inaccuracy of that initial guess is lost in the new workup that appears to provide "the answer."

Most people are uncomfortable with uncertainty, but this is particularly the case for the medical student whose premedical training and preclinical training were focused on certainty: Evaluation was often based on multiple-choice exams with "correct answers." Those students who studied arts and humanities were judged in a more subjective fashion, based on essays and research papers, which revealed the student's ability to understand abstract concepts and to express themselves rationally and critically. The criteria for grading were understandings of concepts and demonstration of adept manipulation of the same. Medical students with strong humanities backgrounds have more experience with uncertainty, but even for them the preclinical years are times of memorization of massive amounts of facts and testing on those facts. During this time their skills for coping with uncertainty often lie dormant, and they too may feel unprepared to face the challenges of uncertainty on clinical rotations.

What is ironic and tragic about this is that the clinician actually lives in a world of guesses, increasingly educated guesses, but guesses nevertheless. With real people in real-life situations, there are too many independent variables for any clinician, or any extant computer, to know with certainty what is "the cause" of an illness, or which is "the right" treatment for that illness. The intellectual process of integration is also idiosyncratic to the specialty of the physicians involved: Surgeons do see things differently from endocrinologists. For the medical student, the integration is a new process, and its accompanying uncertainty discomfiting. Fox classifies the students' uncertainty into three types: (1) the uncertainty inherent in the students' "incomplete mastery" of Western medicine, e.g., the complexities of thyroid function testing take more than one glance before the results can be analyzed correctly; (2) the uncertainties inherent in medicine as a discipline, e.g., the ongoing clinical trials for the treatment of various cancers demonstrate the lack of a definitive treatment strategy for these cancers; and (3) the uncertainty about which uncertainty is applicable in any given situation (Fox, 1989). Regarding the first two types of uncertainty, my biochemistry professor used to describe the dichotomy as "it is known, I do not know" versus "it is not known." For a student, knowing on which side of the dichotomy a given answer lies is nearly impossible. The modeling that occurs on most rotations is more aimed at hiding unknowing than exploring it.

In Case 3-4, James transcribed the certainty that the ID consulting team expressed in their discussion into the consult note in the patient's chart. Some of this certainty stemmed from his inexperience and his lingering assumption that most of the time there is one correct answer to the questions asked in clinical medicine. When the team members, especially the senior resident and fellow, spoke with conviction, James reveled in the clarity of their recommendations; it was a joy finally to be part of "it is known." Unfortunately, that clinical "certainty" was colored by specialty loyalties, lending the recommendations a deeper intensity than the simple facts allowed, and a much deeper intensity than was politic.

As a system, the large teaching hospital is not characterized by smooth communication patterns between all specialties. The competition for research funding, clinical and office space, "good students" for residencies, and patient revenues contributes to intense "clan" rivalry between specialty departments. Communication patterns reify the loyalties typical of turf wars. Attending physicians in academic centers rarely discuss openly differences of opinion across specialty barriers in view of their supervisees. More common is the somewhat pejorative or condescending discussion with the "home team" of the way the other specialty team or "LMD" (local medical doctor) handled the case. As a consequence, many graduating residents are ill prepared for fruitful discussions that are possible in the less rarefied atmosphere of the community hospital.

Comfort with uncertainty comes later now than it did when Fox studied medical students. Often, physicians don't develop it until they have been in practice for many years. Many factors contribute to this developmental delay. The expanding knowledge base means that more time in training is spent with facts than with patients. The expanding technology allows for more facts to be collected about each patient. Finally, Americans have increasingly unrealistic expectations of their medical system. They have begun to believe the medical system's "PR." After all, hospitals issue press releases about how modern medicine can keep 500-g babies alive and transplant livers. Since medicine can do so much, the implication for the physician in training is that their uncertainty must be of the "it is known, I do not know" variety. Apparently, those of us in medical education have systematically obscured from our students and ourselves that there are only two things in medicine that are absolutely certain. The first is that every patient (and every physician) dies. The second is that no pregnancy lasts forever. Everything else is at best a "current truth," not a permanent one.

## CASE 3-5

*Rosa dreaded her first night of call as an intern, but it went smoothly, with her senior resident helping with the things about which she was uncomfortable. The second night seemed less daunting. However, it turned out to be very busy, with everything taking her three times too long. The senior resident on call, Michael, helped her talk to an elderly man with pneumonia about whether he would want to be resuscitated, and guided her through writing the "do not resuscitate" order. A few hours later his blood gases became a bit confusing, but she remembered about how to give oxygen to patients with COPD, and after an agonizing 20 minutes with the lab sheet, made her decision about adjusting his oxygen, and stumbled off to bed. The next morning the old man's primary care physician, Dr. Walker, approached her about her care of his patient in the 3 hours before his death. Dr. Walker gently pointed out Rosa's mistake, noting that it probably was not what killed him.*

*Medical students in surgery spend most of their time holding retractors, often from a vantage point where they can see nothing but the backs of blue-robed surgeons and terrifying OR nurses. As the procedure ends, sometimes they are flattered by being required to cut sutures after knots are tied. Surgeons are more than a bit idiosyncratic in their preferences regarding the preferred length of suture left beyond the knot, and one individual may seem, particularly to the uninitiated, to be inconsistent in her or his preferences, sometimes growling "too long," and at other times, "too short."*

*So, the story goes that one day a particularly bold medical student responded to the surgeon's impatient "Cut!" with an obsequious "Do you want this one cut too long or too short?"*

*Medical students on their surgery rotations find this story very funny.*

## FACING MISTAKES

Mistakes in medicine are very difficult to talk about. Physicians are human beings, so of course they make errors. On the other hand, physicians' mistakes have lethal potential, and so are viewed as intolerable. This quandary is particularly acute for the physician trainee, who presumably makes more mistakes than the experienced physician and is less certain whether those mistakes are because of the inherent difficulty of the problem or personal ignorance.

After 18 months of observing surgeons in an academic community hospital, Charles Bosk developed a typology of medical errors and delineated the consequences of mistakes for physicians at different levels of the hierarchy (Bosk, 1979). He recognized two general categories of mistakes: what he called "errors in technique" and "moral errors." Errors in technique can be "technical" or "judgmental" and moral errors can be "normative" or "quasinormative."

Technical errors are mistakes in performance of medical care. While they may not be minor, they are forgivable, in part because they are inevitable in trainees. Examples such as incorrectly tied sutures that lead to a wound dehiscence, a slip of the scalpel, or a pneumothorax because of an attempted subclavian catheter placement are all simple technical errors. Technical errors continue to be forgivable if they are reported to supervising physicians and addressed promptly. In addition, they shouldn't be repeated. The practical rationale for these criteria is that rapid revelation of error allows for prompt corrective measures to minimize the complications induced: packing of the wound, repair of the tissue, or placement of the chest tube can be effected swiftly. Ideally, the supervising resident will know about the blunder and will have initiated the corrective action before the attending is told. The pressure to have begun repairing the mistake before the attending finds out about the error is intense, but any delay in reporting the unforeseen event must be invisible.

Single technical mistakes are considered a natural consequence of inexperience as well as the solution for that inexperience. A mistake is made, the correct action is taught, and the mistake is not repeated. Though the one patient has suffered, if the student learns from the experience, future patients will be spared the suffering. On the other hand, a pattern of similar mistakes leads to a different conclusion: that the trainee is not learning. Since the assumption is that all students and house staff are bright, well prepared, and immune to the effects of sleep deprivation, repeated errors seem to indicate that the trainee lacks motivation to learn. Some are said to "not care enough about the patient." These failings fall in the realm of what Bosk designates as "moral errors."

Judgmental errors are mistakes made in decisions about a course of treatment. Since medical students and house staff rarely have complete independence in their decision making, they rarely make serious judgmental errors. Rosa's mistake in Case 3-5 could be seen as an example of an error in judgment that had serious consequences. Like the attendings in Bosk's study, Dr. Walker saw her error as serious but within the realm of intern mistakes. (As we shall later see, she made the additional normative moral error of not calling for help when she was uncertain.) Dr. Walker assumed that she was careful but inaccurate in her decision to turn down the old man's oxygen, and generously acknowledged that the patient may have died even if she had responded more appropriately. He did not react as to a "moral error" in the way Bosk describes.

According to Bosk, moral errors happen when the "surgeon has, in the eyes of others, failed to discharge his role obligations conscientiously" (Bosk, 1979). The assumption is that the physician, or trainee, doesn't care enough about the patient, the other colleagues on the team, or the profession of medicine to do the best job she or he can. Accurately diagnosing a moral error is more complicated than understanding what technical and judgmental mistakes are. Communication about moral errors is less explicit and the criteria for moral errors are often more idiosyncratic.

Bosk separates moral errors into the normative and quasinormative. The former term encompasses mistakes with which any of the surgeons would have taken issue. He uses the latter term to describe the "breaches of standards of performance that ... are eccentric and attending-specific" (Bosk, 1979). Both types of moral errors are dealt with quite differently from technical errors. Where the errors in technique are met with specific correction and monitoring for patterns, a single normative or quasinormative error can bring down a public shaming on the offender. Technical errors are seen as reflecting the inexperience of the trainee; moral errors are seen to reflect character flaws such as dishonesty or not caring about the patient or the team. Supervisors respond to moral errors by scolding the offender ("What this patient needs is a *real* physician"), by sarcastically instructing in excruciating detail, and by publicly forbidding further independence until remedial work has been performed.

The most explicit normative rule is "no surprises." "No surprises" means that the physician in charge of any individual trainee is kept informed of changes in the patients' status so that he or she is not blindsided by a problem. The rule applies all the way down the hierarchy: The attending expects no surprises from the chief resident's performance, the chief resident expects none from the junior residents, and on down the line. If the intern caring for a laboring woman fails to inform the supervising physician soon enough for her to arrive before the delivery, that is a surprise. If, as in Case 3-5, the intern fails to ask for help when the patient gets sicker, and patient care suffers, that too is often seen as a normative error. If not calling for help was interpreted by Dr. Walker as indicative of overconfidence or sloppiness, Rosa would have been more forcefully reprimanded to "get her attention." In this instance, Dr. Walker chose to view her mistake as a judgmental error. He does not impugn her character or motivation, but corrects her, checking that she understands her mistake.

Quasinormative errors are even more difficult to predict. By definition, what is considered standard procedure by one attending or in one institution is considered "wrong" in another. The apocryphal medical student in Case 3-6 is suggesting that his error, whether "too long" or "too short," will be a quasinormative one. The concrete difference between one way of closing a surgical wound and another is more obvious than the distinction between one antibiotic regimen and another, so quasinormative errors are probably easier to distinguish on surgical services than on medical or pediatric services. Strong opinions are not, however, limited to surgeons. Doing something the correct way on the wrong service may be seen as a judgmental error or as a moral error in the sense that the offending house staff has assumed that he has better judgment than the supervising resident or attending. This would reveal the character flaw of excessive pride, and a public reprimand would be deemed necessary to ensure no repetition.

Since the "no surprises" rule is clear, and the consequence is a dreaded public dressing-down, why do normative errors still occur? Because it is an equally clear though less explicit rule that "doing" things independently is both the mechanism of learning and the signal that progress has been made. "See one, do one, teach one" is the traditional methodology of medical education. Supervising a trainee takes considerably longer and is more difficult and more anxiety producing than doing the procedure or patient evaluation oneself, a fact trainees often don't quite believe. If the trainee seems to be taking too long, or asks for too much supervision, she will not get the opportunity to practice and will fall further behind in acquiring skills. The trainee then has two motivations to avoid calling for help: loss of an opportunity to learn and loss of face, which means she has not yet learned all that was expected. The supervisor, on the other hand, wants to allow as much independence as is safe because independent performance is highly valued in physicians.

The dynamic within the trainee when faced with these two conflicting rules is almost never discussed across hierarchical lines. Performance expectations are seldom specified in advance. Medical students and house staff compare their performances to the chief residents' or attending physicians'—both unrealistic standards for comparison. Since the feedback they usually receive is vague and rarely based on direct observation of performance (Bucher & Stelling, 1977; Ende, 1983), they rely on these grandiose external or inadequate internal standards. These inappropriate expectations mean that the students and house staff usually feel inadequate and overwhelmed. Exacerbating this is their chronic fatigue, which saps their psychological reserves (Eberle, 1988; Gordon *et al.*, 1986; Smith *et al.*, 1986). Some trainees have trouble discussing their confusion even with peers and end up feeling lonely and stupid. Since the punishment for a publicly found mistake is blame, and asking for help too much may curtail their learning opportunities, trainees often retreat within themselves and learn to keep secrets.

Successful keeping of secrets has obvious dangers for patients, and less obvious risks for students and house staff. Secrets kept about developmentally normal mistakes are particularly insidious: They prevent the reality check offered by a peer or supervisor who points out the inappropriateness of using more advanced physicians as standards of comparison. Peers can and should help each other sort out the technical and judgmental errors from the moral errors. They often do not have the experience to differentiate between normative and quasinormative; more experienced house staff must provide this information. Bosk's study was done in the mid-1970s and since then more attention has been paid to how medical students are treated. The harshness of the shaming he describes has been condemned, but still occurs (Hundert *et al.*, 1996; Sheehan *et al.*, 1990). His typology of errors provides a vocabulary that is useful in discussions aimed at making sense of the system's responses to mistakes. Occasionally, an attending can articulate the difference between the general and the idiosyncratic, but such a degree of self-revelation to subordinates in the hierarchy is delicate and can further confuse the trainees.

It is crucial for students and house staff to continue to speak about their confusions within peer groups and with supervisors, like Dr. Walker in Case 3-5, who have demonstrated their willingness to examine the reality of mistakes in medical education. Although Bosk delineated his typology of technical and moral errors as though the distinctions were clear, his clarity may have resulted from his being an outsider, a sociologist. Many of the errors classified by the surgery teams he observed as normative could also have been simple errors in technique or judgment. Most medical trainees do care about their patients but many become so stressed that they have trouble caring about much of anything, much less attending to all of their patients' needs. If "not caring" is the result of being overwhelmed and not having personal physiologic needs met, it is a normal response, a coping mechanism, not a moral failing (Eberle, 1988). Shaming is not an effective or ethical teaching technique. Yet, as has been demonstrated (Bosk, 1979; Daugherty *et al.*, 1998; Hundert *et al.*, 1996), it is frequently used in place of one. In its use of blame and scolding as coercive techniques of behavior control, medical education mimics a neglectful and abusive family system (McKegney, 1989).

Healthy survival in such a system necessitates breaking the rules about keeping secrets, making judicious, but not paranoid, choices of confidants. Sandra's supervisor (Case 3-3) questioned her in a way that allowed her to describe the "mistake" that had upset her, and was able to teach from the incident in a way that inspired Sandra to push her own limits. Sharing enough so that no one stays alone with fears and uncertainties helps prevent the ego-destroying doubts that prevent learning. Rosa's mistake was treated as an error in judgment by her supervisor, as it should have been. Though she was not shamed for her error, she will feel guilt and sadness, both of which should be shared. Trusted colleagues must form the "compassionate community" that Howard Brody describes as crucial to our ability to attend "to the sufferings of ... patients" (Brody, 1992, p. 267). Open communication is risky in any large system with a history of discomfort with uncertainty. Though medicine is ultimately a discipline steeped in uncertainty, it still seems to hold omniscience as a realistic goal (Dubovsky & Schrier, 1983). Treating uncertainty as the exception rather than the rule contributes to the difficulties found in distinguishing normative and quasinormative errors. When residents and attending physicians can explain their opinions as either widely applied standard operating procedure or idiosyncratic preferences, the important consistencies will become apparent and students will know what to remember for the long haul.

## McKEGNEY'S RULE

*You are* not *competent to assess your own performance (or anyone else's) when you are post call. No, you aren't. Put it away somehow by writing it down, suppressing it, or anything else. You can dump it on someone if you need to, but* do not *process it. You'll do nothing useful and may get hurt. Come back to it the next morning.*

## CASE 3-7

*Olga (finally at the end of her internship!) notices that some of the lab results from the hospital are missing from the clinic chart of one of the patients she is seeing that afternoon. She is sure that it is in medical records and just hasn't been filed, so she goes into medical records to get the reports. Marie, the medical records tech, insists that all loose filing is up to date, and feels that Olga is accusing her of not keeping up. Olga continues to ask to get the records from the hospital, and things escalate.*

*Marie ends up crying, feeling that Olga tried to make a fool out of her in front of everyone. Olga ends up being talked to by the Clinic Manager and is furious. It is not clear to her or to her advisor whether the fury is because she feels that the information she needed should be in the chart when she, the physician, needed it, or because she feels that she was asking gently and that Marie overreacted.*

## CASE 3-8

*It is midnight and David has been sent to draw blood on Mrs. Hussein—she insisted on "Mrs."—for cardiac enzymes. As he moves quietly in the half-light, arranging the tourniquet and the Vacutainer tube, she querulously asks, "Young man, are you practicing on me?"*

## CASE 3-9

*Calvin is finally finishing his internship. He thought it would never end. Next month he will be expected to teach, but how can he? He feels that this has been the longest, most grueling year of his life, but he dreads his first night of call as a G2, the questions that the G1s will have, and responsibility for the patients! He feels he doesn't know enough, that all the other soon-to-be G2s are better prepared than he, that something awful will happen, and his incompetence will be discovered. He considers asking for more rotations as a G1, but is nauseated at the thought of a longer internship, and more nauseated at the shame he would feel at admitting his inadequate knowledge.*

## ADAPTING TO THE IDENTITY

In all training programs, fledgling professionals go through several transitions of identity between their initial "lay" status and being a professional "with all its privileges and obligations." One of the overarching quandaries in the acculturation process is the contrast between the values espoused by the profession and the reality that the trainees experience in their clinical training. Though some schools have introduced "white coat ceremonies" to highlight the values of compassion and humility that we want to reinforce and nurture in our students, the structures of medicine and medical education teach very different lessons about hierarchy and privilege. As Wear (1998) puts it, "Consequently, students may experience their medical education as one built around inconsistencies between what is touted as desirable and the unacknowledged or unquestioned enactments of privilege and exclusion in medical institutions and in the delivery of health care."

This privilege is not only passed on by the behavior of attending physicians toward, for example, clerical staff, but also during the less formal interactions with patients, staff, and formal systems within the training programs. Patients who refuse to believe the more experienced nurse, but acquiesce to the green intern, reinforce the hierarchical power of the role. Hospital policy requiring that the physical therapy orders be written and signed by a physician reinforces the nonsensical notion that the physician trainee knows what is best for the patient's rehabilitation needs. Clinics that establish goals and operating systems without collaboration with the communities that they are supposed to serve should not blame their patients for not availing themselves of the medical care offered. All of this militates against learning true teamwork and true collaboration with patients. And all of it is incorporated in some way into the identities of trainees bound for the most privileged positions in the medical hierarchy. "As they learn the knowledge and skills of doctoring, medical students also recognize and internalize the social and economic divisions of power and authority in medicine, including who fits where, who does what, and who gets the most reward" (Wear, 1997).

Before full acculturation, disequilibrium occurs at each transition with uncertainty about how many of the privileges are deserved and how many of the obligations can be met. This can be an opportunity for bringing the informal instruction about medical hierarchy to consciousness, but the acquisition of privilege and obligation makes for such awkward moments that survival, rather than learning, becomes the priority. A significant number of trainees end up with their feet in their mouths over this each year. After being mere students for so long, they are caught between the desire to have the privilege and ignorance of the power, and its limitations, which accompany this change in status.

Olga is caught between wanting the physician's privilege of not having to hunt things down for herself and not wanting the obligations and the power to do harm that come with that privilege. Olga has spent years watching her teachers assume that things will be taken care of for them; that their view of the world is universally held; and that other ways of doing things are just not right. Power often accrues before the interaction between privilege and obligation is clear to the trainee, a nasty situation. Before the power accrues, whining is irritating to nonphysician staff. After the power is recognized, that complaining becomes threatening and hurtful: same people, same behavior, different meaning. Olga's assumptions about how outpatient medical records are organized, her desire for privilege, and her assumption that her complaining will not challenge anyone are evidence of her unconsciousness of the reality of her situation. The other possibility is that she is acting maliciously, but this is far less common than ignorance about the nuances of balancing privilege and obligation. Learning useful lessons from this incident will take careful work and explicit discussion of the roles of power, privilege, and personal goals for relationships within the medical system.

These systemic paradoxes can have an impact on all aspects of training. For students focused on education as a preprofessional process, being accepted to medical school is like approaching the top of a steep slope of a mountain. At first it appears to be very near the summit. As one clambers over what appears to be the final lip, one discovers that a taller and steeper slope is still ahead. The first 2 years of medical school are generally grounded in the familiar process of classroom study, examination, and grading based on those exams. The small sliver of the "privilege" that accompanies putting on the short white coat excites the neophyte, while trying to stuff the tools of the trade in its pockets frustrates.

As they begin the clinical rotations, the role of physician begins in earnest. For students who have come straight through school, this is probably their first professional role and the recurrent adolescence of the highly educated is in its penultimate stage. For students who have had other professions, their chosen regression to adolescence and apprenticeship is nearing the end. For all, as the excitement fades, confusion encroaches: How do I introduce myself to patients? How do I respect patients' rights to have experienced care and at the same time learn enough to provide good care when I'm done? What is my role on this team, anyway?

## CRITERIA FOR GOOD FEEDBACK AND EVALUATION

*1. Feedback and evaluation should be given respectfully and in relative privacy.*
*2. Feedback should be phrased in descriptive, nonevaluative language.*
*3. Evaluation should be based on explicit criteria, consistently applied.*
*4. Feedback and evaluation should be based on firsthand, direct observations whenever possible.*
*5. Feedback and evaluation should be about behaviors that are changeable, not personality characteristics or inferred motivations.*
*6. Feedback and evaluation should be expected, timely, and limited in quantity.*

*(Adapted from Ende J: Feedback in clinical medical education. JAMA 250:777–781, 1983.)*

As a medical student, to be called "doctor" holds a thrill tinged with dishonesty. One is not yet a doctor, and truthfulness demands that the distinction be acknowledged. Excessive emphasis on student inexperience is unfair to both the student and the patient, since it increases anxiety without increasing safety. A compromise must be reached. The term "medical student" is actually confusing to many patients; after all, nurses and PT students study "medicine" in the minds of some outside the medical professions. Introducing oneself as a "student doctor" seems to be clear to most English speakers in the United States. It has the advantage of being free of jargon, acknowledges the training status of the student, and indicates which training program he or she is in.

So, what should David in Case 3-8 say? On the one hand, fairness and honesty demand that he acknowledge his relative inexperience but not undermine both himself and the patient by harping on it. There is probably no one right answer. Different schools and hospitals will have cultural norms that need to be respected. Discussing this with fellow medical students and house staff will clarify local norms. Lying about one's inexperience rarely works anyway, as patients are very attuned to the demeanor of those who may cause them pain. In addition, lying reinforces the trainee's sense that not knowing is somehow shameful, rather than being "appropriate for gestational age," perpetuating further the pattern of secret keeping that hampers learning. For both the trainee and the patient, clarifying the degree of supervision and naming the supervisor ("I am the student doctor working with Dr. Senior Resident") can provide reassurance based on honesty and trust. Many trainees, at many levels of training, express fear that their inexperience will be discovered. Medical students fear that their less-than-perfect understanding of the basic sciences will be glaringly obvious on rounds. The meaning attached to these errors depends on many factors: the ego strength of the student, the atmosphere on the ward team, and whether the supervising physician employs "pimping" to exert power (Brancati, 1989). In situations where supervision does not include direct observation of patient care, secret self-awareness of knowledge gaps engulfs the sense of mastery over what is known. Their sense is that they have successfully fooled everyone for a time, but that they are impostors who will eventually be discovered and ejected from the profession.

Printed in black and white, the fear sounds melodramatic. This "impostor" syndrome is more common among women than men, but there is considerable overlap. Because of the decline in bedside ward rounds as technical information is relied on more and more for diagnosis, students and residents are observed even less than previously. Since they know they have not been directly observed, they find their superiors' evaluations arbitrary and actively discount them. Bucher and Stelling's (1977) study showed that without feedback based on direct observation, trainees use internal criteria, sometimes idiosyncratic, for evaluating their own performances. Unfortunately, more recent work (Hundert *et al.*, 1996) demonstrates that unrealistic expectations and faulty feedback persist.

Calvin in Case 3-9 is scared for at least two reasons. He faces a role transition with an abrupt increase in independence and responsibility. Without adequate feedback regarding the specifics of his performance, he does not know whether he is sufficiently well trained to take on his new responsibilities. When he is on call his first night as a G2, he will be surprised at how much he has learned in the last year, and he will discover that he is not alone in the hospital. Once he is over the top of the steep slope of internship, he can see ahead. Not only is there another slope, but there are climbers ahead of him who can be consulted about the right path to take.

Obtaining clearer feedback before the transition can facilitate the awareness that progress has been made. Ideally this feedback has two parts: first, individualized feedback focusing on the trainee's "next steps" in his or her own developmental task, and second, evaluative information focusing on how the trainee compares to others at the same level of training. Structuring this feedback is difficult from the trainee's position of relative powerlessness, but the trainee is the one who is motivated to obtain the specific information needed about his performance. Since most teachers in medicine did not have clear, specific feedback during their training, they are unfamiliar with giving it. It can shock teachers to have students ask for specific information, but particularly those immediately higher in the hierarchy will usually answer the questions if they are limited in quantity and posed explicitly: What is one thing you think I do well? What is something I need to work on? And, how would you suggest I do it differently? If needed, handing the supervisor a copy of Ende's article (Ende, 1983) will clarify the request.

Some of the anxiety of adopting the identity of "physician" can be alleviated by more specific information. If the feedback is provided properly about behaviors, rather than inferred personality characteristics, performance is separated from identity and self-worth. This is a crucial process for maintaining health as a physician. If one chooses to "be" a physician, rather than choosing to "practice" medicine, one is far more vulnerable to the devastation that results from physician error and patient morbidity and mortality. After all, the mortality rate is eventually 100%. Healthy physicians are not sanguine about illness and death, but they must recognize that they have worth as human beings outside of their roles as physicians.

For trainees, especially in a university rather than a community hospital setting, the distance from their teachers mitigates against learning much about how "grown-up" physicians maintain their "detached concern" (Fox, 1989). Medical students in particular are so awash in their uncertainty about whether something is known, Fox's third category of uncertainty, that they can't get a perspective on how their observations of their teachers relate to their own goals. After all, relatively few students and house staff will be attending physicians in teaching hospitals when they finish their training. Programs that use community physicians as part-time teachers do much to bridge this gap. The community physician provides a model for balancing life and work without the perplexing intrusions of research, tenure, and university politics that affect university-based physicians. Students and residents may not be able to articulate what is distracting their teachers from patient care and teaching, but they recognize the orbital distortion induced by academic gravitational forces. Contact with community physicians clarifies which sources of the distraction are part of university life and which are inherent in medical practice.

## CASE 3-10

*Philip couldn't help but join the other interns in gossiping about Tina and Dr. Hank Corcoran, the cardiologist. He feels that, as an intern, she is being singularly stupid to "date" an attending physician old enough to be her father, and a married one at that. It is true that he only does morning report occasionally to fill in when one of the regular internists is gone, so he isn't technically her supervisor, but it still doesn't seem right.*

*Philip has noticed that since she and Dr. Corcoran began making eyes at each other, Tina has stopped going out for pizza and beer with the other interns and the ER nurses. Corcoran seems underfoot all the time on the medicine units, but he isn't very open to questions about patients, unless Tina is the one asking the questions. Philip is furious with Corcoran for giving Tina special attention, and angry with Tina for agreeing to pay the price. She probably thinks she is in love with him. Doesn't she know he's going to drop her as soon as he is bored? Why doesn't Arthur Stein, the department chair, take Corcoran aside and tell him to keep his pants zipped? Philip thinks Dr. Stein would have to be blind to not notice what's occurring.*

## CASE 3-11

*Gail is finishing her fellowship year in geriatrics. Most of her clinical time has been spent caring for the elderly, but she has had two sessions a week in the family practice clinic, where 28-year-old Beth became her patient 10 months ago. Beth has had over a dozen physicians in the last 5 years: internists, a gynecologist or two, three neurologists, an orthopedist, and a handful of psychotherapists. Gail carefully sent for old records, and Beth's first progress notes are in volume three, the first two volumes being full of scratchy copies of handwritten notes from the clinicians who responded to the release of information forms. All of her visits with Beth confuse Gail: She can't figure out why the patient came to the clinic. Beth always shows up for her appointments with long lists of concerns and authorization forms to be completed and "walks in" at other times without an appointment. On the other hand, she clearly isn't taking her anticonvulsants: The last time she was brought into the ER seizing, her blood level was negligible. The time before that, her level was in the therapeutic range and should have prevented the seizure. Her last neurologist said that her family physician could handle her anticonvulsants, effectively dumping her in Gail's lap. Her current neurologist thinks that Beth has psychogenic seizures, and that's why the meds don't work.*

*Gail feels saddled with tasks beyond her expertise. She feels that Beth is dependent on her, expecting Gail to organize her transportation and housing as well as her anticonvulsants. In addition, Beth has begun to comment on Gail's increasingly obvious pregnancy, which makes Gail very uneasy for reasons she cannot articulate. In a visit when Gail tried to make a clear contract with Beth about how many visits and phone calls per week were feasible, Beth dropped the comment that she now lives near Gail and walks by her house every other day. This rattled Gail so much that she didn't finish their discussion of the contract. Gail talked to Dr. Landau, one of the faculty who is known for her skill in caring for difficult patients. Gail asked Dr. Landau for advice, or permission to terminate as Beth's physician, anything to help her feel less trapped. Beth's comments about Gail's pregnancy and Gail's house frighten her. She is afraid that Beth will "do something." She doesn't feel she has the right to quit as Beth's physician unless Beth breaks a specific contract. In discussion with Dr. Landau, she realizes that she has taken on social worker as well as physician functions, that Beth can't always tell which professional is right to handle which problems, and that Gail can direct her to more appropriate professionals. She also realizes that she has not told her husband about her anxiety about this unstable patient walking by their house, and resolves to bring him in on her decision making. The fear dissipates some as her goals of her relationship with Beth are clearer to Gail, but none of her discussions with Dr. Landau can completely eliminate the feeling that Beth is constantly pulling at the hem of Gail's white coat.*

## FINDING THE BOUNDARIES

In Case 3-10, Philip is in a quandary: He feels profoundly uncomfortable with Tina's romantic relationship with Hank Corcoran, but isn't sure it's any of his business. In some ways, he sees their relationship as between consenting adults, but on the other hand, their relationship seems wrong. Some of the interns are whispering about it among themselves, but no one is talking to Tina, and there has been no official response from the department head. If we apply the family metaphor introduced at the beginning of this chapter, this cross-generational love affair looks like incest between uncle and niece.

Very few writers have discussed sexual relationships between trainees and teachers in medicine. Recognizing the power inequities and the potential for exploitation, a number of universities have addressed relationships between students and teachers with varying degrees of proscription. How these rules should apply to physicians in training and their supervisors is unclear. The guidelines regarding intraoffice romance developed for businesses are also not quite pertinent. House staff are often students and always employees, but they are employed by the hospital, not the department chair. In university and business settings, mixing a direct supervisory relationship, especially if it involves job or academic performance evaluation, with a romantic relationship is the most taboo of dual relationships because one person's power to consent is assumed to be compromised (Peterson, 1992). In the medical system, the supervisory lines are less rigid; attending physicians have variable supervisory and teaching roles within their own departments and other departments within the hospital or university. House staff are in a unique position; they are neither students who are vulnerable to the whims of their professors, nor are they full-fledged physicians. On the other hand, their professional status is still very dependent on the evaluations of their supervisors.

In Case 3-10, the incest metaphor falls apart in several ways. Tina is not a child, she is a grown woman. Dr. Corcoran is not her blood relative, and not her direct supervisor. On the other hand, she is isolated by the time demands of internship and vulnerable because of the stresses of internship in ways that are not true of an attending physician (Gordon *et al.*, 1986). She is also vulnerable to his authority and privilege, even if he does not have direct supervision over her. The isolation of the couple from her social context, the other interns, the mixture of resentment and pity felt by the uninvolved "siblings," and the silence and blindness on the part of the parental generation are all typical patterns found in families with incest.

Close mentoring in educational settings is a personal as well as a professional process. Good teacher–student relationships involve support aimed at developing the helping professional. Healing professionals need emotional balance and reserves in order to be with their patients in illness and pain. Like Dr. Walker and Dr. Landau, good teachers do not stick to teaching just the facts, they bring their selves, with their human forgiveness and compassion to aid their students in expanding their own forgiveness and compassion. In an isolated system like the teaching program, this educational intimacy can be confused with an emotional or sexual one. Exploitation occurs when two crucial precepts are ignored. First, the teacher–student relationship is essentially asymmetrical, and must be. Second, the goal of the relationship is the benefit of the student. When the relationship is operating for the benefit of the "instructor" more than the benefit of the student, the relationship has become exploitative. In a functional teaching relationship, teachers certainly benefit. Helping a student become a fine physician is personally as well as professionally satisfying. Being part of another human being's growth is a real high, and we teach because of that high. To avoid even inadvertent exploitation, our sources for meeting our own needs for love, self-esteem, and sex must be outside of our teaching and patient care relationships (Bograd, 1992; Peterson, 1992).

In addition to the educational intimacies inherent in medical education, the hierarchy is temporary. The "generations" are so short as to seem almost arbitrary. In Case 3-11, Gail is distressed because Beth is a challenging patient and because she is near enough to Dr. Landau's "generation" that she won't get a simple answer. In a few months, Gail and Dr. Landau will both be "parents" and the asymmetry of their relationship will be more a function of their personal relationship than of the hierarchical teacher–student relationship. Dr. Landau will begin to consult Gail at times, and they will gradually become colleagues.

Within the medical education "family," Gail is functioning like a young adult still living at home. She is board certified and capable of practicing on her own, but has chosen to continue her training to obtain more expertise. At some level, she feels she should be able to make it on her own without help. Part of her worry is in anticipation of the upcoming time when she thinks she won't have Dr. Landau to ask for advice. In actuality, she will have senior partners in practice who will be available for consultation, and Dr. Landau will welcome telephone consultations from Gail as she has from other residents who graduated before her. As noted in the section on "Adapting to the Identity," Dr. Landau's clarifications that Beth is challenging, that Gail is not incompetent because she is having difficulty, and that Dr. Landau will not disappear off the face of the earth on the day Gail graduates are all reassuring, even when they won't fix things.

The reasons that Beth is difficult to care for are myriad. As this is not a neurology textbook, this discussion will focus on the challenges in the physician–patient relationship rather than the diagnosis and treatment of "pseudoseizures." As trainees move from their identities as laypeople to professionals, they acquire the habits and values of the profession. As noted earlier, they distance themselves emotionally in order

## APPROACHES BY PATIENTS OR COLLEAGUES AND TEACHERS FOR ROMANTIC OR OTHER INTIMATE RELATIONSHIPS NECESSITATE DIFFERENT RESPONSES

*Your interest is a factor, but does not really affect the appropriate initial response.*

*The appropriate response to patients is "No" followed by something about how romantic relationships are against the rules (Gabbard & Nadelson, 1995). Further explanation will sound like an invitation to negotiate, but this is not negotiable. When you feel sexual attraction for a patient, tell a colleague (Neher, 1999). Often the simple telling is enough to dissipate the excitement. In small towns, where everyone is a patient, the situation may be different, but not without consultation.*

*With colleagues or teachers, if the role situation is what makes you uncomfortable, then you can say you need to think about it. Which means that you need to talk about it. If you are just not interested, "No" or Miss Manners's, "No, thank you" are obviously appropriate.*

to keep a cool head in the presence of death and pain. They become more comfortable with probabilities rather than certainties, and recognize mistakes as (dreaded) learning opportunities. As Fox described, they begin to develop detached concern (Fox, 1989). Medical students often have the role of intermediary between the "real doctors" on their teams and the patients because they are only partly trained and therefore only partially acculturated. In this role, their empathy with and understanding of the patient is often greater than that of their senior colleagues. Medical student explanations of phenomena are frequently more understandable to the patient than professorial explanations. This makes sense. Patients are more likely to ask their real questions of the student, who is less intimidating and who spends longer with them than more senior members of the team because the students simply take longer to do their tasks. In addition, the students have a better memory of the transition between not knowing and knowing.

One of the hazards of this proximity of understanding between students and patients is that with the narrower gap, the emotional boundary between patient and student is less well defined. That boundary need not be huge, but its existence will become increasingly important as the trainee gains more responsibility. The empathy that is crucial to providing humane care is a double-edged sword. If the distinction between professional and patient is obscured, the asymmetric intimacy that is the kernel of the healing relationship will be lost. The development of boundaries is often via denigration of patients, as exemplified by the term "gomer" in *The House of God* (Shem, 1978). This method is simplistic and falls naturally in the hierarchy and privilege of the physician's role, but is unethical and ultimately undermines the physician's humanity. If patients come to be seen as so markedly "the other," students, and the physicians they will become, will have joined an abusive hierarchy. For medical students, keeping the necessary, but not excessive, asymmetry is difficult, but is also an essential part of learning how to create and maintain a therapeutic relationship.

With some patients, boundary maintenance is fairly easy. They have expectations of what the medical professionals in their lives can and cannot do. They have sufficient emotional and intellectual resources to obtain consultation about medical issues and look to other resources in their social circles or public services to meet their other needs. For families with catastrophic or chronic illnesses, the medical consultation may be quite global in its scope: Do I need to make out my will? Can we have sex? Will my dad need to live with us? But even when the consultation is global with respect to the patient's world, it is restricted with respect to the physician. The relevant part of the physician's world is that which includes the physician–patient relationship. How much of the physician is revealed within that relationship is variable, depending on the community norms, the style of the physician, and the specifics of that physician–patient relationship.

As Gail observed in Case 3-11, some facts about the physician's life are impossible to keep private, like advancing pregnancy. Gail generally felt comfortable with patients' comments on her pregnancy, but with Beth something was different. Beth's incapacity, whether because of intellectual deficits or personality disorder, to structure the relationship from her end left Gail to deal with an emotional as well as a medical morass. Gail's goal of being open and responsive to her patients' needs backfired. Her tactic of being patient-centered in her care is the appropriate ideal for a physician. Her advancing skills left her open to the chaos of Beth's life. Dr. Landau's greater experience with patients with boundary problems provided her with an algorithm for structuring the relationship and bringing the chaos to a level with which Gail could cope. Gail is left with the discomfort inherent in choosing to stay in a clinical relationship with someone who cannot tell where the limits of the asymmetric intimacy should lie. By consulting with someone else, she can make sense out of the chaos and define her own working parameters. She can also learn about her own counter-transference, in this case regarding the sense of physical vulnerability associated with pregnancy and her own tendency to face her fear without consultation or support.

When working to maintain appropriate boundaries with "difficult patients" such as Beth, or "difficult attendings" like Dr. Corcoran, it is important to keep five simple guidelines in mind (McKegney, 1993):

- Don't do it alone.
- Get a life.
- Don't do it alone.
- Take it seriously, but *not* solemnly.
- Don't do it alone.

Although these guidelines appear obvious, implementing them breaks many of medicine's family rules.

## CONCLUSION

As noted throughout this chapter, the essential tactic for healthy development in the medical family is to break the rule about secrets, whether those secrets are about feelings, uncertainty, or errors. Emotions can't be controlled and will not be denied. Strong feelings are inevitable, not evil. They can immobilize the neophyte or can be the source of insight and empathy when acknowledged, discussed, and addressed. Uncertainty is likewise the clinicians' home territory, albeit an uncomfortable dwelling. Despite the challenges of time constraints and technocracy that are so much a part of modern medicine, physicians in training come to know that they often will not know what will happen next, and may never know why. Mistakes are human, learning from them is expected, and the pain of making them can be ameliorated by avoiding blame. Professional identity formation involves traversing problematic paradoxes of ideals and realities of the medical system. The identity transitions are easier if taken stepwise, with support from peers and trusted mentors. Clear boundaries in relationships with patients, colleagues, and supervisors don't always come easily. We each need to know our own identities, accept our feelings, and make choices about our behavior, keeping in mind the goals of the relationship. And when in doubt, get a consult.

Like adults who are recovering from child abuse, the process of becoming a physician has many stages. Though an individual proceeds from one step to the next, the path is more of a spiral than a direct ascent. The first step is to remember the incidents. The second is telling the stories, which may also be an inextricable part of remembering. One colleague had to elaborate on the 35-year-old story from his internship several times before he remembered the "punch line" that had injured him. A simple recitation of the facts is not sufficient, the feelings evoked need to be revealed; apparently irrelevant details can hold the key to emotional content. Next, we must let go of responsibility for having been hurt. Lastly, refusing to deny our perceptions and avoiding blame, we take up the challenge of doing it differently with students, colleagues, staff and patients (McKegney, 1989). These tasks seem daunting, but with the companionship of friends and colleagues, becoming a physician is the process of becoming more fully oneself.

*Sam Hines (medical student) and Ray Leo (intern) are reporting to the senior resident, Petra Cahill, about the night's many admissions. After discussing the two admissions to the intensive care units, they briefly summarize the admittedly incomplete workup of the woman with abdominal pain who was transferred from the ER to the medicine floor at 7:00 AM, an hour ago. Petra hears that Sam has not yet done a pelvic examination on the patient, and promptly tears into him, implying that his evaluation will reflect his "incompetence." Ray tries to defend Sam, pointing out how busy they have been, the unavailability of a nurse to chaperone the pelvic at change of shift, and that Petra is being inappropriately cruel.*

1. Who is who in this medical "family"? If Sam is the "kid brother," what role does Ray have? and Petra?
2. What dysfunctional family behavior patterns are evident in this story?
3. How can Sam and Ray soothe their injured self-esteem?
4. What would be the potential problems or solutions if Sam or Ray tried talking to the chief resident about Petra's threats about Sam's evaluation?

*Lois Janda just joined the Department of Ob/Gyn after finishing her residency in another state. On her third month as ward attending she supervised G1s and G2s from her own department and a G2 from the family practice program, Frank Gagne. She found him very attractive, and he seemed to respond in kind. They chat, briefly because of his schedule, over lunch whenever they run into each other in the cafeteria. About 3 weeks after the end of the rotation, he asks her out for dinner.*

1. Is it right for Lois to accept Frank's invitation? Why or why not?
2. If they become romantically involved, would you see this relationship as "incestuous"?
3. Would it make a difference if she were older? if the sex roles were reversed?
4. How would your assessment of the relationship be different if she were one of the family practice faculty?

*Esther is working with Dr. Lawler for her fourth-year outpatient pediatrics rotation. The next patient is a 5-year-old, Greg Rollin, brought in by his father for a kindergarten physical. Esther introduces herself to them as "the student doctor working with Dr. Lawler" and asks if she can begin the office visit while Dr. Lawler finishes some phone calls. Mr. Rollin replies, "Of course, anything for a girl as cute as you." Esther feels put down, but isn't sure if she feels worse about being a medical student or about being a woman.*

*When she presents the case to Dr. Lawler before they go back in the room to see Greg, she mentions his father's remark. Dr. Lawler apologizes to Esther for Mr. Rollin's poor boundaries and at the end of the visit he takes Mr. Rollin aside and tells him that his comment to Esther was inappropriate.*

1. Should Esther have made a comment to Mr. Rollin herself? Why or why not?
2. What elements in Dr. Lawler's handling of the situation contributed to Esther's feeling respected? as a medical student? as a woman?
3. If a patient makes a similar comment to Esther when she is a third-year resident, how might her response be different? How does her process of identity formation contribute to the difference?

*Larry Martin is on his first clinical rotation as a third-year medical student, the family practice inpatient service. Constance Orvieti is his G2, and Patrice Haas is the attending. The second day on rounds, after Constance finishes presenting the case, Dr. Haas asks Larry about the differential diagnosis of lung nodules based on chest x-ray appearance. He is very flattered, and does his best to cover the bases. When she starts pushing him to rank the most likely diagnoses for the patient admitted last night, he feels confused and trapped. He doesn't remember ever reading anything that specific in the pathology textbook. Dr. Orvieti stares at the wall, and Larry can't tell whether she is ashamed of him because he doesn't know or if she doesn't know the answers to Dr. Haas's questions either.*

1. *Which dysfunctional family behavior patterns do you see in this case?*
2. *What are the sources of Larry's uncertainty?*
3. *How can he get a sense of what expectations are realistic for him at his stage of training?*

## CASE 5

*After the resuscitation, Dr. Kim Pierce felt like she was going to cry right there in front of everybody. On one level, she knew that the baby's apnea was not something she could have prevented. After all, she wasn't called until 10 minutes or so before the delivery, and she ran from the pediatric call room to L&D as fast as she could. The obstetrician handed her the blue baby, and she intubated and bagged him until he got pinker, and put in the umbilical line. Despite all that, he was still limp and making no respiratory effort when the team from the university Level III nursery arrived 20 minutes later.*

*Later that morning in the office, she told the story to her partners, George and Sharon, not sure of what she was looking for. She just needed to tell someone. And she cried, and they hugged her, and she went on with her day.*

1. *Has Kim failed to develop "detached concern"? What behaviors suggest that she has or has not?*
2. *What factors influenced Kim's decision to let herself cry where she did?*
3. *How do you express strong feelings? How do you adapt to the constraints inherent in the medical system?*
4. *What elements of place and characteristics of companions provide you with the safety you need to get emotional support?*

## RECOMMENDED READINGS

Bosk CL: *Forgive and Remember: Managing Medical Failure*. Chicago, University of Chicago Press, 1979.

Bosk is a medical sociologist who spent 18 months studying how surgeons respond to error. This complete write-up of his study is dense, but offers the unique outsider's eye on medical ritual.

Ende J: Feedback in clinical medical education. *JAMA* 250:777–781, 1983.

Ende succinctly delineates criteria for effective feedback and evaluation.

Fox RC: *The Sociology of Medicine: A Participant Observer's View*. Englewood Cliffs, NJ, Prentice–Hall Inc, 1989.

Renee Fox has been studying medicine for over four decades; many of her insights into how physicians are trained and cope with their training and practice are summarized in this book.

McKegney CP: Medical education: A neglectful and abusive family system. *Fam Med* 21:452–457, 1989.

In this theoretical discussion, the metaphor of a family system is applied to medical education.

Sheehan KH, Sheehan DK, White K, *et al.*: A pilot study of medical student "abuse." *JAMA* 263:533–537, 1990.

This paper reports on one of the first formal surveys of medical student abuse.

Smith AC, Kleinman S: Managing emotions in medical school: Students' contacts with the living and the dead. *Soc Psychol Q* 52:56–69, 1989.

One of the few recent observational studies of medical student acculturation illuminates coping strategies over the course of training.

Wear D: Professional development of medical students: Problems and promises. *Acad Med* 72:1056–1062, 1997.

An overview of professional development of medical students, focusing on how the structures of medical education often work directly against teaching the moral values that it espouses.

## REFERENCES

Bograd M: The duel over dual relationships. *Fam Ther Networker* 16(6):33–37, 1992
Bosk CL: *Forgive and Remember: Managing Medical Failure*. Chicago, University of Chicago Press, 1979.
Brancati FL: The art of pimping. *JAMA* 262:89–90, 1989.
Brody H: *The Healer's Power*. New Haven, Conn, Yale University Press, 1992.
Bucher R, Stelling JG: *Becoming Professional*. Beverly Hills, Calif, Sage Publications, Inc, 1977.

Daugherty SR, Baldwin DC, Rowley BD: Learning, satisfaction and mistreatment during medical internship: A national survey of working conditions. *JAMA* 279:1194–1199, 1998.

Dubovsky SL, Schrier RW: The mystique of medical training. *JAMA* 250:3057–3058, 1983.

Eberle S: A progressive agenda for family practice residency training. *Fam Syst Med* 6:371–384, 1988.

Ende J: Feedback in clinical medical education. *JAMA* 250:777–781, 1983.

Epstein RM, Morse D, Frankel RM, Frarey L, Anderson K, Beckman HB: Awkward moments in physician–patient communication about HIV risk. *Ann Intern Med* 128:435–442, 1998.

Fox RC: *The Sociology of Medicine: A Participant Observer's View*. Englewood Cliffs, NJ, Prentice–Hall, Inc, 1989.

Gabbard GO, Nadelson C. Professional boundaries in the physician–patient relationship. *JAMA* 273:1445–1449, 1995.

Gordon GH, Hubbell FA, Wyle FA, Charter RA: Stress during internship: A prospective study of mood states. *J Gen Intern Med* 1:228–231, 1986.

Harper G: Breaking taboos and steadying the self in medical school. *Lancet* 342:913–915, 1993.

Hundert EM, Douglas-Steele D, Bickel J: Context in medical education: The informal ethics curriculum. *Med Educ* 30:353–364, 1996.

Lassetter J: Educating interns: All in a day's work. *RN* 47:85–86, 1984.

McKegney CP: Medical education: A neglectful and abusive family system. *Fam Med* 21:452–457, 1989.

McKegney CP: Surviving survivors: Caring for patients who have been victimized. *Prim Care Clin North Am* 20:481–494, 1993.

Neher JP: Time and tide. *Arch Fam Med* 8:270–271, 1999.

Novak DH, Epstein RM, Paulsen RH: Toward creating physician-healers: Fostering medical students' self awareness, personal growth and well being. *Acad Med* 74:516–520, 1999.

Peterson MR: *At Personal Risk: Boundary Violations in Professional–Client Relationships*. New York, WW Norton & Co, Inc, 1992.

Sheehan KH, Sheehan DK, White K, Leibowitz A, Baldwin DC: A pilot study of medical student "abuse." *JAMA* 263:533–537, 1990.

Shem S: *The House of God*. New York, Dell Publishing Co, Inc, 1978.

Silver HK, Glicken AD: Medical student abuse: Incidence, severity, and significance. *JAMA* 263:527–532, 1990.

Smith AC, Kleinman S: Managing emotions in medical school: Students' contacts with the living and the dead. *Soc Psychol* Q 52:56–69, 1989.

Smith JW, Denny WF, Witzke DB: Emotional impairment in internal medicine housestaff: Results of a national survey. *JAMA* 255:1155–1158, 1986.

Smith RC: Unrecognized responses and feelings of residents and fellows during interviews of patients. *J Med Educ* 61:982–984, 1986.

Stein LI: The doctor–nurse game. *Arch Gen Psychiatry* 16:699–703, 1967.

Wear D: Professional development of medical students: Problems and promises. *Acad Med* 72:1056–1062, 1997.

Wear D: On white coats and professional development: The formal and the hidden curricula. *Ann Intern Med* 129:734–737, 1998.

Wolf TM: Perceived mistreatment and psychological well-being of graduating medical students. *Psychol Health Med* 2:273–284, 1997.

## CHAPTER 4

# Being a Physician

*John L. Coulehan*

## CASE 4-1

*In 400 B.C. on the Greek island of Kos a young man consulted a physician because of shaking fevers and chest pain. He had gotten sick with cough and fever several weeks earlier, seemed to get better, but then the illness recurred. The physician observed his patient in a kindly but businesslike manner. The patient was a thin man, breathing rapidly, and splinting the left side of his chest. There was a deep look of fear in his eyes, hollowed cheeks, a grimace of pain. The patient sat on a stool, facing away from the light. There was a broad, soft lump over one area of the lower rib cage, appearing warmer and redder than the surrounding skin. When he shook the young man, the physician expected to hear "a wave and a noise," but there was no sound. He took this to be a sign of pus in the chest. An assistant smeared the back of the young man's chest with a thin, watery slip of clay. At the place the clay dried first, the warmest point, the physician made an incision and quickly inserted a hollow tin tube. Brownish fluid began to drain. An assistant secured the tube. It remained in place draining fluid for several days while the patient's fevers disappeared. Meanwhile, the physician prescribed a liquid diet, herbs, and purgatives for his very weak, but grateful, patient (modified from Majno, 1975, pp. 156–157).*

## EDUCATIONAL OBJECTIVES

1. To present and discuss the concept of a moral phenomenology of medical practice
2. To list and illustrate the character traits or characteristics associated with satisfaction in medical practice
3. To discuss and illustrate possible abuses of power in the physician–patient relationship, especially boundary violations, or inappropriate intimacy
4. To discuss and illustrate conflicts of interest in the physician–patient relationship
5. To present psychological and social factors that may, in some cases, lead to professional stress, emotional numbness, and burnout
6. To explicate the physician's moral and professional obligations to an impaired colleague

Case 4-1, written nearly 2500 years ago, is easily understandable to the modern reader. While the specific methods may differ, the physician's role and behavior are remarkably contemporary. The Hippocratic physician used his hand, his mind, and his heart to help the young man recover. Hand, heart, and mind. Together, these words signify the calling and the full personal commitment that has characterized the profession of medicine throughout history. While the manifestations and proportions of each have changed with changing times, hand, mind, and heart are all essential to medicine. In ancient Greece, the physician used his hands to gather data and to intervene, as in the case above. He understood the physical findings within a mental framework that explained illness as a natural phenomenon, rather than a random or supernatural occurrence. For example, Hippocratic physicians tasted the patient's urine to determine its sweetness in cases now known as diabetes mellitus, and they explained epilepsy as an imbalance of humors, rather than a message from the gods. The physician's heart was also committed to healing. Medicine was a life work dedicated to helping others, not just another craft or business. In the Hippocratic *Precepts* the author was explicit about the connection between caring and medicine: "For where there is love of man, there is also love of the art." And, of course, the *Epidemics* contains the best-known (albeit distorted) of all the Hippocratic sayings: "As to diseases, make a habit of two things—to help, or at least to do no harm."

Mind and hand have not always necessarily been synergistic in the history of medicine (King, 1970). After the Roman era, rational theories were long emphasized at the expense of the "hand" or empirical dimension. For example, the comprehensive theory of physiology and medicine developed by the Roman physician Galen was fossilized during the Middle Ages and used as the basis of medical practice for nearly 1500 years. The Christian era in Europe was associated with the ascendancy of religious values at the expense of skeptical thinking and natural science. Authority replaced observation as a source of truth. While Galen himself was a keen observer, his system became an unquestioned authority that stifled subsequent genera- tions' creativity and investigation. Later theorists tinkered with Galen's theory by developing gizmos and codicils to update it. Other physicians, however, rejected rational systems that didn't seem to jive with reality. These empiricists, like the seventeenth century Englishman Thomas Sydenham, confined themselves to recording systematic clinical observations, rather than trying to figure out the big picture (King, 1970). In the eighteenth and nineteenth centuries, hand and mind began again to work together, leading to the development of modern medicine.

Medicine's heart has endured, though, despite the vicissitudes of mind and hand. By "heart," I mean the personal experience of medical practice, as well as the physician's motivation and commitment. These, too, have varied according to history and culture. For example, the Common Era brought an infusion of Judeo- Christian values, which transformed and deepened the Greek and Roman virtues of medicine. In the realm of the heart, however, there are striking similarities between today's practitioner and Hippocrates, who wrote: "The dignity of a physician requires that he should look healthy, and as plump as nature intended him to be.... He must be clean in person, well-dressed, and anointed with sweet-smelling unguents that are not in any way suspicious.... In appearance, let him be of a serious but not harsh countenance.... The physician must have at his command a certain ready wit, as dourness is repulsive both to the healthy and to the sick" (Jones, 1923). Sounds pretty familiar, doesn't it?

In this chapter, I want to investigate medicine as a practice of the heart. What is it like to be a physician? How does it feel? What are the satisfactions, the stresses, the motivations? Some might argue that these topics are too vague to discuss in a meaningful way. Medicine is so complex and fragmented that generalities about "doctoring" may no longer be anything but platitudes. A pathologist and nuclear medicine specialist. An anesthesiologist and occupational medicine specialist. A staff internist in an HMO and a solo practitioner in Wyoming. What do these women and men have in common? There appear to be more differences than similarities among specialties. Moreover, medical practice is changing so rapidly that doctoring in five or ten years will undoubtedly be experienced much differently than today.

Nonetheless, though change is hard upon us, there are commonalties in doctoring that might be called the moral phenomenology of medical practice. These features include elements of motivation, character, psy- chology, skills, satisfaction, and moral legitimacy. In the next section I present a sketch of this phenomenol-

**Table 4.1**
Phenomenology of Professionalism in Medicine

Empathy
Engagement versus detached concern
Tenderness
   Benevolence or altruism
   Compassion
   Caring
Steadiness
   Duty
   Fidelity
   Courage
Practical judgment
Humility or self-effacement
Honesty
Fidelity
Playfulness, humor, creativity

ogy (see Table 4.1). In later sections I focus on the potential for abuse of power and conflicts of interest in medicine. Finally, I describe serious health risks, including burnout and substance abuse, that sometimes arise from the demands of medical practice.

## CASE 4-2

*In 1972 TP was the physician assigned to an Indian Health Service facility that served a large boarding school, as well as several thousand Navajo people scattered over 400 square miles of arid steppe in northern Arizona. He and his wife lived with their two young children in a trailer nestled in a stand of cottonwood trees near the clinic. TP would frequently see 70 to 80 patients in a day, many of whom were quite ill, but some of whom had merely come to "town" to socialize a few hours at the trading post and pick up a bottle of "big red pills" for their aches and pains. As the day progressed, he would see an amazing variety of patients: tuberculosis, pneumonia, conjunctivitis, acute rheumatic fever, mitral stenosis, broken bones, alcoholism, an epidemic of hepatitis.*

*Sometimes TP would walk home at the end of the day with his heart singing, "This is the life for me!" He felt like he had accomplished a lot. His work was interesting, important. The patients liked him. Other days he would trudge home feeling dull, angry, incompetent, and overworked. Many patients simply wouldn't take their medicines. Screaming kids got on his nerves. His medical backup was some 60 miles away. He felt he was being manipulated. Because few people in the community had phones and everyone knew where the physician lived, patients would appear at TP's trailer at all hours of the night and weekends—mothers with sick kids, drunks beaten up on the way home from bars in Holbrook. The administrator at the regional hospital said, "Well, you should just turn those people away. Don't treat them. Clinic hours are nine to five." TP couldn't turn patients away, but often on weekends he and his family would drive 3 hours to Flagstaff to stay in a cheap motel, cook their meals on a Coleman stove, and sleep gratefully without the threat of a staccato knock at midnight.*

# EXPERIENCE, VIRTUE, AND
# SATISFACTION IN MEDICAL PRACTICE

In Case 4-2, TP was learning what it means to be a physician not from a textbook, in the abstract, but in the day-to-day events that make up a life. He was discovering that his life wasn't entirely his own anymore: He had obligations to patients, to the Navajo community, and to the medical profession itself. Sometimes the thought of these duties made him grateful and proud. Yet, at other times they seemed insufficient to alleviate his fatigue or quench his anger. Early in medical school, students tend to romanticize the power and virtue of medicine. Later, when they begin the day-to-day experience of taking care of patients, they sometimes become cynical when the reality doesn't live up to their expectation. Medicine as a profession is difficult, complex, personally demanding. Often, the answers are unclear and the physician's ability to help is limited. In medical practice one encounters suffering that is unfair, intractable, and meaningless. The physician experiences the thrill of healing, but also feels the impotence of failure. She experiences the gratitude of some patients, but also encounters anger, ignorance, and dislike. It is easy to become cynical if you approach medicine with messianic expectations, or without much understanding of your own motivation, needs, and limitations.

## Engagement, Empathy, Enjoyment

Most surveys show that physicians derive considerable satisfaction from taking care of patients. For example, in one study of California physicians, 80% indicated satisfaction with their jobs and over 90% reported enjoying their relationships with patients. Interestingly, nearly two-thirds (63%) characterized their work as "fun," a telling observation in this period of considerable significant change and presumed stress in medicine (Chuck *et al.*, 1993). Satisfaction with medical practice requires that you enjoy its day-to-day activities. An abstract sense of "doing good" by helping others is not enough. When asked about their motivation, applicants to medical school usually say they like science, they want to help people, and they enjoy interacting with others. These three motivations come in different mixtures and sizes. All are necessary, but enjoying "working with people" is the most basic. Both scientific interest and humane motivation are mediated through encounters with patients, families, colleagues, and other health workers.

In Case 4-2, the joys of TP's practice came from his successful interactions with patients. These may have been successful in one or more of a variety of ways—medically (the patient got better), intellectually (the case was interesting), emotionally (the patient's response was personally gratifying), or socially (he simply enjoyed interacting with the patient). At this point in his career, TP did not have the opportunity to experience some of the other major satisfactions of medicine; for example, he had very little financial reward, prestige, or sense of power. Conversely, most of TP's dissatisfactions arose from unsuccessful physician–patient encounters. In his case, cultural difference played a major role. TP anticipated a clear separation between his personal and professional life, but the Navajo community was unused to that type of distinction. Likewise, Navajo patients had trouble understanding the need to keep taking medication once they were feeling better. They believed that the real cause of illness was an underlying personal disharmony that could only be cured by a Navajo *haatali* or medicine man. Thus, they sought out traditional healing ceremonies as well as Anglo medications. When the appropriate ceremony had been performed, they believed there was no point in continuing to take the Anglo pills.

Yet, despite such cultural differences, much of the time TP understood how his patients were feeling and he was able to "connect" with them. They, in turn, felt that he really cared about them, even though he knew little about their culture. In other words, TP's successes were based as much or more on his care and feeling of *empathy* as they were on technical knowledge.

Empathy is a chameleon concept; various observers describe its colors quite differently (Aring, 1958; Basch, 1983; Hoffman, 1984; Spiro, 1992; Zinn, 1993). Some writers emphasize its *intellectual* or *cognitive* aspect, arguing that empathy is primarily a type of knowledge about other people's feelings and experience; in other words, a method of projecting yourself into their place. Getting under their skin, so to speak. We learn what others are thinking or feeling by interpreting various verbal and nonverbal cues. Some people are better at this than others. At one end of the spectrum, there are autistic persons who seem unable to form this type of human connection. In fact, autism can almost be defined as a global lack of empathy. People who choose medicine as a career tend to be closer to the other end of the continuum. They enjoy interacting with other people and, therefore, might well be expected to have a high natural degree of empathy.

Some writers stress the *affective* aspect of empathy (Halpern, 1993; Spiro, 1992). They argue that you can't know how a patient is feeling in a given situation without, in some sense, actually experiencing that feeling yourself. Let's say a patient comes to see you for treatment of chronic osteomyelitis in his left foot, a condition he developed as a result of stepping on a nail while working at a construction site. His antibiotic treatment has been intermittent and ineffective because of financial and personal problems: his wife left him, his business went bankrupt. You can tell by dozens of signs—the way he sits, the look on his face, the tone of his voice—that he is depressed, frustrated, angry, even overwhelmed. These conclusions are hypotheses (tentative knowledge) about his condition, yet at the same time they are associated with feelings. You obviously don't feel as depressed or overwhelmed about the situation as he does, but you do feel something. You are not a detached observer. This affective aspect of empathy is an essential component of a physician's experience.

A third definition focuses on the *skills* required to be empathic. This operational approach says, "Look, let's not be vague. Let's take the mysticism out of empathy. What we're really talking about here is a set of interactive skills." In this sense, empathy results from developing good eye contact, active listening, facilitative responses, and other communication techniques. The physician can learn to be more empathic, simply and precisely, by acquiring and perfecting these skills (Coulehan & Block, 2001).

Finally, some writers place empathy on the level of *virtue* (Reich, 1989). The relationship between sympathy, empathy, and compassion is a complex topic that cannot be covered here, but it is important for us not to confuse empathy itself with the motivation or personal attributes that lead a person to develop empathy. In medicine the motivation is presumed to be good or virtuous: benevolence, care, compassion, sympathy. I discuss these motivations in the next section. One may, however, have nonvirtuous motivations for developing empathy. Consider the con artist, for example, who wins people's trust because of his charismatic skills, but then uses their trust for his own nefarious ends. Consider also the charismatic cult leader who drives his followers to destruction.

The affective nature of empathy leads to a curious paradox between engagement and detachment in medicine. Medical educators have long taught that physicians should learn to keep their distance from patients (Aring, 1958; Becker, Geer, Hughes, & Strauss, 1961; Blumgart, 1964; Fox, 1957). This stance of emotional detachment has been called *clinical distance* or *detached concern*. William Osler explored this issue when he wrote that physicians should adopt a "judicious measure of obtuseness" by which they become relatively "insensible" to the slings and arrows of their involvement with patients. He called this ability *aequanimitas*, the virtue by which physicians maintain the inner calmness required in their work (Osler, 1932).

Why is emotional detachment thought to be necessary? For two reasons: first, it protects physicians doctor from being overwhelmed by their patients' pain and suffering. The layperson who faints at the sight of blood becomes an accomplished surgeon at least in part by learning to "disconnect" from the emotional side of the experience. Perhaps in this context "barrier" is a better metaphor. While physicians might be physically close to their patients, they must (metaphorically) put on protective clothing, gowns and masks, to shield them from emotion. This barrier begins in gross anatomy laboratory and develops over many years of socialization in the culture of medicine. The second reason for detachment is the belief that it protects the patient, because an emotional response may lead to biases in clinical judgment which compromise patient care.

Rather than pairing the terms *detachment* and *concern* to describe the physician's professional stance, I prefer to borrow the words *steadiness* and *tenderness* from Thomas Percival. In his *Medical Ethics* (1803), this British Enlightenment physician discussed the tension between objectivity and subjectivity in medicine when he enjoined physicians to "unite tenderness with steadiness" in their care of patients. Under "steadiness" Percival included the intellectual virtue of objectivity or reason, along with the moral virtue of courage or fortitude. By "tenderness" he meant humanity, compassion, fellow-feeling, and sympathy. These are sentiments, moral virtues, and, to use more contemporary terminology, complex emotional attitudes. In another place, Percival contrasted the "coldness of heart" that often develops in practitioners who do not cultivate these virtues with the "tender charity" the moral practice of medicine requires. The ability to combine tenderness and steadiness in physician–patient interactions requires *emotional resilience*, rather than emotional numbness.

Fortunately, in Case 4-2, TP's practice situation was such that he could not become detached. Whatever he learned in medical school about keeping his professional distance was soon forgotten. He fully experienced his emotions and those of his patients. Thus, he was faced with the necessity of developing an emotional resilience that would allow him to practice medicine objectively, while still being open to the subjective component of each interaction.

---

### CASE 4-3

*SR is a 40-year-old oncologist who belongs to a small group practice in a medium-sized midwestern city. SR also directs the Cancer Center at the local hospital. He is known in the medical community as a very aggressive physician who takes pride in saying that he never gives up on a patient. When a patient dies he considers it a personal defeat. He frequently speaks up in support of concepts like palliative care and hospice, but in practice he rarely uses them because he is convinced that his patients are "fighters" who want a "full-court press." SR's medical colleagues are divided in their assessment of his practice style. Some like to refer patients to him because they know he provides the most aggressive and up-to-date chemotherapy available. Others are concerned because of his reputation as an aggressive, no-nonsense physician who focuses "too much on the tumor, too little on the patient."*

## Benevolence, Compassion, Caring

The relief of suffering is a fundamental goal of medicine. However, the ability to implement this goal by prolonging life is a relatively new phenomenon. Throughout most of history, physicians didn't have the tools to cure disease or prolong life, except perhaps in a few surgical situations, such as amputation of a gangrenous limb. Sometimes you'll hear physicians say, "The chief moral obligation of physicians has always been to preserve the lives of their patients as long as possible." This type of statement might be made in the context of end-of-life care, when a physician is trying to explain his or her reluctance to honor a patient's wish to discontinue life-sustaining therapy. It is useful to remember that such statements are anachronistic. In fact, since in the past the *cure* of illness and extension of life were so infrequent, the chief moral obligation in medicine was always to comfort and *care* for one's patients.

The image of a physician sitting by a patient's bedside is one of the most compelling representations of medical caring. Figure 4.1 is a reproduction of *The Roads of Doctor Chekhov* by the Russian artist, A. P. Shepelyoka. Anton Chekhov (1860–1904), one of the giants of world literature, was also a physician, who continued to practice medicine and work in public health even after he had achieved great success as a writer. In fact, he served for many years as a general practitioner to the villagers around his country home at Melikhovo. *The Roads of Doctor Chekhov* captures an imaginary scene in which Chekhov is making a house call. He sits on his young patient's bed, comforting her with his left hand, while having turned to look at her mother, with whom he speaks seriously. The physician's mien is reserved and proper, but also engaged and reassuring. A shaft of light shines into the dark room through the window drapes—perhaps a suggestion of hope.

The term *care* is used in two ways in medicine. Its external dimension consists of the sequence of things physicians do for patients, the aggregate of professional services they perform. In this sense care is a list of items or behaviors. "He received the best medical care" often means he received everything the latest technology had to offer. The internal dimension of care, on the other hand, is the personal quality or emotional attribute that motivates the physician to perform the services in the first place. Another word for this internal aspect of care is *compassion*. People who choose to become physicians do so in large part because of a general commitment to help others (benevolence), but they are unlikely to be satisfied with medicine in the long run unless they also have compassion for individual suffering people, many of whom are bothersome, unpleasant, or even downright unlikeable.

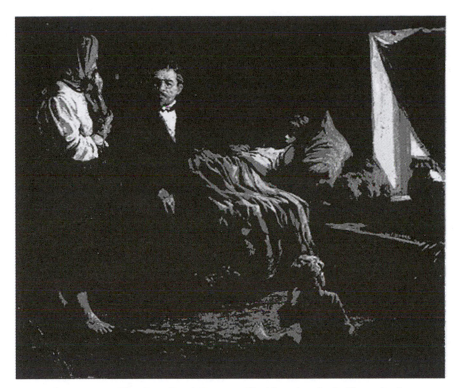

**Figure 4.1.** *The Roads of Doctor Chekhov* by A. P. Shepelyoka.

The psychologist Carl Rogers listed three attributes he believed essential in any healing relationship. These therapeutic core qualities are empathy (already discussed), genuineness or honesty (discussed below), and unconditional positive regard (Rogers, 1961). Positive regard is the ability to suspend your moral or personal judgment about the patient's behavior, to set aside your negative feelings (if you have some) and work in the patient's best interests. Positive regard is a function of compassion, based on an understanding of human connectedness: we are all ultimately in the same boat, we all make mistakes, we are all in need of help. Compassion, like any virtue, can grow or diminish over time. Physicians become more compassionate by practicing empathy and trying to do the best job they can. Alternatively, compassion can be largely "snuffed out" if external stress, the emergence of other priorities, or professional burnout lead the physician to approach patients as objects, rather than subjects.

In Case 4-3, instead of caring for his patients, SR seems to be marching to a different drummer. The word *march* is appropriate. SR approaches medicine as if it were a war: Disease is the enemy, the physician is a warrior, the goal of medicine is to fight and conquer disease. We often use metaphors or models in describing the physician–patient relationship. Robert Veatch, for example, wrote about the *priestly model*, in which the physician controls the access to healing power, while the patient has no say in the matter and is kept in the dark; and the *engineering model*, in which the physician acts like a technician or engineer, while the patient functions as a broken machine (Veatch, 1972). William May analyzed the metaphors of physician as parent, fighter, technician, and teacher (May, 1983). Each of these metaphors implies a different type of relationship. If the physician is considered a parent, for example, patients must be treated like children. This implies a benevolent despot who acts in the patient's best interest without consulting the patient, or even against his wishes (*paternalism*), much the same as in Veatch's priestly metaphor.

The military metaphor is particularly popular today. Witness the "war against cancer" and our frequent characterization (as in Case 4-3) of good patients as "fighters." When SR's colleagues comment that "he treats all his patients aggressively," many of them, at least, are paying him a compliment. Or at least a mixed compliment. Aggressive in tumors means bad, but in physicians it generally means good. We train physicians to fight, to hold on, never to yield. "Don't back down," we tell our students, "treat your patients aggressively. Take risks. Push to the limit. You must often inflict new damage—incisions, tubes, toxic medications—to conquer your patient's disease and alleviate his pain." Unfortunately, if disease is the enemy and the physician is a warrior, the patient, to continue the metaphor, tends to be thought of as a battlefield rather than a person.

Sometimes we admire aggressiveness in physicians even when, as in Case 4-3, it conflicts with other important values, like compassion or honesty. Naked aggression would make more sense, of course, if medicine were literally a war. In some traditional cultures, the warrior role is, in fact, almost literal. Shamans in central Asia believe that serious illness is caused by spirit possession. To cure the patient the healer must fight the spirit and vanquish it. Likewise, Navajo Singers (*haatali*) believe that some sickness is caused by soul-loss. In these cases the medicine men are obliged to wrestle with dark powers in order to restore their patients' souls to harmony. For these traditional healers, medical practice is a perilous enterprise that puts them at personal risk. If they prove weaker than their opponent, they might, in fact, be injured or destroyed. Interestingly, a threat of injury also exists in scientific medicine: The aggressiveness and emotional distance implied by the war metaphor may can lead physician-warriors into the cycle of professional stress, abuse of power, and burnout.

Each of these metaphors sheds some light on the physician–patient relationship, but also casts a shadow. While capturing one characteristic of illness or healing, it fails to account for other features. It takes several such images to sketch the whole truth about medicine. However, some metaphors are far more useful than others. In particular, those that capture basic medical values like empathy, care, and compassion, e.g., physician as parent, friend, or teacher, ought to be emphasized more than those that embody less humane values, e.g., physician as warrior or technician. Veatch characterizes the ideal physician–patient relationship as a contract model, while May uses the term *physician's covenant*.* Both of these are grounded in compassion and respect. Both specify duties far more complex than winning a war. SR might have chosen a career in oncology because he wanted to "beat" cancer, but he needs to learn that aggression is justified only in the service of compassion.

## CASE 4-4

*LC is taking care of an elderly patient with multiple medical problems, including a stroke that left her with right-sided paralysis, and aortic stenosis, i.e., narrowing of the aortic valve in her heart. She begins to complain of fatigue and shortness of breath. LC examines her two or three times over a period of several weeks and orders some diagnostic tests. The findings on physical examination, as well as the results of an echocardiogram, convince her that the patient's symptoms are the result of severe depression, precipitated by her stroke. She tells the patient and her family that the heart problem is not responsible. Despite antidepressant treatment, the patient continues to get worse and winds up in the Emergency Department where the cardiology consultant concludes that she has "critical" and life-threatening aortic stenosis. This could have been diagnosed and treated several weeks ago, but LC simply made a mistake.*

## Practical Judgment, Humility, Honesty

Problem solving is part of the joy of medicine. Physicians are blessed almost every day with the personal and intellectual satisfaction that comes from helping to solve significant human problems. No wonder medical school applicants say that the intellectual stimulation of medicine is one of the profession's most attractive

---

*May contrasts "covenant" with "contract," stressing the connotation of gift and indebtedness in the former. To him "contract" exemplifies the marketplace. On the other hand, Veatch uses the marriage contract as an example of a contract that is really a covenant. To him the two models are similar. This controversy is important here only in that both writers stress the donative and fiduciary nature of the relationship.

features. Among practicing physicians, the satisfaction of solving medical problems is one of the major motivations for a medical career (Schwenk *et al.*, 1989). It is exhilarating to make an obscure diagnosis or to discover that your patient has the classic findings of a disease you just read about. In fact, some students believe that generalist practice must be less stimulating than subspecialty practice because the latter provides more intellectual challenge by "going deeper" into a specific field. The generalist, this line of reasoning goes, doesn't have any really interesting cardiac or GI patients; only a cardiologist or gastroenterologist is equipped to manage them. This, however, is a misconception on two accounts. First, patients with complex medical problems probably have more need for a primary care physician than patients with minor complaints because they need someone to coordinate their care and help them focus on maintaining function and a healthy perspective. Second, primary care, perhaps counterintuitively, can be more stimulating than a subspecialty because the human problems that patients present in ordinary practice are often more difficult, and certainly every bit as challenging, as diseases dealt with by subspecialists.

The flip side of a profession that revels in problem solving is uncertainty. All diagnostic and therapeutic decisions are, in a sense, experiments. As we evaluate patients we formulate hypotheses, refine the hypotheses, test them, and try to confirm them by seeing what happens when we embark on a certain course of action. While we may take into consideration benefits, risks, probabilities, clinical experience, pathophysiological knowledge, and opinions of experts and peers, medical decisions are still based on hypotheses. These may at times be very well supported, but they are still not certain. Is disease X really causing the patient's symptoms? Will medication Y really help relieve the symptoms? Learning to accept and work within uncertainty is a major part of the physician's professional education. Expert knowledge about a particular disease or specialty is not enough. Sound *clinical judgment* also requires a logical, empathic, and honest approach to decision making within a framework of uncertainty.

Renee Fox distinguished three types of uncertainty in medicine: the physician's incomplete mastery of available knowledge, inadequacy of the state of the art itself, and uncertainty of where the boundary lies between the two (Fox, 1957). LC, in Case 4-4, relied on an imperfect test, the echocardiogram, in deciding that her patient's symptoms were more related to depression than to aortic stenosis. Is that a state-of-the-art error or a culpable mistake? Should she have pursued another test or consulted a cardiologist? In a case like this it is difficult to know the answers; you can always second-guess when a bad result occurs. The important issue here, however, is to understand that physicians have to learn to deal with their mistakes.

Because misjudgments and mistakes are inevitable in medicine, *humility* (or self-acceptance) and *honesty* are especially important character traits. When we talk about honesty in medical ethics, it is usually with reference to how much to tell our patients. How do we tell patients "the bad news"? When should we withhold information? Should we ever lie to patients? Such discussions are grounded in the tension between our respect for autonomy and the (usually wrong) perception that sometimes truthfulness may not be in the patient's best interest. However, honesty with oneself precedes honesty with patients. Self-delusion is rampant everywhere, but physicians are perhaps particularly vulnerable for a variety of reasons. Our motives are noble; our mistakes, after all, are usually made in the interest of helping others. We carry high responsibilities and work long hours—again in the interest of our patients. Society looks to us as authorities and pays us lots of money and high respect. Following this line of reasoning, it is easy to embrace into the comforting delusion that our decisions are always justified and our errors minimal.

In Case 4-4, LC's misjudgment as to the importance of her patient's aortic stenosis was an understandable mistake. After all, the clinical findings were conflicting. The echocardiogram suggested that the aortic valve narrowing was not as severe as it ultimately turned out to be. Yet, the patient was harmed. Could LC have done a better job? Perhaps so, perhaps not. Regardless, it is essential that she accepts responsibility for making the misjudgment. In his 1905 valedictory address to the medical students at McGill University, William Osler said, "Learn to play the game fair, no self-deception, no shrinking from the truth; mercy and consideration for the other man, but none for yourself, upon whom you have to keep an incessant watch" (Osler, 1932).

Honesty with oneself leads, as night leads to day, to humility or *self-acceptance*. John F. Christensen (1992) and his colleagues published a study of physician mistakes under the perceptive title, "The Heart of

Darkness: The Impact of Perceived Mistakes on Physicians." These investigators interviewed 11 community hospital physicians about errors they had made in caring for patients. These physicians reported two main strategies for coping with mistakes. One was problem-focused: They used the opportunity to obtain new knowledge and learn from the mistake. The second strategy was emotion-focused: They shared their feelings with their spouses, colleagues, or sometimes the patients involved. Being truthful with the patient or family was a particularly helpful way of dealing with the mistake, although the process itself was extremely anxiety-provoking. While this emotion-focused strategy was seen as beneficial, the physicians complained that there was too little support for it in medicine. Peer review structures, like Morbidity and Mortality Conferences, tend to be solely problem-focused. Colleagues often tend to minimize feelings or give facile reassurance, rather than thoughtful emotional support. In addition to these specific ways of coping, the investigators also found that physicians who accepted medicine's limited control over illness and acknowledged the inevitability of making mistakes were better able to understand and profit from their own errors.

## CASE 4-5

*On "ethics rounds" a subintern in medicine presented the case of an HIV patient with pneumocystis pneumonia just transferred to the MICU. The patient was agitated, delirious, coughing, and gasping for breath. The students on the unit expressed their concern about their own risk of infection. Although they used universal precautions, they were still uncomfortable with the slim chance that they might contract HIV. "After all," one said, "it seems like we're always drawing blood or putting in another line."*

*We began to discuss the physician's ethical obligation to treat HIV patients. Our talk soon gravitated to the medical school's policy that students be required to participate in the care of patients suffering from HIV. "Coercive," one of them called this policy. "It infringes on our basic rights," another said. In fact, most of the students believed the policy to be wrong.*

*"I don't have any problem with treating AIDS patients," one of them said. "I think it's the right thing to do for me, but you can't force someone else to treat a patient if she doesn't want to."*

*"There's too much risk," another claimed. "It's an individual decision. Every doctor has the right to treat or not treat whomever he pleases."*

## Discipline, Fidelity, Courage

The emergence of the HIV epidemic in the early 1980s led to a reexamination of the concepts of fidelity and courage in medicine (Daniels, 1991). However, an exclusive focus on the a physician's duty to provide care despite the risk of infection obscures the need for fidelity and courage in all aspects of medical practice. It is true that HIV brings back into focus the profession's ethical tradition that requires heroism in the line of duty. This tradition is reflected in the AMA's Code of Ethics. History, however, presents us with a more sober and realistic view of physician behavior. Some physicians have acted selflessly and courageously in times of plague, others have fled from the danger. Courage, like other virtues, must be viewed in light of competing values. It seems unreasonable to hold that physicians are morally required to take great risks for their patients, thereby sacrificing their own lives and harming their loved ones. On the other hand, fidelity to our patients, in the case of already-established relationships, and fidelity to the profession itself, in the case of sick people who have no physician, demands that we take smaller degrees of risk as part of our professional obligation. The risk of infection with communicable diseases, like tuberculosis and hepatitis B, is an expected and reasonable occupational hazard.

The emergence of HIV made risk to health workers highly visible because of HIV's mysterious (at least, initially) and fatal nature. Nonetheless, the probability of patient-to-physician transmission through finger-stick or mucosal contamination is very low, especially with the use of universal precautions. There is now a wide consensus that the level of risk in caring for HIV patients is well within the reasonable range, even for surgeons. Therefore, physicians have a duty not to refuse to treat patients on the basis of their HIV status. The medical student in Case 4-5 was wrong: Physicians do not necessarily have the right to treat or not treat whomever they choose (see Daniels, 1991, for a further discussion of this complex topic).

The issue of fidelity to patients and the requirement for courage in medical practice is actually much more pervasive than the risk of communicable diseases. Fidelity means sticking with the patient even when the going gets tough: when treatment isn't working, when the cancer is bound to be fatal, when the patient is angry and demoralized. Fidelity also means serving as the patient's advocate in various interactions with employers, managed care organizations, insurance companies, state agencies, and so forth. Sticking with patients through the ordinary ups and downs of illness requires a certain amount of courage, a willingness to put your reputation on the line for the patient. The good physician doesn't hide behind job descriptions or bureaucratic limits when the interests of her patient are at stake. She is willing to dive in and do what she can. This day-to-day courage is far more important to medical practice than is the occasional act of heroism.

---

## CASE 4-6

*In the lobby of a University Health Center sat an architectural model of the Center as it will look in fifteen years. Beside the model, a group of curious people watched a videotape on which a soothing baritone voice announced that he is about to reveal "tomorrow's medicine today." The model showed existing buildings in dull gray, but demonstrated the future in various brighter colors: a basic science building anchored in the clouds, a magnificent new patient care tower, an extraordinary subterranean parking facility. The hypnotic voice described dramatic achievements in organ transplantation and nuclear magnetic resonance, new ways of treating cancer by "enhancing the body's own immune response," comprehensive programs in sports medicine and in geriatric care. The tape showed physicians, nurses, and technicians going about their serious business with very serious expressions. A radiologist stared mournfully at an impressive machine. A nurse frowned at an IV infusion pump.*

*As medical students and house officers passed through the lobby, they frequently stopped to joke about this heavy-handed promotion film. For weeks the elevators were full of humorous comments about their friends and professors shown on the tape, and about the aura of pomposity and self-importance the tape conveyed.*

## Playfulness, Humor, Creativity

Physicians have always tried to balance the heavier aspects of their work with humor. Hippocrates, for example, cautioned physicians to adopt a serious and respectable mien, but also warned that they be witty, because "dourness is repulsive both to the healthy and to the sick." Even in these days of dramatic change in the profession, surveys show that the great majority of physicians enjoy their work and characterize it as "fun." The media, of course, portray medicine as an extremely serious business, indeed: a constant treadmill of life-and-death decisions, a volatile mix of fatigue and principle, emotion and science. No wonder physicians are tempted to take themselves too seriously and become humorless and self-important.

One type of humor often encountered in medicine is *gallows humor*, the pervasive joking we do about the ugliness and pain of clinical situations. Joking about one patient's horrible wound or another patient's bad breath is a type of defense mechanism. Professional distance allows us, at least momentarily, to defuse our own bad feelings by objectifying patients and making light of them. Gallows humor tends to be indiscriminate, however. We sometimes poke fun at our teachers, colleagues, and subordinates as well. The emotional intensity of medical training, combined with long hours and chronic fatigue, promotes this type of defense—sharp, sarcastic wit as a way of coping with one's feelings, thereby avoiding having to "feel" them. The problem with gallows humor is that it can become a pernicious habit, rather than just an occasional emotional outlet. If used extensively, it can lead to permanent detachment and emotional numbness.

A more healthy type of humor is based on empathy and compassion. Medical practice makes us privy to more human foibles and personal stories than are encountered in most other professions. One of its biggest lessons is, or ought to be, that we are all basically in the same boat: "There, but for the grace of God, go I." Humor based on this understanding is gentle, rather than sarcastic; it tends to connect us, rather than separating us. Yet it still serves the helpful function of looking obliquely, rather than directly, at our pain, anger, anxiety, or sadness, thereby helping us to cope with these feelings. Case 4-6 illustrates another form of humor. The young physicians in this case enjoyed making light of the fund-raising tape because they well understood how fallible the Health Center's professionals were and had little patience with the air of omnipotence the tape conveyed. They turned the discrepancy between their real-life knowledge of medicine and the tape's pomposity into a fertile source of humor. Not taking oneself too seriously is an important habit for physicians to acquire.

## CASE 4-7

*The Chief of Medicine at a world-renowned Medical Center was held in great awe by the medical community at large, but he was despised and feared by his nurses, medical students, and house officers. He commonly harassed, exploited, and humiliated them on daily rounds. In some cases he would tell students that they shouldn't become physicians because they are too "ignorant" or "unobservant." His temper was legendary, leading him, at times, to throw patient charts to the floor and stomp out of rounds when someone had forgotten an important laboratory value. It was well known that when the Chief himself made mistakes, he generally blamed them—often in public—on his assistants. Interestingly, former students and residents sometimes look back on their time with the Chief and romanticize it; they tend to visualize him as a hero of the days when medicine was stronger and more rigorous than it is today.*

## THE PHYSICIAN'S POWER

The relationship between physicians and patients has traditionally been viewed as benign and caring, a fiduciary relationship in which a stronger, more knowledgeable party (the physician) agrees to provide medical assistance to a weaker, more vulnerable party (the patient). More contemporary models of the patient–physician relationship stress reduction of the power imbalance by means of joint decision making, patient education, and informed consent. In today's prevalent marketplace metaphor, the physician becomes simply a "provider" who puts a certain type of service on the market; the patient is a "consumer" of this service. A related metaphor considers the physician to be a technician or engineer who provides technical assistance according to the patient's specifications. It is true that enhancing the patient's power, particularly the right to make informed choices about treatment, has been an extremely important development in U.S. medicine over the last 40 years. Yet this development should not obscure the fact that physicians continue to wield tremendous power and that, in fact, there is an intrinsic imbalance of power between physician and patient (Brody, 1992).

In *The Healer's Power* Howard Brody considers three types of medical power (Brody, 1992, pp. 16–17). The first is the *Aesculapian* power that physicians have by virtue of their knowledge and training. This is the impersonal content of medicine, the knowledge and skills peculiar to the profession. A second type is the *charismatic* power that physicians wield based on their personal qualities and interpersonal skills. Characteristics like empathy, compassion, fidelity, honesty, courage, and practical judgment contribute to this type of authority. Comments like "He has a wonderful bedside manner!" or "She has truly mastered the art of medicine!" reflect one's charismatic power. Finally, physicians have enormous *social* or *cultural* power. Part of this arises from the fact that society gives the medical profession authority to determine what counts as illness and medical disability. Illness exempts people from certain social obligations and gives them access to benefits. In turn, the ill person is expected to act in specified ways, e.g., follow the physician's orders, try to get better, and the like. Thus, physicians hold the power to determine whether a patient's experience or behavior constitutes "illness," rather than, for example, laziness, cheating, or moral failure. This social power generally leads to high prestige and socioeconomic status. It also has a spillover effect in that physicians' opinions in nonmedical areas like education, social welfare, and politics tend to be weighted more heavily than they deserve.

Power in the physician–patient relationship can be viewed as a drama in which "the extraordinary power of sickness to make patients susceptible to change at all levels of the human condition is matched by the equal power of this benevolent relationship with its unseen but powerful connection" (Cassell, 1991, p. 73). Thus, the physician's power is necessary to combat (note the war metaphor) the enemy and to strengthen the weakened victim. Power should be used solely for these purposes. However, the physician's power may also be abused. One type of abuse is when physicians use social power to gratify their own emotional needs. In Case 4-7 the Chief of Medicine, a narcissistic, emotionally immature man, was abusing his position in the social system of the profession itself. He typically enhanced his own sense of self-worth by attacking and diminishing those under his professional control. Unfortunately, the socialization process in medicine during the middle part of the twentieth century tended to foster this pattern. Medical education was, and is still, hierarchical in nature; trainees were expected to work long hours with little immediate reward, except for the privilege of working with certain "great" clinicians; and these senior clinicians had often devoted their lives to climbing the ladder in a medical social system that gave them few emotional outlets. As physicians were socialized into the "culture of medicine," they began to excuse the Chief's behavior as an example of necessary rigor. They reinterpreted the past as not so bad because it was, after all, their past and they turned out to be good clinicians. Future physicians, they reasoned, would benefit by passing through the same type of initiation.

## CASE 4-8

*A surgical subspecialist saw large numbers of patients for whom he regularly prescribed narcotics, barbiturates, and benzodiazepines in large quantities. One morphine-addicted nurse had gone to him for years as her primary care physician. After completing a detoxification program, she admitted that many years previously she had learned from her classmates in nursing school that this physician would prescribe whatever was requested. In return for yielding to his sexual advances, he had been providing her with morphine and diazepam for more than a dozen years.*

## Boundaries, Intimacy

This case of a surgeon who sold narcotics prescriptions and sexually exploited his patient illustrates egregious abuse of power in the physician–patient relationship. The surgeon's state-regulated authority to prescribe controlled substances (Aesculapian power) allowed him to engage in the profitable exercise of selling prescriptions for narcotics and other psychotropic drugs. In this he betrayed his professional commitment to prescribe only "that method of treatment which, according to my ability and judgment, I consider for the benefit of the patient" (Hippocratic Oath). Moreover, he may well have used his personal charisma and the social power of his position to manipulate this particular patient and others like her.

This case also raises the issue of intimacy and *boundaries* in the physician–patient relationship. How close a personal relationship may we as physicians develop with our patients? In some cases we may feel sexually attracted to patients. Strong transference may lead patients to feel especially attracted to their physicians. Though the American Academy of Psychiatry strongly condemns the practice, surveys have shown that 5% or more of psychiatrists admit to having had sexual relations with patients. While sexual intercourse between patients and physicians has been discussed most openly in psychiatry, it certainly can, and does, occur in all fields of medicine. Physicians who engage in this type of behavior have tried to justify it in one of two ways. Some argue that the sexual relationship is therapeutic for the patient. This implies that the physician is sufficiently in control (i.e., powerful) to use his or her sexual urge as an instrument. Thus, the physician's claim that he or she is trying to help the patient is simply an appeal to medical power. In fact, the physician is preying on the patient's vulnerability and gratitude.

The second type of justification is an appeal to love: the physician is, in fact, in love with the patient; the patient, in love with the physician. This assertion of love, insofar as it can be separated truthfully from the imbalance of power issue, goes counter to the heart of the physician–patient relationship. Physicians must maintain some standard of objectivity, despite their closeness and connection to patients. Earlier in the chapter I rejected the term *detached concern* because it suggests emotional numbness rather than the emotional resilience that is required for good patient care. I suggested rather that we use more heartfelt, less sanitized words to describe the physician's professional stance: the balancing of steadiness with tenderness. Steadiness is essential for objective decision making. Intimate personal relationships with patients undermine steadiness and impair medical care. Thus, physicians typically ought not to provide medical care for their own parents, spouses, and children. Of course, the level of steadiness required, and therefore the appropriateness of treating family members, depends on how much is at stake in the given situation. Thus, a pediatrician treating his child for an ear infection is far different from a husband treating his wife for multiple sclerosis. Because the need for objectivity in clinical judgment precludes intimate relations, the claim that sex with patients is justified because of "love" is either self-delusion or indicates a willingness to enter a situation in which objective decision making will be impaired.

## CASE 4-9

*Dr. FD and her colleagues in Sunnydale Internal Medicine Associates are considering whether they should enroll as participating physicians in EconoCare, a for-profit managed care organization in their state. Managed care is rapidly growing in their area. If Sunnydale Internal Medicine Associates does not participate, the group may well lose a large portion of its patients. In reviewing the contract, Dr. FD notes that it includes the requirement that participating physicians agree not to reveal to their patients any disagreements they might have with EconoCare policy, or to recommend therapeutic options that are not covered by EconoCare. Dr. FD believes that such "gag rules" are unethical and recommends that the group not join, unless EconoCare is willing to change the contract language.*

## CONFLICTS OF INTEREST

Professional conflicts of interest arise in medicine, first, because the patient's and physician's interests are not identical; and, second, because medicine is a social system in which many other parties play a role: employers, insurance companies, governmental agencies, and so on. Many people today have a romantic idea that the physician–patient relationship in the past was free of such conflicts. Not so. However, the "business" of medicine and conflicting professional obligations are now more visible than they were in the past because health professions are more complex and their impact on society greater. I want here to sketch three foci of potential professional conflict: managed care arrangements, where financial incentives may cause physicians to offer less than optimal care; and ownership of health facilities and defensive medicine, where financial incentives may cause physicians to provide unnecessary care.

## Managed Care, HMOs

We tend to think that in the traditional physician–patient relationship, as exemplified by fee-for-service private practice, the physician acted solely in the patient's best interest, while submerging his own needs and desires. The subsequent availability of health insurance brought a third party into this relationship. Until the late 1980s this third party was largely a facilitator and passive observer, providing reimbursement for services the physician ordered. Neither the patient nor physician had to worry much about money; the patient obtained needed care and the physician was paid for services rendered. In such a setting it was inevitable that "more" would tend to be "better." These dynamics resulted in unnecessary surgery and overutilization of services (Franks *et al.*, 1992). Such overutilization represents a type of conflict of interest that we don't usually consider: patients systematically exposed to excess risks and costs. These errors of commission are often just as damaging to the patient's interest as errors of omission.

The pressing need for cost control has dramatically changed the role of the third party. In *managed care* arrangements, the health insurer decides which services are justified in a given setting, and restricts access to specialty referral and testing. In the last decade, managed care has grown to become the predominant method of healthcare financing in the United States and has largely replaced the traditional fee for service model. This movement has brought the generalist physician back to center stage as the coordinator of care because patients usually have to obtain approval from their primary physician in order to be eligible for specialty services. Ideally, the primary care physician provides preventive services and manages most acute and chronic medical problems. Such a system is more rational, efficient, and cost effective than an open market in which people choose specialist physicians according to the symptoms they develop.

However, the strengths of managed care can also be viewed as weaknesses, as in an optical illusion when a beautiful vase becomes two old crones staring at one another. The "management" in managed care limits the patient's autonomy in choosing providers. In practice, the primary physician becomes a *gatekeeper*, who at times is forced to take an antagonistic role when patients request medically unwarranted services or referrals. In fact, some HMOs provide monetary incentives for primary care physicians *not* to refer to specialists, thereby introducing a financial conflict of interest with patients. Managed care arrangements also limit physician autonomy. Physicians may only be able to refer to certain specialists who have contracts with the patient's managed care plan. Case 4-9 illustrates one particularly unethical requirement that some managed care organizations have used to restrict physician autonomy. In this case, the physician clearly becomes an agent of the corporate entity, required to conceal from patients relevant information about therapeutic options. In reaction to such practices, some state legislatures have passed laws prohibiting "gag rules" and other restrictive practices. For example, in the early 1990s many managed care programs permitted mothers only 24 hours of hospital stay after delivering their infants, arguing that discharge after 24 hours is perfectly safe for mother and baby in the large majority of cases. Nonetheless, in some cases serious health problems are missed. The widespread popular disaffection with "drive-through deliveries" led to state mandates that require insurance programs to allow a minimum of 48 hours of postnatal inpatient care.

Managed care does not necessarily conflict with good patient care, nor with physician satisfaction, and the physician's duty to be an advocate for his or her patients doesn't disappear in this new environment. The obligation to provide the best care we can may sometimes run afoul of managed standards. A test or treatment that the physician considers essential may be disallowed by the insurance program. Advocacy then demands that the physician explain the situation to the patient; appeal the decision; and even recommend that the patient obtain the service despite nonapproval. This process takes time, energy, and negotiating skill. It may not be the cup of tea for a traditionalist who says, "That's not why I went to medical school." However, solidarity with the patient demands that such skills be developed.

## Defensive Medicine

The term *defensive medicine* is usually used to describe a pattern of practice that is strongly influenced by the desire to avoid malpractice liability. Instead of making clinical decisions based solely on benefits and risks to the patient, the physician considers perceived liability risks in the decision making process. Many studies demonstrate that physicians do, in fact, alter their practices in response to the threat of liability. The emergency medicine physician, for example, may routinely order CT scans on all head injury patients, even if clinical circumstances do not warrant the scan. Similarly, the internist or neurologist may order an MRI on all patients who present with headache, knowing, of course, that the vast majority of such scans are not clinically justified. In one study internal medicine residents reported "defensive medicine" as the main reason for ordering 8% of laboratory tests and 14% of x-rays in their practice (Dewar, 1994). Defensive medicine is thought to be a particular problem in the United States because of the excessive number of malpractice suits.

Reynolds and colleagues estimated the total annual cost of defensive medicine in the United States to be about 10 billion dollars (1984–1995 data), representing nearly 11% of expenditures for physician services (Reynolds *et al.*, 1987).

Defensive medicine constitutes a professional conflict of interest because it leads physicians to compromise their patients' best interests due to liability risk to themselves. Malpractice liability is discussed more thoroughly in Chapter 17, "Reducing Malpractice Risk," of *A Guide to Clinical Expertise*. Here, however, I want to make three points about defensive medicine as it relates to the psychology and phenomenology of medical practice. First, the specter of liability is not always a negative influence. So-called "defensive" measures may sometimes improve the quality of medical practice. For example, in some studies physicians report spending more time with patients, hiring more office staff, and obtaining more complete informed consent because of the threat of malpractice liability (Dewar, 1994). Whatever the initial motivation for adopting these measures, it seems likely that they may result in better patient care. Medicine is no longer a solitary profession in which practitioners practice independently, assured of noninterference by colleagues or the state. Peer review and other quality control measures are now the norm. In the United States the pervasive fear of malpractice appears to serve as a mechanism of social control that in some ways enhances and in other ways works to the detriment of patient care.

Second, fear of liability is only one of several factors that contribute to the overuse of laboratory tests and therapeutic interventions. Surveys in Britain and the Netherlands, where malpractice litigation is far less frequent than in the United States, have demonstrated similar patterns of overutilization (Dewar, 1994; Veldhuis, 1994). In these studies, fear of peer disapproval, physician discomfort with medical uncertainty, absence of clear guidelines for appropriate care, and a tendency to adhere to the "technological imperative," i.e., the availability of a new technique tends to make its use appear desirable, were all listed as factors contributing to overutilization.

Physicians have an emotional commitment to action. They are often tempted to act even in situations when they know, or ought to know, that simply watching and waiting would most benefit the patient. Similarly, while the probability of reducing medical uncertainty by performing a certain test might be very small, the desire to reduce uncertainty is often great enough to cloud a physician's probabilistic reasoning. For this reason *errors of commission* in medicine have typically been considered less blameworthy than *errors of omission*. The resident knows that if she performs an unnecessary bone marrow test on a patient with mild anemia she is less likely to be humiliated at Morning Report than if she fails to perform the bone marrow test when the Chief of Medicine actually thinks it was indicated. Physicians often talk of ordering certain tests "for completeness sake." A right upper quadrant ultrasound may confirm the physician's clinical impression of cholelithiasis, but the physician may also order an abdominal CT scan, just in case. While the first test explains the clinical findings, the second is performed solely for the sake of completeness. For these reasons, defensive medicine is, in fact, synergistic with the medical tendency to err on the side of doing too much.

Third, good physician–patient interaction is, in fact, the best defensive medicine. For some years now malpractice insurers have sponsored seminars for physicians on how to reduce their risk of being sued. A major reason for these seminars is to improve physician communication skills. An empathic, compassionate approach with good interactive techniques leads to better diagnosis and therapy. This approach also enhances patient satisfaction. Satisfied patients generally do not bring malpractice suits against their physicians. In fact, if an adverse outcome of care occurs, the strongest predictor of a malpractice action being brought against the physician is a pre-existing poor physician–patient relationship (Beckman *et al.*, 1994; Vincent *et al.*, 1994).

## CASE 4-10

***Dr. Mark Korsakoff is a neurologist on the medical staff of your hospital. Last year he assumed a large debt when he joined several other physicians in purchasing an MRI machine and establishing***

*a new diagnostic center (Health Scan Inc.) near Suburban Mall. Health Scan initiated a major advertising campaign including frequent commercials on local television stations. Consumers were urged to contact Health Scan ("where we offer you the most advanced new scanning equipment") if they had headaches, injury, joint pain, or other persistent symptoms. The enterprise has been very successful, so successful in fact that the hospital administrator, Mr. R. Tape, complained that Health Scan Inc. was siphoning off patients and reducing the volume of MRI use at the hospital's diagnostic facility. You are aware that some of the medical staff are unhappy with Korsakoff and a little envious because of his glittering financial success.*

## Diagnostic Facilities

While physicians who work in HMOs and other institutional settings may experience pressures to underutilize medical services, physician entrepreneurs who own diagnostic and other medical facilities tend to overutilize services by too frequent referral of patients for tests or procedures. This type of conflict of interest may seem at first to compromise patient care less than practice arrangements that promote fewer referrals and less testing. After all, here the error, if there is one, lies on the side of being more careful and doing tests "just in case," even if they are not technically indicated.

Many studies, however, have shown that physicians who own facilities overutilize them. The AMA's Council for Health Policy found that approximately 10% of physicians in the United States have ownership interests in diagnostic laboratories, hospitals, nursing homes, or other facilities that might involve self-referral. Moreover, for important classes of services, "patients of physicians who self-refer have higher utilization rates than other patients" (Council, 1992). For example, self-referring physicians sent patients to obtain laboratory testing at a 45% higher rate than other physicians. Another study concluded that physicians with a financial interest in imaging facilities referred patients for diagnostic studies 4.0 to 4.5 times more frequently than did other physicians (Hillman *et al.*, 1990).

As a result of such studies, the AMA Council on Ethical and Judicial Affairs recommended in 1992 that "physicians should not refer patients to a health care facility outside their office practice at which they do not directly provide care or services when they have an investment interest in the facility." The main exception to this recommendation is in cases where "there is a demonstrated need in the community for the facility and alternative financing is not available." The bottom line is that, consciously or unconsciously, financial self-interest conflicts with patient interest in these situations. Thus, self-referral at the very least gives the appearance of impropriety; at worst it is a blatantly unethical practice. The federal government has accepted this professional judgment by creating Medicare regulations against referral to self-owned facilities.

In Case 4-10 Health Scan Inc. was in the MRI business to make money. There is nothing in the case to suggest that the hospital's scanning facilities were overburdened, inadequate, or inconvenient to patients. As a neurologist, Dr. Korsakoff would naturally refer many patients for MRI studies. The decision about whether or not to get an MRI for a patient with headaches or dizziness is a complex one; different neurologists might decide differently. Nonetheless, data indicate that physicians like Korsakoff who own such facilities order many more MRIs than other physicians.

## CASE 4-11

*Dr. AT has practiced oncology in a small northeastern city for 20 years. He initially belonged to a small group practice, but has been working on his own for the last 5 years. Dr. AT is well known for his aggressive approach to treatment, his commitment to patients, and his willingness to teach medical students from State University. He has always prided himself in the ability to work 16 hours a day for the benefit of his patients. Since his divorce 6 years ago, Dr. AT has had little contact with his three children because they moved with their mother to another city. Dr. AT used to be active in various church groups, but no longer finds the time to get involved. In fact, his friends have been worried about him for the last couple of years. To them, he seems tired, irritable, distant, and somewhat depressed. Newer members of the hospital staff have never seen the optimistic and energetic man AT used to be.*

## SATISFACTION, PROFESSIONAL STRESS, AND BURNOUT

There are two paradoxes built into the U.S. folk image of the kindly general practitioner who loved his profession, worked long hours, was permanently on-call, and became the town's font of humane wisdom. The first has to do with the limits of medical power. During the early twentieth century, physicians had far fewer tools and far less ability to alter the natural history of disease than their counterparts in the 1900s. The friendliness, accessibility, wisdom, and moral authority that characterize our image of general practitioners in the "good old days" contain a healthy mixture of fact and fiction. Nonetheless, the cultural belief that those "old days" were better than today is somewhat paradoxical, given the their lack of medically effective tools and technology.

The second paradox has to do with the character of the physician. Kindly, yet firm. Intensely practical, yet committed to virtue. Accessible at all hours of the day and night. Married to his practice, yet also a family man. Always having the time to share part of himself with patients, friends, or students. From where did this prodigious level of energy come? The truth is that few flesh-and-blood physicians ever really met this cultural standard. Physicians have always had to juggle the stresses of their personal and professional lives, hopefully managing to achieve a satisfactory and healthy outcome.

Some surveys indicate that most physicians are satisfied with their work and feel professionally fulfilled (Baker & Cantor, 1993; Chuck *et al.*, 1993). Other surveys reveal more evidence of physician disaffection (Cohen *et al.*, 1990). Nonetheless, in recent years there has been a perception of widespread dissatisfaction in the medical community (Glick, 1990; Schroeder, 1992). Physicians have been speaking out more than in the past about their personal and professional concerns: heavy work load, long hours, fatigue, bureaucratic interference, alienation from families and social networks, commercialization of medicine, difficult physician–patient relationships, and the expense and stresses of medical education. More recently, managed care and other arrangements that limit physician autonomy add to the dissatisfaction. In some specialties, oncology and emergency medicine, for example, physicians are highly vulnerable to emotional exhaustion and burnout. In one study, 46% of Canadian emergency physicians reported medium to high levels of emotional exhaustion while feeling low levels of personal accomplishment (Lloyd *et al.*, 1994). In a survey of U.S. oncologists, over half expressed some sense of professional burnout (Whippen & Canellos, 1991). In Case 4-11 one particular oncologist, Dr. AT, appears to be heading toward burnout, if he is not already there. Long hours, time pressure, and on-call commitment are important stressors in medicine, although the need to maintain medical knowledge and repeated exposure to life-and-death situations also create stress (Richardson & Burke, 1991). Among oncologists the most frequent reason cited for emotional exhaustion was insufficient personal or vacation time. Other factors cited were continuous exposure to fatal illness, frustration with limited therapeutic success, and reimbursement problems.

Some observers argue that internal factors are responsible for most physician dissatisfaction. Glick, for example, argues that today's physicians experience a greater sense of entitlement than past physicians did, corresponding to the rampant growth of entitlement and "rights" in our general culture (Glick, 1990). Moreover, Glick claims that there has been a change in the type of feedback that physicians consider satisfying. This change creates dissonance between physicians and patients. The patient is looking to feel better and to be treated in a personal and supportive way. However, the physician, especially the subspecialist, no longer looks for his or her satisfaction in the give-and-take of human relationships, but concentrates on achieving disease-oriented goals. This often involves technical matters that are only indirectly of interest to the patient.

While the dynamics that Glick outlines are undoubtedly present in today's medicine, providing service and interacting with people remain sources of satisfaction for most physicians. Burnout occurs not so much

HIGH CAREER EXPECTATIONS
STRONG MOTIVATION
↓
LONG WORK HOURS
EXPENDITURE OF PHYSICAL AND EMOTIONAL ENERGY
PHYSICIAN BECOMES:
Depleted
Detached
Depersonalized
In Denial
↓
BURNOUT
Reduced social involvement
Feelings of victimization
Feelings of lack of accomplishment
Focus on money and power
Disruptive behavior
High malpractice risk

**Figure 4.2.** The physician stress and burnout cycle.

because people find themselves in the wrong profession, but because they fall into a vicious cycle of internal and external factors that leaves them emotionally exhausted. Figure 4.2 summarizes this cycle. First, physicians begin with high career expectations. These include both internal (caring, curing, intellectual stimulation) and external (status, financial rewards) goals. To accomplish their goals, physicians expend large amounts of physical and emotional energy. In doing this, they become are vulnerable to the five "D's" of emotional stress: depletion, detachment, depersonalization, denial, and depression. A sense of being drained or depleted first manifests itself in social life. The physician simply doesn't feel that he or she has time and energy for family or friends, for personal or social causes. This leads to emotional detachment from family and friends, as well as from patients. In Case 4-11 Dr. AT illustrates this continuum. In the process of depersonalization, patients may be treated as objects—organs, body parts, or "the gallbladder in room 1017." Because of their high expectations of themselves, physicians are often reluctant to admit that things are not going well. While most learn to cope with mistakes in clinical practice, it is more difficult to admit failure to meet personal goals. The need for objectivity in medicine may also lead to emotional numbness, which creates an internal barrier (denial) to experiencing one's own feelings and personal needs.

Finally, the physician may reach the stage of emotional burnout and depression with diminished social attachments; feelings of inadequacy, cynicism, and victimization; and proneness to disruptive behavior, chemical dependency, depression, and suicide. Because burnout adversely affects professional performance as well, the physician is also more vulnerable to malpractice suits. In Case 4-11 Dr. AT is irritable, withdrawn, and depressed. What effect do you think this has had on his ability to care for his patients?

Table 4.2 presents a list of risk factors or early signs of emotional distress that lead to burnout. Many of these factors can be summarized by the term *indispensable person syndrome*. Personality characteristics that foster good medicine can also become distorted if not counterbalanced by other qualities. For example, a passion for helping others, the desire always to do a good job, and willingness to accept responsibility are all qualities of a good physician. These can be distorted, however, by the grind of practice into messianic and perfectionist patterns of behavior. The indispensable physician values high achievement, but wants to go it alone. While they can't say "No" to new responsibilities, neither can they rely on others to help them accomplish the work. It is difficult or impossible to ask for help. Yet the indispensable physician is often angry because he or she is always giving, while others are always taking.

An important factor in maintaining good professional and personal health is to avoid becoming indispensable. Listen carefully to the advice that *you* typically give to fatigued and harried patients: Be sure to

**Table 4.2**
Risk Factors for Physician Burnout

Is highly motivated to succeed
Likes to be considered indispensable
Likes to work alone
Has difficulty saying "no"
Chronic sense of work overload
Dislikes accepting help from others
Dislikes delegating responsibility
Dislikes discussing problems
Dislikes discussing feelings
Externalizes blame
Personal identity merges with professional identity
Has little time for family and friends.

take time for yourself. Enjoy your family. Go on vacations. Develop outside interests. Slow down. Change your schedule so that you have time for exercise and meditation or other relaxation techniques.

## CASE 4-12

*AK was a subintern in surgery at University Hospital. She was on call with SD, a second-year resident. Unexpectedly, SD took advantage of an early evening lull to leave the hospital for a quick dinner. When he returned, the senior resident sent him to speak with Mrs. L., a 70-year-old woman who had been admitted through the emergency room and was scheduled for an exploratory laparotomy the next morning. AK accompanied SD to the patient's room. She noticed that SD had alcohol on his breath. His manner was strangely uninhibited and jocular in dealing with Mrs. L., who appeared agitated and a bit confused. His preop interview and examination were hurried and superficial. When Mrs. L. seemed ambivalent and continued to ask questions he had already answered, SD became impatient and said, "Look, you need this goddamn operation. Just sign the forms!" Embarrassed, Mrs. L. signed.*

*The next day at the operation, AK noted that SD was subdued, but as far as she could tell, assisted the surgeon quite adequately. However, disturbed by his behavior the night before, AK took the opportunity to talk with LR, another surgical resident, who reported that SD graduated near the top of his class in a very competitive medical school. During his internship there had been a story of a "driving while intoxicated" (DWI) incident, but SD simply joked about it. More recently, LR had heard that SD's long-time relationship with a woman he had known since medical school broke up in a somewhat violent and disturbing way. She knew no details. His clinical work was generally good, but he was often rather avuncular and distracted on morning rounds.*

*LR suggested that AK relate the incident with Mrs. L. to the surgery residency director. AK wasn't sure what to do.*

## ────── AM I MY BROTHER'S KEEPER? THE IMPAIRED PHYSICIAN

There is good evidence in Case 4-12 that SD was drinking while on duty (alcohol on his breath), that his performance was significantly impaired (rude and angry behavior), and that he had a history of prior alcohol abuse (DWI). When presented with the story of SD, however, medical students have great difficulty trying to figure out what AK's responsibility is. Part of this difficulty arises from AK's status as a medical student. In the hierarchical field of medicine, persons on lower levels may well believe that they should not take it on themselves to judge the behavior of their higher colleagues. After all, reporting SD's behavior may somehow damage their grade or their chance for a good recommendation. However, this also illustrates a more general concern: Whistle-blowers have a rather ambiguous position in our society. We supposedly admire them. We tout their integrity and courage. Yet, at the same time there the concept of "telling" on our colleagues or friends is a little repugnant to us, evoking memories of childhood breaches of trust and tattletales. In SD's case the feature that generally tips the balance for students is the observation of alcohol on his breath. This is the "smoking gun" that eventually leads students to say that AK should report SD to the residency director. Many argue that they would first confront SD and give him a chance to seek help voluntarily for his presumed drinking problem. Others defer a personal confrontation because of the power imbalance between AK and SD.

The American Medical Association is unambiguous about a physician's responsibility regarding impaired colleagues: "A physician should expose, without fear or favor, incompetent or corrupt, dishonest or unethical behavior on the part of members of the profession." This statement from the AMA's *Current Opinions of the Judicial Council* (1984) specifies a wide range of impairment, as well as other immoral or unprofessional conduct. Our moral obligation in this regard is based both on (1) individual integrity and commitment to patient welfare and (2) allegiance to the community of professionals to which we belong. In return for the trust and privileges it receives from the community, the medical profession must set and monitor its own standards of professional behavior. Yet, Case 4-12 illustrates the dynamics that have led to a poor record in the medical profession of monitoring incompetence, substance abuse, and unprofessional behavior.

Physicians may become unable to perform their duties for a wide variety of reasons, including disease, mental illness, dementia, and substance abuse. The syndrome of burnout contributes directly because it may be a factor in mental illness, and indirectly through demoralization and lowering of personal standards. The term *impaired physician* is usually used, however, to refer to impairment as a result of substance abuse or chemical dependency. To quote Dr. Richard Blondell, "Without help, physicians who become chemically impaired face the possibility of premature death and may cause harm to their patients. Knowledgeable physician colleagues are the most significant factor in any strategy to prevent these tragic events" (Blondell, 1993).

In the past physicians have often been reluctant to confront and openly challenge their impaired colleagues. This situation is well illustrated in William Carlos Williams's wonderful story "Old Doc Rivers" (Williams, 1984). Doc Rivers is a compassionate, dedicated physician who for 30 years has taken care of anyone in town who needed help, "doing something, mostly the right thing, without delay and of his own initiative." Rivers's patients are "a population in despair, out of hand, out of discipline, believing in the miraculous." Everyone knows, however, that Rivers has a tragic flaw: dope addiction. The narrator of the story (another physician) believes that the addiction arose from Rivers's inability to set limits on pouring himself into the medical work. He thinks that the problem reflects more the flawed world of human suffering than the physician's personal shortcomings. He and the other physicians in town clearly admire Rivers, even though they have serious questions about his behavior. Sometimes, for example, Rivers passes out during operations. The narrator's wife asks, "Why do you physicians not get together and have his license taken away?" But the narrator reflects, "I doubted that we could prove anything. No one wanted to try." In the end Rivers kills a patient by compressing her strangulated hernia, but none of his colleagues reports him. The story demonstrates a mistaken understanding of professional ethics, in which admiration for, and solidarity with, the man outweigh one's duty to help a colleague and prevent harm to his patients.

In chemical dependency, individuals habitually use a mood-altering substance despite adverse consequences. Most authorities believe that the prevalence of such dependency among physicians is roughly the same as in the general population (Centrella, 1994). Some studies suggest, however, that patterns of alcohol and drug use are different in that physicians more frequently abuse controlled drugs like opiates and benzodiazepines because of the opportunity for self-prescription, while less frequently using illegal drugs like cocaine and psychedelics. Overall, the AMA estimates a lifetime prevalence of 6–8% for alcohol abuse and 1–2% for other drug abuse or dependence. Each year about 100 deaths of U.S. physicians are directly attributed to chemical dependency. Certain specialties appear to be at higher risk than others for chemical dependency, including anesthesiology, emergency medicine, psychiatry, and family practice (Centrella, 1994).

**Table 4.3**

Signs of Chemical Dependency among Physicians

| Risk factors and early signs | Late signs |
|---|---|
| Alcoholic family members | Family dysfunction |
| Regular use of alcohol | Depression |
| Drinking to relax or sleep | Drinking while "on call" |
| Drinking while studying | Auto accidents |
| Drinking alone | Memory impairment |
| Frequent intoxication | Needle marks |
| Cigarette smoking | Missed work |
| No religious affiliation | Negativism |
| High grades in medical school | Poor patient care |

Table 4.3 lists a number of risk factors for chemical impairment, as well as signs and symptoms of established dependency. As is the case with other professionals, impaired physicians tend to "protect" their work performance as long as possible, even after family and other personal relationships have suffered. However, because chemical dependency is a progressive disorder, clinical judgment and physician–patient relationships eventually suffer. The fact that professional impairment tends to occur in the late stages of dependency complicates early diagnosis and treatment, at least on the basis of professional monitoring. Physicians may discuss their concerns with friends and colleagues on a strictly personal basis, but if such help is turned down (e.g., the physician denies there is a problem), there is often reluctance to take the next step and report the impaired physician to appropriate professional or state authorities. This approach almost ensures that patients will be harmed, perhaps seriously, before intervention occurs. Case 4-12 illustrates a middle ground in which effective action might be taken prior to serious injury. SD had clear evidence of drinking while on duty and subsequent inappropriate behavior. The harm in this case may have been relatively small (rudeness to a patient), but certainly sufficient to warrant reprimand and investigation of alcohol abuse.

The medical profession has generally taken a therapeutic, rather than a punitive, approach to physician impairment. Many state and local medical societies have organized voluntary and confidential programs that promote treatment for impaired physicians and monitor their subsequent performance. In some cases these programs have a nonvoluntary component in that continued medical staff privileges might be linked to successful completion of rehabilitation. While the medical society's goal is to rehabilitate the physician, the state licensure board's main goal is to protect the public. Thus, the licensure board traditionally responds to physician misconduct by limiting or revoking the medical license. However, these goals are not mutually exclusive and in many jurisdictions a good working relationship has developed between professional societies and state licensure boards (Blondell, 1993).

Treatment for chemically dependent physicians is most effective when it involves the support of colleagues, includes well-defined intervention goals, is based on documentation of specific impaired behaviors, and begins soon after the crisis situation that has precipitated intervention (Centrella, 1994). Initial detoxification, which usually lasts about 1 month, may involve either outpatient or inpatient treatment. Extended care of 6 months or more may be required in some cases. An essential part of any long-term therapeutic plan is a mechanism for monitoring future professional performance. Overall, physicians who enter drug rehabilitation programs have better treatment outcomes with less recidivism than the general population of drug abusers, with reported recovery rates without relapse ranging up to 84% (Centrella, 1994).

## CONCLUSION

The virtues, pleasures, and responsibilities of being a physician are closely intertwined. While medicine is rapidly changing in many respects, certain features of medical practice endure. The major goals of medicine include caring for the sick and relieving their suffering. These goals can generally be accomplished only in the context of interpersonal relationships. Thus, the patient–physician relationship lies at the core of the physician's responsibility (competent, trustworthy care), skill development (empathic communication), and professional satisfaction (helping, social interaction, problem solving). In particular, clinical empathy, a complex skill that has cognitive, affective, and motivational components, is an essential ingredient for effective medical practice. Personal qualities important in doctoring include benevolence, compassion, caring, practical judgment, honesty, humility, discipline, fidelity, courage, playfulness, humor, and creativity.

Physicians are powerful by virtue of their medical knowledge, social role, and personal qualities and interpersonal skills. Patients are vulnerable by virtue of their illnesses and lack of knowledge. Physicians should use medical power to promote the interests of their patients. In some cases, however, physicians abuse their power or otherwise engage in activities that conflict with their patients' best interest. Engaging in intimate relationships with patients is a clear example of abuse. Conflict of interest may manifest itself in unnecessary or inadequate medical care. Physician ownership of health facilities and defensive medicine are associated with provision of unnecessary services. Managed care arrangements may sometimes lead to less than adequate medical care by restricting appropriate services.

Most physicians enjoy their work and find it personally and professionally fulfilling. The dynamics of medical practice, however, may lead to chronic emotional stress and, eventually, to burnout. Physicians sometimes deplete themselves emotionally, detach from family and friends, depersonalize their patients, deny their problems, and become depressed. Physicians who consider themselves indispensable and fail to make "space" for self and family are particularly vulnerable to burnout. Burnout harms not only physicians, but their families and patients as well. Abuse of drugs or alcohol is another possible response to emotional stress. While the prevalence of substance abuse among physicians approximates that in the general population, the pattern of drug use differs with specialty. Physicians have a professional duty to help their impaired colleagues. The first step toward helping impaired physicians is to identify them and facilitate appropriate treatment. Professional organizations, in concert with state agencies, work to foster a therapeutic response that helps physicians while minimizing harm to their patients.

# CASES FOR DISCUSSION

## CASE 1

*Dr. Heigh Tech seems to have it all. After completing an orthopedic surgery residency at a prestigious medical center, he joined a well-known multispecialty group practice. Over the next few years his practice grew by leaps and bounds. His aggressive surgical approach and good outcomes led to referrals of "hard cases" from all over the region. Initially, Tech loved his work. His colleagues had trouble understanding how he could be so consistently pleasant and enthusiastic, given his characteristic 12- to 14-hour workdays. He seemed always ready to help others, but he never accepted any help in his own practice. More recently, however, Tech has begun to complain about overwork: He never gets to take a vacation; patients won't leave him alone; as soon as he leaves the hospital, everything goes to pot; his wife just doesn't seem to understand how much pressure he's under. "I don't know why other people can't pull their share of the work!"*

1. *Discuss the satisfactions and dissatisfactions Dr. Tech finds in medical practice.*
2. *Discuss personality characteristics that may make Dr. Tech vulnerable to professional burnout.*
3. *Where do you think Dr. Tech is on the stress–burnout cycle? What would you advise Dr. Tech to do at this point?*

## CASE 2

*Your patient DK has chronic osteoarthritis of his knees. After a spurt of yard work last week, he developed severe pain and swelling of his right knee. You diagnose inflammation and a small effusion secondary to osteoarthritis. You plan to inject a corticosteroid preparation to reduce the inflammation. However, you accidentally use the wrong vial and inject methylprogesterone instead. Later, the nurse brings the mistake to your attention when she notices the empty vial. (This medication has no beneficial effect on arthritis; on the other hand, a single intra-articular injection is probably not harm-*

*ful.) Three days later DK returns for his scheduled follow-up visit. He tells you that his knee is "100% better." In fact, you note that the erythema and swelling are largely gone.*

1. *What type of mistake is this? Would you consider it a culpable error? Explain.*
2. *Should you have tried immediately to call DK and explain the mistake to him? What would you say?*
3. *Let's say you were unable to reach DK. Now that he has returned to your office and his arthritis is "100% better," what should you do?*

## CASE 3

*At 74 years old Dr. T is still going strong. He practices obstetrics–gynecology full-time, including a full surgical schedule. He is well known among the staff for his high energy and gruff manner. Dr. T is definitely not "politically correct": he calls a spade a spade, and his positions on social mores are "Victorian," as one of his younger colleagues put it. Dr. Agra, a new general internist on staff, comments to you that she would never refer a patient to Dr. T because he is "incompetent and abusive to women." In conversation, Dr. Agra reports that Dr. T doesn't seem to understand newer concepts of endometriosis and premenstrual syndrome. Moreover, he refers to patients as "girlie." In the last couple of years you have heard other physicians make remarks about Dr. T's somewhat outdated medical concepts, but his patients, who are mostly older women, seem to love him. You have, however, heard several patients in your practice make negative comments about Dr. T's personality and skills. You wonder if the old guy is still competent.*

1. *Discuss how you would go about evaluating the competence of a practicing physician.*
2. *Should physicians be required to pass periodic evaluations tests of their knowledge and skills? Should physicians be required to retire at a certain age? Please explain.*
3. *What should you or other members of the hospital medical staff do at this point to help Dr. T or his patients?*

## CASE 4

*You are a 45-year-old female urologist in a large staff model HMO. HS is a 38-year-old patient with chronic prostatitis. He also suffers from anxiety attacks and depressive episodes since his wife died in a tragic accident 4 years ago. As part of your medical care, you spend time giving him supportive counseling. You have the feeling that he is physically attracted to you, as you are to him. At one point he asks you out for lunch, but you refuse, explaining that your work schedule would not permit it. A couple of months later, the computer software company HS works for switches to a different health insurance program, so that your services are no longer covered. He calls you the next month and tells you that he has arranged to see a urologist in the new plan. He also tells you that he really enjoys your company and asks you out to dinner, noting that it would be "okay" since you are no longer his physician.*

1. *Is the physician–patient relationship compatible with close friendship or intimacy with patients? Where does one draw the line?*
2. *Describe some of the dynamics that might lead HS to be attracted to you, his physician. What might lead you to be attracted to him? Would these dynamics be different if you were a male gynecologist and he were a woman with endometriosis?*
3. *Are there professional or moral reasons not to "get involved" with HS while he is still your patient? What about now? When does he stop being your patient? That is, when do the dynamics described in question #2 no longer exist or become morally irrelevant?*

## CASE 5

*One of your young colleagues in anesthesiology, Dr. Ernest Barr, has had a difficult year, having just gone through a bitter divorce. Because of the divorce he moved from upstate New York to your town and joined the medical staff in your hospital about 8 months ago. Recently, he has appeared more distant and withdrawn than usual. While he has never seemed very social, he is now outright irritable. He has also uncharacteristically called in sick several times in the last few weeks, necessitating last minute changes in the operating room schedule. You have never heard any complaints before about the quality of Dr. Barr's medical care, but you recently noted him to fall asleep briefly during an operation and, later, to make a mistake in medication dosage. Fortunately, the error was caught and corrected by the assisting nurse anesthetist. You mention this incident to a fellow surgeon who reports a similar occurrence the previous week during a cholecystectomy. In that case, the patient became hypotensive for no apparent reason and the surgeon suspected an anesthesia error. You wonder what is going on with Dr. Barr and whether you should try to do something about it.*

1. *Dr. Barr's performance seems to be impaired. What are the possible reasons for this? List the features of the case that suggest each one.*
2. *What should be done? Do you, as a colleague on the medical staff, have any responsibility to do something? If so, why?*
3. *Barr denies any problems when you raise the issue with him. He tells you to mind your own business. He reminds you that we all sometimes make mistakes. What should you do next?*
4. *Describe the epidemiology and characteristics of substance abuse among physicians.*
5. *Describe the two systems available to sanction unprofessional behavior. Which system would you now approach in Dr. Barr's case? Why?*

## RECOMMENDED READINGS

Brody H: *The Healer's Power.* New Haven, Yale University Press, 1992.

> In this book Howard Brody investigates the nature, sources, and implications of the physician's power. Acknowledging that this power has both positive and negative sides, Brody develops a medical ethic based on the interactive process of doctoring. Chapter 16 on "The Physician's Character" is an excellent discussion of virtues in medicine.

Cassell EJ: *The Nature of Suffering and the Goals of Medicine.* New York, Oxford University Press, 1991.

> In this book Eric Cassell investigates the human meaning of suffering and develops an understanding of medical practice in which relieving that suffering is a major goal.

Williams WC: *The Doctor Stories.* Compiled by Robert Coles. New York, New Directions, 1984.

> This book brings together many of William Carlos Williams's short stories about taking care of patients. They illustrate many of the experiences, virtues, and abuses of doctoring discussed in this chapter. In particular, "Old Doc Rivers" is a fine story about an impaired physician.

## REFERENCES

Aring C: Sympathy and empathy. *JAMA* 167:448–452, 1958.

Baker LC, Cantor JC: Physician satisfaction under managed care. *Health Affairs* 12(suppl): 258–270, 1993.

Basch MF: Empathic understanding: A review of the concept and some theoretical considerations. *J Am Psychoanal Assoc* 31:101–126, 1983.

Becker HS, Geer B, Hughes E, Strauss A: *Boys in White: Student Culture in Medical School.* Chicago, University of Chicago Press, 1961.

Beckman HB, Markakis KM, Suchman AL, Frankel RM: The doctor–patient relationship and malpractice. Lessons from plaintiff depositions. *Arch Intern Med* 154:1365–1370, 1994.

Blondell RD: Impaired physicians. *Primary Care* 20:209–219, 1993.

Blumgart HL: Caring for the patient. *N Engl J Med* 270:449–456, 1964.

Brody H: *The Healer's Power.* New Haven, Yale University Press, 1992, pp 26–43.

Cassell EJ: *The Nature of Suffering and the Goals of Medicine.* New York, Oxford University Press, 1991.

Centrella ML: Physician addiction and impairment—Current thinking: A review. *J Addict Dis* 13:91–105, 1994.

Christensen JF, Levinson W, Dunn PM: The heart of darkness: The impact of perceived mistakes on physicians. *J Gen Intern Med* 7:424–431, 1992.

Chuck JM, Nesbitt TS, Kwan J, Kam SM: Is being a doctor still fun? *West J Med* 159:665–669, 1993.

Cohen AB, Cantor JC, Barker DC, Hughes RG: Young physicians and the future of the medical profession. *Health Aff (Millwood)* 9:138–148, 1990.

Coulehan JL, Block MR: *The Medical Interview: Mastering Skills for Clinical Practice.* Philadelphia, FA Davis Co, 2001.

Council on Ethical and Judicial Affairs, American Medical Association. Conflicts of interest. Physician ownership of medical facilities. *JAMA* 267:2366–2369, 1992.

Daniels N: Duty to treat or right to refuse? *Hastings Cent Rep*, March–April 1991, pp 36–46.

Dewar MA: Defensive medicine: It may not be what you think. *Fam Med* 26:36–38, 1994.

Fox RC: Training for uncertainty, in Merton RK, Reader GG, Kendall P (eds): *The Student Physician.* Cambridge, Mass, Harvard University Press, 1957, pp 207–241.

Franks P, Clancy CM, Nutting PA: Gatekeeping revisited—Protecting patients from overtreatment. *N Engl J Med* 327:424–429, 1992.

Glick SM: From *Arrowsmith to The House of God,* or "Why Now?" *Am J Med* 88:449–51, 1990.

Halpern J: Empathy: Using resonance emotions in the service of curiosity, in Spiro H, *et al* (eds): *Empathy and the Practice of Medicine.* New Haven, Yale University Press, 1993, pp 160–173.

Hillman BJ, Joseph CA, Mabry MR, Sunshine JH, Kennedy SD, Noether M: Frequency and costs of self-referring and radiologist-referring physicians. *N Engl J Med* 323;1604–1608, 1990.

Hoffman ML: Interaction of affect and cognition in empathy, in Izard CE, Kagan J, Zajonc RB (eds): *Emotions, Cognitions, and Behavior*. London, Cambridge University Press, 1984, pp 103–131.

Jones WHS: From "The Physician" and "Decorum." *The Works of Hippocrates*, Cambridge, Mass, Harvard University Press, 1923.

King L: *The Road to Medical Enlightenment 1650–1695*. New York, American Elsevier, 1970, pp 1–14.

Lloyd S, Streiner D, Shannon S: Burnout, depression, life and job satisfaction among Canadian emergency physicians. *J Emerg Med* 12:559–565, 1994.

Majno G: *The Healing Hand*. Cambridge, Mass, Harvard University Press, 1975, pp 156–157.

May WF: *The Physician's Covenant*. Philadelphia, Westminster Press, 1983.

Osler W: *Aequanimitas*. New York, McGraw-Hill, ed 3, 1932. "Aequanimitas," pp 27–32; "The student life," pp 395–423.

Reich W: Speaking of suffering: A moral account of compassion. *Soundings* 72:83–108, 1989.

Reynolds RA, Rizzo JA, Gonzalez ML: The cost of medical professional liability. *JAMA* 257:2776–2781, 1987.

Richardson AM, Burke RJ: Occupational stress and job satisfaction among physicians: Sex differences. *Soc Sci Med* 33:1179–1187, 1991.

Rogers CR: The characteristics of a helping relationship, in Rogers CR (ed): *On Becoming a Person: A Therapist's View of Psychotherapy*. Boston, Houghton Mifflin Co, 1961, pp 39–58.

Schroeder SA: The troubled profession: Is medicine's glass half full or half empty? *Ann Intern Med* 116:583–592, 1992.

Schwenk TL, Marquez JT, Lefever RD, Cohen M: Physician and patient determinants of difficult physician–patient relationships. *J Fam Pract* 28:59–63, 1989.

Spiro H: What is empathy and can it be taught? *Ann Intern Med* 116:843–846, 1992.

Veatch RM: Models for ethical medicine in a revolutionary age. *Hastings Cent Rep* 2:5–7, 1972.

Veldhuis M: Defensive behavior of Dutch family physicians. Widening the concept. *Fam Med* 26:27–29, 1994.

Vincent C, Young M, Phillips A: Why do people sue doctor? A study of patients and relatives taking legal action. *Lancet* 343:1609–1613, 1994.

Whippen DA, Canellos GP: Burnout syndrome in the practice of oncology: Results of a random survey of 1,000 oncologists. *J Clin Oncol* 9:1916–1920, 1991.

Williams WC: *The Doctor Stories*. Compiled by Robert Coles. New York, New Directions, 1984.

Zinn W: The empathic physician. *Arch Intern Med* 153:306–312, 1993.

## CHAPTER 5

# The Physician in Literature

*William Monroe and John L. Coulehan*

## CASE 5-1

*An unconventional country doctor renowned for his ability to heal difficult cases was brought by some friends to a village to see a blind man who had not been helped by traditional treatments. Concerned about the interest his arrival had created, the doctor took the man to a place outside of town where they could be free of curiosity-seekers. There the doctor treated the patient—by putting spittle on his eyes. The man's sight was improved but not entirely restored: to him, people looked like trees, walking. After a second treatment the grateful patient could see clearly. The doctor asked him to return to his home without telling the townspeople how he had been cured.*

## EDUCATIONAL OBJECTIVES

1. Identify five ways that physicians have been understood and portrayed in Western culture
2. Understand how you are likely to be perceived by your patients and by society as a whole
3. Draw on, through literature, a wider range of experiences and a broader repertoire of responses available to you as you begin your clinical practice
4. Evaluate, with sound and subtle distinctions, your virtues (and vices) and those of your fellow physicians

## INTRODUCTION

Many readers will recognize Case 5-1 as a retelling of Mark 8:22–26, "The Blind Man of Bethsaida." It is a good way to begin a chapter on "The Physician in Literature" because it reminds us that the best-known stories about a gifted healer, at least in the West, are the New Testament accounts of Jesus of Nazareth. During the Roman occupation of Palestine, there were many teacher-healers—"teacher" is the literal translation of the Latin word *doctor*—who promised to produce "signs and wonders." Stories about these teachers often depicted healers with dazzling powers of prophecy and rejuvenation. They were prophetic

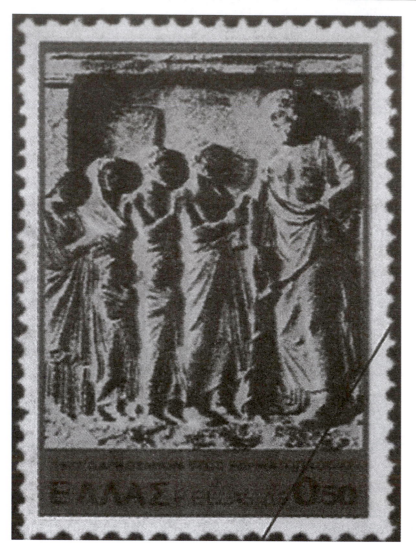

*Postage stamps are ubiquitous reminders of the values of the societies that issue and circulate them, and they often feature physicians, medical scientists, and medical situations. Asklepios, a Greek demigod and the son of Apollo, is called the first physician. Worshipped as both a hero and a god, he was, in the words of Homer, "a great joy to mortals, a soother of evil pains."*

figures, magicians really, who could raise the dead and make the sun darken in the noonday sky. They were eager to have their powers proclaimed far and wide by their followers.

Jesus provides us another model of the physician-healer. We notice first in this short but famous passage that Jesus is not wholly successful the first time he treats the blind man. Some commentators have seen intentional humor in Mark 2:24: When the blind man says he sees "people looking like trees and walking," it may be an ironic commentary on the grandiose claims made for other prophetic healers of the first decades of the Common Era. In any case, Jesus repeats the treatment, and when the man can see distinctly, sends him home telling him to avoid the rumor-mongering crowds of the village. Jesus does not want his healing powers publicized.

Like it or not, any physician practicing in Europe or the Americas will have Jesus of Nazareth as one of his or her forebears. Indeed, there are a multitude of figures from both sacred and secular literature whose presence in our collective imagination contributes to our images and expectations of physicians, even today. Medicine, like other professional practices, is a social and cultural encounter as well as a scientific or biomedical intervention. It is important, therefore, that a good clinician not only understand biomedical procedures but also the many cultural expectations that patients, and society generally, have of physicians.

Physicians, like other professionals, perform within a cultural theater. They are not merely operatives, functionaries, or bureaucrats; they are, well, physicians, and people have opinions, apprehensions, and even prejudices about them. We are all familiar with doctor jokes, the social and economic status of physicians, and the power and prestige associated with the medical profession generally. These sources of conventional wisdom about doctors are not merely amusing (or frustrating); they actually lay the groundwork, they create the field or background with which or on which physicians must do their work. It would seem clear, then, that the best practitioners will understand how physicians have been (and can be) understood and socially constructed through stories, plays, and poems.

In addition to helping you understand how physicians have been and are perceived, reading literature about physicians and medical situations will expand the range of experiences that you will be able to draw on as a practitioner. Throughout our careers we will get to know physicians whose clinical skills and mental agility make us want to emulate them. We will also meet others whose abuse of substances, brusque treatment of patients, or inattentiveness to detail will inspire some combination of anger, pity, and contempt. In any case, we will be making judgments about our peers and colleagues and about the medical situations we encounter. At the least, reading literature about physicians multiplies the number of such encounters, thus increasing the range and density of a physician's experience with other physicians and with medical situations.

More than that, literary works are constructed to focus a reader's attention on the challenges, conflicts, and dilemmas inherent in any given situation so that the reader takes away not just an awareness but also an opinion, an evaluation, an attitude toward the situation. And an attitude, as the literary theorist Kenneth Burke says, is an "incipient act, a leaning or inclination" (Burke, 1969, p. 50). Experiencing literary works does more, therefore, than merely increase our knowledge of medical situations and the virtues of the physicians acting on and within them. Literary works, read with a certain level of openness and engagement, can actually modify the repertoire of responses available to a physician—and thus modify the capacities of that physician. By incrementally modifying knowledge, capacities, and attitudes, stories about medicine can reconfigure the characteristics and virtues of physicians (Monroe, 1998, pp. 22–23).

## CHAPTER ORGANIZATION

This chapter will be laid out thematically rather than chronologically or generically. It will begin with the Physician as Savior, take a look at the Physician as Scientist and the Physician as Detective, consider Physician Burnout and the Incompetent/Impaired Physician, and end with a consideration of "The Compleat Physician."

### CASE 5-2

*A young doctor, just out of medical school, worries about his competence as he begins his first assignment in a rural community hospital. His anxiety is compounded by the fact that his predecessor in the town was a physician of extensive experience and skill, respected and loved by everyone. One of his first patients is a young girl who has been brought to the hospital by her mother and grandmother. The girl is experiencing labored breathing and seems terrified. The young doctor quickly determines that the girl has diphtheria, a common killer of children at the time, and that the disease has already reached the stage of tracheal obstruction. He maintains his calm demeanor despite the anger he feels at the patient's mother and grandmother, who have waited 5 days before bringing in the child.*

## FEMALE PHYSICIANS IN LITERATURE

*Sarah Orne Jewett, "A Country Doctor"*
*Elizabeth Stuart Phelps, "Doctor Zay"*
*Annie Nathan Meyer, "Helen Brent, M.D."*
*William Dean Howells, "Dr. Breen's Practice"*
*Virginia Woolf, "The Years"*
*Steward Massad, "Change"*
*Marge Piercy, "Homage to Lucille, Dr. Lord-Heinstein"*
*Susan Mates, The Good Doctor*
*Safiya Henderson-Holmes, "Snapshots of Grace"*
*Perri Klass, Other Women's Children*

*With the girl on the verge of death, the doctor decides that only an emergency tracheotomy can save her—but the grandmother distrusts doctors and the mother initially refuses treatment. The doctor loses his calm demeanor, denouncing the grandmother's advice, threatening the mother with her child's death, and finally begging her to consent to the procedure. Despite his aggressive insistence, he remains uncertain of his skills and fears that he might actually kill the little girl if he attempts the procedure. Under intense pressure from the doctor, the mother finally agrees, and he quickly and expertly performs a tracheotomy. He has saved the child.*

# THE PHYSICIAN AS SAVIOR

"The Steel Windpipe" by Mikhail Bulgakov is a classic tale of the physician as savior. Probably most physicians, like other members of the helping professions, are motivated at least in part by stories such as Bulgakov's. We want to be heroes; we want to be the one who saves the day. We also realize intuitively that heroic action requires the whole person, that it takes more than mere technical training to resolve a crisis. Knowledge and skills are necessary, to be sure, but not sufficient. The young physician also needs courage, quick thinking, sensitivity, and the ability to function despite conflict, pressure, and strong emotions.

Bulgakov suggests a connection between the character of the newly minted physician and his successful intervention to save the child. The safe path would have been a more conventional, less risky, course of treatment. If he had then lost the patient, the death would have occurred within the safe haven of an established protocol. But he puts his self-esteem as well as his reputation on the line for the benefit of the little girl. His actions truly are heroic. He is victorious. The child lives.

*Diphtheria is an infection of the upper respiratory tract caused by* Corynebacterium diphtheriae. *It was a common illness during the first half of the twentieth century until immunizations began following World War II. Diphtheria primarily attacks children. It begins like a common cold with a runny nose, and after a day or two the nasal discharge may become purulent (containing pus). The throat and the tonsils become red and swollen, covered with a whitish-gray membrane. The membrane thickens and extends up into the nose and down into the throat, involving the trachea. The neck tissues swell and the patient has trouble swallowing and breathing. Within a week, the patient may become comatose and die. For many who survive, the heart and peripheral nerves may remain inflamed for several months.*

*In Williams's era, the mortality rate for diphtheria was 30–50%. Today we treat diphtheria patients with penicillin and an antitoxin to* Corynebacterium diphtheriae *toxin, and very few die from this disease.*

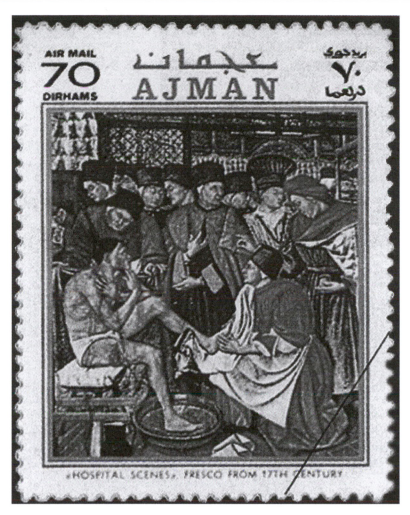

*Since ancient times, the laying on of hands has been associated with the art of medicine.
Here, the comfort and curative power of the human touch suggests a different kind of
savior—the humble servant rather than the heroic interventionist.*

Literature also provides us with tales that suggest the complexity and potential dangers of the physician-as-savior role. One of the more famous in this category is "The Use of Force" by the physician William Carlos Williams. In this story a physician arrives at a rundown tenement—yes, at one time, doctors did make house calls—where he encounters two concerned parents and his patient, a recalcitrant little girl. The mother explains that the girl has had a fever and sore throat. The physician naturally decides that he should have a look and asks the 12-year-old to open her mouth and say "Ahh." She will not comply. Over the next several minutes the physician becomes more and more exasperated as he tries one method and then another to get the child to open her mouth. Finally, to the horror of the parents, who, he thinks, have allowed the child to control the situation, he pries a spoon between her teeth while she kicks and fights. The physician has discovered the culprit, and it is exactly what he suspected. The patient has diphtheria. This is the secret that she had fought so hard to keep.

The stories of Bulgakov and Williams show a similar pattern. Both involve children with diphtheria in need of emergency care; both contain solicitous parents who are serious impediments or, at the least, of no help and in the way; and both stories culminate with the aggressive, even violent, intervention of the

*Have television physician dramas, feature films, and popular literature given us a realistic picture of just how powerful and heroic physicians typically are? Or do they suggest, perhaps erroneously, that physicians are dramatic rescuers of those in crisis?*

physician. But here the similarities cease, for "The Steel Windpipe" depicts a hero who saves a child from a death from disease compounded by ignorance and lethargy, while "The Use of Force" reveals a physician who has apparently lost control of his emotions and is intent on dominating his patient as well as the situation. The imagery used by Williams, who was a prominent "Imagist" poet of the Modernist period (1910–1945), evokes struggle and resistance on the part of the patient and sexual arousal and satisfaction on the part of the physician. Some readers have even suggested that an alternate title for the story, one that reveals the author's underlying concerns, would be "The Rape of the Throat." In any case, Williams is trying to achieve quite sobering and cautionary effects in his readers: Rather than being heroic, he suggests that "macho" intervention can spring from a need to dominate and control. As a physician himself, Williams was well positioned to suggest that powerful interventions are sometimes motivated less by the well-being of the patient than by the psychological needs of the physician.

## CASE 5-3

*Disturbed by the ignorance and suffering that he sees everywhere, a brilliant physician becomes passionately committed to using his biological research to explain the nature of living matter and to create a more perfect human being. He pursues his goal not by means of genetic engineering, but by reconstructing a creature using human body parts. Working in a sequestered laboratory and proceeding against the advice of his colleagues, he is eventually able to confer life on the creature; but he suddenly becomes appalled at what he has done, suffers what amounts to a mental collapse, and abandons his now living, but monstrous, creation. By the time he returns, some weeks later, the creature has escaped. Rejected by humanity at large as well as his maker, the creature becomes destructive and kills a number of people close to the physician. In the end, the physician finally assumes responsibility for his experimental work by luring the creature far out onto the Arctic ice, thus killing them both.*

## THE PHYSICIAN AS SCIENTIST

Most of us will recognize this as the case of Dr. Frankenstein, one of the most famous physician-scientists in Western literature. In 1814, Mary Wollstonecraft, a passionate 17-year-old English girl, ran away to Switzerland with poet Percy Bysshe Shelley, whom she married in 1816. While in Switzerland and while barely out of her teens, she created the Frankenstein story as her contribution to a literary game played by the circle of literati who had gathered in the mountains. Subsequently the book took on a life of its own, becoming one of the most successful novels of the nineteenth century; over the years it has inspired scores of films, plays, and stories, some of them distinguished in their own right. Perhaps one reason for the fascination we have with the Frankenstein story springs from the hubris that Dr. Frankenstein displays when he disrupts the natural order of the world. His obsession with scientific achievement is not mitigated or balanced by larger social or ethical concerns. Yet we do well to remember that Dr. Frankenstein's intentions are good: His objective is to improve humankind, not to harm. As a model of an "overreacher," Dr. Frankenstein has become a widely recognized icon in our culture.

But the question remains, how can we determine who is a Frankenstein and who is a beneficial, cutting-edge researcher? Is *Frankenstein* merely an outdated story, motivated by a hysterical fear of science, or does

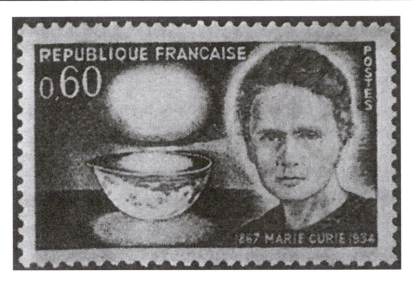

*Marie Curie devoted her life to medical research, sharing the Nobel Prize in Physics with her husband for their studies of radioactivity. After her husband's death, she won a second Nobel Prize, in Chemistry, for isolating polonium and radium. During World War I she trained physicians to use radium to fight cancer and to produce x-ray images of the human body.*

it have something to tell us about certain kinds of research? Some argue that all medical research is ultimately good for humanity, because it extends the range of our knowledge. But what are the social and ethical implications of the human genome project, of cloning, and of genetic engineering generally? The medical research undertaken by the Nazi doctors, some of whom were respected physicians, is one historical instance that raises questions more troubling even than Shelley's fiction. Frankenstein's monster, it would seem, is still with us.

A recent work of literature about medical research gone awry is *Miss Evers' Boys*, a play by physician-writer David Feldshuh. Feldshuh, drawing on James H. Jones's historical study, *Bad Blood*, creates a chilling depiction of a United States Public Health Service project officially known as the Tuskegee Study of Untreated Syphilis in the Negro Male. Working in the interest of medical science, well-intentioned physicians withheld penicillin and earlier forms of treatment from their patients in order to observe the long-term effects of syphilis. There is an obvious racial dimension to the play in that a white government pursues an ethically dubious research study on black subjects. But complicating the race issue is the active participation of a historically black institution, a black physician-scientist, and a dedicated black nurse—the "Miss Evers" of the play's title. For their part in the experiment, her "boys" receive useless injections, a certificate of appreciation from the public health service, and a burial at government expense when they die. The story is a shocking one and seems, like *Frankenstein*, to belong in another time and place; but the 40-year-long Tuskegee Study was only suspended when Jean Heller, an Associated Press journalist, broke the story in 1972.

Stories of scientific medicine gone awry are troubling, but fortunately they represent the exception rather than the rule. In the popular media, the scientist is almost always depicted as a force for good. And since the marriage of science and medicine a century ago, medical scientists have become powerful role models in both fiction and reality. In television and film, for example, physicians almost always succeed in developing a miraculous antidote in time to save the ship, or the world, from the fatal disease. In general, the culture looks to wise and able doctor-scientists for relief from almost any earthly, or unearthly, calamity.

One early classic that in many ways defined the role of the doctor-scientist is Henrik Ibsen's *An Enemy of the People*. Ibsen creates the character of Dr. Robert Stockman whose devotion to the scientific method brings him into conflict with the parochial interests of local politicians and businessmen. Ibsen's play was written during the late nineteenth century, when eminent bacteriologists like Louis Pasteur and Robert Koch were able to show that communicable diseases could be transmitted by microorganisms, sometimes in food and drinking water. Dr. Stockman, a devotee of the new science, is the leading physician in a resort town in southern Norway. The town depends on the tourism generated by its local spa, but when Dr. Stockman sends a specimen for a bacterial culture, he finds that the water is badly contaminated. From that moment, Stockman never questions his duty as a physician and as a scientist: he informs the community leaders that the spa must be closed to protect the public health.

Because Dr. Stockman has been well liked and respected, his stand on the health risks of the spa takes his colleagues by surprise. They present various arguments in an effort to persuade him to change his mind. There will be grave economic damage to the entire community; local investors will lose money; workers in the town will lose their jobs; other spas in the region will capitalize on the bad publicity. Regardless of what others say, Stockman is determined to do the right thing, to close down the baths, even though it means losing the support and respect of the town's VIPs and the companionship of his friends. By the end of the play, Stockman has paid a heavy price for his whistle-blowing: He has lost his job and been labeled "an enemy of the people," an ironic fate for a medical scientist trying to faithfully, and intelligently, serve the people.

Occasionally writers will contrast the compromises inherent in the practice of medicine with the purity of scientific research. *Arrowsmith*, Sinclair Lewis's 1925 novel, is the most important work in American literature dealing with the potential antagonism between medical practice and the high-minded pursuit of scientific truth. Lewis develops the plot so that young Martin Arrowsmith will eventually have to choose between the ideals represented by his two medical school mentors: T. J. H. "Dad" Silva, the exemplary clinician, and Max Gottlieb, the scientific researcher. At the outset of his career, Arrowsmith chooses private practice in North Dakota, then public health work in Iowa. These jobs provide him an income and allow him to marry, but he proves to be ill-suited for clinical work. Gottlieb had predicted Arrowsmith would never last as an ordinary physician, and he happily arranges for his protégé to join him at a prestigious research institute in New York.

Gottlieb, who has studied with Louis Pasteur and Robert Koch, the German physician and bacteriologist, characterizes the scientific calling as "intensely religious" and insists that Arrowsmith must give up any attachment to "that American bitch-goddess Success" if he wants to be a true scientist. Eventually Arrowsmith has an opportunity to prove his mettle as a researcher when he is sent to a plague-ridden Caribbean island to test the efficacy of a new drug. But after arriving on the island, Leora, his long-suffering wife and companion, contracts the disease and dies. Arrowsmith, devastated by her death, gives up the controlled scientific experiment that he had planned and administers the drug to everyone on the island. He returns to New York a scientific failure but a popular hero. Soon he remarries a New York socialite and is in due course offered the directorship of his mentor's research institute. Sensing that he is on the verge of settling down and selling out, Arrowsmith declines the offer and leaves his new wife to pursue pure research as an independent scientist in the forests of Vermont. Thus does Lewis set up a competitive dichotomy between clinical practice, with its promise of financial gain, and a proudly independent approach to medical research, utterly free of the corrupting marketplace. The dichotomy may seem somewhat forced, and Lewis has never been thought of as a subtle or complex thinker. But the competition between research and clinical practice still creates tension within the world of medicine, and, indeed, within the lives of individual physicians.

## CASE 5-4

*A young woman in good health dies in the ancestral home of her stepfather, a physician with a scandalous past and an uncontrollable temper. The authorities are mystified and can offer no*

*The tension between what is taught and what is practiced is as severe today as it was in Sinclair Lewis's day.*

*Consider the following common clinical practices:*
- *Not letting patients leave the office without a prescription in hand, whether they need one or not.*
- *Prescribing antibiotics for colds.*
- *Prescribing the latest, most expensive medications when over-the-counter medicines would work just as well.*
- *Treating patients according to tradition rather than evidence-based medicine.*
- *Emphasis on dramatic, resource-intensive procedures.*
- *Neglect of proven public health practices such as immunizations and prenatal care.*
- *Reliance on pharmaceutical sales representatives rather than medical journals for treatment protocols.*

*Consider the following problems with medical research:*
- *Most research takes place in tertiary medical centers where subjects of the research are not typical of the general population or of the population visiting a primary care physician.*
- *Most research is sponsored by pharmaceutical companies that have a vested interest in the outcome.*
- *The pressure to publish results in an overload of retrospective research of dubious value.*
- *Research findings are often split into "the smallest publishable unit" to achieve a higher quanity of publications.*

*explanation for the woman's death. The woman's twin sister, now living in the room where her sister died, fears for her own life. She decides to seek the help of a specialist. The specialist takes a full history from the living sister and does his own thorough examination of the premises. He agrees with her that the circumstances point to a cause of death both sinister and mysterious, and he decides to spend the night in the room where her sister died. Using his unique powers of observation and inference, the specialist discovers the cause of death: To the utter astonishment of all, the stepfather has trained an exotic viper to crawl down a bell rope into the bed of his victim. Thus had he dispatched his stepdaughter; but this time, the snake, startled by the fierce attack of the specialist, returns the way it had come and delivers a fatal bite to its physician-trainer. The stepfather, who had coveted the inheritance of both girls, is now dead; and the twin sister, who had the good sense to consult the specialist, is now free to marry.*

## THE PHYSICIAN AS DETECTIVE

Many will recognize this case as one of the adventures of Sherlock Holmes, not himself a physician but the fictional creation of a physician, Sir Arthur Conan Doyle. Conan Doyle wrote a number of "doctor tales," but he is best known as the imagination behind the world's most famous detective. In this particular tale, "The Adventure of the Speckled Band," the criminal is himself a physician, and his medical knowledge and analytical thinking enable him to effect an especially insidious murder. Describing the killer Holmes has this cogent observation: "When a doctor does go wrong he is the first of criminals," Holmes says. "He has nerve and he has knowledge." But "The Speckled Band" is exceptional: Usually the only physician in a Sherlock Holmes story is the loyal but unimaginative sidekick, Dr. Watson. In this story as in the others, Conan Doyle directs our primary attention to the detective, with his problem-solving cogitations, and the detective is,

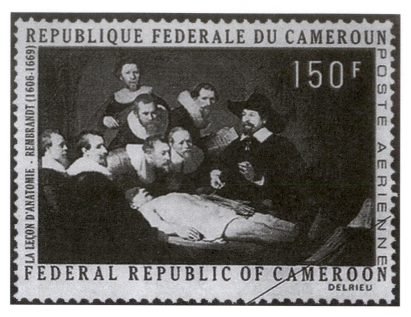

*"The Anatomy Lesson of Dr. Nicolas Tulp" is one of Rembrandt's acknowledged master-pieces. In it we see a physician, impeccably dressed, dazzling his contemporaries by revealing the interior of a cadaver's forearm and hand.*

technically speaking, not a physician. Why, then, do we consider a Sherlock Holmes tale in a chapter on the physician in literature?

Certainly Holmes is a figure who, like a physician, has both nerve and knowledge. In fact, many Sherlock Holmes aficionados believe that the character of the master detective is based on a real physician, Dr. Joseph Bell, who was one of Conan Doyle's professors at the University of Edinburgh. Dr. Bell was renowned for his amazing powers of analysis and inference. Let us then conceive of Holmes not merely as a detective addressing himself to criminal acts, but as a brilliant diagnostician seeking the underlying cause of some human evil. Once we accept this equivalence, it is easy to see similarities between the world's greatest detective and a physician particularly skilled at diagnosis. Both are concerned with bringing to light those underlying causes that are hidden from plain view. Both rely on unusual, even uncanny, powers of observation and inference. Both bring great experience and practical judgment to their cases. Both are "specialists" who are called in only when routine methods have failed—Holmes, after all, is called the world's first consulting detective.

Conan Doyle, however, was not the originator of the classic detective story. That distinction belongs to Edgar Allen Poe, who created the detective genre as we know it with two seminal stories, "The Purloined Letter" and "The Murders in the Rue Morgue." In these stories, as in the still more popular Sherlock Holmes series, Poe and Conan Doyle develop a sequence of observation, hypothesis generation, and hypothesis testing that is recognizable as the basic formula for medical diagnosis. Of course, the similarity is most striking when the underlying cause of the evil is mysterious and when the diagnostician demonstrates both

*What are the consequences of focusing attention primarily on the diagnostic process? Is a correct diagnosis the ultimate goal of a physician?*

brilliance and detachment—Sherlock Holmes and Auguste Dupin, Poe's detective, maintain an aristocratic, almost supercilious distance from their "patients." Whether the riddle be who committed the murder or what is causing the illness, there are always clues (symptoms or test results) confronting a determined investigator with a difficult challenge. Eventually, sometimes almost instantly, he properly interprets the signs and solves the riddle.

To achieve the desired result, the detective-diagnostician must bring to bear what John Cawelti calls "the poet's intuitive insight and the scientist's power of inductive reasoning"—qualities proper to a first-rate physician (p. 93). Indeed, certain "doctor virtues" (determination, attentiveness to detail, insight, and interpretive skill) can be found to varying degrees in twentieth-century detective-heroes such as Hercule Poirot, Dr. Gideon Fell, Mr. Campion, Lord Peter Wimsey, Nero Wolfe, Adam Dalgliesh, and many others. By simple analogy, these brilliant diagnosticians are, to borrow a phrase from a famous play by Moliere, "physicians in spite of themselves."

## CASE 5-5

*An elderly professor of medicine is driven to evaluate his life when he learns he is suffering from a terminal illness. He is revered by generations of younger physicians and can look back on a career of unparalleled professional accomplishment. Yet he considers himself a fraud. He believes that he has failed as a husband and a father and is convinced that "something vital, something really basic" is missing from his life.*

## PHYSICIAN BURNOUT

The physician described in the case above is Dr. Nikolai Stepanovich, the protagonist of Anton Checkhov's "A Dreary Story," first published in 1889. Chekhov, himself a physician, continued to practice medicine long after he had achieved resounding success as a writer. This particular story, though published in 1889, has a contemporary feel: Sometimes the enormous expectations laid on physicians and the day-to-day demands of medical practice gradually wear down a physician's commitment. The result is a condition that we all know as "burnout." The theme of Chekhov's story, the need to find meaning and fulfillment in life, is a need we can all relate to. In a sense, the objective reality—whether Dr. Stepanovich really is a failure—is irrelevant. He experiences himself as an isolated and fragmented person. There appears to be no one he can turn to for support and no one to ease his burden. Like those physicians who tend to intellectualize their personal problems, he has suppressed his emotions to maintain a sense of control. When self-sufficient persons confront burnout or depression, they often have difficulty seeking emotional support from others.

Chekhov confronted the dark side of medical practice again in "Ward No. 6," published in 1892. Dr. Ragin is also an older physician, but unlike Dr. Stepanovich, the academic physician, he is a practitioner. Ragin has spent the last 20 years as the physician in charge of a provincial district hospital. During the early years, he was energetic and enthusiastic about his work. He made hospital rounds daily, worked long hours in the clinic, and tried to keep up with the latest medical developments. As time went on, however, Ragin began to perceive the "palpable futility" of his work. Eventually he becomes convinced that nothing he does makes any difference. The hospital is poorly equipped and out-of-date, yet Ragin decides that it would be a waste of time to try to remedy the situation. He also begins to withdraw emotionally. He rarely makes hospital rounds, he avoids the clinic, and he frequently disappears to his study where he reads books and drinks beer undisturbed for hours on end. He becomes a fatalist, believing that "dying is the normal and legitimate end of us all." With few personal friendships and little professional energy, he learns to divert himself by holding long conversations with a man named Gromov, a paranoid intellectual who is incarcerated in Ward 6, the lunatic ward of the hospital. Faced with Ragin's strange behavior and ongoing dereliction of duties, the town

*Have you or someone you know experienced "burnout"? Have you, despite your making it
this far, perceived yourself as a failure? Are there habits that can be developed during
medical school that might prevent future burnout?*

council finally takes action and replaces him. Ragin decides to take an extended leave from his professional duties, and when he returns from his travels, the new superintendent tricks him into visiting Ward No. 6 again, where he is promptly incarcerated as a lunatic. A few days later Ragin has a stroke and dies.

It is difficult to draw a simple moral from a tale like Chekhov's. But if we want to identify a flaw in Dr. Ragin that leads to his professional and mental collapse, it may be his tendency to embrace abstraction, while avoiding the concrete and the particular. He doesn't seem to connect with his patients, or with other persons at all. Nor apparently does he understand that he has a responsibility to make that connection. His observation that "dying is normal" is a valid abstraction, but one that does not take into account the real suffering of individual patients and their loved ones. His reading does not help him empathize with his patients, but is rather a symptom of his narcissistic sense of superiority and isolation. He realizes that he has become emotionally numb, but never quite understands that his withdrawal constitutes an abandonment of his professional duties, however he may rationalize his inaction.

## CASE 5-6

***Impressed with reports of the achievements of modern science, a pretentious pharmacist encourages a town doctor to attempt a form of corrective surgery with which he is unfamiliar. The would-be patient, a stable boy with a clubfoot, is not keen on having an operation. At first the doctor also hesitates, but when his wife points out the value of a successful operation for his reputation and the significant financial benefits for his practice, he goes along. Initially the surgery to straighten the foot seems to be a success, but in a few days the boy develops gangrene. A physician with more surgical experience is called from another town and must amputate the leg to save the boy's life.***

## THE INCOMPETENT/IMPAIRED PHYSICIAN

Initially this case may, like Shelley's *Frankenstein*, seem outdated. As inhabitants of the twenty-first century, we may feel confident that medicine has moved far beyond the doltish errors of mid-nineteenth-century provincial France, which is the setting for this episode from Gustave Flaubert's *Madame Bovary*. But have we really left incompetencies, inattentiveness, and conflicts of interest so far behind? The Institute of Medicine, an arm of the National Academy of Sciences, estimates that about 98,000 Americans die every year as a result of medical mistakes—more than from breast cancer, highway accidents, or AIDS. And when physicians double as investors in the medical devices they develop, use, promote, or evaluate, conflict of interest issues come to the fore. Like Homais, the pharmacist in Flaubert's 1857 novel, physicians can still become enamored with the inflated promises of revolutionary techniques and protocols.

One of the few benefits of the managed care revolution may be reducing the inclination to do too many (new) procedures. The greater temptation these days is to ration or withhold procedures, even when they are clinically indicated. Whether it relates to doing unnecessary procedures or withholding beneficial ones, this episode from *Madame Bovary* reminds us that physicians can be susceptible to pressures external to the case itself—personal, financial, and professional pressures that can compromise medical judgment and endanger patients.

In "Old Doc Rivers" William Carlos Williams provides a number of perspectives on a gifted but reckless and impaired physician. Rivers, renowned for his uncanny diagnostic insights, is also a good example of the paternalistic physician, for he practices medicine as a unilateral activity, often without his patients' consent or even their awareness. Most of the time his actions are beneficial, as when he quickly amputates, with bandage scissors, the badly damaged arm of a laborer who has been "clipped" by a trolley car. But on another occasion a boy approaches him in a public saloon about an abscess on his neck. Without a word of warning Rivers takes a scalpel out of his vest pocket and makes a swipe at the abscess. The boy jerks backward in fear when he sees the knife coming at him and, wounded by the blade, runs from the place "bleeding and yelling." We also learn that on occasion Rivers will do operations that are not clinically indicated, such as the time he did a tonsillectomy on one of his protégés; and he has also been known to remark that a woman needs only half her organs—"the others were just a surgeon's opportunity" (p. 36). Most disturbingly, Old Doc Rivers is dependent on what the narrator calls "dope," a category that includes alcohol, morphine, and cocaine. An indulgence that may have started as mere recreation eventually becomes necessary for basic clinical functioning. While doing a surgical procedure, Rivers would sometimes "retire for a moment (we all knew why), return, change his gloves, and continue. The transformation in him would be striking. From a haggard old man he would be changed 'like that' into a resourceful and alert operator" (p. 18).

Again, it would be easy for us to discount the actions of Williams's Doc Rivers as just the antiquated habits of a very bad physician. In fact, alcoholism and substance abuse are as prevalent today in the physician population as in the U.S. population at large. According to Eugene Boisaubin, "Anonymous surveys of American physicians, from academic medical centers to rural communities, show consistent rates of 12 to 15 percent over the course of a career, and 8 percent at any one time." Thus, it is likely that approximately 50,000 physicians in the United States currently meet the American Medical Association criteria for substance abuse. Boisaubin points to certain personality attributes, such as reliability, conscientiousness, and the desire to achieve as attributes that can, ironically, suggest a predisposition for psychopathologies. Physicians can be "too hard on themselves," leading to a sense of inferiority, or, conversely, overconfident in their abilities, leading to a sense of omniscience and indestructibility.

Williams's story is particularly effective at developing the potential connection between physician paternalism and physician psychopathology. There is not a simplistic cause-and-effect relationship, but there may be a pattern of mutual reinforcement between substance abuse and physician paternalism. For example: The illusion of indestructibility and the reality of superior technical knowledge allow the gifted physician to live and practice "on the edge" by taking actions that others recognize as risky and dangerous. Substance abuse further reinforces the illusion by producing a euphoric sense of prescience and capacity, thus confirming the physician's overconfidence in his extraordinary powers. And naturally, if one has extraordinary powers beyond the ken or comprehension of mere mortals, then it must be completely appropriate to take an aggressive, unilateral, paternalistic approach to clinical practice. "Frightened, under stress, the heart beats faster, the blood is driven to the extremities of the nerves, floods the centers of action and a man feels in a flame." Thus does Williams describe the effects of drugs on his exhausted physician, who is overextended and overmatched by the relentless working of sickness among the poor. "That's what Rivers wanted, must have wanted" from the substances to which he resorted more and more often as his skills deteriorated, his practice waned, and his life spiraled out of control.

As in many of his stories, however, Williams creates an equivocal situation in "Old Doc Rivers." This hard-working GP has many virtues, including a sharp diagnostic eye, extensive experience, and tough

---

*In a recent survey of emergency physicians, one-quarter described themselves as burned out or impaired due to drugs, alcohol, or mental illness. Nearly one-quarter reported that they planned to leave emergency medicine within 5 years (Doan-Wiggins et al., 1995).*

determination: When he had assessed a situation, the narrator tells us, "he didn't founder. He made up his mind and went to it" (p. 18). It is true that Rivers crosses the line on many occasions and that some patients die under his care, perhaps unnecessarily. But he saves the lives of countless others, most of them the working poor who are barely able to compensate him for his trouble. Rivers is not an evil figure; he is a talented physician who is ultimately done in by a combination of arrogance and indulgence. While Williams depicts a particular physician in a particular place and time, the unhappy combination of qualities that we find in Old Doc Rivers has not disappeared from the world of medicine.

## CASE 5-7

*Substituting for his boss, an assistant to a senior professor of medicine makes a house call on a young woman whose family owns a factory in a suburb of Moscow. The patient is chronically ill with palpitations, insomnia, and "nerves." When the physician examines her, he can find no physical basis for her symptoms and brusquely dismisses her complaints. The young woman's mother invites the physician to stay overnight, and he accepts. During the evening, he meanders around the factory buildings, ruminates on the plight of the workers, and, with a flash of insight, connects the oppressive environment with his patient's illness. He realizes that the monstrous social and economic system weighs heavily on his patient and that these conditions are as insupportable for her as they are for the oppressed workers in her family's factory. With his perspective thus altered, the physician revisits the young woman, validating her symptoms and telling her that they are actually signs of a healthy sensitivity.*

## CONCLUSION: "THE COMPLEAT PHYSICIAN"

How can symptoms of illness be considered signs of life? In the case above, based on Chekhov's 1898 story "A Case History," the physician, Dr. Korolyov, experiences a significant change between his first and second visits to the patient. In the second visit, having seen the factory as a heartless, grinding, dehumanizing machine of poverty, he experiences a stronger connection to his patient, and this connection leads him to behave with more gentleness and compassion. The patient responds to his compassion by revealing her own sense of the basis of her invalidism, admitting that she has "no illness" but is really "weary and frightened" of life. Korolyov decides that her symptoms are actually appropriate responses to the existential suffering and moral injustice of the oppressive world in which she lives. One might even say that to be completely healthy in such a world would be its own form of sickness.

The change in Korolyov can be characterized as a movement from detached concern to compassionate solidarity and illustrates the healing power of a good doctor–patient relationship. After he understands better the entire biopsychosocial situation (see Chapter 20, "The Family System"), Korolyov is able to approach the patient with more empathy and understanding. He continues to recognize the importance of sound clinical data in making an accurate diagnosis, but he is also sensitive to the patient's feelings. His overnight stay and his exploration of her environment allow him to view his patient's story in a broader context, to adopt a more holistic perspective. He opens himself to an imaginative appreciation of the environment's dehumanizing and "diseasing" force. He is then able, by a further imaginative leap, to "recognize" and validate his patient in a different, deeper, and more meaningful way.

Albert Camus's novel *The Plague* presents another compassionate and virtuous physician in the character of Bernard Rieux. The critical public health situation is reminiscent of that in Ibsen's *An Enemy of the People*, though the setting is northern Africa rather than Norway. Dr. Rieux is practicing in the Algerian city of Oran when he begins to notice the first isolated cases of fever and swollen buboes. He carefully observes his patients, records the clinical data, and connects his clinical observations to the fact that carcasses of dead rats have suddenly become apparent throughout the city. When a group of officials meet to discuss the

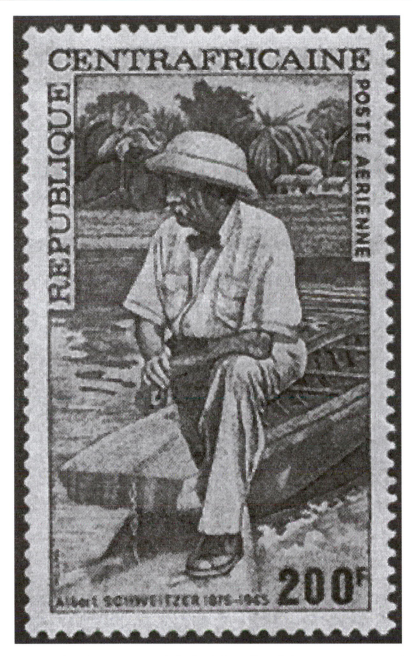

*At the age of 30, the already accomplished scholar Albert Schweitzer moved to Africa with his wife to establish a hospital for the treatment of leprosy and sleeping sickness. In 1952 he received the Nobel Peace Prize for his contributions to the improvement of the human condition.*

crisis, Dr. Rieux argues that they are faced with an epidemic of bubonic plague that is out of control, and, like Ibsen's Dr. Stockman, he has the courage to advocate a very unpopular course of action. He insists that the emergency requires the quarantine of the entire city—no one in, no one out—until the epidemic runs its course. Though this is in many ways a more radical recommendation than simply closing a city spa, Rieux's knowledge and force of character carry the day.

Like Stockman, Korolyov, and many other physicians in literature, Dr. Rieux is portrayed as a vibrant, compassionate human being and a paragon of integrity. As the plague gains momentum, Rieux throws himself into fighting the epidemic. He has no serum or antibiotic that will cure the disease, but he knows that bubonic plague is transmitted to humans by fleas that pick up the bacillus from rodents. So Rieux forms volunteer sanitary squads to canvas the city, cleaning up garbage and exterminating rats. Though he has no cure to offer his patients, the physician works night and day caring for and comforting plague victims, visiting them in their homes and putting himself at personal risk. While others fret and philosophize ("Is the plague a punishment for our sins?") or try to save their own skins by escaping from the city, Rieux never wavers from his role as steadfast clinician. He embodies a simple faith in the necessity of gestures of healing, even when the clinical prognosis is doubtful. As author, Camus validates Rieux's dogged commitment to healing by depicting the physician's physical, intellectual, and emotional hardiness in the face of the "diseases" of superstition, confusion, and hysteria.

Rieux's tireless and courageous work represents a twentieth-century analogue of the physician as heroic healer. As Anne Hudson Jones explains, "the heroic physician as a character type begins to appear in Western literature around the mid-nineteenth century … reaches its peak in the 1930's and 1940's … and is in decline by the 1970's" (p. 8). Yet Rieux remains an image of what we might call, following Isaak Walton, "The Compleat Physician" (Walton & Cotton, 1903). While Rieux cannot succeed in eradicating the plague—just as we cannot eradicate disease and eliminate death—he can and does do his part as a physician and as a human being. He accepts the "responsibility to work and fight for the communal good," as Jones says, and provides a compelling image of heroism for those who struggle against AIDS and other intractable diseases with relatively ineffective methods (p. 16). Thus, Rieux is not a classic hero in the sense cf a fighter whose only measure of success is victory over an opponent. As he himself insists, "there's no question of heroism in all this. It's a matter of common decency" (p. 150).

*The Plague* anticipates by half a century the reluctant admission that medical practice has its limitations. Today we are more ready than we were in the optimistic 1950s to acknowledge some of the hard realities about the precarious nature of individual and public health. Except for pieces with simplistic, triumphalist plots, literature about physicians almost always includes loss and limitation. Stories like those we have surveyed in this chapter, when they are doing their work, may well affect a physician (or medical student) reader in the same way that his experience in the factory town affected Chekhov's Dr. Korolyov. By allowing us to see underlying causes of illness and contextual factors that challenge the physician and complicate clinical practice, literature can help make the world of medicine more refined, compassionate, and, in the end, personally rewarding.

## CASES FOR DISCUSSION

## CASE 1

*Several students were in a coffee shop drinking double-shot lattes and discussing how medicine is represented in the media. A fourth-year medical student said, "It's awful. Medical shows like* ER *and* Chicago Hope *give people the wrong idea … it's not all action and life-and-death decisions, most of medicine is pretty routine." But her friend, a graduate student in literature, replied, "What do you mean? Nowadays there are lots of programs that show real-life medicine, like* The Operation, *or* Paramedics, *or* Trauma: Life and Death in the ER … *no script, no actors, they tape the real thing. So people can experience the real scoop. The public knows what goes on."*

1. *Do television series like* The Operation *and* Paramedics *capture the "real" texture of medicine? If so, what makes them more "real" than traditional medical dramas? If not, explain why.*
2. *What is the role of narrative (story) in medical practice? Compare the patient narratives in a fictional drama like* ER *with a real-life drama like* Trauma: Life and Death in the ER.
3. *Discuss the evolution of images of physicians on television. How do earlier programs like* Marcus Welby, Ben Casey, *and* Dr. Kildare *differ from some more recent physician portrayals?*

## CASE 2

*Dr. Jones is a co-investigator in a major research program studying brain metabolism in substance abusers. He and his colleagues utilize a complex protocol of PET (positron emission tomography) to localize brain activation at different stages in the detoxification process. Dr. Jones also serves as a primary care physician at the drug rehabilitation center from which most of the study subjects are recruited. The protocol requires that volunteer subjects remain off all medications, including sedatives, to suppress their withdrawal symptoms, for 24 hours prior to the PET procedure. Dr. Jones explains that he has no problem judging whether it is safe to withhold medications in any of his patients (who are also subjects), because he clearly distinguishes his therapeutic and research roles.*

1. *What are the advantages and disadvantages of combining clinical research and patient care in the same portfolio? Can you ethically serve as the responsible physician for one of your research subjects?*
2. *How would Dr. Martin Arrowsmith have analyzed this situation?*
3. *Are substance abusers in a rehabilitation program a vulnerable population? Can you envision ways in which their participation might be coerced? How does this scenario compare or contrast with the Tuskegee experiment?*

## CASE 3

*Consider the case of Dr. Heigh Tech, whom you met in Chapter 4 (Cases for Discussion, Case #1). It is now 2 years later. Dr. Tech has made several surgical misjudgments, in two cases leading to major malpractice suits. His behavior has caused great concern among his colleagues. He seems morose, angry, and unpredictable. He no longer plays any role in hospital committees. Ever since his divorce last year, Dr. Tech has taken to disappearing, for a day or even 2 days at a time, sometimes when he is scheduled to be on-call. A few of his friends have tried to engage him in conversation, but he denies that there is anything wrong. "Nothing's wrong with me," he says. "Medicine has gone to hell. That's the problem."*

1. *How would you characterize Dr. Tech's clinical condition and professional condition at this point? How does this relate to his situation 2 years earlier?*
2. *Compare Dr. Tech's situation with that of Dr. Ragin in "Ward Number Six." What are the similarities? What are the differences?*
3. *In "Old Doc Rivers" most of the other physicians rallied behind Doc Rivers, despite his obvious impairment. Why do you think that the medical staff is not rallying behind Dr. Heigh Tech?*

## CASE 4

*Dr. Susan Delvecchio practices in a semirural community adjacent to a national laboratory noted for its outstanding work in nuclear physics. When routine water monitoring revealed that a small amount of tritium (a radioactive isotope of hydrogen) has seeped into the local water supply, officials from the laboratory put out a statement assuring the community that the minute concentration of tritium is harmless. However, the citizens are outraged, claiming that an "epidemic of cancer" in their community is caused by radioactivity from the laboratory's reactors. The community petitions Dr. Delvecchio to help lead the fight to have the laboratory shut down. Laboratory officials claim that epidemiological studies show the region has no higher rate of cancer than expected. Indeed, Dr. Delvecchio has reviewed these studies and agrees with their findings. She also realizes that Vacation Paradise, a national conglomerate, has plans to open a resort and casino in the area, but may be frightened away by persistent rumors about radioactivity in the water and soil.*

1. *In what ways does this situation parallel that of Dr. Stockmann in* An Enemy of the People? *In what ways is it different?*
2. *How could Dr. Delvecchio best serve the interests of her patients and the community? Would this be a heroic course of action?*
3. *Imagine the cooling system failed and there was a major meltdown at the laboratory's reactor, spewing a Chernobyl-like cloud of radioactivity into the atmosphere. How do you think Dr. Rieux in* The Plague *would react to such a catastrophe?*

## CASE 5

*Because so many Americans experience unsatisfactory interactions with their physicians, the popular media recently have taken an interest in doctor–patient communication. One case in point is a video documentary presenting examples of medical school courses designed to teach students how to be more empathic. A segment of this video shows a woman with neurofibromatosis (NF) speaking to a large group of medical students. (NF is a genetic disorder that results in numerous fibrous tumors developing all over the body. John Merrick, the title character in the play* The Elephant Man, *probably suffered from NF.) After the talk, the woman takes off her blouse so the students can see the tumors on her chest and back. With the woman's permission, a number of students come up and hug her. At least one student is so uncomfortable with this violation of privacy that he leaves the classroom. Most students, however, appear to feel that it is perfectly appropriate for the patient to strip in front of them (and the camera), and for them to show their "empathy" by hugging the half-naked woman.*

1. *Today the camera's eye is ubiquitous. Is privacy a relevant concept here? What would you say to the medical student who requested that the viewing be in a more private setting?*
2. *Do you believe that hugging a half-naked person is a good way to demonstrate empathy? Explain.*
3. *If a person voluntarily agrees to "go public" with his or her sad story or medical condition, is it possible to exploit that person? Explain.*

## RECOMMENDED READINGS

Aull F: *The On-Line Database of Literature and Medicine: An Annotated Bibliography.* New York, New York University Medical Center, 1996.

A useful compilation of summaries and annotations of many of the works that have become part of the literature and medicine canon. Includes several indexes—by genre, keywords, ethnicity, gender, and so on—to the literary works. The database is regularly updated and available online at http://mchip00.nyu.edu/lit-med/lit-med-db/literature.html.

Belli A, Coulehan J (eds): *Blood & Bone: Poems by Physicians.* Iowa City, University of Iowa Press, 1998.

An anthology of 100 poems by the best contemporary physician-poets. These poems show the practice of medicine as a poetic act, that of witnessing human suffering, and that this experience cannot be expressed fully in scientific terms.

Downie RS: *The Healing Arts: An Oxford Illustrated Anthology.* Oxford, Oxford University Press, 1995.

An anthology intended to illustrate that there can be tools other than scientific ones for dealing with illness. Downie suggests that such tools and the skills needed for using them can be learned from the arts, and he includes the visual and musical as well as the literary.

Gordon R (ed): *The Literary Companion to Medicine: An Anthology of Prose and Poetry.* New York, St. Martin's Press, 1996.

This compilation consists of 50-plus excerpts, for the most part, of longer works such as *Middlemarch, Madame Bovary,* and *War and Peace.* A compendium of pieces about physicians, and often by physicians.

Reynolds R, Stone J (eds): *On Doctoring: Stories, Poems, Essays.* New York, Simon & Schuster, Inc, 1991.

As the title suggests, stories, poems, and essays, mostly complete, by and about physicians and medical situations. Includes short biographical notes preceding each of the selections and a score of illustrations, reproduced in black and white.

## REFERENCES

Boisaubin E: The impaired physician. *The Chronicle: The Newsletter of the Institute for the Medical Humanities 17*(1):1,5, Spring 1999.
Bulgakov MA: The steel windpipe, in *Diaboliad and Other Stories.* Bloomington, Indiana University Press, 1972.
Burke K: *The Rhetoric of Motives.* Berkeley, University of California Press, 1969.
Camus A: *The Plague.* New York, Modern Library, Inc, 1948.
Cawelti JG: *Adventure, Mystery, and Romance: Formula Stories as Art and Popular Culture.* Chicago, University of Chicago Press, 1976.
Chekhov A: *Ward Number Six and Other Stories.* Oxford, Oxford University Press, 1988.
Doan-Wiggins L, Zun L, Cooper MA, Meyers DL, Chen EH: Practice satisfaction, occupational stress, and attrition of emergency physicians. Wellness Task Force, Illinois College of Emergency Physicians. *Acad Emerg Med* 2(6):556–563, 1995.
Doyle AC: The adventure of the speckled band, in *Sherlock Holmes: The Four Novels and the Fifty-Six Short Stories Complete,* ed 2. New York, Clarkson N Potter, Crown Publishers, 1975.
Eichenwald K, Kolat G: When physicians double as business men. *New York Times,* A1, C16–17, November 30, 1999.
Feldshuh D: Miss Evers' Boys. New York, Dramatists Play Service, Inc, 1995.

Flaubert G: *Madame Bovary*. New York, Modern Library, Inc, 1918.

Ibsen H: *An Enemy of the People*. London, Faber, 1997.

Jones JH: *Bad Blood: The Tuskegee Syphilis Experiment*. New York, Maxwell Macmillan International, 1993.

Jones AH: *The Heroic Physician in Literature: Can the Tradition Continue?* Louisville, KY, American Osler Society, 1994.

Lewis S: *Arrowsmith*. New York, Harcourt, Brace & World, 1952.

Monroe W: *Power to Hurt: The Virtues of Alienation*. Chicago, University of Illinois Press, 1998.

Poe EA: *The Complete Tales and Stories of Edgar Allan Poe*. New York, Random House, Inc, 1975.

Shelley MW: *Frankenstein, or, The Modern Prometheus*. Oxford, Oxford University Press, 1998.

Walton I, Cotton C: *The Compleat Angler*. New York, Scott-Thaw, 1903.

Weiss R: 98,000 Americans die yearly from medical mistakes, report says. *Houston Chronicle*, 2A, November 30, 1999.

Williams WC: *The Doctor Stories*. New York, New Directions Books, 1984.

## CHAPTER 6

# B. Key Skills

# Interviewing as Clinical Conversation

*Kathleen A. Zoppi*

*(Student knocks and enters the examination room)*

STUDENT:   *Hi, Mr. Arredondo?*
PATIENT:   *Yes, that's me.*
STUDENT:   *I'm Vijay Patel, a fourth-year medical student, and I'm working with Doctor Black today. I'm here to do a history and physical. Is that all right with you?*
PATIENT:   *Yes, that's fine.*
STUDENT:   *Good, then, let me sit down and ask you some general questions first. How have you been feeling since you last saw Dr. Black?*

## EDUCATIONAL OBJECTIVES

1. Describe the purposes of clinical conversations
2. List the components of communication that can be observed during the interview, including nonverbal cues, topic offerings, follow-ups, and types of responses
3. Describe ways of observing and altering the process of the interview to improve communication with patients
4. Elicit the basic components of the medical history from patients
5. Describe the similarities and differences between a clinical conversation and social conversation
6. Describe a patient-centered approach to interviewing
7. Identify the advantages of a patient-centered approach for patient health outcomes

## INTRODUCTION

No skill is more crucial to physician effectiveness than the ability to interview patients. The medical interview has been described as the "cornerstone of the diagnostic process" (Stillman & Swanson, 1987). In

Case 6-1, it is clear that in the first few seconds of interaction, the student has both gathered important information about the patient's symptoms and created rapport with the patient, obtaining permission to work with him. These opening interview skills are important, as they facilitate the acquisition of more information later in the interview. Furthermore, Balint (1964) has referred to the physician's skill at interviewing as "the drug 'doctor' "—complete with "undesirable and unwanted side-effects"—indicating the therapeutic value of allowing patients to express fully the problems that are troubling to them and that may or may not be related to the disease. For each patient, the process used to elicit information, arrive at a diagnosis, negotiate treatment, or plan the next visit may be a little different, but knowledge of some common principles about communication with patients will help the physician to effectively interact with each patient.

What makes an interview good? Dr. Gayle Stephens (1994) referred to a good interview as a "clinical conversation," where the goals are to focus on the patient's needs, to improve the patient's health, and to enable the physician to serve as a health consultant to the patient. Physicians and patients probably have different ideas about what makes a "good" interview: Physicians want to get enough information from the patient to accurately understand the patient's illness; patients want to understand why they are ill, whether their illnesses will go away or become worse, and what they can do about their problems. Physicians want to understand the nature of symptoms and the disease that causes them; patients want to understand their illness and suffering, and why it has happened to them. These differences may set up diverging goals for the interview that can cause competition between the patient's and physician's agenda. Part of a good interview is accomplishing a reasonable joint agenda in the amount of time available for the visit.

The quality of the physician–patient interaction also has important consequences for both the clinician and the patient. Physicians who enjoy their interactions with patients are more likely to listen well and to feel more satisfied with their practices (Mechanic, 1992; Suchman *et al.*, 1993). Patients who feel they were able to communicate their problems are more likely to show improvement in symptoms (Greenfield *et al.*, 1985; Headache Study Group of the University of Western Ontario, 1986), are more likely to return to the same physician (Hansson *et al.*, 1988), and are less likely to sue (Lester & Smith, 1993; Levinson *et al.*, 1997). There may be physiological benefits to satisfying interviews for both patients and physicians as well, including lowered blood pressure and heart rate (Lynch, 1985). In addition, patients who communicate effectively with physicians about the nature of the problem and the treatment are more likely to follow a treatment plan (Ley, 1988), which will presumably improve their health and functioning. In particular, the active involvement of patients in creating a plan, called reaching common ground, is key to improved health status (Stewart *et al.*, 2000).

## Comparison between Social Conversations and Clinical Conversations

An important step in having good interaction with patients is keeping a clear understanding about the similarities and differences between clinical and social conversations. *Social conversations* are cooperative ventures, characterized by mutual control and reciprocity. Social conversations can range among many topics and can include many emotions. Both participants expect to disclose information about themselves, and each is expected to display interest and regard for the other's disclosures. The purpose of the social conversation is to enhance a relationship, to make a decision, to engage in a ritual, or to end or close a relationship. Participants in conversation usually ask questions of each other in about equal proportions, they each speak and listen about half the time, and they usually match each other in amount of disclosure, rate of speech, and nonverbal behavior (Cappella, 1994).

Similarly, physicians and patients in *clinical conversations* exert mutual control over the interview and respond to each other's bids and cues. They also may match each other's nonverbal behaviors, such as posture, gesture, rate of speech, volume, and intonation—often unconsciously. However, in contrast to social conversations, there is marked inequity in clinical conversations in terms of who talks and who listens, who discloses personal information, who asks questions, and who raises and closes topics. In clinical conversations, while many of the same cooperative principles apply, it is important to note that the focus of the conversation is on the patient's problem, illness, or concern; the goal of the interaction is to arrive at some resolution of the concern, or a plan to treat it; the physician does not disclose as much as the patient and is more likely to talk longer and to ask more questions than the patient. These differences, in addition to the patient's potential physical and psychological dependence on the physician for technical advice and understanding because of illness, fear, or incapacity, are what distinguish clinical conversations from social conversations.

<hr>

## CASE 6-2

*Tom, a third-year medical student, is in the ambulatory clinic. It is his first day of seeing patients. He picks up the chart from the door, on which the nurse has written that the patient is there because of a "sore throat." The data sheet indicates that the patient is a 19-year-old male college student. His temperature and blood pressure are normal. Tom knocks on the door and enters the room.*

DOCTOR: *(Standing) Hello, Matthew.*
PATIENT: *(Seated on examination table) Hi.*
DOCTOR: *(Still standing) I see you have a sore throat today. How long have you had it?*
PATIENT: *A few days.*
DOCTOR: *Have you had a fever or chills?*
PATIENT: *(Not making eye contact) No.*
DOCTOR: *Any drainage in the back of your throat?*
PATIENT: *No.*
DOCTOR: *You haven't been coughing then?*
PATIENT: *(Squirming on the table) No.*
DOCTOR: *(Reaching for a tongue depressor) Let's take a look then....*
*Elapsed time = 17.78 seconds*

# FUNDAMENTAL INTERVIEW SKILLS

## How the Interview Should Be Started

In our culture, greetings and introductions are ritualized exchanges: People say hello and introduce themselves, usually shaking hands and gauging their physical distance prior to sitting down and beginning to talk about anything more important. Physicians can and should use many of the same social rituals in an encounter with a patient to help set a comfortable pace and tone to the conversation. In most nonemergency situations, clinical conversations are similar to social conversations. The clinician would greet the patient, introduce herself, and invite the patient to sit comfortably while speaking. The provider might also begin a brief social conversation, for example, about the weather, or sport, or some current event, prior to the real "medical business" at hand. When no social exchange occurs, interviews can get off to a difficult start, as in Case 6-2.

Instead, ideally, an interviewer would acknowledge the patient's identified reason for the visit (the sore throat), but would seek to establish a relationship early in the visit and would allow the patient to identify any other concerns early in the conversation. Both the patient and physician would make themselves comfortable, both socially and physically, before beginning the business of the encounter. Notice the differences between the previous interaction and the following:

DOCTOR: Hello, I'm Tom, a third-year medical student working with Dr. Smith today. What do you prefer to be called?
PATIENT: (Seated in chair) My name is Matthew, but I like to be called Matt.
DOCTOR: (Extends hand for a handshake) Nice to meet you, Matt.

PATIENT:   (Shakes hand, makes eye contact) Nice to meet you, too.

DOCTOR:   (Sitting on stool and placing chart on desk) What would you like to tell me about yourself?

PATIENT:   Well, I'm here because I've got a big basketball game this Friday night, and my coach is worried I won't be able to play. I've been pretty tired and rundown for a couple of weeks, and now I've got a bad sore throat. I'm a starter, and this is the last game before the playoffs, and I'm really worried I won't be able to play the whole game.

Elapsed time = 31.97 seconds

What differences exist between the initial parts of these two interviews? The initial part of the second interview, which lasted about 10 seconds longer than the first, helped Tom know what the patient prefers to be called, that he's pretty concerned about being ill and potentially missing a game, that he's been sick for a few weeks, and that he only recently developed a sore throat. In comparing the two approaches to the interview with Matt, also notice that there are a number of directions each interviewer could proceed after the initial part. With the additional information acquired in the second interview, the physician might think about anemia, infectious mononucleosis, HIV infection, or cardiomyopathies, rather than centering on the more common cause of sore throat in teenagers, viral pharyngitis and "strep throat."

## How to Hear What the Patient Says and Listen to the Meaning

In the two versions of the interview in Case 6-2, the difference between the physical act of hearing and perceptive listening is obvious. The first interviewer physically heard the patient's complaint. He has a sore throat. But did Tom know why Matt was there? What was his actual reason for coming? Do healthy people usually go to a physician after having a sore throat for a few days? Why did he come today, rather than yesterday or tomorrow? Was it just the first time he could get an appointment? Why does Matt's reason for being there matter? Does it affect the treatment plan or recommendations?

In the second version of the interview, it is clear that Matt's concern is not just about having a sore throat, but about how it might affect his ability to play in an important basketball game. He is also quite concerned about his stamina, and his coach is worried, too. It is possible that an interviewer could ask a number of questions that would help uncover these concerns, including "Who else is worried about your illness?" and "Are you having any other problems or symptoms?" The simple act of listening and not interrupting the patient early in the interview results in relatively more data about the problem, with less additional work on the part of the interviewer.

In fact, an interview style that assumes that patients have concerns beyond the chief complaint, sometimes not related directly to symptoms, has been termed a *patient-centered approach*. Patient-centered interviewing involved elicitation of both the symptoms and the patient's perceptions about illness (What does the patient believe is causing the illness? What kinds of worries or concerns does the patient have about the illness?) and patient preferences about treatment. This kind of approach relies on several key interview skills: The physician facilitates the early and complete expression of the patient's problem, uses cues and clues from the patient's behavior to identify other concerns or expressions of feeling about the problem, and asks the patient for preferences regarding follow-up or treatment. Patient-centered care respects the values and preferences of the patient in the course of delivering skillful medical care. It has been linked to improved outcomes of care, including higher patient satisfaction, greater reduction of patient distress, and improved health status.

Good perceptive listening by the physician is one of the most elusive and sought-after skills, and is possibly the best psychotherapeutic tool in a physician's repertoire. But true listening, without interruption, is a rare occurrence in the first few minutes of the interview. A study of 74 visits to an internal medicine clinic demonstrated that in 69% of visits, physicians interrupted patients after the mention of only one concern, within an average time to interruption of 18 seconds. In instances when patients were allowed to complete their thoughts, the average time they spoke was about 1.5 minutes (Beckman & Frankel, 1984). When this study was replicated recently, the average interruption was at 23 seconds (Marvel *et al.*, 1999), and interruptions were associated with patients disclosing their concerns late in the interview, often prolonging it.

## LISTENING CAREFULLY

*Active listening is a skill that requires constant attention, simultaneously, to what is expressed by the other person (verbally, nonverbally), to what is not said, and to your own reactions and responses to the interaction. In a medical interview this may require more focused energy than a more passive, conventional way we tend to listen in social situations. If a friend were telling you about a problem, and you were really concerned about understanding what was wrong, you might listen more actively, with greater attention to the words and mannerisms of the person, fewer questions or changes of topic, and a greater focus on the key expressions the person shared.*

It is often difficult to listen if patients seem confused, vague, or unnecessarily descriptive in their use of language. The interviewer may feel confused, bored, impatient, or angry. "It is important to remember that the emotional reactions of the clinician during the interview may be as important a cue about the patient as what is said. Attention to the cues and clues patients offer is key to good patient-centered interviewing: patients may repeat phrases, look particularly distressed, or even ask questions that indicate their true (underlying) assumptions about their illness" (Lang *et al.*, 2000). Often, what the physician feels while listening perceptively is similar to the unspoken feelings of the patient. If the physician feels sad, it may be that the patient also feels sad. One of the great advantages of having clinical conversations while a medical student is that a student is often better at listening than is a physician later in training. Patients will often share important information with students they will not tell their physicians, simply because students are better listeners.

## How to Define the Medical Student's Role

One of the most difficult aspects of interviewing patients during medical school is the ambiguous role the student has in delivering care. While a medical student is part of a healthcare team, her role is also that of a learner. The team may value input about the patient and may include what is told to them by the student in her notes and treatment plan. Unfortunately, medical student input is often not asked for or disregarded if it is offered. A student may, as indicated earlier, hear information from the patient or the family that others do not know and that is important to the patient's treatment. Students may witness treatment of patients that they perceive to be inappropriate or insensitive. And during all of these interactions, the student may be treated by

## ATTENDING TO CUES AND CLUES (Lang *et al.*, 2000)

*Research on patients who tell physicians their concerns has indicated a few types of cues and clues that might indicate patients have additional worries or symptoms they haven't yet identified to you. They include:*
- *Repetition of words or phrases*
- *Presence of other people (if not usual)*
- *Stories, especially about someone else's illness*
- *Offering hypotheses*
- *Additional symptoms, whether they appear to be associated or not*
- *Speech dysfluencies (hesitations, pauses)*
- *Slow response to questions*

*Example: Early in the interview, patient says, "I really, really want to get rid of this pain before things get busy at work." Patient later says, "Work is really going to get busy." A simple follow-up question, "Tell me more about what's going on at work," would likely yield important clues to the patient's concerns.*

## MALPRACTICE AND COMMUNICATION (Levinson *et al.*, 1997)

*The threat of malpractice is pretty frightening to a medical student, or any physician! In the clinical practice of medicine, it is impossible to get it right every time, and many students fear that any error can result in malpractice suits. It is important to know that communication with patients may be a more powerful predictor of malpractice suits than the actual commission of errors. In a study of over 1000 interactions between patients and physicians, it was found that no-claims physicians in primary care were more likely to educate patients, to facilitate patients' questions, and to laugh and use humor more.*

the patient as the person who is responsible for the treatment plan. Patients may address the student as "Doctor," while the student feels she is still a learner, trying to integrate a great deal of information into organized clinical skills.

Adhering to a few simple rules should help students meet these challenges. Students should always identify themselves truthfully as medical students when they begin to talk with patients. If the student is practicing interviewing and is not having a clinical conversation as part of the patient's team, that should be stated explicitly. If a patient asks a student not to tell his physician something, the student should identify herself as obligated to talk with the physician about it, but encourage the patient to tell the physician on his own. The student may also ask the attending physician or resident how he wishes to be informed of what was learned from the patient. It is often the case that the student may learn crucial information, and the patient may benefit from its inclusion in the treatment plan.

### CASE 6-3

*Nancy, a second-year student, is on rounds with the family practice attending physician and a resident. The team is seeing Nellie Hatter, a 65-year-old woman who is lying across her bed at an angle when they enter the room. She greets the team "Hello, doctors!" and is smiling. Nellie's attending physician begins to ask her how she slept, and whether she is comfortable.*

DOCTOR:    *Did you have a good night last night?*
PATIENT:    *Yes, I slept just fine. I feel much better than last night.*
DOCTOR:    *You were in bad shape when you came in. Your blood sugar was over 600 when we saw you in the emergency room. Why do you think that happened?*
PATIENT:    *I don't know. My husband gives me my medication every morning before I eat. I'm sure I had it yesterday. Maybe it's due to stress ...*

### DEFINING YOUR ROLE TO THE PATIENT

*In the course of the interview with the patient, you will introduce yourself and set expectations about your role as part of the medical team. Sometimes patients don't understand differences among students, residents, or other caregivers. So tell the patient explicitly who you are and why you are there:*
    *"Hi, I'm Martha Jones, a second-year medical student, and I'm working with Dr. Bluefield. He has asked me to come talk with you about what's bothering you, as part of my training in working with patients. Are you willing to talk with me? I won't be taking care of you all the time; this is for my education."*

In interviewing this patient, how is it decided what to ask next? Questions could be asked about the patient's insulin dosage, and how her husband remembers to give her the shot:

**DOCTOR:**    Could be. Does your husband give you the shot at the same time every morning?

This line of questioning would help determine if the patient is receiving her medication. These questions might also yield some information about their relationship, about the husband's memory, and about her dependence on him for her care. The provider could also pick up her lead about what she thinks caused her blood sugar to be high:

**DOCTOR:**    Stress? Why do you think this could be due to stress?

This question might cause the patient to think her "theory" about stress was subject to scrutiny, and not valid. A similar, yet simpler, approach to following the patient's lead would be:

**DOCTOR:**    Stress? Tell me more about your stress.
**PATIENT:**    Well, yesterday, my son and daughter-in-law and I had some words … they live in the downstairs of our house. She's a nurse, and she and my son moved in last year when he lost his job in California. I'm a Jehovah's Witness, and don't like her drinking and smoking.

Simple repetition of the patient's last words can often be an encouraging response to help the patient continue with a particular train of thought. In this case, following the patient's lead resulted in a clearer understanding of what the patient believed affected her blood sugar, as well as some potential resources or impediments to her follow-up care after discharge from the hospital. This information did not directly exclude other causes of

---

## FUNNELING VERSUS FOLLOWING THE PATIENT'S DIRECTION

*Students might think about how the asking of specific questions, one following another, is a way of obtaining increasingly precise information. Funneling is a technique used to obtain, through successive iterations, more detailed data from a respondent in an interview.*

*Example:*

  **STUDENT:**    *So the pain started yesterday?*
  **PATIENT:**    *Yes, about 2 o'clock*
  **STUDENT:**    *Was it sharp or dull?*
  **PATIENT:**    *Sharp, like a knife.*
  **STUDENT:**    *Was it continuous or intermittent?*
  **PATIENT:**    *It started and stopped.*
  **STUDENT:**    *What made it stop?*

*A probe can sometimes accomplish the same goal in a less directed, interrogation-like approach:*

*Example:*

  **PATIENT:**    *… so after lunch, I felt this pain in my side, like a sharp knife.*
  **STUDENT:**    *You say it felt like a sharp knife. Tell me more about what that felt like …*
  **PATIENT:**    *It just felt like someone was sticking a hot knife into my side, and then it went away after a few minutes …*

*Notice that in each case, the same data are gained; in the second example, the patient actually offers additional (potentially relevant) data about the sensation of heat, not obtained using the funnel.*

*Funnel questioning is useful when respondents are not forthcoming, or unable to respond to open-ended questions.*

her high blood sugar, e.g., infection or a skipped dose of insulin, but did give additional information not available through the first approach of questioning.

## How a Physician Should Respond to Patients' Expressions of Feelings

In Case 6-3, the patient gave a clue that she was concerned about the effects of stress on her health. Though she did not appear upset—she was smiling and said she rested well—she did offer what she was thinking on why she had become ill. A wise conversationalist, whether in a social or clinical interaction, will attend to the other person's last remark before changing the subject. For this patient, her worries about her family may have contributed to her physical illness and admission, and may even seem more troubling to her than her hospitalization.

Patients often do not express their feelings directly, even when they are quite distressed. It is important to notice what patients do not say, as well as what they do say. In Case 6-2, when Tom talked with Matt, he might have noticed that Matt looked flushed and avoided eye contact when asked what was wrong. As he reached for a tongue depressor, Tom might have even tried to have some cheery conversation about the local professional team's latest basketball win, and might have noticed that Matt seemed withdrawn or sullen. It is sometimes a useful strategy to observe nonverbal cues or facial expressions and to comment on them directly:

TOM:     I notice that you aren't talking too much and that you look uncomfortable when I ask you questions …

Sometimes such direct observation or reflection can help the patient identify feelings and trust that the physician is willing to hear more about what is of concern. Occasionally, patients will surprise physicians with strong feelings or expressions about their illnesses, their families, or other physicians. It may take the provider aback to have such an intimate or powerful statement made when questions have barely been asked of the patient at all. And yet, the powerful role of the physician/healer can evoke strong confidences. Sometimes just listening to a patient's expression about her worries, without intervening, and without judging, can be more difficult than "doing," and infinitely more valuable to the patient. The student's own emotional response to a patient's feelings can also be a useful clue about what's going on with the patient (Epstein, 1999).

## How Timing and Pacing Can Be Gauged

Medical lore places a value on quick, efficient, concise interviews that lead to an accurate diagnosis. However, few of *your* conversations with patients will (initially) feel quick and efficient. One of the important arts of the interview involves the rhythm of the interview, the timing and pacing of the patient's speech, the pauses and silences, the changes of topic, the nonverbal communication, the physical examination, the social conversation, and the farewells. The physician often inadvertently matches the natural rate of speech and movement of the patient, and sometimes wishes the patient would slow down or speed up. It is clear that people in ordinary conversations match their speech and movements to each other more and more as the conversation progresses, but it is often useful to deliberately pay attention to, and try not to match the patient's rate of speech, gestures, or movements. If a patient seems anxious, it may be useful to slow down and see if this also slows the patient's speech. If it does not affect the patient, this failure to change may be useful diagnostic information. If a patient seems very sad, speaking slowly and painfully quietly, it may be inappropriate to overcompensate by smiling, telling jokes, and talking quickly, but it may be useful to change the rate and tone to see if the patient's affect changes when talking about something happy or enjoyable.

It is critical as an interviewer to become familiar with, and aware of, one's own predisposition as a speaker. A provider from a family of fast-talking, interrupting, simultaneous speakers may overwhelm patients whose natural speech patterns require that they wait several seconds after the physician is done speaking before beginning to speak themselves. No one speech pattern is necessarily better or worse than others, but awareness of when style is a catalyst and when it is a barrier to good interaction is integral to the development of a clinical conversationalist.

# What to Do Next

One of the hardest developmental tasks of the clinical conversationalist is to structure the interaction, maybe by using a checklist of questions (such as a review of systems checklist) while trying to maintain a normal conversational flow and paying attention to the patient's cues. It is normal to feel torn between these two tasks, and there is no easy solution to the dilemma. The useful principle to remember is equifinality: There are many ways to get there from here! Studies of medical interviewing have shown that highly focused short interviews can be just as effective in gathering information and creating patient well-being as longer, more rambling interviews. The key principles for effective interviews that collect pertinent information and satisfy concerned patients are: they allow patients time to express their worries, fears, or needs; they seem relaxed and unhurried, even if they are not actually very long; they enable patients to express, either verbally or nonverbally, some emotions; they enable physicians to respond to the emotions expressed by patients; and they enable patients to leave the interview knowing more about what's wrong and what to do about it than at the start. In addition to gathering sufficient information about the present illness and past medical history, these are the key ingredients to a good clinical conversation. Each patient's clinical presentation will dictate whether asking a few questions and moving to a physical examination, or talking for a while and rescheduling the physical, is the better approach.

## How the Physical Examination Is Navigated

The physical examination, and the ritual laying on of hands, is one of the primary defining features that distinguishes the clinical conversation from other professional encounters. Touch, outside of a handshake or a shoulder pat on closing, is unlikely to occur with a minister, lawyer, or accountant, whereas touching by the physician of the patient during an examination is an integral part of the visit. Apart from the diagnostic acumen required to distinguish among heart and lung sounds or to palpate and feel physical changes in organs and muscles, the physical examination is a socially challenging experience for both patient and physician. It is useful to make some social gesture to establish contact, such as a handshake, prior to the nonreciprocal touch of the physical examination. It may also be useful for the physician to assist the patient in being seated and getting comfortable for the physical examination, if the patient is elderly or needs such help. The physical examination should be described and prefaced for the patient, not just done to the patient. This might involve the physician saying, "And now I'm going to listen to your heart and lungs...." And physical findings should be described to the patient, who otherwise may misinterpret a squint and silence as cues that something in the breath sounds is horribly wrong. "Your heart and breathing sound perfectly normal." Such feedback is probably better than attempting to distract the patient with social small talk, especially if the patient is anxious. However, if one begins to offer evaluative feedback during the examination and then stops, this may offer the patient an opportunity for the patient to assume that something is wrong as well (Heritage, in Heritage & Maynard, in press). Thus, students are encouraged to think carefully before speaking while examining the patient. During the physical examination it may be a good time to ask further questions related to the area of the examination, however, since patients may more easily recall symptoms when being touched (e.g., while palpating the abdomen, asking "So you said you have this pain every morning?"). The physical examination should be focused on the systems/regions related to the patient's concerns, unless a full history and physical is being completed (see Chapter 8 on the physical examination).

## How the Agenda Can Be Better Managed

Patients often come to the physician with many concerns, which may not be of equal importance. A patient who is concerned about his teenaged daughter, his earache, and the pain in his chest might prioritize what he wants to discuss differently than the physician. He may spend time initially discussing his daughter, whereas the physician may want to focus initially on the chest pain as the most ominous symptom. In this case, a useful skill to practice is the overt identification of priorities. The physician may wish to state clearly that there is a limited amount of time, e.g., 20 minutes, and her desire to know the patient's greatest concern. Planning for a return visit within a short period of time to finish what could not be completed today may be important, as may agreeing with the patient about what can be postponed. This kind of negotiation over the agenda is similar to the negotiation of a plan but may initially seem more difficult because it requires stepping back from the interaction to notice what needs to be discussed.

## Why Discussing the Diagnosis Is Important

Once the physical examination is completed and the history is taken, the physician may recognize the need for more data to confirm her thinking. This may require that some lab test be performed, which may be as simple as a blood test, or may be more extensive and invasive testing. While being uncertain about a diagnosis and gathering more evidence may be routine work for the physician-scientist, such uncertainty may contribute greatly to the patient's anxiety. Tests and procedures are seldom routine for patients, and each one may require a different amount of explanation. It may, for example, be common for patients to have their blood drawn, but to have an MRI or a CT scan can be very frightening. It is important for the physician to help prepare the patient for what she can expect from the experience so the patient will come to the test or procedure less anxious and more cooperative. It is also useful to explain to patients what data the tests may offer, and how the results will contribute to the physician's thinking about what is wrong, and when it may be possible to make a diagnosis about the patient's condition.

---

### CASE 6-4

*Dr. Moyer is a first-year family practice resident. Her patient, Albert Fuller, is ready to go home from the hospital. He is a 66-year-old male who was admitted for treatment of blood clots in his left leg. Dr. Moyer's chief resident planned to send him home on anticoagulants, with a home health nurse scheduled to draw blood weekly to check his clotting. The chief resident just received a page from the social worker, saying Mr. Fuller has refused to take his prescription, and he doesn't want a nurse visiting him at home. The resident asks Dr. Moyer to go to the floor to find out what the problem is.*

---

## How a Treatment Plan Should Be Discussed

Construction of a treatment plan and negotiating that plan with patients will be discussed in detail in Chapter 11, but in Case 6-4, it would be useful to know a few pieces of information. It would be helpful to know from Mr. Fuller what he thought was wrong with him, and how he thought it might best be treated. If he thinks that his leg was swollen because he bumped it, and it's better now, he won't be likely to accept a long-term treatment plan. It would also be useful to know when and how the resident discussed the plan for discharge with Mr. Fuller, and with any relevant family or friends. Asking Mr. Fuller what his understanding was of what was to happen after he left the hospital and what he or others thought about the plan may also help. Verifying Mr. Fuller's understanding and correcting any misunderstandings are always useful. If, in fact, he disagrees with the resident's plan, it is possible to start negotiating knowing what Mr. Fuller has in mind, and by listening carefully to him, Dr. Moyer may be able to negotiate a plan that meets both Mr. Fuller's health needs and his provider's concerns.

## How the Interview Should Be Closed: Planning for the Next Visit

Most interviews will end naturally with the physician and patient finalizing plans for follow-up and treatment. Ask the patient to review, either by repetition or by acknowledgment, the plans for medications, tests, follow-up visits, or treatments. Ask the patient if there are questions or unfinished business before beginning to stand up, closing the chart, or saying good-bye. It is not uncommon for patients to present "doorknob" agendas: When the physician's hand is on the doorknob, ready to exit, patients may have one or more important unresolved concerns that they want to discuss. This pattern can best be averted by asking patients early in the visit about any other concerns, prior to setting the agenda for the day's visit; sometimes even this careful checking will not prevent a last-minute concern. "Doorknob" concerns may be important enough to warrant reopening the discussion, such as with a patient who says she's had trouble breathing the past few days. On the other hand, it may be possible to discuss the problem at an upcoming visit. If the problem can be postponed until the next visit, it is still important for the clinician to acknowledge the patient's concern, while not completely resolving it.

Say good-bye to patients in a way that allows them to return with a sense that the conversation has been important. Assure them of how they can contact you in case of an emergency, and touch or shake hands prior to departing.

## CONCLUSION

This chapter described the important behaviors of interviewers who are engaging in a clinical conversation with patients. Key behaviors were reviewed, including greeting the patient, attending to the patient's comfort, attending to the patient's chief concern, completing the parts of the medical history and physical examination, and closing the interview. The importance of a patient-centered approach, attending to the patient's words, affect, and nonverbal cues, was stressed. Patient-centered interviewing, especially working with patients toward common ground about treatment, results in improved patient satisfaction and health.

The importance of key components of the physician–patient relationship such as empathy, responsiveness to feelings, shared control, and timing and pacing was also reviewed. Social and clinical conversations were contrasted. Research on the development of interviewing skills indicates that, like any physical examination skills, they require rehearsal and practice. Practice may involve role-playing or interviewing with friends or, better still, taping (either audio or video) encounters with actual patients and reviewing those tapes to observe what you do well and what might need improvement.

## CASES FOR DISCUSSION

### CASE 1

*A patient comes to the family practice center. The nurse has written on the chart note that she is there for a sinus infection. You enter the room, seeing a well-dressed woman in a suit. You greet her, introduce yourself, and ask her how she is. She begins to cry.*

1. *What could you do or say next?*
2. *If the physician says, "What's wrong?" and the patient responds, "Never mind. I'm here for sore throat," how should the physician proceed?*
3. *Should the physician proceed to ask the patient about her sinus symptoms?*

### CASE 2

*You are running late in your afternoon on the ward, and you receive a new admission. Your resident tells you to interview the patient; you begin to go to the room. Before you get there, the nurse for the unit grabs your sleeve, rolls his eyes, and says, "This one is a real doozy. You have no idea what a problem he will be. He's already made two of the nursing students angry."*

1. *What would be the best strategy for beginning this clinical conversation?*
2. *Why should you be especially aware of any feelings you experience on talking to the patient?*
3. *Assuming this patient talks rapidly and loudly, why would you want to use a matching style? A complementary style?*

## CASE 3

*You are a medical student on the family medicine service. You enter a room to take a history of a patient who was just admitted. He is lying in bed, with his gown high above his waist, no underwear on, and no covers.*

1. *What do you say first?*
2. *How would your clinical conversation differ from social conversation under some circumstances?*
3. *How could you let the patient know, without shaming or embarrassing him, that you need him to respect you during the interview?*

## CASE 4

*You are in the clinic and your next patient is a 13-year-old boy who is accompanied by his mother. The reason for the visit is the boy has been having trouble sleeping. When you ask him why, he explains that he often wakes in the middle of the night and screams, sweating and flushed. Usually, his parents come to get him, and he sleeps the rest of the night with them. His mother reports that this has been happening more frequently lately, especially since she was told she needed surgery on her shoulder.*

1. *What do you ask next in order to understand what is happening to this boy?*
2. *Given that a 13-year-old boy is not the world's best conversationalist, under what conditions would you want to interrupt him? Let him talk?*
3. *How would you prepare the boy (and mother) for physical examination behavior during this encounter?*

## CASE 5

*You are in the family practice center, and interviewing a new patient. She is a 35-year-old mother of three. She seems happy and relaxed as you talk but when you begin to ask her about her marriage, she avoids eye contact and gives shorter answers.*

1. *What reasons might a patient begin to change her demeanor?*
2. *How might you reflect to your patient your observation that her affect and eye contact changed?*
3. *The patient responds to your conversation by saying, "I'm fine. My marriage is fine." What hypotheses might you hold in mind for future visits?*

# RECOMMENDED READINGS

Balint M: *The Doctor, His Patient, and the Illness*. New York, International Universities Press Inc, 1964.

Balint was a British psychoanalyst who worked with general practitioners on their feelings about their patients. In this classic work, he describes the relationship between the patient and the physician as a potential source of healing, comparing the physician's style of interaction to a drug, implying that the interview style is just as therapeutic as the medication prescribed.

Billings JA, Stoeckle JD: *The Clinical Encounter*, ed 2. Chicago, Year Book Medical Publishers Inc, 1999.

This is one of the most comprehensive and thorough references on the medical interview. The chapter on "Eliciting Information for Diagnosis and Management" is a compendium of questions and approaches to the basic history and physical, and offers an excellent range of options for students and residents who desire examples.

Meador C: *A Little Book of Doctor's Rules*. Philadelphia, Hanley & Belfus, 1992.

A delightful compendium of aphorisms distilled from Dr. Meador's own clinical practice. He offers key rules for working with patients that are useful for students and experienced clinicians alike.

# REFERENCES

Balint M: *The Doctor, His Patient, and the Illness*, ed 2. New York, International Universities Press Inc, 1964.
Beckman H, Frankel R: The effect of physician behavior on the collection of data. *Ann Intern Med* 101:692–696, 1984.

Cappella JN: The management of conversational interaction in adults and infants, in Knapp JL, Miller GR (eds): *Handbook of Interpersonal Communication*, ed 2. Beverly Hills, Calif, Sage Publications, 1994, pp 380–418.

Epstein RM: Mindful practice. *JAMA* 282(9):833–839, 1999.

Greenfield S, Kaplan S, Ware J: Expanding patient involvement in care. *Ann Intern Med* 102:520–528, 1985.

Hansson R, Remondet JH, Obrochta D, Bell L: The dissatisfied medical patient: Predictors of intent to change doctors. *Med Times*, pp 97–101, 1988.

Headache Study Group of the University of Western Ontario. Predictors of outcome in headache patients presenting to family physicians. *Headache* 26:285–294, 1986.

Heritage J, Maynard DW: Practicing medicine: Talk and action in primary care encounters. Cambridge, Cambridge University Press (in press.)

Lang F, Beine K, Floyd M: Clus to patients' explanations and concerns about their illness. *Arch Fam Med* 9(3):222–227, 2000.

Lester G, Smith S: Listening and talking to patients: A remedy for malpractice suits. *West J Med* 158:268–272, 1993.

Levinson W, Roter DL, Mullooly JP, Dull VT, Frankel RM: Physician–patient communication: The relationship with malpractice claims among primary care physicians and surgeons. *JAMA* 277(7):553–559, 1997.

Ley P: *Communicating with Patients*. London, Croom Helm Ltd, 1988.

Lynch J: *The Language of the Heart*. New York, Basic Books Inc, 1985.

Marvel MK, Epstein RM, Flowers K, Beckman HB: Soliciting the patients' agenda: Have we improved? *JAMA* 281(3):283–287, 1999.

Mechanic D: Health and illness behavior and patient practitioner relationship. *Soc Sci Med* 34(12):1345–1350, 1992.

Stephens G: A family doctor's rules for clinical conversations. *J Am Board Fam Pract* 7:179–181, 1994.

Stewart M, *et al*: The impact of patient-centered care on patient outcomes. *J Fam Pract* 49(9):796–804, 2000.

Stillman PL, Swanson DB: Ensuring the clinical competence of medical school graduates through standardized patients. *Arch Intern Med* 147(6):1049–1052, 1987.

Suchman A, Roter D, Green M, Hepkin M, and The Collaborative Study Group of the AAPP. Patient satisfaction with primary care office visits. *Med Care* 31(10):83–92, 1993.

# Taking a History

*Elizabeth Steiner*

*Mrs. Melinda Harrison, a 54-year-old woman, has just moved to this area. She comes to the office of Dr. Sarah Johnson to establish care and for a "complete physical." Dr. Johnson knocks, enters the room, and addresses the patient.*

DR. JOHNSON:    *Good afternoon, Mrs. Harrison. Welcome to our practice. I'm looking forward to getting to know you.*

MRS. HARRISON:    *Hello, Dr. Johnson. I'm so concerned about so many things. I hope you'll have time to talk to me about all of them.*

DR. JOHNSON:    *I'm glad you told me that you have several concerns. We'll do our best to address them during this visit and other visits if necessary.*

MRS. HARRISON:    *Oh good!*

DR. JOHNSON:    *Today we'll start by taking a complete history so I can learn all about you. First, I'd like to know more about your concerns. Tell me about them.*

MRS. HARRISON:    *Well, of course I'm having a terrible time with hot flashes …*

## EDUCATIONAL OBJECTIVES

1. Discuss interviewing techniques that facilitate history taking
2. Detail the components of a complete history
3. Describe a patient's pain complaint in an organized and concise fashion
4. State the difference between a complete history and a problem-focused history
5. Address issues of special situations: children, adolescents, pregnant women, the elderly, the mentally disabled

## INTRODUCTION

Taking a history, whether that of a new patient or of an established patient with a new problem, is the physician's first and perhaps the most revealing step in the diagnostic process. Understanding the skills

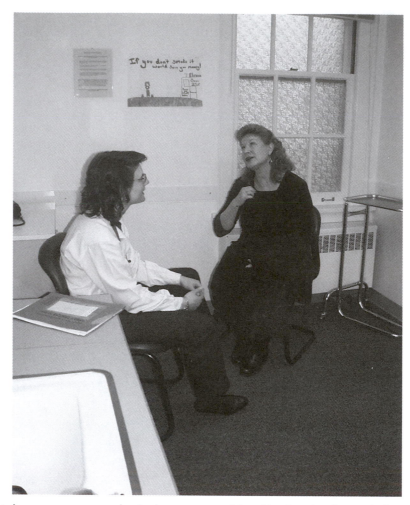

**Case 7-1.** Dr. Johnson uses open body language as Mrs. Harrison's physical discomfort becomes evident.

required during a clinical conversation (Chapter 6) is indispensable; equally important is the physicians' awareness of what they need to learn about patients to help them improve their health.

At a time in medical history when diagnostic techniques based on laboratory assays are increasingly available, physicians can understandably challenge the significance of the medical history. Sometimes patients forget what they know; they may misreport; they may even conceal important elements while revealing matters that seem only tangential to their health. How reliable, how useful are their histories?

In fact, a well-designed medical history provides a solid foundation for all subsequent diagnostic and treatment decisions. Patients are whole human beings; illness or health affects the totality of their bodies and emotions. By listening carefully to patients' versions of their medical and surgical histories, their social and family histories, their accounts of work and leisure, physicians can learn a great deal about the specific circumstances that have brought them to the office. Physicians need to hear the unspoken assumptions or fears that lie beneath the patients' comments; they need also to be able to read their patients' gestures and body language. Listening skills must be combined with speaking skills; physicians need to know how to ask and restate questions, how to follow up on answers to those questions, and how and when to press patients to give fuller or more explicit answers.

Since patients are not the same, no single technique of taking a medical history will fit all situations. Yet the necessary information can be elicited and recorded in a systematic way, so that the passage of time between one medical visit and the next will not erode the physicians' understanding of their patients. Also, physicians do not practice in a vacuum; their colleagues, nurses, and other health professionals need to understand the patient as well. A complete history will help the medical team coordinate its treatment, and help patients continue the treatment once the physician discharges them. Such a history will allow physicians to note changes in patients' health, and to act early to forestall medical difficulties.

As many chapters in this volume point out, the skills that physicians need are developed through a lifetime of practice. What may seem excessively formal at first will become natural and easy as physicians interact with infants and the elderly, with those who are stable, those who are disturbed, and those who are angry, despondent, fearful, or uncomprehending. Each interview with a patient teaches physicians more about the patient and about themselves as physicians. This chapter will help begin the process of taking useful and dependable medical histories.

## INTERVIEWING SKILLS

The previous chapter gives excellent examples of the medical interview as a clinical conversation, and points out strengths of good interviewing technique and weaknesses related to poor technique. In this section, we will discuss some of the more concrete aspects of interviewing, including open versus closed questions, body language, seating arrangements, normalizing language, and putting patients at ease.

As noted in Chapter 6, practitioners (physicians or students) must introduce themselves, and must ensure that patients are addressed in the way they are most comfortable. Generally speaking, it is always safer to take a more formal approach with adult patients, using their surnames until invited to address them by their given names. With children, one must take care to learn if they have a preferred nickname, and conversely, not assume that longer names are automatically shortened to a common nickname.

In the vast majority of situations, the open-ended question yields more information and more patient satisfaction than the closed-ended (yes/no answer) question. In addition, open-ended questions do not necessarily add time to the interview. Consider the following scenarios. In each case, Jane, a fourth-year medical student, is taking a history from Alan, a 20-year-old male with abdominal pain.

| | |
|---|---|
| JANE: | Alan, do you have pain in your abdomen? |
| ALAN: | Yes. |
| JANE: | Can you show me where it is? |
| ALAN: | (pointing to his right lower quadrant) It's right here. |
| JANE: | Did it start there, or somewhere else? |
| ALAN: | It started around my belly button, and moved there. |
| JANE: | Did it start today? |
| ALAN: | No, yesterday evening … |

Time elapsed: 18 seconds

Or …

| | |
|---|---|
| JANE: | Alan, tell me about your pain. |
| ALAN: | Well, it started yesterday evening with some nausea, and discomfort around my belly button. By this morning, it was more like pain down here (pointing to his right lower quadrant). |

Time elapsed: 10 seconds

In the second scenario, Jane got more information, in less time, and Alan felt more in control of the interview process, which increases his satisfaction with the encounter. There are clearly circumstances in which the closed-ended question is useful, and these will be considered later in the chapter.

## CASE 7-2

*Dr. White is talking with Sandra, a 15-year-old patient who complains of generalized fatigue.*

SANDRA: *I don't know, some days I just feel as if I don't have anything good in my life. I'm just tired and miserable all the time.*

DR. WHITE: *You know, people who feel that way sometimes think about hurting themselves. Have you had any such thoughts?*

SANDRA: *Well, sometimes I wonder what would happen if I took a bunch of pills.*

Normalizing language, as illustrated by Dr. White in Case 7-2, allows the physician to ask potentially difficult or embarrassing questions in a way that puts the patient more at ease, and increases the likelihood that the patient will give an honest response. In Case 7 - 2, Dr. White uses normalizing language to elicit Sandra's thoughts of self-harm. Sandra may have been too embarrassed to answer honestly if Dr. White had asked, "So, are you thinking about killing yourself?" instead.

Finally, the physician's body language, seating arrangements, and the patient's level of undress will all affect the effectiveness of the history taking process. Physicians should maintain open body language, and if possible, should take a history sitting at the same level as the patient. The dynamic between patient and physician alters significantly if the patient is already in a gown, on the exam table, before the history is taken. Ideally, the patient should be sitting in a chair, with street clothes on, when the physician enters the room to take the history.

## THE COMPLETE HISTORY

When a patient presents for a complete history and physical examination, or is admitted to the hospital for almost any reason, the most important task is taking a thorough history. As previously discussed, how you take the history can set the stage for all future interactions with the patient, and can often mean the difference between appropriate care and delayed care. In this section we will review the details of a complete history, along with mnemonics that can help you remember some of the many important pieces of a complete history. Developing a systematic way of taking a history will ensure that you do not forget to cover any part.

Over the years, physicians have developed a standard order for the complete history, and this is the order we will use here. While at times it may seem restrictive to use a standard format, doing so allows the reader to follow the history easily, and enhances communication among health care providers. Every written page of the history should be placed in the correct location in the patient's chart and should contain the patient's full name, date of birth, and medical record number if relevant. Notes should be legible, dated (and timed, if in the hospital), and signed with the writer's name and level printed under the signature (e.g., Andrew Gordon, MS 1).

Finally, patients are often unclear about details of their history, or may omit important points through forgetfulness or embarrassment. Other sources of information, including medical records from other providers, hospital discharge summaries, and family members, can add substantially to the complete history.

### Identification and Chief Complaint

Every history should begin with a standard introductory sentence. The sentence should contain the patient's name, sex, age, ethnicity or race, and the identity of the person giving the history. For example, "Amelia Anderson, a 78-year-old Italian-American woman, presents today with her daughter, Betty Johnson, who is the primary informant for the history." Alternatively, if the patient can provide the history herself, the last part might say "... with her daughter, Betty Johnson, and provides a clear history herself." While including race or ethnicity may not be relevant in all cases, it can provide important clues about specific illnesses to which the patient might be vulnerable (e.g., thalassemia in patients of Mediterranean origin), about ways they might respond to treatment (e.g., African-Americans respond well to diuretics for hypertension), or about counseling that might be relevant (e.g., preconception counseling about Tay–Sachs disease for an Ashkenazi Jewish couple). Lastly, the patient's chief complaint, the symptoms that caused the patient to seek medical care, should be mentioned.

## History of the Present Illness (HPI)

The longest section of the history is the HPI. In this section, you must convey in a concise, complete way all of the major issues for the patient at this time. Generally, in addressing each concern, you should include some variation on the "OPQRST" mnemonic (see Table 7.1). When asking about the patient's complaints, it is particularly important to use open-ended questions, allowing the patient to describe the symptoms in his or her own words. If the patient can't provide specific details, it is reasonable to offer choices ("Is the pain sharp or dull? Is it worse before you eat or after, or doesn't eating affect it?"). Clearly, the OPQRST mnemonic will not apply precisely to every complaint, but you can modify this useful tool as circumstances indicate.

In this section you should also include information about relevant Past Medical History (PMH), Past Surgical History (PSH), Family History (FH), and Occupational or Social History. For example, if Mrs. Anderson complains of chest pain, relevant history in this section would include previous heart or lung disease, family history of heart disease, her smoking history, and what is known about her lipid levels.

## Allergy/Intolerance

Accurate and complete documentation of allergy and intolerance is critical to patient care. The list should include both true allergies (reactions such as urticaria, angioedema, and laryngospasm), as well as intolerance (nausea, headache, or other mild symptoms). Many patients will state they are "allergic" to a medication when in fact they have some intolerance to it. Physicians should help patients understand the difference between allergy and intolerance. Documenting intolerance as an allergy can limit therapeutic options unnecessarily. You should inquire about both allergy and intolerance to medications, foods, and environmental allergens (e.g., bees, dust mites). State clearly for each irritant whether the patient has an allergy or intolerance, and what symptoms the patient experienced.

## Current Medications

Many substances qualify as medications, including prescription drugs, over the counter (OTC) medications, herbal preparations, and nutritional supplements. A comprehensive list of all such substances the patient uses currently (and sometimes within the past 6 months) permits accurate evaluation of possible interactions and adverse effects. The list should include strength, frequency, and indication for the medication, as well as the name of the healthcare provider who recommended the medication. Many patients consult multiple health care providers, including alternative practitioners, but may be reluctant to tell that information to a new physician. This is an ideal time to use normalizing language to elicit this information. "Mrs. Anderson, many patients get some healthcare from providers such as chiropractors or naturopaths. We can

**Table 7.1**
OPQRST Mnemonic

| | |
|---|---|
| O—Onset | Date/time of onset of complaint. Can be specific date, or duration in days, weeks, etc. |
| P—Provocative/or palliative factors | What makes the symptom better or worse? Medications, body position, certain foods or environments? |
| Q—Quality | Describe the symptom. For pain symptoms, is it sharp, dull, achy, burning, etc.? |
| R—Region/radiation | Where is the symptom located? Does the pain radiate to another area? |
| S—Severity | How bad is it (a one-to-ten rating system can be helpful)? Does the severity vary or remain constant? |
| T—Timing | When does the symptom occur (time of day, related to eating or certain activities, etc.)? |

all help you better if we work together. Do you see any other physicians or alternative healthcare providers? If so, what are their names and what medications or supplements have they prescribed for you?" If patients seem unsure of the details of their medications, ask them to bring all of their medications, in the original containers, to their next visit.

## Immunization Status

Immunization records are an important part of any patient's medical history. Children require an extensive series of immunizations, and the recommendations for these change almost annually. As a result, you must inquire specifically about a child's immunization history, including types of immunizations, and number of doses of each. If possible, make a photocopy of the child's official immunization record for the chart. For adults, document dates of tetanus, influenza, pneumococcal, and hepatitis A and B immunizations. For women, document rubella immunity as well. Childhood illnesses such as varicella, measles, and mumps should also be documented, either by immunization or by clear history of the disease.

## Past Medical History

The Past Medical History (PMH) provides a comprehensive overview of any significant past health events. It should include recurrent acute illnesses (e.g., streptococcal pharyngitis), chronic illnesses (e.g., diabetes), all hospitalizations, and the gravity, parity, and menstrual history for women. For each item, include the date (year is usually adequate), and any relevant information such as location (e.g., what city or hospital). It is also helpful to include related diagnostic procedures. Some physicians address habits such as tobacco, alcohol, and drug use in the PMH, while others do so in the Social History (see below). Information related to a woman's menstrual and reproductive history can be included in the PMH or in the Review of Systems (see below).

Generally, we present the PMH in outline form, rather than narrative (see Table 7.2). The PMH will give important clues about potential health risks or the etiology of current symptoms, and thus you should always take the time to discuss it thoroughly with the patient.

## Past Surgical History and Hospitalizations

The Past Surgical History (PSH) states in outline form all surgical procedures and hospitalizations the patient has undergone. Again, the information should include the date, indication, and geographic location of the procedure or hospitalization. If relevant, you should reference the PMH for indication (e.g., 1997 Coronary Artery Bypass Grafting (3 vessels) 2nd to #3.1 above, San Bernardino, CA).

**Table 7.2**
Past Medical History Sample

1.0 Hypertension (dx 1975)
2.0 Tobacco abuse 60 pack-year history, quit 1997
3.0 Coronary Artery Disease (dx 1988) 2nd 1.0 & 2.0 above
    3.1 Anterior Myocardial Infarction 1997—San Bernardino, CA
        3.1.1 Angiography 1997 3 vessel disease, diffuse small vessel disease
    3.2 Mild Congestive Heart Failure (last echocardiogram 1998 LVEF 40%)
4.0 Chronic Obstructive Pulmonary Disease 2nd 2.0 above (dx 1990)
    4.1 Chronic Bronchitis
    4.2 Pneumonia 1995
5.0 Degenerative Disc Disease L5-S1
    5.1 MRI 1996

# Social History

The Social History (SH) forms a cornerstone of patient care. By obtaining a complete SH, you and other physicians will understand the patient as a whole person, rather than as a set of unrelated medical problems. The SH also provides important information about activities that may predispose the patient to various illnesses and problems.

Taking a thorough SH requires patience, good interviewing skills, and a matter-of-fact approach, since patients may perceive many of the topics in the SH as "too personal" or the provider as being judgmental about the patient's behavior. Again, the use of normalizing and prefatory language will help the patient understand that your interest is in understanding the patient as a whole person, and achieving an accurate assessment of her health status. An opening statement such as "Now we're going to talk about parts of your life that aren't strictly medical, but reflect who you are as a whole person and aspects of your life that might affect your health. Some of these questions may seem very personal, but we ask them of all our patients, and your honest and complete answers will allow us to care for you better." The components of a complete SH and suggestions about ways to ask for the information are listed in Table 7.3.

# Family History

The Family History (FH) provides important information about genetic risks the patient may have for various diseases. The FH should include current age/age at death and all significant health issues for grandparents, parents, siblings, and children. Especially in the case of established office patients, developing a genogram that reflects both FH and social interactions or tensions between the patient and family members will allow you to see patterns more clearly, and remember key aspects of the patient's social situation.

# Review of Systems (ROS)

The ROS concludes the complete history. In the ROS, you inquire about any aspect of the patient's physical or emotional health not previously discussed. Again, the style of interviewing will determine the success of obtaining a complete ROS. Since the ROS is long, and can present multiple options to the patient, you must be sure to preface these questions with a comment such as "Now we're going to talk about you from head to toe, to be sure we haven't missed anything important. I'll be asking lots of questions, but if I go too fast, or you don't understand a question, please be sure to stop me." In asking these questions, you must

**Table 7.3**
Social History

| Topic | Question to ask |
| --- | --- |
| Marital/living status | Do you have a spouse or domestic partner? Who lives at home with you? Are there other significant people in your life I should know about? Any pets? |
| Occupation/education | Do you work outside the home? What jobs have you held? Are you exposed to any toxic substances? How do you feel about your work? What is the highest level of education you completed? |
| Hobbies | What do you enjoy doing in your free time? |
| Cultural identification | How do you identify yourself culturally or ethnically? In what ways is this identification important to you? |
| Spirituality | Tell me about important spiritual or religious aspects of your life. How do your religious practices interact with your healthcare? |
| Tobacco use | Do you now or have you in the past used any tobacco products? If so, what, how much, and for how long? |
| Alcohol use | How much alcohol do you drink (quantity, frequency, how long, and any abuse)? |
| Drugs | What recreational or street drugs do you use now or in the past (get details)? |
| Sexual activity | Do you have intimate physical contact with men, women, or both? How many partners have you had in your lifetime? What concerns do you have about your sexual activity? (Sexually transmitted diseases should be listed under PMH or ROS.) |

present each one individually, rather than as a list, which can be confusing. For example, when discussing constitutional signs and symptoms, ask "Have you noticed any changes in your weight? What about night sweats?" rather than "Have you noticed night sweats, weight changes, fever, chills, or increasing fatigue?" In this way, when the patient responds yes or no to a question, you'll know which question is being answered. The ROS is the only time in the interview process when the closed-ended question is preferred, since you want to be sure you have covered all relevant areas. For any positive response, you will then ask more detailed questions to understand the problem thoroughly. Again, while the list below notes medical terminology, you should "translate" those terms to lay language when asking the questions. Often, you may omit some questions from the ROS as circumstances dictate, but you should cover every area at some level.

*General*: fever, chills, malaise, usual weight, weight change (unintentional), fatigue
*Diet*: restrictions (by choice, religion, or intolerance), general style
*Endocrine*: polydipsia, polyuria, heat or cold intolerance, skin or hair changes
*Hematologic*: bruising, fatigue, lymphadenopathy, easy bleeding, transfusions
*Head and neck*:
  General—headaches (review OPQRST if yes), syncope, severe head injury
  Eyes—change in vision, diplopia, visual field loss, photophobia, pain, floaters, last exam
  Ears—tinnitus, hearing loss, infections, dizziness/vertigo
  Nose/sinuses—allergies, frequent infections, discharge, sense of smell, nosebleeds
  Mouth/throat/neck—dental history/last exam, sores, recurrent pharyngitis, dysphagia, change in voice, swelling/lumps
*Respiratory*: asthma/wheezing, dyspnea, pneumonia, recurrent bronchitis, asbestos exposure, chronic cough
*Cardiovascular*: chest pain, cyanosis, peripheral edema, orthopnea, exercise tolerance
*Gastrointestinal*: change in appetite or food tolerance, pain, change in bowel habits (pain, frequency, character), blood in/on stool, nausea/vomiting, gastroesophageal reflux, jaundice, dysphagia, fecal incontinence
*Genitourinary*: urinary frequency/urgency/pain/incontinence/nocturia/infections, sexually transmitted diseases, sexual function and concerns
  Males—penile discharge, erectile dysfunction, dribbling, testicular pain or lumps, hernias, contraceptive needs
  Females—menstrual history (menarche, frequency, menopause age, amount of flow, symptoms), reproductive history, contraceptive use history and current needs, intermenstrual bleeding, breast lumps/discharge, vaginal discharge
*Musculoskeletal*: fractures, arthritis, joint pain/swelling, bony deformity, weakness
*Neurologic*: vertigo, paresthesias, sensory loss, seizures, syncope, tremors, memory loss, weakness or paralysis
*Psychiatric*: depression, anxiety, irritability, sleep disturbances, general mood, verbal, sexual, or physical abuse

## CASE 7-3

*Jonathan Wilson, a 19-year-old patient, comes into the office complaining of a rash. As Muhammed Alasharifi, a second-year medical student, prepares to go in the room, the medical assistant tells him that the patient seems very nervous, and reluctant to answer questions. Muhammed notes from the chart that Jonathan has just finished his first year at college.*

MUHAMMED: *Hello, Jonathan. I'm Muhammed Alasharifi, a second-year medical student. I'll be talking with you first today, before Dr. Baker joins us.*
JONATHAN (sitting with arms folded, not making eye contact): *Umm, Hi.*
MUHAMMED: *What brings you to the office today?*
JONATHAN: *Well, I have this rash, and I'm kind of worried about it.*
MUHAMMED: *Tell me more about your worries.*
JONATHAN: *I'm worried something I did might have caused it.*

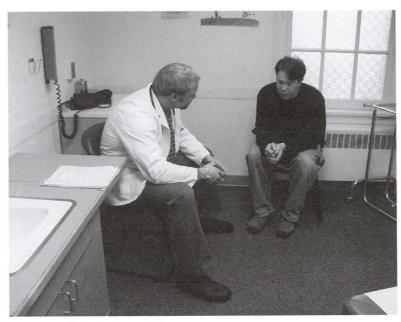

**Case 7-3.** Note Jonathan's closed body language, reflecting his nervousness. Muhammed's welcoming manner should overcome this soon.

MUHAMMED:       *Oh. Often patients know a lot about what's going on with them. What do you think might have caused your rash?*
JONATHAN: **(unfolding his arms):**       *Umm, I'm not really sure …*
MUHAMMED:       *Well, since rashes can be caused by lots of things, how about if you and I sort it out together? I'm going to ask a lot of questions, some of which may seem quite personal, but they're all important in sorting out your problem …*

## THE PROBLEM-FOCUSED HISTORY

Established patients often present to the office with acute problems. In these situations, the physician will take a modified, or problem-focused history (PFH). Again, the HPI forms the cornerstone of the PFH, since through it the physician will learn about problems, eliciting all of the elements of the OPQRST mnemonic as modified for that problem. For example, in the case of the rash "T" might refer not only to when the rash started, but whether it changes relative to heat or cold or various exposures. "Q" might include questions about color, itchiness or pain, blanching, and texture.

When taking a PFH, the physician should particularly inquire about relevant travel, occupational factors (e.g., wrist pain in a data clerk might represent carpal tunnel syndrome), social factors, sexual history, and similar episodes in the past. The PFH should also include focused versions of the PMH, PSH, and FH.

### CASE 7-3 (continued)

*Jonathan has told Muhammed that the rash started about a week ago, is not itchy, and seems to be spreading from his leg all over his body.*

MUHAMMED:       *Jonathan, tell me about any new experiences in the weeks before the rash started.*
JONATHAN:       *Umm, like what?*

MUHAMMED (sensing Jonathan's unease, and realizing that this is an appropriate time for closed questions):   *Did you do any traveling?*

JONATHAN:   *No, except coming home from college in Connecticut.*

MUHAMMED:   *How about using any new soaps or body care products?*

JONATHAN:   *Don't think so, unless my mom uses some different detergent.*

MUHAMMED:   *Have you had any intimate physical contact with women or men over the past months?*

JONATHAN:   *Umm, well, you promise you won't tell my folks but that's what I'm worried about ...*

*Note that Muhammed, sensing Jonathan's reluctance, started with more neutral questions and slowly moved into more personal areas as Jonathan opened up. As a result of this approach, and using nonjudgmental language and tone, Muhammed arrives at the source of Jonathan's concern.*

### CASE 7-4

*Janice Brown is a 17-year-old girl who has seen Dr. Ellen Hayes since birth. Today, Janice presents with concerns about her menstrual periods, which have been irregular lately. Dr. Hayes's nurse notes on the chart that Janice seems more anxious than usual. Janice comes to the visit with her mother, also a patient of Dr. Hayes.*

DR. HAYES:   *Good morning, Janice, good to see you. Hello, Mrs. Brown.*

JANICE:   *Hello, Dr. Hayes.*

MRS. BROWN:   *Dr. Hayes, Janice is worried about her periods. They aren't very predictable, and she has some discomfort with them.*

DR. HAYES:   *Thanks for getting us started, Mrs. Brown. Why don't we let Janice tell us as much as possible first, then you can add any details after she's done ...*

## SPECIAL SITUATIONS

Many patients present special challenges when taking a history. The physician must often modify both interviewing techniques and the content of the interview to reflect the individual circumstances of the patient. Some of the most common examples of these special situations include taking a history from children, adolescents, pregnant women, the elderly, the mentally disabled, and patients whose primary language is different from that of the physician. In this section, we will review the basics of taking a history from each of these types of patients . For a more detailed review of this area, consult some of the suggested readings at the end of this chapter.

## Children and Adolescents

Children and adolescents require both a different interview technique and the inclusion of different topics in the history from adult patients. Clearly, a 5-year-old may not be able to provide a complete history independent of his parent. However, any child who talks can provide useful information about a health problem if queried correctly. When interviewing young children, the closed question becomes a more important part of the process. For example, you might ask a 4-year-old to point to "the place on your tummy where it hurts." Asking children about their problems directly helps develop trust between the physician and the child, starts the learning process about being responsible for one's own health, and shows the child that the physician respects him or her as an individual. Dr. Hayes, in Case 7-4, acknowledges Mrs. Brown's contribution, but also makes it clear that she wants to hear from Janice first.

Confidentiality is another critical issue with older children and adolescents. Each state has its own laws about confidentiality with minors. Often, reproductive health issues in adolescents can be kept confidential from the parents, as opposed to general health problems. However, medical students and physicians must be aware of the law in their own state.

Physicians must work with adolescents to create a safe environment in which the patient will discuss issues confidentially. In an established physician–patient relationship, conversations about confidentiality can start as early as age 8 or 9. A typical conversation Dr. Hayes might have had with Janice at age 10 and her mother might sound like this:

**DR. HAYES:** Janice, you're getting to an age where most kids have a lot of questions. I hope you'll always go to your parents first, but we all know that can be awkward sometimes.

**MRS. BROWN:** That's for sure!

**DR. HAYES:** It's reassuring for parents and kids to know that I can be a safe, trustworthy adult who can answer questions for you. It's even OK to come see me just to talk. If you do, I want you and your folks to understand the rules about confidentiality. That means what I will tell your parents and what I won't tell them.

**MRS. BROWN:** I'm glad we're talking about this with Dr. Hayes, Janice.

**DR. HAYES:** Janice, anything you and I talk about privately will stay private unless you give me permission to tell your parents. That means even things like sexual activity, or if your friends are encouraging you to try alcohol or drugs.

**JANICE:** Really? You won't tell them unless I say it's OK?

**DR. HAYES:** Yes. There are two exceptions. If I'm worried that you're likely to hurt yourself or hurt someone else, then I have to tell them right away. Otherwise I'll encourage you to talk to them about everything, but I can't tell them without your permission.

**MRS. BROWN:** I agree with Dr. Hayes, honey. I hope you'll talk with us, but you can always come to her with any questions and I'll respect your confidentiality too. I'd much rather you get good information from her!

It is important, therefore, to give children time alone with the physician at every visit, starting at around age 8, to allow them time to discuss "private" issues with you. As a trusting relationship develops, children and adolescents will reveal significant information about themselves if asked in a nonjudgmental fashion. This relationship will allow the physician to elicit critical information about friendship patterns, accident prevention behaviors (e.g., bicycle helmet and seat belt use), risk behavior (tobacco, alcohol, and drug use, sexual activity), and school performance issues. In addition to direct questioning, a written confidential history can provide a springboard for discussion of a wide range of issues with adolescents (Cavanaugh, 1986).

## Pregnant Women

When obtaining a history from a pregnant woman, the physician must include all aspects of the complete history as noted above, and must also focus on some special issues. Areas of particular importance in this situation include previous obstetric history, occupational and environmental exposures, genetic history for both the patient and the father of the baby, and a detailed social history that includes the emotional response of the patient and her family to the pregnancy, and her risk for domestic violence (which increases during pregnancy, especially if the pregnancy is unplanned).

## The Elderly

Too often, interviews with elderly patients begin like this:

### CASE 7-5

*Mabel Robinson, 80 years old, comes in to see Dr. Matthew Simpson to establish care. She lives alone, but her daughter, Laura Nelson, accompanies her to the visit.*

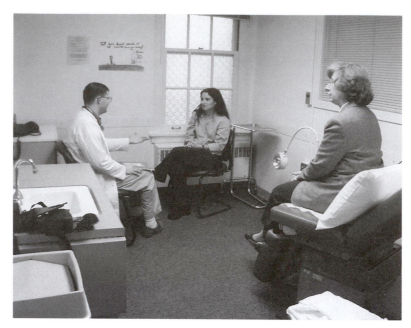

**Case 7-5.** How *not* to take a history from an elderly patient!

DR. SIMPSON:     *Hello, Mabel, I'm Dr. Simpson. It's nice to meet you.*
MRS. ROBINSON:     *(looking uneasy) Hello, Dr. Simpson.*
DR. SIMPSON:     *(turning to Mrs. Nelson) What brings your mother into the office today?*
MRS. NELSON:     *Well, Doctor …*

Elderly patients have a variety of special needs during the history-taking process. Of utmost importance is the need to be treated with respect. Too often physicians treat elderly patients as children, with inappropriate familiarity and indirect history taking through a relative. In Case 7-5, Mrs. Robinson's discomfort stemmed both from Dr. Simpson's use of her first name, and from his questioning of her daughter, rather than herself. Such behavior by the physician immediately forms a barrier between physician and patient that hinders effective care.

Histories from elderly patients should address several areas of unique concern. Functional assessment (see Chapter 16), nutritional status, financial independence (can they afford medications, food, and so on), depression, and alcohol use all require close attention. It is also appropriate to obtain a sexual history from elderly patients, as this aspect of their lives can affect their sense of well-being, and is often ignored. Immunization status and preventive screening (e.g., mammography and flexible sigmoidoscopy) history should be evaluated.

Finally, physicians must address issues related to patient autonomy such as advance directives for healthcare. The primary care physician has an obligation to understand, document, and respect the patient's wishes regarding level of care, heroic measures, and preventive screening.

## Bilingual Interviews

In the United States, the ethnically diverse population virtually guarantees that physicians will have patients in their practices who do not speak English well. These patients present multiple difficulties during the history-taking process, including use of interpreters (with inherent translation inaccuracies), cultural differences, and conflicting perceptions of disease and illness between the patient and the physician. Frequently, interpreters do not translate accurately or completely (Ebden *et al.*, 1988). They may paraphrase the question or the response, leave out details of the response, or report inaccurately if they believe that the question or response is culturally or personally embarrassing to the patient. The latter is especially true when the interpreter is a relative of the patient, as is often the case. While family members often serve as interpreters, they are more likely to omit information, change answers, and blur the true meaning of questions to avoid embarrassment. If at all possible, one should use a professional medical interpreter, familiar with both English medical terminology and the appropriate terms in the patient's primary language. Clear communication with the interpreter about the need to translate fully everything the patient says will enhance the history substantially. Finally, physicians should frame questions as if they are asking the patient directly. "Tell me more about your pain" affords the patient more respect than asking the interpreter "Can she tell me about her pain?"

## The Mentally Disabled

Improved healthcare and a trend toward deinstitutionalization of people with mental disabilities or pronounced psychiatric illness bring more of these patients into mainstream medical practice. These patients present challenges related to emotional maturity, language skills, personal world-view (in essence analogous to cultural differences), and their previous experiences with healthcare. Above all, the physician must accord them the same respect as any other patient. Patients with significant effects from either mental disabilities or pronounced psychiatric illness will often be accompanied by a caregiver of some sort to medical visits. In this case, we can compare the interview to that with a child or a very elderly person. The physician should clarify the role of the caregiver in the patient's daily life. How knowledgeable is the caregiver about the patient's daily routine? Generally, both the patient and the caregiver have important information to contribute, and the physician must question each directly.

## CONCLUSION

This chapter covers a wide range of material related to taking a thorough history. The complete history was outlined in detail, and a variety of special circumstances were reviewed. Physicians can gain a lot of information that allows formulation of a fairly complete differential diagnosis if they take histories with care. Equally important, the process of taking a history allows the physician to establish a rapport with the patient that will form the foundation of the healthcare relationship. Both verbal and nonverbal information becomes apparent during the interview, and both are critical to the complete picture the physician is painting of patients as whole people.

Learning to take histories effectively is a lifelong process. In the first years of medical school, the process feels stilted, but as students develop a sense of the flow of the history, they become more aware of nuances in the context of the interview. During residency and then in practice, one's history-taking skills are constantly refined based on experience and continuing education. Taking a good history can be one of the most rewarding experiences for physicians, because it provides so many opportunities to makes diagnoses, establish rapport, and identify areas that require further attention (e.g., prevention). This chapter can serve as a reference throughout the training process to remind learners of specific areas of questioning.

## CASES FOR DISCUSSION

### CASE 1

*A patient comes in complaining of fever, aches, and a sore throat for 3 days. You know that he is active with a church youth group that often travels for events.*

1. *What questions would you ask about recent travel or other exposures?*
2. *How would you elicit any specific concerns he might have about his illness?*
3. *What would you ask as a pertinent past history?*

## CASE 2

*You introduce yourself to a new patient as a medical student. Despite your good body language and appropriate verbal cues to the patient, she answers you in short phrases, minimizes eye contact, and sits with a closed posture.*

1. *What issues might this patient bring to the visit, in terms of her medical history, her possible diagnoses, and her previous relationships with physicians?*
2. *How would you approach these issues with her?*
3. *How should you proceed if she remains uncommunicative?*

## CASE 3

*You are taking a complete history from an elderly patient with a complicated PMH and PSH. In addition, he is hard of hearing, has a fairly poor memory, and speaks at length in response to every question.*

1. *Which techniques of interviewing might help most with this patient?*
2. *What other resources might be available to help get accurate information about this patient?*
3. *What are some of the pitfalls in interviewing this patient? How could you avoid these pitfalls?*

## CASE 4

*A woman presents for her first prenatal visit. Early in the interview, you realize that she is already about halfway through her fourth pregnancy. She seems unconcerned about the fact that she has presented for care so late in her pregnancy.*

1. *Why might she have presented so late? How could you elicit that information in a nonjudgmental way?*
2. *What questions should you ask her about her past history that relate specifically to her obstetric history and potential risk factors for this pregnancy?*
3. *What might you say to encourage her to be more attentive to her health and that of her unborn child?*

## CASE 5

*A 9-year-old boy presents for a routine well-child visit. His father accompanies him.*

1. *Discuss ways to address issues of confidentiality with the boy and his father.*
2. *What specific issues are children this age facing? What would you ask the boy to get information about these issues?*
3. *If he is not engaged in the interview process, what techniques could you use to establish good communication with him?*

# RECOMMENDED READINGS

Carlat DJ: The psychiatric review of symptoms: A screening tool for family physicians. *Am Fam Physician* 58(7):1617–1624, 1998.
   A detailed guide for any provider seeking to take a thorough psychiatric history.
Coulehan JL, Block MR: *The Medical Interview: Mastering Skills for Clinical Practice*, ed 3. New York, FA Davis Co, 1997.
   Excellent reference for interviewing skills appropriate to a wide range of clinical settings and diverse patient groups.
Fields SD: History-taking in the elderly: Obtaining useful information. *Geriatrics* 46(8):31–35, 1991.
   Resource for specific areas of questioning and potential barriers that might exist in interviewing elderly patients.
Green M: Interviewing children and adolescents. *Patient Care*, September 30, 1986, pp. 76–90.
   Good review of both interviewing techniques and specific questions to ask children and adolescents.

Lax MB, Manetti FA, Klein R: Recognizing occupational disease—Taking an effective occupational history. *Am Fam Physician* 58(4):935–944, 1998.

> Very good tables regarding specific complaints and their potential occupational origins. Screening questions about occupational illness.

Tomlinson J: Taking a sexual history. *Br Med J* 317:1573–1576, 1998.

> A well-written, practical, detailed article on a very difficult topic. Good illustrations and sidebar examples emphasize key points.

# REFERENCES

Cavanaugh RM: Obtaining a personal and confidential history: An opportunity for prevention *J Adolesc Health Care* 7:118–122, 1986.
Ebden P, *et al*: The bilingual consultation. *Lancet* 1851:347, February 13, 1988.

## CHAPTER 8

# Physical Examination

*Diane L. Elliot and Linn Goldberg*

## CASE 8-1

*Mrs. R. had delayed finding a new physician for almost a year. Finally, she could not refill her medications without a physician's prescription and made an appointment. She had heard good things about this physician, but the first visit made her anxious. She wondered what it would be like.*

*After escorting her into the examination room, the nurse asked Mrs. R. to put on a gown. She had been waiting for 20 minutes when the physician entered. Dr. B. was running late, as a noon business meeting had become bogged down in administrative decisions. There were no last-minute cancellations, and the afternoon schedule was full. It was now 3:30 PM, and Dr. B. was about 30 minutes behind. Pulling the chart off the door rack, Dr. B. read that Mrs. R. had moved to this area about a year ago and now needed refills on her blood pressure medicines. The nurse had recorded her blood pressure as 145/85 mm Hg.*

*The interaction between Mrs. R. and Dr. B. lasted about 15 minutes. Dr. B. measured her blood pressure, then auscultated her heart and lungs. Mrs. R. had not offered any specific complaints or concerns, and Dr. B. had her sign consents for release of information to obtain prior records, ordered some laboratory tests, refilled her medications, and scheduled her for a return appointment. Dr. B. anticipated that the history would be more focused after an opportunity to review old records and laboratory studies. Dr. B. wished that they could have spent more time establishing rapport and getting to know each other, but nothing seemed urgent.*

*Mrs. R. was glad that the visit was short. However, Dr. B. seemed so rushed that she felt uncomfortable raising her concerns. She had expected to have a checkup and a more thorough examination. Her former physician had done a "complete examination" every year. She wondered whether Dr. B. was someone she could trust in a crisis.*

## EDUCATIONAL OBJECTIVES

1. List, describe, and provide a rationale for maneuvers performed during a "screening" physical examination

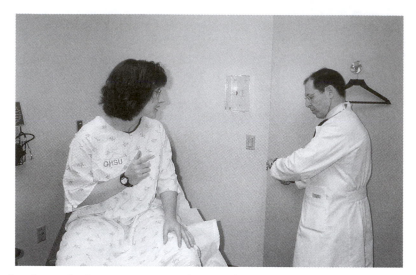

**Mrs. R. waiting for doctor in the exam room.** The initial visit can cause anxiety for the patient and may set a tone for subsequent visits.

2. List unique aspects of examining children and how the physical examination process or findings might differ for a child's physical examination
3. Describe the limitations of physical assessment and methods to decrease examination unreliability
4. Describe how the physical examination affects the physician–patient relationship
5. Describe unique issues related to the breast, pelvic, and genitourinary examination and relate means to minimize patient distress during these examinations

# INTRODUCTION

The physical examination is a constant dimension of physician–patient interactions. Although medical knowledge and laboratory assessment are advancing rapidly, the techniques of inspection, percussion, auscultation, and palpation have not changed. Physical examination abilities are critical skills for assessing patients and are of lasting value. When surveyed, practicing physicians indicated that competence in the physical examination and medical interview ranked most important among a long list of clinical abilities (Kern *et al.*, 1985).

In this chapter, we present a rationale for learning a specific physical examination sequence and the content and order for a "screening" examination. Assessment issues unique to pediatric patients are reviewed. In addition to detecting and defining illness, physical assessment also functions to meet patient expectations and enhance physician–patient rapport. We outline "therapeutic" functions of the examination and review components that require high physician sensitivity.

## CASE 8-2

*M. S. was beginning her third year of medical school. This was her first rotation on the inpatient service. Last year, she practiced components of the physical examination in her weekly preceptor experience. Still, she was not sure what the resident had meant when he asked her to do "a complete H and P." She had hoped to watch the intern examine a patient before she had to do one.*

*Her preceptor, the physician whose office she'd visited weekly last year, rarely did a complete examination. In that ambulatory setting, the examiner focused on aspects relevant to the patient's*

151

BASIC GUIDELINES
FOR THE SCREENING
PHYSICAL
EXAMINATION OF
ADULTS

*complaints or maneuvers known to be useful in screening for illness. She thought about her music lessons. It seemed like she had learned different passages but had not played the whole composition from beginning to end. She wanted to be able to play the piece by heart and not require her physical diagnosis textbook while examining a patient.*

*Feeling awkward, M. S. resolved to practice the complete sequence several times on her roommate before the next admitting day. She needed to memorize an examination sequence. Interpreting findings, deciding when to perform additional maneuvers, paying attention to the patient, and maintaining rapport gave her much to think about during the examination. She could not learn to improvise until she had mastered the basic "composition" of the physical examination.*

## Why Learn a Particular Examination Sequence?

The physical examination's sequence is designed for efficiency and patient comfort. For example, beginning the examination with attention to a patient's hands and measuring vital signs permits continued eye contact and is less threatening than an initial examination of the eyes and ears. The examination's order progresses from "head to toe," and each anatomic area follows the pattern: inspection, percussion, auscultation, and palpation. This progression permits using information in subsequent examination procedures. For example, percussion of the liver's lower border is used to determine where to palpate for its edge; the eye examination begins with inspection of the external eye structures, followed by assessing visual acuity. Reduced acuity might lead to a more thorough definition of visual fields and additional time observing the optic disk, vessels, and background retina. Patient comfort and examination efficiency are assisted by minimizing position changes and clustering aspects performed with the patient in different positions (sitting, supine, and standing).

# BASIC GUIDELINES FOR THE SCREENING PHYSICAL EXAMINATION OF ADULTS

The following is a suggested sequence for the well-patient "screening" physical examination. Maneuvers are outlined in Table 8.1. Although several physical examination texts provide detailed information on examination maneuvers (Bickley *et al.*, 1998; Greenberger & Hinthorn, 1993; Novey & Novey, 1998; Seidel, 1999; Swartz, 2001; Willms *et al.*, 1994), most do not include recommendations for an expedient "screening examination." This probably reflects lack of any order's proven superiority. Suggested sequences, similar to items in Table 8.1, are included in compressed physical examination guides (Macklin *et al.*, 1994; Novey & Novey, 1998).

The physical examination commences with the examiner washing her hands, which cleans and warms them. Patient contact begins by touching the patient's outstretched hands and observing the upper extremities. This initial nonthreatening maneuver allows assessment of the patient's reaction to physical contact.

## Vital Signs

Vital signs are assessed by palpating the radial pulse for 15 seconds to determine heart rate and rhythm. If irregularities are detected, palpate for a longer interval and establish whether all beats are peripherally transmitted by auscultation of the precordium while palpating the radial pulse. Assessing respiration involves observing or palpating chest movement as unobtrusively as possible, such as while seeming to palpate the pulse or auscultate the precordium. Measuring height, weight, and temperature also is done prior to the examination or early in its sequence.

Blood pressure can be measured with the patient seated or reclining, and in each position, the artery measured should be at the level of the heart. The examiner should select a blood pressure cuff with a width about 20% greater than the diameter of the arm. Cuffs that are too small can give falsely high readings. The examiner should establish the systolic pressure by inflating the cuff while palpating the radial artery, rapidly

**Table 8.1**
Suggested Physical Examination Sequence

Approach the seated patient to perform the following:
  General inspection, state of nutrition, and apparent age
  Vital signs (pulse, blood pressure, respiratory rate)
  Inspection of hands and fingernails
  Inspection of scalp and face
  Inspection of scleras and conjunctivas
  Visual acuity
  Pupil reaction to light (consensual and direct)
  Funduscopic examination
  Inspection external ears
  Otoscopic examination of tympanic membranes
  Hearing
  Inspection of nasal mucosa
  Inspection of oropharyngeal mucosa
Move behind or beside the seated patient to perform the following:
  Palpation of anterior cervical or supraclavicular nodes
  Palpation of thyroid gland
  Palpation of each carotid artery
  Percussion of spine and posterior lung fields
  Auscultation of posterior lung fields
Ask the patient to recline supine and cover torso and legs with a drape. Ask the patient to pull up the gown so that the chest is exposed and
    perform the following:
  Inspection of breasts
  Palpation of breasts and axillary nodes, with the woman's hands behind her head
  Inspection of neck veins and estimation jugular venous pressure
  Palpation of precordium
  Auscultation of precordium
  Auscultation of carotids
Patient remains supine, gown is lowered, and drape positioned to reveal the patient's abdomen
  Inspection of abdomen
  Auscultation of abdomen and over the abdominal aorta, renal, and iliac arteries
  Percussion of abdomen and liver span in the midclavicular line
  Assess for splenomegaly by percussion of upper left quadrant during deep inspiration
  Light abdominal palpation
  Palpation of right upper quadrant for liver edge during inspiration
  Deep abdominal palpation of all four quadrants
  Palpation of inguinal, femoral, and axillary nodes (if last not performed during breast palpation)
Patient's gown is lowered further and drape is positioned to:
  Inspect lower extremities
  Palpate lower extremity pulses and assess for edema
Patient resumes the sitting position (if indicated, supine and seated blood pressure can be performed at this time)
  Assess remaining cranial nerves (visual fields to confrontation [III]; facial sensation, muscles of mastication [V]; facial movement
    [VII], palate movement and phonation [IX, X]; shoulder shrug [XI]; and tongue movement [XII])
  Stretch reflexes: triceps, brachioradialis, patella, Achilles
  Patient stands down from the table to demonstrate gait
Genital and rectal examinations are performed as final maneuvers (patient dresses after this aspect of the examination)
  Males stand for inspection of penis and palpation of the scrotum contents and inguinal ring; patient turns to face the examination table
    for digital prostate and rectal examination
  Females (who emptied their bladder prior to beginning the physical examination) are positioned for the pelvic examination

deflating it when the pulse is no longer palpable. This initial determination of systolic pressure guides subsequent cuff inflation during auscultation of the pressure. The examiner reinflates the cuff to about 20 mm Hg above the palpated systolic pressure, the stethoscope is placed firmly over the brachial artery (medial to the tendon of the biceps muscle), in the antecubital fossae, and then the cuff is deflated while listening.

# HEENT (Head, Eyes, Ears, Nose, and Throat)

The examiner faces the patient for the majority of the HEENT evaluation. The examiner assesses the sclera and conjunctiva of each eye by asking the patient to look upward, while retracting the lower lid

153

BASIC GUIDELINES
FOR THE SCREENING
PHYSICAL
EXAMINATION OF
ADULTS

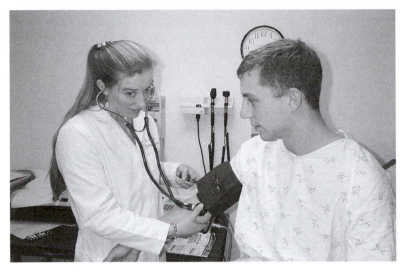

**Taking BP.** Wrap an appropriately sized cuff around the arm. Quickly inflate the cuff while palpating the radial pulse to determine an estimate of systolic pressure. Rapidly deflate the cuff. Reinflate the cuff to 20 mm Hg above the systolic pressure and gradually deflate the cuff while listening with the diaphragm over the brachial artery in the medial antecubital fossa.

downward. Vision is evaluated early in the examination using a near vision card or wall chart and while the patient wears any corrective lenses. Detecting abnormalities of visual acuity can result in additional time spent on other aspects of the eye examination.

Extraocular movements are evaluated as the patient fixes gaze on the examiner's finger. The examiner should ask the patient to look into the distance and then at the patient's finger held 8 inches from the nose, while observing for pupillary constriction and convergence. When observing the pupillary response to light, the examiner inspects for pupillary constriction in the same eye and the consensual response by the ipsilateral pupil.

For the ophthalmoscope examination, the patient should be positioned at a height comfortable for the examiner and the room darkened to increase pupillary dilation. The examiner holds the ophthalmoscope with the right hand and uses the right eye when examining the patient's right eye. The examiner should use the left

*In 1998, the definition of obesity was changed to be based on the Body Mass Index (BMI), which is weight in kilograms divided by (height in meters)$^2$. Using BMI, rather than height–weight charts, allowed direct comparison of adults with different heights and frame sizes. Also, talking about BMI may be less emotionally charged than discussing weight or percentage of body fat. With this new definition, more than half of U.S. adults are classified as overweight or obese, and that percentage grows each year. With a BMI greater than 27, 7 out of 10 adults will have high blood pressure, diabetes, or abnormal lipid levels.*

| BMI | Weight Category |
|---|---|
| *less than 18.5* | *underweight* |
| *18.5 to 24.9* | *normal (healthiest weights)* |
| *25 to 29.9* | *overweight (may harm health, especially if there are other risks for heart disease)* |
| *30 to 40* | *obese (definite health risks)* |
| *more than 40* | *extreme obesity (major health risks)* |

*Orthostatic changes refer to a comparison between the pulse and blood pressure when supine and when standing. It takes several seconds for the autonomic nervous system reflexes to respond and normalize blood pressure, and allowing adequate time (at least 3 minutes) for equilibration is important when assessing for an orthostatic change. Volume depletion of at least 20% and autonomic insufficiency can both cause a drop in blood pressure when standing.*

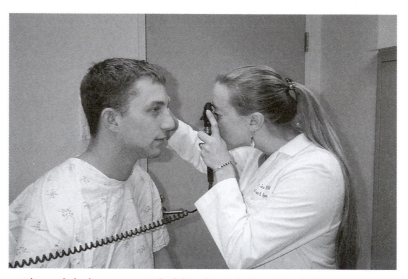

**Ophthalmoscopy.** The ophthalmoscope is held in the right hand and the examiners use their right eye when examining the patient's right eye. Placing the thumb along the brow steadies the head, allows the examiner to know the head position, and prevents the ophthalmoscope from inadvertently touching the globe. Positions are reversed for the left eye.

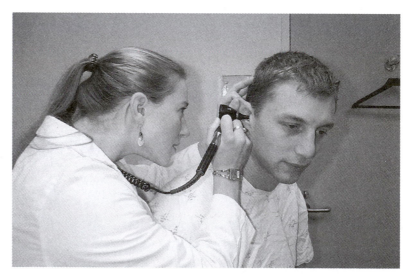

**Otoscope.** The external ear canal is directed anteriorly. Holding the scope in a hand that also rests on the patient's head permits steadying the instrument. It also allows the hand, scope, and head to move as a unit, which can avoid injury, if the patient makes a sudden head movement.

**155**

**BASIC GUIDELINES
FOR THE SCREENING
PHYSICAL
EXAMINATION OF
ADULTS**

*Hearing loss occurs in a third of elderly individuals, and screening for its presence is recommended among this group. Asking whether a "hearing problem" affects aspects of their life and pure tone audiometry are used to assess hearing. The usual clinical means to check hearing, such as whispered voice, finger rub, or watch tick, have not been well studied as to their test characteristics.*

hand and left eye when examining the patient's left eye. From a position of about 15 inches from the patient and about 15 degrees lateral to the patient's line of vision, the examiner shines the light beam on the pupil to elicit the "red reflex." To observe the anterior eye structures, positive diopters (black numbers) are used. The examiner moves slowly toward the patient's eye, bringing the optic disk into focus by adjusting the lens disk. The examiner assesses the disk and retinal vessels, and then asks the patient to look directly at the light, so that the macula (located two disk diameters lateral to the optic disk) can be observed.

The examiner should inspect and palpate the auricles and posterior auricular regions. By gently pulling the auricle upward, backward, and slightly away from the skull, the examiner can insert the otoscope speculum in a downward and forward position and observe the tympanic membrane and canal. To observe the nasal mucosa, septal location and integrity, the examiner is positioned in front of the patient and gently inserts the short wide nasal speculum through each nostril, while inspecting the nasal passages.

The examiner should inspect the lips, all surfaces of the tongue, gingiva, palate, and buccal mucosa. To examine the floor of the mouth, the examiner asks the patient to touch the "roof of your mouth," with the tip of the tongue. To visualize the posterior pharynx and palate movement, the examiner presses a tongue blade firmly down on the patient's nonprotruded tongue and asks the patient to say "ah."

The head and neck contain several node-bearing areas for palpation: (1) preauricular nodes in front of the ears, (2) occipital nodes at the posterior base of the skull, (3) anterior cervical nodes in front of the sternomastoid muscle, (4) posterior cervical nodes posterior to the sternomastoid muscle, and (5) supraclavicular nodes above the clavicle and in the angle formed by the clavicle and the sternomastoid muscle.

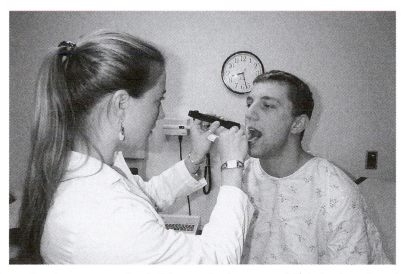

**Mouth.** With the patient's tongue resting in his mouth, the tongue blade is placed on the posterior third of the tongue and pulls the tongue forward to better reveal the posterior pharynx.

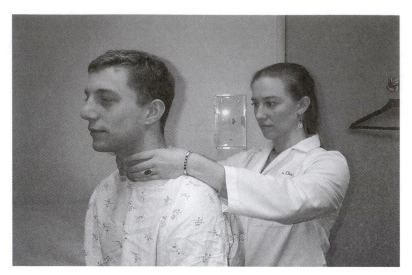

**Thyroid.** The thyroid can be palpated from the patient's front or back. Swallowing elevates the pharynx, and the gland may be felt moving upward under the examiner's fingers.

The examiner can palpate the thyroid gland while standing in front or in back of the patient. The thyroid gland lies across the trachea below the cricoid cartilage, with the lateral lobes curved around the sides of the trachea. From the front, the thyroid is displaced to one side by using the thumb to apply pressure on the thyroid cartilage. With the opposite hand, the thyroid can be palpated between the thumb (held in front of the sternomastoid) and the second and third fingers placed behind the sternomastoid. The procedure should be repeated for the opposite side. From behind the patient, the procedure is similar, except that the thyroid cartilage is displaced with the second and third fingers. The thumb of the opposite hand is behind the sternomastoid muscle, and the second and third fingers palpate the gland. The examiner can palpate and auscultate the carotid arteries during the HEENT examination or defer this portion until examining the heart and blood vessels.

## Chest and Back

Moving behind the patient (if not already in that position for the thyroid examination), the examiner palpates the vertebral spinous processes. To examine chest wall movement, ask the patient to inhale deeply, while observing the extent and symmetry of respiratory movement. The examiner should percuss the posterior lung fields and then auscultate the posterior and lateral lung fields, using the diaphragm of the stethoscope. The patient should be asked to breathe deeply through the mouth. A similar sequence is followed for the anterior lung fields.

## Breast

For the breast examination, a woman should be sitting and undressed to the waist. The examiner inspects both breasts, then asks the patient to recline, with her hands behind her head. The examiner should

*The French physician René-Théophile-Hyacinthe Laënnec was born in 1781. In 1816 he invented the stethoscope. Initially he used rolled up paper, which eventually became a foot long cylinder of wood. Laënnec coined many of the terms used to describe auscultatory lung findings. He died of tuberculosis at age 45. It is easy to remember the stethoscope's inventor as it hangs around "Le Neck."*

157

BASIC GUIDELINES
FOR THE SCREENING
PHYSICAL
EXAMINATION OF
ADULTS

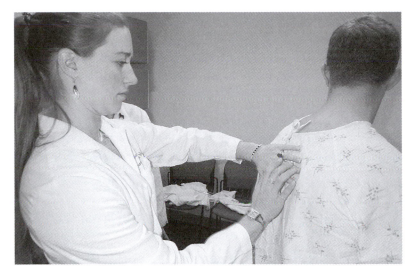

**Lungs.** Percussion prior to auscultation may alert the examiner to areas of dullness or hyperresonance.

systematically examine all four quadrants and the tail of each breast, using a uniform pattern to ensure a complete examination. A man's breasts should be examined in a similar manner, if a male has breast complaints or when gynecomastia is present on inspection.

## Axillary Lymph Nodes

The examiner should ask the patient to relax the upper extremity and place the cupped fingers of her hand into the patient's armpit. The right hand palpates the left axilla, and the left hand palpates the right axilla. With the examiner's hand moving slowly down over the surface of the ribs, the fingers palpate axillary tissue as it is compressed against the chest wall. The technique is repeated with the examiner palpating outwardly against the humerus. After palpating the axilla, the examiner should rewash her hands.

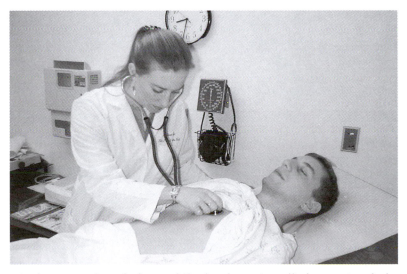

**Heart.** The gown is drawn up from below, while the drape is pulled up to just below the area being examined. Routinely auscultate in the four valvular areas with the diaphragm and with the bell.

To estimate venous pressure, the patient is positioned so that the meniscus or highest point of internal jugular vein oscillation is visible along the sternomastoid muscle. The vertical distance (perpendicular to the floor) between this point and the sternal angle plus 5 cm is the venous pressure in centimeters of water.

Appropriate draping maintains patient comfort. To minimize exposure, the gown is brought up from below, and the drape positioned inferior to the area being examined. With the patient supine, the examiner observes the precordium, then palpates the following areas of the chest wall: (1) aortic area (second intercostal space to the right of the sternum), (2) pulmonic area (second and third intercostal spaces to the left of the sternum), (3) tricuspid area (left lower sternal border), and (4) mitral area [apex or fifth intercostal space in the left midclavicular line where mitral murmurs and left ventricular sounds (S4, S3) are heard best]. All four areas are auscultated with the diaphragm and bell. When using the diaphragm (for high-pitched sounds), it should be pressed firmly onto the chest. When using the bell (for low-pitched sounds), it should be applied lightly, with only enough pressure to produce an air seal between its rim and the chest.

# Abdomen

The examiner should lower the drape and gown to expose the abdomen and inspect its contour. For descriptive purposes, the abdomen is divided into four quadrants (right upper quadrant, left upper quadrant, right lower quadrant, left lower quadrant) by two imaginary perpendicular lines crossing at the umbilicus. In addition, the "epigastrium" (the region between the right and left upper quadrants directly inferior to the sternum) also is used in describing abdominal findings.

The examiner should auscultate the abdomen, while listening for: (1) the frequency and character of bowel sounds, (2) an aortic bruit (in the midline, above the umbilicus), (3) renal artery bruits, and (4) bruits in the two iliac arteries. Following auscultation, the examiner percusses lightly in all four quadrants to assess the distribution of tympany and dullness. The examiner begins liver percussion in the right midclavicular line at midchest level, percussing downward until reaching the upper border of liver dullness. In the same line, percuss upward from the level of the umbilicus, until reaching the lower border of liver dullness. To assess for splenomegaly, the examiner percusses in the lowest intercostal space in the left anterior axillary line. The examiner then asks the patient to take a deep breath and percusses again. When the size of the spleen is normal, the percussion note remains tympanitic.

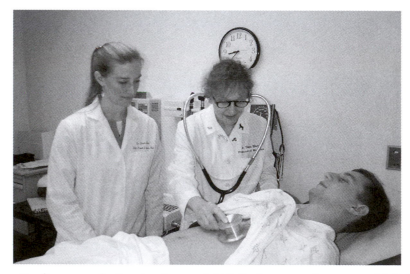

**Big stethoscope.** Cardiac auscultation is a learned skill. Early on, students may think that more senior clinicians are using a special stethoscope.

**159**

BASIC GUIDELINES
FOR THE SCREENING
PHYSICAL
EXAMINATION OF
ADULTS

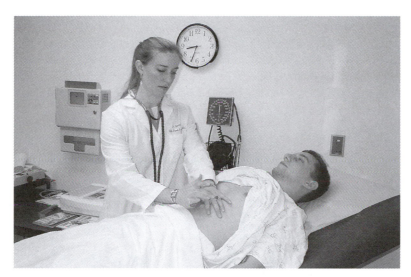

**Abdominal exam.** Resonance superior to the left lower costal margin, when the patient has inhaled deeply, makes significant splenomegaly unlikely.

Palpation begins with light pressure in all four quadrants, followed by deeper palpation. The examiner watches the patient's face to monitor for expressions of discomfort. Using the palmar surfaces of the fingers, the examiner palpates to identify masses or areas of tenderness. The epigastrium should be palpated deeply to delineate the margins of the aorta. To palpate the liver, the examiner places her right hand on the right lower quadrant, pressing gently in and upward. The patient then takes a series of deep breaths, while the palpating hand is moved upward toward the right costal margin. As the patient inhales, the liver edge may be felt as it descends to meet the examiner's fingers.

To examine the spleen, the examiner's right hand is placed at the lower border of the left rib cage, while gentle pressure is exerted upwards and toward the back, as the patient takes a deep breath in and out. The examiner may wish to repeat the examination while the patient lies on his right side. In this position, gravity may bring the spleen forward and medially into a more easily palpable position.

## Lower Extremities

The examiner inspects both limbs from the groin to the toes, noting symmetry, color, skin texture, hair distribution, venous pattern, and whether there is edema. To assess for pitting edema, the examiner presses firmly for up to 15 seconds behind the medial malleolus, over the dorsum of the foot or on the anterior tibia.

The examiner should palpate the following pulses: (1) femoral, (2) popliteal (behind the patient's knee; the patient's knee should be slightly flexed, and the examiner should press the fingertips deeply into the popliteal fossa slightly lateral to the midline), (3) posterior tibial (posterior to the medial malleolus), and (4) dorsalis pedis (dorsum of the foot midway between ankle and toes, between the extensor tendon of the first toe and second toe). In addition, the inguinal lymph nodes in the groin, which drain the lower limbs, conveniently are palpated when evaluating the femoral pulses. The examiner also auscultates the femoral pulses for bruits.

## Reflexes

Reflexes routinely assessed are the biceps, brachioradialis, patellar (knee jerk), and tendoachilles (ankle jerk). The biceps (C5–C6) is examined with the patient's elbow bent at about 90 degrees with his hand relaxed in his lap. The examiner places her thumb against the biceps tendon on the inside of the elbow and taps the thumb with the reflex hammer. The brachioradialis reflex (C5–C6) is performed with the forearm pronated,

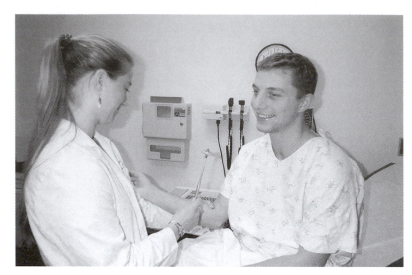

**Reflexes.** To make the hammer strikes consistent, use the hammer's weight to direct its movement and allow the hammer to pivot in the examiner's hand.

and the tendon is struck approximately 4 cm proximal to the radial styloid process. The triceps reflex (C6–C8) is accomplished with the elbow flexed, with the upper arm supported by the examiner or with the patient's hands on the hips. The tendon is struck above the elbow.

For the lower extremities, the patellar tendon (L3–L4) is tapped firmly just below the patella, checking for extension of the knee. With the patient sitting, the examiner's fingers support the patient's dangling foot in mild dorsiflexion, tapping the Achilles tendon ( L5–S1) just above the heel while observing for plantar flexion at the ankle. Gait is evaluated while the patient walks across the room, turns, and returns. The patient is observed for posture, balance, and symmetry of arm swing and leg movements.

## GU Examination

The pelvic and male GU examination are the concluding examination aspects. Men usually are positioned standing with the examiner seated on a stool, to palpate the penis and scrotal contents. Then, the patient faces the examination table for the digital examination. For the pelvic examination, women are in the lithotomy position, with their heads elevated at approximately 30 degrees. These examination components require unique attention to patient comfort, and they are discussed further later in this chapter.

### NORMAL VITAL SIGNS FOR SELECTED AGES

| Age | Heart rate | Blood pressure (normal range is ±15 mm Hg) | Respiratory rate |
|---|---|---|---|
| newborn | 140 | 40/20 | less than 40 |
| 6 months | 130 | 80/45 | 25 to 35 |
| 1 year | 130 | 95/65 | 20 to 30 |
| 5 years | 100 | 100/65 | 12 to 25 |
| 10 years | 75 | 100/65 | 12 to 25 |
| 15 years | 70 | 125/75 | 12 to 18 |

# Assessment of Pediatric Patients

161

BASIC GUIDELINES
FOR THE SCREENING
PHYSICAL
EXAMINATION OF
ADULTS

The physical examination of a child emphasizes milestones of growth and development, preventive healthcare, assessment of the social situation, and providing education to the family (see Tables 8.2 and 8.3). The physical examination is preceded by the examiner and child becoming acquainted, to decrease apprehension associated with the visit. This also allows observation of the interactions between the child and the parent. Clothing should be removed gradually to keep children warm and decrease their stress. During the examination, it is best to begin with areas that will be tolerated easily, rather than adhere to a set sequence. For instance, the ear and throat examination may be saved for last.

The vital signs include charting weight, height, and head circumference, for comparison with standard charts of growth rate. The child's general appearance should be assessed for nutritional status, posture, and gait. Blood pressure measurements require careful attention to cuff size and recognition that normal values differ among age groups. Physical examination components and preventive care aspects unique to pediatric assessment are listed in Tables 8.2 and 8.3.

## Rationale for an Explicit Examination Sequence

Memorizing and adhering to a specific physical examination sequence and using a standard form on which to record findings increase students' ability to consistently perform an efficient examination (Antonelli, 1993). The examination sequence is recapitulated in writing up the examination (Table 8.4a). When studied, learning an explicit pattern decreases students' anxiety when assessing patients and the time needed for the interaction (Klachko & Reid, 1975).

Physical examination abilities, as with any skill, are improved by practice. Medical educators have identified the types of errors examiners make when assessing patients (see Table 8.5) (Wiener & Nathanson, 1976). Two of the three errors are improved by memorizing a specific examination routine. In addition, abilities are enhanced by watching others perform examinations, practicing maneuvers, and obtaining feedback on technique. Reviewing a patient's findings and their interpretation also will calibrate an individual's assessment abilities.

**Table 8.2**
Pediatric Physical Assessment

Vital signs
Chart height, weight, and head circumference; appropriate cuff size for BP assessment; adjust "normal" heart rate and blood pressure for age

Inspection
Skin lesions, bruises, unusual marks (signs of child abuse or neglect); complete skin exam in teens with exposure to sunlight, family history of skin cancer or dysplastic or congenital nevi

HEENT
Visual acuity; evidence ocular misalignment and amblyopia; hearing assessed at 18 months if not previously tested and repeated annually if positive family history or condition predisposing to deafness; dentition and oral hygiene; reactive adenopathy common among children, and of concern when localized or nodes 1.5 cm

Chest
Among small children, respiratory rate (and to a lesser degree heart rate and blood pressure) can vary widely and be influenced by illness and emotion, record whether child was crying during the exam; use the small diaphragm or bell for chest ausculation; observe spine contour for evidence of scoliosis; Tanner stage and breast exam with girls

Cardiac
Until age 7, PMI at or left of midclavicular line, systolic ejection murmurs ("flow" or innocent murmur) and S3 can be normal findings

Abdominal
Liver, spleen, kidneys can be palpated in normal infants, liver often palpable in young children

Genitalia
Males: evidence of hypospadias, undescended testes, hydrocele, and hernia; females: pelvic exam if sexually active

Extremities
Newborn hip dislocation; gait; assess back for scoliosis

Neurologic
Observation of motor skills; gait; be alert for evidence of behavioral or learning disorders, depressive symptoms and suicide risks (such as divorce, alcohol or other illicit substance use, serious medical disorders and bereavement)

**Table 8.3**
Developmental and Preventive Care of Children

| Age | Growth-development | Immunization | Education |
|-----|-------------------|--------------|-----------|
| Newborn to 2 weeks | Lifts head, responds to noise, regards face, follows to midline, turns head side to side | Hepatitis B #1 | Diet: breast, formula, vitamins, fluoride<br>Accident prevention: handling, falling, car seats<br>Behavior: sneezing, hiccups, startle reflex<br>Guidance: spoiling, sib rivalry, pacifier, no bottle in bed, passive smoking |
| 2 months | Vocalizes, lifts head 45°, smiles responsively, follows past midline, kicks | Hepatitis B #2<br>Inactivated polio vaccine (IPV) #1<br>Hemophilus influenza B (Hib) #1<br>Diphtheria/pertussis/tetanus (DPT) #1<br>Heptavalent pneumococcal conjugate vaccine (PC7) #1 | Diet: breast, formula, vitamins, iron, fluoride<br>Accident prevention: car seats, toys, rolling over<br>Behavior: crying, thumb sucking<br>Guidance: where sleeping, colds, taking temperature, acetaminophen/sponging, babysitters |
| 4 months | Lifts head 90°, squeals and laughs, follows 180°, head steady when sitting, grasps rattle, rolls over one way | IPV #2<br>Hib #2<br>DPT #2<br>PCV7 #2 | Diet: breast, formula, weaning, new foods<br>Accident prevention: falling, aspirations, car seats, sharp objects<br>Behavior: drooling, teething<br>Guidance: where sleeping, babysitters, calling physician |
| 6 months | Pulled to sit without head lag, reaches for object, rolls over both ways, smiles spontaneously, sits briefly alone, gums object | Hep B #3<br>IPV #3<br>Hib #3<br>DPT #3<br>PCV7 #3 | Diet: cereal, weaning, no whole milk, new foods<br>Accident prevention: playpen, poisoning, safe highchair, childproof home<br>Behavior: stranger and separation anxiety<br>Guidance: schedule (bedtime/awakening), teething, offer cup, no bottle in bed |
| 9 months | Sits without support, feed self cracker, transfers object from one hand to the other, turns to voice, bangs two cubes, creeps and crawls | | Diet: mashed table foods, finger food, cup<br>Accident prevention: no nuts, candy, or popcorn, electrical outlets, stairs, stove, hot water, car seat, pool<br>Behavior: sitting, crawling, wants to stand<br>Guidance: where sleeping, colds, taking temperature, acetaminophen/sponging, babysitters |
| 12 months | Stands momentarily, walks while holding, plays pat-a-cake, mama and dada, thumb–finger grasp, holds cup to drink | Measles–mumps–rubella (MMR) #1 | Diet: mashed table foods, finger foods, cup<br>Accident prevention: no nuts, candy, or popcorn, electrical outlets, stairs, stove, hot water, car seat, pool<br>Behavior: pulls to stand, nightmares<br>Guidance: consistent discipline, appetite |
| 15 months | Stands and walks alone, builds tower with two cubes, plays pat-a-cake, takes lid off container, drinks from cup | Hib #4<br>DPT #4<br>PCV7 #4<br>Varicella (if lack of reliable history of chickenpox) | Diet: table food, milk (1 pint to 1 quart/day), vitamins, candy<br>Accident prevention: childproof home, matches, stove, bathtubs, teach hot and cold<br>Behavior: self-feeding, simple games<br>Guidance: temper tantrums, family play, masturbation, shoes, bottle, do not start toilet training |
| 18 months | Mimics household chores, stacks three blocks, walks well, climbs, mama, dada, and three words, indicates wants without crying | | Diet: 3 meals per day and snacks<br>Accident prevention: street, refrigerator-freezer, electrical outlets, hot water<br>Behavior: independence/autonomy (''No''), likes action<br>Guidance: toilet training, reading to, temper tantrums, discipline |

**Table 8.3**
(*Continued*)

| Age | Growth-development | Immunization | Education |
|---|---|---|---|
| 24 months | Kicks ball, points to body parts, simple household tasks, stacks six blocks, scribbles, handles spoon well, plays hide and seek, runs well, walks up and down stairs, two-word sentences | PCV7 (single dose, if not previously immunized and older than 24 months) | Diet: 3 meals per day and snacks<br>Behavior: rough and tumble play, sharing<br>Guidance: toilet training, peer play, TV programs, dental care |
| 3 to 6 years | Buttons up (4.2 years), copies square (4.4 years), recognizes 3 colors (4.9 years), hops on 1 foot (4.9 years), throws ball | IPV #4<br>DtaP (acellular pertussis) #5<br>MMR #2 | Diet: 3 meals per day and snacks<br>Accident prevention: street sense, seat belts<br>Behavior: imitates adults, dresses and undresses, brushes teeth<br>Guidance: TV programs, school, bedwetting, separation, chores, attention span |
| 6 to 11 years | School progress, grade achievement, sports, peer relationships, hobbies, stress | Tetanus booster (Td) | Discipline, home conflicts, sex education, contraception, masturbation, smoking, alcohol, drugs, seat belts, helmets |
| 12 to 18 years | | Varicella (if not immunized and lack a reliable history of chickenpox)<br>Varicella #2 (at least 4 weeks following initial dose)<br>Hepatitis B series can be administered to all children and adolescents not previously immunized | |

## CASE 8-3

*S. Y. had a different preceptor each quarter this year. Although all practiced in an ambulatory setting, their "new patient assessment" varied in what examination components were included. Even the same physician did not do the same examinations with each new patient. S. Y. wanted to understand that variability. However, she was reluctant to ask her preceptor about these inconsistencies, because of concern that these questions would challenge Dr. T.'s competence. S. Y. wondered what strategy she would use for a complete examination when assigned to the clerkships.*

## WHY DO PHYSICAL EXAMINATIONS DIFFER?

Although most medical students learn similar physical examination skills, practicing physicians differ in their choice and sequence of maneuvers. That variability has been documented using standardized patients (SPs). SPs are individuals trained to portray a patient, and interactions with SPs are a method to evaluate an individual's patient assessment abilities. To observe what physicians actually do, consenting primary care practitioners were visited by an SP, masquerading as a new patient. Despite consistency in the patient's history, the evaluations varied from 5 to 60 minutes in length, and the recommended examination components performed ranged from 16 to 89% (Carney *et al.*, 1993).

Variability among physicians reflects their preferences, visit circumstances, and patient characteristics. For example, the chance detection of an unusual abnormality might bias an examiner to continue that maneuver, despite evidence that it is not a useful part of the examination. Time limitations and anticipation of follow-up examinations also can influence the choice of examination components. In addition, patient

**Table 8.4a**
Example of Written Physical Examination

Vital signs: weight = 162 lb   height = 68 inches (reported, not measured)
   BP = 178/94 right = left arm sitting   pulse = 78 regular
General appearance = healthy appearing, muscular man, neatly groomed, in no distress, looking stated age
Skin = clear except for 2 × 2-cm tattoo of heart left buttock; no striae, ecchymosis; nails normal
Heard = normocephalic, atraumatic; facial features normal in size and proportion
Eyes = conjunctiva clear, anicteric; no proptosis or lid lag
   PERRL, EOM full, no sustained nystagmus
   20/30 both eyes corrected by near card
   visual fields full to confrontation
   fundi normal A:V ratio at 1:2, no AV nicking, no hemorrhages or exudates; disk margins sharp, cup to disk ratio normal
Ears = canals clear, TMS normal light reflex
Nose = septum midline and intact, membranes normal, no discharge
Mouth = teeth in good repair, oropharynx clear
Neck = supple, full ROM; no thryoid gland appreciated, trachea midline, no adenopathy
Nodes = no nodes palpable in cervical regions, axillae, inguinal areas
Chest = normal chest configuration, 4 cm of diaphragmatic excursion bilaterally, clear to percussion and auscultation bilaterally without
   rales or wheezes
Cardiac = jugular venous pressure @ 6 cm water
   carotids brisk bilaterally, without bruits
   PMI discrete in 5th intercostal space just medial to the midclavicular line
   S1 normal, S2 physiologically split
   no murmurs or extra sounds
Breasts = no gynecomastia or tenderness
Abdomen = flat; bowel sounds present, no bruits; normal percussion resonance; soft, nontender; liver 10 cm in rt. midclavicular line, edge
   not palpable
   no spleen or masses palpable
Genitourinary = normal male genitalia, circumcised, no scrotal masses, no hernias
Rectal = normal rectal tone, prostate smooth and not enlarged, no masses, hemoccult negative stool
Extremities = radial, femoral, popliteal, posterior tibial and dorsalis pedis pulses all present and symmetric
   no clubbing, edema, or evidence of joint deformities
Cranial nerves = I not tested
   II see Eyes
   III, IV, VI EOM intact
   V facial sensation intact and symmetric, jaw strength normal
   VII facial expression normal
   VIII see Ears
   IX, X uvula midline, gag and phonation normal
   XI normal shrug
   XII tongue symmetric in midline
Reflexes = 2+/= @ biceps, patella, Achilles
Sensation = vibratory sense normal both feel (only sensation I assessed)
Coordination and gait = walks briskly, with symmetric arm swing; able to tandem walk
Mental status = alert, appropriate, fluent speech, normal affect, intellectual functions not further assessed

characteristics can affect which examination maneuvers are performed. For example, it has been shown that obese women are less likely to receive a pelvic examination than are nonobese women.

## CASE 8-3 (continued)

*S. Y. had been reluctant to ask Dr. T. about variability in examination components. However, the preceptor had encouraged the student's questions, and finally, S. Y. related her observations about how examinations varied. The observation led to an interesting discussion about what was known about each examination component's utility, which were advocated by different groups, and how Dr. T. came to include certain parts of the examination. The student brought the issue up with her classmates, and they shared similar experiences. Her physical assessment group even talked about a* project to observe their preceptors, gather information on what was done, and define variability in the "screening" examination.

165

WHY DO PHYSICAL
EXAMINATIONS
DIFFER?

## How Useful and Accurate Are Specific Examination Maneuvers?

In recent years, investigators have focused on the utility of physical assessment maneuvers in identifying illness (Fitzgerald, 1990; Hayward *et al.*, 1991; Sox, 1994). Studying the physical examination components has been a challenge, as it is difficult to assemble large numbers of appropriate patients, recruit clinicians with similar training, and compare findings against a "gold standard." Table 8.6 lists information about examination maneuvers and whether sufficient evidence exists to recommend them for a well-patient screening examination. "Not recommended" means the component was considered, but evidence supporting its performance was weak. "Not considered" indicates the maneuver was not evaluated by the authors or an expert panel.

Few patient encounters are exclusively "well-patient" or "screening" examinations. Most interactions are shaped by both the patient's complaints and the prevalence of disorders in the patient's demographic group. For example, an individual complaining of dyspnea would receive close attention on the cardiac and pulmonary examinations, because those systems are likely to reveal the complaint's etiology. A teenager being seen for a "sports physical" would be assessed for abnormalities of joint range of motion, an examination aspect that might not otherwise be performed. Using the history to select examination components is analogous to relying on a patient's history and physical examination findings to select laboratory tests and evaluate results in the context of the prior probability of disease.

### CASE 8-4

*Presenting a patient's history and physical examination at the bedside made the student, N. S., feel uneasy. N. S. was concerned that he might say something that the patient would misinterpret or find embarrassing. However, the attending physician demanded bedside rounds, and the student had practiced the presentation with the team's senior resident. The student was surprised when the attending asked the patient a question identical to his and received a different answer. And, he was embarrassed when he could not remember the liver span in centimeters, as he only had written "normal." His uneasiness was heightened when the murmur he had heard the night before was not heard on rounds. He wondered what had gone wrong and what he could do to avoid these events happening again.*

## Why Don't Examiners Agree on Their Physical Examination Findings?

Clinicians frequently disagree about physical examination findings. Agreement between observers (interobserver reliability) relates to patient factors, examiner influences, and the clinical setting (see Table 8.7) (Department of Clinical Epidemiology and Biostatistics, McMaster University, 1980a; Koran, 1975). The reliability relates to how much confidence or diagnostic certainty can be placed on a finding.

Percent agreement is not an accurate index of interobserver agreement. Disagreement is measured better by concordance, which takes into account both the "true" agreement of observers and the amount of agreement that would occur by chance. Table 8.8 presents an example illustrating the difference between percent agreement and concordance (measured by the kappa statistic). After examining the same 100 men (85 of whom have true prostate enlargement), two different examiners' findings are shown. The percent agreement is misleadingly high because of the high prevalence of the abnormality.

When evaluating studies of physical examination reliability, look for measures of concordance. The kappa statistic is often used (Maclure & Willett, 1987), and a kappa of +1 is perfect agreement, 0 is chance agreement, and −1 is total disagreement. When used to assess interobserver agreement, a kappa greater than

**Table 8.4b**
Abbreviations Used in the Medical Write-Up

| | | | |
|---|---|---|---|
| AAA | abdominal aortic aneurysm | GC | gonococcal |
| ABG | arterial blood gas | GI | gastrointestinal |
| ac | before meals | GSW | gunshot wound |
| ADL | activities of daily living | gtt | drops |
| AI | aortic insufficiency | GU | genitourinary |
| AK | above the knee | HBP | high blood pressure |
| AMA | against medical advice | H & E | hemorrhages and exudates |
| AMI | acute or anterior myocardial infarction | HEENT | head, eyes, ears, nose, and throat |
| AP | anterior and posterior | h/o | history of |
| AS | aortic stenosis | HPI | history of present illness |
| ASA | acetylsalicylic acid (aspirin) | HTN | hypertension |
| ASAP | as soon as possible | Hx | history |
| ASVD | atherosclerotic vascular disease | I & D | incision and drainage |
| A & W | alive and well | IM | intramuscular |
| BBB | bundle branch block | IMI | inferior myocardial infarction |
| BE | barium enema | IV | intravenous |
| BID | twice a day | IVC | inferior vena cava |
| BK | below the knee | IVP | intravenous pylogram |
| BM | bowel movement | JVD | jugular venous distension |
| BMI | body mass index | JVP | jugular venous pressure |
| BP | blood pressure | Ks | kidneys |
| BPH | benign prostatic hypertrophy | KUB | kidneys, ureters, and bladder |
| BRBPR | bright red blood per rectum | LLQ | lower left quadrant |
| BRP | bathroom privileges | LMP | last menstrual period |
| BS | bowel sounds | LOC | loss of consciousness |
| Bx | biopsy | LOL | little old lady |
| CA | cancer | LP | lumbar puncture |
| CABG | coronary arterial bypass graft | L, S, Ks | liver, spleen, and kidneys |
| CAD | coronary artery disease | LLQ | left lower quadrant |
| CBC | complete blood count | m | murmur |
| CBG | capillary blood glucose | MCL | midclavicular line |
| CC | chief complaint | MI | myocardial infarction or mitral insufficiency |
| C, C, E | cyanosis, clubbing, and edema | MR | mitral regurgitation |
| CHD | congenital heart disease | MS | mitral stenosis or multiple sclerosis |
| CHF | congestive heart failure | NAD | no acute distress |
| CNS | central nervous system | NC/AT | normocephalic and atraumatic |
| C/O | complaint of | NKDA | no known drug allergies |
| COPD | chronic obstructive pulmonary disease | NPO | nothing by mouth |
| C-section | Cesarean section | N/V | nausea and vomiting |
| CSF | cerebrospinal fluid | O × 3 | oriented to person, place, and time |
| CVA | cerebrovascular accident | OD | ocular dexter or right eye |
| CVP | central venous pressure | OR | operating room |
| CXR | chest x-ray | OS | ocular sinister or left eye |
| D & C | dilation and curettage | OTC | over the counter |
| DIP | distal interphalangeal | OU | both eyes |
| DJD | degenerative joint disease | P & A | percussion and auscultation |
| DM | diabetes mellitus | pc | after meals |
| DNR | do not resuscitate | PE | physical examination |
| DOE | dyspnea on exertion | PERRL & A | pupils equal, round, and reactive to light and accommodation |
| DT | delirium tremens | | |
| DTR | deep tendon reflex | PHx | past history |
| DVT | deep venous thrombosis | PI | present illness |
| Dx | diagnosis | PID | pelvic inflammatory disease |
| ECG/EKG | electrocardiogram | PMI | point of maximal impulse |
| ENT | ear, nose, and throat | PND | paroxysmal nocturnal dyspnea |
| EOM | extraocular movements | po | per os or by mouth |
| ETOH | alcohol | PRN | give as needed |
| FHT | fetal heart tones | PTA | prior to admission |
| F Hx | family history | PUD | peptic ulcer disease |
| FUO | fever of undetermined origin | PVD | peripheral vascular disease |
| g | gallop (S3 or S4) | Q | every |

Table 8.4b
(*Continued*)

167

WHY DO PHYSICAL
EXAMINATIONS
DIFFER?

| QHS | at bedtime | S/P | status post (following) |
|---|---|---|---|
| QID | four times a day | STAT | immediately |
| qns | quantity not sufficient | STD | sexually transmitted disease |
| QOD | every other day | Sx | symptom |
| r | rub | T & A | tonsils and adenoids |
| RA | rheumatoid arthritis | TAH & BSO | total abdominal hysterectomy and bilateral |
| RAD | reactive airway disease (asthma) | | salpingo-oophorectomy |
| RCM | right costal margin | TB | tuberculosis |
| RF | rheumatic fever | TIA | transient ischemic attack |
| RLQ | right lower quadrant | TID | three times a day |
| R/O | rule out | TM | tympanic membrane |
| ROM | range of motion | TMJ | temporomandibular joint |
| ROS | review of systems | UA | urinalysis |
| RUQ | right upper quadrant | UCD | usual childhood diseases |
| Rx | treatment | UGI | upper gastrointestinal radiograph |
| s | without | URI | upper respiratory infection |
| SC | subcutaneously | UTI | urinary tract infection |
| SCUT | some current urgent tasks | VD | venereal disease |
| S & CVAT | spine and costovertebral angle tenderness | VS | vital signs |
| SEM | systolic ejection murmur | VT | ventricular tachycardia |
| SH | social history | WD/WN | well developed and well nourished |
| SL | sublingual | WNL | within normal limits |
| SLE | systemic lupus erythematosus | W/U | workup |
| Sn | sign | x | except |
| SNF | skilled nursing facility | yo | years old |
| SOB | shortness of breath | | |

0.6 is substantial agreement, 0.2 to 0.6 is fair to moderate agreement, and less than 0.2 is slight or poor agreement.

## Examiner Factors

A physician's clinical performance is not constant, and that variability is a source of examination unreliability (Table 8.7). This inconsistency has been shown by having interns read ECGs when tired and when well rested. Their skill in interpreting ECG rhythms varied with the amount of rest they had (Asken & Raham, 1983). Among busy clinicians, fatigue, transient physical limitations, such as a serous otitis affecting hearing, and other distractions can impact on physical assessment abilities.

Table 8.5
Types of Physical Diagnosis Errors

Technique and detection
    Causing patient discomfort or embarrassment
    Improper use of instruments or performance of the examination
    Failure to perform part of the examination
    Missing a finding
Detection and interpretation
    Reporting a finding that is not present
    Incorrect identification or interpretation of findings
    Lack of knowledge or use of confirming signs
Recording
    Forgetting to record a finding
    Illegible handwriting, obscure abbreviations, or improper terminology
    Recording an interpretation, rather than the findings

**Table 8.6**
Recommended Physical Examination Practices for Adults

| | Comments | Canadian Task Force | U.S. Preventive Services Task Force (1989) | Oboler and LaForce (1989) | American College of Physicians |
|---|---|---|---|---|---|
| Blood pressure | Affected by cuff size and arm position, elevation due to a "white coat" hypertension can lead to misinterpretation | At least every 5 years, and after age 65, every 1 to 2 years | At least every 1 to 2 years, and annually after age 65 | At least every 1 to 2 years | At least every 1 to 2 years and annually if risk factors for coronary artery disease |
| Height and weight | | If adolescent, women of low socioeconomic status, or unusual dietary habits | Every 1 to 3 years after age 40, and annually after age 65 | Every 4 years | Not considered |
| Visual acuity | Record best corrected vision | Not considered | Annually after age 65 | Annually after age 60 | Not considered |
| Hearing | Most accurately assessed using audioscope | After age 18, if noise exposure | Annually after age 65, and begin at age 19 if noise exposure | Annually after age 60 by audioscope | Not considered |
| Oral cavity | Assess both mucosa and dentition | After age 65 or after age 18, if uses tobacco | After age 18, if uses tobacco or alcohol | Not recommended | Annual dental exam; mouth exam not recommended |
| Skin inspection | Higher risk if excess sun exposure, dysplastic nevi, >6 moles more than 5 mm in diameter, or family history of melanoma | Annually after age 18 if excess sun exposure or dysplastic nevi | After age 18 if excess sun exposure, dysplastic nevi, or history of skin cancer | Evaluate for dysplastic nevi at initial visit; annually for high-risk patients | Not considered |
| Auscultate carotids | Bruits are marker for ASVD; bruit absence does not exclude stenosis | Not recommended | If risks for ASVD or symptoms of cerebrovascular disease; every 1 to 3 years after age 40, and annually after age 65 | Not recommended | Not considered |
| Breast | Reinforce self-exam skills and that mammography adds to detection rates | Annually after age 40, and after age 35 if family history of breast cancer | Annually after age 40, and after age 35 if family history of breast cancer | Annually after age 40, and after age 35 if family history of breast cancer | Annually after age 40, and after age 35 if family history of breast cancer |
| Chest exam | | Not considered | Not considered | Not recommended | Not considered |
| Cardiac | Important component for "sports physical," as asymmetric septal hypertrophy is most common cause of sudden death among young athletes | Not considered | Not considered | Auscultate for valvular disease at initial visit and when age 60 | Not considered |
| Abdomen | | Not considered | Not considered | Palpate for abdominal aortic aneurysm annually in men over 60 | Not considered |

**Table 8.6**
*(Continued)*

| | Comments | Canadian Task Force | U.S. Preventive Services Task Force (1989) | Oboler and LaForce (1989) | American College of Physicians |
|---|---|---|---|---|---|
| Stool occult blood | | Not recommended unless family history of colon cancer, then annually after age 40 | Annually after age 50 | Annually after age 50, and begin at age 40 if family history of colon cancer | Annually after age 50, and begin at age 40 if family history of colon cancer |
| Lymph nodes | | Not considered | Not considered | Not recommended | Not considered |
| Musculoskeletal exam | | Not recommended | Not recommended | Back exam not recommended | Not considered |
| Bimanual pelvic examination | | Not considered | Cervical cytology every 1 to 3 years; routine pelvic exams not recommended | Cervical cytology if sexually active, after 2 negative annual cytological exams, cervical cytology at least every 3 years; palpation of ovaries not recommended | Pelvic exam not considered; cervical cytology every 1 to 3 years |
| Digital prostate palpation | American Cancer Society and National Cancer Institute recommend annually after age 50, and if increased risk for prostate cancer, at age 40 | Not recommended | Not recommended | Not recommended | Not recommended |
| Mental status | Several studies document that dementia is often missed | Not recommended | Not recommended | Not recommended | After age 65 |

In addition, practitioners often record "interpretations," rather than specific examination findings. These inferences lose objective clinical information and can be misinterpreted. For example, "no hepatomegaly" conveys less information than recording the liver's percussion span. A normal-sized 8 cm liver could enlarge 2 cm and its size would still be "normal." Similarly, writing "normal mental status" omits results of specific mental status components and assumes examiners share common tests and standards.

**Table 8.7**
Causes for Clinical Disagreement

Examiner
    Biologic variation in the senses
    Tendency to record inferences or classifications rather than evidence
    Bias from prior experiences
    Incorrect use of diagnostic tools
Patient
    Biologic variation in organ systems
    Changes related to illnesses' natural history and management
Setting and equipment
    Disruptive examination environments
    Malfunction or absence of examination equipment

**Table 8.8**
Calculating Agreement and Concordance
of Two Physicians' Examination Findings

|  |  | Observer B's findings | | |
|---|---|---|---|---|
|  |  | Abnormal | Normal |  |
| Observer A's findings | Abnormal | 75 | 10 | 85 |
|  | Normal | 9 | 6 | 15 |
|  |  | 84 | 16 | 100 |

Results when 100 men were examined by two observers. For 75 + 6 patients, both observers agreed, and 10 + 9 individuals were called abnormal by only one observer. Percent agreement = (75 + 6) ÷ 100 = 0.81 (81%). However, the calculated kappa = 0.18 (slight or poor agreement).

Prior experiences and biases also influence clinicians' interpretation of findings. The effect of bias was shown when investigators trained two female patients to present the same information concerning their chest pain. When the first woman was dressed in a business suit and calmly articulated her symptoms, half of the physicians felt that she needed further diagnostic studies. However, when the second woman was dressed less "professionally" and appeared more flamboyant in her manner, only 18% advised further testing, despite identical verbal information. Although risk factors and description of symptoms were similar, the patient's style and physicians' interpretation of the patient's style affected management (Birdwell *et al.*, 1993).

## Patient Components

Biologic variability can account for inconsistency of physical assessment findings (Table 8.7). For example, pleural and pericardial rubs vary with patient position, and distribution of rhonchi can change after a deep cough. The effects of medication, for example, using a narcotic analgesic, and other treatments further compound physical findings' inconsistency.

## Examination Setting

The clinical environment impacts on the examination reliability. Background noise level and examination equipment affect one's ability to perform portions of the examination and recognize abnormalities. For example, "white coat hypertension" can be resolved in a more relaxed setting. Detecting jaundice or pallor in a dimly lit room and auscultating cardiac findings in a noisy clinic are difficult. Time constraints, lack of ancillary help, and a high examination table can result in assessing paretic individuals in their wheelchairs, rather than on the examination table, which could influence the examiner's findings.

### CASE 8-4 (continued)

*N. S. could have decreased the chance that physical assessment findings would vary by minimizing effects of the patient, examiner, and setting. As he reflected back on the patient encounter, N. S. remembered that his examination had been interrupted twice to deal with other issues. He may not have focused his full attention on the interaction. He decided that, in the future, he would record precise findings. Because the student had limited clinical experience, he was not subject to its bias. However, he recognized that examinations recorded in the old chart biased his assessment. Next time, he would reexamine the patient prior to attending rounds and compare his results with other examiners. In addition, he was convinced that it was time to buy a better stethoscope.*

**171**

HOW DOES THE
PHYSICAL
EXAMINATION
AFFECT THE
PHYSICIAN–PATIENT
RELATIONSHIP?

**Table 8.9**
Strategies Minimizing Clinical Disagreement

Examiner limitations minimized by
    Practicing skills and calibrate the examination with a broad range of findings
    Seeking corroboration of key findings (repeating oneself and examination by others)
    Asking "blinded" (nonbiased) examiners to assess the patient
    Confirming key clinical findings with appropriate tests
    Reporting evidence rather than inferences
Patient limitations minimized by
    Repeating assessments to evaluate tempo of an illness and expected changes
Setting limitations minimized by
    Matching the environment to the diagnostic task
    Establishing appropriate rapport prior to the examination
    Using appropriate examination tools

## What Can Examiners Do to Reduce Examination Variability?

There are several ways to reduce clinical disagreement and increase an examination's reliability (see Table 8.9) (Department of Clinical Epidemiology and Biostatistics, McMaster University, 1980b). It often is useful to ask a colleague to repeat portions of the history or physical examination to confirm findings. The second examiner assesses the patient with limited historical information, to remove the effects of bias.

Relating findings to a "gold standard" also will refine an examiner's abilities. For example, comparing the examination for ascites with an abdominal ultrasound, chest findings with the radiograph, and cardiac auscultation with echocardiographic findings increases an examiner's abilities. In addition, repeatedly assessing patients over time acquaints practitioners with the potential variability of findings.

## CASE 8-5

*During hospital rounds, things moved quickly. T. J. knew his role as third-year clerk was to preround and obtain vital signs, review the chart for any new developments, and be prepared to briefly report his findings. Although he did not say much on rounds, T. J. tried to observe all he could about patients and others on the team. The staff physician, Dr. T., always checked a patient's pulse as the first thing. He usually would check the right radial pulse with his left hand, while using his right hand to clasp the patient's right hand. Dr. T. had related that it was something that he began doing as a resident and continued to do. He felt that it was a way to make physical contact and connect with the patient, rather than directly go to examining the wound. T. J. was trying different styles and ways to interact, and this was one that he wanted to try.*

## HOW DOES THE PHYSICAL EXAMINATION AFFECT THE PHYSICIAN–PATIENT RELATIONSHIP?

The physical examination provides information and enhances physician–patient rapport. Study of physician–patient interactions indicates that time spent on the physical examination is positively correlated with patient satisfaction (Robbins *et al.*, 1993). Extrapolating from studies of the interview, maintaining patient comfort, avoiding patient embarrassment, and demonstrating facility with the examination enhance patient satisfaction. Having a clear rationale for performing specific physical examination components can help explain to a patient why examination items were omitted or performed.

Physical contact during the examination may have therapeutic benefits. Touch also can have adverse effects. When objectively assessed, more touching during an office visit correlated with lower patient

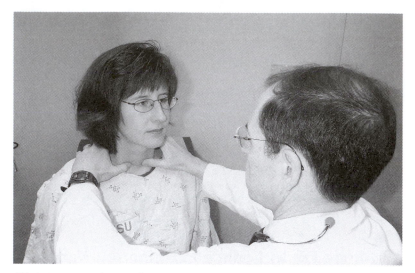

**MD at bedside.** Clinicians may have idiosyncratic features of their bedside exams. Understanding the rationale for different components allows students to adopt selected aspects, as they develop their own examination patterns.

satisfaction (Larsen & Smith, 1981). However, these investigators did not differentiate new from follow-up visits nor determine whether the touch was a response to patient distress. Nevertheless, the findings show that nonverbal actions can negatively influence the physician–patient relationship.

## CASE 8-6

*Ms. F. did not like these annual examinations, but she knew that they were important. Now that she was in her 40s, she had some questions about "menopause." The nurse had asked her to remove her clothing, and she waited in the room dressed only in a gown, with a paper drape across her lap. She was surprised when Dr. K. entered the room with a student, although she had seen the sign concerning medical students being in the office. Perhaps the surprise on her face resulted in Dr. K.'s attempt at humor as he prepared for the pelvic examination and asked, "Did you remember to bring your cervix?"*

## WHICH PHYSICAL EXAMINATION COMPONENTS REQUIRE SPECIAL ATTENTION TO PATIENT COMFORT?

The breast, pelvic, and genitourinary examinations are most likely to result in patient embarrassment and feelings of vulnerability. These examinations require special attention to patient comfort. Physicians also

---

*The use of "manual therapy" or "therapeutic" touch has generated extensive literature and national and international organizations to share experiences (Carruthers, 1992; Fishman et al., 1995; Krieger, 1979). Data substantiating the use of touch primarily are anecdotal, and these techniques' utility has not been assessed rigorously.*

---

173

WHICH PHYSICAL
EXAMINATION
COMPONENTS
REQUIRES SPECIAL
ATTENTION TO
PATIENT COMFORT?

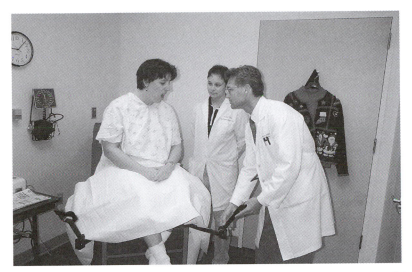

**Woman, MD, and student in exam room on table with stirrups.** Certain aspects of the exam require extra attention to patient comfort.

report anxiety when performing these examinations. Examiner distress has been shown to decrease when these feelings are acknowledged as common and discussed with colleagues (Lang, 1990). Talking about these feelings is preferable to more maladaptive behaviors, such as avoiding the examination or attempting inappropriate sexual humor.

## Pelvic and Genitourinary Examination

In the last 15 years, gynecologic teaching associates or standardized patients have taught the complex motor and verbal skills of the pelvic and breast examination (Beckmann *et al.*, 1992; Wallis *et al.*, 1983). Teaching associates are similar to SPs, in that their examination findings are known, and they can provide feedback on an examiner's skills. Teaching associates also educate students and provide explicit instruction on students' examination abilities. Importantly, teaching associates can teach and discuss appropriate verbal and nonverbal behaviors during performance of the history and physical examination.

Features of a pelvic examination that reduce women's anxiety include obtaining a history while the patient is dressed, rather than when she is disrobed on the examination table (Weiss & Meadow, 1979). Distress is decreased further by performing the examination in an unhurried manner and informing patients about findings (Weiss & Meadow, 1979). Monitoring a woman's comfort is facilitated by elevating the head of the examination table. Allowing a woman to dress before discussing findings reduces her feelings of vulnerability.

Physicians' practices vary concerning the presence of a chaperon during the pelvic examination. This variability is paralleled by surveys of patients' preferences (Patton *et al.*, 1990; Penn & Bourguet, 1992). Although women did not want a chaperon with a female examiner, approximately half preferred one with male examiners. When being evaluated by a male examiner, women (especially teenagers) should be given the option of a chaperon.

## Breast Examination

An examiner's actions during the breast examination are important for detection of abnormalities. It is an opportunity to review breast self-examination recommendations and technique. This review should not be limited to women who admit a lack of skill, as research documents that women's self-rating has a low correlation with their measured abilities (Stratton *et al.*, 1994).

The breast examination can influence a woman's behavior regarding self-examination and her adherence to recommendations for mammography. The factor most affecting mammography rate is the physician's personal recommendation and enthusiasm about mammography's importance (Fox *et al.*, 1994; Friedman *et al.*, 1994; Johnson & Meischke, 1994). Paradoxically, studies indicate that an increase in self-examination skills may decrease the rate of mammography. To avoid this result, the examiner should emphasize that self-examination adds to mammography. A normal self-examination does not negate mammography's utility and vice versa.

## Male Genitourinary Examination

The U.S. Preventive Services Task Force recommends a genitourinary examination for men with a history of cryptorchidism, orchiopexy, or testicular atrophy (U.S. Preventive Services Task Force, 1989). However, most individuals with a testicular malignancy have none of these risks, and others recommend that this procedure and education about testicular self-examination be included during all routine examinations (Vogt & McHale, 1992).

Unlike the pelvic examination, male patients' reactions to a genitourinary examination have not been well studied. Current recommendations are an extension of findings from women's pelvic examinations. Men differ from women in their preference for chaperons during the examination. When studied, 46% of female adolescents wanted a chaperon during the pelvic examination; however, male teens preferred that no chaperon be present during the genitourinary examination (Penn & Bourguet, 1992).

## CONCLUSION

Physical examination abilities are important for confirming diagnostic impressions, detecting abnormalities, documenting progression of illness, and enhancing the physician–patient relationship. As with any diagnostic test, or maneuver, physical assessment has its limitations. Being aware of those limits can allow minimizing factors that decrease examination reliability. A beginning student benefits from learning a basic examination sequence. The basic sequence will remain constant, and it forms a framework on which practitioners will refine their patient assessment abilities throughout their careers.

## CASES FOR DISCUSSION

### CASE 17

*Mr. T. is a 58-year-old man complaining of leg pains. His history is remarkable for 12 years of diabetes and 8 years of hypertension. A. S. is a second-year student working with his preceptor, and he has first contact with Mr. T. today. The student was thinking that seeing this patient was "great," as he had learned about diabetic neuropathies just last week. The student began with a neurologic examination, including assessment of light touch and vibratory sense. He finished the neurologic assessment with gait testing and a Romberg test. While Mr. T. got back on the examination table, A. S. rewashed his hands, then obtained vital signs and began the head and neck examination. After the abdominal examination, the student asked the patient to stand for the rectal. While Mr. T. returned to the table, the student washed his hands again and completed his examination of the extremities and peripheral pulses.*

1. *A. S. thought that the "money" (that is, the examination that was most likely to have findings related to the patient's complaint) was in the neurologic examination. What is wrong with that approach?*
2. *Why is it useful to learn a specific physical examination sequence?*
3. *How do you think the examination was perceived by Mr. T.?*

## CASE 2

*Y. R. is a man who just turned 40 years old, and at the insistence of his wife, he comes in for a "checkup." He also is motivated to make the appointment because a neighbor his age had died recently of a myocardial infarction. Mr. R. has not seen a physician for many years. He has no history of medical problems, and he is feeling well. You are about to begin the physical examination.*

1. *What aspects of the physical examination are of "proven" value for Mr. R.?*
2. *What aspects of the physical examination would you perform? Why?*
3. *How could you define what aspects of the examination Mr. R. thinks would or should be performed? How can you avoid accomplishing that task without appearing as though you don't know what to do? What would you say or do if after completing what you think is indicated, Mr. R. asks, "Is that all you're going to do? I had wanted a complete exam."*

## CASE 3

*The student reentered the examination room with her preceptor. She had explained that Ms. P. was at the clinic for follow-up of her treatment for hypertension. Today, the student had measured the blood pressure as 160/90 mm Hg. The physician began by rechecking the pressure and called out a value of 132/80 mm Hg. He also auscultated the patient's precordium, and holding the diaphragm of the stethoscope to Ms. P.'s chest, he handed the student the earpieces, saying, "Do you hear this systolic murmur?"*

1. *Did the student take the blood pressure incorrectly?*
2. *What factors contribute to unreliability of the examination and how might they relate to this situation?*
3. *The student listened, but couldn't hear a murmur. She did hear the preceptor advising her to "listen hard." What are the student's options in the situation? If she says that she can't hear a murmur, will the patient think that the preceptor is an ineffective teacher?*

## CASE 4

*The student was aware of universal precautions to prevent transmission of HIV disease. Ms. J. (an asymptomatic patient who is HIV positive) had no open skin lesions, but the student had fingertip eczema, with plaques and cracking of his fingertips. The student wondered whether he should put on gloves before beginning the physical examination.*

1. *Should the student put on gloves? How might their use affect Ms. J.?*
2. *How does physical contact affect the physician–patient relationship? How could it enhance the relationship? How might it adversely influence physician–patient rapport?*

## CASE 5

*R. D. is a 2-year-old boy who is brought in by his mother for follow-up of otitis media. It is his third episode this winter. You do not know it, but the mother particularly is worried, as she just saw a TV show that investigated a young boy's death during myringotomy tube placement. R. D. is rambunctious during the history, and his mother lets him make a mess of the examination room. He squirms during the examination and won't cooperate with the otoscopic assessment. He keeps shaking his head and turning away from you.*

1. *Give examples of how a toddler's behavior and parent interactions would provide "diagnostic information" for the physical assessment.*
2. *What could have been done to make the examination easier? Should you comment on the child's behavior? How would you do that?*

## CASE 6

*H. D. is a 14-year-old boy whom you are seeing at your preceptor's office. He is here for a "sports physical" examination, which often includes a GU examination to identify two descended, normal testes (at least that's what F. D., a first-year student, thinks she remembers). Things start out well, and the student thinks her prolonged small talk with H. D. will make the examination easier. However, when she reaches the point for the GU examination, H. D. says, "No way."*

1. *What aspects of the interaction influenced H. D.'s reaction (both positively and negatively)?*
2. *What could have been done to make the patient's reaction less likely? The only other male on the clinic staff was a high school work study student. Should the student have gotten him as a chaperon?*

## RECOMMENDED READINGS

Bickley LS, Hoekelman RA, Bates B: *Bates' Guide to Physical Examination and History Taking*, ed 7. Philadelphia, JB Lippincott Co, 1998.

> Initial edition was published in 1974; it provides explicit guidelines on physical examination maneuvers. The text is large and bulky, and it is similar in size to several other books (such as Seidel, 1999; Swartz, 2001; Willms *et al.*, 1994); a videotape series and a pocket-sized edition ("baby Bates") also are available.

DeGowin RL, Brown DD: *DeGowin's Diagnostic Examination*. New York, McGraw–Hill Book Co, 1999.

> Original edition was by Richard DeGowin's father, and the book is in its seventh edition; this 4- by 6-inch soft-backed book is organized by systems and findings; its structure makes it an efficient, useful source for looking things up but not as helpful when trying to learn the examination.

Elliot DL, Goldberg L: *The Clinical Examination Casebook*. Boston, Little, Brown & Co, 1996.

> This book does the best job of bridging the gap between the basic physical examination guides and medical textbooks (we might be biased); brief patient vignettes, accompanied by a narrative text and tables, show how patient assessment is used to define abnormalities.

Macklis RM, Mendelson ME, Mudge GH Jr: *Introduction to Clinical Medicine: A Student-to-Student Manual*. Boston, Little Brown & Co, 1994.

> Several different paperback books attempt to meet the needs of beginning clerks; along with physical examination information, they contain advice about ward routine, presenting cases and medical "workups."

## ANNOTATED REFERENCES

Antonelli MA: Usefulness of a data-collection form in learning physical diagnosis. *Acad Med* 68:171, 1993. (Brief letter that reviewed students' write-ups and found standard history and physical exam forms were useful and not a "crutch.")

Asken MJ, Raham DC: Resident performance and sleep deprivation: A review. *J Med Educ* 58:382–388, 1983.

Beckmann CRB, Lipscomb GH, Williford L, *et al*: Gynecological teaching associates in the 1990s. *Med Edu* 26:105–109, 1992. (The authors point out the unique advantages to this teaching method: immediate firsthand feedback on abilities, and a relaxed and supportive learning environment; they also caution that budget constraints may compromise this educational strategy.)

Bickley LS, Hoeklman, RA, Bates, B: *Bates' Guide to Physical Examination and History Taking*, ed 7: Philadelphia, JB Lippincott Co, 1998.

Birdwell BG, Herbers JE, Kroenke K: Evaluating chest pain. *JAMA* 153:1991–1995, 1993.

Canadian Task Forces on the Periodic Health Examination: The periodic health examination: 2; 1987 update. *Can Med Assoc J* 138;619–628, 1988.

Carney PA, Dietrich AJ, Freeman DH Jr, Mott LA: The period health examination provided to asymptomatic older women: An assessment using standardized patients. *Ann Intern Med* 119:129–135, 1993. [98 physicians (one-third IM and two-third FM) were visited by a standardized patient for a check-up; physician–patient interactions varied from 5 to 60 minutes (average 28 minutes), and percentage of the recommended examination components varied from 16 to 89%.]

Carruthers A: A force to promote bonding and well-being: Therapeutic touch and massage. *Prof Nurse* 7:297–300, 1992. (This author briefly reviews therapeutic touch.)

Department of Clinical Epidemiology and Biostatistics, McMaster University: Clinical disagreement: I. How often it occurs and why. *Can Med Assoc J* 123:499–504, 1980a.

Department of Clinical Epidemiology and Biostatistics, McMaster University: Clinical disagreement: II. How to avoid it and how to learn from one's mistakes. *Can Med Assoc J* 123:499–504, 1980b. (These two articles present information about measures of clinical disagreement, why it happens, and methods to reduce its occurrence.)

Fishman E, Turkheimer E, DeGood DE. Touch relieves stress and pain. *J Behav Med* 18:69–79, 1995. (This study is one of the few trials of therapeutic touch.)

Fitzgerald FT: Physical diagnosis versus modern technology—A review. *West J Med* 152;377–382, 1990. (The author presents information about limitations of specific aspects of the physical examination.)

Fox SA, Siu AL, Stein JA: The importance of physician communication on breast cancer screening of older women. *Arch Intern Med* *154:2058*–2068, 1994. (The investigators identified factors related to whether women obtain screening mammography; the physician's recommendation and enthusiasm for mammography were important variables relating to mammography rate.)

Friedman LC, Nelson DV, Webb JA, *et al*: Dispositional optimism, self-efficacy, and health beliefs as predictors of breast self-examination. *Am J Prev Med* 10:130–135, 1994. (The three leading reasons for not performing breast self-examination were "forgetting or too busy," "fear of finding something," and "do not know how.")

Greenberger NJ, Hinthorn DR: *History Taking and Physical Examination: Essentials and Clinical Correlates*. St. Louis, Mo, Mosby–Year Book, 1993.

Hayward RSA, Steinberg EP, Ford DE, *et al*: Preventive guidelines: *Annals of Internal Medicine* 114:758–783, 1991. (The authors present an extensive review and comparison of recommendation from A.C.P., Canadian Task Force, and others.)

Johnson JD, Meischke H: Factors associated with adoption of mammography screening: Results of a cross-sectional and longitudinal study. *J Women's Health* 3:97–105, 1994. (Researchers found that the single most influential factor for having a mammogram was a physician's recommendation.)

Kern DC, Parrino TA, Korst DR: The lasting value of clinical skills. *JAMA* 254:70–76, 1985. (The authors surveyed graduates and found that practitioners felt that clinical skills, including physical diagnosis abilities, received inadequate emphasis during housestaff training.)

Klachko DM, Reid JC: The effect on medical students of memorizing a physical examination routine. *J Med Educ* 50:628–630, 1975. (This study documents the utility of memorizing a specific examination sequence.)

Koran LM: The reliability of clinical methods, data and judgements (two parts). *N Engl J Med* 293:642–646, 695–701, 1975. [In part 1, the author reviews data on interobserver agreement for physical examination aspects; part 2 presents agreement concerning diagnostic procedures (such as electrocardiograms and radiographs).]

Krieger D: *The Therapeutic Touch*. New York: Simon & Schuster Inc, 1979. (The author is a noted teacher of this skill, and she describes techniques for detecting illness and enhancing a practitioner's healing abilities.)

Lang F: Resident behaviors during observed pelvic examinations. *Fam Med* 22:153–155, 1990.

Larsen KM, Smith CK: Assessment of nonverbal communication in the patient physician interviews. *J Fam Pract* 12:481–488, 1981.

Macklis RM, Mendelson ME, Mudge GH Jr: *Introduction to Clinical Medicine: A Student-to-Student Manual*. Boston, Little Brown & Co, 1994.

Maclure M, Willett WC: Misinterpretation and misuse of the kappa statistic. *Am J Epidemiol* 126:161–169, 1987.

Novey DW, Novey D: *Rapid Access Guide to Physical Examination*. Chicago: Mosby. Year Book, 1998.

Oboler SK, LaForce FM: The periodic physical examination in asymptomatic adults. *Ann Intern Med* 110:214–226, 1989.

Patton DD, Bodtke S, Horner RD: Patient perceptions of the need for chaperones during the pelvic exams. *Fam Med* 22:215–231, 1990. (Survey of patients that found about half had no preference concerning an examiner's gender, and those with a preference, preferred female examiners. With a female examiner, patients did not want a chaperon, and with a male examiner, a chaperon was preferred by approximately 65% of women.)

Penn MA, Bourguet CC: Patients' attitudes regarding chaperones during physical examinations. *J Fam Pract* 35:639–643, 1992. [These authors analyzed the effects of patient gender, physician gender and patient age (teenagers versus adults); they found that, although most patients did not care whether a chaperon was present, 29% of adult women and 46% of adolescents preferred a chaperon when examined by a male physician; unlike young women, male teens preferred not to have a chaperon present during the genitourinary examination.]

Robbins JA, Bertrakis KD, Helms LJ, *et al*: The influence of physician practice behaviors on patient satisfaction. *Fam Med* 25:17–20, 1993. (These investigators found that being examined was one of the three items that correlated with patient satisfaction.)

Seidel HM, (editor): *Mosby's Guide to Physical Examination*. St. Louis, Mo, Mosby–Year Book, 1999.

Sox HC Jr: Preventive health services in adults. *N Engl J Med* 330:1589–1595, 1994. (Summary of recommendations from the Canadian Task Force on the Periodic Health Examination, U.S. Preventive Services Task Force, and the American College of Physicians; specific discussions focus on breast, colon, and prostate cancer screening.)

Stratton BF, Nicholson ME, Olsen LK, *et al*: Breast self-examination proficiency: Attitudinal, demographic, and behavioral characteristics. *J Women's Health* 3:185–195, 1994. (Less than a third of women practice breast self-examination, and self-report of skills is not an accurate assessment of a woman's abilities.)

Swartz MH: *Textbook of Physical Diagnosis: History and Examination*. Philadelphia, WB Saunders Co, 2001.

U.S. Preventive Services Task Force. *Guide to Clinical Preventive Services: An Assessment of the Effectiveness of 169 Interventions*. Baltimore, Williams & Wilkins Co, 1989.

Vogt HB, McHale MS: Testicular cancer. Role of primary care physicians in screening and education. *Postgrad Med* 92:93–101, 1992. (The authors point out that testicular cancer is an illness of young adults and review the role of the physician and self examination in detecting the examinations.

Wallis LA, Tardiff K, Deane K: Evaluation of teaching programs for male and female genital examinations. *J Med Educ* 58:664–666, 1983.

Weiss L, Meadow R: Women's attitudes toward the gynecologic practices. *Obstet Gynecol* 54:110–114, 1979. (Women's distress is related to anxiety, vulnerability, and humiliation. The authors present specific suggestions for the examiner, including talking to a patient during the examination, allowing patients to change into clothes before discussing findings, and using language that is appropriate for the patient.)

Wiener S, Nathanson M: Physical examination. Frequently observed errors. *JAMA* 236:852–855, 1976.

Willms JL, Schneiderman H, Algranati PS: *Physical Diagnosis: Bedside Evaluation of Diagnosis and Function*. Baltimore, Williams & Wilkins Co, 1994.

## CHAPTER 9

# Appropriate Use of Laboratory Tests

*Victoria S. Kaprielian*

## CASE 9-1

*A 20-year-old white woman presents to her physician's office complaining of increasing nonproductive cough for 1 week. She reports a low-grade fever (100°F) and malaise, but no other respiratory symptoms. In addition, in the past 2 days she's developed some chest pain with coughing. She is otherwise healthy, does not smoke, and is on no medications except an over-the-counter cough syrup, which has given little relief. She has no personal or family history of asthma or other lung problems. On physical examination, she appears slightly uncomfortable but in no distress. Her temperature is 99.5°F, and HEENT assessment is unremarkable except for slight erythema in the oropharynx. Lung examination reveals scattered rhonchi, but no rales or wheezes, including on forced exhalation.*

*The physician suspects the patient has atypical pneumonia or bronchitis. He orders a chest x-ray, the results of which are unremarkable, and a blood count, which shows a slightly elevated number of white blood cells. After a positive cold agglutinin study confirms the likely diagnosis, he prescribes a course of erythromycin.*

## EDUCATIONAL OBJECTIVES

1. Describe three reasons for performing diagnostic tests
2. Discuss two guiding principles for selection of laboratory tests to be used in patient care
3. Describe appropriate uses of common basic laboratory tests, including complete blood counts, urinalyses, electrolytes, and simple x-ray studies
4. Demonstrate awareness of the costs and risks inherent in diagnostic testing
5. Discuss the influences of disease prevalence and test sensitivity and specificity on interpretation of test results
6. Demonstrate understanding of the concepts of positive and negative predictive value, and their application in the use of diagnostic tests
7. Given a case scenario, suggest diagnostic studies necessary and appropriate for the care of the patient described

In the past, physicians in the United States practiced in an environment of seemingly endless resources. Any diagnostic test or approved treatment could be used for any patient, with little regard for cost to the patient or the system. Students and residents were rarely faulted for ordering unnecessary studies, but frequently criticized for not ordering tests of even marginal potential utility. Studies were commonly ordered "just to know," even if they would have little or no impact on treatment or prognosis. In Case 9-1, for example, $150 worth of studies only confirmed the physician's initial impression, and did not change the treatment or outcome.

The realization that our resources are not limitless has prompted dramatic change in the U.S. medical environment. Managed care has come forward as the predominant system for providing care while limiting costs. In this system, physicians are discouraged from performing or ordering any but the most helpful and necessary studies. In order to prepare to practice in such an environment, today's physicians in training must develop a very cost-conscious approach. There are two major steps in the appropriate use of laboratory tests and other studies. The first, selection of studies, requires careful consideration of alternatives and thinking ahead to the potential usefulness of results. The second step, interpretation of results, requires understanding of several basic principles of epidemiology.

## CASE 9-2

*A 21-year-old man presents to his physician with a history of physical examination results essentially identical to those of the patient in Case 9-1. The physician orders no tests, and prescribes a course of erythromycin.*

## SELECTION OF STUDIES

Tests may be used for three basic reasons:

1. To screen for subclinical disease in asymptomatic individuals
2. To identify or clarify diagnoses in symptomatic individuals
3. To monitor status of known disease

In order to select studies and use them appropriately, clinicians should be certain of the reason for ordering tests in the specific patient under consideration. This chapter will focus primarily on the use of tests to pursue a diagnosis; see Chapter 17, "Health Promotion and Disease Prevention," for discussion of the use of studies for screening of asymptomatic individuals. The differences between Cases 9-1 and 9-2 raise several questions. Are laboratory tests or x-rays necessary for the care of these patients? What studies are available for the physician to order? How might they influence the treatment plan? The patient is clearly symptomatic and the precise diagnosis is uncertain, so the first physician orders an x-ray and blood tests. The second physician considers whether further testing is needed before treatment. The history and physical examination are consistent with an atypical pneumonia. A complete blood count (CBC) is commonly done in this situation, as it was in Case 9-1. However, it is unlikely to change the diagnosis or treatment plan. Ordering a chest x-ray is also an option, but findings in atypical pneumonias are inconsistent, and in the absence of other risk factors, an unexpected finding is highly unlikely. Therefore, a course of erythromycin may be prescribed empirically, based on clinical findings only. This inexpensive and effective treatment will adequately treat the several most likely causes of the patient's illness (mycoplasma pneumonia, pneumococcal pneumonia, and acute bronchitis), so absolute identification of the causative organism is unnecessary. In telephone follow-up, the patient reports rapid improvement on the medication. On reexamination 2 weeks later, his symptoms are totally resolved and his lungs are clear.

This chapter proposes two questions to be used as the guiding principles of the approach to choice of laboratory tests. Before performing or ordering any study, the student or physician should consider the following:

1. Will the results of this study affect the plan of care for this patient?
In Case 9-2, both the CBC and chest x-ray were decided against because the physician felt the treatment would, in all likelihood, have remained the same regardless of the results.

2. Is this the least invasive and least costly means of getting the necessary information?
If a study meets the criterion of influencing the plan, then the physician must decide whether an alternative study may be preferable because of lesser risk or cost. For example, bronchoscopy can be very useful in the assessment of some lung infections, and in Cases 9-1 and 9-2 could provide specimens to more accurately determine the causative organism. However, the risks, patient discomfort, and costs involved in this procedure preclude its use except in cases in which less invasive methods fail to provide the necessary information. These questions will be discussed in more detail and applied in the following sections.

## CASE 9-3

*A 34-year-old married woman presents to her physician with a 1-day history of urinary frequency, urgency, and dysuria. These symptoms closely resemble those she had with two prior episodes of uncomplicated cystitis, most recently 18 months ago. She has no fever, back pain, nausea, or other symptoms. Her LMP was 2 weeks ago and normal. On examination, she has mild suprapubic tenderness and no CVA tenderness.*

# Will the Results Influence the Plan?

The first decision a physician must make in appropriate use of laboratory tests is whether to use them at all. Before ordering or performing any study, it is the physician's responsibility to decide what will be done with the results, by answering the following questions:

- What relevant results could this test provide?
- If the results are positive (or abnormal), what will I do?
- If the results are negative (or normal), what will I do?

If the answers to the last two questions are different, the test may be worthwhile. If they are the same, it probably is not.

Case 9-3 demonstrates this well. In this case, the history and examination are classic for uncomplicated cystitis in an otherwise healthy, sexually active woman. This diagnosis is common (and indeed, the patient has had prior episodes) and not likely to indicate more serious disease, especially in the absence of frequent recurrences. The physician appropriately considers ordering a urinalysis and/or culture, and decides against both. A 3-day course of trimethoprim–sulfamethoxazole is prescribed, and the patient's symptoms resolve without difficulty.

Consider these tests individually.

## Urinalysis

A urinalysis (UA) is actually a set of tests performed on a single urine specimen. Its typical cost is approximately $20. The UA can provide a variety of useful information:

1. Specific gravity—a measure of urine concentration, which indirectly provides information as to the patient's hydration status.
2. pH—indicates the degree of acidity or alkalinity of the urine.
3. Color and clarity—these are subjective judgments made by the technicians and are not always useful.
4. Dipstick results—a set of colorimetric reactions on sticks manufactured specifically for this purpose, testing for the presence of glucose, protein, blood, ketones, and other items in the urine. This is often used as a screen to determine whether microscopic examination is worthwhile.
5. Microscopic examination of sediment—the urine is spun in a centrifuge, and the clear supernatant is poured off, leaving a sediment of cells and solids. This is examined and the results quantified in terms of elements seen per high-power field. Important elements include:
   a. White blood cells (WBCs)—greater than 5 generally suggests infection.
   b. Red blood cells (RBCs)—normally not present; in the absence of menses, considerable numbers of RBCs may indicate infection, inflammation, or presence of tumor or stones.
   c. Casts—presence of multiple casts suggests renal disease, either pyelonephritis or glomerulonephritis of some type.

In Case 9-3, a UA could document pyuria (presence of WBCs), but the patient's symptoms are classic enough that the diagnosis is clearly likely and empiric treatment could be recommended even in the absence of many white cells. Similarly, it could show casts, but without fever or costovertebral angle (CVA) tenderness, the likelihood of ascending infection is vanishingly small. A high specific gravity may indicate that the patient needs to increase her fluid intake, but this can be safely recommended without the test results. Therefore, it is appropriate and acceptable to treat without the test. If symptoms had not resolved as anticipated, or if any indications of more extensive infection developed, the patient would return and tests could be performed at that time. This should not, however, be taken to infer that testing is never necessary for assessment of urinary tract infections. If the patient in Case 9-3 had diabetes mellitus or a history of structural abnormality in the urinary tract, she would be at increased risk for complications, and testing would be important. Similarly, if symptoms included fever and/or flank pain, the possibility of ascending infection would be more significant, and a UA would be warranted to look for indications of this (i.e., the presence of casts). Every patient and each incident must be considered individually.

## Urine Culture

There are two common forms of urine cultures: the office screening culture and the formal culture with sensitivities.

The office screening culture, also commonly called a dipslide, is a relatively inexpensive ($20), semiquantitative method of determining bacterial content in the urine. A small plate coated with growth medium is dipped into the urine specimen and incubated for 24 hours. The density of colonies on the plate is then used to estimate the bacterial concentration, by visual comparison with illustrative photos. This provides evidence of the presence of bacteria, but does not identify the organism(s) present, nor can it indicate the response of these bacteria to specific drugs. The office culture is most useful when an equivocal UA requires clarification, or as a test of cure after treatment. In a formal urine culture with sensitivities, a measured amount of urine is plated on a growth medium and incubated. Colonies are counted to provide quantitation of the bacterial concentration. These colonies are further tested and replated on various media to identify the specific organism(s) present. Plating of the organism with various antibiotic-containing disks allows measurement of the sensitivity of the organism to specific antibiotics. This more costly study ($55) is a necessary step in the care of high-risk patients and those with recent antibiotic or hospital exposure, to rule out the presence of resistant organisms that might not respond to the usual antibiotics used to treat urinary tract infections (UTIs).

In Case 9-3, the patient is a healthy woman with no known risk factors for complications. In this situation, the vast majority (80%) of UTIs are caused by *Escherichia coli* (Chew & Finn, 1999), a common intestinal organism, and therefore a urine culture is unnecessary. This organism is typically responsive to a number of common antibiotics, including trimethoprim–sulfamethoxazole, as was used in this case.

As noted earlier, however, differences in the patient's history and risk factors could make more intensive evaluation necessary. If she had been diabetic or had a history of complicated UTIs, UA and some form of culture would be appropriate. If she had been recently hospitalized or catheterized for any reason, identification of the infecting organism and documentation of its sensitivity to the chosen antibiotic would be necessary.

## CASE 9-4

*A 12-year-old boy is brought in by his father, who reports that the child twisted his right ankle while playing basketball with friends yesterday. The child noted immediate pain and left the game; they used ice and Tylenol last night, but he's still unable to bear weight on the leg because of pain in the ankle. He is otherwise healthy, and has no history of significant injuries to this limb in the past. On examination, the right ankle shows substantial swelling and ecchymosis laterally, around and below the malleolus. The child reacts strongly to any palpation of the lateral malleolus or the areas adjacent to it. With coaxing, he demonstrates a limited range of motion in all directions, and will stand lightly on the foot, but cannot bear enough weight to walk on it. The physician orders an x-ray series of the right ankle (AP lateral and oblique views—see Fig. 9.1), with contralateral views for comparison. These are negative for fracture; the initial diagnosis of second-degree ankle sprain is made. Treatment includes brief immobilization (3 days), ice, anti-inflammatory medication, and an exercise rehabilitation program.*

## Bone X-Rays

Of course, appropriate use of laboratory tests does not always mean nonuse. Case 9-4 illustrates a situation in which x-ray studies of two joints are necessary for proper assessment of injury to only one joint.

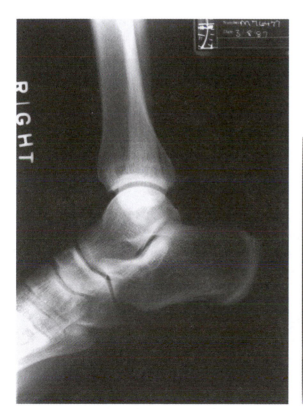
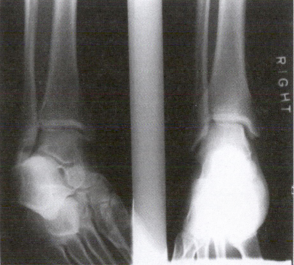

**Figure 9.1.** Ankle radiographs. Standard series, including AP, lateral, and oblique views.

In this case, the physician is faced with the determination of whether the boy has sustained a soft-tissue injury or a fracture. The differentiation is important, since early mobilization is desirable for the former, but prolonged immobilization may be necessary for the latter. Simple x-rays of the bones (i.e., "plane films") can clearly show the bony anatomy and clarify the presence or absence of fracture.

A complicating factor in this case is the age of the patient. Twelve-year-old boys have not yet reached full skeletal height, and thus have cartilaginous growth plates at the epiphyses of many bones. Since cartilage is radiolucent (i.e., allows x-rays to pass through it), x-rays cannot directly show injuries to growth plates. Views of the opposite (uninjured) limb are used for comparison, and growth plate injuries can be indirectly identified by asymmetries in the width of the lucent band and/or position of the bones on either side.

As always, a careful history and physical examination are necessary before the decision to order studies can be made. Several findings, if present, can indicate the increased likelihood of bony injury and should encourage consideration of radiographic study:

- Visible deformity of a limb or joint
- Tenderness that is greater over bone than over soft tissue
- Inability to bear weight (lower limbs)
- Pain out of proportion to apparent injury

These general principles have been more precisely delineated for ankle injuries in the Ottawa rules (see Table 9.1, adapted from Stiell, 1994). In Case 9-4, both the bony tenderness and the child's inability to bear weight on the injured leg support the need for study.

Since growth plate injuries are difficult to identify by physical examination alone and can have significant impact on later growth, x-rays are often important in evaluation of injuries in children. Once the growth plates have closed (age 16–18 in girls, 18–20 in boys), examination-based criteria are more important in determining whether radiographic studies are indicated.

X-rays increase in importance again when evaluating injuries in patients at the other end of the age spectrum. In the elderly, osteoporosis or malignancy can lead to fractures with minimal or no causative trauma. In addition, the inflammatory response to bony injury is often less in the elderly than might be expected, so fractures may not be remarkable on physical examination except for tenderness. Therefore, physicians should have a lower threshold for ordering radiographic studies of injuries in the very old and the very young.

## CASE 9-5

*A 40-year-old male smoker is in for his third visit about upper abdominal pain. About 7 weeks ago he presented with a classic history of burning epigastric pain before meals and late at night, relieved with eating or antacids. Given his smoking, frequent use of ibuprofen, and moderate alcohol intake,*

**Table 9.1**
Ottawa Ankle Rules[a]

An ankle x-ray is only necessary if:
    1. There is pain near the malleoli *and*
    2. Either of these findings:
        a. Inability to bear weight to walk four steps (both immediately and in the emergency room)
        b. Bone tenderness at the posterior edge or tip of either malleolus

[a] Adapted from Steill: *JAMA* 269:1127–1132, 1993.

*the physician felt the pain was most likely acid-peptic in origin, and prescribed 6 weeks of H2 blocker therapy. The patient took his ranitidine as prescribed, but did not decrease his use of cigarettes, ibuprofen, or alcohol. His pain disappeared as long as he took the medication, but returned promptly when he ran out of it last week.*

*At this point, the physician feels a study is warranted to determine if ulcers are indeed present, and to help guide choice of further therapy. He considers upper gastrointestinal (GI) endoscopy versus GI x-ray series, and discusses the options with the patient.*

## Is There a Better Way to Get the Information?

The decision as to which test is optimal is often a difficult one, without absolute right or wrong answers. As in this case, the alternatives are usually not equivalent, and the physician and patient must balance issues of cost and risk against the degree of accuracy and precision needed. In Case 9-5, the x-ray study and the endoscopy each have advantages and disadvantages, and the physician felt that neither was absolutely preferable over the other. Allowing the patient to make the choice is often the best course in this situation. Consider each of these studies in more detail.

### Radiographic Contrast Studies

The upper GI series is one of a class of radiographic studies that use a contrast medium to visualize the structures in question. Since soft tissues and organs are generally radiolucent, plane films without added contrast are of limited use in examining soft tissues. To expand on the information obtainable, radiopaque contrast media of various types can be injected or ingested before the films are taken. The x-rays are blocked by the contrast, and thus the structures containing the contrast are clearly visible on the resulting films. For an upper GI series, the patient drinks a contrast medium (usually containing barium), which allows the esophagus, stomach, and duodenum to be visualized. By using fluoroscopy, taking films with the patient in various positions, and compressing various structures by external pressure, the radiologist can examine the lining of these structures in fair detail, demonstrating the presence or absence of masses, ulcerations, or strictures.

While patients may complain about the chalky texture and taste of the contrast, this study is generally much less uncomfortable for the patient than an upper endoscopy. Its typical cost of $350 is also less than that of the fiberoptic study. However, this test also involves considerable x-ray exposure, which may be a long-term health risk, and its ability to detect ulcer disease (sensitivity; later in this chapter) is less than that of endoscopy.

### Endoscopy

Upper endoscopy is the visual examination of the esophagus, stomach, and first segment of the duodenum by the use of a fiberoptic scope. The endoscope, a long flexible tubelike instrument about 2 cm in diameter, is introduced through the mouth and guided into the desired structures with direct visualization. This does not generally involve radiation, but often requires sedation to minimize patient discomfort from triggering of the gag reflex. The cost (approximately $900) is substantially greater than that of an upper GI series. The endoscope can be used to obtain biopsies and specimens for culture, if indicated.

Endoscopy can be used to examine many other organs. With scopes specifically designed for each, properly trained physicians may examine the sigmoid colon (sigmoidoscopy), the entire colon (colonoscopy), the lungs (bronchoscopy), the nasopharynx and larynx (nasopharyngoscopy), the bladder (cystoscopy), and the uterus (hysteroscopy). In addition to biopsies, some of these scopes allow removal of lesions in their entirety (e.g., colon polyps), eliminating the need for surgery. Developments in this field are ongoing, and the availability of smaller scopes is rapidly expanding the possibilities for diagnosis and intervention.

None of these studies is without risk, however. Whenever a scope is introduced, there is risk of damage to

## OBTAINING INFORMED CONSENT

*Invasive procedures such as endoscopy require informed consent. Informed consent is much more than a patient signing a form. It is a process, to ensure that patients are appropriately involved in clinical decision making. The process of informed consent involves several steps:*

*1. **Discussion***

*Despite the ever-present time pressures, full discussion of the issues is essential. The physician or other healthcare professional obtaining consent must make sure that patients realize they can and should participate in decision making. Discussion should include a clear description of the clinical issue, and the nature of the decision to be made. The possible courses of action (including the option of taking no action) should be discussed, along with the potential risks, benefits, and uncertainties of all of these options.*

*2. **Assessment of the patient's understanding***

*The person obtaining consent should check with the patient to make sure that the discussion has been understood. Asking patients to restate what they have heard is a useful strategy, and will reveal subtle misconceptions that may not otherwise be apparent.*

*3. **Determination of the patient's preference***

*Patients should be asked for their opinion and how they would like to proceed. It should be clear to patients that it is acceptable for them to disagree with the recommendation, or to ask for more time to consider.*

*4. **Documentation***

*As in much of clinical medicine, "if it isn't documented, it wasn't done." A chart note should describe the elements of the discussion, the patient's decision, and the plans to proceed.*

*Adapted from: Sugarman J: 20 Common Problems: Ethics in Primary Care. New York, McGraw-Hill Health Professions Division, 2000.*

the internal organs. Perforation of a hollow viscus is possible, especially if the wall is weakened by ulceration or tumor. This is a serious complication that often requires major surgery for repair.

In Case 9-5, the patient had multiple risk factors for duodenal ulceration, including his use of tobacco, alcohol, and ibuprofen. The physician did not feel strongly that biopsies or cultures were necessary. Either study would be likely to provide the desired information as to whether or not an ulcer was present. In skilled hands, the risks of the procedures are acceptable, though more acutely evident for the endoscopy. Since the physician cannot always predict patients' priorities in such a situation, it is appropriate to involve them in the decision. This patient, having heard a friend last year describe endoscopy as "the worst thing I've ever been through," was most concerned about potential discomfort, and opted for the radiographic study. The upper GI series showed a duodenal ulcer and no other abnormalities. With continued ranitidine, avoidance of ibuprofen, and efforts by the patient to discontinue alcohol and tobacco use, the symptoms resolved completely.

## CASE 9-6

*A thin 63-year-old woman comes in for a routine check of her hypertension. She takes 12.5 mg of hydrochlorothiazide daily, as she has for years, without any problems. Her blood pressure today is 130/84; she brings with her several outside readings with systolic levels of 124 to 138 mm Hg, and diastolics of 80 to 84. She also was tested for potassium level last week at the physician's request; the lab reports the result as 5.6 meq/liter (normal 3.5–5.0).*

*Since the elevated potassium level is completely unexpected, the physician decides to repeat the test. Knowing that changes in renal function can affect potassium levels, she decides to get a chemistry panel to check that also. The results come back in 2 days:*

*Sodium    144 meq/liter (normal 135–145)*
*Potassium    4.0 meq/liter (normal 3.5–5.0)*
*Chloride    100 meq/liter (normal 98–107)*
*Creatinine    1.0 mg/dl (normal 0.6–1.2)*
*BUN    18 mg/dl (normal 8–20)*
*Glucose    103 mg/dl (normal 60–115)*

## INTERPRETATION OF TEST RESULTS

When a physician decides to order a study, she must then analyze the results. This case illustrates important points to consider when interpreting test results:

1. Unexpected results may be mistakes
2. No test is perfect
3. Always consider results in the context of the specific patient

## Unexpected Results May Be Mistakes

The initially elevated potassium level of the patient in Case 9-6 is completely unexpected. Patients on diuretics such as hydrochlorothiazide lose potassium at a higher rate than normal. Periodic checks are often done to look for low levels. Without potassium supplements, elevated levels are highly unusual. Thus, the step of repeating the test is critical before any action is taken. The normal result on the second study is reassuring and within the range of expectation.

What is a "normal" test result? For most tests with numerical results, the normal range is defined statistically as a 95% confidence interval. That is, if a population of healthy people were tested, for tests with a normal statistical (bell-shaped) distribution of results, 95% of the results would fall within the designated "normal" range (plus/minus two standard deviations from the mean; see Fig. 9.2). By definition, this means that 5% of the normal population will have results outside the range defined as normal. Therefore, not all values outside the normal range indicate pathology. This is most often true for results that are just outside the range in asymptomatic individuals. The physician must think carefully about any abnormal values and their relevance to the patient in question before deciding that they indicate a problem.

What was the cause of the first result in Case 9-6? We may never know exactly, but there are several possibilities. Since the repeat test fell within the reference range, it is unlikely that this patient is one of those 5% at the extremes of the normal distribution. There may have been chemical error or artifact in the analysis. Specimens or results may have been mixed up with those of another patient. If the phlebotomy was difficult, there may have been hemolysis in the sample tube; since intracellular potassium levels are much higher than extracellular levels, hemolysis can cause significantly elevated results. Finally, the patient might have had a true but temporary rise in her potassium level, especially if she uses KCl-containing salt substitutes and missed a few doses of her medication. If careful history regarding diet and medication use makes the last of these unlikely, one can generally attribute the value to error or artifact.

In general, with the exception of emergency situations where time is of the essence, it is prudent to recheck unexpected results before making major decisions based on them. Most labs have protocols that require recheck or verification by dilution for substantially abnormal values; however, since that would not eliminate the chance of a contaminated or mislabeled specimen, it is often important to repeat the study on a new specimen as well.

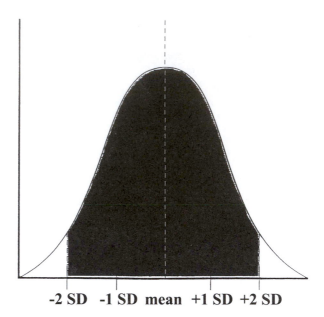

**Figure 9.2.** Bell-shaped distribution of normal results, illustrating 95% of values falling within two standard deviations (SD) of the mean.

## Electrolytes

Electrolyte levels are very commonly ordered blood chemistry studies. These include the concentrations of sodium, potassium, chloride, and bicarbonate ions in the blood, usually the serum poured off a clotted specimen. These results can be used individually and in combination for a variety of purposes and calculations, which are beyond the scope of this chapter. Abnormal electrolyte levels can reflect dehydration, acid–base imbalances, and endocrine abnormalities.

Potassium levels are frequently affected by antihypertensive medications. Because of this, and the ion's critical role in cardiac physiology, monitoring of potassium levels is important for patients with cardiovascular disease on medications.

The set of electrolytes described here is an example of what is commonly referred to as a "panel." Specified lists of chemistry tests can be ordered in sets including as few as 2 or as many as 24 or more separate assays. The ordering convenience of these panels is tempting and has led to routine use of multichem panels for a variety of weak indications. In addition to the monetary cost of the panels themselves, these may lead to unexpected "abnormal" values requiring further assessment. Statistically, if 20 or more tests are performed on a normal individual, at least one result will fall outside the reference range and require further testing to determine its significance (or lack thereof). Thus, one should order only those tests necessary, and use caution in the selection of panels of tests.

## BUN and Creatinine

The blood urea nitrogen (BUN) and creatinine levels are indirect measurements of renal function. Since both of these substances are waste products normally cleared by the kidneys, their blood levels rise when kidney function deteriorates. Normal kidneys have substantial excess capacity, however (a person can survive quite well with the functional capacity of less than half of one normal kidney); these tests do not become abnormal until renal function is greatly impaired. Other tests must be used to detect early stages of kidney impairment.

Loss of kidney function can affect a multitude of other blood chemistries, including potassium, calcium, phosphorus, and magnesium. As noted earlier, when serum potassium rises unexpectedly, it is reasonable to check BUN and creatinine levels to rule out renal failure as the cause.

## CASE 9-7

***A physician reviewing lab reports notices identical results for two of her patients.***

***Mr. Smith, a 50-year-old healthy white man, had requested a "blood test for prostate cancer" after reading a magazine article about it. Despite reassurances that his negative family history and other factors put him at low risk, he insisted, and the physician had agreed to order a prostate-specific antigen (PSA) level.***

***Mr. Jones, a 70-year-old healthy black man, had expressed concern about prostate cancer because his brother had recently died at age 71 of that disease. Since his race and family history placed him at high risk for prostate cancer, the physician had recommended PSA screening, and the patient agreed.***

***Both patients have PSA levels of 6 ng/ml (normal 4). Does this result have the same significance for both of these men?***

# No Test Is Perfect

Every laboratory test has its own characteristics and limitations. No test is 100% accurate. As described in Case 9-6, even when perfectly performed, a test may indicate disease in a patient who is, in fact, normal (called a false-positive result). Similarly, a test may appear normal in a patient with disease (called a false-negative result). The frequency of these results is used to define certain epidemiologic terms that are essential in proper interpretation of test results.

Given two possible categories of test results (positive/abnormal and negative/normal) and the presence or absence of disease, all possible results from a single test can be placed in one of four cells in a 2 × 2 table, as illustrated in Fig. 9.3. We will use this 2 × 2 table to define a few terms, and then apply them to Case 9-7.

## Sensitivity and Specificity

*Sensitivity* describes the ability of a test to detect the disease in question. It is defined as the *percentage of patients with the disease who correctly test positive*. Using the 2 × 2 table in Fig. 9.3,

**sensitivity = true positives/(true positives + false negatives)**

A test with high sensitivity will miss few cases of disease (few false negatives).

| | disease | no disease |
|---|---|---|
| test positive | true positive | false positive |
| test negative | false negative | true negative |

**Figure 9.3.** Structure of a 2 × 2 table of test results.

*Specificity is the percentage of patients without the disease who will correctly test negative.* From the 2 × 2 table in Fig. 9.3, it is calculated as

**specificity = true negatives/(true negatives + false positives)**

A test with high specificity will rarely give an abnormal result in the absence of disease (few false positives).

Sensitivity and specificity are characteristics of the test assay itself. Obviously, it is desirable to have tests with both high sensitivity and high specificity. Because of practical limitations, that is not always possible. Improving sensitivity often results in a decrease in specificity, and vice versa. For example, the distribution of PSA results may be illustrated as in Fig. 9.4.

The selection of the cutoff point for the upper limit of normal determines the sensitivity and specificity of the test. If point A is used, very few patients with disease are missed (those to the left of the cutoff), so the sensitivity is high. This is achieved, however, at the cost of including a large number of patients without disease (to the right of the cutoff), which lowers the specificity. Specificity can be raised to 100% by using point C as the cutoff, but then many patients with disease will be missed, lowering the sensitivity. Usually a point in between (such as point B) is used, allowing a limited number of both false positives and false negatives.

In current practice, PSA testing is usually used in combination with digital rectal examination when screening for prostate cancer. Recent estimates place the sensitivity of this combination (using the cutoff of 4 ng/ml PSA) at 87%, and specificity at 83% (Meyer & Fradet, 1998).

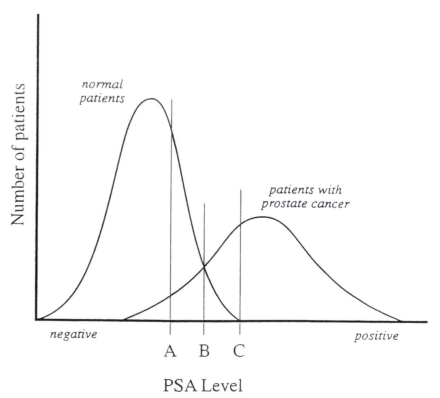

**FIGURE 9.4.** Hypothetical distribution of PSA results in patients with and without disease (see text for explanation).

In clinical situations, even more important than sensitivity and specificity is the concept of predictive value. Faced with an abnormal test result, the physician needs to know the likelihood that the patient truly has disease. Similarly, when results are normal, the provider needs to know the likelihood that the patient is truly disease-free. These likelihoods depend on the prevalence of the disease (the number of persons with the disease) in the population being tested.

*Positive predictive value (PPV) is the probability that a person has the disease, given a positive test result.* From the 2 × 2 table in Fig. 9.3, this is calculated as

**PPV = true positives/(true positives + false positives)**

*Negative predictive value (NPV) is the probability that, given a negative result, the patient is free from disease.* This is calculated as

**NPV = true negatives/(true negatives + false negatives)**

Let us return to Case 9-7 to see how these are affected by disease prevalence.

Mr. Smith is in a low-risk group for prostate cancer. Available prevalence data are limited, because determination of absolute values would require biopsy or autopsy results on a large asymptomatic population. Age-specific estimates (from autopsy studies) place the prevalence of prostate cancer in 50-year-old men at 15%, in 70-year-olds, 39% (Coley *et al.*, 1997). More detailed breakdowns by risk factors are not available. For the purpose of illustration, let us assume that the prevalence in a group of men comparable to Mr. Smith (white 50-year-olds without family histories of prostate cancer) is approximately 15%. Using the sensitivity and specificity estimates given above, the hypothetical 2 × 2 table shown in Fig. 9.5 can be constructed for this population. The positive predictive value of Mr. Smith's PSA result is 47.5%. On the other hand, the negative predictive value of a normal result in this population is 97.3%. In low-risk populations, the test is much more able to correctly predict the absence of prostate cancer than its presence.

Mr. Jones is in a high-risk group, given his age, race, and family history. If we assume a prevalence of 50%, the hypothetical 2 × 2 table for this population is as shown in Fig. 9.6. The positive predictive value for Mr. Jones's result is 83.7%. The negative predictive value of a normal result would be 86.5%. In a high-risk population, a test is better able to rule in disease, and less able to exclude it.

The use of PPV and NPV illustrates the importance of careful consideration of disease likelihood before deciding to order a study. If the prevalence of the disease is very low, even a good test will more often give false-positive than true-positive results.

|  | prostate cancer | no cancer | Total |
|---|---|---|---|
| PSA positive (>4) | 13,050 | 14,450 | 27,500 |
| PSA negative (<4) | 1,950 | 70,550 | 72,500 |
| Total | 15,000 | 85,000 | 100,000 |

**FIGURE 9.5.** Hypothetical 2 × 2 table for PSA screening of prostate cancer in a low-risk population.

| | prostate cancer | no cancer | Total |
|---|---|---|---|
| PSA positive (>4) | 43,500 | 8,500 | 52,000 |
| PSA negative (<4) | 6,500 | 41,500 | 48,000 |
| Total | 50,000 | 50,000 | 100,000 |

**FIGURE 9.6.** Hypothetical 2 × 2 table for PSA screening in a high-risk population.

## CASE 9-8

*A 27-year-old type I diabetic patient has been hospitalized for cellulitis of the left forearm resulting from a cat bite. At his initial presentation, he had a temperature of 39°C; his WBC count was 19.8 thousand/mm³ (normal 5–10) with 32% bands on manual differential. After 2 days of i.v. antibiotics, he is afebrile, and the swelling and erythema are much decreased. Repeat blood count shows WBCs 15.4 thousand/mm³ with a differential of 87% polys, 2% bands, 10% lymphs, and 1% monos. His fasting glucose is 135 mg/dl (normal 60–115), in comparison with 312 mg/dl at admission.*

## Consider Results in the Context of the Patient

All test results must be interpreted in the context of the clinical situation of the particular patient being tested. In Case 9-6, the patient's medication history made the initially elevated potassium level unbelievable, and the repeat level confirmed the clinician's suspicions. In Case 9-8, the second set of WBC and glucose results, while clearly outside the normal range, signify a substantial *improvement* for this patient. These cases illustrate the importance of considering the clinical situation and the patient's past lab values in interpreting results.

Case 9-8 illustrates the importance of looking at trends rather than isolated values. A WBC count of 15.4 is well above normal, and could be worrisome, especially for a diabetic patient. A clinician seeing this result for a patient on i.v. antibiotics could become concerned about the effectiveness of the drug treatment. However, in comparison with the result of 19.8 two days earlier, this actually shows substantial improvement and confirms that the treatment is working well. Similarly, while the fasting glucose of 135 is higher than desirable, it is much better than the previous level of over 300.

### Complete Blood Count

The CBC is a set of counts and measurements of blood cells of various types. This analysis is generally performed by an automated hemocytometer. While the specific values provided may differ slightly between institutions, all CBCs generally include:

1. *White blood cells* (WBC)—the number of white blood cells, in thousands per cubic millimeter (normal 5–10). Elevated values generally indicate infection or some other stressed state. Abnormally low values may occur with immunosuppressed states.

2. *Red blood cells* (**RBC**)—the number of red blood cells in millions per cubic millimeter. Because women lose blood monthly with menses, the reference range for this and several other blood measurements is determined by gender (normal 4.5–6 for men, 4–5.5 for women). The RBC count can be helpful in assessment of anemia, but is used less often than the following two values.

3. *Hemoglobin* (**Hgb**)—the concentration of hemoglobin in grams per deciliter of whole blood (normal 14–18 for men, 12–16 for women). This value is decreased in anemia and hemoglobinopathies.

4. *Hematocrit* (**Hct**)—the percentage of blood volume filled by red blood cells (normal 40–54 for men, 37–47 for women). This can be determined without a Coulter counter by centrifuging a small tube of blood and comparing the height of the RBC column to the total height of the fluid in the tube. This is an important value in assessment of anemia and blood loss.

5. *Mean cell volume* (**MCV**)—the average volume of RBCs in the sample (normal 80–100 fl). Cells are abnormally small in iron deficiency, lead poisoning, and hemoglobinopathies (e.g., sickle cell, thalassemia, hereditary spherocytosis). Heavy smoking, alcoholism, and vitamin deficiencies can increase cell size.

6. *Mean cell hemoglobin* (**MCH**)—the average amount of hemoglobin in each RBC, in picograms. This is influenced by both the size of the cell and the concentration of hemoglobin inside it.

7. *Mean cellular hemoglobin concentration* (**MCHC**)—the average concentration of hemoglobin in the RBCs, in grams per liter. This and the MCH are decreased in iron deficiency, hemoglobinopathies, and other states impairing hemoglobin synthesis.

8. *Platelets*—the number of these tiny cells, in thousands per cubic millimeter. Since these are the shortest-lived of all blood cells, platelet counts are often a reflection of bone marrow activity; they can fall during acute illness, and rebound thereafter. If their number becomes extremely low, the risk of bleeding is increased.

An adjunct to the CBC that is often requested with it is a "differential"—a delineation of the proportions of the different types of WBCs present. While automated estimates are available, most physicians prefer a manually performed count, since current technology does not allow the same precision in automated counts. Proportions of specific cell types may help in interpretation of abnormal WBC counts, or show infection even in the presence of a normal total number of WBCs. Reference ranges vary by age; normal values shown below are for adults.

- Segmented neutrophils (also called polys or segs)—normally 37–80% of the total; increases in the percentage of these cells suggest bacterial infection.
- Band neutrophils (bands)—an immature form, normally not seen in peripheral blood except in the presence of infection or stress.
- Lymphocytes (lymphs)—normally 10–50%; increases suggest viral infection.
- Monocytes (monos)—normally 0–12%.
- Eosinophils (eos)—normally 0–7%; may be increased in allergic states.
- Basophils (basos)—normal cells usually seen in small numbers (0–1%).
- Other immature forms, such as myelocytes, metamyelocytes, and blasts, may be seen in leukemias or perhaps in times of extreme physiologic stress.

In Case 9-8, the presence of a large number of bands in the first blood count indicates the presence of severe infection. While some bands are still present in the follow-up count, the decrease in their proportion reassures us that the treatment is effective, and the patient is improving.

## Glucose

The blood glucose (BG) is perhaps the most frequently used chemistry test. Elevated glucose is the hallmark of diabetes mellitus, and this test is used in both the diagnosis of this disease and the monitoring of known diabetic patients. It may be performed on venous blood using a laboratory chemistry analyzer. Patients may also monitor their own levels at home using an electronic glucometer; these utilize colorimetric reactions from a drop of blood, obtained by fingerstick, on a test strip to provide reasonably precise measurements of whole blood glucose levels. While the fingerstick measurements are less reliable than venous blood testing, the convenience and capability of monitoring at multiple times each day make this test an essential part of modern diabetes management.

Glucose values in a single individual vary greatly over the course of the day, based on timing in relation to oral intake; therefore, it is best measured in the morning after an overnight fast. In Case 9-8, the patient's first fasting glucose was dramatically elevated, as a result of the acute infection. As the infection improved, so did his fasting BG, though it was still higher than desired at the second testing.

# CONCLUSION

Appropriate use of laboratory tests requires consideration of the characteristics of each individual patient and of the tests in question. In selection of laboratory tests and other studies, always make certain that whatever you choose will make a difference in the patient's care, and be sure that the test is the optimal (including most cost-effective) choice for your purpose. In interpretation of results, be aware of test and population characteristics that influence the reliability, accuracy, and meaning of the results. Finally, before acting on results, always be sure they correlate with the clinical situation.

# CASES FOR DISCUSSION

## CASE 1

*A 12-year-old girl is brought in by her mother, who reports that her daughter is complaining of a sore throat. The child has had a runny nose and sore throat for 3 days, and she seems to be feeling a bit worse today. She's been drinking fluids well, but solid food is uncomfortable to swallow. The child is otherwise healthy, and has no significant chronic or past illnesses. On examination she has a temperature of 99.7°F; her throat is red but the remainder of the results of her examination are normal. The mother expresses concern that this might be strep throat.*

1. *What possible diagnoses are you considering?*
2. *What tests might be used? What are the pros and cons of each?*
3. *If your suspicion of strep is low, which test is best suited to reassuring the mother?*

## CASE 2

*An 88-year-old woman is brought in by her husband because she's "not feeling well." The woman says that for the past 2 days she's felt tired and not very hungry, but she can't define any more specific symptoms. Her husband says she's also not thinking quite clearly as usual, being a little more forgetful. She's generally a remarkably healthy woman. She's on no medications except a multivitamin. Her chart indicates she's been treated in the past 5 years for one episode of pneumonia, and one UTI. Physical examination is unrevealing, except that she doesn't look quite as well as she usually does.*

1. *What possible diagnoses are you considering?*
2. *What tests might be helpful?*
3. *Urinary tract infections are a very common cause of general decline in elderly women, and don't always present with symptoms relative to the urinary tract. How might this change your approach?*
4. *Is a urine culture indicated in this case? If so, are full identification of the infecting organism and sensitivities needed?*

## CASE 3

*A 23-year-old man comes in reporting that he twisted his knee playing soccer yesterday. While running, he attempted to make a sharp turn, and had immediate pain and a single pop in his right knee. He had to stop playing, and went home and put ice on it. This morning it's swollen and hurts to bend, and he can only walk with a limp. He's never had trouble with the knee before.*

1. *What possible diagnoses are you considering? Which are most likely?*
2. *Will plane films help to differentiate between the likely diagnoses?*
3. *What physical examination findings might make you want x-rays of the knee?*
4. *Might other radiographic studies be helpful?*

## CASE 4

*Two patients come in independently requesting HIV tests. The first is a recently married 34-year-old woman, who has told you previously that she's used some i.v. drugs in the past and had multiple sexual partners before getting married. The second is the same age and married 10 years; she and her husband each had one prior partner before their marriage, and neither has a history of drug abuse or extramarital sexual contact. Neither woman has any symptoms, nor have they been tested for HIV before.*

1. *How would you classify the risk levels of these two patients? What other information might you need?*
2. *What tests are currently used to test for HIV? What is known about their sensitivity and specificity?*
3. *Before ordering the tests, what would you discuss with the patients about interpretation of the results?*
4. *Both results are negative. How might your discussion of this differ between the two patients?*

## CASE 5

*A 69-year-old man presents reporting he had several episodes of visible blood in his stool about a week ago. This was painless and not associated with any other symptoms. It has now resolved and his bowel movements are normal. He's had hemorrhoids before, but notes that this bleeding was different. Neither he nor his family have any history of colon cancer or polyps, but he is overweight and doesn't eat a very healthy diet.*

1. *What diagnoses are you considering?*
2. *What studies could help in determining the cause of the bleeding? What are their risks and costs?*
3. *Assuming his physical examination is negative, how might you proceed?*

# RECOMMENDED READINGS

Grossman ZD, Katz DS, Santelli ED, *et al.*: *Cost-Effective Diagnostic Imaging: The Clinician's Guide*, ed 3. St. Louis, Mo, CV Mosby Co, 1995.

> A concise and usable discussion of appropriate selection of radiographic studies, with cost information. While the authors occasionally recommend studies in situations with low likelihood of findings, they otherwise promote a very rational approach.

Mulley AG: The selection and interpretation of diagnostic tests, in *Primary Care Medicine: Office Evaluation and Management of the Adult Patient*, ed 3. Philadelphia, JB Lippincott Co, 1995.

> A concise review of the necessary epidemiologic principles and their application in determining and revising diagnostic probabilities.

Nicoll D, McPhee SJ, Chou TM, Detmer WM (eds): *Pocket Guide to Diagnostic Tests*, ed 2. Stamford Conn, Appleton & Lange, 1997.

> A convenient pocket-sized reference on the use and interpretation of various tests.

Pagana KD, Pagana TJ: *Mosby's Manual of Diagnostic and Laboratory Tests*. Mosby–Year Book, 1998.

> Alphabetically arranged handbook of tests, including explanation of the physiology, contraindications, and procedural steps. Necessary patient education is specifically addressed for each.

Speicher CE: *The Right Test: A Physician's Guide to Laboratory Medicine*, ed 3. Philadelphia, WB Saunders Co, 1998.

    A compact, easy-to-read, and well-referenced paperback reviewing issues from the physician's point of view. The introduction is a detailed discussion of general principles, including evidence-based medicine in selection of laboratory tests.

## REFERENCES

Chew LD, Fihn SD: Bacterial infections of the urinary tract in women, in Rakel R, *Conn's Current Therapy 1999*, ed 51. Philadelphia, WB Saunders Co, 1999, pp 677–681.

Coley CM, Barry MJ, Fleming C, Mully AG: Early detection of prostate cancer, Part I: Prior probability and effectiveness of tests. *Arch Intern Med* 126:394–406, 1997.

Meyer F, Fradet Y: Prostate cancer: 4. Screening. *CMAJ* 159:968–972, 1998.

Stiell IG, McKnight RD, Greenberg GH, *et al.*: Implementation of the Ottawa ankle rules. *JAMA* 271:827–832, 1994.

Sugarman J: *20 Common Problems: Ethics in Primary Care*. New York, McGraw-Hill Health Professions Division, 2000.

## CHAPTER 10

# Making a Diagnosis

*John P. Langlois*

*Dr. Nolan, a family physician in private practice, began using her diagnostic skills almost as soon as she awoke. At 6:00 am the hospital called telling her that Mr. Siddiqui, a 64-year-old patient on the telemetry unit who had been diagnosed with a myocardial infarction yesterday afternoon, was having an unusual cardiac rhythm that the nurses were having trouble interpreting. After a few quick questions to assess that the patient had a stable blood pressure and no signs of shock and to be sure that supportive measures of oxygen and intravenous fluids were in place, she ordered an electrocardiogram (ECG) and headed for the hospital. During the 10-minute ride she reviewed in her mind the diagnostic possibilities. On arrival she found a stable patient with a rapid heart rhythm (tachycardia) with a wide complex on the ECG. Through an organized and stepwise approach she was able to correctly diagnose and treat Mr. Ingle's ventricular tachycardia while arranging for his transfer to the intensive care unit.*

*After a quick breakfast she completed her hospital rounds, including a complete history and physical on a new patient admitted with abdominal pain. After a hectic start to the day Dr. Nolan has a full schedule at the office. She was 30 minutes late getting to the office but has made up a little time on her first 3 patients: an OB recheck at 38 weeks, a truck driver with hypertension, and a child with a fever and otitis media. She has an additional 9 patients on her morning schedule and 14 for the afternoon. She takes a deep breath and prepares to see her next patient.*

## EDUCATIONAL OBJECTIVES

1. Identify and describe the basic characteristics of four diagnostic methods—exhaustive, algorithmic, pattern recognition, and hypothetico-deductive
2. List the major steps in the hypothetico-deductive approach to clinical reasoning
3. Identify several pitfalls and optimizing strategies for each step
4. Define the concept of differential diagnosis and discuss its usefulness

Clinical practice presents a challenge of a widely varying spectrum of patients and problems with which to deal. Behind each door is an unknown, a question in search of an answer, and before the door is opened, the possibilities of what that answer will be are nearly endless. The patient may present for a simple health maintenance visit or with symptoms suggesting an acute myocardial infarction, a simple cold, or a complication of AIDS. In addition, the first-contact physician often sees diseases present for the first time and in their earliest and most confusing stages. It is in the "front line" trenches of patient care that well-developed skills for making an efficient and accurate diagnosis are essential, as in Case 10-1. A practicing physician is continually challenged to use every technique available to make the correct diagnosis for her patient.

There are a number of techniques that physicians use to arrive at the correct diagnosis (Curtis, 1993; Sloane *et al.*, 1997). One technique that is often taught early in medical school is the *exhaustive* method, where every possible question is asked and every available piece of data is collected and organized to help arrive at the diagnosis. In Case 10-1, Dr. Nolan's admission history and physical included the components of a complete workup—chief complaint, history of present illness, past medical history, current medications, allergies, family history, social history, review of systems, vital signs, complete physical, laboratory values, x-ray results, assessment, and plan. Although this degree of completeness is important for the hospitalized patient, she does not have the luxury of time or the energy to be able to employ that method for every patient on today's schedule.

A second method is the *algorithmic* method. In this approach, the decision options are already laid out based on a proven strategy. The physician then follows the steps making decisions at preselected branch points, based on the clinical data available. Dr. Nolan used this method this morning in assessing and caring for Mr. Siddiqui by following an Advanced Cardiac Life Support (ACLS) algorithm for tachycardia (Fig. 10.1) that she had learned in her residency. Unfortunately, algorithms have not yet been developed for all medical problems, and many presentations are too complex to lend themselves well to this approach.

A third diagnostic method is *pattern recognition*. In this technique a pattern of clues or clinical characteristics trigger a memory response in the physician of something that he had seen or learned previously. Dr. Nolan used this technique when she recognized a brown rash on the cheeks and forehead of her pregnant patient as melasma, a skin change related to the increased estrogen level in pregnancy. Pattern recognition takes considerable clinical experience, and often the clues are partial and may be too incomplete to trigger awareness of the pattern.

The technique that is used most often by physicians is the *hypothetico-deductive* method. In this method clues and hunches are used in a systematic way to guide a focused inquiry and the development of a rank-ordered list of hypotheses. This list is known as a differential diagnosis or "diff." The method consists of a series of steps, some of which occur essentially simultaneously (see Fig. 10.2). Each of these steps has distinct characteristics, potential pitfalls, and possible shortcuts. By optimizing each step, avoiding the pitfalls, and taking advantage of any shortcuts, the physician can arrive efficiently and accurately at the correct diagnosis.

The systematic but problem-focused nature of the hypothetico-deductive method particularly lends itself to the primary care setting, where the population and their potential medical issues represent a broad spectrum of problems. Diagnosis of these "undifferentiated patients," who are not preselected into an organ-specific clinic population, requires a high level of diagnostic skill. The purpose of this chapter is to review in detail the characteristics, pitfalls, and shortcuts in each step of this approach to making the diagnosis in order to help you to be a more efficient, accurate, and skillful diagnostician.

## CASE 10-1 (Part II)

*The next patient is a 58-year-old woman named Betty with a complaint of "cough" as recorded by the nurse. Vital signs are recorded as: temperature 100.2°F orally, blood pressure 138/92 mm Hg,*

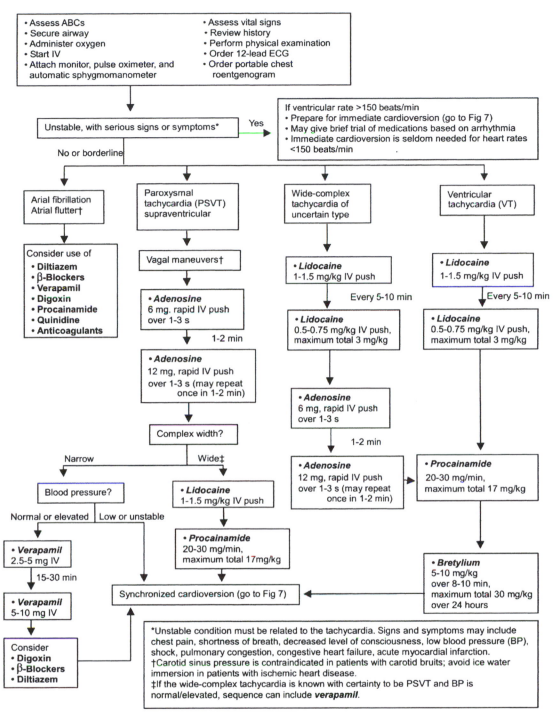

**Figure 10.1.** Tachycardia algorithm. Reprinted with permission from: Emergency Cardiac Care Committee and Subcommittees, American Heart Association. Guidelines for cardiopulmonary resuscitation and emergency cardiac care, III. Adult advanced cardiac life support. *JAMA* 268:2223, 1992.

*pulse rate 60 beats per minute, and 20 respirations per minute. While reviewing the chart outside the door, Dr. Nolan hears a persistent cough. As she enters the room she sees a tired-looking woman who has just finished a spasm of coughing. She has already begun the diagnostic process and has developed some initial hunches to help direct and focus her approach to making the correct diagnosis.*

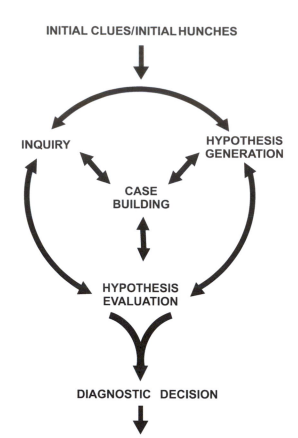

**Figure 10.2.** Schematic of the steps in the hypothetico-deductive process.

## INITIAL CLUES/HUNCHES

Even before Dr. Nolan has asked Betty a single question, she has used available clues and observations to form initial hypotheses that focus and organize her approach. Before obtaining these early data, the diagnostic possibilities were nearly endless. Now the clinician has an initial list of possibilities. Although not all clinicians will admit to forming hunches quite this early in the encounter (before the patient is seen), forming hunches occurs very early and guides further steps in the reasoning process. Table 10.1 outlines the characteristics, pitfalls, and shortcuts of this first step in the hypothetico-deductive method.

**Table 10.1**
Initial Clues/Initial Hunches

Characteristics
   Early information leads to very early hypotheses
   Involves initial rapid focusing
   Gives initial direction to encounter
Pitfalls
   Premature closure
   Failure to recognize patients' true reason for seeking medical care
   Failure to clarify initial confusion (e.g., "What do you mean by 'diarrhea'?")
Shortcuts
   Always generate more than one initial hunch
   Clarify chief complaint
   Ask yourself, "Why now?"

Isn't the clinician "jumping to conclusions" by forming a list of diagnoses before laying eyes on the patient? Jumping to conclusions is a potential pitfall in this step of the diagnostic process. If the clinician places too much value on a single diagnosis and he is unwilling to consider other options, this will subvert the diagnostic process. An example of premature closure is when a physician, during a flu epidemic, assumes that a patient with a fever and achiness automatically has the flu and is unwilling to consider or to look for evidence of other possibilities, such as pneumonia or pyelonephritis. These initial hunches must be flexible and expendable, as the situation requires. Note that the plural *hunches* is always used. By developing more than one initial hunch, you automatically make it difficult to become overly focused on one idea.

Initial clues can be misleading. Early in the diagnostic process the clinician must be alert and be prepared to change his approach. For example, a male patient may be embarrassed to tell the female nurse that the true reason for his visit is sexual dysfunction, and may instead give "headache" as a chief complaint. Beginning the visit with an open question such as "What brings you to the office today?" may elicit the patient's true agenda.

It is imperative that the clinician clarify the reason for coming into the office, but, at times, the patient's stated reason for coming may not seem to make sense. If the patient has had mild, occasional headaches for 6 months, why has he come to the office today? In these situations it may be useful to ask yourself, "Why now?" The patient may recently have learned of a co-worker who has been diagnosed with a brain tumor. The terminology used by the patient can be misleading. A patient's idea of "diarrhea" may be very different from the medical definition, and your diagnostic approach must vary accordingly.

Numerous potential pitfalls in this stage of the diagnostic process can be avoided by working at being clear and accurate about the reason why the patient is presenting. At this point, the clinician should have more than one early diagnostic "hunch" that will direct the next steps in the diagnostic process.

---

## CASE 10-1 (Part III)

*Dr. Nolan's initial hunches about Betty's illness are bronchitis versus reactive airway disease. After confirming the patient's chief complaint of "cough," she questions the patient about her recent history. The patient reports that she began getting sick about 10 days ago. At first she thought it was a chest cold that would pass, but it has not gotten better. The cough is nonproductive (no phlegm), "hacking," and seems to be worse at night when she lies down. She has tried a humidifier and cough medicine but they don't seem to help. Initially there was some nasal congestion but this resolved after 2 days. The patient states she has noticed some wheezing and that her chest feels tight. She does not have a history of asthma or allergies. No one at home has been sick but several people at the office have been sick with similar symptoms. Their illness did not last this long. When asked if there are any other symptoms associated with this illness, the patient reports that her feet have been swelling a little more than usual. The patient speaks in short but complete sentences. Dr. Nolan notices a smell of tobacco smoke and a quick glance at the chart reveals a history of hypertension for which the patient is taking captopril, an angiotensin converting enzyme (ACE) inhibitor, 50 mg twice a day.*

## THE DIAGNOSTIC CYCLE

It is at this point that the clinical reasoning process appears to become very complex and to appear almost random and haphazard. The concept of a stepwise, definable process seems to break down. The reason for this apparent chaos is that several steps are occurring almost simultaneously. Once a question is asked (inquiry), the answer is used to evaluate the existing hunches (hypothesis testing). In addition, the answers to the questions can generate additional possibilities (hypothesis generation). These hypotheses bring new questions to mind and the cycle continues. At the same time the clinician is modifying her differential diagnostic list as well as generating an abbreviated summary of the clinically relevant history (case building). The result is a

## BRONCHITIS OR REACTIVE AIRWAY DISEASE?

*Many problems in medicine are so close in presentation that clinicians must use their clinical reasoning skills to sort them out. This is true of bronchitis and reactive airway disease, but an understanding of the pathophysiology can help.*

*Acute bronchitis is the result of an infection of the small airways in the lung or bronchi. The infection is caused by viral organisms in the majority of cases, but bacteria or atypical organisms such as mycoplasma have been implicated. As the body fights off the infection the resulting inflammation results in swelling, increased mucus production, and sometimes irritability or spasm of the smooth muscles in the wall of the bronchial tree. Symptoms can include those of the infection (malaise and possibly fever) as well as symptoms of the inflammation (cough, phlegm, and wheezing). The wheezing can respond to bronchodilator medications such as those used in asthma. A cough may persist for several weeks after the acute episode.*

*Reactive airway disease (or asthma) also involves inflammation of the bronchial tree, but in this case the inflammation is due to allergy or other environmental triggers. The inflammation results in swelling, mucus production, and irritability of the smooth muscles of the airways—the same as acute bronchitis. Once the inflammation is present, relatively minor irritations such as dust, exercise, or cold air can trigger an attack. An infection such as a viral bronchitis can trigger an attack as well. Symptoms include difficulty breathing, wheezing, and cough either alone or in combination. Bronchodilators will help symptoms briefly, but the key to treatment is suppression of the inflammation. Regular doses of an anti-inflammatory medication, such as an inhaled corticosteroid, is the cornerstone of therapy.*

*As can be seen, there are many similarities between bronchitis and reactive airway disease. A careful history and physical examination, careful follow-up of persistent symptoms, and a healthy index of suspicion will help you sort out this diagnostic dilemma.*

### References

Curtis P: Respiratory tract infections, in Sloane PD, Slatt LM, Curtis P, Ebell MH (eds): *Essentials of Family Medicine.* Baltimore, Williams & Wilkins Co, 1997, chap 35.

Vura-Weis DE: Asthma and chronic obstructive pulmonary disease (COPD), in Sloane PD, Slatt LM, Curtis P, Ebell MH (eds): *Essentials of Family Medicine.* Baltimore, Williams & Wilkins Co, 1997, chap 19.

series of interdependent events occurring rapidly (see Fig. 10.2) and, in some experienced physicians, nearly subconsciously. Although it may seem confusing when taken as a whole, by analyzing each component individually, a method for understanding and optimizing each step will become clear.

## Inquiry

With the first question a cascade of events is started, initially guided by the starting hunches (see Table 10.2). There are specific strategies and types of questions that are employed. A *search* strategy employs questions that are aimed toward obtaining specific information. During initial questioning, Dr. Nolan was obtaining specific information on the present illness by means of an organized approach. A look back at the case will show that she obtained information on the following areas of importance related to the symptom of cough: duration, quality, exacerbating or relieving factors, therapeutic attempts, and associated symptoms. This was not accidental, but a deliberate attempt to obtain as complete an understanding of the primary symptom by intentionally asking questions on the short list of symptom characteristics she felt was relevant. The list of relevant issues may vary depending on the type of symptom. For example, a list for a complaint of pain might include: duration, quality, location, radiation, changeover time, exacerbating/relieving factors, associated symptoms, and therapeutic attempts. Note that this list could be used for any type of pain—chest pain, head pain, foot pain—and that not every clinician's approach need be exactly the same. The systematic

**Table 10.2**
Inquiry

Characteristics
  Guided by hypotheses
  Two techniques of inquiry that give initial direction to encounter:
    • Search—seeking additional data to support or refute existing hypotheses
    • Scan—randomly or routinely ordered questions to explore further
Pitfalls
  Limited focus on one hypothesis
  Too much random or routine choice of items
  Rigidity of style or approach
Shortcuts
  Gather data in blocks, a series of questions that clarify a complaint
  Choose and develop high-yield questions
  Be flexible in approach, e.g., do early physical for complaint of rash

gathering of a block of needed information can make processing of the data easier and makes it less likely that an important facet of the history will be missed.

A *scan* strategy is also used. The purpose of this inquiry is to explore other clues or hypotheses that have not been brought to light by more focused questions. Scan strategies include random exploration of other systems, or a more ordered but routine "review of systems" approach to questioning. Open-ended questions can be useful in scanning for additional information. Dr. Nolan asks the vague question, "Have you noticed any other symptoms that we haven't discussed yet?" and learns about the foot swelling, a new clue that may be important.

## Hypothesis Testing

The majority of Dr. Nolan's questions in Case 10-1, Part III, were of the "search" type. This is characteristic of a mature and efficient reasoning style. The questions asked are carefully thought out and designed to clarify important points of the history and to "test" the existing hypotheses. When we think of tests in medicine, we are quick to think of laboratory tests or imaging studies. It is important to remember that questions are tests and have similar characteristics of sensitivity, specificity, and predictive value. The questions that you ask of patients are the principal means you have to evaluating and ordering your hypotheses to make the correct diagnosis of your patient.

With what questions did Dr. Nolan begin to evaluate her initial hypotheses? Even her initial series of questions, which clarified the details of the chief complaint, provided clinical information that will help in ordering hypotheses. For example, the 10-day duration of the illness makes a pure viral process less likely. This protracted time course and the nonproductive nature of the cough diminish the likelihood of a typical bacterial process, such as a pneumococcal infection. After getting these initial data, she focuses on the hypotheses she has developed by asking questions related directly to reactive airway disease or asthma and infectious causes or exposures. Table 10.3 outlines the characteristics of the hypothesis testing process.

Questions can be used in several ways to evaluate hypotheses, each involving a different strategy (Kassirer & Gorry, 1978). In the strategy of *confirmation*, a question is used to *elicit a finding that supports the disease*. An example is to ask about exertional chest pain to evaluate the possibility of stable angina, the presence of which supports the diagnosis of stable angina.

A second strategy is *elimination*, where *the absence of a finding goes against the presence of a disease*. The same example of chest pain can be used: If exertional chest discomfort is not reported, then stable angina is less likely. Note that the phrase *less likely* is used. Just as there are false-negative lab test results, there are few answers to medical questions that are 100% sure. It is best to base your decisions on several corroborating factors.

**Table 10.3**
Hypothesis Testing

Characteristics
    Each question is a test of existing hypotheses
    There are several strategies for hypothesis testing:
        • Confirmation—presence of finding supports disease
        • Elimination—absence of usually present finding goes against presence of disease
        • Discrimination—discriminates between two or more hypotheses
        • Exploration—a search for evidence of the disease in other systems
Pitfalls
    Inaccurate data
    Overreliance on the weight of evidence
Shortcuts
    Use carefully selected high-yield questions
    Consider and optimize the accuracy of the data

# HOW DO CLINICAL REASONING SKILLS MATURE?

*When you work closely with a clinician/preceptor, their reasoning may not seem to follow all of the steps of the clinical reasoning process as described in this chapter. How does clinical reasoning change as a clinician gathers more experience? Research into clinical reasoning has begun to shed some light on these changes.*

*Research shows that although there is significant similarity in the approach to clinical problems for students and experienced clinicians, there are some differences (Neufeld et al., 1981). Both groups employ a similar number and timing of diagnostic hypotheses, weigh findings against hypotheses in a similar manner, process findings and multiple hypotheses in a parallel manner, and use questions and the physical exam to a similar extent. Differences were found in the level of content and how specific the diagnostic hypotheses were between the groups. This was found to be the best predictor of diagnostic outcome and was correlated closely with increasing education and experience.*

*Testing of theoretical assumptions about clinical problem-solving skills leads to some paradoxical results. For example, it has been assumed that the expert will gather more of the significant, critical, or essential data than the novice will. Instead, studies have shown that experienced clinicians may gather the same amount or less of these data than an early clinical reasoner. Some tests of clinical reasoning skills show minimal differences in problem-solving performance measures relative to final-year medical students or beginning residents and experienced clinicians. In some cases an apparent decline in performance measures has been noted. This is counter to expectations and to the actual clinical performance of the groups. Third, errors in diagnosis made by experts have been assumed to be the result of inattention to detail, lack of knowledge, or shortcuts. It would then be expected that errors would more likely occur when experts make quick decisions. Studies in "visual" specialties of radiology and dermatology appear to contradict this by showing an association of errors with longer time spent viewing the case. Can these discrepancies be explained by a change in the way that clinical reasoning skills evolve?*

*Research suggests that the advanced clinician develops an efficient strategy that combines different components of more than one clinical reasoning style. A combination of "pattern recognition" and the "hypothetico-deductive model" appears to be active. The vast cumulative experience of the busy physician allows the development of illness scripts or patterns that incorporate the essential features of an illness as well as variations from the norm. As information is gathered, a smaller amount of data may be required to trigger a diagnosis for the experienced clinician, whereas the novice may need more pieces of the puzzle to create the same picture. Expert clinical reasoners may also use instance scripts in*

## HOW DO CLINICAL REASONING SKILLS MATURE? (Cont.)

*which particular patients and their illnesses are used in a rapid and highly efficient matching process comparing these scripts to new cases in order to diagnose new cases. Physicians have been shown to retain and employ vivid memories of cases for 20 years or more.*

*The development of scripts and the integration of pattern recognition in hypothetico-deductive clinical reasoning could explain some of the observed discrepancies described above. The fact that expert problem solvers gather less of the "essential" data than novices could be related to earlier triggering of the correct diagnosis by use of a highly refined illness script or instance script honed by years of practice. It is possible that some studies that show a decline in some aspects of reasoning skills with experience are not recognizing that not gathering all the data before making an accurate decision is more efficient and at least equally effective. The fact that more errors seem to be made when more time is spent may indicate that, in these instances, there is not a script to match the problem and both novice and expert must revert to the more time consuming and less efficient and accurate hypothetico-deductive model.*

*Experiments and theories are just beginning to shed more light on the fascinating and complex functioning of the clinical problem solver. The mind of the clinician will continue to reveal unique answers and questions. In the meantime, it is your duty to hone your reasoning processes to the finest edge possible.*

### References

Neufeld VR, Norman GR, Barrows HS: Clinical problem solving by medical students: A cross-sectional analysis. *Med Edu* 15:315–322, 1981.

Schmidt HG, Norman GR, Boshuizen HPA: A cognitive perspective on medical expertise: Theories and implications. *Acad Med* 65(10):611–621, 1990.

A third strategy for hypothesis testing is *discrimination*. In this approach, the answer to a *question can discriminate between two or more hypotheses.* A very useful "discriminating" strategy in the patient complaining of "dizziness" is to differentiate "lightheadedness" from true vertigo. One approach is to ask, "Does the room seem to spin around during these episodes, such that you have to hang onto something to keep from falling?" (If the patient can tell you which direction the room is "spinning," that is even more convincing!) Determining that the patient's dizziness is true vertigo results in a very different list of possible hypotheses from a symptom of lightheadedness or near syncope.

A fourth questioning strategy is exploration, where the goal is to *search for evidence present in other organ systems that may support the hypothesis.* In a patient who presents with a complaint of fatigue, the hypothesis of hypothyroidism may be considered. Proper evaluation of this hypothesis will involve exploration of many organ systems, asking about skin changes, changes in voice, excessive menstrual flow, constipation, and so forth. A number of disease processes may have a primary symptom involving one organ system, but additional supporting findings may be revealed when other systems are explored.

Hypothesis testing does have its pitfalls. The most common is inaccurate data. Both patient and laboratory may unintentionally mislead the clinician. As a result, it is wise to use a variety of strategies in evaluating your hypotheses. Sometimes the weight of evidence can seem greater than it is in reality when two or more tests demonstrate the same finding. An example from radiology may illustrate this point best. A patient with abdominal pain is shown to have gallstones on an ultrasound study. The diagnosis of cholecystitis (gallbladder inflammation) as the cause of the pain is not made more likely if the gallstones are also seen on an abdominal CT scan, as both studies only reveal the same data by a different technique. Evidence of a blocked duct and inability to visualize the gallbladder on a nuclear medicine study does give new information and lends additional support to the diagnosis. A large number of positive tests, or a number of positive answers to similar questions, may not lend additional support to the hypothesis if they reveal the same information in a different way.

All questions are not created equal. As seen in the examples here, some questions have a very high yield of useful information. A single, well-asked, carefully selected "high-yield" question can dramatically change your differential diagnosis list. Learning high-yield approaches that have worked for others and developing your own list of quality questions to use in commonly encountered clinical situations will improve your diagnostic efficiency. In addition, well-developed interviewing and interpersonal skills will improve the sensitivity and specificity of your questions.

# Hypothesis Generation

At the same time that questions are being asked and hypotheses are being tested, new data result in the generation of new hypotheses (see Table 10.4). Any question has the potential to both evaluate and generate hypotheses simultaneously. Dr. Nolan asked about other symptoms associated with Betty's illness in Case 10-1, Part III, and got a history of foot swelling, raising the new hypothesis of congestive heart failure (CHF), which can present with coughing and wheezing. This would be an important diagnosis not to miss since CHF would not be expected to go away on its own or to respond to treatment for reactive airway disease or bronchitis.

Hypotheses may be generated by clues other than responses to questions. During a medical encounter, the physician is being literally bombarded with information such as sights, sounds, smells, emotional affect, body language, and so on. Dr. Nolan made a note of the patient's speech pattern as a manifestation of difficulty breathing at rest. Also, the smell of tobacco smoke raises the hypothesis that an exacerbation of an underlying chronic obstructive pulmonary disease (COPD) may be the cause of the patient's symptoms. One side effect of an ACE inhibitor is a cough; so another hypothesis is generated from a new source.

Valuable sources of clues, and hence hypotheses, may be overlooked at times. In fact, medical students are often concentrating so hard on the next question that much of these valuable data are missed. Experienced clinicians may be so adept at using these data that they occur nearly automatically and are incorporated into their thinking without their conscious awareness. Cultivating and practicing an awareness of these other clues is a valuable clinical tool.

As with the other steps in this clinical reasoning process, there are potential pitfalls in the hypothesis generation step. Never generating the hypothesis that is the correct diagnosis is the end result of these pitfalls. Missing key clues is one pitfall. The significance of an essential bit of information may not be apparent to the inexperienced clinician who has not yet learned that a patient's complaint of seeing "flashing lights" may be a warning symptom of an impending migraine or of a tear in the retina. Key clues for common and important

**Table 10.4**
Hypothesis Generation

| |
| --- |
| Characteristics |
|     Additional data leads to new hypotheses |
|     Data are only clues when their significance is recognized |
|     Data may come from many sources |
| Pitfalls |
|     Missing key clues |
|     Not developing a broad enough differential |
|     Familiarity can cloud vision |
| Shortcuts |
|     Use all sources of available data |
|     Learn and watch for clues |
|     Be alert for familiarity bias and other biases |
|     Use differential diagnosis broadening tools, when needed |

**Table 10.5**
Differential Diagnosis Broadening Tools

Have you considered …
    Common diseases?
    Uncommon presentations of common diseases?
    Life-threatening/serious/treatable diseases?
    Rare diseases?
Anatomical approach
    What structures are in the region that could produce the symptoms?
Pathophysiologic approach
    V—vascular
    I —inflammatory
    N—neoplastic
    D—degenerative
    I —intoxication
    C—congenital
    A—autoimmune
    T—trauma
    E—endocrine
Infectious agents (smallest to largest)
    Viruses
    Rickettsias
    Bacteria
    Spirochetes
    Fungi
    Parasites
Don't forget the great imitators …
    Syphilis, tuberculosis, HIV/AIDS, pulmonary embolus

diseases can be learned and their use in generating hypotheses practiced by producing broad differential diagnosis lists.

Failure to produce a broad enough differential is another pitfall. But how can you tell when it is broad enough, or how can you work to make it broader when you have run out of questions and ideas? There are a number of strategies that can help when you need to broaden your differential (see Table 10.5). An anatomical approach to the cause of a problem may be useful (Byyny & Adams, 1981), using your knowledge of the anatomy of the symptomatic area and the diseases of those structures to help broaden your differential. For example, if the complaint is right upper quadrant abdominal pain, you can start with skin problems that might cause pain (such as early shingles, even before the rash), move to musculoskeletal chest pain, then consider diseases of the lower lung, liver, gallbladder, duodenum, pancreas, back, and so on. This systematic approach can help you discover possibilities that you might not have considered.

Another approach to broadening the differential is to use a pathophysiologic approach to the symptom (Byyny & Adams, 1981). Consider each of the classes of disease. For example, could an infectious process be responsible for the symptom of right upper quadrant pain? Could it be a traumatic process? An inflammatory process? A congenital process? Continue until you have considered all of the major types of disease process. Since this list can be rather long and you want to consider all potential causes, some people have developed mnemonics to help (see Table 10.5). Note that the first letter of each word in the pathophysiology list combines to make a single word (Collins, 1987). Whatever strategy you use, use one that you will remember and be able to use consistently. Some of the unusual infectious causes of disease such as rickettsias or parasites may not jump readily to mind. Organizing a list of infectious agents in order of size (see Table 10.5) and reviewing it may help bring to mind some of the more unusual causes of a symptom complex (Collins, 1987).

Some diseases are confusing, with multiple and varied manifestations that can mimic many other diseases. These have been referred to as the "great imitators," and the classic representatives are syphilis and tuberculosis. A modern addition to this list is HIV and AIDS. Characteristic of all of these diseases is their subtlety, especially in the early stages of disease, and their wide range of manifestations. If you do not consider them often, you will likely miss an opportunity to diagnose them early. You may want to customize your list of "imitators" and not just rely on the classics. Pulmonary embolus can have varied and subtle presentations and early recognition is very important. Mononucleosis (Epstein–Barr virus infection) is another candidate for the list. This list can be used in reviewing your diagnoses to see if any of these masqueraders might warrant consideration. Another approach is to learn several key clues for each of these diagnoses and look often for those clues, when the clinical situation is appropriate.

Bias on the part of the clinician is another potential pitfall in generating hypotheses. A bias may be negative—for example, a reluctance to take seriously a patient who may have exaggerated symptoms in the past. It may also be positive—for example, not wanting to consider cancer as a possibility in someone of whom you are very fond. This bias is called a *familiarity bias* and is one important reason why physicians should be very cautious when evaluating friends, colleagues, employees, or family members. There are many who would advocate avoiding these situations completely, but that is not always possible. Biases can be very subtle in their effects on the clinical reasoning process. Awareness of their presence or the possibility of their presence is a first step, and a willingness to get impartial help is essential.

## Case Building

If the diagnostic cycle of three processes occurring together seems too complicated, there is a fourth component that is simultaneous with inquiry, hypothesis testing, and hypothesis generation. This component of the process is called *case building*. The human brain, although the most efficient data processing instrument known, has its limitations. For example, evidence suggests that clinicians can only maintain up to seven active hypotheses on their differential diagnosis list (Kassirer, 1989). Likewise, there are limitations to the amount and detail of data that can remain under active consideration, although this is harder to quantify. Case building is a technique that streamlines and condenses the clinical material. The clinician almost naturally assembles the key facts and clues about the case, in such a way that a brief concise summary is usually possible.

A look at an example of case building will help to shed some light on the process. Table 10.6 demonstrates how this "thumbnail sketch" is continually evolving during a clinical encounter. During her last weekend on call, Dr. Nolan was called to see a patient who presented to the emergency room with severe shortness of breath. If you could read her mind every 10 to 30 seconds during the encounter, the results might look something like Table 10.6. After the chief complaint Dr. Nolan's next key clues are visual: that the patient cannot lie down without worsening of his shortness of breath (orthopnea) and that his neck veins are distended [jugular venous distention (JVD)]. To keep her sketch manageable, she takes these three clues and collapses them into the category "symptoms of congestive heart failure." The timing of the symptoms is a key clue. Sudden onset of CHF is usually caused by an acute insult to the heart. Focused questions lead to the history of recent chest pain. In this acute and unstable situation, rapid progress to a focused physical examination followed by an ECG is appropriate. These additional clues are added and are then collapsed into a hypothesis of a ruptured papillary muscle—The part of the heart to which the chordae tendineae are attached to hold the mitral valve in position is weakened by the heart attack and breaks loose. This hypothesis will be further tested

**Table 10.6**
Case Building: An Example

Middle-aged man with shortness of breath
Middle-aged man with shortness of breath, orthopnea, and JVD
Middle-aged man with symptoms of CHF
Middle-aged man with new-onset symptoms of CHF today
Middle-aged man with new-onset symptoms of CHF today, with history of chest pain 2 days ago
Middle-aged man with new-onset symptoms of CHF today, with history of chest pain 2 days ago, and new murmur
Middle-aged man with new-onset CHF, history of chest pain, new murmur, and ECG C/W recent anterior myocardial infarction
Middle-aged many with new-onset CHF, recent anterior MI, and possible ruptured papillary muscle

# PAPILLARY MUSCLE RUPTURE
# AND ACUTE CONGESTIVE HEART FAILURE

*The case described in the discussion on Case Building illustrates how knowledge of detailed anatomy and physiology can help explain an unusual case presentation. The mitral valve in the heart is responsible for keeping the blood in the powerful left ventricle from returning to the left atrium and lungs when the heart contracts. The two leaflets of the valve are supported from this pressure by strong* chordae tendineae *(Fig. 10.3) and these are attached to a papillary muscle arising from the inner wall of the left ventricle. During a myocardial infarction (MI) or "heart attack" these small muscles can be damaged by decreased blood flow and oxygen. This can occur even with relatively small heart attacks. The muscle may take 1 to 2 days to weaken and rupture. This explains the delay from the episode of pain to the onset of respiratory distress in our case. A new murmur or abnormal heart sound may be heard. The dysfunction of the valve and even the tip of muscle flailing back and forth with each beat of the heart can be seen on an ultrasound examination of the heart or echocardiogram.*

*Once the muscle has ruptured, half of the valve can no longer function. The forceful stream of blood that should have gone to support the body is now, in part, directed backward into the lungs. This results in a reduction of blood flow to the vital organs of the body and increased congestion of blood and fluid in the lungs. This condition is called* congestive heart failure. *This term is confusing to patients and families as many think of*

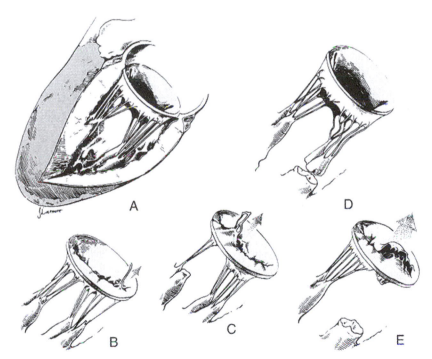

**Figure 10.3.** Mitral regurgitation after MI due to papillary muscle rupture. (A) Normal annulus, chordae, leaflets, and papillary structures. (B) Ruptured posterolateral chordae with mild back flow through mitral valve (mitral regurgitation). (C) Partial rupture of head of anterolateral papillary muscle with moderate mitral regurgitation. (D) Complete rupture of the posteromedial papillary muscle. (E) Severe mitral regurgitation due to papillary muscle rupture. Reprinted with permission from: Camacho MT, Muehrcke DD, Loop FD: Mechanical complications, in Julian DG, Braunwald E (eds): *Management of Acute Myocardial Infarction*. London, WB Saunders Ltd, 1994, p 307.

# PAPILLARY MUSCLE RUPTURE
## AND ACUTE CONGESTIVE HEART FAILURE (Cont.)

*heart failure as a stopping of the heart. Heart failure refers to the pumping function of the heart no longer being sufficient to meet the needs of the body. This can come on slowly, but in this case, with a sudden loss of function in a major valve in the heart, the symptoms of congestive heart failure including* dyspnea *(shortness of breath) and* orthopnea *(increase in difficulty breathing while lying flat).*

*Papillary muscle rupture is a rare complication of heart attack, but it is an extremely serious condition requiring quick recognition and prompt action. By using your knowledge of anatomy and physiology, and solid history and physical examination skills, you will be able to use your clinical reasoning to put the picture together and get the patient the help that is desperately needed.*

### Reference

Braunwald E (ed): *Heart Disease: A Textbook of Cardiovascular Medicine*, ed 5. WB Saunders Co, Philadelphia, 1997, pp 1243–1244.

as a stat echocardiogram is ordered and a call to a cardiologist is made while emergency stabilization of the patient occurs.

Case building is assembling the key facts and clues in a case and simplifying and modifying them as new information develops in order to keep the complexity of this case description manageable. The resulting sketch is longer and more complex than when the case started, but because of condensation of several facts into an interim hypothesis, it is not merely a sequential list of all data obtained. This process does have potential problem areas (Table 10.7). As mentioned previously, not obtaining or recognizing key facts or clues will affect the quality and utility of the case description. Inquiry, hypothesis evaluation, and hypothesis generation all feed into and affect the quality of the case building process. The more effective and efficient the clinician is in these steps, the more relevant and useful the summary will be.

The step in case building where several steps or clues are combined or condensed is another potential source of problems. If the reasoner combines clues incorrectly, an error occurs. For example, if a physician sees a person who is suddenly unable to move her arm and leg on one side, condensing this presentation to a "hemiparesis" may be appropriate, but to automatically label this a "stroke" may be incorrect. The differen-

**Table 10.7**
Case Building

| |
|---|
| Characteristics |
|     "Case building" is a system to manage data |
|     Streamlining and condensation of facts |
|     The reasoner retains relevant high-priority data |
|     Generation of a thumbnail sketch that is added to and modified |
| Pitfalls |
|     Missing key points |
|     Condensation bias |
|     Narrowing of focus too early |
| Shortcuts |
|     Keep your thumbnail sketch true to the facts |
|     Avoiding condensing the hypothesis too early |
|     Be careful not to throw out potential valuable data |

tial for a hemiparesis may include stroke, but there are other possibilities that should be considered, such as a spinal cord lesion or injury. This type of error is called a *condensation bias*. In order to avoid it, it is important to maintain an adequate differential diagnosis and to be careful not to overinterpret available data.

---

### CASE 10-1 (Part IV)

*Further questions by Dr. Nolan reveal that Betty denies paroxysmal nocturnal dyspnea—suddenly awakening with the feeling of shortness of breath, a symptom associated with CHF. She reports some shortness of breath with exertion. The patient attributes her foot swelling to sitting up in a chair at night because she coughs more when she lies down. She denies shortness of breath with lying down (orthopnea). There is no history of chest pressure or chest pain. Her only risk factor for heart disease is high blood pressure, which has been well controlled. The patient has been taking captopril 50 mg twice daily for her blood pressure for 2 years. She does not smoke and has not smoked in the past, but her husband smokes in the home and it aggravates the cough.*

*A focused physical examination confirms the absence of nasal congestion and postnasal drip. Wheezes are present with forced expiration on lung examination and physical signs of pneumonia or CHF are absent. A peak flow determination of 275 liters per minute demonstrates that the patient is able to move air somewhat less rapidly than expected, indicating a mild to moderate airway obstruction. An albuterol nebulizer treatment, to administer a bronchodilating medication directly to the airways, is given by the nurse as a therapeutic trial while Dr. Nolan sees her next patient. Twenty minutes after the treatment, the peak flow has increased to 325 liters per minute. Dr. Nolan has made a diagnostic decision and returns to the patient to inform her and to begin planning and implementation of treatment.*

## A Diagnostic Decision

In most clinical encounters a moment arrives where the clinician makes a diagnostic decision. The preceding steps with their pitfalls and shortcuts are all directed at getting you to this point effectively and efficiently, but how do you know when you have arrived? Unfortunately, there is no bell or alarm that goes off when you have gathered enough information to alert you that all of the important pieces of information have been obtained. The diagnostic decision occurs when uncertainty about the diagnosis has been reduced to an acceptable level for the clinician (see Table 10.8).

How does the clinician reach a decision? There are some tools that are commonly used. The first is the *representativeness heuristic*, a process where the clinician matches his patient's symptoms with a classic or textbook description of disease (Reigelman, 1991). The basis for this process occurs during the hypothesis testing phase, where the physician is obtaining specific data to compare and contrast hypotheses and to compare these hypotheses to the characteristics of disease processes that he has learned. There are a number of pitfalls with this process. Not every disease has "read the textbook." Patients often present with incomplete or modified disease manifestations. This problem can be especially significant in primary care, where patients often present early, before the "classic" manifestations described in the textbooks are detectable. An uncommon presentation of a common problem occurs more often than a rare disease.

Physicians must be alert to the marked variation that may occur in the presentation of the same disease process in different patients. One patient with a myocardial infarction may have severe, crushing substernal pain radiating to the jaw and left arm, associated with nausea, sweating, and palpitations. Another patient with the same amount of damage to the same area of the heart may present with a vague complaint of "chest discomfort, like heartburn." The "disease" is the same but the "illness" is a function of the patient's personal, biologic, and emotional response to the process. Patients may intentionally or unwillingly engage in denial and fail to openly convey critical information necessary to make the diagnosis. Awareness of this

**Table 10.8**
A Diagnostic Decision

Characteristics

  A diagnosis requires that the cause, the disease, and the clinical manifestations fit together and have an adequate and coherent explanation

  Reasoner decides that there are enough data to adequately reduce uncertainty

  Diagnostic decision usually made by 10 minutes into the visit

  Representativeness heuristic—a matching process where reasoner matches patient's symptoms with those of classic or textbook descriptions

  Principle of parsimony—put together as many of the clues as possible into one disease process

Pitfalls

  Patient may present with incomplete or modified disease manifestations

  Patient may engage in denial or fail to convey the key points

  A disease process uncovered may not be the one involved in production of the symptoms, e.g., gallstones and RUQ pain, hemorrhoids and rectal bleeding

Shortcuts

  Acknowledge any uncertainty that remains in the diagnosis

  Maximize and evaluate the reliability of the data

  Find out what the patient's concerns are

  Provide a "safety net" for the patient

---

possibility and, if available, prior knowledge of the patient and his response to disease can help to overcome this pitfall.

Another useful approach in making the diagnosis is the *principle of parsimony*, the process of trying to put together as one disease process the clinical manifestations of the patient (Reigelman, 1991). In some cases it may appear that the patient has more than one disease process occurring, as in a patient with burning on urination and a sore ankle, where both problems may be caused by Reiter's syndrome. Another patient with pelvic and right upper quadrant pain may seem to have two separate processes but actually has pelvic inflammatory disease with perihepatitis (the Fitz–Hugh–Curtis syndrome). Searching for a potential explanation for all of the symptoms with one diagnosis forces you to broaden your differential and consider disease processes that affect multiple sites and systems. An obvious pitfall for the principle of parsimony is the fact that a patient may have more than one disease occurring simultaneously. Two common diseases occurring simultaneously may be more likely to occur than one very rare disease.

Dr. Nolan employed both approaches to making a diagnostic decision in Case 10-1. Her initial hunches of "bronchitis versus reactive airway disease" continued to remain near the top of her differential diagnosis list, although by the end neither fit a "classic" or typical case description. The acute onset, associated fever, and exposure to others with similar symptoms support a diagnosis of bronchitis, but the long duration of the illness and the documented presence of bronchial obstruction do not fit with the typical case. On the other hand, although evidence of wheezing and reversible bronchospasm support the diagnosis of reversible airway disease, new-onset asthma in an older adult without a significant allergic history is unusual, and the acute onset and presence of an elevated temperature are not supported. Fortunately, Dr. Nolan is able to use the principle of parsimony in this case. Occasionally, an infectious bronchitis can trigger bronchospasm and a symptom complex similar to asthma in a patient without an allergic history or other prior evidence of lung disease, asthmatic bronchitis. For Dr. Nolan, this is the most adequate and coherent explanation that best combines the cause, the clinical manifestations, and the disease, an essential definition of the diagnosis.

Can physicians be 100% sure of their diagnosis? In many clinical situations this is not possible. Reasonable doubt often persists despite the most effective diagnostic process. Awareness of this residual uncertainty is essential. Often a "final diagnosis" might best be considered a "working diagnosis." It is incumbent on the physician to create a "safety net" for the patient in order to reduce the risk to the patient of residual uncertainty. The "safety net" might consist of a scheduled follow-up visit to assess efficacy of the

# WHAT IS REITER'S SYNDROME?

*There are many diagnostic situations in which what appear to be unrelated and distant manifestations can be linked by a single diagnosis. Reiter's syndrome is one of these diagnoses.*

*Reiter's syndrome (or reactive arthritis) is a constellation of signs and symptoms that appear shortly after certain infections of the genitourinary or gastrointestinal tract. The syndrome was first described in 1916 as a symptom triad of nongonococcal urethritis, conjunctivitis, and arthritis after an episode of bloody diarrheal illness. It was later discovered to be caused by* Shigella, Salmonella, *and* Campylobacter *infections of the GI tract as well as sexually acquired infections of the genital tract, usually* Chlamydia trachomatis. *The majority of cases occur in young males.*

*Reiter's syndrome can have many clinical manifestations. Arthritis is common and occurs most commonly in the lower extremities. Sixty-one percent of patients also have low back pain and the specific symptom of heel pain. Nearly half have symptoms of irritation of the urethra (such as burning with urination and discharge) and a third have symptoms of conjunctivitis or "pink eye." In addition to these classic symptoms, the syndrome can include skin rashes on the palms and soles, on the end of the penis, and in the mouth. With all of these possible findings it should be no surprise that this condition can be tricky to diagnose.*

*Reiter's syndrome is felt to result when the initial infection triggers an immune reaction in the body that attacks the body's own tissues (an autoimmune disease). This helps explain why there are so many findings in so many places. The disease process usually runs a 3- to 12-month self-limited course. By being alert to this and other conditions that have many possible presentations and disparate findings, you can more readily diagnose your patients and provide them the help that they need.*

### Reference

Arnett FC: Reactive arthritis (Reiter's syndrome) and enteropathic arthritis, in Klippel JH (ed): *Primer on the Rheumatic Diseases*, ed 11. Atlanta, Arthritis Foundation, 1997, pp 184–188.

---

therapy, instructions to the patient on what to expect from the therapy, and when to call if symptoms are not improving or getting worse. Physicians and patients must learn to live with some uncertainty, but the negative impact can be minimized by careful and thoughtful planning and communication.

## CASE 10-1 (Part V)

*Dr. Nolan reenters Betty's examination room to find her appearing more comfortable and coughing less. A brief lung examination reveals improved air movement and less wheezing. Dr. Nolan informs Betty of the diagnosis of asthmatic bronchitis, and relates this to her symptoms and the improvement seen with the nebulizer treatment. She writes a prescription for an albuterol metered dose inhaler, two puffs 15 minutes apart, every 4 to 6 hours, and instructs her in the correct use of the inhaler. Another prescription is written for enteric-coated erythromycin, 333 mg to be taken with food three times a day for 7 days. Betty is informed of the possible side effects of stomach irritation from the erythromycin and jitteriness from the albuterol. She is encouraged to avoid exposure to her husband's cigarette smoke, and states that she has already planned to have him smoke outside. She is asked to call if her symptoms worsen or are not significantly better in the next day or two and to come back for a follow-up visit in 5 days. Betty demonstrates understanding of the instructions and leaves the office more comfortable, both physically and emotionally.*

## WHAT IS THE FITZ–HUGH–CURTIS SYNDROME?

*While studying medicine one is in effect learning a new language. Not only are there technical and anatomical terms, but many conditions have the names of the person or persons who first discovered them attached. These are called* eponyms. *Although there has been a recent tendency to avoid eponyms, the student of medicine will undoubtedly be confronted by them from time to time.*

*The Fitz–Hugh–Curtis syndrome was named for the three physicians who described it. The syndrome is a complication of pelvic inflammatory disease (PID). PID results from inflammation when a sexually transmitted infection such as gonorrhea or chlamydia sets up a polymicrobial inflammation of the cervix, uterus, fallopian tubes, and surrounding structures. Usually the symptoms of PID are localized to the pelvis but from time to time the infection spreads within the abdominal cavity and causes inflammation of the liver capsule. Rarely the syndrome has been seen in men and in these cases it is felt that the infection spreads through the bloodstream. The liver capsule has lots of nerve endings and is very sensitive.*

*Fitz–Hugh–Curtis syndrome (better labeled "PID with perihepatitis") presents a challenge to the clinical reasoner. At times it presents as both pelvic pain and right upper quadrant pain. In these cases one might be tempted to invoke two simultaneous disease processes to explain the findings. Sometimes the pain in the right upper quadrant can be so severe as to overshadow the pelvic symptoms. An awareness of the syndrome, a couple of focused questions, and a pelvic examination will help avoid the false trap of pursuing gallbladder disease, ulcer, or hepatitis as possible causes.*

*Although Fitz–Hugh–Curtis syndrome sounds like one of those "zebras" that are never seen, it is common enough that a primary care physician who cares for a sexually active population could expect to see several cases in his career. Now that you have PID with perihepatitis to put on your differential, you will be able to dodge the diagnostic pitfalls it brings with it.*

### Reference

Roy S: Pelvic infection, in Mishell DR, Brenner PF (eds): *Management of Common Problems in Obstetrics and Gynecology*. Boston, Blackwell Scientific, 1994, pp 391–399.

# CONCLUSION

We have examined the steps in the hypothetico-deductive reasoning process. Beginning with some initial hunches, we have analyzed our way through a whirlwind of inquiry, hypothesis testing, and hypothesis generation—each part feeding off and contributing to the others in a complex circular waltz. As if this was not enough, at the same time it was necessary to build and modify a brief but accurate and complete outline of all of the pertinent facts and maintain and modify a list of possible diagnoses. Eventually this process reduced diagnostic uncertainty to an acceptable level and a diagnosis was selected, a complex process in itself. It is no wonder that for many years the clinical reasoning process was seen to be too complex to describe and teach.

The reasoning process needed to make the correct diagnosis can seem to be an overwhelming quagmire of simultaneous processes, gaping pitfalls, and shortcuts that appear to have as many limitations as they have benefits. When taken step by step, each component can be learned, practiced, and optimized to improve the success and efficiency of the whole process. The lists of characteristics, pitfalls, and shortcuts outlined here are not intended to be comprehensive or complete. They are intended to serve as examples, as bricks for a foundation that you will build on, both consciously and unconsciously, throughout your medical career.

## HOW TO BECOME AN EXPERT IN CLINICAL REASONING

*How does one become highly skilled in the vital function of clinical reasoning? In some aspects of medical practice and in other areas of life, focusing highly on the skill itself may be the best path. The surgical specialist chose to focus on a narrow part of the spectrum of the surgical world to achieve a very high level of competence in that area. The sub-subspecialty of eye muscle surgery is an example of this. Athletes usually focus on the specific skills of one area of their sport in order to achieve their goals. To become an excellent right fielder in baseball, one hones a defined set of skills. Is it sufficient to focus on the steps of the problem solving process in order to become an expert diagnostician?*

*Clinical reasoning cannot be viewed as an isolated set of skills or techniques that is sufficient for high-level clinical competence. It is an integration or focal point of a much larger set of competencies (Neufeld et al., 1981):*

1. *Knowledge and clinical experience. Development and continual fine-tuning and adjustment of a huge and constantly changing and expanding personal database is a key component to success. This is the result of ongoing study and experience.*
2. *Interpersonal skills. The expert clinical reasoner must be able to establish rapport with the patient and maintain high-quality communication. This forms a strong foundation for the diagnostic as well as the therapeutic process.*
3. *Interviewing and physical examination skills. The ability to skillfully obtain accurate data from the patient and the physical examination is essential in producing the data that drive the reasoning process. These "basic" clinical skills continue to be vital to the skilled clinical reasoner and clinician.*
4. *Clinical reasoning skills. Though not sufficient in itself, a facility with the component techniques of clinical reasoning and the pitfalls and shortcuts of these techniques is vital.*

*The aspiring student who works hard to become a well-rounded and highly developed clinician—with a high level of knowledge, interpersonal skill, and finely tuned history and physical examination skills—clearly lays the foundation needed to become an excellent clinical reasoner and diagnostician.*

### Reference

Neufeld VR, Norman GR, Barrows HS: Clinical problem solving by medical students: A cross-sectional analysis. *Med Educ* 15:315–322, 1981.

There is more to making the right diagnosis than following a collection of steps. Clinical reasoning brings all of your medical knowledge and experience, all of your skill at interviewing and physical examination, all of your interpersonal skills and insights, in essence your entire being, and uses these to bear on the problems of your patient. As you gain increased knowledge, skills, and experience in all facets of medicine, it will contribute to your ability to make the correct diagnosis.

There is an old joke: "Why do they call it the 'practice' of medicine? Don't doctors ever get it right?" Like many jokes, there is more than a grain of truth. There is always room for continued growth and improvement as a physician, a continual search to learn from your experiences and to do better the next time. Physicians' diagnostic skills may not peak until their mid-50s. I believe that a majority of these physicians would tell you that they are still trying to improve their skills, to learn more and to do better the next time. As you progress in your medical career, I encourage you to follow their example and keep "practicing," in the fullest sense of the word.

## CASE 1

*Outside of the examination room, you pick up the chart of Mr. Black, a 42-year-old man whose chief complaint is "headache." According to the chart, he has a history of hypertension. And his blood pressure today is 180/110 mm Hg. The lights are off in the room and you find Mr. Black lying on the examination table.*

1. *What clues have you identified in the scenario above?*
2. *List several initial hunches that could guide your initial questioning and reasoning.*
3. *What are some potential pitfalls at this early stage of this encounter?*

## CASE 2

*Mr. Antonelli is a 50-year-old truck driver who was last seen in your office 5 years ago for a broken ankle. The nurse obtained the chief complaint of a "sore shoulder," and the patient states that it has been sore off and on for 6 months. It usually bothers him after he has played catch with his son and is not particularly painful. The examination reveals normal strength and range of motion with minimal tenderness over the bicipital tendon on the right.*

1. *What are your hypotheses at this point?*
2. *Are there clues that may suggest that "shoulder pain" may not be his primary reason for coming to the office?*
3. *What questions might help you uncover an alternative reason for this visit?*

## CASE 3

*Ms. Clay is a 21-year-old woman who complains of abdominal pain. Pain has been present for 2 days but has worsened this morning and is located in the right lower quadrant. She vomited once last night and feels nauseated and has not eaten. Her last menstrual period was 5 weeks ago. She is a junior in college and works part-time as a cashier in a bookstore. She smokes a half pack a day, drinks occasionally on weekends, and denies illicit drug use. She is sexually active in a long term, monogamous, heterosexual relationship.*

1. *What hypotheses have you formed from the above information?*
2. *Using the differential diagnosis broadening tools (anatomic approach, pathophysiologic approach, "great imitators"), see if you can expand your differential.*
3. *What additional questions would you ask now to test your hypotheses?*
4. *Write a thumbnail sketch of this case in one or two lines that would quickly and accurately communicate the essentials of this case to a colleague.*

## CASE 4

*Abbie is a pretty 2-year-old child you had delivered and cared for. You are called to the emergency room to see her because she had a 1-minute, generalized seizure this evening. She was confused and lethargic for several minutes after the event, and was found to have a temperature of 104.2°F rectally. She was given acetaminophen and taken to the ER. On examination she is quiet but alert, has a right otitis media (middle ear infection), and does not have a stiff neck.*

1. *What are your current hypotheses?*
2. *What additional history would you obtain now? Physical examination? Laboratory studies?*
3. *Would you obtain a lumbar puncture (spinal tap) on this patient? What are the risks and benefits of doing it? Of not doing it?*
4. *Are there any potential sources of bias that you need to be aware of in making your clinical decisions?*

# CASE 5

*Mr. Diorio is seen in the office as a work-in patient for acute chest pain. The pain occurred in his left anterior chest while he was at work. He smokes a pack of cigarettes a day, is 40 pounds overweight, and is very concerned that he is having a heart attack because his mother and father both have a history of "heart trouble."*

1. *What is your differential diagnosis at this point?*
2. *What additional information is needed to give you a complete clinical description of his pain? Of his risk factors for cardiovascular disease?*
3. *On completion of his history, physical, and review of an ECG, you are 95% certain that this patient has musculoskeletal chest pain from lifting at work. Recognizing that there is a 5% chance that you are wrong, how would you deal with that uncertainty in caring for this patient?*

## RECOMMENDED READINGS

Kassirer JP, Kopelman RW: *Learning Clinical Reasoning.* Baltimore, Williams & Wilkins Co, 1993.

> This text includes a very detailed description of the clinical reasoning process, backed up by a series of excellent clinical cases, each illustrating a specific point. Appropriate for early clinicians as well as more advanced clinical reasoners.

Rakel RE (ed): *Essentials of Family Practice*, ed 2. Philadelphia, WB Saunders Co, 1998.

> This general, primary care-oriented text presents much of its clinical content in problem-oriented chapters, focusing on clinical cases. This helps readers improve their knowledge base, while testing their current knowledge and problem-solving skills.

Reigelman RK: *Minimizing Medical Mistakes: The Art of Medical Decision Making.* Boston, Little Brown & Co, 1991.

> This is a very readable book, filled with practical hints and tips that are illustrated by realistic clinical examples. Recommended as a next step in reading about practical clinical reasoning techniques.

## REFERENCES

Byyny RL, Adams K: The logic of clinical problem solving: Differential diagnosis, in Beck P (ed): *Cases in Clinical Reasoning.* Chicago, Year Book Medical Publishers Inc, 1981, pp 14–15.

Collins RD: *Differential Diagnosis in Primary Care.* Philadelphia, JB Lippincott Co, 1987, pp xii–xiii.

Kassirer JP: Diagnostic reasoning. *Ann Intern Med* 110:894, 1989.

Kassirer JP, Gorry GA: Clinical problem solving: A behavioral analysis. *Ann Intern Med* 89:248–249, 1978.

Reigelman RK: *Minimizing Medical Mistakes: The Art of Medical Decision Making.* Boston, Little Brown & Co, 1991, p 73.

Sloane PD, Curtis P, Ebell MH, Fischer M, Ives TJ, Newton WP: In Sloane PD, Slatt LM, Curtis P, Ebell MH (eds): *Essentials of Family Medicine.* Baltimore, Williams & Wilkins Co, 1997, p 207.

## CHAPTER 11

# Instituting Treatment

*Jeff Susman*

*D. G., a 68-year-old gentleman, presents with nocturia and increasing urinary urgency. He is on no medications and has been in good health. He must get up at night at least every 2 hours and finds it difficult to sit through an entire meeting without making a hasty exit for the restroom. He must strain to initiate urination and has found the urinary stream to be less forceful. D. G. presents to his physician asking if anything can be done to alleviate his distressing symptoms.*

## EDUCATIONAL OBJECTIVES

1. Understand the issues relevant to instituting patient-centered medical therapy
2. Describe the negotiation of treatment with the patient, including the balancing of benefits, harms, and costs of therapy in today's healthcare environment
3. Discuss the role of the family and community in treatment decisions
4. Describe the importance of the balance between patient and physician needs with regard to therapy decisions
5. Define the role of watchful waiting, trials of therapy, and "n of 1" trials
6. Discuss the factors influencing the initiation of treatment
7. Describe how uncertainty affects treatment decisions and the trade-offs this entails
8. Outline methods for enhancing adherence with medical therapy

## INTRODUCTION

The decision to institute treatment should be made thoughtfully and in concert with the patient. This decision is ideally based on a combination of physician, patient, and family preferences and an educated estimate of likely outcomes (Table 11.1).

**Table 11.1**
Issues to Consider When Initiating Treatment

Patient preferences
Efficacy of treatment (including effects on disease outcome, function, patient well-being)
Treatment alternatives (including lifestyle modification, integrative approaches, and nonpharmacological interventions)
Potential drug–drug interactions
Harms of treatment
Natural history of problem when untreated
Cost of treatment
Concomitant medical problems
Age
Gender
Cultural and ethnic factors (e.g., acceptability of treatment, coherence with cultural norms)
Social issues (e.g., social support, living circumstances)
Need for monitoring and follow-up
Ways to enhance adherence

An accurate history including the functional and psychosocial impact of the problem, a targeted physical examination, and judicious ancillary testing will help inform decision-making. In Case 11-1, D. G. is found to have a history of significant lifestyle compromise and a physical examination consistent with BPH. There is no suggestion of prostate cancer. Further workup would be prudent.

## CASE 11-1 (continued)

*D. G.'s physician administers the American Urological Association Symptom Index (Fig. 11.1; McConnell et al., 1994).*
*D. G. scores in the severe range. A physical examination including a focused neurological examination is remarkable only for an enlarged, smooth prostate. Results of urinalysis and serum creatinine are normal. D. G. is eager to begin therapy immediately, "Anything which will allow me to make it through my conference calls."*

In some instances, the physician may choose to observe the natural history of a problem, so-called "watchful waiting." For example, a physician may choose to closely follow a patient with fatigue, arthralgias, or mild mood disturbance rather than immediately performing an elaborate workup or instituting aggressive treatment. In Case 11-1, however, D. G. clearly desires immediate treatment.

## CASE 11-1 (continued)

*D. G.'s physician discusses treatment options including surgery or the initiation of an alpha blocking agent or finasteride. While the success rate for surgery is greater, D. G. opts for a trial of medication given the potential complications of surgery (McConnell et al., 1994). Terazosin is chosen (Table 11.2).*

When therapy is begun, the physician should initiate measures to enhance adherence and guarantee follow-up. In Case 11-1, the physician has asked D. G. to keep track of serial symptom scores. An office nurse checks with D. G. after 1 week to confirm that he is tolerating the terazosin without undue side effects. An office follow-up visit is scheduled in 1 month. At that point therapy will be reassessed and modifications made. The clear plan for follow-up and measurable outcomes of therapy should allow an accurate assessment of therapy.

| Questions to be answered | AUA Symptom Score (Circle 1 number on each line) | | | | | |
|---|---|---|---|---|---|---|
| | Not at all | Less than 1 time in 5 | Less than half the time | About half the time | More than half the time | Almost always |
| 1. Over the past month, how often have you had a sensation of not emptying your bladder completely after you finished urinating? | 0 | 1 | 2 | 3 | 4 | 5 |
| 2. Over the past month, how often have you had to urinate again less than 2 hours after you finished urinating? | 0 | 1 | 2 | 3 | 4 | 5 |
| 3. Over the past month, how often have you found you stopped and started again several times when you urinated? | 0 | 1 | 2 | 3 | 4 | 5 |
| 4. Over the past month, how often have you found it difficult to postpone urination? | 0 | 1 | 2 | 3 | 4 | 5 |
| 5. Over the past month, how often have you had a weak urinary stream? | 0 | 1 | 2 | 3 | 4 | 5 |
| 6. Over the past month, how often have you had to push or strain to begin urination? | 0 | 1 | 2 | 3 | 4 | 5 |
| 7. Over the past month, how many times did you most typically get up to urinate from the time you went to bed at night until the time you got up in the morning? | 0 (None) | 1 (1 time) | 2 (2 times) | 3 (3 times) | 4 (4 times) | 5 (5 times or more) |

Sum of 7 circled numbers (AUA Symptom Score): _____

**Figure 11.1.** American Urological Association symptom index for benign prostatic hyperplasia. From Barry, Fowler, O'Leary, *et al*: The American Urological Association symptom index for benign prostatic hyperplasia. *J Urol* 148:1549–1557, 1992.

**Table 11.2**
Balance Sheet for BPH Treatment Outcomes

| Direct treatment outcomes | Surgical options | | | | Nonsurgical options | | |
|---|---|---|---|---|---|---|---|
| | Balloon dilation | TUIP | Open surgery | TURP | Watchful waiting | Alpha blockers | Finasteride |
| 1. Chance for improvement of symptoms (90% confidence interval) | 37–76% | 78–83% | 94–99.8% | 75–96% | 31–55% | 59–86% | 54–78% |
| 2. Degree of symptom improvement (percent reduction in symptom score) | 51% | 73% | 79% | 85% | Unknown | 51% | 31% |
| 3. Morbidity/complications associated with surgical or medical treatment (90% confidence interval), about 20% of all complications assumed to be significant | 1.78–9.86% | 2.2–33.3% | 6.98–42.7% | 5.2–30.7% | 1–5% Complications from BPH progression | 2.9–43.3% | 13.6–18.8% |
| 4. Chance of dying within 30–90 days of treatment (90% confidence interval) | 0.72–9.78% (high-risk/elderly patients) | 0.2–1.5% | 0.99–4.56% | 0.53–3.31% | 0.8% chance of death ≤90 days for 67-year-old man | | |
| 5. Risk of total urinary incontinence (90% confidence interval) | Unknown | 0.06–1.1% | 0.34–0.74% | 0.68–1.4% | Incontinence associated with aging | | |
| 6. Need for operative treatment for surgical complications in future (90% confidence interval) | Unknown | 1.34–2.65% | 0.6–14.1% | 0.65–10.1% | | 0 | |
| 7. Risk of impotence (90% confidence interval) | No long-term followup available | 3.9–25.4% | 4.7–39.2% | 3.3–34.8% | About 2% of men age 67 become impotent per year. Long-term data on alpha blockers are not available. | | 2.5–5.3% (also decreased volume of ejaculate) |
| 8. Risk of retrograde ejaculation (percent of patients) | Unknown | 6–55% | 36–95% | 25–99% | 0 | 4–11% | 0 |
| 9. Loss of work time (days) | 4 | 7–21 | 21–28 | 7–21 | 1 | 3.5 | 1.5 |
| 10. Hospital stay (days) | 1 | 1–3 | 5–10 | 3–5 | 0 | 0 | 0 |

[a]Source: McConnell JD, Barry MJ, Bruskewitz RC, et al.: Benign Prostatic Hyperplasia: Diagnosis and Treatment. Quick Reference Guide for Clinicians. Rockville, MD, Department of Health and Human Services, Public Health Service, Agency for Health Care Policy and Research. AHCPR Publication No. 94-0583.

Attention should also be paid to the unique needs of special populations, including elders, patients with chronic illnesses, and individuals whose cultural or social background may impact their treatment. A 27-year-old homeless drug addict with AIDS may have significant difficulties adhering to a multidrug treatment regimen. Significant social, psychological, and medical supports would be required to achieve optimal therapy.

Thus, each individual poses a unique challenge when instituting treatment. The physician must balance the patient's needs and preferences, the likelihood of benefits and harms, and the costs and functional impact of therapy.

## CASE 11-2

*J. B., a 44-year-old black male, presents with lightheadedness, fatigue, and blurred vision. His history is positive for polydipsia and polyuria. His father suffered a heart attack at age 57, and his mother has a history of diabetes mellitus and hypertension. The patient smokes two packs of cigarettes per day. On physical examination his blood pressure is 140/92 mm Hg, weight 84 kg, and height 5 feet 7 inches. The rest of the examination results are normal. Initial laboratory testing discloses a blood glucose of 302 mg/dl, a total cholesterol of 257 mg/dl, a low-density-lipoprotein (LDL) cholesterol of 154 mg/dl, and a high-density-lipoprotein (HDL) of 35 mg/dl. Other laboratory results are normal.*

## TREATMENT INITIATION

## Deciding to Begin Treatment

The decision if and when to begin treatment bears careful consideration. When a patient presents to the physician, active intervention is not always necessary. Indeed, many patients simply want reassurance that the condition will spontaneously remit. For example, the patient with a cold or a minor injury often warrants such an approach.

In other conditions, only certain patients need active treatment. For a patient presenting with a sore throat, the decision to treat is based on the probability of the individual having a streptococcal infection, since the results of a throat culture usually take 1 to 2 days. Certain features are associated with an increased or decreased probability of streptococcal infection. For example, the presence of tender cervical adenopathy, fever, tonsillar exudate, and lack of cough increase the likelihood of streptococcal infection to 42.5% based on an overall prevalence of group A streptococcal pharyngitis of 10% (Centor *et al.*, 1986). Centor and colleagues recommend empiric treatment when the clinical signs predict a probability of streptococcal infection greater than 47% without testing, in order to optimize outcomes, including the prevention of rheumatic fever, the quicker resolution of symptoms, and the avoidance of unnecessary antibiotics. If the patient has none of the above features, the likelihood of a strep infection is less than 3% (Centor *et al.*, 1986). Most physicians and patients would defer therapy in such patients given the low probability of infection.

The decision to initiate therapy will be influenced by the seriousness of the problem and its prevalence. For example, a physician is apt to initiate anticoagulant therapy for a 68-year-old who presents with pleuritic chest pain, a tender calf, atrial fibrillation, and mitral valvular disease. In this instance, the possibility of a serious disease, pulmonary embolism, is high, as the patient has multiple findings making this diagnosis more likely. On the other hand, a well 27-year-old who presents with upper respiratory symptoms and pleuritic chest pain would be far less likely to have a pulmonary embolism. Few physicians would begin anticoagulant therapy for this individual without further evidence.

In practice, many factors influence therapy. A physician's previous experience, particularly critical incidents where a treatment had a spectacularly good or bad result, may overshadow reason. For example, if the above-mentioned 27-year-old who presented with pleuritic chest pain ultimately had an occult neoplasm and a pulmonary embolism, the physician might be much more aggressive in evaluation and treatment. Many physicians will poorly estimate the prevalence of disease states and the potential benefits and harms of treatment. Indeed, such outcomes are often unknown in the typical office setting. Finally, patients clearly influence physician choices of therapy.

Even in instances where the physician believes treatment is of low probable benefit, some patients may request therapy. It is not unusual for a patient (or the patient's parent) to "demand" treatment despite a low probability of benefit. In the end, there are trade-offs of costs, the possibility of adverse outcomes, and the use of unnecessary medication or procedures (DeNeef, 1987). Such decisions become dependent on a subjective weighing of patient preference. Most practitioners would acquiesce to treatment when the harms are relatively infrequent or of limited magnitude. Where each practitioner draws this line is an individual decision.

The decision to initiate any treatment is even more complex in individuals, such as J. B. in Case 11-2, with a chronic disease such as diabetes mellitus. In the patient with diabetes mellitus, the threshold for treating hypertension may be lower because of the synergistic effect of hypertension and diabetes mellitus in accelerating renal and vascular disease. In a frail elder, the decision to treat mild hyperglycemia may be forestalled because of the risks of hypoglycemia and limited benefits. In Case 11-2, treatment appears warranted; the question is which options to use and how to begin.

## CASE 11-2 (continued)

*In discussion with the patient, J. B. is willing to meet with the dietitian. J. B.'s physician suggests that his wife join this meeting since she does most of the cooking, and J. B. agrees. An appropriate diet is prescribed. The patient is also willing to use his lunch hour to play basketball at the gym where he works. He does not want to quit smoking at the present time. After discussing the options of beginning insulin versus an oral hypoglycemic agent, J. B. responds that "I would rather be dead than on the needle."*

## Tailoring Treatment Decisions

Once a decision to initiate treatment is made, the focus and form of therapy should be tailored to the patient. In Case 11-2, J. B. has expressed important preferences concerning treatment. Understanding the patient's perspective can enhance adherence to a treatment plan (Cohen-Cole, 1991). Moreover, the physician treating the patient with multiple problems would be advised to ascertain the issues of most interest to the patient. Thus, in an initial visit, recommendations to quit smoking, lose weight, reduce salt intake, limit fat intake, exercise, begin insulin, and begin an antihypertensive medication would be overwhelming and all would likely be ignored. A more effective strategy would be to have a discussion concerning the options for treatment and their potential harms and benefits. It should be remembered that negotiating a plan for care in patients with chronic problems often takes time and usually occurs over a series of visits.

## CASE 11-2 (continued)

*After 3 months of dietary therapy, J. B.'s physician places J. B. on glipizide 5 mg daily and schedules a return visit in 1 month. At that time his BP is 136/86 mm Hg, glucose 215 mg/dl, and his weight is down 2 kg. He has been very compliant with diet, a fact corroborated by his spouse.*

In some cases, a long-term physician–patient relationship built on trust allows the physician and patient to mutually agree on a treatment plan that was initially untenable. For example, in the treatment of depression, many individuals are loath to initiate antidepressant medications. In one poll, 70% of individuals would take a medication for a headache while only 12% would take an antidepressant (Roper Reports, 1986). Recent investigations suggest that physicians actively negotiate with patients with regard to the "right" time to begin antidepressant therapy (Susman *et al.*, 1995). Moreover, many practitioners will use "watchful waiting" or a "tincture of time" approach. In managing minor depressive symptoms, many physicians indicated that they followed patients to see if their mood disturbance resolved or worsened, and initiated further treatment on this basis. Thus, continuity of the physician–patient relationship is important.

The initial response to treatment in Case 11-2 has been successful. By respecting the patient's wishes to concentrate on diet modification rather than smoking and respecting his concern about injections and prescribing an oral hypoglycemic agent, patient trust and initial treatment progress have been accomplished. While alternative or additional therapy may be appropriate in the long run, rapport building is important when treating any patient, especially an individual with a chronic disease.

## CASE 11-2 (continued)

*J. B. returns after 2 months. He is continuing on a program of diet and exercise modification. He is happy with his slimmer self, having lost 3 more kg. His BP is 138/87 mm Hg, glucose 225 mg/dl, and an initial HbA$_1$C 11.4%. J. B.'s physician continues to discuss the importance of diet and exercise, gently reminds him about smoking cessation, and schedules a follow-up in 1 month. He will have his blood pressure checked weekly at a worksite clinic and report on his home-monitored blood glucose to your office nurse.*

## Nonpharmacologic Treatment Modalities

While sometimes relegated to second-class status, nonpharmacologic therapy can be effective for many conditions. Nonpharmacologic approaches have important places in the management of such common disorders as hypertension, hyperlipidemia, and diabetes mellitus (weight control, diet, exercise, smoking cessation), mood disorders (counseling), and even conditions such as obstructive sleep apnea [weight control and nasal continuous positive airway pressure (CPAP)]. While lifestyle modification may prove challenging, it is important to set reasonable goals for therapy and allow time for these interventions to be effective. A potential pitfall for physicians is urging patients to make multiple lifestyle changes simultaneously in a very short time. When patients are "unsuccessful," the physician will then place them on an alternative pharmacologic treatment because of the "failure of conservative therapy." Again, a longer-term perspective, months to years as in J. B.'s case, should be taken.

## CASE 11-2 (continued)

*J. B. follows up in a month accompanied by his wife. He appears to be doing excellently based on his physical examination and laboratory results: BP today is 128/80 mm Hg and at work all readings have been under 134/86 mm Hg. His blood glucose level is gradually decreasing with the most recent readings between 104 and 210 mg/dl. Nonetheless, J. B.'s physician senses some unresolved problems. After some initial pleasantries, it turns out that Mrs. B. is quite concerned because of problems in their marital relationship. J. B. has had gradually increasing problems with erectile dysfunction, getting and maintaining an erection, over the past year. He is quite embarrassed and says that he still loves his wife very much, but "things just don't seem to work like they used to." While a comprehensive review of systems had been performed as part of the initial evaluation, his physician is not surprised to have "missed" this issue.*

## Arranging Follow-Up

An important part of initiating therapy is scheduling follow-up. Follow-up can be done by phone, in the office by another staff member, at the home, or at another community venue. For example, in Case 11-2, J. B. is asked to attend a worksite program so that further data can be gathered on his blood pressure control, and so as to maintain regular contact with the office nurse. Other common follow-up providers might include visiting nurses, home health aides, and physical therapists. Particularly for individuals who are older or require protracted skilled care, such as prolonged antibiotic therapy, home visits may be important. Many worksites have programs emphasizing wellness, occupational issues such as back care, and employee assistance programs for individuals with substance abuse or mental health problems. A large number of volunteer and community agencies offer programs, support groups, and educational materials. Moreover, as in J. B.'s case, adequate follow-up allows the physician to support the patient through difficult lifestyle changes and enhances adherence to recommendations.

## Initiating Treatment Is an Ongoing Issue

It is not uncommon for a richer understanding of a patient's medical and psychosocial problems to unfold over time (Cohen-Cole, 1991). Even direct questioning about a particular issue, such as sexual problems, may fail to elicit the full story until a patient and his family gain trust in the physician, as in Case 11-2. Thus, initiating treatment is an ongoing process that requires careful vigilance to changes in the patient's status and demeanor and thoughtful mobilization of the involvement of the family and significant others.

Office systems can also play an important role in supporting the physician in decisions to monitor and initiate changes in therapy (Pommerenke & Weed, 1991). For example, flow sheets can be quite helpful in monitoring the course of a chronic illness. Peak expiratory flow rates can be monitored in patients with asthma, $HbA_1C$ measurements followed in patients with diabetes mellitus, and blood pressure determinations tracked in those with hypertension. Nursing staff can complete inventories geared to specific problems. In Case 11-2, an office nurse could inquire about foot and skin care, monitor hypoglycemic episodes, and monitor regular ophthalmologic evaluation. A midlevel practitioner or nurse may play a key role in education and monitoring of chronic illness. Staff can also use questionnaires or instruments to screen for certain conditions and guide the physician to consider the initiation of treatment. For example, the Beck or Zung depression inventories or PRIME-MD instrument may be helpful to initially uncover those with depressive symptoms who might benefit from a more complete history and physical (Fig. 11.2) (Depression Guideline Panel, 1993).

More and more evidence suggests that developing an office environment that promotes health is an important part of medical care.

### CASE 11-2 (continued)

*After taking further history and in consultation with J. B., his physician offers a urology evaluation for his impotence. He is scheduled for follow-up in 3 months. During the next months, J. B. learns more about diabetes mellitus by attending meetings of the local chapter of the American Diabetes Association. He learns about a program through the local hospital for patients with diabetes and enrolls. The local nurse, dietitian, endocrinologist, and retinal specialist discuss the importance of preventive care and a stable long-term relationship with a primary care physician.*

**Zung Self-Rating Depression Scale**

| Name _____<br>Age _____ Sex _____ Date _____ | None OR<br>a Little<br>of the Time | Some of<br>the Time | Good Part<br>of the Time | Most OR All<br>of the Time | |
|---|---|---|---|---|---|
| 1. I feel down-hearted, blue and sad | | | | | |
| 2. Morning is when I feel the best | | | | | |
| 3. I have crying spells or feel like it | | | | | |
| 4. I have trouble sleeping through the night | | | | | |
| 5. I eat as much as I used to | | | | | |
| 6. I enjoy looking at, talking to and being with attractive women/men | | | | | |
| 7. I notice that I am losing weight | | | | | |
| 8. I have trouble with constipation | | | | | |
| 9. My heart beats faster than usual | | | | | |
| 10. I get tired for no reason | | | | | |
| 11. My mind is as clear as it used to be | | | | | |
| 12. I find it easy to do the things I used to | | | | | |
| 13. I am restless and can't keep still | | | | | |
| 14. I feel hopeful about the future | | | | | |
| 15. I am more irritable than usual | | | | | |
| 16. I find it easy to make decisions | | | | | |
| 17. I feel that I am useful and needed | | | | | |
| 18. My life is pretty full | | | | | |
| 19. I feel that others would be better off if I were dead | | | | | |
| 20. I still enjoy the things I used to do | | | | | |

SDS RAW SCORE

SDS INDEX

**Figure 11.2.** Zung Self-Rating Depression Scale (Zung, 1965, 1974). From Zung WWK: A self-rating depression scale. *Arch Gen Psychiatry* 12:63–70, 1965.

# Using the Healthcare Team

Many times, a team or collaborative approach to care is useful. Judicious consultation and referral can help provide comprehensive state-of-the-art care. By acknowledging the strengths of the healthcare team, both within the primary care office and in the greater community, a patient can receive support from a group of experts, coordinated by the primary care physician. Good communication, mutual respect, and an open mind make for added value in collaborative care.

## CASE 11-3

*A. S., a 74-year-old male, has a history of benign prostatic hypertrophy, mild congestive heart failure, and diabetes mellitus. He is widowed and lives at home. His medication regimen consists of glyburide 10 mg daily and enalapril 5 mg daily. Following the death of his wife last year, A. S. has gradually withdrawn from his social activities. He no longer plays cards at the senior center, has given up tending his vegetable garden, and complains he is just too tired to engage in outside activities. He goes to bed at 9 PM, awakens at 4 or 5 AM, and tends to nap during the day. He just doesn't feel like cooking. He denies being depressed, but allows he just isn't interested in life anymore. While he has thought it would be a relief to "have it all over with," he denies active suicidal intent. His physician makes a presumptive diagnosis of depression. After discussion, A. S. is willing to initiate antidepressant therapy, "Anything to alleviate this fatigue, but I'm not going to some shrink."*

## MAKING INFORMED TREATMENT DECISIONS

### Initiating Treatment with Concomitant Medical Conditions

In Case 11-3, A. S. is willing to initiate pharmacologic treatment for his depression. Now, the physician must initiate treatment with a holistic care plan in mind. Such planning should consider the patient's overall medical status, risk for medication-induced side effects, and the costs of therapy. A recent summary of the literature suggests that counseling and medication are equally efficacious in the treatment of mild depression (Depression Guideline Panel, 1993). In this instance, the patient has clearly decided against formal counseling and is willing to initiate antidepressant therapy. His current conditions may significantly influence the choice of antidepressant. Common tricyclic antidepressant side effects include sedation, anticholinergic problems, postural hypotension, and cardiac problems.

With A. S.'s history of heart failure—diabetes mellitus, which might predispose to orthostatic hypotension; and benign prostatic hypertrophy—it would appear he is at risk for tricyclic-induced side effects. Probably the best tricyclic choice for A. S. is nortriptyline (Pamelor), which has relatively low anticholinergic and cardiac side effects. Newer antidepressants also avoid most of these potential problems. For example, the selective serotonin reuptake inhibitors, e.g., fluoxetine (Prozac), paroxetine (Paxil), and sertraline (Zoloft), have little or no anticholinergic and postural problems and low potential for cardiac problems (Shaughnessy, 1995).

---

### CASE 11-3 (continued)

*Based on these considerations, A. S.'s physician decides to prescribe fluoxetine. The physician performs an initial Beck inventory and hopes to see a drop in score of at least 10%. The physician explains that unlike other medications, fluoxetine takes approximately 4 to 8 weeks to become effective. Potential side effects such as wakefulness are described and the physician suggests A. S. begin at 10 mg, each morning. A. S. is told that up to 70% of individuals improve on their initial antidepressant and the physician schedules a phone call in 3 days to discuss any progress. If the patient notices any significant problems or increasing depression, he is advised to call immediately.*

A. S. calls within an hour. "I tried to get that medicine and my insurance plan won't cover it. I decided I would just go ahead and buy it, but what is it made of—gold? I can't afford to take it!" Sheepishly, A. S.'s physician apologizes and ascertains that paroxetine is covered under the patient's managed care plan.

### Recommendations on Initiating Therapy

On initiation of any therapy, certain guidelines should be followed. A clear explanation of the medication's intended action and possible side effects is important. Many medications have significant drug–drug, drug–disease, or drug–nutrient interactions. Clear prescribing instructions should be given, including when the dose is to be taken and under what conditions. The initial course of treatment should be outlined and plans for follow-up should be arranged. Guidelines for earlier follow-up should be given. In many patients, an "n of 1" trial is initiated: An intervention is tried and a principal outcome measure is monitored before and during therapy (Kazdin, 1982). In Case 11-3, the effect of an antidepressant on A. S.'s Beck score will be monitored. Occasionally, the physician may choose to withdraw therapy and see if the intervention truly accounts for the noted improvement in outcome.

# ORTHOSTATIC HYPOTENSION

## Definition

*Orthostatic or postural hypotension is a drop in blood pressure associated with a change to a more upright posture. It is typically defined as a drop in the systolic blood pressure of 20 mm Hg or diastolic blood pressure of 10 mm Hg when going from a lying to a standing position. Classically, the pulse should rise, although this change is inconsistent, particularly in older individuals who have autonomic dysfunction.*

## Diagnosis

*In checking a patient for orthostatic hypotension, it is important for the patient to be lying long enough for blood volume to equilibrate. It is prudent to have the patient lying down for 10 or 15 minutes before measuring the lying blood pressure and pulse. Then ask the patient to rise to a standing position. This change in posture (as opposed to simply sitting) will be the most likely to provoke an orthostatic change. Be ready to break a patient's fall! Immediately take the patient's blood pressure and pulse. Repeat these measurements after 1 and 5 to 10 minutes. Some patients will demonstrate a late fall in blood pressure.*

## Differential Diagnosis

*Drugs*
> *Diuretics*
> *Antidepressants and antipsychotic agents*
> *Antihypertensives*
> *Parkinsonian agents*
> *Sedatives/hypnotics*

*Intravascular Volume Depletion*
> *Blood loss*
> *Diarrhea*
> *Adrenal insufficiency*

*Neurologic Disease*
> *Autonomic neuropathy (e.g., associated with diabetes, amyloid)*

*Other*
> *Pregnancy*
> *Prolonged bed rest*
> *Sympathectomy*

## Management

*Management depends on the cause. For drug-induced orthostatic changes, a change in dose or medication is often indicated. In cases of intravascular volume depletion, volume replacement and disease treatment are pursued. Support stockings, salt supplements, mineralocorticoids (e.g., fludrocortisone), and other medications are used to treat clinically significant orthostatic hypotension.*

## MANAGED CARE FORMULARIES

*Many managed care organizations (MCOs) will have a specific formulary or group of drugs that are approved for use and payment through their plans. The theory is that restricting drug choice will allow more appropriate prescribing and decrease costs of care. Some formularies have been constructed from an "evidence-based medicine" viewpoint and attempt to establish the most appropriate drug choices within a given drug class or rational approaches to managing common problems. On the other hand, the choice of drugs may be driven by deals struck between managed care companies and pharmaceutical manufacturers, often through an intermediary called a pharmacy benefits manager (PBM). For example, the PBM might negotiate with the manufacturers of different selective serotonin reuptake inhibitors (SSRIs) to obtain the best price by agreeing to preferentially use a given agent. Managed care organizations might then place the "preferred" drug on the formulary and cover the full cost of this selected drug (less a small copay). The MCO might allow the prescription of other SSRIs but pass on more of the expense of these "alternative" agents. Formularies, and prior authorization, are also used to control access to expensive therapies such as growth hormone and agents to treat HIV infection.*

## Considering Costs

In today's medical environment, cost is an important aspect of medical care. Unfortunately, calculating costs can be challenging. It is important to consider not only the actual medication cost, but also the cost of monitoring and ongoing medication management and from whose perspective costs are being viewed. Clearly, from A. S.'s perspective, a medication that is not covered under his insurer's formulary will be personally quite expensive and, without clear evidence of differing efficacy, of unwarranted expense. The "Red Book" is a list of average wholesale prices (AWP) and can be useful in considering drug acquisition costs. However, other costs are important to consider. For example, will drug levels or laboratory tests need to be monitored, and will follow-up visits or procedures be needed? Moreover, total costs are significantly related to real-world effectiveness as opposed to theoretical efficacy (Wilson, 1992). For example, reserpine is quite inexpensive and is effective as an antihypertensive. However, its side effect profile may lead to discontinuation or medication-induced problems. Similarly, in a study evaluating the relative effectiveness of imipramine and desipramine, older tricyclic antidepressants, versus fluoxetine, a newer SSRI, patients randomized to fluoxetine were more likely to receive adequate treatment when compared with the tricyclics (Simon *et al.*, 1994). Finally, in today's world of managed care, from whose perspective costs are accrued becomes an important ethical issue. Many plans place the physician at risk for expenses. Under such a plan, a practitioner could choose a less costly medication at the expense of patient convenience or side effects. Thus, consideration of costs is an important part of practicing medicine today.

## CASE 11-3 (continued)

*A. S. returns after 8 weeks. He says his fatigue is improving and he has noticed a significant improvement in his sleep routine. He is thinking about returning to the senior center to play cards. He is grateful to his physician for her ongoing help.*

## Enhancing Adherence

Methods to enhance adherence are an important part of initiating and maintaining therapy (Table 11.3).

Adherence is compliance with the clinician's instructions and may be influenced by the patient's motivation; the problem being treated; the medication's benefits, harms, and costs; and the quality of the

**Table 11.3**
Selected Factors Enhancing Adherence

| |
|---|
| Simplify instructions |
| Provide written instructions at appropriate comprehension level |
| Discuss common side effects and their treatment |
| Enhance patient's feeling of self-control and choice |
| Provide tools for self-monitoring |
| Understand the disease from the patient's perspective; understand their conception of illness and treatment |
| Develop ways to help reinforce therapy |
| Address barriers to therapy |
| Simplify the treatment regimen |
| Involve family members and significant support partners |
| Schedule follow-up |
| Regularly seek patient feedback |
| Limit the number of medications |
| Set clear treatment goals and assess progress regularly |

physician–patient relationship. Nonadherence is very common; for example, up to 50% of individuals with hypertension are not taking their medication at the end of 1 year of treatment. Adherence may be improved by simplifying instructions, simplifying medication regimens, discussing common side effects, enhancing the patient's feeling of self-control and choice, understanding the illness from the patient's perspective, providing the tools to implement self-monitoring, and developing ways to enforce therapy or deal with barriers to ongoing treatment (Ruffalo *et al.*, 1985). In Case 11-3, prescribing a medication once a day, providing written instructions, involving caregivers and significant others, discussing side effects before and during therapy, and continuing to explore the patient's feelings were all done to enhance adherence.

## CASE 11-4

*G. M., a 32-year-old factory worker, presents with low back pain. He said he injured his back on the job while working on the assembly line. He is responsible for tightening two bolts and installing a filter in a truck assembly plant. He has had shooting pains down his right leg and complains of some mild tingling. He denies bowel or bladder complaints and says that other than the pain, his strength is unchanged. He denies any other medical problems, constitutional symptoms, drug abuse, risk factors for HIV infection or immunocompromise, or trauma.*

*On physical examination, G. M. is in some obvious discomfort. The straight leg raise is equivocally positive on the left and positive at 35 degrees on the right. He has a minimally diminished ankle reflex on the right, and diminished light touch and sensation on the lateral aspect of the right foot. Results of the rest of the examination are unremarkable.*

*Dr. C. M. makes the presumptive diagnosis of an S1 radiculopathy and begins to discuss treatment options when the patient inquires, "You mean to tell me you aren't going to do an x-ray, aren't recommending bed rest, and won't authorize traction and a TENS unit like the last time I was out?"*

# DEALING WITH UNCERTAINTY AND BALANCING SCIENCE WITH HUMANITY

## Dealing with Uncertainty and the Use of Clinical Policies

Medical practice changes. What was once accepted as dogma falls aside with the acquisition of new knowledge. While traditionally, patients were placed on strict bed rest, put in traction, and offered a wide variety of exotic therapies, recent literature has demonstrated the lack of effectiveness of such interventions for patients with back pain (Bigos *et al.*, 1994).

One of the great challenges for the family physician is keeping up with the medical literature. Especially when medical practice has changed significantly, or different physicians' practices vary widely, the clinician may look for help in making informed decisions. Many organizations, such as the Agency for Health Care Policy and Research (AHCPR), are developing clinical policies, practice parameters, or practice guidelines. These policies provide explicit summaries of the literature, including the latest in diagnosis and management strategies. Moreover, the policies currently available through the AHCPR, covering conditions ranging from low back problems to pressure sores, are accompanied by well-written patient guides. As discussed, a key task in initiating therapy is to negotiate with patients and address their understanding of their illness. A clinical policy, therefore, not only can help guide physician decision-making, but also can support patient adherence and improve education (see Chapter 22, "Development of Clinical Guidelines").

---

### CASE 11-4 (continued)

*The physician shares the AHCPR low back problems patient brochure with the patient. She explains that bed rest is recommended for no longer than 4 days, that there is no evidence that traction is helpful, and that a TENS unit is of unproven benefit in the treatment of acute low back pain. Although G. M. is skeptical, he is willing to discuss options recommended as effective. The physician decides together with G. M. to try a nonsteroidal anti-inflammatory drug (NSAID) and to touch base over the next couple of days.*

*After 48 hours, however, the pain has increased and the patient notices increasing numbness. He goes to his local chiropractor and experiences significant relief of his discomfort after a week of manipulative therapy. He returns to his physician's office in 2 weeks saying he continues to have pain, but found it impossible to take the NSAID because of stomach upset. The manipulative therapy has helped somewhat, but there is still considerable numbness. The physician discusses further options and decides to switch the medication to acetaminophen and instructs the patient to apply cold packs at home. After 7 weeks, the patient continues to experience pain and activity limitation. He continues to have numbness and the results of his physical examination, while stable, are consistent with an S1 radiculopathy. A CT scan of the spine discloses an L5–S1 herniated disk with S1 nerve root entrapment. The physician offers referral to a spinal surgeon, who after discussing options with the patient, recommends chymopapain treatment.*

## Sharing Uncertainty with Others

It is important for the primary care physician to maintain continuity of care both in the initial treatment phases and during any ongoing consultations or referral. Decisions to order further diagnostic tests or treatments should be based on the patient's response to therapy, his ongoing preferences, and the opportunity to influence the course of illness. The vast majority of patients with low back problems, even with radiculopathy, recover uneventfully (Bigos *et al.*, 1994). Initiating treatment requires a knowledge of the natural history of the disease in question, an understanding of the effect of various treatment strategies, and the trade-offs of each. While surgery for herniated disks is effective, the long-term outcome for most patients following more conservative therapy is the same. The question becomes how much does the patient value

---

### CHYMOPAPAIN THERAPY

*Chemonucleolysis or dissolving of herniated disk material can be achieved with chymopapain injection with the goal of relieving pressure on the nerve root. While chymopapain has been shown to be effective when compared with saline injections in randomized controlled trials, it is not as effective as diskectomy. Moreover, the occurrence of serious side effects, including life-threatening anaphylaxis and transverse myelitis, has diminished the enthusiasm for this intervention.*

shorter-term improvement at the risk of a surgical complication. In this instance, the surgeon has recommended a treatment option that has significant risks and is not as effective as other surgical options such as diskectomy (Bigos *et al.*, 1994).

Again, the physician should be able to act as an advocate and interpreter for the patient and family members with consultants. In Case 11-4, the physician might suggest other treatment options that are more appropriate and act as an intermediary between the patient and the surgeon.

## CASE 11-4 (continued)

*After a standard diskectomy, the patient continues to have pain and applies for workmen's compensation. G. M. says that he is fed up with his job and things are not going well at home, either. In fact, G. M. is drinking up to 12 bottles of beer each day and he and his wife are nearing a divorce. Assessment of the physical examination is remarkable for multiple pain behaviors but there are no new findings. A follow-up MRI is unremarkable, and the orthopedic consultant says there is nothing further to be done: "He will just have to live with it." The patient wonders if he should be placed on Percodan or a stronger medication.*

## Unproven or Risky Treatments

Unproven or even risky treatments are sought by some individuals, especially those with chronic or incurable diseases. It is important for the physician to react to such patients with equanimity, offer support and hope, and suggest more appropriate alternative measures. Individuals such as G. M. in Case 11-4 with chronic pain or concomitant psychiatric problems offer special challenges to the physician. When initiating ongoing therapy, such circumstances test the mettle of even the most experienced clinician. Clearly negotiating boundaries of care, working with a multidisciplinary team, and developing an empathetic but firm approach are needed. Involving the family, co-workers, and significant others in an intervention can be more effective than trying to treat such patients alone.

## CASE 11-4 (continued)

*G. M. returns after undergoing counseling and working with a multidisciplinary pain management team. After much self-reflection, he has retrained for another job, moderated his alcohol use, and patched up his marriage. He is extremely grateful for his physician's help, and grateful that his father, B. M., has come for evaluation of his own back problems. B. M. is 78 years old and has had increasing back problems over the past 3 months. Other than a history of prostate cancer, B. M. has been remarkably well. He has noted a 10-pound, unintentional weight loss over the past month. Physical examination is remarkable for some tenderness at the L2 vertebra.*

*The physician is concerned about B. M.'s history of prostate cancer, unintentional weight loss, and back tenderness. The physician's worst fears are confirmed when a bone scan and subsequent MRI discloses metastatic cancer, presumably from the prostate.*

---

### INFORMED CONSENT

*Informed consent is a process—not a form, document, or signature—that details the purpose of an intervention, its benefits and harms, and potential alternatives in a noncoercive environment, in terminology a patient can understand. The signature of a form only serves to document this process and provide evidence of active authorization for an intervention.*

---

## MULTIDISCIPLINARY TEAMS

*Multidisciplinary teams are used for a variety of patients including individuals with diabetes, pain, and premature neonates. By assembling a team of experts, it is hoped that a more holistic assessment and management of patients can occur. Individuals with specialized expertise are then available to help patients more comprehensively.*

*As an example, consider the patient with chronic back pain. A multidisciplinary team might consist of specialists in family medicine, orthopedics, physical therapy, neurology, neurosurgery, psychiatry, chiropractic, acupuncture, occupational medicine, physical medicine, and a host of complementary therapies. The patient might complete a thorough traditional medical evaluation, undergo an assessment for mental health problems, consult with a variety of experts in pain management, explore "work-hardening" exercises, enhance communication between the patient and family, and work with occupational therapists on work site modification.*

## Treating Special Populations

When initiating therapy the physician must remember to assess the whole patient, her personal history, and unique background. This assessment should consider the epidemiology, culture, and beliefs of the patient and her community. For example, the astute clinician in Case 11-4 recognized the different epidemiology of back pain in B. M. While his son's presentation was similar, B. M. has a much higher risk of having a serious underlying cause of his back discomfort.

In elders, the physician must consider changes in the distribution, absorption, metabolism, protein binding, pharmacokinetic, and pharmacodynamic action of medications. For example, the half-life of benzodiazepines may be significantly longer in elders. Elders may also have significant comorbidities that make them susceptible to medication side effects. Moreover, they may lack the social supports, sensory or motor facilities, or capability to adhere to optimal therapy.

Functional outcomes become increasingly important, rather than curative goals, in the elderly (see Chapter 16, "Functional Assessment"). While a diuretic may improve blood pressure, the precipitation of orthostatic hypotension and falls, a common side effect, could be devastating. Modifying cardiac risk factors, such as cholesterol, may have less influence on a patient's longevity and significantly impact a patient's quality of life.

Other special populations have important needs. For example, in today's diverse society, understanding the patient's cultural, ethnic, and racial background can also be crucial. An individual with G6PD deficiency will be intolerant of certain medications. A Jehovah's Witness may refuse blood products on religious grounds. An elderly Czech farmer may have certain dietary preferences. And an individual who is homeless will face significant barriers to adhering to many treatment regimens. Understanding the patient's needs and sociocultural perspective is important to tailoring therapy appropriately (Helman, 1994).

## CONCLUSION

The decision to institute therapy should be considered judiciously. Many patients will warrant watchful waiting. Others will benefit from nonpharmacologic treatment. The initiation of therapy will depend on the seriousness of the problem, the probability of treatment success and complications, and patient preference. In many cases, a series of treatment options will be outlined and an initial therapy chosen.

When beginning treatment, measures to enhance adherence and plans for follow-up should be enacted.

The physician should set outcome goals and discuss ways to monitor for possible complications. Involving the patient in treatment will enhance adherence. The partnership between the clinician and patient is important to ongoing treatment success.

Special care should be paid to the patient's unique needs. Many patients will have preexisting conditions, extenuating social or economic circumstances, or particular ethnic or cultural preferences. Acknowledging and respecting these differences will also enhance adherence to treatment. By carefully considering the whole patient, the astute physician can help guarantee favorable outcomes.

# CASES FOR DISCUSSION

## CASE 1

*P. M., a 25-year-old i.v. drug abuser, presents because of fatigue, night sweats, and an oral rash. During the course of the history, the physician learns he has had multiple same-sex partners and has been engaging in "risky" sexual activities, i.e., is at high risk for sexually transmitted diseases. P. M. has had a positive HIV test. On physical examination the physician finds an oral rash suggestive of candida infection and generalized adenopathy. A CD4+ lymphocyte count is 150 cells/ml.*

1. *Does this patient have AIDS?*
2. *When should treatment with antiretroviral therapy be started? Does such therapy forestall the development of AIDS, prolong an asymptomatic phase, or increase life span?*
3. *Are there particular illnesses to which this patient is susceptible? What interventions are appropriate to prevent these illnesses?*
4. *What nonpharmacologic treatments should be instituted?*
5. *What role do family, community support groups, and other counseling resources play in this patient's treatment?*

## CASE 2

*J. M., a 36-year-old woman, presents with a 3-month history of a distinct mass in her right breast. She has a history of fibrocystic changes and underwent aspiration of a benign breast mass 3 years ago. Her mother and a sister have a history of breast cancer. Examination discloses a discrete 2-cm mass in the right upper quadrant of the right breast. An attempt at aspiration is unsuccessful.*

1. *What further diagnostic evaluation, if any, would you recommend before instituting treatment in this patient?*
2. *How would your recommendations differ if the patient were 26 or 76? If the patient had no family history of breast cancer? If the mass first appeared 2 weeks ago?*
3. *If the mass turned out to be an adenocarcinoma, and there was no evidence of distant metastasis, what options would you recommend? Construct a list of the pros and cons of various treatment options.*

## CASE 3

*D. C., a frail 89-year-old, presents with urgency, hesitancy, and difficulty maintaining a good urinary stream. The patient has a history of moderate Alzheimer's disease, diagnosed 3 years ago; coronary artery disease and congestive heart failure; osteoarthritis; and diabetes mellitus. Evaluation by your urologic consultant discloses prostate cancer with an equivocal area of bony metastasis to the spine on bone scan. The patient's daughter has flown in from California and wants to know what you recommend as treatment.*

1. *What factors influence treatment decisions in this patient?*
2. *What is the natural history of prostate cancer in this patient?*
3. *How would you make treatment decisions for a cognitively impaired individual?*
4. *What if the patient had never clearly expressed wishes regarding treatment and your judgment concerning the best course of action differed from the daughter's?*

## CASE 4

*L. S., a 64-year-old with mild Parkinson's disease and diabetes mellitus, presents to your office having "passed out." The patient is a vice president at a major corporation and a vigorous and mentally sharp individual. He was rising to go to the bathroom yesterday evening when he "fainted," just missing hitting his head on the nightstand. He said he didn't really lose consciousness, but felt light-headed. He returned to bed, rested, and after sitting up for a short period of time, was able to make it to the bathroom without incident. His wife was away on a business trip, but on her return, "made him" come to your office for assessment. She is quite concerned, and wonders if his heart is acting up. The patient takes levodopa/carbidopa 100/25 TID and glipizide 5 mg po qd. Examination reveals an alert, cooperative gentleman in no distress.*

- *BP 130/70 mm Hg, pulse 67/minute, respirations 12/minute*
- *HEENT: normal*
- *Neck: supple, no bruits*
- *Lungs: clear to A and P*
- *Cor: S1, S2, no murmurs, clicks, or rubs*
- *Periphery: remarkable for minimal distal sensory peripheral neuropathy in toes*
- *Results of neurologic examination are normal except for a slight tremor and minimal rigidity in the upper extremities*
- *HbA$_1$C is 8.1%, results of the chemistry profile and EKG are normal*

  1. *What is the differential diagnosis in this patient?*
  2. *How useful is the clinical history and examination in narrowing down the possibilities?*
  3. *Are there are any other historical or physical findings you would seek?*
  4. *How much further evaluation (if any) is prudent?*
  5. *What would you tell this patient about driving or operating his Rototiller this spring?*
  6. *How likely is the patient to experience another "spell"?*

## CASE 5

*A 17-year-old high school gymnast presents to the office with a painful right ankle. She fell off the parallel bars earlier today and now complains of discomfort and swelling along the lateral aspect of the ankle. She believes she bent her ankle inward, but is not sure. She is extremely upset because the state tournament is tomorrow.*

*On examination there is obvious swelling and early bruising. There is pain on palpation in a diffuse area along the lateral aspect of the ankle. There is no point tenderness along the posterior edge or tip of either malleolus. There is no tenderness at the base of the metatarsals or at the navicular. The patient limps, but can cautiously bear weight with assistance.*

  1. *Did this patient break her ankle? Did she sprain her ankle? Do you remember the anatomy of the ankle ligaments?*
  2. *Is an x-ray needed? Will treatment be influenced by the findings on x-ray?*
  3. *Are there some guidelines that might help in ordering an x-ray?*
  4. *How would you manage this patient?*

## CASE 6

*A 7-year-old presents with earache. An examination discloses a red ear with a poorly movable tympanic membrane. You believe the patient has otitis media.*

  1. *What factors would you consider in initiating therapy?*
  2. *What are the costs of various alternative treatments?*
  3. *How would you deal with a parent requesting an effective, but costly, pharmacologic treatment when less costly alternatives were available?*

## RECOMMENDED READINGS

Brody DS: The patient's role in clinical decision-making. *Ann Intern Med* 93:718–722, 1980.

Clearly articulates the primary role of the patient in clinical decision-making.

Erhardt LR: The essence of effective treatment and compliance is simplicity. *Am J Hypertens* 12:105S–110S, 1999.

    Despite clear evidence concerning effective treatment of coronary heart disease, current clinical practice falls short of established guidelines. This article reviews factors influencing physician adherence to guidelines and patient adherence to medications.

Helman CG: *Culture, Health and Illness*. London, Butterworth–Heinemann, 1994.

    A classic work of medical anthropology describing the interaction of culture, well-being, illness, and disease.

Hilfiker D: *Healing the Wounds: A Physician Looks at His Work*. New York, Viking Penguin, 1987.

    An insightful, often heartwrenching look at an individual's practice, including the challenges of diagnosis and treatment and facing the limits of knowledge and ability.

Kehoe WA, Katz RC: Health behaviors and pharmacotherapy. *Ann Pharmacother* 32:1076–1086, 1998.

    Suggests factors influencing health-related behaviors and how to address them in practice.

Lutfey KE, Wishner WJ: Beyond "compliance" is "adherence". Improving the prospect of diabetes care. *Diabetes Care* 22:635–639, 1999.

    Argues for a patient-centered approach to care that recognizes influences on patient behavior and ways to enhance therapeutic adherence.

Pauker SG, Kopelman RI: Some familiar tradeoffs. *N Engl J Med* 331:1511–1514, 1994.

    This article describes the decision-making process used to initiate anticoagulant therapy, including the trade-offs balanced in management. The clinical problem-solving series in *NEJM* is an excellent resource for thinking about the initiation of therapy.

# REFERENCES

Bigos S, Boyer O, Braen G, *et al*: Acute Low Back Problems Guideline Panel. *Acute Low Back Problems in Adults. Clinical Practice Guideline. Quick Reference Guide No. 14*. Rockville, Md, US Department of Health and Human Services, Public Health Service, Agency for Health Care Policy and Research, AHCPR Publication No. 95-0643, 1994.

Centor RM, Meier FA, Dalton HP: Throat cultures and rapid tests for diagnosis of group A streptococcal pharyngitis. *Ann Intern Med* 105:892–899, 1986.

Cohen-Cole SA: *The Medical Interview: The Three-Function Approach*. St. Louis, Mo, Mosby–Year Book Inc, 1991.

DeNeef P: Selective testing for streptococcal pharyngitis in adults. *J Fam Pract* 25:347–353, 1987.

Depression Guideline Panel. *Depression in Primary Care*. 1993.

Helman CG: *Culture, Health and Illness: An Introduction for Health Professionals*. London, Butterworth–Heinemann Ltd, 1994.

Kazdin AE: *Single-Case Research Designs*. London, Oxford University Press, 1982.

McConnell JD, Barry MJ, Bruskewitz RC, *et al*: *Benign Prostatic Hyperplasia: Diagnosis and Treatment. Quick Reference Guide for Clinicians*. Rockville, Md, US Department of Health and Human Services, Public Health Service, Agency for Health Care Policy and Research. AHCPR Publication No. 94-0583, 1994.

Pommerenke FA, Weed DL: Physician compliance: Improving skills in preventive medicine practices. *Am Fam Physician* 43:560–568, 1991.

Roper Reports. Report to Medicaid: What people do for minor health problems. New York, Roper Organization, 1986, pp 86–88.

Ruffalo RL, Garabedian-Ruffalo SM, Pawlson LG: Patient compliance. *Am Fam Physician* 31:93–100, 1985.

Shaughnessy AF: Considerations in antidepressant therapy. *Fam Pract Recertif* 17:31–37, 1995.

Simon GE, Von Korff M, Katon WJ: Balancing cost and effectiveness of antidepressant drugs in primary care: A randomized trial. Presented at the eighth annual NIMH international research conference on mental health problems in the general health care sector, Sept 7–9, 1994, McLean, Va, pp 72–73.

Susman JL, Crabtree BF, Essink G: Depression in rural family practice: Easy to recognize, difficult to diagnose. *Arch Fam Med* 4:427–431, 1995.

Wilson DM: Assessment of an intervention in primary care: Counseling patients on smoking cessation, in Tudiver F, Bass MJ, Dunn EV, Norton PG, Stewart M (eds): *Assessing Interventions: Traditional and Innovative Methods*. Beverly Hills, Calif, Sage Publications Inc, 1992, p 139.

## CHAPTER 12

# Recordkeeping and Presentation

*William M. Chop, Jr.*

## CASE 12-1

*Trembling, Mr. Madigan opens the door of his home to Dr. Harrison. Mr. Madigan's wife Mary is deathly ill with fever and shortness of breath. Dr. Harrison examines her, diagnoses pneumonia, and drives her to a small-town hospital in the next county.*

*After a bumpy ride, Dr. Harrison presents Mrs. Madigan's case to Dr. Bell, a physician practicing at the county hospital. A few words about Mary's past poor health and her difficult life on a run-down old farm help complete the picture for Dr. Bell and the night nurse, who both commit the story to memory. No paper records are exchanged. The physician examines Mrs. Madigan and gives verbal orders to the nurse, who helps the new patient into a bed on the ward. Dr. Bell writes the patient record by simply recording Mrs. Madigan's name and diagnosis in the ward's large ledger book. She miraculously survives the pneumonia, and after 3 weeks of prayer, care, and fresh air her husband takes her home. Dr. Bell records the final outcome of the case on the same line of the same ledger, and the case is closed. Her hospital record consists of one line of text. The year is 1911.*

## EDUCATIONAL OBJECTIVES

1. Discuss users and uses of patient records
2. Explain the advantages and disadvantages of source-based and problem-oriented records
3. Given a patient encounter, author a data base, a problem list, and an assessment and plan
4. Given a patient encounter, write an untitled "SOAP" note and a true problem-oriented record, and explain the advantages and disadvantages of each
5. Explain the advantages and disadvantages of traditional, problem-based, and newspaper-style case presentations
6. Given a patient encounter or record, a particular audience, and a purpose, give a verbal presentation that efficiently and effectively conveys the patient's story and achieves the purpose for that audience
7. Produce accurate, honest records and presentations that favorably portray each patient as a person worthy of empathy and care

Skills in recordkeeping and presentation add leverage to other clinical skills. The process of preparing records and presentations yields insight into a patient's case, protects against clinical oversights, and provides feedback that will advance clinical expertise. Recordkeeping and presentation are primary means by which general and case-specific medical knowledge and wisdom are transmitted over time and space to other physicians. The ability to capture and transmit the story of each patient is fundamental in maintaining the professional literature and preserving the art of medicine.

Writing about patient cases is an ancient medical tradition, but in the past it was done only infrequently, mostly to support investigation and education rather than to support direct patient care. The one-line record of Case 12-1 was typical in small rural hospitals. Today, patient records are authored mainly because they are so helpful in the care of individual patients. But they have also become complicated, and are now multicomponent documents with many users and uses. The ability to maintain medically useful patient records is one of the hallmarks of a good physician. This chapter will help develop strong skills in understanding, using, and keeping patient records.

The importance of excellent oral presentation skills has also grown during the twentieth century. Presentations of a patient's case remain an important part of the grand tradition of medicine, especially in medical education settings. In the past, physicians had a slower pace and a relatively small menu of available diagnostic modalities and treatments. Simple communications sufficed. Dr. Harrison's presentation to Dr. Bell in Case 12-1 was simple and direct compared with the frequent, rapid, and concise communication of patient information needed today. Consultation and teaching also depend heavily on quality verbal presentations of patient cases. This chapter will focus on the importance of strong skills in listening to and presenting patient cases.

In approaching these subjects, remember that charting and presentation skills depend on medical knowledge and experience. An excellent patient record or presentation will only result from excellent data collection and analysis. Do not become discouraged if it is initially difficult to produce smooth, useful records and presentations.

## CASE 12-2

*Mrs. Smith thoughtfully completed the health forms. She listed her diabetes mellitus, her hypertension, and the births of her children. She explained her possible allergy to sulfa drugs. On the review of systems form she checked the appropriate boxes and explained all of the symptoms she was experiencing. The nurse took her vital signs and complaints, and led her to an examining room.*

*Dr. Susan Jones picked up the chart of this new patient from the rack on the examination room door, and began to read it. New patient ... 47-year-old woman ... diabetes mellitus ... hypertension ... makes a living as an artist. She entered the examination room, and started the visit. After the visit, Dr. Jones wrote a two-part prescription form, gave the original to Mrs. Smith, and filed the copy in the chart. She had Mrs. Smith sign releases to get records from her previous physicians. She completed the problem list in the chart, filled in the top of the flow sheet with a preventive health plan, and wrote the new medication and dose at the bottom. She then dictated a progress note. The next afternoon, after the transcribed progress note returned, Dr. Jones reviewed and signed it, and a nurse placed it in Mrs. Smith's chart. When copies arrived from Mrs. Smith's previous physicians, Dr. Jones reviewed them, updated the chart with a brief note, and filed them in the "old record" section. Two weeks later, Mrs. Smith's insurance company requested a copy of her chart, and it was sent. A month later Mrs. Smith's chart was randomly selected by the clinic's quality assurance committee for review. It passed. Three months later the chart was reviewed as part of a retrospective research study of antihypertensive medications. When Mrs. Smith returned for a sprained ankle 4 months later, Dr. Jones's detailed note allowed her partner to more quickly appreciate Mrs. Smith as a person, and to take better care of her and her family.*

Sigurdsson describes the purpose of patient records simply, stating that they are "aids to the treatment of the patient," "instruments of teaching, learning, and research," and "a source of statistics," and warns that "the ultimate test of a system for collecting and handling data in primary health care should be whether such a system helps us to understand better the special relationship between healer and patient; not just the interaction between the two, but the relationship itself in its full sociocultural context" (Sigurdsson, 1984). Physicians view patient records as confidential information covered by the Hippocratic oath, wherein "whatever, in connection with my professional practice, or not in connection with it, I may see or hear in the lives of men which ought not to be spoken abroad I will not divulge, as reckoning that all such should be kept secret." However, a large number of third parties to the patient–physician relationship now vie for access to medical records. The Council on Scientific Affairs of the American Medical Association (1993) cites seven categories of users and 13 broad uses of patient records. This chapter focuses mainly on the role patient records play in patient care and the patient–physician relationship, but a brief discussion of the full spectrum of important users and uses for patient records will help to set the stage.

At its essence, the patient record is a tool to facilitate the complex process of caring for patients in sickness and health. The process of care involves many people, including patients, families, students, residents, physicians, consultants, nurses, educators, researchers, psychologists, lab technicians, radiology technicians, insurance companies and other third-party payers, financial staff, managers, reviewers, licensing and accrediting agencies, and professional associations. All of these people interact with the patient, the patient record, and each other, in different ways, and for many purposes, as illustrated in Case 12-2.

The most obvious purpose of the patient record is to serve as a memory device to foster continuity of care. Even when a patient sees only a single physician, that physician cannot afford to rely on simple memory for all of the important details about that particular patient. At a second visit the physician uses the record to gain a clinical and personal foothold based on the information recorded at the first visit. Even in less desirable clinical settings where the patient sees a new physician at each visit, good records help each different physician to gain a more rapid and complete understanding of the patient as a person and of the patient's medical needs. Through each physician's contribution, a historical record for the future is maintained that is much more accurate and comprehensive than memory.

The record helps clinicians to visualize the patient's clinical situation to support intelligent diagnosis and treatment. Even if no illness is identified, a record helps the physician to assess and manage health risks in providing preventive care to both individual patients and communities.

Patient records document the patient's case management for billing and legal purposes. Because of legal and economic pressures, an unfortunate line of thinking has been allowed to arise in medical management circles that "if it's not documented, then it didn't happen." Of course this statement is not true, but without a medical record that documents and justifies a physician's bill to the patient, bureaucrats will claim that the physician did not actually render a service, or that the service was unnecessary, and that the bill was at best a mistake and at worst fraud. Also, if a patient feels that a physician was negligent and sues the physician, the patient record is considered objective evidence of what actually happened. Physicians are especially sensitive to the tension between the need for records to be concise and clinically relevant and the need for records to serve these somewhat arbitrary legal purposes. Misunderstandings arise from this area of tension when people who have a single-minded view of the patient record do not appreciate the multiple priorities of the physician.

Patient records also are a window into a physician's past experiences. Records are ideal for use in teaching and in gathering research information. Records support case-based reasoning in which specific past cases help solve new cases and collections of past cases are used to formulate future practice guidelines. Utilization review, quality assurance, and licensing entities use patient records to assess physician performance, and medical students and residents are constantly evaluated through their patient recordkeeping.

Finally, in considering the ubiquitous nature of patient records in healthcare today, it is critical to remember the Hippocratic admonition that *patient information must be kept confidential*. Those clinically caring for the patient should have access to the entire patient record, but no third party should be permitted to access the record without the explicit permission of the patient, and then only on a need to know basis. All parties accessing the record must carefully protect patient confidentiality, and not permit any transfer of patient information without the patient's explicit consent.

---

### CASE 12-3

*First the intern, then the chief resident, and finally the pediatric floor nurses interviewed the mother and poked and prodded the little girl late into the night. Five hours later the sun was rising. The on-call team assembled at morning report to present their admission of the 6-year-old girl with pneumonia and a pain crisis resulting from sickle-cell disease. Soon afterward, James Johnson, MSII, the medical student assigned to the service, was dispatched to introduce himself, examine the patient, and write a problem-based progress note. The student read the admission H&P, examined the patient, and wrote this "untitled SOAP note":*
3/27/2000 0815 Student Note

(S)ubjective: *Pain is decreased in legs and feet. Still complaining of pain in her right chest when she coughs. Not hungry this morning, but thirsty and drinking juice.*

(O)bjective: *Vital signs: T 101.0° F, HR 115, BP 100/54, RR 34. Medications: Oxygen 28% mask, IV: D5;X4NS at 100 ml/hr, oral morphine, cefazolin 300 mg IV q8h. Input 800 ml, output 300 ml urine, no bowel movements. General: Alert, fussy but cooperative. Lungs: Patient splinting the right side of chest. Decreased breath sounds, dullness and rales are noted in the right posterior lung field. Heart: Tachycardic; regular rate and rhythm; no murmurs, gallops, or rubs. Abdomen: BS normal, no tenderness, masses, or hepatosplenomegaly. Extremities: Tender diffusely in the legs. Lab: Pending.*

(A)ssessments: *(1) right lower lobe pneumonia; (2) sickle-cell disease with pain crisis.*

(P)lans: *Continue hydration, antibiotics, morphine, oxygen, and check lab.*

## Type of Information and Records

Medical information about a patient may be discovered through direct observation or from another source, such as the patient, a parent, a nurse, another physician, or a previous medical record. The information may pertain to health or disease, to one or more systems, and to one or more pathologic conditions. Medical information of any type from any source is subject to various biases.

In the past patient records were almost exclusively "source oriented," arranged according to the source authoring or providing the information. This orientation did not facilitate analysis of patient problems very well, so another method of structuring the same data base, called the problem-oriented medical record (POMR), was developed by Weed (1968) and is still in extensive use. The essential element of the POMR system is the *titled progress note*. A data base is collected and recorded, and then a separate note is written for each problem identified. Each problem-oriented note is comprised of relevant history, physical, and lab data abstracted from the patient information data base, followed by an assessment of its significance, and by a three-part plan detailing the diagnostic, therapeutic, and educational options needed to address that problem. A list of active and inactive problems is kept at the front of the chart to serve as a table of contents to the dated, titled notes in the chart. Since each problem is separately addressed and recorded along with supporting data, analysis, and plan, the logic and thinking behind the plan is quite evident for each problem. Other recordkeeping systems that do not abstract history, observations, assessment, and plan for each problem into a single context do not clearly and overtly reveal the thinking and logic behind the plan.

### Untitled SOAP Notes

In Weed's problem-oriented system, the note describing each problem is arranged by history ("Subjective"), physical and laboratory findings ("Objective"), Assessment, and Plan. These problem-based notes have thus become known as "SOAP Notes." If a patient has five problems addressed at a single visit, then, after the data base has been recorded, five separately titled SOAP notes should be written—one for each problem. The essence of the POMR is not the arrangement of information in a SOAP fashion, but *titled progress notes*—a clinical data base abstracted into data pertinent to problems and indexed to a problem list. But ironically the SOAP arrangement has become more popular than titled progress notes. Many physicians who write notes arranged in a SOAP fashion think that they are using problem-oriented records, when in fact they are not. Case 12-3 exemplifies such an *untitled SOAP note*.

It is so easy for physicians to gravitate toward the use of untitled SOAP notes that they deserve to be discussed explicitly. Although physicians are continually "foraging for data" in caring for patients, constant time pressure limits the opportunity to optimally synthesize additions to the patient record (Tang *et al.*, 1994). At each patient encounter, information tends to be gathered in a parallel fashion, not by problem. A physician may also obtain data from other sources, such as the current chart, an old chart, a nurse's clipboard, a family member, the patient, the laboratory computer, a verbal report from a radiologist, and so forth. All of this information must be collated and considered in addressing the patient's problems. It seems natural to record this information as it is collected in a source-oriented data base, but after doing so, many physicians find it burdensome to duplicate portions of the data in the separately titled problems of a true problem-oriented system. Instead the data base is followed by a simple list of assessments and a simple list of plans that are not tied to the data base. Anyone reading the record is forced to glean from the data base any information that would seem to support the assessments and plans. In untitled SOAP notes the thought process behind the assessment is not well preserved.

In summary, untitled SOAP notes are not ideal, but they are often used, are often adequate, and are often the best record that a physician can be expected to produce given the intense time pressures of medical practice. A well-constructed and defended POMR is ideal because it preserves both the data and the rationale of the clinician's diagnoses and plans, but it involves redundancy and increased effort.

## CASE 12-4

*Later that morning the student made rounds with the chief resident, who showed him how to rewrite the note in problem-oriented fashion so that the thinking and decision-making process would be displayed more clearly. The chief advocated using "History" and "Observations" instead of "Subjective" and "Objective" because they were more accurate terms.*

**3/27/2000 0815 Medical Student Note**

**Problem #1: PNEUMONIA, RIGHT LOWER LOBE**

    **History:** *Still complaining of pain in her right chest when she coughs.*

    **Observations:** *Vital signs: T 101.6° F, HR 115, BP 100/54, RR 34. On oxygen 28% mask and cefazolin 300 mg IV q8h. Lungs: Patient splinting the right side of chest. Breath sounds are decreased and dullness and rales present in the right posterior lung field, and clear elsewhere.*

    **Assessment & Plan:** *Pneumonia clinically is slightly better, and does not seem to have spread. Patient has not developed respiratory distress. Almost certainly bacterial. Sputum studies pending. Initial films without effusion, but risk of emphysema present.* **Diagnostically,** *get sputum studies, CXR tomorrow to document response and exclude effusion.* **Therapeutically,** *continue cefazolin and oxygen, add respiratory therapy.* **Educationally,** *try to keep patient and parents informed about progress.*

**Problem #2: SICKLE-CELL DISEASE WITH PAIN CRISIS**

**H:**     *Pain is decreased in legs and feet. Not hungry this morning, but thirsty and drinking juice.*

**O:**     *Medications: Oxygen 28% mask, oral morphine, hydration per problem #3. Heart: Tachycardic with regular rate and rhythm with no murmurs, gallops, or rubs. Abdomen: BS normal, no tenderness, masses, or hepatosplenomegaly. Extremities: Tender diffusely in the legs.*

**A/P:**     *Pain improved. No evidence of other complications thus far. No current diagnostic plans.*

*Therapeutically, continue hydration, oxygen, and morphine as necessary. Treatment of pneumonia should also help. No educational plans at present.*

**Problem #3: FLUID/ELECTROLYTES/NUTRITION**

**H/O:** *Drinking fluids well, not hungry. IV: D5;X4NS at 100 ml/hr. Input 800 ml. Output 300 ml urine, no bowel movements. Good skin turgor. Electrolyte panel pending.*

**A/P:** *Not dehydrated, but has higher fluid requirement due to fever, increased respiratory rate, and need for hydration due to sickle crisis. Diagnostically, obtain pending electrolyte panel now and daily while on IV to guide additional IV fluids. Watch input and output. Therapeutically, continue IV but encourage oral intake. Decrease IV rate as oral intake increases.*

## The Titled HOAP Note

The medical student in Case 12-4 could see that more work was involved in authoring the titled progress notes of the problem-oriented medical record, but after writing precisely about each problem, he had a better understanding of his patient's situation, an easier time following the patient's course, and an easier time presenting the case to his attending physician. The revised note also revealed his thinking much more clearly to his supervisors.

Case 12-4 also illustrates how physicians sometimes write progress note assessments and plans in proper POMR fashion, but take another short-cut and do not write a separate source-oriented data base. Instead, data are included only in the problem-oriented abstracts of the data base supporting each related assessment and plan. This method preserves both data and logic, and is concise, but may make the data harder to find. Usually this method is used only for progress notes where less data are recorded, or when a data base has been previously recorded in the chart, perhaps by another physician. Compared with untitled SOAP notes, titled notes are superior sources for verbal presentations. But although this system encapsulates each problem unto itself, the lack of a source-oriented data base as in Case 12-4 forces another clinician foraging for data to read each individual problem until the information of interest is located. If the results of a chest examination and x-ray are only recorded under the problem "TB exposure" and not in a data base, then a cardiologist evaluating the patient for chest pain must read the TB problem in order to find a description of the chest examination. Moreover, the use of a titled note implies that there is no need to search the data base for additional support. Therefore, if a titled note incompletely abstracts the supporting information from the data base, it can make a case look artificially weak. An untitled SOAP note might actually be preferable to a poorly written titled note.

Since physicians are not always able to produce an ideal POMR, how should charting be approached? In general, physicians should strive toward an ideal POMR by using clinical judgment to create the most important "views" of each case. Ideally there should be an overall data base, a view by problem, perhaps a view by medication, a chronological view, and so forth. Much of this involves writing the same information over and over in different parts of the chart, although a computer-based record system may obviate this chore. Sometimes a mere reference to another part of the chart, e.g., "see Social History," is sufficient. Redundancy is expensive in terms of physician and transcriptionist time, so in reality only the most useful redundancies can be incorporated into charts. It is up to physicians to do this in a clinically meaningful manner. As long as physicians honestly attempt to address the needs of potential future audiences, useful charts generally are produced.

# Charting

The term *charting* is used by physicians to refer to the maintenance of a patient record in a chart. A chart is an integrated record that includes a number of preprinted forms, dividers, and other devices to improve the utility of the information we record. Although there are many different types of charts, physicians typically use two types.

*Hospital charts are episodic*, typically covering only one discrete episode of care over one block of time. Such charts tend to be divided into many sections, sometimes 15 to 20. Typical sections are admission history and physical, orders, progress notes, vital signs, nurses' notes, consultations, lab, radiology, ECG, and so forth. This format is convenient for people who deal with only one aspect of patient care, because they can focus on only that section of the chart. Chart subdivisions may also make it easier to follow trends; for example, a physician can flip through the radiology section to see how an infiltrate is progressing on serial chest x-ray reports. However, storage of these records all over the chart in a source-oriented manner makes it difficult for physicians to view a case chronologically by problem. For this reason, results stored in other sections are often transcribed by the physician into the daily physician progress notes, permitting the progress notes to stand more coherently by themselves. All too often, however, physicians fail to record all meaningful results tied to specific problems. Reviewing such a chart is difficult and time-consuming. It is clinically unreasonable to expect physicians to transcribe and comment in the progress notes on every single test and study reported elsewhere in the chart, but at least the significant results should be referred to and discussed.

Unlike hospital charts, *outpatient charts are not episodic*, but cover the patient over time through periods of health and disease. Charts in an outpatient primary care setting typically have five to ten source-oriented sections. The sections might be progress notes, intake forms and flow sheets, lab and x-ray results, consultations, and so forth. A number of special forms are used to facilitate long-term continuous care of the patient. (Figs. 12.1–12.3). Usually, some forms called *intake forms* are completed by the patient, such as a survey of past medical history and a written review of systems. While it may be suboptimal to rely on these forms instead of a personally taken history, these forms prime the patient's memory and serve as an excellent starting point for discussion.

Progress notes are the key component of the outpatient primary care chart. They are supported by lab tests, radiographs, outside reports and records, and other third-party paperwork filed chronologically. Problem lists and flow sheets are especially important components of the outpatient chart. These are preprinted forms, usually with grids, on which to record problems, medications, and important serial observations like blood pressure and target lab values. Preventive interventions can also be tracked easily with a flow sheet.

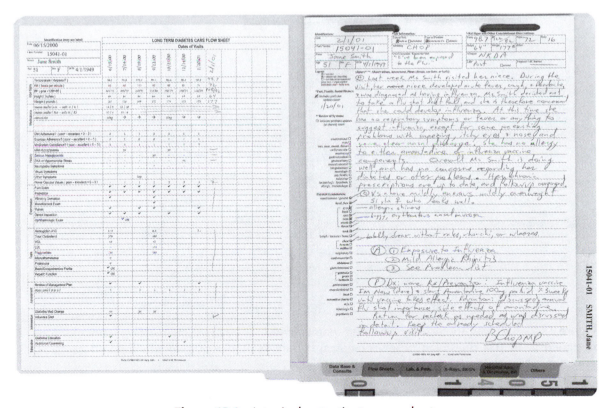

**Figure 12.1.** A typical outpatient paper chart.

**Identification:**

Date

Chart Number

Name

| Age | Sex | DOB |
|-----|-----|-----|

**Legend:**
☑ = normal
☒ = abnormal (describe)
☐ = not taken/not examined
plain text = organ system
**bold italic text** = body area

**\*Past, Family, Social History:**

☐ Includes pertinant
   updates since:

**\*\*Review of Systems:**

☐ Includes pertinant updates
   (as shown) since:

constitutional ☐
eyes ☐
ears, nose, mouth, throat ☐
cardiovascular ☐
respiratory ☐
gastrointestinal ☐
genitourinary ☐
musculoskeletal ☐
integumentary ☐
neurologic ☐
psychiatric ☐
endocrine ☐
hematologic, lymphatic ☐
allergic, immunologic ☐

**Physical Examination:**
constitutional / general ☐
*head, face* ☐
eyes ☐
fundi ☐
ears ☐
nose ☐
mouth ☐
throat ☐
*neck* ☐
lymph / immune / heme ☐
*chest* ☐
*breasts* ☐
*axillae* ☐
respiratory ☐
cardiovascular ☐
*abdomen* ☐
gastrointestinal ☐
*genitalia* ☐
*groin* ☐
*buttocks* ☐
genitourinary ☐
musculoskeletal ☐
*back* ☐
*extremities (each)* ☐
skin ☐
neurologic ☐
psychiatric ☐

**Visit Information:**

| Type of Visit ☐ walk-in ☐ scheduled | Type of Problem ☐ acute/acute f/u ☐ chronic |
|---|---|

Attending

Chief Complaint / Reason for Visit

**Vital Signs and Other Constitutional Observations:**

| Temp | BP | Pulse | Resp |
|------|----|-------|------|
| Height | Weight | Other | |

Allergies

| LMP ☐ normal | Pregnant? / BC Method |
|---|---|

**History\* \*\*, Observations, Assessment, Plans** (dictate, use form, or both):

©1995 B Chop MD   •   Used with Permission

**Figure 12.2.** Charting forms are often used, particularly in outpatient charts. This particular form is designed to help a physician observe medical documentation requirements imposed by the U.S. government. It can be completed by hand, but it is also compatible with dictation transcribed onto self-stick paper.

**Identification (may use label)**

Date 06/15/2000

Chart Number 15041-01

Name Jane Smith

Age 51 | Sex F | DOB 4/1/1949

## LONG TERM DIABETES CARE FLOW SHEET
### Dates of Visits

| | | 6/15/00 | 7/14/00 | 8/19/00 | 9/12/00 | 10/25/00 | 12/14/00 | 1/20/01 |
|---|---|---|---|---|---|---|---|---|
| **Vital Signs** | Temperature ( degrees F ) | 98.1 | 98.8 | 102.5 | 99.1 | 98.6 | 98.4 | 98.4 |
| | HR ( beats per minute ) | 82 | 80 | 110 | 90 | 90 | 85 | 78 |
| | BP ( goal <120/<80 ) | 165/92 | 155/90 | 150/92 | 134/85 | 130/79 | 130/75 | 128/78 |
| | Height ( inches ) | 64 | 64 | 64 | 64 | 64 | 64 | 64 |
| | Weight ( pounds ) | 181 | 176 | 169 | 172 | 174 | 173 | 175 |
| **Medications** | Human Insulin (AM – units N / R ) | 18 / 8 | 22 / 10 | | | | | |
| | Human Insulin ( PM – units N / R) | 10 / 4 | 12 / 6 | | | | | |
| | atorvastatin | 10mg | → | → | → | 20mg | → | → |
| | | | | | | | | |
| | | | | | | | | |
| **History** | Diet Adherence? ( poor – excellent = 0 – 3 ) | 0 | 2 | 1 | 3 | 3 | 2 | 2 |
| | Exercise Adherence? ( poor – excellent = 0 – 3 ) | 0 | 2 | 0 | 0 | 1 | 1 | 2 |
| | Medication Compliance? ( poor – excellent = 0 – 3 ) | 3 | 3 | 3 | 3 | 3 | 2 | 3 |
| | Mild Hypoglycemia | - | yes | - | - | yes | - | - |
| | Serious Hypoglycemia | - | - | - | yes | - | - | - |
| | DKA or Hyperosmolar Illness | - | - | - | - | - | yes | - |
| | Neuropathy Symptoms | - | - | - | ? | - | - | - |
| | Visual Symptoms | - | - | - | - | - | - | - |
| | Other Symptoms | | | hosp | | | | |
| | Home Glucose Values ( poor – excellent = 0 – 3 ) | - | 1 | 1 | 2 | 2 | 3 | 3 |
| **Examination** | Foot Exam | ✔ | ✔ | ✔ | ✔ | ✔ | ✔ | ✔ |
| | Inspection | ✔ | ✔ | ✔ | ✔ | ✔ | ✔ | ✔ |
| | Vibratory Sensation | ✔ | | | ✔ | | | |
| | Monofilament Exam | | | | ✔ | | | |
| | Pulses | ✔ | | ✔ | ✔ | | | ✔ |
| | Dental Inspection | ✔ | ✔ | ✔ | | ✔ | | ✔ |
| | Ophthalmologic Exam | | ✔ OK | | | | | |
| **Tests** | Hemoglobin A1C | 11.9 | | | 8.5 | | | 7.1 |
| | Total Cholesterol | 270 | | | 180 | | | |
| | HDL | 40 | | | 42 | | | |
| | LDL | -- | | | 114 | | | |
| | Triglycerides | 756 | | | 165 | | | |
| | Microalbuminemia | 0 | | | | | | |
| | Proteinuria | 0 | | | | | | |
| | Basic/Comprehensive Profile | ✔ OK | | | | | | |
| | Hepatic Function | ✔ OK | | | | | | |
| **Assessment** | Review of Management Plan | ✔ | | ✔ | | | | ✔ |
| | Stress Level ( 0 to 3 ) | 3 | - | 2 | 2 | 2 | 1 | 2 |
| | | | | | | | | |
| | | | | | | | | |
| **Intervention** | Diabetes Med Change | yes | | yes | yes | | | |
| | Influenza Shot | ✔ | | | | | | |
| | | | | | | | | |
| | | | | | | | | |
| **Education** | Diabetes Education | ✔ | | | | ✔ | | |
| | Nutritional Counseling | ✔ | | | | | ✔ | |

©1984-2001 B Chop MD.   •   Used with Permission.

**Figure 12.3.** Flow sheets are especially helpful in caring for patients with chronic conditions. Some flow sheets are generic, and require the physician to specify the information important to track. Other flow sheets are designed for a specific chronic condition, like diabetes, so in addition to providing a view of data over time, they also help the physician to remember to address important recurring issues.

## OUTPATIENT PAPER CHART ORGANIZATION

*Outpatient paper charts have a number of features as shown in Figure 12.1. Most have colored tabs corresponding to the chart number so that it is easy to recognize if a chart has been filed on the wrong shelf. On the inside cover there is often room for a problem list and/ or flow sheet, as shown in Fig. 12.2. They are kept accessible since they enhance the physician's ability to view the big picture, to spot information trends over time, and to solve clinical problems. Their use also provides a redundancy and reduces the chance that important information will be missed. There is usually a clip to hold punched papers in place, and a series of tabbed dividers that make it easier to file reports in the correct section, and to find reports when reviewing the chart. The progress notes may be dictated and transcribed, or handwritten, possibly on a special form, as illustrated in Fig. 12.3. The notes are often kept in reverse chronological order so that the latest notes are on top and easy to read and write. Laboratory reports, radiology reports, and outside consultation notes are filed under specific tabs.*

Problem list forms allow physicians to list the patient's major problems for quick reference and review during follow-up visits. It is important that these forms actually be used. *If they are not kept consistently up to date, they will not be trusted, they will not be referred to, and it is even less likely they will be maintained.*

The form and function of charts have important implications for medical care (Donnelly, 1988). For example, there are some parts of the data base that tend to be collected or updated infrequently, and other parts that are updated almost every time the patient comes to the office. A patient's living conditions may be recorded only once, if at all, on a sheet kept in the back of the chart, whereas a patient's blood pressure may be recorded at the top of each visit. Bias may result from this, since the physician may concentrate on the medical information close at hand rather than look back into the chart to find something of greater importance to the patient's care. To ensure that such a problem receives due attention, many physicians record any significant aspect of a patient's data base in the problem list. If "very poor housing" is recorded as a problem on the problem list, it will be far more likely to receive due consideration from the physician as plans are made at future visits.

Bias also occurs because of the artificial subjective–objective dichotomy introduced by Weed's problem-oriented medical record. In reality the distinction between subjective and objective information is fuzzy. Usually the story of the patient, the history, is the most important and useful part of the data base. Yet by definition the patient's story is considered "subjective." Ironically, some physician observations contain considerable subjectivity, but are classified as "objective." Use of the latter term obscures the physician's fallibility and humanity. Instead of "SOAP," Donnelly and Brauner (1992) advocate thinking and writing in terms of "HOAP," meaning, "History, Observations, Assessments, Plans," an example of which is given in Case 12-4. *History* is a more honorable term than *subjective*. It makes it clear that the patient's observations, the previous observations of the current physician, and the observations of other physicians and institutions all belong together in the history section. The *observation* section is reserved only for the current observations of the authoring physician, including current lab results and tests.

The subjective–objective dichotomy so entrenched in the SOAP mnemonic has also been reinforced by a change in the meanings of the terms *symptoms* and *signs*. Modern use of the term symptom refers to an abnormal phenomenon experienced by an individual. A sign is an abnormality discovered by the physician during an examination. However, prior to 1900 the term symptom generally referred to "any manifestation of a disease whether perceived by a patient or a physician" and sign to "a perception that led to a meaningful inference about the patient and his or her disease." Signs were considered to be symptoms with meaning. It was not the source of information that distinguished between these two (Donnelly & Brauner, 1992). Nonetheless, in modern usage symptoms are recorded in the history or subjective section of the data base and progress notes; signs noted by others are also recorded in the history or subjective section; and only the observations of the authoring physician are recorded in the observation or objective section.

## CASE 12-5

*It was a hectic afternoon in the student clinic. Maria Brown, MSII, was feeling rather stressed. She walked to examination room No. 2, slipped the thick chart quietly out of the rack on the door, and opened the chart of Margaret Green, another patient she'd never met. She scanned down the problem list: obesity, diabetes mellitus, hypertension, ethanolism, tobaccoism, depression, and many more. The flow sheet showed a series of elevated blood pressure readings, and a series of equally elevated glucose readings. At least ten medications were on the flow sheet, most no longer active. And then, on the top progress note, she read the final note written by the outgoing MSIV assigned to Ms. Green. It began, "This is a difficult, noncompliant 47-year-old alcoholic who comes to clinic frequently with multiple somatic complaints." The other notes indicated many attempts to diagnose and treat her complaints, most of which failed. The new patient intake forms that Ms. Green had completed 3 years ago were sparsely completed and were not helpful.*

*Maria dreaded seeing a "difficult, noncompliant alcoholic," but she took a deep breath, letting it out slowly. She cleared her mind of distractions, pictured Ms. Green as a suffering, perhaps confused person, and set a learning goal for herself for this visit: find out who Ms. Green the person really is. With a calm demeanor she entered the room, allowed her patient to speak without interruption, and addressed her concerns. She gleaned from the chart that several preventive interventions were overdue. A plan was negotiated. Soon the visit was complete, with a recheck scheduled in 2 weeks. As Ms. Green left, she told Maria that it was the first visit where anyone really listened to her.*

*Sitting at the physician's workstation, Maria completed the chart, adding new problems to the problem list: illiteracy, loneliness, grief, poverty. She would scarcely be able to address these problems as a student physician, but now they wouldn't be forgotten. And she added a neatly printed picture of Ms. Green's life to the chart as insurance against a future student dreading her patient on a future hectic afternoon: "Margaret Green is a pleasant 47-year-old woman. She was orphaned as a baby and was raised in a series of foster homes. She was physically and mentally abused in many of the homes, until finally at the age of 13 a woman took her in who loved her, cared for her, and adopted her. Since she was hard of hearing she did poorly in school, finally dropping out at age 16 because she could not keep up and because so many children made fun of her. For the next 20 years she was employed cleaning buildings but after she turned 40 her adopted mother suddenly died. Her health deteriorated, and she quit working...." Maria paused, sad at seeing such a story in black and white, but pleased that Ms. Green's chart was no longer "poisoned."*

## Reviewing Patient Records

It is important to be skilled in reviewing patient records. Unfortunately, physicians and especially new students of medicine frequently do not review patient charts adequately. Osheroff *et al.* (1991) found that 52% of patient care-related questions arising in an internal medicine teaching program "requested a fact that could have been provided using the patient record or hospital information system." Students should review the patient record more effectively prior to seeing patients and prior to presenting those patients to other physicians. Reviewing charts is also an effective way to learn about writing charts. In a thick patient chart there are frequently three or four notes that prove to be especially helpful. Look carefully at these key notes, decide what it is about them that makes them especially helpful, and when appropriate, try to emulate them.

There is almost always some type of record to review before seeing a patient. Even when the patient is new, it is likely that some sort of intake history form has been completed. Remember that the physician is responsible for the information the patient discloses on intake forms. If a patient writes that she is taking birth control pills, but the physician fails to read it and prescribes an antibiotic that reduces the effectiveness of those pills, then the patient may become pregnant. The same thinking applies to information in previous progress notes in the clinic chart. The physician must consider those notes during the current episode of care. Review the chart and be up to date on the patient before entering the examination room.

Reviewing the chart does not mean reading the entire chart. If previous authors have been keeping up with problem lists and problem-oriented notes, medication lists, and flow sheets, then it is easy to review the patient's chart. Often a previous note summarizes important past information in such a way that both data and thinking are reliably preserved. Sometimes, though, the previous notes are sparse and disorganized, requiring the physician to "read between the lines," and "forage for data" in the patient intake forms, past notes, and old records.

The method used to review a chart also depends to some extent on the review's purpose. If the patient already has a physician and presents to a Saturday morning walk-in clinic with an acute sore throat, then a review of past abdominal surgeries is unnecessary. However, an infectious disease specialist must carefully search the entire patient record for clues when consulted about a patient with fevers that remain unexplained despite a well-directed workup.

In learning to review charts, notice helpful and unhelpful features and take a lesson from them. Legible handwriting and typed notes speed chart review. A complete data base is important, but an excessive volume of redundant normal observations can obscure important past observations and inhibit chart review. When problem lists, medication lists, and flow sheets are not maintained, they cannot be trusted as a condensed representation of the patient's case, so the physician is forced to review the entire chart.

It is helpful to adopt a consistent agenda to try to extract *functional* information about the patient from the chart. Review the activities of the patient—occupation, hobbies, exercise, typical days. A note documenting that a patient is a volunteer who delivers meals to homebound people 3 days a week says something important about the patient and establishes a baseline that can be used as a basis for comparison later. Reviewing patient activities will also raise awareness of how often physicians neglect to record functional information. *Too often it is impossible to tell from a chart how a patient is really doing.* Two patients may have virtually identical charts from a disease standpoint, yet one is doing very poorly in life, while the other scarcely notices poor health. The lack of a good record of function makes it very difficult to effectively address a patient's needs.

Finally, take special notice of how the patient record is able to either humanize or dehumanize the patient. Prior to reading a chart and entering an examination room, each physician should "suspend judgment" so that she is prepared to interact with the patient as a person in need and not as an abstract "case." If the chart berates the patient or inappropriately leads a reviewer to conclude that the patient is "difficult," as in Case 12-5, there is a risk the physician will be "poisoned" by that information and establish a less satisfactory relationship than would have occurred if the chart had portrayed the patient more humanely. Patient records should ideally establish that the patient is a person with a life and family who should be treated with respect and compassion. However, many progress notes are simply sterile; often little social history has been recorded other than something like, "smokes two packs per day." Before meeting any patient, shake off any "poison" noted in the chart by scanning for narratives that establish the patient as a person. Take time to read the social and family histories, and scan the progress notes for "stories" about the patient. Enter the examination room prepared to be compassionate and empathetic. And if the chart does not contain an adequate narrative of the patient as a person, add one!

# Authoring Patient Records
## General Considerations in Authoring Records

An important clinical skill is authoring excellent patient records in an efficient manner. The author of a patient record creates a legacy that may follow the patient the rest of her life and represents the author's skills and logic in a form that may be reviewed and used by many future physicians. The record is a literary work and a tool specifically designed to benefit that patient in the future. Consequently, physicians have a profound responsibility to be complete, accurate, precise, and concise—and an equal responsibility to present the patient as a person worthy of respect. It's a difficult and time-consuming task. Physicians in primary care specialties can easily spend 5 to 10% of their working time authoring patient records.

Patient records must be legible, so they should be typed whenever possible. Many physicians find that dictating notes for later transcription is both faster and less expensive. Dictating is faster, captures more detail, and is compatible with computerized record systems. The time saved can then be devoted to other activities. Dictated notes are more comprehensive. It is much easier and faster to dictate the flourishes and details that establish the patient as a person, and to leave a clear starting point for the next patient encounter. Future physicians can review typed notes much more easily and quickly. Physicians typically review transcribed dictation and sign it before placing it permanently in the patient's chart. Although this requires the physician to handle the chart a second time, it also provides a second chance to think about the patient and notice any potential problems with the previous care. Unfortunately, students commonly are not taught how or permitted to dictate, mainly because of expense and the need for a promptly completed chart for preceptors to review and sign. However, today's more powerful computer hardware makes computerized voice recognition software systems effective for entering text and controlling a computer system. There are no transcription costs and notes are completed in "real time," making them an excellent tool for students of medicine. As they continue to improve they will virtually eliminate conventional dictation systems.

It is always important to know and document the sources of information and opinion about the patient. A major write-up such as an admission history and physical examination should reference the source of information and its estimated reliability. When the source is a person, such as the patient or the patient's parent, that person is called an "informant." Histories are not taken, but created. The author of the history— the "historian"—is the physician, established by a signature at the end of the write-up.

When the source of information is a "third party" such as lab or x-ray reports, or records from another facility, be sure to verify the information with names, ID numbers, dates, and times. Be sure to date, time, and sign all notes. Physicians with illegible signatures should type or print their name underneath. If the note occupies more than one physical sheet of paper, then sign at the end of each sheet and note that the write-up is continued to another page. Record the date and time on each continuation page.

Any changes made to the medical record must leave an "audit trail" by writing any new information; crossing out incorrect information with simple lines that leave the old information legible; and dating, timing, and signing the change. In many cases an explanatory addendum can be added to a chart, but sometimes it's safest to directly edit an old note. For example, if a patient develops a drug allergy it might be good to note it, with the current date, on previous notes that stated "no allergies." In cases known to concern litigation, however, it is best not to make any changes, even if they are signed and dated, without first discussing it with a lawyer.

In using patient records, remember that they must remain accessible. For that reason, most facilities do not permit records to be taken off premises for any reason. It is preferable to make a photocopy if the record is truly needed elsewhere. For the same reason, all charts not in proper storage should be left out in the open where they can be seen. They should never be hidden in a drawer, a cabinet, or a locked room. Forms and papers important to the record must be handled carefully, preferably by fixing any loose forms in the chart. Each sheet of paper should have the patient's unique chart identifier written on it so that if it is separated from the chart, it can be refiled later. The addition of photographs of the patient to the chart can serve as a useful patient identifier with the advantage that they simultaneously add a human dimension to the patient's record. Computer-based patient record systems may be accessible from a wide variety of locations, but have their own security issues. If using such a system, be especially careful to guard your password and to secure the system whenever you leave a workstation so that someone else does not access the workstation with your identity to violate confidentiality, to change records, to order tests in your name, or worse.

## CASE 12-6

**3/15/2000 1640 Resident Admission Note (RAN)**

*ID: Jane Smith is a 51-year-old patient from Smallville, Texas. She is a commercial artist, mainly a painter, married with four children, three still living at home. She has hypertension and adult-onset diabetes mellitus. This is her first hospital admission since her youngest child was born. The history is obtained from the patient, who is a reliable informant, and by phone from Dr. Susan Jones, her attending family physician.*

*CC: "I'm coughing up blood and my chest hurts." She is admitted by Dr. Jones for treatment of a right lower lobe pneumonia.*

*HPI: Mrs. Smith felt well until about 8 days ago when she developed fever, chills, headache, body aches, sore throat, and nonproductive cough. She began taking over-the-counter cold medications and acetaminophen. After 2 days she went to see her family physician, Dr. Susan Jones, who diagnosed influenza A and prescribed amantadine 200 mg STAT followed by 100 mg twice a day. Her glucose was normal. By the next day she began to feel better and her fever resolved. She continued to have a dry cough until 2 days ago when she began to feel achy again and began coughing up small amounts of yellow sputum. Yesterday chills and fever reappeared and a pain in the lateral right chest developed that was worse with coughing and deep breathing. Her discomforts continued today and she also began to feel somewhat short of breath. At about 10 AM, she started coughing up dark blood. The appearance of the blood frightened her so she came to the emergency room (ER). After evaluation in the ER, Dr. Jones was called, and she admitted the patient.*

*Mrs. Smith smoked one pack per day for 15 years, but quit 10 years ago as a health measure. She has no history of pneumonia, lung disease, TB, cancer, or asbestos or other exposures; there is no history of coagulopathy. She has never had either influenza or pneumococcal vaccines.*

*The hemoptysis was especially frightening to Mrs. Smith because her brother has lung cancer. She feels embarrassed that she did not seek attention earlier. She is tired of having to worry about her health and take medications, so she just kept hoping that this problem would go away.*

*PMH:*

*1.* **Diseases:**

**Diabetes mellitus:** *15 years ago she developed polyuria and fatigue, was found to have a fasting blood glucose of 286 mg/dl, and was diagnosed with adult-onset non-insulin-dependent diabetes mellitus. She weighed 223 pounds at the time. She took the news positively and went on a diet (2500 calories per day), began taking an oral hypoglycemic, and learned to check her own glucose values. She began a water aerobics class, which she continued up until last year. Her very best friends are all members of this class. Her weight dropped to 145 pounds and she was able to stop taking the oral hypoglycemic. In the last year she has been nursing her ill brother frequently, and had to stop her aerobics classes. Her weight rose to 169 pounds, glucose into the low 200 range, she developed polyuria, and last month Dr. Jones recommended that she resume glyburide 5 mg every morning. Her glucose readings then decreased to the 120 mg/dl range, but when she became ill they increased again to the low 200 range. She is unaware of any complications of her diabetes mellitus, and sees an ophthalmologist annually.*

**Hypertension:** *Diagnosed 15 years ago at the same time her diabetes mellitus was discovered. She has always taken a diuretic, no apparent side effects, with good blood pressure control.*

*2.* **Trauma and Operations:** *None significant. G4P4 with four normal vaginal deliveries.*

*3.* **Transfusions:** *None.*

*4.* **Immunizations:** *Had usual childhood immunizations. No hepatitis B series. No influenza or pneumovax.*

*5.* **Medications:**

*Glyburide 5 mg qd for the last month for diabetes mellitus, no side effects.*

*HCTZ 25 mg qd for 15 years for hypertension, no side effects.*

*Amantadine 100 mg bid for influenza A, currently on day #6, no side effects.*

*Acetaminophen recently for pain and fever, and an over-the-counter cold medication.*

*6.* **Allergies:** *Long ago a sulfa medication caused a "rash."*

*Family History:*

*Grandparents: Paternal grandfather died, 87, old age; paternal grandmother alive, 86, has diabetes mellitus, hypertension, hypothyroidism, lives out of state; maternal grandfather died, 74, stroke; maternal grandmother died, 73, colon cancer.*

*Parents: father died, 60, heart attack, emphysema; mother died, 70, kidney infection, diabetes mellitus.*

*Siblings: Brother age 53, alive with terminal lung cancer, hypertension.*

*Children: Bill, 20, attending college 100 miles away; Adam, 17; Amy, 16; Lisa, 15. All are in good health. There is no history of other cancers, congenital diseases, TB, mental disease, or any other serious diseases.*

*Social History:*

*Mrs. Smith was born and raised in a suburb of Dallas, attended the University of Texas graduating with a degree in art. Her parents and brother later moved to Smallville, so she settled there also. She lived at home and was employed in commercial art until she married 21 years ago. When her children all were in school she went back into commercial art, lately working out of her home. Her husband is in a stressful construction job presently. She has remained monogamous. She considers her marriage good but not very supportive. Her children are very active in school activities.*

*Hobbies are reading and sculpture—she makes metal welded statues and has a lot of noise exposure from a grinder—has not done much in the last year.*

*Habits: Drinks at least 12 cups of drip coffee per day. Drinks alcohol only occasionally. Smoked one pack per day cigarettes for 15 years, but quit 10 years ago as a health measure. No illicit drug use.*

*Has been very preoccupied with caring for her terminally ill brother who has lung cancer. He lives in Mrs. Smith's guest room. She does not want to be here in the hospital because she is afraid he will need her help. She handles all his medication, feeds him all his meals, bathes him, and does some respiratory therapy. Caring for him is very time-consuming.*

*She has always tried to minimize her own health needs. She grieved quite a bit when diagnosed with diabetes mellitus, but soon accepted the need to take better care of herself, so she quit smoking and started water aerobics classes and a weight loss program. When she began caring for her brother she was forced to quit her classes. She gained weight, her diabetes mellitus became symptomatic again, and she became discouraged. Her husband is very stressed himself, and provides little help. She refuses to ask her children to help her. Most of her friends were in her aerobics class and she has no one to talk to now. She used to attend church, and does pray about her situation, but stopped going about 6 months ago.*

*ROS (review of systems):*

*General/Systemic: gained about 25 pounds over last year; generally tired lately; no hot or cold intolerance; no abnormal bleeding.*

*HEENT: No visual problems, sees ophthalmologist; thinks her hearing is a little worse, has had much noise exposure to metal grinder, did not use hearing protection; occasional hay fever symptoms; sees dentist, no current dental problems.*

*Neck/Nodes: No lumps or pain.*

*Chest/Breasts: No chest pain except as in HPI; checks breasts a few times a year, but has never had a mammogram, no lumps or discharge noted.*

*Respiratory: No breathing problems except as in HPI.*

*Cardiovascular: BP typically runs around 135/85 on her diuretic; no chest pain except as in HPI; no palpitations, dyspnea (except as in HPI), orthopnea, or paroxysmal nocturnal dyspnea. No claudication or edema.*

*GI: no nausea, vomiting, heartburn, dysphagia, diarrhea, constipation, hematemesis, hematochezia, melena.*

*GU: sometimes she loses urine when she coughs; last menstrual period 6 weeks ago; has had some hot flashes over the last year and menses have been irregular, not on hormones; Pap smear 3 years ago was normal, has never had an abnormal one; no hematuria, dysuria, frequency, but has had some polyuria lately.*

*Musculoskeletal: no muscle or joint pain or swelling except (1) for years has had tight, tense neck and headaches when she works a lot at her art; currently not flared; and (2) has tingling, paresthesias, and some pain in her right wrist and forearm worse when she is working a lot.*

*Neurologic: as per musculoskeletal section above, otherwise no loss of consciousness, tremors, seizures, or neurosensory changes.*

*Skin: a bit dry recently; no rashes or lesions.*

*Psychiatric: has had difficulty falling asleep and early morning awakening for at least a year; appetite has been increased and she eats to relax; frequent crying spells for no particular reason; does not enjoy any activities anymore; no past diagnosis or treatment for depression; denies suicidal ideation.*

*PE (physical examination):*

*Vital signs: T 102.5F, BP 150/92, HR 110, RR 32; wt 169 pounds, ht 64 inches.*

*General: alert, oriented, ill woman who tries to be helpful; initially dyspneic but improved with oxygen.*

*HEENT: no head trauma; no facial tenderness; pupils equal, round, and reactive to light and accommodation; extraocular muscles intact without nystagmus; fundi with some arteriolar narrowing; nose congested; TMs and canals clear, hearing grossly intact but perhaps a bit hard of hearing; mouth with good dentition, pink mucosa with normal lips, tongue, and throat.*

*Neck: supple; full range of motion; no jugular venous distention; carotid upstrokes normal without bruits; no thyromegaly.*

*Nodes: no abnormal nodes appreciated in neck, supraclavicular, axillary, epitrochlear, or inguinal areas.*

*Breasts: no masses, skin changes, retraction, or discharge.*

*Chest: mildly increased AP diameter, no tenderness; tachypneic, no retractions but splinting right chest; breath sounds slightly decreased diffusely; no wheezing, rales, rhonchi, or dullness except for the right lower posterior lung field which is dull to percussion and has tubular breath sounds and rales.*

*Heart: mild tachycardia with S1, single S2, and no murmurs, gallops, or rubs appreciated.*

*Abdomen: BS normal; soft, nontender; liver 8 cm by percussion; no masses or splenomegaly.*

*Genital: externally normal, vagina normal, cervix multiparous, bimanual with normal uterus size and position, no adnexal enlargement or tenderness appreciated. Pap smear taken, result pending.*

*Rectal: normal tone, no masses; stool brown, occult blood negative.*

*Neurological: normal mental status; cranial nerves 2–12 intact; deep tendon reflexes at biceps, triceps, patellar, and Achilles are 2+ bilaterally; motor examination intact in mass, tone, and strength; sensory examination intact to light and sharp touch, but mild vibratory loss in feet bilaterally; gait and coordination intact; Romberg and Babinski signs absent.*

*Skin: fair skinned with actinic changes on face and shoulders, but no lesions noted; skin somewhat dry.*

*Lab: chest x-ray shows a dense right lower lobe infiltrate without effusion, otherwise normal. Remainder of lab tests are pending.*

*Problem List:*

1. *Pneumonia, right lower lobe, postinfluenza*
2. *Diabetes mellitus, adult-onset*
3. *Hypertension, chronic essential*
4. *Obesity*
5. *Perimenopausal*
6. *Stress urinary incontinence, palpable bladder*
7. *Hearing loss, mild, history of noise exposure*
8. *Depressive syndrome, etiology undetermined*
9. *Psychosocial stress*
10. *Excessive caffeine use, 12 cups coffee per day*
11. *Actinic skin*
12. *Breast cancer prevention*
13. *Allergic to sulfa medications*

*Assessments/Plans:*

**Problem #1: PNEUMONIA, RIGHT LOWER LOBE, POSTINFLUENZA**

H/O:   *By history patient had an influenza syndrome that improved with treatment, but later flared with a productive cough, hemoptysis, pleuritic chest pain, fever, and dyspnea. On examination she is febrile, tachypneic, splinting her right chest, and has signs of right lower lobe consolidation. Chest x-ray confirms a right lower lobe infiltrate.*

A/P:   *This is likely a secondary bacterial pneumonia, possibly caused by Streptococcus pneumoniae, Haemophilus influenzae, or Staphylococcus aureus. The hemoptysis in this context is consistent with pneumonia, but must be watched carefully. At risk for development of empyema. Plan to check pending lab, including sputum Gram stain. Start broad-spectrum IV antibiotics, pulmonary toilet, pain meds to help her cough and breathe more deeply. Monitor carefully. See orders. Since patient is a former smoker and has a family history of lung cancer will need to be sure infiltrate improves and resolves completely and is not related to a tumor. Also needs pneumococcal vaccine and annual influenza immunizations.*

**Problem #2: DIABETES MELLITUS, ADULT-ONSET**

H/O:   *Began as an adult 15 years ago (per PMH) and initially required oral hypoglycemic, later was controlled by diet (2500 calories per day) and exercise (water aerobics), but patient stopped exercising, gained weight, became symptomatic, and 1 month ago reinstitution of oral hypoglycemic. Has not had obvious complications. On examination (undilated) has no diabetic retinopathy, but does have palpable postvoiding bladder and loss of some vibratory sensation in feet. Blood glucose pending.*

A/P:     *Overall patient has had a fairly benign course because of her previous efforts. Control has been worse in the last year, mostly for psychosocial reasons, and probably glucose is even worse now because of the stress of the pneumonia. Plan to monitor and control glucose acutely, and to address the psychosocial problems to try to permit patient to resume diet and exercise program.*

**Problem #3: HYPERTENSION, CHRONIC ESSENTIAL**

H/O:   *Mild hypertension for 15 years on diuretic without side effects or complications. Current blood pressure 150/92. Fundal examination shows arteriolar narrowing. Lab pending.*

A/P:   *Hypertension has been mild and controlled by history, and there is scarcely any evidence of end-organ damage. Nonetheless, because she also has a positive family history and diabetes mellitus she is at even higher risk for strokes and heart disease, so it is important to control her BP. Plan to continue the diuretic and consider starting an aspirin per day to reduce risk of strokes and heart attacks.*

**Problem #4: OBESITY**

H/O:   *Has gained weight over the last year as discussed in #2 above. Thyroid gland normal.*

A/P:   *Probably the weight gain was related to the effects of lifestyle changes and possibly depression, but because patient has also had dry skin and fatigue, hypothyroidism should be ruled out. Plan to address the psychosocial issues, encourage proper diet and exercise, and check thyroid function tests.*

**Problem #5: PERIMENOPAUSAL**

H/O:   *Lately has had irregular menses and hot flashes, age is compatible with menopause.*

A/P:   *May be menopausal. At risk for osteoporosis. Continued estrogen would be beneficial from a cardiovascular standpoint, also. However, obesity or thyroid could also be affecting menses. Plan to check thyroid function tests, and Pap smear for estrogen index. Will consider estrogen replacement with patient after hospitalization.*

**Problem #6: STRESS URINARY INCONTINENCE, PALPABLE BLADDER**

H/O:   *Longstanding problem, off and on. Four vaginal deliveries.*

A/P:   *May be related to childbirth, but may be retaining urine because of diabetic neuropathy and may be at risk of infection. Could also be related to menopause. Anticholinergic effects of whatever cold preparation she is currently taking could have contributed too. Plan to check pending lab including urinalysis, and treat as indicated. Also will quantitate postvoid residual with bladder ultrasound.*

*Problem #7: HEARING LOSS, MILD, HISTORY OF NOISE EXPOSURE*

*H/O:* Becoming hard of hearing and has excessive noise exposure without protection.

*A/P:* Hearing loss may well be related to noise exposure. Will quantitate as outpatient, and recommend hearing protection. Will make sure patient able to hear discussions during this hospitalization.

*Problem #8: DEPRESSIVE SYNDROME, ETIOLOGY UNDETERMINED*

*H/O:* Anhedonia, sleep disturbance, appetite changes, crying spells, much stress and grief related to her terminally ill brother. Appears depressed, denies suicidal ideation.

*A/P:* Depressive syndrome. May be situational and there are several other problems that could be related such as possible hypothyroidism or menopause. She is also acutely ill. Depression could be important if it caused loss of control of diet and exercise and exacerbated her diabetes mellitus. Plan to observe carefully, discuss with patient, and consider treatment after acute problems have stabilized.

*Problem #9: PSYCHOSOCIAL STRESS*

*H/O:* See social history.

*A/P:* Stress is definitely contributing to the deterioration of this patient's health. Initially, if agreeable to family and brother will ask hospice program to consult for additional support of brother.

*Problem #10: EXCESSIVE CAFFEINE USE, 12 CUPS COFFEE PER DAY*

*H/O:* 12 cups of drip coffee per day chronically.

*A/P:* At risk for caffeine withdrawal headaches and dysphoria while here. May be contributing to sleep disturbance, also. Allow reduced amount of coffee, and encourage patient to reduce amount more.

*Problem #11: ACTINIC SKIN*

*H/O:* Fair skinned with significantly actinic skin, face and shoulders.

*A/P:* At risk for skin cancers. Encourage sunscreen use, limit solar exposure. Needs regular skin examinations.

*Problem #12: BREAST CANCER PREVENTION*

No risk factors and examination normal, but due for baseline mammogram. Will obtain while here.

*Problem #13: ALLERGIC TO SULFA MEDICATIONS*

Will not use sulfa drugs, and will be careful with related compounds.

*Signature*

## The History and Physical Examination

Traditionally one of the first clinical tasks medical students face is to author a complete history and physical examination on a patient being admitted to the hospital. Case 12-6 represents such a write-up. Students now participate in outpatient clinical experiences much earlier in medical school. In outpatient settings a "complete H & P" is rarely done at a single visit. However, it remains the standard for an ideal *initial* data base, even for outpatients.

The complete patient data base should include identifying information, a chief complaint, a history of the present illness, a past medical history (including meaningful descriptions of current and past medical conditions, operations, medications, allergies, risk factors, and other important historical information), a family history, a social history, a review of systems, a physical examination, and the results of lab and other special studies. The history and observation data base is followed by a problem list, and then by a note for each problem excerpting, in SOAP or HOAP fashion, the supporting history and observation data from the data base, with narrative assessments and plans for diagnosis, therapy, and patient education, as outlined in Table 12.1. Any risk factor identified should be included in the problem list and addressed in the assessments and plans.

**Table 12.1**
Traditional Format for the History and Physical Examination

| Component | Information included |
|---|---|
| Heading | Date, Time, Type of Note |
| ID | Patient identification, Informant/Source of history, Estimate of reliability |
| CC | Chief Complaint |
| HPI | History of Present Illness |
| PMH | Past Medical History |
| | Disease (active and past), trauma, and operations (chronologically)—describe all relevant details |
| | Other relevant risk factors and problems |
| | Transfusions |
| | Immunizations |
| | Medications (significant past, currently prescribed, currently OTC) |
| | Allergies/adverse reactions |
| FH | Family History (includes ethnic, genetic, and familial risk factors) |
| SH | Social History (personal profile, support systems, travel history, exposure and occupational history (including hobbies), health promotion habits, substance use/abuse, sexual history, etc.) |
| ROS | Review of Symptoms |
| PE | Physical Examination |
| Lab | Laboratory tests, x-rays, etc. |
| Problems | Problem list (including "health maintenance") |
| A/P | Assessments and Plans for each problem |
| Signature | |

## CASE 12-7

*The resident who admitted Mrs. Jane Smith, Case 12-6, gave the following comprehensive presentation at a busy morning report session. Note the strategic omissions and summarizations.*

*"For our next admission I would like to present Mrs. Jane Smith, who is a 51-year-old woman admitted to Dr. Jones's service for pneumonia. She is a married 51-year-old from Smallville, Texas, employed as a commercial artist. She has hypertension and adult-onset diabetes mellitus. This is her first hospital admission since her youngest child was born. History is obtained from the patient, who is reliable, and by phone from Dr. Susan Jones, her attending family physician.*

*"She presented to the emergency room stating that her chest hurt when she breathed and that she was coughing up blood. She felt well until 8 days ago when she developed a fever, chills, headache, body aches, sore throat, and dry cough. She began taking over-the-counter cold meds. After 2 days she went to see her family physician, Dr. Jones, who diagnosed influenza A and prescribed amantadine. Her glucose was in good control. By the next day she began to feel better and her fever resolved. Two days ago she developed myalgias and the cough became productive. Yesterday she developed chills, fever, and right lateral pleuritic chest pain. Today she felt dyspneic and at 10 AM started coughing up some dark blood. The appearance of the blood frightened her so she came to the emergency room.*

*"She has a 15 pack-year smoking history, quitting 10 years ago as a health measure. She has no history of pneumonia, lung disease, TB, cancer, or asbestos or other exposures; there is no history of coagulopathy. She has never had either influenza or pneumococcal vaccines.*

*"The hemoptysis was especially frightening to Mrs. Smith because her brother has lung cancer. She feels embarrassed that she did not seek attention earlier. She is tired of having to worry about her health so she just kept hoping that the problem would go away.*

*"Her past medical history is remarkable for 15 years of diabetes mellitus. At first it was treated with oral meds, then she lost a lot of weight and was able to control it well with diet and exercise. A year ago she had to quit her aerobics class to care for her brother. She started gaining weight and a*

*month ago Dr. Jones had to start her back on glyburide. She also has a history of hypertension well controlled for 15 years on hydrochlorthiazide.*

*"Family history includes diabetes mellitus, hypertension, stroke, MI, and colon and lung cancer. Her husband and children are well. Socially she is a commercial artist whose husband is in a stressful construction job. One child is in college, and three are at home, ages 17, 16, and 15. She drinks 12 cups of coffee per day. It's significant that she is preoccupied with caring for her terminally ill brother who has lung cancer and now lives in the patient's guest room. Caring for him is very time-consuming and stressful. Her support systems are poor at present.*

*"Her review of systems is most significant for a 25-pound weight gain over the last year. She's not exercising, has increased appetite, and finds herself eating to relax. She also has difficulty falling asleep, early awakening, frequent crying spells for no particular reason, and inability to enjoy the activities she used to like.*

*"On examination this is an alert but ill woman who is cooperative. She was initially dyspneic, but improved with oxygen. She was febrile at 102.5 F, with BP 150/92, HR 110, and RR 32. She is 5 feet 4 inches tall and mildly obese at 169 pounds. Her head and neck were normal. No abnormal nodes were appreciated. Her chest was nontender with a mildly increased AP diameter. She was tachypneic, with no retractions but splinting her right chest. Breath sounds were slightly decreased diffusely and no wheezing, rales, rhonchi, or dullness were present except for dullness, tubular breath sounds, and rales in the right lower posterior lung field. The only other remarkable examination findings were a palpable bladder, mild vibratory sensation loss in the feet, and actinic skin. Her chest x-ray confirmed a right lower lobe infiltrate without effusion. Other lab is pending.*

*"Mrs. Smith has the following problem list:"*

*The resident then gave the full problem list from Case 12-6, and then presented the history, observations, assessment, and plan for the most important problems of pneumonia, diabetes, depressive syndrome, and psychosocial stress. The final summation was as follows:*

*"I will be pleased to elaborate on any of the less relevant problems that I was only able to mention. In summary, Mrs. Smith is a functional, hardworking woman admitted with a severe, acute postviral right lower lobe bacterial pneumonia and adult-onset diabetes mellitus that is no longer in dietary control because of the effects of psychosocial stress and possible depression. I will be happy to entertain questions."*

---

# CASE PRESENTATIONS

## Types of Case Presentations

While patient records are relatively audience independent, presentations are always audience dependent. Although there are audiences and situations where a complete data base is presented, verbal presentations are usually brief, and present a developed point of view, not just a recitation of information. The style of presentation also depends on the clinical situation. An admission presentation made by a new medical student will tend to be much more comprehensive than a presentation made at rounds on a patient who has been in the hospital for several days.

Early in clinical training, medical students are often expected to give "complete presentations." These often are the equivalent of reading the written history and physical examination since the goal is to verify that the student has collected and analyzed a complete data base on the patient. After gaining experience, presentations will be shortened by omitting findings that are not positively or negatively relevant to the patient's problems. While rotating with a subspecialty, students are often asked to focus only on findings pertinent to that subspecialty.

The purpose of a presentation also determines the style and depth. "Morning report" presentations (Fig. 12.4) are often conducted as much for academic as for communication purposes. Therefore, the cases are often presented as unknowns, mainly concentrating on data, with the attending physician asking questions to cause the audience to think about the diagnostic possibilities. Another type of morning report is simply to

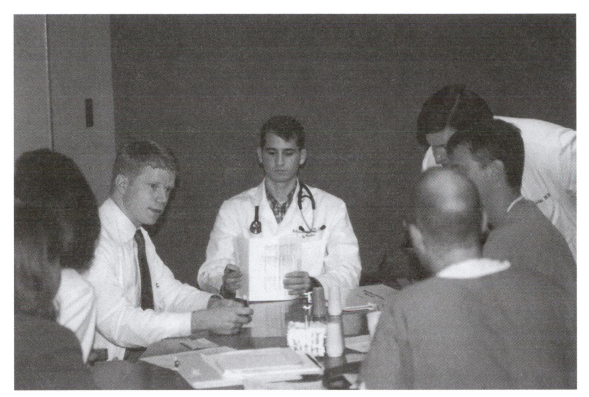

**Figure 12.4.** At "morning report" a student presents his latest patient to the hospital team.

present information most pertinent to the case to launch a discussion of the diagnoses or problems. Often this type of presentation is like reading the assessment and plan without the data base. A brief overview of the patient is given, followed by a presentation of each problem, the data supporting that problem, and the plans for that problem.

Other presentations involve routine work rounds and "checking out" a case to another physician who is going to assume care of the patient for the night or the weekend (Fig. 12.5). These presentations are problem oriented, brief, and focus on pitfalls and plans. Presenting to consultants is another important skill. A presentation to a busy consultant should give the most important information first and then add the details. Do not present the patient as an "unknown" where the consultant must keep listening and waiting for the punch line. Tell the consultant who is calling, and then what, why, and how, followed by who, where, and when. It is very helpful to listen to experienced physicians present cases in order to learn how to present salient points of a patient's story without boring the audience with a recitation of irrelevant details.

## Giving Case Presentations

Case presentations are fun for those who are prepared, but stressful for the unprepared. Develop skill in both planned and spontaneous case presentations. Know the importance of each particular presentation for patient care, for education, and for grades! Know the purpose of the presentation and the intended audience. Consider rehearsing the presentation either actually or mentally. Be prepared to deliver the presentation the audience needs and expects.

Presentations should be short, no longer than 5 minutes, even for complicated cases. According to Cutler (1985), "A case presentation should consist of sifted, selected, and processed data and must be delivered in a lucid, brief, precise manner. It ought to include only the most important positive findings and a few pertinent negatives." There may be instances when for the purpose of educational gamesmanship students are expected

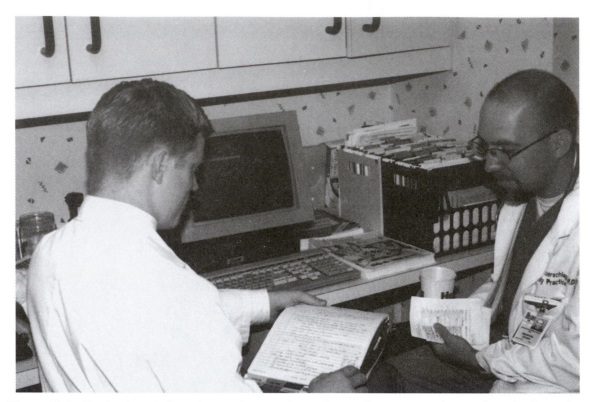

**Figure 12.5.** During hospital work rounds, a student refers to the patient's chart as his Chief Resident listens to his case presentation.

to present a case as an "unknown," without selling the audience on any particular diagnosis. However, in most situations simply present a cogent argument supporting the best positions and refuting any less plausible alternative positions.

The best way to decide what information needs to be presented, given the requirement for brevity, is to "think backwards." Each diagnostic or therapeutic plan should have a supporting problem or diagnosis. For each significant problem or diagnosis identified and excluded, be able to identify the historical, clinical, and lab observations that provide a rationale for including or excluding that diagnosis or problem. These data, along with a general description of the patient and the vital signs, are the *core case data*. Present only the core case data, the problems and plans they support, and nothing else. If these data are reduced to compact, technical language, it is quite likely that the entire case can be presented in 5 minutes or less, as was done by the resident in Case 12-7.

Decide whether to do a traditional presentation, a problem-oriented presentation, or a "newspaper-style" presentation for a busy consultant. If a full problem-oriented assessment and plan has already been written using excerpts from the data base, then the case can be directly presented by problem from that write-up. If the traditional format is to be used in which the core case data are presented followed by the problem list and plan, then the core case data from each problem must be combined back into one abbreviated data base that can be presented as a unit. Case 12-7 was presented in this manner. It is a good idea for presenters to have something written as a guide, especially if tired or distracted. It can be helpful to "highlight" the core case data on a photocopy of the write-up, so that only core data are presented, in order, as a unit. Notecards or other working notes are also helpful. Neither the traditional nor the problem-oriented approach is difficult if the case has already been written up and the core case data are selected by working backwards. The newspaper-style presentation to a consultant is different and will be discussed separately.

Begin the presentation with a brief description of the patient that sets the stage for the audience to regard the patient as a person and not just a case. Mention the informant and the reliability of the information. State the chief complaint in the patient's exact words if they facilitate understanding of the case, but if clinical judgment indicates no distortion would result, it is acceptable to restate the chief complaint more succinctly. For hospitalizations the reason for admission is stated up front, as the resident did in Case 12-7, although some attending physicians prefer not to hear the reason for admission until the plan is discussed.

After the opening of a traditional presentation, go through all of the core case data in the same order that they would appear in the patient record. Stick strictly to the core case data that were selected by working backward through the case. Follow the HOAP arrangement, presenting the history, personally made observations, and tests. After presenting the data, give the problem list, followed by a separate assessment and plan for each significant problem.

Do not let the audience erroneously think that the presentation is jumping around, as may happen if the patient's history includes historical observations or tests. Make it obvious that they are historical. For example, after presenting most of the history, say, "After Mrs. Bennett's arrival at the ER, she was evaluated by Dr. Casey, who observed that Mrs. Bennett was tachypneic and splinting her right chest. He ordered a chest x-ray that showed a right lower lobe effusion, so prior to calling us, he performed a thoracentesis removing 250 ml of pus." If instead it was simply stated that a chest x-ray and thoracentesis were done, without mentioning Dr. Casey, it might appear that the presentation skipped straight from history to observations. Someone would probably interrupt wanting the rest of the history, the vital signs, and the examination.

After the opening of a problem-oriented presentation, launch right into the problem list, starting with the problem related to the chief complaint. State the entire list, then for each problem germane to the presentation, describe its specific core history, observations, assessment, and plan. Include the general description of the patient and the vital signs with the first problem, even if they are not particularly important to that problem, because it helps in portraying the patient as a person and because the vital signs are always relevant to the overall case.

Conclude either type of presentation by summarizing the case. Restate the most important problems and plans to help consolidate major points of the case, and help the audience focus on the meat of the case instead of on whatever minor details were presented last. The goal should be to present all of the core case data and analyze them so well that the audience is left speechless, without questions!

Skill in less formal types of presentations will develop naturally, but the "newspaper-style" presentation is especially worth discussing. It is an "all business" type of presentation designed to present specific facts and requests as efficiently as possible. It is used most often with consultants. Like it or not, there are always some consultants who will seem intimidating. Others are very busy and preoccupied. By knowing the patient's core case data and following a few simple rules, even medical students can be confident and do quite well at presenting to consultants.

If a consultant likes cases presented in a certain manner, then present them that way. Otherwise, use the newspaper-style presentation format. Imagine a general surgeon who is paged while beginning a cholecystectomy. A nurse dials the number on a speaker phone. An intern answers, and launches into a story, "We've got a patient, Mrs. Green in room 315, who is a 65-year-old female with diabetes mellitus and hypertension who was admitted with a right cerebral infarction. We've had a lot of trouble controlling her hypertension." By this time the surgeon is annoyed. It is not even clear why the intern is calling so it's especially unclear what data are important to try to catch from the intern's presentation. The surgeon is also occupied with the operation and wants the intern's presentation to get to the point. It would have been much better if the intern had said, "This is Dr. McCoy with the resident service. We would like to consult you on a patient who may have a perforated duodenal ulcer. May I tell you about the case?" With permission granted, the intern continues, "At exactly 6 AM this morning the patient suddenly developed intense epigastric pain that is now generalized. The abdomen is silent, rigid, and has rebound. Abdominal x-rays are pending. The patient is tachycardic and has

# ELECTRONIC MEDICAL RECORD SYSTEMS

*Electronic medical record (EMR) systems have yet to achieve their promise. They have been around since the 1960s, but recently computers have become advanced enough to make electronic records practical for busy physicians. While a full discussion of emerging EMR systems is well beyond the scope of this chapter, some brief comments are in order.*

*It is important to recognize that EMR systems may not make physicians more* efficient; *rather, they are tools intended to make physicians more* effective, *and to help physicians do things that could not or would not be done otherwise. An EMR system should do more than emulate a paper chart.*

*There are many systems available and they are anything but standardized. Some use completely proprietary software and run on machines located in the physician's office. Other systems are provided by "Application Service Providers" or ASPs, and will run the physician module in a Web browser, and depend on a fast and secure Internet connection. This moves much of the computer maintenance outside the physician's office, but sends patient information far and wide and has raised privacy concerns. Most EMR systems introduce a lot of complexity into a medical practice.*

*In the academic family practice center where I work, for example, we have 36 residents, 12 faculty physicians, medical students, and several specialists who together conduct about 70,000 outpatient visits a year. Over 100 support people including nurses and clerks are also involved with medical records. Often several people need access to the chart at the same time. Managing paper charts effectively in such a setting is quite difficult. But a computer system is even harder. First, a central infrastructure is needed. A computer department takes responsibility for maintaining large central data-base servers that are kept running and backed up and secure. These are networked to hundreds of personal computers hard wired to offices, charting areas, nursing stations, and every exam room, and connected with wireless technology to laptops and outside hospitals. All must be maintained. Our lab has hardware and programs that provide two-way connections to the medical record system. The scheduling, billing, and transcription departments also have connections. Each physician and clinical employee has to be trained to use the system well, including the new people who come along from year to year. We all will soon be faced with frustrating federal mandates regarding medical record operations. There are many more technical considerations, but overall, it's safe to say that operating an EMR system is a mammoth task. Moreover, when compared on the whole with paper charts, the EMR system probably consumes more physician time, not less. Yet there are still many reasons to use an EMR system.*

*The EMR system permits many people in many locations, even in distant hospitals, to read a chart simultaneously. The notes are all legible. The EMR system promotes accurate prescribing, and it checks drug interactions. It promotes good, secure clinical communications about a patient, including electronic delivery of the results of tests and studies, and accurate, recorded communications between members of the healthcare team. It provides for the use of consistent charting methods with reminders and prompts, warnings about allergies, and automatic graphing of clinical data. It also maintains a detailed clinical data base that, with the proper reporting software, can be used to answer many types of research questions. Features like these can make physicians more effective. In the early twentieth century, before there were paved roads and gas stations and repair shops, it was anything but convenient to own an automobile. But it was obvious that the automobile would someday do important things that the horse could never do, so the automobile advocates persisted despite the temporary inconvenience. When the bugs were worked out of it and when standardization arrived, the transition to the automobile fully hit its stride. People began to reap the benefits, and eventually despite the loss of the aesthetics of horse-powered transportation, automobiles became the norm. But if we knew then what we know now about getting railroaded by technology, would we have been more careful designing traffic systems and laws and automobiles? And will we be just as cautious as we adopt more and more electronic tools in medicine?*

a low-grade fever. She's 65 and has already been in the hospital for a week because of a right cerebral infarction and hypertension. We feel she needs a surgical opinion as soon as possible."

This type of presentation gives the most important and dramatic facts first, up front. It's very efficient to listen to this type of presentation, even when busy and preoccupied. Moreover, after only three sentences the preoccupied surgeon has enough information to tell the intern that it would be best to call someone else.

# VOICE RECOGNITION SYSTEM

*One of the biggest problems with EMR systems has been data input. Often EMR systems contain "templates" for entering routine patient data. Sometimes the consistency and speed of a template can be good. But often templates reduce individuals to a common and bland denominator, and fail to capture "the voice of the patient." A richly worded individualized narrative remains the gold standard for medical records, but it can be a problem to enter it into the computer. Not everyone types. Only a few people type as fast as they can talk. Transcription services are expensive and sometimes slow. Would you like your computer to obey your verbal commands and type neatly while you dictate? Good news. Voice recognition (VR) systems for medical charting are practical with today's computer hardware and software—sometimes.*

*In the past, VR systems had to be extensively "trained" for a particular person's voice. Today's systems are speaker independent, require far less training, and produce fairly accurate output even when used by different people. Older systems also required the speaker to pause between each word, but today's systems recognize continuous speech.*

*Modern VR systems type the correct word partly by recognizing the vocabulary context in which a word is used; therefore, they can correctly transcribe a statement like the following, which uses the homonyms "two," "to," and "too": "Two woman were going to the fair but they became too tired and went home." However, when the speaker uses a large specialized vocabulary such as that employed by family physicians, the VR system loses the ability to make use of vocabulary context clues; therefore, special medical vocabulary software modules that add a medical dictionary and context clues to medical speech are needed. Without a medical vocabulary module, practically every medical word is replaced by incorrect lay terms, and the correction and training required makes medical dictation a time-consuming and frustrating process. And unfortunately, medical modules are very overpriced and seem to cost in the range of ten times as much as the general-purpose VR system they support.*

*Since voice recognition systems type faster than most people, even poor typists can produce neat, readable notes without the expense and turnaround time of using a human transcriptionist. However, VR systems still make mistakes and have several problems. They generally require an expensive noise-reduction microphone and still perform poorly in noisy environments. They have more problems with small, common words like "no ifs, ands, or buts" than they do with large, unique words. They may combine a long word and a small word into a wrong word. They may add and drop words. They never make spelling mistakes because they only type words that appear in their dictionaries; instead, they may substitute a correctly spelled but wrong word, an error that cannot be detected with a spelling checker. (Some of the resulting correctly spelled nonsentences are hilarious, but others are medically dangerous if uncorrected.) Overall accuracy rates range from 95 to 99%, which is not as good as it sounds. Proofreading and retraining during dictation requires concentration and adds yet one more intellectual demand to the family physician's busy day. But because of types of hard-to-notice errors made by VR systems, dictating (perhaps with a handheld device) with the intent to proofread, correct, and train later, can be equally demanding. Moreover, the audio provided by handheld digital recording devices is highly compressed and poorly suited for voice recognition, making the error rates even higher.*

*At the moment, although it still requires a dedicated physician in the right type of practice to make a medical VR system function well, the state of the art is advancing so quickly that there is little doubt that these systems will soon replace conventional medical transcription as the best way to produce richly worded, professional narratives of clinical encounters.*

Computer systems approaching that described in Case 12-8 are a reality today in some practices (Fig. 12.6). Even more sophisticated systems are on the way. The future of patient records and case presentations is exciting. Computer systems make it possible to easily record, classify, and store large amounts of detailed patient information, to view that information in creative, helpful ways; and to share and communicate information with others involved in the care of the patient. A whole new series of skills will be needed by the physicians who participate in the medical informatics revolution and in computer-based patient record systems. It will be up to those physicians to create record templates, initiate clinically desirable practice guidelines, present patients and charts over video links, and otherwise initiate the features of record systems in a humane, professional manner that preserves the art and humanity of medicine.

Authoring patient records and presenting cases are skills critical to a physician's career. Over a career, much time and energy is spent authoring and reviewing patient records. There are important technical considerations involved in optimally using and creating patient records and presenting cases. It is equally important, however, that records remain confidential and portray a true and accurate story of each patient as a person.

# CASES FOR DISCUSSION ────────────────────────────────

## CASE 1

*A previously healthy 40-year-old man is paralyzed from the shoulders down because of a motor vehicle accident. During his acute hospitalization his problems included spinal shock, urinary retention, two operations on his neck, pulmonary edema, pneumonia, kidney infection, fecal impaction, bedsores, and depression. He has health insurance through an HMO, disability insurance through his employer, and is suing the person who caused the accident. After he is more stable he is transferred to a rehabilitation unit where he receives physical and occupational therapy. When he returns home he requires home visits.*

1. *Who are some of the most important users of this gentleman's patient records?*
2. *What are some of the important uses for his patient records?*
3. *How could inadequate or distorted records adversely affect this patient?*

## CASE 2

*A physician wrote the following untitled HOAP note:*

*H: 6-year-old here because of right ear pain and fever for 3 days. Also, chronically has runny nose and rubs eyes a lot. Has chronic itchy rash on arms. Developed a new rash on chest last week. Severely sunburned on face recently. Has wheezing problems during soccer; has been out of previously prescribed medications for 6 weeks including albuterol and cromolyn sodium inhalers because mother thought they were no longer needed. Overdue for immunizations. No known medication allergies.*

*O: Fussy, well-hydrated. T 101.9F. Bags under eyes. Left TM clear, right TM bulging and red. Nose with boggy, weepy nasal mucosa. Neck supple. Lungs with diffuse end-expiratory wheezing, otherwise clear. Skin with scaly, secondarily excoriated patches in the flexor areas, and ringlike scaly reddish lesions on torso. The torso lesions have hyphae on KOH preparation.*

*A: #1—Acute otitis media (OM), right*
*#2—Allergic rhinitis*
*#3—Atopic dermatitis*
*#4—Tinea corporis (ringworm)*
*#5—Sunburn*
*#6—Asthma, mildly flared off meds*
*#7—Needs immunizations*

P: #1—Amoxicillin 250 mg tid 10 days for OM
#2—Clemestine fumarate 1.34 mg bid for allergic rhinitis and atopic dermatitis
#3—Clotrimazole cream applied bid for tinea corporis
#4—Albuterol and cromolyn inhalers qid for asthma
#5—Recheck in 14 days and as needed

1. How could the above note be rearranged into a true problem-oriented note?
2. What are the advantages and disadvantages of this note compared with a problem-oriented version?
3. What are the three components of an excellent plan section? Which are missing in the above note?

## CASE 3

An elderly male patient arrives at the emergency room unconscious. According to family members, over the last week he gradually became more lethargic. They were unable to arouse him that morning. Many interrelated diagnoses are noted on old charts, including ethanolism, alcoholic liver cirrhosis, ascites (fluids in the peritoneum), coronary artery disease, hypertension, prostatic hypertrophy with history of urinary retention, and several others. He is on a long list of medications. A family member reports the patient had rectal bleeding yesterday. A nasogastric tube is inserted, and gross blood is found in the stomach. The case is so complex and the patient so critical that it seems best for the intern to appraise the chief resident about the case before fully evaluating the patient.

1. What approach should the intern take in presenting the situation to the chief? Why?
2. How should the intern present the case in consulting a busy gastroenterologist about the GI bleeding?

After additional study, it is confirmed that the patient has hepatic encephalopathy precipitated by bleeding esophageal varices. At morning report the next day the intern wants the audience to mentally work through the differential diagnosis of the initial presentation.

3. What approach should the intern use for the presentation at morning report? Why?

All problems are addressed, and the patient is ready for discharge. To better convey the patient's current status, the intern decides to call the out-of-town family physician who will assume care for the patient.

4. How might the intern best present this complex case to the physician assuming care?

## CASE 4

A medical student picks up a chart in clinic to review prior to a visit, notes the two problems ethanolism and hypertension, and reads the previous note written by a resident who previously saw the patient:

Subjective: Anxious, demanding 49-year-old alcoholic hypertensive who returns wanting more medication refills. Noncompliant with propranolol. Denies being on any other medications. Claims she's not drinking. Complains of insomnia and fatigue. Unemployed. Sits around all day apathetic and doing nothing.

Objective: Dirty 49-year-old woman with rotten teeth but no alcohol on breath.

1. What could the effects of such a note be on the patient's care?
2. How could the above note be revised to portray the patient truthfully but more positively?
3. What steps could the student take to keep from being "poisoned" by this note even before meeting the patient?

## CASE 5

A group of primary care physicians using paper records has become busier and busier and must expand its capabilities. The group's main priority is to continue to provide excellent, comprehensive, personal care to its large number of patients and families. At the same time, the group wants to be able to practically review its own medical records in order to conduct quality assurance and community research activities and to become more effective in providing preventive care services. To accomplish its goals, the group has decided to convert to a computer-based patient record system. In deciding what system to use, some physicians are extremely concerned that the new system not disturb the patient–physician relationship. Some are concerned that the system capture the true stories of their patients rather than forcing the use of simplistic boilerplate stories preprogrammed into the system. Others want all of the convenience features of such a system, such as chart sharing, electronic communications between all members of the healthcare team, interfaces to lab equipment and the hospital, and so forth.

1. *How should this group best balance the needs and desires of the patients and physicians in deciding how to implement a computer-based patient record system?*
2. *Where should terminals for the system be placed? In examination rooms? In workstations outside the examination rooms? Both? How might terminal placement affect charting and the patient–physician relationship?*
3. *What are some of the risks and benefits of implementing a computer-based patient record system?*

## RECOMMENDED READINGS

Cutler P: *Problem Solving in Clinical Medicine: From Data to Diagnosis*, ed 3. Baltimore, Williams & Wilkins Co, 1998.

This entire book is a medical gem. I recommend reading it cover to cover toward the end of the second year of medical school to prepare for intense clinical activity. Although Cutler advocates a more detailed and lengthy data base than is generally practical, his material on records and presentation is as wise and helpful as the rest of the book. The second edition (1985) of this book contained fewer cases but was much more extensive in discussing records and presentation.

Donnelly WJ: Righting the medical record: Transforming chronicle into story. *JAMA* 260:823–825, 1988.

This is a readable and important article that makes a strong case for including "the voice of the patient" in the medical narrative. As information technology advances, clear thinking like Donnelly's is needed to provide a defense against those who would have us produce illness narratives using only sparse, limited language that can be processed even by unsophisticated computer systems.

Orient JM: *Sapira's Art and Science of Bedside Diagnosis*, ed 2. Philadelphia, Lippincott Williams & Wilkins, 2000.

This book magnificently lives up to its title. It is useful to the medical student, but will remain a good friend throughout one's career. It presents an uncompromisingly Hippocratic view of our profession and of patient–physician relationships. The sections on recordkeeping are detailed to the extreme. Few physicians will live up to the standards in this book, but the vision of excellence it portrays is a wonderful guide for those striving to be the best.

## REFERENCES

Council on Scientific Affairs, American Medical Association: Users and uses of patient records: Report of the Council on Scientific Affairs. *Arch Fam Med* 2:678–681, 1993.

Cutler P: *Problem Solving in Clinical Medicine: From Data to Diagnosis*, ed 2. Baltimore, Williams & Wilkins Co, 1985, p 199.

Donnelly WJ: Righting the medical record: Transforming chronicle into story. *JAMA* 260:823–825, 1988.

Donnelly WJ, Brauner DJ: Why SOAP is bad for the medical record. *Arch Intern Med* 152:481–484, 1992.

Osheroff JA, Forsythe DE, Buchanan BG, Bankowitz RA, Blumenfeld BH, Miller RA: Physicians' information needs: Analysis of questions posed during clinical teaching. *Ann Intern Med* 114:576–581, 1991.

Sigurdsson G: The medical record in general practice: Where art and science meet. *Scand J Prim Health Care* 2:113–116, 1984.

Tang PC, Fafchamps D, Shortliffe EH: Traditional medical records as a source of clinical data in the outpatient setting. *Proc Annu Symp Comput Appl Med Care* 575–579, 1994.

Weed LL: Medical records that guide and teach. *N Engl J Med* 278:593–657, 1968.

## CHAPTER 13

# C. Advanced Skills

# The Difficult Clinical Conversation

*Kathleen A. Zoppi and Catherine P. McKegney*

*Dr. Wang's first patient of the day is a 39-year-old woman, Tonya Miller, who has vaginal discharge and a weight loss of 70 pounds (from 178 pounds to 108 pounds) over 2 months. She is divorced and has no children. She lives alone, and has no family members in town. Dr. Wang begins to ask about her past medical history, which includes a tonsillectomy as a child. The patient reports nothing unusual in her history except recently persistent fatigue.*

## EDUCATIONAL OBJECTIVES

1. Describe situations or topics that may contribute to difficult clinical conversations
2. Describe possible helpful responses to difficult conversations with patients
3. Describe and demonstrate insight regarding patients or situations that are difficult because they evoke particular responses from the student, which may be related to difficulties or family issues of the learner
4. Describe resources for managing the feelings patients evoke in the student
5. Describe common patterns in difficult encounters
6. Define content and relational aspects of communication processes

## INTRODUCTION

When Dr. Wang saw Ms. Miller in Case 13-1 for the first time, many different diagnostic possibilities came to her mind, including infection, inflammation, nutritional deficiencies, gastrointestinal disease, or malignancies. But Dr. Wang had a funny sense of missing something important, and that this patient's picture was more complicated than it appears. She considered running some tests to rule in, or rule out, certain possibilities.

DR. WANG: I'm curious about what you think might be causing you to lose weight. Do you have any ideas?

MS. MILLER: No. I'm eating the same as I have been. I think maybe it's because I've been nervous lately.

DR. WANG: Nervous. Tell me more about being nervous.

MS. MILLER: I don't know, I just feel jumpy all the time. Like something is about to happen. But everything is just fine. So I don't know what's wrong.

DR. WANG: Has anything changed in your life recently?

MS. MILLER: No. Like what?

DR. WANG: Changes at home?

MS. MILLER: No.

DR. WANG: Changes at work?

MS. MILLER: No.

DR. WANG: Any new stresses that you can think of?

MS. MILLER: No, none. I think I'm fine, it's just my stomach and this diarrhea that are slowing me down.

DR. WANG: Well, I think that we need to find out a little more about why you're having this weight loss. I'd like to order some blood tests for starters, and to see you back next week. Is that okay with you?

MS. MILLER: That's fine.

---

### CASE 13-1 (continued)

*Ms. Miller's lab tests came back, and showed she had normal liver function test results, and her thyroid test results were normal. She was slightly anemic. Dr. Wang has a funny feeling of something missing. She asked Ms. Miller to begin some nutritional supplements, and return in 2 weeks.*

In Case 13-1, what one might *not* know about the patient may be as useful to the diagnosis and treatment as what one *does* know about her. In this chapter, we will try to outline frequently encountered difficult interviewing situations, and offer some ways of working within them to better meet the goals of caring for the patient while maintaining balance and poise. We will describe these difficult situations using a relational model of communication in clinical conversations.

## WHAT MAKES AN ENCOUNTER DIFFICULT?

An interaction between patient and physician can become difficult when both parties feel (or are) unable to understand the other (Starfield *et al.*, 1981); when there is incongruity between the patient's and physician's goals or values (Taylor, 2000; Waitzkin, 1991); or when the patient and the physician battle for control (Suchman, 1998). Sometimes difficulties arise because patients and physicians treat each other as though they were significant people, such as parents or teachers, from each of their past experiences, rather than as the people they are now. Such difficulties related to countertransference (the physician's feelings toward the patient) or transference (the patient's feelings toward the physician) can distort the relationship and create difficult communication (Stein, 1985). This phenomenon may mean that caring for an elderly female patient is more difficult for a physician who had difficulties with his grandmother, and easier for a physician whose grandmother died at a younger age. The physician's own life cycle stage may also affect her ability to care for patients, either because the experience is "too close to home" or because of inexperience with the stage the patient is in at the time (see Chapter 20). Each physician will find different types of patients who push his or her buttons: One of the key skills to managing difficult encounters is to use self-awareness of what kinds of patients or problems are likely to "push one's buttons" (see Table 13.1), and then to employ strategies to use that knowledge for the patient's improved care and one's own professional development (Ellis, 1983). This self-knowledge and the skill to use this self-knowledge does not happen automatically: Real improvement in

**Table 13.1**
A Taxonomy of Difficult Patient–Physician Interactions

| Difficult topics or situations | Patient characteristics | Relationship characteristics | Person of the physician |
|---|---|---|---|
| Giving bad news | Personality disorders | Patient–physician value differences | Family-of-origin issues |
| End-of-life issues | Resistance to change/readiness to change | Countertransference or transference issues | Physician life cycle stage |
| HIV risk | Psychological difficulties, including anxiety, depression, somatization | | Personal psychological difficulties |
| Sexuality/sexual behaviors | | | |
| Chemical dependencies or other addictions | | | |
| Violence | | | |
| Incest or sexual abuse | | | |
| Rape | | | |
| Multiple family members in conflict | | | |

interactions with patients takes concerted effort (Epstein, 1999). The experienced clinician will become increasingly sensitive to feeling her buttons being pushed, will hear a "warning bell" earlier in the interaction, and will seek help from colleagues or teachers.

## Relational Communication in Difficult Clinical Conversations

In any interaction between two people, there are two levels of message exchange: One is at the content level, where the message is encoded in words or nonverbal cues such as gestures. Sometimes communication difficulties occur when people misunderstand each other at the content level: They do not clearly understand each other's words or cues. However, more often difficulties arise when there are differences between what is said and what is meant or interpreted. This difference between message and meaning occurs at the relational level, in which nonverbal cues, context, or relationship history may be congruent with, or may contradict, the content level of the message. Suppose that two longtime friends are talking, and one comments to the other: "Hey, nice haircut!" If this message is delivered with a straight face, a sincere expression, and unwavering eye contact, it may be heard by the recipient as a compliment. However, imagine a relationship where both parties frequently tease each other. If the speaker uttered the same words (content) but instead rolled his eyes and smirked, the meaning (relational) level would be different. The first instance would have been a compliment, where the content and relational levels were congruent, but the second an insult, where content and relational levels contradicted each other. In any interaction, meaning is created and negotiated at the relational level, and often this level is more important than the content or what is actually said.

In the course of clinical conversations, noticing what is occurring at the relational level is critical for understanding and resolving difficult interactions. In the process of attending to the patient's relational message, the physician may be able to choose a different way of responding than usual. In noticing that the patient is saying he is angry, but that his voice is whiny, it is possible to acknowledge his need for reassurance rather than responding with anger or defensiveness. In addition, noticing what relational messages the physician is giving, through body language, facial expression, distance, or movement, is important, particularly when the physician is using herself as a diagnostic and therapeutic instrument to improve the health of the patient. One of the inherent contradictions in medical education is the admonition to use yourself as a diagnostic tool, attending to your own feelings as a barometer of the interaction (Balint, 1964), while much of the experience in medical school trains one to ignore internal feelings and reactions. Throughout this chapter, we will identify situations in which both the patient's and the physician's feelings contribute to the quality of the interaction: Neither person is free from affecting the interaction. Paying close attention to when patients evoke certain feelings can be one of the best (and most challenging) ways of learning about what issues or problems in your own life are important or unresolved. It is also useful to include more sources of information, including family members, nursing staff, or others who can help provide missing pieces of the puzzle.

---

## CASE 13-1 (continued)

*Dr. Wang was stumped by Ms. Miller's problems: She'd been in practice 7 years, and was still not able to figure out the linkages among Ms. Miller's weight loss, anemia, fatigue, "jumpiness," and generally normal lab test results. She met with Ms. Miller one day in her examination room, and Ms. Miller's sister was with her.*

> DR. WANG:     *Well, I'm glad you are both here today. I'm quite concerned that you, Ms. Miller, are still not feeling well, and that we can't seem to find what's wrong. I wonder if there is anything that I've missed, or that we haven't talked about.*
>
> SISTER:     *Well, I've been wondering that too. She's been sick for 5 months, and she looks weak and tired.*
>
> DR. WANG:     *Ms. Miller, your sister seems to be very concerned about how you have been feeling. Is there anything you haven't told me that might affect how you are feeling?*
>
> MS. MILLER:     *Yes, I guess I have been worried that when I used coke several years ago, that might be affecting me now.*
>
> DR. WANG:     *I think that is very important information. Tell me more about how you used when you did.*
>
> MS. MILLER:     *Well, I used to do tricks to get my drug …*
>
> SISTER:     *And it was up until 5 years ago that she was really messed up…*

In Case 13-1, Ms. Miller presents the physician with a difficulty: Should Dr. Wang ask specific questions about her sexual history, drug and alcohol use, or other health habits which might or might not offer clues about her current illness? The nagging sense that something is missing in the picture of the patient's problem might have been one identifying clue that the patient's health habits should be part of the discussion. In this case, the physician's pursuit of her own sense of discomfort led to a greater understanding of the patient as well as of the possibility that she had risks of exposure to HIV (human immunodeficiency virus).

## The Physician's Own Reaction as a Clue

The physician's response to the patient while carrying on a clinical conversation can be a useful source of data. While it is difficult for a physician to simultaneously listen to the patient, pay attention to the interaction, and monitor herself, it may be most worthwhile for the physician to use her own reactions as a source of data. In Case 13-1, the physician was not clear about what feelings were evoked by Ms. Miller, but was clear (and communicated this to the patient) that she was confused and needed to ask some questions again. The systematic repetition of parts of the history may help confirm the feelings evoked the first time, or may help resolve what was unclear during the preceding interview.

Skilled clinicians will notice their own feelings at the same time as observing the patient's behaviors. If one feels overcome with sadness, and this sadness is only present when the clinician is with the patient, it may be that the patient is sad, or that something about the patient's situation has triggered some sadness in the clinician and may be a useful clue about what's going on with the patient. An angry patient in the office may be a very angry, rageful person in many situations. The physician may be only one of many recipients of her anger. Knowing this, through talking with her about other parts of her life, may actually help the physician understand her anger and work with her more easily, with more empathy for her as a person.

It may also be helpful to tune in to what the patient is *not* saying, such as when a patient says she is doing just fine, and isn't upset about the death of her sister, but the longer the physician is in the room, the sadder and more lonely the physician feels. Sometimes the physician who is attuned to the patient's clues may detect feelings the patient isn't even aware of yet; for example, perhaps the patient is smiling tensely as she talks about her husband working long hours, but her fists are tightly clenched, betraying anger she may be feeling. It may be therapeutic for the physician to merely reflect the incongruity observed; for example, by stating, "I noticed that you said your marriage was fine, but when you talked about your husband, your fists were clenched."

Finally, a physician's emotional response may provide useful clues about who in the physician's life the patient represents: perhaps the gray-haired sweet lady reminds the physician of his grandmother, or the angry patient brings up memories of an aunt who was disliked. The recognition of the countertransference, or the feelings evoked by the patient, is important to separating fact from fiction. The care of the patient depends in part on the physician's ability to *accurately* recognize the patient's needs and behaviors, rather than assuming the patient is like another person from the past. This accurate perception cannot be accomplished if a physician reacts unconsciously, unaware that his reaction is really a reaction to a patient or other person from the past.

Often, the awareness of a particular countertransference toward a patient can be a clue about undiscovered features of the patient which may be useful in working more constructively with that person. For example, in Case 13-1, the physician may reflect that Ms. Miller reminds her of her college roommate, whom she likes a great deal. However, this resemblance begins to dissolve as Dr. Jones gets to know the patient better, and sees the differences between the real patient and the one initially perceived.

## CASE 13-2

*Ms. Karen Brodie is a 55-year-old woman who was admitted to the inpatient service with a concussion and a broken arm. She stated that she fell down the stairs in her house after tripping over a pet. An x-ray of her fractured arm is consistent with an injury caused by a blow to the forearm with a large object. She is cooperative until the interviewing resident tries to ask questions about her fall. She becomes sullen and silent and tells him it is none of his business.*

MS. BRODIE: *I already told you what happened.*

RESIDENT: *Yes, but I think it is important to be sure about what really happened so we don't treat you the wrong way. I think this injury looks more like you were hit than like you fell down the stairs.*

MS. BRODIE: *Well, you're wrong. I told you the truth. Why can't you just take care of me?*

RESIDENT: *How can you expect me to take care of you when you aren't telling me what really happened?*

## When the Patient and Physician Differ in Their Agendas: Readiness to Change

When confronted with a patient who is not interested in divulging more of her history, the physician may be tempted to stop questioning, out of respect for the patient's privacy and perhaps out of fear of evoking the patient's anger. In effect, Ms. Brodie in Case 13-2 is saying, "Just take care of me, don't ask me why..." (Ness & Ende, 1994). And yet, without additional questioning, it may be unclear what really happened to the patient to cause her injuries. However, confronting Ms. Brodie directly, implying that she was lying, would likely be counterproductive. On the other hand, accepting her story without questioning might allow her to go home to a potentially violent situation, where the harm done to her next time might be even worse (see Chapter 32).

In fact, each year 2–8 million women in the United States experience physical violence in their homes, which often escalates after the woman seeks medical attention (Sassetti, 1993). Thus, it is important to proceed deliberately but carefully in gathering information and in documenting information gathered, because such data may also be used later in police or legal proceedings. Since the patient and physician may begin the encounter with different goals for the relationship, attending and identifying the relational levels of the interaction may be important when negotiating with the patient.

One important beginning point is for the physician to negotiate the relationship and responsibilities with the patient prior to obtaining a detailed history. Ms. Brodie will be very concerned about the confidentiality of what she tells the physician. Thus, it is important to clarify with her the privacy afforded her in the patient–physician relationship. It is also important for her to know what is written within the medical record, and who might have access to the record, including insurers and third-party reviewers.

It is also necessary for the physician to understand, and to work with the patient, in a manner that empowers positive behavioral change but does not presume readiness. In other words, the patient may not even be contemplating leaving her husband, whereas the physician thinks that leaving is the only possible positive move the patient could make. Such a dyssynchrony will inevitably result in discord. A more productive encounter may result if the physician acknowledges to the patient her concerns, and offers openness to helping the patient to change when she feels able to do so. (Rollnick *et al.*, 1999).

Beginning with some general screening questions as part of a routine psychosocial history can be useful when assessing whether a person is likely the object of abuse. It is crucial that the interviewer maintain a calm, nonreactive nonverbal stance: It may be helpful to put down pen and paper and take a relaxed listening posture.

RESIDENT:     Tell me about the people who live in your house.
MS. BRODIE:     Well, there's my husband, my two teenagers, and our dog, Max.
RESIDENT:     How do they all get along?
MS. BRODIE:     Okay most of the time.
RESIDENT:     What about the rest of the time?
MS. BRODIE:     Well, the kids fight like they all do, and my husband gets mad and takes it out on me.
RESIDENT:     How does he do that?
MS. BRODIE:     Well, he yells and throws things around a lot.
RESIDENT:     Do you ever feel that you and your children are not safe?
MS. BRODIE:     Well, sometimes.
RESIDENT:     That must be hard for you.
MS. BRODIE:     I'm used to it.

It might be tempting to move more quickly here, to ask the patient whether she has ever considered leaving her husband, or whether today's injuries represent an outburst by her husband. It is important to attend to signs of discomfort, since the patient has just indicated that the abuse she described is not a big problem for her. The wise physician will move along at the patient's pace, or gently leave the door open to return to the topic later.

RESIDENT:     Do you feel you would be safe if you went home today?
MS. BRODIE:     I guess so.
RESIDENT:     What could you do to feel safe?
MS. BRODIE:     I guess I could take the phone number of the hotline and keep the car keys outside so I could leave if I need to....

The therapeutic benefits of seeing the physician as a resource, not another (albeit psychological, not physical) dominator, is critical to the patient's improvement. Since domestic violence is a disease that often escalates when the patient makes a move to become independent of the abuser, it is critical for the physician to acknowledge and support the patient in her attempts to move slowly enough to be on solid ground with each new step.

Confrontation of the patient who seems to be giving contradictory information can also be a useful therapeutic strategy. This must be handled gently and respectfully, but it helps the physician to better understand what help the patient is seeking.

PHYSICIAN: The last time I saw you, you told me your husband was drinking a lot and hitting you. Today, you are saying he's fine and you are doing well. I'm curious about how this has changed since we last spoke.

MS. BRODIE: Well, it's better than it was. I just want it all to be okay right now, all right?

PHYSICIAN: I want it to be okay, too. But in case it isn't okay again, I also want you to know I am here to help you if you want me to.

MS. BRODIE: I know that. Thank you. I just hope he can behave well enough that I don't have to move out. I'll let you know how we're doing.

## CASE 13-3

*Mr. Fisher is a 68-year-old man with end-stage renal disease. He has had several visits to the nephrologist, who has said that there was nothing more that could be done for him. He has had dialysis three times each week for the past 4 years. His children, who are married and live close by, take turns driving him to the appointments. Mr. Fisher is increasingly disoriented and unable to care for himself. He was admitted to the hospital and needs a complete history and physical. The nephrologist did not discuss the prognosis with the patient or his children but felt the primary care physician should begin to help them prepare for his death. The patient's family physician is out of town. Dr. Monon, a first-year resident, is assigned the care of Mr. Fisher. He is startled by the resemblance of the patient to his own grandfather.*

DR. MONON: *How are you feeling today, Mr. Fisher?*

MR. FISHER: *Fine. Where am I?*

DR. MONON: *You are in the hospital. Do you know what day it is?*

MR. FISHER: *It's Sunday. Can I go home now?*

DR. MONON: *Not yet. We are still concerned about why you were sick yesterday. Do you remember coming to the hospital?*

MR. FISHER: *No. My son comes to see me every Sunday. I need to be home when he comes ...*

## Talking about Terminal Illness

There are some major difficulties facing the physician, Dr. Monon, who treats Mr. Fisher in Case 13-3. When caring for an unfamiliar patient, it is often hard to assess what behavior is normal and routine and what is unusual and the result of stress or illness. In Case 13-3, an additional source of difficulty is that the patient and family are not aware of the seriousness of his illness or its likely terminal outcome. This lack of awareness not only affects them in their decision-making about the aggressiveness of treatment but likely also affects the physician and how open she feels she can be with the family. Some of what may need to be discussed with this patient and family involves code status and about anticipating the death of the patient. Mr. Fisher's confusion makes communication more problematic: It would be easiest and best to talk directly with him; what presents difficulty is that he seems to be able to be oriented at some times and not others. The physician would be prudent to document the waxing and waning of mental status through a series of mini-mental status examinations at each visit to demonstrate improvement or decline (see Fig. 13.1). In addition to the difficulties of talking with the patient about his diagnosis and prognosis, it is difficult to manage and help support the family members in their feelings about their father's impending death. And yet, in order to help the family cope and plan appropriately, it will be necessary to help them decide, with Mr. Fisher, how he wishes to be treated and what kind of care he'll receive. All of these issues are complicated by the countertransference of the physician, who is reminded of his own grandfather when he talks with Mr. Fisher. The physician finds himself feeling more emotional and sad, and even more angry when one of the patient's sons wishes aloud that his father would just die quickly and quietly. After talking with a behavioral preceptor, Dr. Monon realizes that his own feelings of wanting to save Mr. Fisher at all costs are related to his feelings for his grandfather and are interfering with his ability to listen to the family members in this situation. He finds greater equilibrium as he listens with greater care to what this family wants for Mr. Fisher.

| Give one point for each correct response | | Score | Points |
|---|---|---|---|
| Orientation | | | |
| 1. What is the | Year | _____ | 1 |
| | Season | _____ | 1 |
| | Date | _____ | 1 |
| | Day | _____ | 1 |
| | Month | _____ | 1 |
| 2. Where are we? | State | _____ | 1 |
| | County | _____ | 1 |
| | Town or City | _____ | 1 |
| | Hospital/nursing home/other building | _____ | 1 |
| | Floor | _____ | 1 |
| Registration | | | |
| 3. Name three objects, taking one second to say each. Then ask the patient to repeat all three. (Give one point for each correct answer. Repeat the answers until patient learns all three.) | | _____ | 3 |
| Attention and calculation | | | |
| 4. Serial sevens: Ask the patient to count backwards from 100 by sevens, as 93, 86, 79, etc. (Stop after five answers; give one point for each correct answer.) Alternative: Spell WORLD backwards. | | _____ | 5 |
| Recall | | | |
| 5. Ask for names of the three objects learned in question 3. (Give one point for each correct answer.) | | _____ | 3 |
| Language | | | |
| 6. Point to a pencil and a watch. Ask the patient to name each as you point. | | _____ | 2 |
| 7. Ask the patient to repeat "No ifs, ands, or buts." | | _____ | 1 |
| 8. Ask the patient to follow a three-state command. "Take paper in your right hand. Fold the paper in half. Put the paper on the floor." | | _____ | 3 |
| 9. Ask the patient to read and obey the following command: "CLOSE YOUR EYES." (Write in large letters.) | | _____ | 1 |
| 10. Ask the patient to write a sentence of his or her choice. (The sentence should contain a subject and an object and should make sense. Ignore spelling errors when scoring.) | | _____ | 1 |
| 11. Ask the patient to copy the design shown. (Give one point if all sides and angles are preserved and if the intersecting sides form a quadrangle.) | | _____ | 1 |
| | | (Total) | (Total) |

FIGURE 13.1. The Folstein Mini-Mental Status Examination. Scores of less than 20 suggest delirium or dementia (organic impairment) or, less commonly, depression or schizophrenia. Adapted with permission from Folstein MF, Folstein SE, McHugh PR: 'Mini-Mental State': A practical method for grading the cognitive state of patients for the clinician. *J Psychiatr Res* 12:189–196, 1975. Copyright 1975, Pergamon Press Inc.

## CASE 13-4

*Ms. Graves is a 35-year-old multiparous homemaker who was referred by her ob-gyn for a routine set of screening tests, including a CBC for anemia, a VDRL, and an HIV screening test. Her ob-gyn felt that routine screening was important for all of his pregnant patients. She is returning to the office today for her test results. Her results indicate she is HIV positive. When the test was discussed with her on her last visit, she expressed no concern at all that she had any risks for exposure to HIV. She and her husband have been married for 10 years; however, 5 years ago, they separated for 3 months. Each had different sexual partners at that time. They since reconciled, had three other children, and have been monogamous. She has had no occupational exposures, has never used i.v. drugs, and cannot recall any exposures to blood or blood products. Today's visit will require discussion of the risks to her and of the 30% likelihood of her child being HIV positive (U.S. Public Health Service, 1995).*

## Sharing Bad News

Sharing bad news affects both the patient and the physician, albeit to a lesser degree. Ms. Graves in Case 13-4, who was not expecting any bad news at all during her otherwise normal pregnancy, is likely to be quite unprepared emotionally and intellectually for the interaction about her test results. She will likely respond with disbelief, anger, shock, or denial. At some point, she will have questions about how the disease was transmitted to her, including questions about her husband and his sexual practices, and their other respective sexual partners. She will have questions regarding what this implies about her health, the health of her child, and the viability of her pregnancy. The physician will feel an urgency to talk about the need for medical follow-up and treatment, and will want especially to talk with the patient about how she can take good care of herself and her family during a stressful time. And yet these subjects cannot be discussed before the patient is ready to hear them and to accept the diagnosis. This process could take weeks, and the physician may feel impatient waiting for the patient to be ready to hear what needs to be done. In addition, timely intervention will help the child, even if the mother's condition cannot be changed. It is difficult for the physician to be empathic, to stay with the patient in her "hell," and to be clear-sighted enough to move forward and help her get the treatment she and her child need.

Much research about sharing bad news acknowledges there is no one best way to deliver such information. However, research by Buckman (1992) and Maynard (1991) offers some guidelines: (1) assessing the recipient as much as possible to know prior to the delivery of bad news what preferences the patient might have, including setting and involvement of significant others or family members; (2) forecasting the bad news, by indicating that what is to follow is bad news, can help briefly prepare the patient for what he is about to hear and acknowledges the effect on the patient of what is about to be told; and (3) not overwhelming the patient with additional information, but rather waiting, silently, for the patient to respond and being patient with that reaction are important to the patient's feeling comfortable in expressing grief, anger, or in asking questions that are most central to him. Physicians often tend to overwhelm patients with data, facts, and probabilities. While this information may be useful to the patient, even precious, it is often delivered in a manner that is more anxiety producing for the patient. If delivered too rapidly or too soon, it may be a way of the physician avoiding the anxiety associated with the patient's grief at hearing bad news.

DR. O'BRIEN: Ms. Graves, I need to talk with you about some bad news from the testing we did the other day.

MS. GRAVES: What is it? Is it my baby? What's wrong?

DR. O'BRIEN: No, it's not about your baby. I told you I was running some other tests, including a test for HIV (human immunodeficiency virus). Your HIV test came back positive, indicating you have the virus that causes HIV disease or AIDS. (Pauses)

MS. GRAVES: Oh my God. I can't believe it. There's no way I could have AIDS! What about my baby?

DR. O'BRIEN:    Your baby has approximately a 30% chance of having the virus. There are some treatments we should talk about which might help you and may prevent the development of the disease in your baby so she cannot have the disease. What are you thinking right now?

MS. GRAVES:    Well, I'm not thinking, I'm so scared, doctor. What can I do? (Begins crying)

DR. O'BRIEN:    (Sits) Let's just sit for a while together. We can do some things to help; and we can talk about those when you are ready.

## CASE 13-5

*Mrs. Coldwell is a 74-year-old woman who has been a patient in the practice for 4 years. She has CHF (congestive heart failure), impaired mobility from arthritis, and has frequently missed scheduled appointments. During her most recent physical examination 6 months ago, she had blood in her stool and was told to have a sigmoidoscopy or colonoscopy within the next month. She said she would schedule the appointment but since has only called for refills of her medication. Her primary physician sent her a certified letter indicating that she needed to come back for a follow-up visit. She told the nurse who called her that she was worried about not being able to pay for the test, and that her cousin who had the test was found to have cancer, followed by chemotherapy before she died.*

## Patients Who Don't Want to Follow a Plan

Patients sometimes have reasons for not accepting medical advice or for not following it despite believing the advice to be useful. These reasons may be rational, such as disagreeing with a physician's assessment or diagnosis of a problem. Patients may be willing but unable to follow treatment recommendations because of lack of money or transportation. They may receive other advice from family or friends that is more influential. Each of these circumstances can challenge the physician, who may feel angry or powerless in the face of the patient's behavior. These feelings can result in a dismissal of the patient, either emotionally or in reality from the practice. The patient who decides that another form of treatment is better, who doesn't seem to trust the physician, may be responding to the physician's lack of clear explanation or to the physician's lack of understanding of the patient's belief system.

Mrs. Coldwell in Case 13-5 had several barriers to seeking treatment, including money for medical care, lack of insurance, and transportation difficulties, but most important was the difference between her goals and those of her physician. She was not certain that she wanted treatment even if she had cancer. Her physician felt obligated to educate her about the consequences of her thinking.

## CASE 13-6

*Ms. Russo is a 38-year-old woman who is a new patient to the practice. She has been treated for borderline hypothyroidism and hyperprolactinemia. She has been taking Synthroid 0.1 mg p.o. q.d. and bromocriptine 0.5 mg p.o. b.i.d. She is concerned because she had an unusually light period 2 weeks ago at the normal time, and yesterday began bleeding heavily and having severe cramps. She is angry because she called her gynecologist and could not get an appointment for 2 weeks. Today, before her appointment, she called and yelled at the front desk receptionist about how long it took her to answer the telephone.*

## Patients Who Are Angry

The physician seeing Ms. Russo in Case 13-6 may fear opening the examination room door and facing Ms. Russo's anger. And it is quite likely that she will be angry for a few minutes. The wise physician will allow the patient to talk, and will just listen for the first few minutes, while the patient relates what's wrong. It will also be important to respond to her emotional expressions of fear, anger, or sadness, acknowledging these as normal and reasonable responses to what has happened to her. It will also be critical to let her complete as much of the story as she is willing to tell, to let her cool down, before moving to the underlying reason for the visit. It is important to not engage in problem solving at the content level about the other physician's office, or in detail about your office staff although feedback from patients is often useful information.

| | |
|---|---|
| DR. JONAS: | Ms. Russo, I'm Dr. Jonas. How are you? |
| MS. RUSSO: | Not so great. I've been trying to get in and get some help about my bleeding, and getting through to my gyn and to your office has been ridiculous. What kind of offices do you run, anyway? You doctors must not really want to actually see patients, do you? I just can't believe you would let me keep on bleeding and not see me right away. |
| DR. JONAS: | You felt you should have been seen right away. |
| MS. RUSSO: | I guess I really was worried. |
| DR. JONAS: | Well, it sounds as though you've had quite an experience. I really do try to see patients and am glad you got in to see me today. Why don't you tell me more about your bleeding? |
| MS. RUSSO: | Okay, well, it started 3 days ago … |

Dr. Jonas in Case 13-6 was wise to allow the patient to express her feelings without letting her "hook" him: He did not react with anger, as often is the most likely response, but rather was able to remember that the patient's anger is *her* feeling, and does not necessarily need to be his as well. The physician was able to reflect the patient's feelings using her words, a simple technique to indicate listening and attention to the patient's words.

## CASE 13-7

*Mr. Chester is a 70-year-old man who has been coming into the office for 6 years. During this time, he has been diagnosed with Alzheimer's disease, which has been progressing. He also has diabetes mellitus and lives alone. Despite his Alzheimer's disease, he has been able to care for himself and has been managing his insulin and his diet. A visiting nurse sees him twice a week. His children, who live out of town, visit each weekend and cook and clean for him. He came to the office today with a blood sugar of 750 mg/dl. The patient is sure that he took his insulin this morning, but cannot tell what day of the week it is.*

## Working with Families

As in Case 13-3, the physician in Case 13-7 needs to document the patient's mental status through a series of examinations. However, including the family as additional historians may offer fruitful data about the course of Mr. Chester's illness and help project the needs for additional care or treatment. A family meeting with the children and Mr. Chester may yield some useful discussion and a decision about how to care for Mr. Chester in the future. The physician who wants to care for the patient must mobilize the entire family around a plan that they can all support. This mobilization entails asking who all of the relevant participants are and inviting them to join the meeting. It is important for the physician to greet each person and to ask each one to talk about what he wishes for the care of the patient. In addition, the physician may find himself involved in trying to negotiate differences among family members, and an important task is clarifying viewpoints for family members without taking sides (see Chapter 20 for working with families).

| | |
|---|---|
| DR. BRUNO: | Thanks for coming today. Your father and I thought it would be good if we could all talk together about what's happening. Why don't we start with you, Mr. Chester; what are your concerns about how you're doing? |
| MR. CHESTER: | Well, I sure hate getting sick enough to come to the hospital. But I ain't goin' to a nursing home either. |

DAUGHTER:    Dad, stop that. We aren't going to put you in a home …

SON:    June, don't say that. Dad, we need to do whatever's best for you. We can't promise that you won't need to go to a nursing home; that's the doctor's decision.

DR. BRUNO:    Well, actually, that's a decision we all will make together today. Mr. Chester, I know we've talked and you don't want to go to a nursing home. But as your doctor, I can't allow you to stay someplace where you're not safe. Lately, you have been sick more often, and I don't feel you can be safe if you live alone. So today we need to talk about having someone live with you in your home, or you living with one of your children, or your moving somewhere safer.

MR. CHESTER:    Okay.

## CASE 13-8

*The last scheduled patient of the day in the clinic is a 25-year-old primagravida artist, Mrs. Munoz, who is 12 weeks into her pregnancy. She and her husband have come to the office for a regularly scheduled checkup. The nurse indicates that neither of the couple speaks English. They have brought the husband's 13-year-old sister along as a translator. This visit requires a pelvic examination, scheduling for an alpha-fetoprotein (AFP) test, and an ultrasound.*

## Language or Communication Barriers

The usual difficulty of explaining a test and the potential results is exacerbated by the language barrier in Case 13-8. It is critical that the patient and her husband understand the reason for the test, and the limits of its interpretation. And yet, without a translation, the interactants may be reduced to communicating through hand gestures and broken phrases while conveying highly technical content. However, the inclusion of a 13-year-old relative as a translator can be difficult and even unacceptable in some cases. The inclusion of a younger relative as a translator is common, and yet it is often unclear what issues can safely be addressed with a family member in the room. Discussion of sexual practices, including needs for a sexually transmitted disease (STD) or human immunodeficiency virus (HIV) check, can become difficult at best. It may be questionable practice to perform a pelvic examination in the presence of a young girl, and yet to cut off communication during the examination can compromise patient care. It may be useful for the physician to include the translator as much as possible in the general history, and for more specific questions or difficult subjects to try to find a translator (or to have the practice use the ATT Language Line for translation) for a subsequent visit. Above all, recognition of the need for professional translation in critical circumstances may require ingenuity and creativity in a more remote medical setting (Witte & Kuzel, 2000).

## CASE 13-9

*A 36-year-old man, Mr. Thomas, is seeing Dr. Sonja Smyth for the first time. He is a healthy man who is requesting a preemployment physical. He has a family history of early MI (myocardial infarction) (his father had an MI at 40) but is otherwise in good health.*

DR. SMYTH:    *Mr. Thomas, I'm Dr. Smyth. How are you today?*

MR. THOMAS:    *Very well, thank you. Please call me Dave.*

DR. SMYTH:    *Thank you Dave. I see you're here for a preemployment physical. Have you had any recent illnesses or problems you'd like to talk to me about?*

MR. THOMAS:    *No, not really, I'm in good health. I'm excited about my new job, and just hope I can meet the right woman in this city …*

DR. SMYTH:    *(noticing that Mr. Thomas is an exceptionally handsome man when smiling) Well, I hope so, too. Tell me more about your move here …*

# Physician Feelings for Patients

The patient in Case 13-9 inspired some feelings in Dr. Smyth that are in conflict with her professional role. While sexual feelings are normal, and occur often in patient–physician encounters, they are not to be acted on. Yet many physicians report engaging in sexual relationships with patients (5–10%, in some studies) despite explicit prohibitions against such contact by the ethical standards of physicians (Council on Ethical & Judicial Affairs, American Medical Association, 1991; Gartrell, 1992). The wise physician will notice such feelings as they arise and will respond to set appropriate limits when necessary, deliberately steering the conversation onto professionally safer ground.

MR. THOMAS:    ... so I hope I can find the right woman here.

DR. SMYTH:    I hope that happens for you, too. Tell me about what illnesses you have had in the past ...

## CASE 13-10

*Laura Boaz, a 21-year-old college student, came to the physician for a checkup 6 months into her first pregnancy. She was very concerned about completing her education, and described herself as sure that she wanted to place the baby for adoption. She had discussed this with her boyfriend, Mark, who was supportive of her desire to have the baby and to seek adoption arrangements. Neither Laura nor Mark had told their parents about the pregnancy. Despite the presence of two of Laura's sisters at college, Laura believed they hadn't noticed that she was pregnant.*

Dr. Potter liked Laura. She and the patient had gone to the same Catholic high school; both of their families went to the same church. They were both the eldest daughters in working-class families, and over the course of the pregnancy shared stories of their families. Dr. Potter respected Laura's decision, and felt Laura was exceptionally mature in the manner she handled her feelings about the pregnancy and her family. After the delivery, Dr. Potter counseled Laura and was satisfied that her patient felt comfortable with the adoption, and was prepared to use abstinence or birth control to prevent another pregnancy. Dr. Potter was dismayed to see Laura on her schedule 8 months later for another prenatal visit, with a due date in 3 months.

# Why the Visit Can Go Too Well

A sneaky aspect of countertransference can occur when patient and physician like each other and relate well: They can assume that they are too much alike, and the physician may not recognize signs of problems or difficulties the patient is not overtly sharing (Stein, 1985). This blind spot can result in insufficient attention and discussion of areas of disagreement between patient and physician, with the result that issues may resurface. In particular, the physician in Case 13-10 felt disappointed with the patient (and ultimately with herself) for not working harder to probe Laura's true feelings and resolution of her problems.

# CONCLUSION

This chapter has focused on the difficulties that may arise between patients and physicians in clinical conversations. Particular types of problems, including misunderstandings at the content level, differences in agendas or expectations, battles for control in the interview, and issues of countertransference, were identified. Specific skills for working with patients who are angry, who have a terminal illness, or who have been abused were identified.

Students who have difficult encounters with patients are encouraged to notice patterns in their encounters and to identify whether those patterns are the result of particular countertransferences or family interactions from the student's past. Ongoing consultation with peers, colleagues, or teachers concerning difficult relationships can be useful in identifying and changing patterns of interaction.

Noticing when conflicts occur between patients and physicians at the content level (such as disagreements or misunderstandings) and when they occur at the relational level (such as battles for control) can help the student determine when a conflict can easily be resolved.

## CASES FOR DISCUSSION

### CASE 1

*You are a fourth-year medical student on call at midnight on the family practice service. You are asked by your supervising resident (who is in the Emergency Room) to do an admitting history and physical on a patient. You enter the room and introduce yourself as a fourth-year student working with the family practice team. The patient says, "Oh, dear, you're too young and cute to be a doctor! I can't wait until you examine me."*

1. *What do you say next to the patient?*
2. *How do you structure the interview (physically, by seating, facial expression, and eye contact) and verbally (by telling the patient what you are going to do) to maintain good rapport with the patient?*
3. *How do your answers differ if the patient is:*
    a. *a 35-year-old woman who is very attractive*
    b. *a 22-year-old man who is very handsome*
    c. *a 76-year-old woman who is not very appealing*
    d. *an 87-year-old man who smells like alcohol*

### CASE 2

*Mr. Graves is a 74-year-old man with end-stage renal disease. He has survived many operations, daily dialysis, but his kidney failure is now untreatable. You are the third-year clerk on the renal service, and Mr. Graves pleads with you to be honest and tell him if he has a chance to live. His son, who is in the room, looks stricken, and tells his father, "Of course you'll be fine, dad...."*

1. *What do you say to Mr. Graves?*
2. *How can you respond to his fears and his son's false reassurance, without contradicting his son?*
3. *Who would you ask for help in working with the patient and his family?*

### CASE 3

*Ms. Cornell is a 27-year-old mother of four who has been seeing your preceptor in the family practice center for 5 years. She has been in good health, with some depression noted 2 years ago, which was successfully treated with medication. She is returning today for a Pap smear and routine annual examination. Your preceptor asks you to see the patient and take a history. When you enter the room, you notice that Ms. Cornell has bruises along her upper arm, and she looks tearful.*

1. *How do you begin the interview?*
2. *How do you ask about the bruises?*
3. *Ms. Cornell says she is fine, but is still crying throughout the conversation. How do you reflect this observation to her?*

### CASE 4

*Tommy Capione is a 6-year-old boy who has been in good health until the past year. Since the beginning of first grade, he has visited the family practice center eight times for a variety of infections. His mother has brought him to the office because he is wheezing and sounds very congested. Tommy is lethargic and disoriented. You begin to suspect that this pattern of infections may be ominous and want to test Tommy for HIV.*

1. *How do you begin to explain the need for an HIV test to Tommy and to Tommy's mother? Do you speak to them together or alone?*
2. *When she protests, saying there is no way for Tommy to have AIDS, how do you respond?*
3. *How do you suggest they discuss the need for the test with Tommy's father, who is at work during the appointment?*

---

## CASE 5

*Mrs. Pink is a 38-year-old woman who has been treated for clinical depression for the past 3 months. She has been on medication and in psychotherapy for problems with her marriage. Her husband is verbally abusive and dominates her. She has wanted to become pregnant, but he has forbidden her to try, saying that she is like a child already and is incapable of taking care of a child. Today, she has come to the office requesting a pregnancy test. The test is positive. She is convinced that the medication she is taking will harm her child and that she should terminate the pregnancy to avoid any further problems with her husband.*

1. *What steps would the physician need to take to talk with the patient?*
2. *How should the physician respond to the patient's returning home to her husband after the visit?*
3. *Mr. Pink calls and demands the physician tell him whether his wife is pregnant or not. How should the physician respond?*

# RECOMMENDED READINGS

Balint M: *The Doctor, His Patient, and the Illness.* New York, International Universities Press Inc, 1964.

> Balint's classic work describes the therapeutic role of the physician's understanding of the patient as a "drug." This chapter is an excellent summary of the ways "difficult patients" ask for help from physicians, and how physicians can work with patient requests.

Brody H: *The Healer's Power.* New Haven, CT, Yale University Press, 1992.

> Discusses the power of healing in the patient–physician relationship and the struggles of working ethically with difficult patients.

Buckman R: *How to Break Bad News.* Baltimore, Johns Hopkins Press, 1992.

> Dr. Buckman, a Canadian family physician, details a systematic, research-based model for giving patients and families bad news.

Candib L: *Medicine and the Family.* New York, Guilford Press, 1995.

> This is a wonderful discussion of the feminist relational view of the patient–physician relationship. The reader will learn how to view relationships in the context of society.

Epstein R: Mindful practice. *JAMA* 282:833–839, 1999.

> The author identifies the qualities of the mindful physician, who is able to maintain simultaneous self-awareness and awareness of the patient.

Frey JJ: The clinical philosophy of family medicine. *AJM* 104(4):327–329, 1998.

> Dr. Frey is a family physician who identifies the ways that difficult situations with patients may actually strengthen the patient–physician relationship.

Newell R: *Interview Skills for Nurses and Other Health Care Professionals.* London, Routledge & Kegan Paul, 1994.

> This book uses a cognitive behavioral model for structuring work with patients, including specific skills for working with emotions, assessing the patient, and helping patients change behaviors.

Peterson M: *At Personal Risk: Boundary Violations in Professional–Client Relationships.* New York, WW Norton & Co Inc, 1992.

> The author compares physicians, psychotherapists, and ministers in an analysis of "traps" in patient encounters that result in boundary violations, including sexual relations with patients/clients.

Rollnick S, Mason P, Butler C: *Health Behavior Change.* Edinburgh, Churchill Livingstone, 1999.

> The authors apply principles of motivational interviewing for behavioral change to health care relationships.

Stein H: *The Psychodynamics of Medical Practice.* Berkeley, University of California Press, 1985.

> A useful introduction to the ideas in this chapter about relationships between patients and physicians.

Taylor TR: Understanding the choices that patients make. *JABFP* March–April 13(2):124–133, 2000.

> The author identifies the many reasons why patients may choose different courses of action than those recommended by their physicians.

Balint M: *The Doctor, His Patient and the Illness*, ed 2. New York, International Universities Press Inc, 1964.

Buckman R: *How to Give Bad News*. Baltimore, Johns Hopkins University Press, 1992.

Council on Ethical & Judicial Affairs, American Medical Association: Sexual misconduct in the practice of medicine. *JAMA* 266:2741–2745, 1991.

Ellis A: How to deal with your most difficult client: You. *J Ration Emot Ther* 1(1):3–8, 1983.

Epstein RM: Mindful practice. *JAMA* 282:833–839, 1999.

Gartrell NK: Physicians report having sex, hearing about sex with patients. *Am Med News* 24:10, 1992.

Maynard D: Bearing bad news in clinical settings, in Dervin B (ed): *Progress in Communication Sciences*. Norwood, NJ, Ablex Publishing Corp, 1991.

Ness D, Ende J: Denial in the medical interview. *JAMA* 272:1777–1781, 1994.

Rollnick S, Mason P, Butler C: *Health Behavior Change*. Edinburgh, Churchill Livingstone, 1999.

Sassetti M: Domestic violence, in Elliott B, Halverson K, Hendricks-Matthews M (eds): *Family Violence and Abusive Relationships*. Primary Care 20(2):289–306, 1993.

Starfield B, *et al*: The influence of patient–practitioner agreement on outcome of care. *AJPH* 71(2):127–131, 1981.

Stein HS: Whatever happened to counter transference? in Stein HF, Apprey M (eds): *Context and Dynamics in Clinical Knowledge*. Charlottesville, University Press of Virginia, 1985.

Suchman A: Control and relation. In Suchman A, Bothelho R, Henton-Walker P: *Partnerships in Healthcare*. Rochester, University of Rochester Press, 1998.

Taylor TR: Understanding the choices that patients make. *JABFP* March–April 13(2):124–133, 2000.

US Public Health Service Recommendations for Human Immunodeficiency Virus: Counseling and Voluntary Testing for Pregnant Women. *Morbidity Mortality Weekly Rep* 44(FF-7):1–14, 1995.

Waitzkin H: *The Politics of Medical Encounters*. New Haven, Yale University Press, 1991.

Witte TN, Kuzel AJ: Elderly deaf patients' health care experiences. *JABFP* 13(1):81–83, 2000.

## CHAPTER 14

# Managing Chronic Illness

*John S. Rolland*

## CASE 14-1

*Janice, a married woman in her 30s with two small children, received the most up-to-date medical treatment and expert surgical interventions during her 4-year bout with cancer. Six months after her physician pronounced her cured, Janice and her husband Sam separated. A prolonged emotional and financially draining divorce and custody battle ensued. Sam drank heavily and became verbally abusive. Both children developed behavioral problems at home and at school that required crisis intervention, bringing this disintegrating family to treatment for the first time.*

## EDUCATIONAL OBJECTIVES

1. Describe a comprehensive family systems model for assessment and clinical intervention with families facing chronic illness and disability
2. Describe the psychosocial demands of illness based on the pattern of: onset, course, outcome, incapacitation, and level of uncertainty
3. Describe the crisis, chronic, and terminal phases of illness, the transitions between phases, and the psychosocial developmental tasks associated with each phase
4. Discuss the interface of illness, individual, and family life cycles; multigenerational legacies of illness and loss; and how these relate to coping and adaptation to chronic illness
5. Describe how health belief systems will affect a patient's or family's response to illness

## INTRODUCTION

The psychosocial strains on a family with a member suffering a serious health condition can rival the physical strains on the patient. A growing body of research is demonstrating that any comprehensive approach to intervention should include the family (Campbell & Patterson, 1995; Weihs *et al.*, 2001). This chapter provides a family systems-oriented model for patients with chronic and life-threatening illness and disability. At the heart of systems thinking is the focus on *interaction*. With physical disorders, particularly chronic

# GLOSSARY

Cohesion. *The degree of emotional bonding between family members. There is great cultural and ethnic variation as to what is considered normative.*

Complementarity. *The degree of harmony in the meshing of family roles, as between husband and wife or partners; to the extent that the roles dovetail satisfactorily, the partners are able together to provide and receive mutual satisfaction from the relationship.*

Disengagement. *A family organization with overly rigid boundaries, in which members are isolated and feel unconnected to each other, each functioning separately and autonomously, with little involvement in the day-to-day transactions within the family.*

Enmeshment. *A family organization in which the boundaries between members are blurred and members are overconcerned and overinvolved in each other's lives, limiting individual autonomy.*

Psychosomatic. *The interplay between psychological and physical phenomena. Traditionally, this term has been used to denote a pathological process, where individual or family psychological distress or dysfunction is expressed through physical symptoms.*

disease, the focus is the interaction of a disease with an individual, family, and other biopsychosocial systems (Engel, 1977, 1980). The Family Systems-Illness Model presented in this chapter places the family as its central reference point (Rolland, 1994a). This choice is made with the recognition that the family is a system influenced heavily by a range of social, economic, institutional, and political forces in the larger environment.

The Family Systems-Illness Model (Figure 14.1) (Rolland, 1984, 1987a,b, 1990, 1994a,b, 1998) is based on a strength-oriented perspective viewing family relationships as a resource, and emphasizing the possibilities for resilience and growth, not just their liabilities and risks (Walsh, 1998). A serious health crisis offers families an opportunity for deepening their relationships.

Families enter the world of illness and disability without a psychosocial map. To master the challenges, families need, first, a psychosocial understanding of the condition in system terms. This means learning the

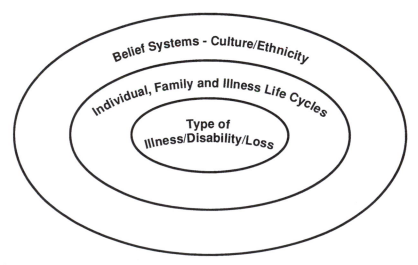

**Figure 14.1.** The Family Systems-Illness Model. Reprinted from: Rolland JS: *Families, Illness, and Disability*, New York, Basic Books Inc, 1994, p. 14.

expected pattern of practical and emotional demands over the course of the disorder, including a time line for disease-related developmental tasks associated with different phases of the disorder as it unfolds. Second, they need to gain a systemic understanding of themselves as a functional unit. Third, an appreciation of individual, couples, and family life cycles helps them stay attuned to the changing fit between the demands of a chronic disorder and emerging developmental issues for the family unit and each member. Finally, families need to understand the beliefs and multigenerational legacies that guide their constructions of meanings about health problems and their relationship to caregiving systems.

This chapter presents this clinical model to provide a pragmatic way of thinking about family coping and adaptation to chronic conditions. This discussion will highlight the interactive processes between the psychosocial demands of different chronic disorders over time and key components of family functioning. Beginning with the expected psychosocial demands of a disorder through its various phases, this chapter will cover family systems dynamics that emphasize: (1) multigenerational patterns; (2) family and individual life cycles; (3) family belief systems (including those associated with culture, ethnicity, and gender); and (4) family factors that facilitate or impede the relationships between patient, family, and health professionals. This normative model emphasizes the goodness of fit between the psychosocial demands of the disorder and the strengths and vulnerabilities of a family. Figure 14.2 depicts one useful way to represent the interface between illness and family.

## CASE 14-2

*Dan and Kathy are a young dual-career couple with two children, aged 3 and 1, living in a large metropolitan area. Kathy had a 2-week history of intermittent double vision, fatigue, and mild numbness and a "heavy feeling" in both legs.*

With persistent symptoms, her internist referred her to a neurologist, who after a quick workup informed the couple that Kathy has multiple sclerosis. Her symptoms respond well to a brief course of steroids. The neurologist has explained the treatment approach to her disease, informed her that the disease is very unpredictable, describing the range of possible complications, and instructed her to contact him immediately if symptoms return.

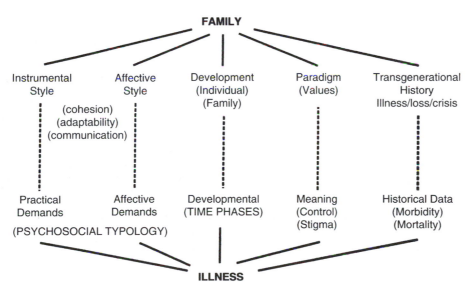

**Figure 14.2.** Interface of chronic illness and the family. Reprinted from Rolland JS: Family systems and chronic illness: A typological model. *J Psychother Fam* 3(3):143–168, 1987.

## MULTIPLE SCLEROSIS

*Multiple sclerosis is a demylinating disease of the central nervous system, characterized by recurrent attacks of focal or multifocal neurologic dysfunction. These attacks occur, remit, and recur seemingly randomly over many years with the disease most commonly beginning in early adult life. Classic features include impaired vision, nystagmus, dysarthria, decreased perception of vibration and position sense, ataxia and intention tremor, weakness or paralysis of one or more limbs, spasticity, bladder, bowel, and sexual problems; and for many, signs of dementia in later stages. The clinical course is highly unpredictable in its overall severity; the frequency, timing, and severity of relapses; and the progression of the disease. Besides disability, a major challenge for patients and their families is living well in the face of the disease's highly unpredictable course.*

Dan, Kathy, and their extended families are terrified. Kathy wonders if her illness will destroy her budding career as a real estate broker, while Dan feels maybe he should take a second job to ensure an adequate income for the family. The couple wonders whether they should cancel their plans to have more children and move out of their recently purchased first home, a three-story old Victorian. Kathy feels insecure about her ability to be an adequate mother if her condition worsens. Her parents feel the couple should move back to their small hometown to be close to their large extended families. Neither Dan nor Kathy has ever lived with a chronic disorder and their parents are in good health. To them, the psychosocial implications of multiple sclerosis are akin to being suddenly transported to a foreign country and living under a permanent, amorphous, and unpredictable "dark cloud."

## ——— PSYCHOSOCIAL TYPOLOGY AND TIME PHASES OF ILLNESS

In order to think in a truly interactive or systemic manner about the interface of the illness and the individual or the illness and the family, one needs a way of describing illness itself in systems terms and a schema that recasts the myriad of biological diseases in psychosocial terms over time. Such a schema must simultaneously remain relevant to the interactions between the psychosocial and biological worlds and provide a common language that transforms or reclassifies our usual medical terminology.

There have been two major impediments to progress in this area. First, insufficient attention has been given to the areas of diversity and commonality inherent in different chronic disorders. Second, there has been a glossing over of the qualitative and quantitative differences regarding how various diseases are manifest over the course of an illness. Chronic conditions need to be conceptualized in a manner that organizes these similarities and differences over the disease course so that the type and degree of demands relevant to clinical practice are highlighted in a more useful way.

The psychosocial importance of different time phases of an illness is not well understood. Clinicians often become involved in the care of an individual or family coping with a chronic illness at different points in the "illness life cycle." Understanding the evolution of a long-term illness is hindered because clinicians rarely follow the family through the complete life history of a disease.

Only a few clinical studies have addressed the importance of broad time phases of illness. One example has been studies that examine the adaptive versus harmful role of denial, loosely defined as one's attempts to negate the existence of a problem, at different points of the disease course. For parents of a child with leukemia, denial may enable them adaptively to perform necessary duties during earlier phases of the illness, but might lead to devastating consequences for the family if maintained during the terminal phase. Likewise, denial may be functional for recovery on a coronary care unit after a myocardial infarction, but harmful if this translates into ignoring medical advice vis-à-vis diet, exercise, and work stress over the long term.

The problems of illness variability and time phases are addressed on two separate dimensions: (1) Chronic illnesses are grouped according to key biological similarities and differences that dictate significantly distinct psychosocial demands for the ill individual and her family, and (2) the prime developmental time phases in the natural evolution of chronic disease are identified.

## Psychosocial Typology

The goal of the psychosocial typology presented here is to create clinically meaningful and useful categories with similar psychosocial demands for a wide array of chronic disorders across the entire life span; it is not intended for traditional medical treatment or prognostic purposes, but for examining the relationship between family or individual dynamics and chronic disease. This typology conceptualizes broad distinctions of the pattern of (1) onset, (2) course, (3) outcome, (4) type and degree of incapacitation, and (5) degree of uncertainty. These categories are hypothesized to be the most psychosocially significant for a wide range of illnesses and disabilities. Although each variable is actually a continuum, it will be described here in a categorical manner by the selection of key anchor points along the continuum.

### Onset

Illnesses can be divided into those that have either an acute onset, such as strokes, or a gradual onset, such as Parkinson's disease. Although the total amount of family adaptation might be the same for both types of illness, for acute-onset illnesses these affective and practical changes are compressed into a short time, requiring of the family more rapid mobilization of crisis management skills. Families able to tolerate highly charged affective states, exchange clearly defined roles flexibly, problem-solve efficiently, and utilize outside resources will have an advantage in managing acute-onset illnesses. The rate of family change required to cope with gradual-onset diseases allows for a more protracted period of adjustment.

### Course

The course of chronic diseases can take three general forms: progressive, constant, or relapsing/episodic. A *progressive* disease (e.g., Alzheimer's disease, emphysema) is one that is continually or generally symptomatic and progresses in severity. The individual and family are faced with the effects of a perpetually symptomatic family member, where disability increases in a stepwise or progressive fashion. This means that a family must live with the prospect of continual role change and adaptation as the disease progresses. Periods of relief from the demands of the illness tend to be minimal. Increasing strain on family caretakers is caused by both exhaustion and the continual addition of new caretaking tasks over time.

A *constant-course* illness is one where, typically, an initial event occurs after which the biological course stabilizes. A single-episode myocardial infarction or spinal cord injury are two examples. Typically, after an initial period of recovery, the chronic phase is characterized by some clear-cut deficit or residual functional limitation. Recurrences can occur, but the individual or family is faced with a semipermanent change that is stable and predictable over a considerable time span. The potential for family exhaustion exists without the strain of new role demands over time.

A *relapsing* or *episodic* course in illnesses like ulcerative colitis and asthma is distinguished by the alternation of stable periods of varying length, characterized by a low level or absence of symptoms, with periods of flareup or exacerbation. Strain on the family system is caused by both the frequency of transitions between crisis and noncrisis and the ongoing uncertainty of *when* a recurrence will occur. This requires a family flexibility for alternation between two forms of family organization. Also, the wide psychological discrepancy between periods of normalcy versus illness is a particularly taxing feature unique to relapsing diseases.

### Outcome

The extent to which a chronic illness is a likely cause of death and the degree to which it can shorten one's life span are critical features with profound psychosocial impact. The most crucial factor is the initial *expectation* of whether a disease is a likely cause of death. On one end of the continuum are illnesses that do not typically affect the life span, such as lumbosacral disk disease or arthritis. At the other extreme are illnesses that are clearly progressive and usually fatal, such as metastatic cancer. There is also an intermediate more unpredictable category, including both illnesses that shorten the life span such as cardiovascular disease, and those with the possibility of sudden death, such as hemophilia. Perhaps the major difference between these kinds of outcomes is the degree to which the family experiences anticipatory grief and its pervasive effects on family life.

When loss is less imminent or certain an outcome, illnesses that may shorten life or cause sudden death provide a fertile ground for idiosyncratic family interpretations (Rolland, 1990). The "it could happen" nature of these illnesses creates a nidus for both overprotection by the family and powerful secondary gains for the ill member. This is particularly relevant to childhood illnesses such as hemophilia, juvenile-onset diabetes mellitus, and asthma (Minuchin *et al.*, 1975, 1978).

## Incapacitation

Incapacitation can result from impairment of cognition (e.g., Alzheimer's disease), sensation (e.g., blindness), movement (e.g., stroke with paralysis, multiple sclerosis), energy production (e.g., cardiovascular disease), and disfiguring diseases (e.g., severe burns) associated with social stigma (e.g., AIDS).

The extent, kind, and timing of incapacitation imply sharp differences in the degree of stress facing a family. For instance, the combined cognitive and motor deficits of a person with a stroke necessitate greater family role reallocation than a spinal cord-injured person who retains his cognitive abilities. For some illnesses, like stroke, incapacitation is often worst at the time of onset and would magnify family coping issues related to onset, expected course, and outcome. For progressive diseases, like Alzheimer's disease, disability looms as an increasing problem in later phases of the illness, allowing a family more time to prepare for anticipated changes. It provides an opportunity for the ill member to participate in disease-related family planning.

By combining the kinds of onset, course, outcome, and incapacitation into a grid format we generate a typology with 32 potential psychosocial types of illness. This grid is shown in Table 14.1.

## Uncertainty

The predictability of an illness and the degree of uncertainty about the specific way or rate at which it unfolds overlay and color the other attributes: onset, course, outcome, and incapacitation. For illness with highly unpredictable courses, such as Dan and Kathy (Case 14-2) with multiple sclerosis, family coping and adaptation, especially future planning, are hindered by anticipatory anxiety and ambiguity about what they will actually have to deal with. Living in the face of threatened loss can be particularly difficult for families like Dan and Kathy, who are in early adulthood or the childrearing phase of the family life cycle. Families unable to put long-term uncertainty into perspective are at high risk for exhaustion and dysfunction.

The complexity, frequency, and efficacy of a treatment regimen, the amount of home- versus hospital-based care required because of the disease, and the frequency and intensity of symptoms vary widely across illnesses, with important implications for individual and family adaptation. Some regimens require significant financial resources and caregiving time and energy (e.g., home kidney dialysis, cystic fibrosis). Treatments least likely to be adhered to are those that have a high impact on lifestyles, are difficult to accomplish, and have minimal effects on the level of symptoms or prognosis (Strauss, 1975). Although they reduce time-consuming dependence on medical centers, home-based treatments place heavier responsibility on patient and family. Therefore, the degree of family emotional support, role flexibility, effective problem solving, and communication in relation to these treatment factors will be crucial predictors of long-term treatment compliance.

It is important to consider the likelihood and severity of disease-related crises and associated family

**Table 14.1**
Categorization of Chronic Illnesses by Psychosocial Type[a]

| | Incapacitating | | Nonincapacitating[b] | |
|---|---|---|---|---|
| | Acute | Gradual | Acute | Gradual |
| **Fatal** | | | | |
| Progressive | | Lung cancer with CNS metastases<br>AIDS<br>Bone marrow failure<br>Amyotrophic lateral sclerosis | Acute leukemia<br>Pancreatic cancer<br>Metastatic breast cancer<br>Lung cancer<br>Liver cancer | Cystic fibrosis* |
| Relapsing | | | Incurable cancers in remission | |
| **Shortened life span, possibly fatal** | | | | |
| Progressive | | Emphysema<br>Alzheimer's disease<br>Multi-infarct dementia<br>Multiple sclerosis (late)<br>Chronic alcoholism<br>Huntington's chorea<br>Scleroderma | | Juvenile diabetes*<br>Malignant hypertension<br>Insulin-dependent adult-onset diabetes |
| Relapsing | Angina | Early multiple sclerosis<br>Episodic alcoholism | Sickle-cell disease*<br>Hemophilia | Systemic lupus erythematosus* |
| Constant | Stroke<br>Moderate/severe myocardial infarction | PKU and other congenital errors of metabolism | Mild myocardial infarction<br>Cardiac arrhythmia | Hemodialysis-related renal failure<br>Hodgkin's disease |
| **Nonfatal** | | | | |
| Progressive | | Parkinson's disease<br>Rheumatoid arthritis<br>Osteoarthritis | | Non-insulin-dependent adult-onset diabetes |
| Relapsing | Lumbosacral disk disorder | | Kidney stones<br>Gout<br>Migraine<br>Seasonal allergy<br>Asthma<br>Epilepsy | Peptic ulcer<br>Ulcerative colitis<br>Chronic bronchitis<br>Irritable bowel syndrome<br>Psoriasis |
| Constant | Congenital malformations<br>Spinal cord injury<br>Acute blindness<br>Acute deafness<br>Survived severe trauma and burns<br>Posthypoxic syndrome | Nonprogressive mental retardation<br>Cerebral palsy | Benign arrhythmia<br>Congenital heart disease | Malabsorption syndromes<br>Hyper-/hypothyroidism<br>Pernicious anemia<br>Controlled hypertension<br>Controlled glaucoma |

[a]Modified from Rolland JS: Toward a psychosocial typology of chronic and life-threatening illness. *Fam Sys Med* 2:245–263, 1984. Reprinted with permission of Family Process Inc.
[b]Asterisks indicate early.

anxiety (Strauss, 1975). A clinician should assess the family's understanding about the possibility, frequency, and lethality of a medical crisis. How congruent is the family's understanding with that of the medical team? Are their expectations catastrophic or do they minimize real dangers? Are there clear warning signs that the patient or family can recognize? Can a medical crisis be prevented or mitigated by detection of early warning signs or institution of prompt treatment? When a patient or family heed the early warning signs of a diabetes insulin reaction or asthma attack, a full-blown crisis can usually be averted. How complex are the rescue operations? Do they require simple measures carried out at home (e.g., medication, bed rest) or do they necessitate outside assistance or hospitalization? How long can crises last before a family can resume "day-to-day" functioning? It is essential to ask a family about its planning for such crises and the extent and accuracy of their medical knowledge. How clearly have leadership, role reallocation, emotional support, and use of resources outside the family been formulated? If an illness began with an acute crisis (e.g., stroke), then assessment of that event provides useful information as to how that family handles *unexpected* crises. Evaluating the overall viability of the family's crisis planning is crucial.

## Time Phases of Illness

In this psychosocial schema of chronic diseases, the developmental time phases of illness are a second dimension. The concept of time phases provides a way for the clinician to think longitudinally and to reach a fuller understanding of chronic illness as an ongoing process with landmarks, transitions, and changing demands. Each phase has its own unique psychosocial developmental tasks that require significantly different strengths, attitudes, or changes from a family. To capture the core psychosocial themes in the natural history of chronic disease, three major phases can be described: (1) crisis, (2) chronic, and (3) terminal. The relationship between a more detailed chronic disease time line and one grouped into broad time phases is diagrammed in Figure 14.3.

### The Crisis Phase

The crisis phase includes any symptomatic period before diagnosis and the initial period of readjustment and coping after the problem has been clarified through a diagnosis and initial treatment plan. This period holds a number of key tasks for the ill member and family. Moos (1984) describes certain universal practical illness-related tasks, including: (1) learning to deal with pain, incapacitation, or other illness-related symptoms; (2) learning to deal with hospital or health clinic environments and any disease-related treatment procedures; and (3) establishing and maintaining workable relationships with the healthcare team. In addition, there are critical tasks of a more general, sometimes existential nature. The family needs to: (1) create a meaning for the illness event that maximizes a preservation of a sense of mastery and competency; (2) grieve for the loss of the preillness family identity; (3) gradually accept the illness as permanent while maintaining a sense of continuity between their past and future; (4) pull together to undergo short-term crisis reorganization; and (5) in the face of uncertainty, develop a system flexibility toward future goals.

During this initial crisis period, providers have enormous influence over a family's sense of competence and the methods devised to accomplish these developmental tasks. The initial meetings and advice given by providers at the time of diagnosis can be thought of as a "framing event." Because families are so vulnerable at this point, clinicians need to be extremely sensitive in their interactions with family members. Who is included or excluded (e.g., patient) from a discussion can be interpreted by the family as a message of how a family should plan their communication for the duration of the illness. One family, accustomed to open, frank discussion, described how the physician came to the mother's hospital room and took the family members to a separate room to inform them that the mother had cancer and discuss the diagnosis. At this vulnerable moment, the family felt that they were being instructed implicitly to exclude the mother in any discussion of her cancer. Providers who in some fashion blame the patient, a family member, or the whole family for an

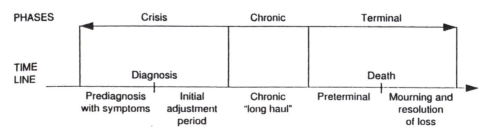

**Figure 14.3.** Time line and phases of illness. Reprinted from Rolland JS: Toward a psychosocial typology of chronic and life-threatening illness. *Fam Syst Med* 2:245–262, 1984.

illness (e.g., delay in seeking an appointment, negligence by parents, poor health habits) or distance themselves from a family may undercut a family's attempt to sustain a sense of competence.

## The Chronic Phase

The chronic phase, whether long or short, is the time span between the initial diagnosis and readjustment period and the third phase when issues of death and terminal illness predominate. This era can be marked by constancy, progression, or episodic change. Thus, its meaning cannot be grasped by simply knowing the biological behavior of an illness. Rather, it has been referred to as "the long haul," or "day-to-day living with chronic illness" phase. Often the individual and family have come to grips psychologically or organizationally with the permanent changes presented by a chronic illness and have devised an ongoing modus operandi. The ability of the family to maintain the semblance of a normal life under the "abnormal" presence of a chronic illness and heightened uncertainty is a key task of this period. If the illness is fatal, this is a time of "living in limbo." For certain highly debilitating but not clearly fatal illnesses, such as a massive stroke or dementia, the family can become saddled with an exhausting problem "without end." Paradoxically, a family's hope to resume a "normal" life cycle might only be realized after the death of their ill member. This highlights another crucial task of this phase: the maintenance of maximal autonomy for *all* family members.

For long-term disorders, customary patterns of intimacy for couples become skewed by discrepancies between the ill member and well spouse/caregiver. Shame-based emotions often remain underground and contribute to "survivor guilt." As one young husband lamented about his wife's cancer, "It was hard enough 2 years ago to absorb that, even if Ann was cured, her radiation treatment would make pregnancy impossible. Now I find it unbearable that her continued slow, losing battle with cancer makes it impossible to go for our dreams like other couples our age." Psychoeducational family interventions that normalize such emotions related to threatened loss can help prevent cycles of blame, shame, and guilt. Also, when physicians inquire about and validate the psychosocial burden of caregivers, especially well spouses, they help prevent the physical burden of the patient from becoming the only currency in family relationships. This approach facilitates families seeing a chronic disorder as a "we" problem rather than solely the domain of the patient, a major contributor to dysfunctional family dynamics when living with serious illness or disability.

Medical care for chronic illnesses is often provided in specialty clinics, where patients and families dealing with similar disorders may develop significant relationships, even in the clinic waiting area. Progression, relapse, or death of another patient can trigger fears of "Will I (we) be next?" and deflate family morale. It is useful for clinicians to inquire about such contacts and offer family consultations.

## The Terminal Phase

The last phase is the *terminal* period including the preterminal stage of an illness in which the inevitability of death becomes apparent and predominates family life. It encompasses the periods of mourning, bereavement, and resolution of loss (Walsh & McGoldrick, 1991). This phase is distinguished by the predominance of issues surrounding separation, death, grief, resolution of mourning, and resumption of "normal" family life beyond the loss. Clinicians should keep in mind recent evidence (Wortman & Silver, 1989) that supports a much broader range of nonpathological grief reactions, somewhat tempering how we use traditional stage theories of loss (Kubler-Ross, 1969).

The transition to this phase is fraught with possibilities for blame, shame, and guilt. The family may blame the medical team for failing to provide a cure, especially if physicians had earlier given an overly optimistic prognosis. The patient and family members may blame themselves or one another for having lost "the battle." This is particularly true of families guided by a strong sense of personal responsibility and control.

As families enter this phase, one of the key tasks is a shift in their anticipation of the possibility of a terminal phase to its probability, and finally its inevitability. Clinicians can function as a guide for families, helping them gently relinquish their hopes for cure, initiate a humane plan for palliative care, and instill hope in developing a pathway for the experience of death. Clinicians should expect intense grieving related to giving up the often protracted struggle to overcome the disease. This is distinct from the experience of anticipatory grief, where family members prepare for the loss of a loved one. Mastery in the chronic phase, which emphasized maintaining autonomy within the constraints of the disorder, must now be redefined in terms of a process of preparing emotionally and practically for death. Similar to the initial crisis phase, families generally need to accept more intense involvement by health professionals. However, the role of the professional and medical technology is geared more toward caregiving, providing physical and emotional comfort, than medical stabilization and improvement. In this sense, families need not only to reinclude health providers more, but also to see their role differently. Clearly, this change of roles is often more challenging for the healthcare team than for the family, because of strong beliefs about professional success being equated with life not death.

For the terminally ill member, the most important needs are controlling pain and suffering, preserving dignity and self-worth, and receiving love and affection from family and friends. When families are coping with anticipatory loss in the final phase of an illness, the quality as much as the quantity of time becomes a priority. Clinicians need to explore a family's fears about the process of dying and about the loss itself. Anticipation of a family member's increasing pain or suffering is often of greater concern that death. This is especially common in longstanding progressive diseases, in which the anticipation of death has been rehearsed many times. Early reassurance about effective means of pain control and informed discussion with the family concerning the ill member's wishes about lifesaving measures can alleviate a major source of anguish. Families face a number of practical tasks in the terminal phase. As distinguished from sharing emotions, families need to decide when and whom to tell about the transition. If they have not decided beforehand, the patient together with key family members need to decide about such things as: the redefinition of family roles in this final stage of an illness; a living will; the extent of medical efforts desired; who has power of attorney if the patient is not competent to make sound decisions; preferences about dying at home, in the hospital, or at hospice; and wishes about a funeral and memorial service.

## Transition Periods

Critical transition periods link the three time phases. Carter and McGoldrick (1998) and Levinson (1986) have clarified the importance of transition periods in the family and adult life cycle literature. Transitions in the illness life cycle are times when families reevaluate the appropriateness of their previous life structure in the face of new illness-related developmental demands. Unfinished business from the previous phase can complicate or block movement through the transitions. Families can become permanently frozen in an adaptive structure that has outlived its utility (Penn, 1983). For example, the usefulness of pulling together in the crisis period can become a maladaptive and stifling prison for all family members in the chronic phase. Enmeshed families would have difficulty negotiating this delicate transition.

The interaction of the time phases and typology of illness provide a framework for a chronic disease psychosocial developmental model that resembles models for human development. The time phases (crisis, chronic, and terminal) can be considered broad developmental periods in the natural history of chronic disease. Each period has certain basic tasks independent of the type of illness. Each "type" of illness has specific supplementary tasks. The basic tasks of the three illness time phases and transitions recapitulate in many respects the unfolding of human development. For example, the crisis phase is similar in certain fundamental ways to the era of childhood and adolescence. Child development involves a prolonged period during which the child learns the fundamentals of life as parents temper other developmental plans (e.g., career) to accommodate raising children. In an analogous way, the crisis phase is a period of socialization to the basics of living with chronic disease, when other life plans are frequently put on hold by the family to accommodate to the illness. Just as the transition from adolescence to adulthood is marked by the relinquishing of a moratorium in order to assume adult identity and responsibilities, the transition to the chronic phase of illness emphasizes autonomy and the creation of a viable ongoing life given the realities of the illness. In the transition to the chronic phase, a "hold" or moratorium on other developmental tasks that served to protect the initial period of socialization/adaptation to life with chronic disease is reevaluated. The separate develop-

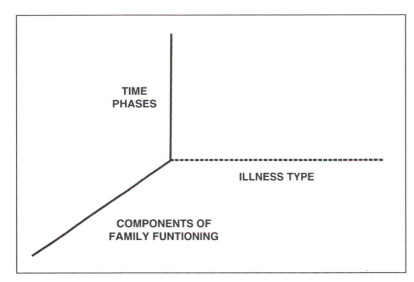

**Figure 14.4.** Three-dimensional model: Illness type, time phase, family functioning. Reprinted from Rolland JS: Chronic illness and the life cycle: A conceptual framework. *Fam Process* 26(2):203–221, 1987.

mental tasks of "living with chronic illness" and "living out the other parts of one's life" must be brought together.

The typology and phases of illness can be combined so that each "psychosocial type" of illness can be thought about in relation to each of the time phases. The addition of a family systems model creates a three-dimensional model (Fig. 14.4). Psychosocial illness types, illness time phases, and components of family systems variables constitute the three dimensions. This model allows consideration of the importance of strengths and weaknesses in various components of family functioning in relation to different disease types and at different illness phases.

## Clinical Implications

By facilitating a clinician's grasp of chronic illness and disability in psychosocial terms, this model provides a framework for assessment and clinical intervention with affected families. The clinician can think with greater clarity and focus. Attention to features of onset, course, outcome, and incapacitation provide markers that focus a clinician's questioning of a family. For instance, acute-onset illnesses demand high levels of adaptability, problem solving, role reallocation, and balanced cohesion. A high degree of family enmeshment might make a family less likely to be able to cope with these demands. Forethought on this issue would cue a clinician toward a more appropriate family evaluation.

The time line of an illness delineates psychosocial developmental stages of an illness, each phase with its own unique developmental tasks. It is important for families to solve phase-related tasks within the time limits set by the duration of each successive developmental phase of an illness. The failure to resolve issues in this sequential manner can jeopardize the total coping process of the family. Therefore, attention to time allows the clinician to assess a family's strengths and vulnerabilities in relation to the present and future phases of the illness.

The model clarifies treatment planning. Taken together the typology and time phases provide a context to integrate other aspects of a comprehensive assessment. Awareness of the components of family functioning most relevant to particular types or phases of an illness guides goal setting. Sharing this information with the family and deciding on specific goals will provide a better sense of control and realistic hope to the family.

This knowledge educates the family about warning signs that should alert them to call on a family therapist at appropriate times for brief goal-oriented treatment.

## CASE 14-3

*Joe, his wife Ann, and their three teenage children presented for a family evaluation 10 months after Joe's diagnosis with moderate-severe asthma. Joe, aged 44, had been successfully employed for many years as a spray painter. Apparently, exposure to a new chemical triggered the onset of asthmatic attacks that necessitated hospitalization and occupational disability. Although somewhat improved, he continued to have persistent and moderate respiratory symptoms. Initially, his physicians had predicted that improvement would occur, but remained noncommittal as to the level of chronicity. Continued breathing difficulties contributed to increased symptoms of depression, uncharacteristic temperamental outbursts, alcohol abuse, family discord, and finally admission to an alcohol detox unit.*

*In my initial assessment, after discharge to outpatient psychiatric treatment, I inquired as to their prior illness experience. This was the nuclear family's first encounter with chronic illness, and their families of origin had limited experience. Ann's father had died 7 years earlier of a sudden and unexpected heart attack. Joe's brother had died in an accidental drowning. Neither had experience with disease as an ongoing process. Joe had assumed that improvement meant "cure." In addition, Joe had a history of alcoholism that had been in complete remission for 20 years. Illness for both had meant either death or recovery. The physician/family system was not attuned to the hidden risks for this family coping with the transition from the crisis to chronic phase of his asthma, the juncture where the permanency of the disease needed to be addressed.*

# MULTIGENERATIONAL HISTORY OF ILLNESS, LOSS, AND CRISIS

Many systems-oriented practitioners have emphasized that a family's present behavior cannot be adequately comprehended apart from its history (Boszormenyi-Nagy & Spark, 1973; Bowen, 1978; Carter & McGoldrick, 1998; Framo, 1992; Walsh & McGoldrick, 1991). Historical questioning is a way to track key events and transitions to gain an understanding of a family's organizational shifts and coping strategies *as a system* in response to past stressors. This is not a cause-and-effect model, but reflects a belief that such a historical search may help explain the family's current style of coping and adaptation. A historical systemic perspective involves more than simply deciphering how a family organized itself around past stressors; it also tracks the evolution of family adaptation over time. Patterns of adaptation, replications, discontinuities, shifts in relationships (e.g., alliances, triangles, cutoffs), and sense of competence are important considerations. These patterns are transmitted across generations as family myths, taboos, catastrophic expectations, and belief systems (Walsh & McGoldrick, 1991). By gathering this information a clinician can create a family genogram (McGoldrick *et al.*, 1999). A chronic illness-oriented genogram focuses on how a family organized itself as an evolving system specifically around previous illnesses and unexpected crises in the current and previous generations. A central goal is to bring to light the adults' "learned differences around illness" (Penn, 1983).

The psychosocial types and phases of illness are useful concepts in the family evaluation. Although a family may have certain standard ways of coping with any illness, there may be critical differences in their style and success in adaptation to different "types" of diseases. A family may show a disparity in their level of coping with one disease versus another, disregarding differences in demands. If the clinician inquires about different types of illnesses (e.g., relapsing versus progressive, life-threatening versus non-life-threatening), she will make better use of historical data. For instance, a family may have consistently organized successfully when faced with illnesses that were not life-threatening, but reeled under the weight of the mother's metastatic breast cancer. Such a family might be particularly vulnerable if another life-threatening illness were to occur. Another family may have experienced only non-life-threatening illnesses and be uninformed about how to cope with the uncertainties particular to life-threatening diseases. Cognizance of these facts will draw attention to areas of strength and vulnerability for a family facing cancer or any life-threatening illness. In Case 14-3, I learned critical family background information, which if it had been incorporated into the initial treatment plan might have averted a family crisis, relapse of alcohol abuse, and hospitalization.

Tracking a family's coping capabilities in the crisis, chronic, and terminal phases of previous chronic illnesses highlights complications in adaptation related to different points in the "illness life cycle." A family may have adapted well in the crisis phase of living with a spinal cord injury, but failed to navigate the transition to a family organization consistent with long-haul adaptation. A rigidly enmeshed family may have become frozen in a crisis structure and been unable to deal appropriately with issues of maximizing individual and collective autonomy in the chronic phase. Another family with a member with chronic kidney failure may have functioned very well in handling the practicalities of home dialysis. However, in the terminal phase their limitations around emotional expression may have left a legacy of unresolved grief. A history of phase-specific difficulties can alert a clinician to potential vulnerable periods for a family over the course of the current chronic illness. The following case illustrates the interplay of problems coping with a current illness, fueled by unresolved issues related to a particular type or phase of disease in one's family of origin.

## CASE 14-4

*Mary, her husband Bill, and their son Jim sought treatment 4 months after Mary had sustained a serious concussion in a life-threatening head-on auto collision caused by the driver of the other vehicle. For several months, there was some concern by the medical team that she might have suffered a cerebral hemorrhage. Ultimately, it was clarified that this had not occurred. Over this time, Mary became increasingly depressed and, despite strong reassurance, continued to believe she had a life-threatening condition and would die of a brain hemorrhage. In the initial evaluation, she revealed that she was experiencing vivid dreams of meeting her deceased father. Apparently her father, with whom she had been extremely close, had died of a cerebral hemorrhage after a 4-year history of a progressive debilitating brain tumor, marked by progressive and uncontrolled epileptic seizures. Mary, 14 at the time, was the "baby" in the family, her two siblings being much older. The family had shielded her from his illness, culminating in her mother's decision that she not attend either the wake or the funeral. This event galvanized her position as the "child in need of protection"—a dynamic that carried over into her marriage. Despite her hurt, anger, and lack of acceptance of the death, she had avoided dealing with her feelings with her mother for over 20 years. Other family history revealed that her maternal grandfather had died when her mother was 7 years old. She had had to endure an open casket wake at home. Her experience of this as traumatic was a major factor in her mother's attempt to protect her daughter from the same kind of memory.*

*Mary's own life-threatening head injury had triggered a catastrophic reaction and dramatic resurfacing of previous losses involving similar types of illness and injury. Therapy focused on a series of tasks and rituals that involved her initiating conversations with her mother and visits to her father's grave.*

The family's history of coping with crises in general, especially unanticipated ones, should be explored. Illnesses with acute onset (e.g., heart attack), moderate-severe sudden incapacitation (e.g., stroke), or rapid relapse (e.g., ulcerative colitis, diabetic insulin reaction, disk disease) demand in various ways rapid crisis mobilization skills. In these situations the family needs to reorganize quickly and efficiently, shifting from its usual organization to a crisis structure. Other illnesses can create a crisis because of the continual demand for family stamina (e.g., spinal cord injury, rheumatoid arthritis, emphysema). The family history of coping with moderate-severe ongoing stressors is a good predictor of adjustment to these types of illness.

For any significant chronic illness in either adult's family of origin, a clinician should try to get a picture of how those families organized to handle the range of disease-related affective and practical tasks. Also, it is important to find out what role each played in handling these emotional or practical tasks. Whether the parents (as children) were given too much responsibility (parentified) or shielded from involvement, such as in the case of Mary, is of particular note. What did they learn from those experiences that influences how they think about the current illness? Whether they have emerged with a strong sense of competence or failure is essential information. In one particular case involving a family with three generations of hemophilia transmitted through the mother's side, the father had been shielded from the knowledge that his older brother who died in adolescence had had a terminal form of kidney disease. Also, this man had not been allowed to attend his brother's funeral. From that trauma he made a strong commitment to openness about disease-related issues with his two sons with hemophilia and his daughters who were genetic carriers. By collecting such information about each adult's family of origin, one can anticipate areas of conflict and consensus. Unresolved issues related to illness and loss can remain dormant in a marriage, and suddenly reemerge triggered by a chronic illness in the current nuclear family (Penn, 1983; Walker, 1983). Penn describes how particular coalitions that emerge in the context of a chronic illness are replications of those that existed in each adult's family of origin. The following case is prototypical:

> If a mother has been the long-time rescuer of her mother from a tyrannical husband, and then in her own family bears a son with hemophilia, she will become his rescuer, often against his father. In this manner she continues to rescue her mother but, oddly enough, now from her husband rather than from her own father.... In this family with a hemophiliac son, the father's father had been ill for a long period and had received all the mother's attention. In his present family, this father, though outwardly objecting to the coalition between his wife and son, honored that relationship, as if he hoped it would make up for the one he had once forfeited with his own mother. The coalition in the nuclear family looks open and adaptational (mother and son), but is fueled by coalitions in the past (mother with her mother, and father with his mother). (Penn, 1983)

The reenactment of previous system configurations around illness can occur largely as an unconscious, automatic process. Further, the dysfunctional complementarity can emerge *de novo* specifically within the context of a chronic disease. On detailed inquiry, couples frequently reveal a tacit unspoken understanding that if an illness occurred they would reorganize to reenact "unfinished business" from their families of origin. Typically, the role chosen represents a repetition or opposite of a role played by themselves or the same-sex parent. A clinician needs to maintain some distinction between functional family process with and without chronic disease. For families that present in this manner, placing a primary therapeutic emphasis on the resolution of family-of-origin issues might be the best approach to prevent or rectify an unhealthy triangle.

Families, like those just described, with encapsulated illness "time bombs" need to be distinguished from families with more pervasive, longstanding dysfunctional patterns where illnesses can become embedded in a web of preexisting fused family transactions. In the traditional sense of "psychosomatic," this kind of severely dysfunctional family displays a greater level of baseline reactivity such that when an illness enters their system, this reactivity gets expressed somatically through a poor medical course or treatment noncompliance. These families lack the foundation of a functional nonillness system. The initial focus of therapeutic intervention may need to be targeted more on pragmatic immediate help rather than family-of-origin work, with more limited therapeutic aims.

A third group of symptomatic families facing chronic disease are those without significant intra- or intergenerational family dysfunctional patterns. Any family may falter in the face of multiple superimposed disease and nondisease stressors that impact in a relatively short time. With progressive, incapacitating diseases or the concurrence of illness in several family members, a pragmatic approach that focuses on expanded or creative use of supports and resources outside the family is most productive.

## THE ILLNESS, INDIVIDUAL, AND FAMILY LIFE CYCLES

To place the unfolding of chronic disease into a developmental context, it is crucial to understand the intertwining of three evolutionary threads: the illness, individual, and family life cycles. The psychosocial typology and phases of illness offer a language to characterize diseases in psychosocial and longitudinal terms, each illness having particular patterns and expected developmental life course. Since an illness *is* part of an individual, it is essential to think simultaneously about the interaction of individual and family development.

The *life cycle* is a central concept for both family and individual development (see Chapter 2). Life cycle means there is a basic sequence and unfolding of the life course within which individual, family, or illness uniqueness occurs. A second key concept is the human *life* structure. Levinson (1986) described life structure to mean the design of a person's life at any given point in the life cycle. This design is made up of an individual's various commitments (e.g., work, family, religious affiliation, hobbies) and the relative importance of each commitment. The life structure mediates transactions between the individual, the family, and the environment. Although Levinson described the individual adult male life cycle, his concepts can be applied to the family as a unit.

Illness, individual, and family development have in common the notion of periods or phases marked by different developmental tasks. For instance, a major task of early adulthood is to establish an independent life structure, typically involving modifications in one's family-of-origin relationships. Levinson (1986) has described five major eras in individual life structure development: childhood and adolescence; early, middle, and late adulthood; and late, late adulthood. Each lasts approximately 20 years.

Levinson noted that these life cycle eras are linked by the alternation of *life structure-building/ maintaining* (stable) and *life structure-changing* (transitional) periods, each lasting roughly 5 to 7 years, during which certain developmental tasks are addressed independently of marker events. The primary goal of a structure-building/maintaining period is to form a life structure and enrich life within it based on the key choices an individual and family has made during the preceding transition period. In a transition period one weighs different possibilities for personal and family life, eventually deciding on and drawing up the blueprints for the next phase.

The delineation of separate periods derives from a set of developmental tasks associated with each. Transition periods are potentially the most vulnerable because previous individual, family, and illness life structures are reappraised in the face of new developmental tasks that may require major, discontinuous change rather than minor alterations. The concept of phases in the family life cycle is particularly useful to the task of integrating illness, individual, and family development. Family life cycle theory has tended to divide development into stages demarcated by nodal events such as marriage or birth of a first child. Carter and McGoldrick (1998) have delineated the following six family life cycle stages: (1) the unattached young adult, (2) the newly married couple, (3) the family with young children, (4) the family with adolescents, (5) launching children and moving on, and (6) the family in later life. Combrinck-Graham (1985) proposes a family life spiral model in which the entire three-generational family system oscillates through time between periods of higher family cohesion (centripetal) and periods of relatively lower family cohesion (centrifugal). These periods coincide with oscillations between family developmental tasks that require intense bonding or high cohesion, such as early child rearing, and tasks that emphasize personal identity and autonomy, such as adolescence. During a higher-cohesion period, both the individual member's and family unit's life structure emphasize internal family life. External boundaries around the family are tightened while personal boundaries between members are somewhat diffused to enhance family teamwork. In the transition to a lower-cohesion period, the family life structure shifts to accommodate goals that emphasize an individual family member's life outside the family. The external family boundary is loosened while separateness between some family members increases.

Several key life cycle concepts provide a foundation for understanding the experience of chronic disorders. The life cycle contains alternating transition and life structure-building/maintaining periods. Further, particular periods can be characterized as requiring either higher or lower cohesion in order to meet psychosocial demands (Fig. 14.5).

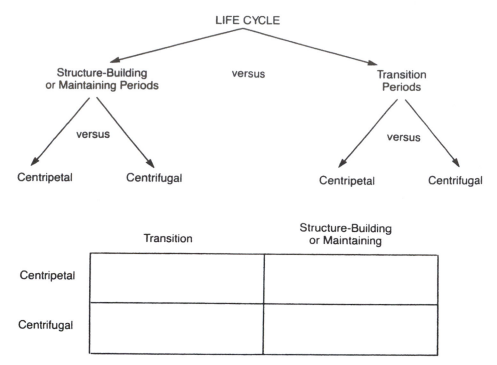

**Figure 14.5.** Periods in the family and individual life cycles. Reprinted from Rolland JS: Chronic illness and the life cycle: A conceptual framework. *Fam Process* 26(2):203–221, 1987.

---

### CASE 14-5

*Vivek and his wife Rajshri presented for treatment 6 months after Vivek had sustained a severe burn injury to both hands that required skin grafting. A year of recuperation was necessary before Vivek would be able to return to his job, which required physical labor and full use of his hands. Prior to the injury, his wife had been at home full time raising their two children, aged 3 and 5. Although Vivek was temporarily handicapped in terms of his career, he was physically fit to assume the role of househusband. Initially, both Vivek and Rajshri remained at home using his disability income to "get by." When Rajshri expressed an interest in finding a job to relieve financial pressures, Vivek resisted and marital strain caused by his injury flared into dysfunctional conflict.*

*Sufficient resources were available in the system to accommodate the illness and ongoing child-rearing tasks. Their definition of marriage lacked the necessary role flexibility to master the problem. Treatment focused on rethinking his masculine and monolithic definition of "family provider," a definition that had, in fact, emerged in full force during this higher-cohesion phase of the family life cycle.*

## Integrating Individual, Family, and Illness Development

A basic question is: What is the fit between the practical and emotional demands of a condition and family and individual developmental tasks and life structures at a particular point in time? How will this fit change as the course of the illness unfolds in relation to the family life cycle and the development of each family member? In general, chronic conditions tend to push individual and family developmental processes toward increased cohesion and transition.

The idea of degrees of cohesion is useful in linking the illness life course to individual and family life

## Periods of Higher and Lower Cohesion

If the onset of an illness coincides with a lower-cohesion period for the family, it can derail the family from its natural momentum. If a young adult becomes ill, she may need to return to the family of origin for disease-related caretaking. Each member's autonomy and individuation are at risk. The young adult's ability to establish a life away from home is threatened either temporarily or permanently. Both parents may have to relinquish interests outside the family. Family dynamics as well as disease severity will influence whether the family's reversion to a high-cohesion life structure is a temporary detour within their general movement outward, or a permanent reversal. A highly cohesive or enmeshed family frequently faces the transition to a more autonomous period with trepidation. A chronic illness provides a sanctioned reason to return to the "safety" of the prior high-cohesion period. For some family members, the giving up of the building of a new life structure already in progress can be more devastating than when the family is still in an earlier phase with more preliminary future plans. An analogy would be the difference between a couple discovering that they do not have enough money to build a house versus being forced to abandon their building project with the foundation already completed.

Disease onset that coincides with a high-cohesion period in the family life cycle (e.g., early child rearing) can have several important consequences. At a minimum, it can foster a prolongation of this period. At worst, the family can become permanently stuck at this phase of development, when the inward pull of the illness and the phase of the life cycle coincide. The risk here is their tendency to amplify one another. For families that function marginally before an illness onset, this kind of mutual reinforcement can trigger a runaway process leading to overt family dysfunction. Minuchin and colleagues' (1975, 1978) research of "psycho-somatic" families has documented this process in several common childhood illnesses.

When a parent develops a chronic disease during a higher-cohesion child-rearing phase of development, a family's ability to stay on course is severely taxed (Rolland, 1999). The impact of the illness is like the addition of a new infant member with "special needs" competing for potentially scarce family resources. In psychosocially milder diseases, as with Vivek and Rajshri (Case 14-5), efficient role reallocation may suffice to keep family development on course. If the disease affecting a parent is more debilitating (e.g., traumatic brain injury, cervical spinal cord injury), its impact on the child-rearing family is twofold. A "new" family member is added, a parent is "lost," and the semblance of a single-parent family with an added child is created. For acute-onset illnesses, when both events occur simultaneously, family resources may be inadequate to meet the combined child-rearing and caretaking demands. This situation is ripe for the emergence of a parentified child or the reenlistment into active parenting of a grandparent. These forms of family adaptation are not inherently dysfunctional. A clinician needs to assess these structural realignments. Are certain individuals assigned rigid caretaking roles, or are they flexible and shared? Are caretaking roles viewed flexibly from a developmental vantage point? For an adolescent caretaker, this means the family being mindful of the approaching developmental transition to an independent life separate from the family. For grandparent caretakers, it means sensitivity to their increasing physical limitations or need to assist their own spouse.

The need for family cohesion varies enormously in different types and phases of illness. The tendency for a disease to pull a family inward increases with the level of incapacitation or risk of death. Progressive diseases over time inherently require more cohesion than constant-course illnesses. The ongoing addition of new demands as an illness progresses keeps a family's energy focused inward. After a functional adaptation has been achieved, a constant-course disease (excluding those with severe incapacitation) permits a family to get back on track developmentally. The added inward pull exerted by a progressive disease increases the risk of reversing normal family disengagement or freezing a family into a permanently fused state.

## CASE 14-6

*Mr. L., aged 54, had become increasingly depressed as a result of severe and progressive complica-tions of his adult-onset diabetes mellitus that had emerged over the past 5 years. These complications included a leg amputation and renal failure that recently required instituting home dialysis on a four times a day basis. For 20 years, Mr. L. had had an uncomplicated constant course, allowing him to lead a full active life. An excellent athlete, he engaged in a number of recreational group sports. Short- and long-term family planning had never focused around his illness. This optimistic attitude was reinforced by the fact that two people in Mrs. L.'s family of origin had had diabetes mellitus without complications. Their only child, a son aged 26, had uneventfully left home after high school and had recently married. Mr. and Mrs. L. had a stable marriage, where both maintained many outside independent interests. In short, the family had moved smoothly through the transition to a more centrifugal phase of the family's life cycle.*

*His disease's transformation to a progressive course coupled with the incapacitating and life-shortening nature of his complications had reversed the normal process of family disengagement. His wife took a second job, which necessitated her quitting her hobbies and civic involvements. Their son and his wife moved back home to help his mother take care of his father and the house. Mr. L., disabled from work and his athletic social network, felt a burden to everyone and blocked in his own midlife development.*

*The essential goal of family treatment in developmental terms centered around reversing some of the system's centripetal overreaction back to a more realistic balance. For Mr. L., this meant a reworking of his life structure to accommodate his real limitations while maximizing a return to his more independent style. For Mrs. L. and her son, this meant developing realistic expectations for Mr. L. and reestablishing key aspects of their autonomy within an illness/family system.*

Relapsing illnesses alternate between periods of drawing a family inward and periods of release from the immediate demands of disease. However, the on-call state of preparedness dictated by many such illnesses keeps some part of the family in a higher cohesion mode despite medically asymptomatic periods, hindering the natural flow between phases of the family life cycle.

One way to think about the phases of illness is that they represent to the family a progression from a crisis phase requiring high cohesion to a chronic phase often demanding less cohesion. The terminal phase, if it occurs, forces most families back into being more inwardly focused and cohesive. The so-called "illness life structure," developed by a family to accommodate each phase in the illness life cycle, is colored by the inherent inward pull of each time phase. For example, in a family where illness onset has coincided with a lower-cohesion phase of development, the transition to the chronic phase permits a family to resume more of its momentum.

### Transition and Stable Periods

Clinicians need to be mindful of the timing of the onset of a chronic illness, with individual/family transition and life structure-building/maintaining periods of development. All *transitions* involve the basic processes of endings and beginnings, generating an undercurrent of preoccupation with death and finiteness (Levinson, 1986). Chronic and life-threatening illness precipitates the loss of the preillness identity of the family. It forces the family into a transition in which one of the family's main tasks is to accommodate the anticipation of further loss and possibly untimely death. When the onset of a chronic illness coincides with a transition in the individual or family life cycle, issues related to previous, current, and anticipated loss will be likely magnified. Transition periods are often characterized by upheaval, rethinking of prior commitments, and openness to change. As a result, those times hold a greater risk for the illness to become unnecessarily embedded or inappropriately ignored in planning for the next developmental period. During a transition period, the very process of loosening prior commitments creates a context for emergence of family rules regarding loyalty through sacrifice and caretaking. Indecision about one's future can be "resolved" by excessive focus on a family member's physical problems. This focus can be a major precursor of family dysfunction in the context of chronic disease. By adopting a longitudinal developmental perspective, a clinician will stay attuned to future transitions and their overlap.

An example can highlight the importance of the illness in relation to future developmental transitions. Imagine a family in which the father, a carpenter and primary financial provider, develops multiple sclerosis. At first, his level of impairment is mild and stabilized, allowing him to continue part-time work. Because their children are all teenagers, his wife is able to undertake part-time work to help maintain financial stability. The oldest son, aged 15, seems relatively unaffected. Two years later, the father experiences a rapid progression of his illness leaving him totally disabled. His son, now 17, has dreams of going away to college. The specter of financial hardship and the perceived need for a "man in the family" creates a serious dilemma of choice for the son and the family. In this case there is a fundamental clash between developmental issues of separation/individuation and the ongoing demands of progressive chronic disability on the family. This vignette demonstrates the potential clash between simultaneous transition periods: the illness transition to a more incapacitating and progressive course, the adolescent son's transition to early adulthood, and the family's transition from the "living with teenagers" to "launching young adults" stage. Also, this example illustrates the significance of the type of illness. A less incapacitating or a relapsing illness (as opposed to a progressive or constant-course disease) might interfere less with this young man's separation from his family. If his father had an intermittently incapacitating illness, like disk disease, the son might have moved out but tailored his choices to remain nearby and thus available during acute flareups. Illness onset may cause a different kind of disruption if it coincides with a *life structure-building/maintaining period* in individual or family development. These periods are characterized by the living out of choices made during the preceding transition period. Relative to transition periods, family members try to protect their and the family unit's current life structure. Diseases with only a mild level of psychosocial severity (e.g., nonfatal, none/mild incapacitation, nonprogressive) may require some revision of individual/family life structure, but not a radical restructuring that would necessitate a return to a transitional phase of development. A chronic illness with a critical threshold of psychosocial severity will demand the reestablishment of a transitional form of life, at a time when individual/family inertia is to preserve the momentum of a stable period. An individual's or family's level of adaptability is a prime factor determining the successful navigation of this kind of crisis. In this context, family adaptability involves the ability to transform its entire life structure to a prolonged transitional state.

For instance, in the previous example, the father's multiple sclerosis rapidly progressed while the oldest son was in a transition period in his own development. The nature of the strain in developmental terms would be quite different if his father's disease progression had occurred when this young man was 26, had already left home, finished college, secured a first job, married, and had a child. In the latter scenario, the oldest son's life structure is in a centripetal, structure-maintaining period within his newly formed nuclear family. To fully accommodate the needs of his family of origin would require a monumental shift of his developmental priorities. When this illness crisis coincided with a developmental transition period (age 17), although a dilemma of choice existed, the son was available and less fettered by commitments in progress. Later, at age 26, he has made commitments and is in the process of living them out with his newly formed family. To serve the demands of an illness transition, the son might need to shift his previously stable life structure back to a transitional state. And, the shift would happen "out of phase" with the flow of his individual and nuclear family's development. One way to resolve this dilemma of divided loyalties might be the merging of the two households.

This discussion raises several key clinical points. From a systems viewpoint, at the time of a chronic illness diagnosis it is important to know the phase of the family life cycle and the stage of individual development of all family members, not just the ill member. This is important information for several reasons. First, chronic disease in one family member can profoundly affect developmental goals of another member. For instance, a disabled infant can be a serious roadblock to a mother's mastery of child rearing, or a life-threatening illness in a young adult can interfere with the spouse's readiness to become a parent. Second, family members frequently do not adapt equally to chronic illness. Each member's ability to adapt and the rate at which they do so is related to the individual's own developmental stage and role in the family. The oldest son in the previous example illustrates this point.

There exists a normative and nonnormative timing of chronic illness in the life cycle. Coping with chronic illness and death are considered normally anticipated tasks in late adulthood. On the other hand, illnesses and losses that occur earlier are "out of phase" and tend to be developmentally more disruptive (Neugarten, 1976). As untimely events, chronic diseases can severely disrupt the usual sense of continuity and rhythm of the life cycle. The timing in the life cycle of an unexpected event, like a chronic illness, will shape the form of adaptation and the event's influence on subsequent development (Levinson, 1986).

The notion of "out of phase" illnesses can be conceptualized in a more refined way. First, since serious diseases demand higher family cohesion, they can be more disruptive to families in a lower-cohesion phase of development. Second, the onset of chronic disease tends to create a period of transition, the length or intensity of which depends on the psychosocial type and phase of the illness. This forced transition is particularly "out of phase" if it coincides with a life structure-building/maintaining period in the individual's or family's life cycle. Third, if the particular illness is progressive, relapsing, increasingly incapacitating, or life-threatening, then the phases in the unfolding of the disease will be punctuated by numerous transitions. Under these conditions a family will need to more frequently alter their illness life structure to accommodate the shifting and often increasing demands of the disease. This level of demand and uncertainty keeps the illness in the forefront of a family's consciousness, constantly impinging on their attempts to get back "in phase" developmentally. Finally, the transition from the crisis to the chronic phase of the illness life cycle is often the key juncture where the intensity of the family's socialization to living with chronic disease can be relaxed. In this sense, it offers a "window of opportunity" for the family to recover its developmental course. Chronic diseases that occur for adults in the child-rearing period can be most devastating because of their potential impact on family financial and child-rearing responsibilities. Again, the actual impact will depend on the "type" of illness and preillness family roles. Families governed by rigid gender-defined roles as to who should be the primary financial provider and caretaker of children will potentially have the greatest problems with adjustment and need to be coached toward a more flexible view about role interchange.

In the face of chronic disease, an overarching goal is for a family to deal with the developmental demands presented by the illness without family members completely sacrificing their own or the family's development as a system. Therefore, it is vital to ask about what life plans had to be canceled, postponed, or altered as a result of the diagnosis. It is useful to know whose plans are most and least affected. By asking a family when and under what conditions they will resume plans, put on hold or address future developmental tasks, a clinician can anticipate developmental crises related to "independence from" versus "subjugation to" the chronic illness. Family members can be helped to resume their life plans, at least to some extent, by helping them resolve feelings of guilt, overresponsibility, and hopelessness and find resources internal and external to the family for more freedom, both to pursue their own goals and to provide needed care for the ill member. The previous case (14-6) of Mr. L., with serious complications from diabetes, and his wife and son is a good example of these developmental challenges.

## CASE 14-7

*Lucy and Tom G., a young couple, have a child Susan, aged 5, who is terminally ill with leukemia. The pediatric oncologist offers the parents the choice between an experimental treatment with a low probability of success or halting treatment.*

*Tom's position is "Let's stop; enough is enough." Lucy, on the other hand, feels, "We must continue; we can't let her die." The couple cannot reach an agreement, and the physician is immobilized. He requests a psychiatric consultation for the couple.*

*When the consultant asks, "What is your explanation of how your daughter got leukemia?" the critical story emerges. Tom basically sees it as bad luck. Lucy, however, has a very different belief. During her pregnancy with Susan, Lucy's father had a heart attack and died several months later from a second episode. Lucy experienced this as a time of great stress and grief, which she feels adversely affected the intrauterine life of Susan. After Susan's birth, by normal delivery, Lucy was still mourning the loss of her father, and feels that this affected the quality of her bonding with Susan and led to a hidden depression in her infant. Further, Lucy had read research linking depression with lowering of the effectiveness of the immune system, which could, in turn, decrease normal surveillance and clearing of cancer cells from the body. She believes this combination of factors caused her child's cancer, and that if she had been a more competent mother, this never would have happened. Lucy said she had never told this story to anyone, because no one had ever asked, and she was very ashamed. She had hoped for a cure so that the whole issue could be resolved. She cannot accept stopping treatment because, to her, it means that Susan's death will be her fault.*

## HEALTH/ILLNESS BELIEF SYSTEMS

Each of us as an individual and as a part of larger systems adopts a value orientation, belief system, or philosophy that shapes our patterns of behavior toward the common problems of daily life in society (Kluckhohn, 1960). Beliefs provide coherence to family life, facilitating continuity between past, present, and future and a way to approach new and ambiguous situations. Depending on which system we are speaking of, this phenomenon can be labeled as values, culture, religion, belief system, world-view, or family paradigm.

Reiss (1981) has shown that families as a unit develop paradigms for how the world operates. One component of the family's overall construction of reality is their set of health/illness beliefs that will determine how they interpret illness events and guide their health-seeking behavior (Rolland, 1987b, 1998). Although individual family members can hold different beliefs, the values held by the family unit may be the most significant.

It is useful to distinguish different levels of meaning about illness that can affect collaboration. Drawing on Kleinman's work (1988), in systems terms, we can distinguish the *biological, human experience of individuals and families,* and *societal* levels of meaning (Fig. 14.6).

Traditionally, health professionals live in the world of biological diseases, focusing their attention on medical diagnosis and treatment. Patients and their families live in the world of their human experience of symptoms and suffering, typically in some symbolic form, that represents a synthesis of biological, personal, family, and cultural meanings. The societal level represents meanings that become associated with a physical problem as a result of larger macrosocial, economic, political, or institutional forces (Olkin, 1999; Sontag, 1978, 1988). For example, some conditions are seen as a reflection of poverty, technological oppression (e.g., pollution), or immoral lifestyle. Diseases common in inner cities, such as lead poisoning, cancer, asthma, and AIDS, can be viewed through this larger societal lens. Belief systems can be conceptualized as the mediator between these levels of meaning, especially as a bridge between the biological level and the human experience and societal levels. Clinicians need to be able to navigate between these levels of meaning.

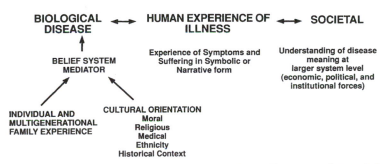

**Figure 14.6.** Levels of meaning. From Rolland JS: *Families, Illness, and Disability: An Integrative Treatment Model.* New York, Basic Books Inc, 1994, p 130.

At the time of a medical diagnosis a primary developmental task for the family is to create a meaning for the illness that preserves a sense of competency and mastery in the context of partial loss, possible further physical compromise, or death. Since serious illness is often experienced as a betrayal of our fundamental trust in our bodies and belief in our invulnerability and immortality (Kleinman, 1988), the creation of an empowering narrative can be a formidable task. Family health beliefs help us grapple with these existential dilemmas of our fear of death, attempts to sustain our denial of death, and attempts to reassert control over unjust suffering and untimely death. At a practical level, belief systems serve as a cognitive map guiding decisions and action.

Our inquiry into and curiosity about family beliefs is perhaps the most powerful foundation stone of effective patient, family, and healthcare professional relationships (Wright *et al.*, 1996). In the initial crisis phase, it is useful for clinicians to inquire about key beliefs that shape families' illness narratives and coping strategies. This means gaining an understanding of a family's overall belief system, of family beliefs brought into play by the strains of a serious health problem, and the meanings associated with the condition itself. A thorough assessment includes tracking beliefs about: (1) normality; (2) mind–body relationship, control, and mastery; (3) meanings attached by a family, ethnic group, religion, or the wider culture to symptoms (e.g., chronic pain), types of illness (e.g., life-threatening disorders), or specific diseases (e.g., AIDS); (4) assumptions about what caused an illness and what will influence its course and outcome; (5) multigenerational factors that have shaped a family's health beliefs; and (6) anticipated nodal points in illness, individual, and family life cycles when health beliefs will be strained or need to shift. Second, a clinician needs to assess the fit of health beliefs within the family and its various subsystems (e.g., spouse, parental, extended family) as well as between the family and the healthcare system and wider culture.

## Beliefs about Normality

A family's beliefs about what is normal or abnormal and the importance they place on conformity and excellence in relation to the average family have far-reaching implications for adaptation to chronic disorders (Rolland, 1994a; Walsh, 1993, 1998). Families' values that allow having a "problem" without self-denigration have a distinct advantage in utilizing outside help and maintaining a positive identity in the face of chronic conditions. Help seeking that is defined as weak and shameful undercuts this kind of resilience. Essentially, in situations of chronic disorders where problems are to be expected and the use of professionals and outside resources is necessary, a belief that pathologizes this normative process adds insult to injury.

Two excellent questions to elicit beliefs about how families define normality are, "How do you think other *average* families would deal with a similar situation to yours?" And, "How would a *healthy* family cope with your situation?" The first question gives a good indication of whether family members have a sense of the range of possible experiences and what is typical. Do they make their comparisons in relation to situations that really have similar psychosocial demands, or are they making unrealistic or unfair ones? A family dealing with the initial phase of a traumatic brain-injured member could do themselves a disservice by comparing their coping ability and strategies with a family facing a seizure disorder. The second question invites a family to share their views about what is healthy or optimal. Like couples that unrealistically describe optimal relationships as problem-free, without conflict or suffering, often families facing chronic disorders have a narrow, romanticized version of healthy adaptation that is unrealistic and leaves them feeling deficient. Descriptions of "Superstar Copers" in the popular literature and the media, while sources of inspiration, can also contribute to families feeling inadequate by comparison.

Families with strong beliefs in high achievement and perfectionism tend to equate normality with optimal. They tend to define normality or successful family functioning in terms of ideal or "problem-free" characteristics. Families that define normality in this way are prone to apply standards in a situation of illness where the kind of control they are accustomed to is impossible. Particularly with untimely conditions that occur early in the life cycle, there are additional pressures to keep up with normative socially expectable developmental milestones of age peers or other young couples. The fact that life cycle goals may take longer or need revision requires a flexible belief about what is normal and healthy. This lack of a comparison group is one reason why self-help groups and networks can be so useful to families dealing with developmentally off-time conditions. They provide a normalizing context.

Successful coping and adaptation are enhanced when a family believes in a biopsychosocial frame for illness that normalizes a psychosomatic interaction. This highlights the importance of the initial "framing event" and whether professionals actively normalize a psychosomatic interplay, thereby helping to counter-act pathologizing family and cultural beliefs. A physician might say, in a hypothetical situation, to a family facing asthma, "Many families notice that asthma is affected by stressful times, but fear that I would view that as a definite sign of psychiatric problems. I want you to know that asthma normally gets worse during the inevitable strains that arise in family life. It is important that you keep me informed about major family stresses so that I can decide with you whether adjusting Susan's medication or finding better ways to reduce stress will be the best approach." This promotes a positive attitude toward the potential role of psychosocial factors in influencing disease course and the quality of life. Rather than a shameful liability, a family can approach a psychosomatic interplay as an opportunity to make a difference and increase their sense of control.

## Mind–Body Relationships

The concept of mind–body relationship has been the subject of discourse and debate for millenia. The term mind–body relationship has come to represent several related but distinct beliefs that are important to differentiate.

First, there is one assumption that the mind and body are separate worlds and that what goes on in each can interactively affect the other. There is tremendous diversity about how this distinction is seen, if at all, and the degree to which the interaction is seen as equal or more a one-way street. Until recently, traditional Western medicine has tended to minimize the potential impact of the mind on the body.

Second, it is useful to distinguish beliefs about the mind as a logical, thinking process that can determine *actions* that may help in healing the body (e.g., seeking medical care, changing diet or activity patterns), from those of the mind as a source of thought or energy that can directly impact body physiology. The latter includes beliefs about the importance of emotional states such as positive attitude, love, anger, humor, or depression on maintaining physical health and promoting or interfering with healing of the body from disease. It includes beliefs about the mind as the locus of responsibility and the role of willpower in affecting the body. Healing practices such as meditation or guided imagery are based on beliefs about the importance of the mind.

Traditional mental health theories and research endeavors have been pathology-based, tending to emphasize character traits or emotional states that affect body chemistry adversely. From this perspective, emotions can affect the body negatively, but possible positive influences of healthy attitudes have been neglected. We need to be aware of our own belief biases, often promoted in our professional training, which is typically based on the study of pathology, disease, or dysfunction.

More recently, the public has been increasingly drawn to popular literature citing the importance of positive attitudes in healing. These practitioners emphasize the unity of mind and body rather than as distinct worlds. Also, they describe healing as a state of being, involving mind and body, rather than in strictly biomedical terms where something is done to the "body." We need to be particularly mindful that families may be more familiar with and open to these positive possibilities, while our own professional thinking remains antiquated and skewed to a more exclusive view of a mind–body relationship that is based on pathology. The danger lies in not inquiring about family beliefs that are more health-promoting. Or worse, based on our own rigid mind-set, which we defend on the basis of the lack of "hard research data," we may communicate to a family our lack of interest in these ideas or even dismiss them as unscientific and unworthy. In the process, we can undermine a possible powerful source of healing, shame a family, and undermine a mutual workable alliance necessary for any effective treatment.

Third, we need to understand beliefs about "mind" and spirit that extend beyond the individual to include family, community, or a higher spiritual force. To what extent do family members see the locus of energy that can both harm the body and heal it as residing in these other parts of the larger ecosystem? Anthropologists have found tremendous diversity in the role of family, community, God, or nature as a source of healing. Such beliefs are typically expressed in the form of rituals. In our society, a family's religious community will often organize a prayer service to promote healing for an ill member. Clinician understanding of family members' beliefs about mind–body relationships provides a foundation for joining with a family and tailoring biopsychosocial treatment strategies more sensitively (Griffith & Griffith, 1994; Walsh, 1999). Areas of strength and vulnerability can be identified, and ways of including the family in a complementary fashion with other treatments can be suggested.

## The Family's Sense of Mastery Facing Illness

It is critical to determine how a family defines mastery or control in general and how it transposes that definition to situations of illness. Some key thinkers about this issue such as Aaron Antonovsky (1979), Antonovsky and Sourani (1988), and David Reiss (1981) have distinguished between a belief in the ability to control life events, such as illness, and beliefs that life events are comprehensible or manageable. Antonovsky refers to the latter as a "sense of coherence." Others see mastery of health problems as similar to the concept of health locus of control (Lefcourt, 1982), which can be defined as beliefs about what influences the course or outcome of an illness. It is critical to distinguish whether a family's belief system is based on the premise of internal control, external control by chance, or external control by powerful others.

An internal locus-of-control orientation means that there is a belief that an individual/family can affect the outcome of a situation. Families with such a belief about their health will endorse such statements as "I am directly responsible for my health" or "If I become sick, I have the power to make myself well again."

An external orientation entails a belief that outcomes are not contingent on the individual's or family's behavior. Families that view illness in terms of chance will agree with such statements as "Luck plays a big part in determining how soon my family member will recover from an illness" or "When I become ill it's a matter of fate."

Individuals who see health control as in the hands of powerful others will see health professionals, God, or sometimes "powerful" family members, rather than themselves, as exerting control over their bodies. They will endorse statements such as "Regarding my health, I can only do what my doctor tells me to do" or "My family has a lot to do with my becoming sick or staying healthy."

A family may adhere to a different set of values concerning control when dealing with a *biological* problem as opposed to other day-to-day issues. Therefore, it is important to assess a family's basic value system first, and then, with increasing specificity, to assess notions about control for illnesses in general, chronic and life-threatening illness, and finally the specific disease facing the family. A family guided normally by an internal locus of control may switch to an external viewpoint when a member develops any chronic illness, or perhaps only in the case of a life-threatening disease. Such a change might occur in a family with a strong need to remain in accord with society's values, a particular ethnic background, or a specific multigenerational experience with life-threatening diseases. One can inquire as to whether a family has any particular beliefs surrounding specific types of illnesses. Regardless of the actual severity in a particular instance, cancer may be equated with "death" or "no control" because of medical statistics, cultural myth, or prior family history. For many, certain types of heart disease with a similar life expectancy as certain forms of cancer could be seen as more manageable because of prevailing cultural beliefs. Imagine a family traditionally guided by a strong sense of personal control. If the paternal grandfather, the powerful patriarch of the family, died at midlife because of a rapidly progressive and painful form of cancer, the family may develop an encapsulated exception to their views about control that is specific for cancer or generalized to include all life-threatening illnesses.

A family's beliefs about mastery strongly affect the nature of its relationship to an illness and to the healthcare system. A family's beliefs about control are a predictor of certain health behaviors, particularly treatment compliance, and suggest the family's preferences about participation in their family member's treatment and healing. In my experience, families that view disease course/outcome as a matter of chance tend to establish marginal relationships with health professionals largely because their belief system minimizes the importance of their own or a health professional's relationship to a disease process. Just as any psychotherapeutic relationship depends on a shared belief system about what is therapeutic, a fit between the patient, his family, and the healthcare team in terms of these fundamental values is essential. Families that express feelings of being misunderstood by health professionals are often referring directly or indirectly to a lack of joining at this basic value level.

The goodness of fit between the family beliefs about mastery and what the medical situation dictates can vary with the phase of the condition and the type of setting (i.e., ICU, outpatient office, hospice). In some illnesses, the crisis phase involves protracted care outside the family's direct control. For instance, the recovery phase after a stroke may begin with an intensive care unit and months of extended care at a rehabilitation facility. This may be stressful for a family that prefers to tackle its own problems with a minimum of outside control or interference. For this family, the patient's return home may increase the workload but allows members to reestablish more fully their values concerning control. A family guided more by a preference for external control by experts will have greater difficulty when their family member returns home. For this family, leaving the rehabilitation hospital may be the most difficult time, because it means the loss of their locus of competency, the professionals caring for them. Health providers' cognizance about this basic difference in belief about control can guide a psychosocial treatment plan tailored to each family's needs.

In the terminal phase of an illness a family may feel least in control of the biological course of the disease and the decision-making regarding the overall care of their ill member. Families with a strong need to sustain their centrality may need to assert themselves more vigorously with health providers. Effective decision-making regarding the extent of heroic medical efforts or whether a patient will die at home, an institution, or hospice requires an effective family–provider relationship that respects the family's basic beliefs.

## The Family's Beliefs about the Cause of an Illness

When a significant health problem arises, all of us wonder "Why me (or us)?" and "Why now?" As illustrated poignantly in Case 14-7, we construct an explanation or narrative that helps organize our experience. The context within which an illness event occurs is a very powerful organizer and mirror of a family's belief system. The limits of current medical knowledge mean tremendous uncertainties persist about the relative importance of a myriad of factors in the onset of disease, and this allows individuals and families to develop highly idiosyncratic ideas about what caused their family member's illness. A family's beliefs about the etiology of an illness need to be assessed separately from its beliefs about what can affect the outcome. One way to gather this information is to ask each family member for his or her explanation of the existence of the disease. Responses will reflect a combination of the current level of medical knowledge about the particular disease in concert with family mythology. Wynne *et al.* (1992) underscore the importance of distinguishing beliefs that are external (such as societal) and viewed as more outside family members' control versus more toxic ones that blame individual family members or the entire family system. Negative beliefs may include punishment for prior misdeeds (e.g., an affair), blame of a particular family member ("Your drinking made me sick"), a sense of injustice ("Why am I being punished? I have been a good person"), genetics (e.g., cancer runs on one side of the family), negligence by the patient or parents (e.g., sudden infant death syndrome), or bad luck. Asking this question can function as an effective family Rorschach, bringing to light unresolved family conflicts.

Attributions about the cause of an illness that invoke blame, shame, or guilt are particularly important to uncover. Beliefs of this nature make it extremely difficult for a family to establish functional coping and adaptation to an illness. In the context of a life-threatening illness the blamed family member is held accountable for potential murder if the patient dies. Decisions about treatment can become confounded and filled with tension. A mother who feels blamed by her husband for their son's leukemia may be less able to accept stopping a low-probability experimental treatment than the angry, blaming husband. A husband who believes his drinking caused his wife's coronary and subsequent death may have a pathological grief reaction and may increase his drinking to mask his profound guilt.

In my clinical experience, families with the strongest, at times extreme, beliefs about personal responsibility and those with the most severely dysfunctional patterns will be those most likely to attribute the cause of an illness to a psychosocial factor. In families with a strong inner locus-of-control, an ethos of personal responsibility guides all facets of life, including the cause of an illness. For these families, a relative lack of acknowledgment of "outrageous fortune" as a factor in illness events can create for these families a nidus for blame, shame, and guilt. For highly dysfunctional families, characterized by unresolved conflicts and intense blaming, attributions of what or who is responsible for an illness often become ammunition in long-term family power struggles.

## Flexible Belief Systems

It is difficult to characterize an "ideal" family health belief about mastery or control. On one hand, a major thesis of systems-oriented medicine is that there is always an interplay between disease and other levels of system. On the other hand, illnesses and phases in the course of disease may vary considerably in their responsiveness to psychosocial factors versus their inherent nature. Distinctions need to be made between a family's beliefs about their overall participation in a long-term disease process, their beliefs about their ability to control the biological unfolding of an illness, and the flexibility with which a family can apply these beliefs. Optimal family narratives respect the limits of scientific knowledge, affirm basic competency, and promote the flexible use of multiple biological and psychosocial healing strategies.

A family's belief in their participation in the total illness process can be thought of as independent from whether a disease is stable, improving, or in a terminal phase. Sometimes, mastery and the attempt to control biological process coincide. A family coping with a member who has cancer in remission may tailor its behavior to help maintain health. This might include changes in family roles, communication, diet, exercise, and balance between work and recreation. Suppose the ill family member loses remission and vigorous efforts to reestablish a remission fail. As the family enters the terminal phase of the illness, participation as an expression of mastery must now be transposed for a successful process of letting go.

The difference between a family experiencing a loss with a sense of competency versus profound failure is intimately connected to this kind of flexible use of their belief system. For instance, it can be helpful if clinicians recognize that the death of a patient, whose long debilitating illness has heavily burdened others, can be a matter of relief as well as sadness to some or all family members. Since a sense of relief over death goes against most conventions in our society, it can trigger massive guilt reactions that may be expressed tangentially through such symptoms as depression and negative family interactions. Clinicians will need to help family members accept, with a minimum of guilt and defensiveness, the naturalness of ambivalent feeling they may have for their deceased member.

Thus, flexibility within the family and the health-provider system may be the key variable in optimal family functioning. Families can view mastery in a rigid, circumscribed way that views biological outcome as the sole determinant of success, or families can define control in a more "holistic" sense where involvement and participation in the overall process is the main criterion defining success. This is analogous to the distinction between "healing the system" and curing "the disease." Healing the system may influence the course or outcome of an illness, but disease outcome is not necessary to a family feeling successful. This flexible definition of mastery permits the quality of relations within the family or between the family and health providers to become more central to criteria of success. It permits the health provider's competence to be viewed from both a technical and a caregiving perspective (Reiss & Kaplan De-Nour, 1989) that is not linked only to the biological course of the disorder.

## Fit among Family, Clinicians, and Health System Beliefs

As family illness beliefs are articulated, a clinician should inquire about the degree of family consensus or congruence among members concerning a particular value, such as health locus of control. This is important because it is a common, but unfortunate, error to regard "the family" as a monolithic unit that feels, thinks, believes, and behaves as an undifferentiated whole.

In assessing the family's level of agreement, one should learn about the family's general tolerance for differences. Is the family rule "We must agree on all/some values" or are diversity and different viewpoints acceptable? Further, clinicians should determine whether the family policy about consensus is adhered to in relation to prevailing cultural or societal beliefs. Can the family hold values that differ from the wider culture? The family's general rule has multiple determinants that include cultural norms, historical context (era of "family consensus" versus each member "doing his/her own thing"), and the beliefs of the adults' families of origin.

A family's rules about consensus can have profound implications for permissible options when a family faces chronic illness. If consensus is the rule, then individual differentiation implies deviance. If the guiding principle is "We can hold different viewpoints," then diversity is allowed. When working with illness-related values in a family where consensus is the rule, attention to the entire family is mandatory. One treatment goal can be to help families negotiate their differences and support the separate identity, needs, and goals of each member. In a family where diversity is permitted there may be greater latitude to work on certain disease-related psychosocial issues with the ill member alone or with other family members without mobilizing family resistance.

Next, it is important to look into the *actual* level of agreement with regard to illness values both within the family and between the family and medical system. How congruent are the family's basic beliefs about control with their illness value system? A family that is uniformly external will generally adapt best if psychosocial interventions are tailored to that fact. On the other hand, a family that generally adheres to an internal locus of control but feels the opposite with a particular disease may, through exploration of underlying issues, be able to change its beliefs about illness. It is critical to keep in mind that beliefs about control refer to a family's beliefs about the importance of their *participation in the total illness process* rather than just their beliefs about a disease's curability.

It is important to analyze differences among family members in terms of illness values. Disparities in two- and three-person relationships involving the ill member are particularly significant. Consider a common situation in which there is a longstanding loyalty conflict for a man caught between his spouse and his mother. Both women vie for his devotion, while he is unable to define boundaries between his family of origin and nuclear family. This dysfunctional triangle may have smoldered for years in a precarious balance when the man develops a slowly progressive and debilitating illness such as multiple sclerosis. If the man and his mother share a strong sense of internal control while his spouse grew up in a family that saw chronic illness as a matter of fate, an unbalancing of this triangle is likely to occur. The smoldering mother–son coalition now reemerges in full force fueled by shared basic beliefs concerning mastery, while the marital couple is driven apart.

The different ethnic backgrounds of the adults in a family may be a primary reason for the kind of discrepancies about illness beliefs that emerge at the time of a major illness (McGoldrick *et al.*, 1996). Differences may occur in such areas as beliefs concerning control; the definition of the appropriate "sick role" for the patient; the kind and degree of open communication about the disease; who should be included in the illness caretaking system (e.g., extended family, friends, professionals); and the kind of rituals viewed as normative at different stages of an illness (e.g., hospital bedside vigils, healing and funeral rituals) (Imber-Black, 1991; Wolin & Bennett, 1984). In families of mixed ethnic heritage, clinicians should assess these areas for consensus, disagreement, and negotiation.

It is common for differences in beliefs or attitudes between family members to erupt at major transition points in the treatment or disease course. For instance, in situations of severe disability or terminal illness, one member may want the patient to return home while another prefers extended hospitalization or transfer to an extended care facility. Since the chief task of patient caretaking is usually assigned to the wife/mother, she is the one most apt to bear the chief burdens in this regard. If this family also operates under the constraint of traditional role assignments where the wife/mother defers to her spouse as the family decision maker, she may not make her true feelings known and may become the "family martyr," taking on the home nursing tasks without overt disagreement at the time critical decisions are made with health professionals. Clinicians can be misled by a family that presents this kind of united front. A careful and perceptive assessment can help avert the long-term consequences to such a family of role overload, resentment, and deteriorating family relationships.

It is essential to assess the fit between the belief systems of the family and the healthcare team. It is basic to a collaborative relationship (Rolland, 1998; Seaburn et al., 1997). The same questions asked of the family are relevant to the medical team. What is the attitude of the healthcare team about its and the family's ability to influence the course/outcome of the disease? How does the health team see the balance between its versus the family's participation in the treatment and control of the disease? If basic differences in beliefs about health locus of control exist, how can these differences be reconciled?

Because of the tendency of most health facilities to disempower individuals and thereby foster dependence, utmost sensitivity to family values is needed to create a therapeutic system. Many breakdowns in relationships between "noncompliant" or marginal patients and their healthcare providers can be traced to natural disagreements at this basic level that were not addressed.

The relative need for consensus will vary according to the type and phase of the illness (Reiss & Kaplan De-Nour, 1989). One point where a good fit of values is usually needed is during the initial crisis period when health providers engage in much high-technology medicine and rapid decision-making and exchange of information, especially if life-threatening circumstances prevail. Teamwork is particularly important. Illnesses characterized by recurrent crises or key transitions have nodal points of stress where the strength of collaborative relationships will be tested.

It is common for differences in beliefs or attitudes to erupt at any life-cycle transition or major nodal transitions in the illness. The murky boundary between the chronic and terminal phase is a good example. The attitudes and behaviors of the medical team can either facilitate or hinder this process for a family. A healthcare team that maintains heroic efforts to avert the death of the patient can convey confusing messages. Families may not know how to interpret continued lifesaving efforts. Especially in cases involving dementia, this can contribute to a family's sense of ambiguity about the ill person's continued role in the family (Boss, 1999). Is there still real hope that should be taken by families as a message to redouble their faith in and support of medical improvement? Do the physicians feel bound to a technological imperative that requires them to exhaust *all* possibilities at their disposal, regardless of the odds of success? Often physicians feel committed to this course for ethical reasons, a "leave no stone unturned" philosophy, or because of fears concerning legal liability. Is the medical team having its own difficulties letting go? Strong relationships with certain patients can be fueled by identifications with losses, often unresolved, in health providers' own lives (McDaniel et al., 1997). Healthcare professionals and institutions can collude in a pervasive societal wish to deny death as a natural process truly beyond technological control (Becker, 1973). Sometimes, endless treatment can represent the medical team's inability to separate a general belief in curing a disease from beliefs about participation (separate from cure) in a patient's total care. Professionals need to closely examine their own motives for treatments geared toward cure rather than palliation, particularly when a patient may be entering a terminal phase. Professionals' self-examination needs to be done in concert with a careful understanding of the family's belief system.

As clinicians, we need to become aware of how our own family background affects our health beliefs and their interactions with families. It is useful for clinicians to take a personal inventory in terms of the kinds of beliefs described in this chapter. Multigenerational beliefs and legacies about illness and loss are particularly important. Areas of strength and vulnerability need to be identified, such as instances of overcoming adversity and unresolved loss issues (McDaniel et al., 1997).

Finally, because information about and linkage to community resources and services is frequently valuable, the clinician must assess how family health beliefs influence their overall illness behavior within a community (Mechanic, 1978). Clinicians need to know the availability of and access to community resources relevant to the management of long-term illnesses. This includes a range of primary, secondary, and tertiary medical, rehabilitation, respite, transportation, housing, institutional, and financial entitlement services. Also, it includes potential psychosocial support from friends, neighbors, and self-help groups, and religious, ethnic, cultural, or other group affiliations. On the family side, one must inquire about a family's prior experience using such resources. Have these experiences been affirming or alienating? To what extent is the family adequately informed about potential outside sources of help? Ignorance may reflect family isolation from the community as a result of such things as geographical distance in a rural setting, lack of education (e.g., literacy), language barrier, poverty, race, and ethnic or religious distinctions from the wider culture. On the other side, a family's willingness to use outside resources may be limited by ethnic/cultural values, certain family dynamics, and their own illness paradigms.

For example, rigidly enmeshed families tend to view the world as dangerous and threatening to their fragile sense of autonomy. Individual autonomy is sacrificed to keep the family system intact. Their beliefs about control will need to be defined within a framework of family exclusiveness that minimizes the role of outsiders. The occurrence of a chronic illness presents a powerful dilemma for these families. The illness may necessitate frequent excursions beyond the family borders or require the inclusion of outside professionals for disease management. Any hope of establishing a viable family–healthcare team relationship depends on exquisite sensitivity to this interplay of dysfunctional family dynamics and their belief system.

## CONCLUSION

This chapter has described a three-dimensional model for looking at the impact of chronic illness on families. On the first dimension, psychosocial "types" of illnesses are created based on combinations of four components: onset, course, outcome, and degree of incapacitation. The second dimension distinguishes three phases in the life history of chronic disease: crisis, chronic, and terminal. The third dimension includes various universal and illness-specific components of family functioning. Particular attention was given to the family health beliefs, multigenerational history of illness, loss, and crisis, and the interface of the individual and family life cycles with chronic disease. This three-dimensional model provides a framework for effective clinical intervention that takes into account the important interactions between illness, individual patients, and their families.

## CASES FOR DISCUSSION

### CASE 1

*José and Leticia, a young, successful dual-career couple in their early 30s, have been married for 4 years, when José, who has had a lifelong mild case of hemophilia, contracts AIDS from a contaminated blood factor infusion he required after a heated discussion with his wife during which he had punched a wall. José, who has an intense belief in personal control and overcoming adversity, decides that he will cure himself within a year. He had always maintained excellent control of his hemophilia, which he inherited through his mother's side of the family.*

*Past family history is significant. José's mother decided to divorce his father when José was 5 years old. Subsequently, his father's business failed, and he committed suicide when José was a teenager. José's mother sees her son as the shining star of the family, who unlike his derided father will be a big success in life. Leticia was an only child; her mother had left Leticia's father when Leticia was a teenager. Her father was described as nice but ineffectual; he had a series of psychiatric hospitalizations for depression. Leticia had tried to help her father, but felt unsuccessful. Leticia sees in José the strong-willed, successful man, who unlike her father had mastered chronic illness (hemophilia).*

1. *Given the family histories, what do you see as the major psychosocial risks for José and Leticia and their marriage? What if José becomes terminally ill, develops a dementia, and cannot be managed at home? What are the possible issues of blame, shame, and guilt? Who else in the extended family might be at risk, and why?*
2. *Given José's beliefs about control and mastery, what are the psychosocial risks given the lethality of his disease? Would you try to intervene and how?*
3. *Discuss the possible strains on José, Leticia, and the marriage of an "off-time" terminal illness.*

4. *What dysfunctional skews could develop between José and Leticia in their roles as patient and well spouse/caregiver?*

5. *How are the psychosocial demands of hemophilia and AIDS similar and different?*

## CASE 2

*You are called by the head nurse for the ICU to intervene with a patient and his mother who were disrupting the unit because the mother insists on staying at her son's bedside. The ICU's customary rules limit family visits to 10 minutes. The patient, Stavros, aged 42, had been admitted with symptoms of intractable angina. He is first-generation Greek-American, married for 15 years to Dana, who is from a Scandinavian background. A longstanding smoldering triangular conflict has existed for the couple in terms of Stavros's divided loyalties between his strong relationship to his family of origin, particularly his mother, and his spouse. On admission, his mother began a 24-hour vigil by her son's hospital bed. Dana greatly resents her mother-in-law's seemingly intrusive behavior. Stavros's mother is critical of what she perceives as Dana's emotional coldness and relative lack of concern. Stavros feels caught between his warring mother and wife and complains of increased symptoms.*

1. *Thinking in terms of different ethnic traditions of the family members, including your own, how would you react to this case? Thinking systemically, how would you approach a consultation with the patient/family?*

2. *Thinking in terms of the intersection of three distinct belief systems—your work setting (hospital and ICU), yourself as a health professional, and your personal cultural/ethnic/family values—how might these affect your strategy with this case? What biases might interfere with your effectiveness? How could you avoid taking sides?*

## CASE 3

*Mrs. L. tells you that she is concerned that her daughter Janice, aged 5, has been compulsively masturbating for the past 3 months, and that this is an indication of sexual abuse. When the child assessment reveals no evidence of abuse, you inquire about other recent stressful events in the family. Only at that point does the mother reveal that her husband had a subtotal gastrectomy 9 months ago because of stomach cancer, and that 3 months earlier he had been rehospitalized for further tests that proved inconclusive. When Mrs. L. is asked what the children have been told, she reports that, after her husband's surgery, they had told the children only that "Daddy had a tummy ache, so the doctors removed Daddy's stomach so he'd feel better." Mrs. L. reveals that she herself worries constantly about her husband's condition, but that he won't come in and won't discuss it, stating that after the surgery, "He was adamant that he did not want ever to talk about it. He went back to work almost immediately, and insisted that everything is fine." Asked if this medical crisis had had any impact on the children, especially Janice, she replies, "Well, she doesn't tell me about any worries. But now that you ask, at dinner every night, when we say grace, Janice prays out loud for Daddy's stomach. But no one in the family comments on this."*

1. *Thinking in terms of healthy family communication in the face of threatened loss, how would you intervene in this case? Who would you try to convene and why?*

2. *In what ways would you handle communication with children differently than with the couple?*

3. *How would you view the husband's personal decision to minimize his problem and keep it private in the context of other symptomatic family members?*

## CASE 4

*Mr. and Mrs. S., both in their early 70s, live alone in their home of 40 years. Mrs. S. has had congestive heart failure for 5 years and more recently a progressive dementia caused by a series of minor strokes. A recent exacerbation of her condition has led to a hospitalization. The family physician feels the couple have reached their limits and has suggested a nursing home placement for Mrs. S. The family includes three adult children, Ann, Joe, and Beth. All live far away, and all are married and raising children. Ann has come to visit her parents during her mother's hospitalization. Family history is significant in that when Mr. and Mrs. S. had their first child, Ann, Mrs. S.'s aging mother, who also had advanced heart disease, had been living with them for several years. At the time, Mr. S. felt that her mother should enter a home while Mrs. S. was strongly opposed. Eventually, Mrs. S. deferred to her husband's wishes. Her mother went to a nearby nursing home and died within a year. Mrs. S. feels the placement hastened her mother's demise and continues to blame her husband for forcing this "cruel decision." The family is in a stalemate about the current dilemma. Mr. S. and Ann are strongly opposed, while Joe and Beth feel the physician's suggestion is correct and necessary.*

1. *How is the multigenerational story of Mrs. S.'s mother critical to understanding this case? How might it affect each family member's feelings about placing Mrs. S. in a nursing home?*
2. *Would you have a family meeting? How would you decide whether to include Mrs. S.? What about Joe and Beth, who are not in town?*
3. *How are gender norms a factor in this case? How might you address them with this family?*
4. *How are life cycle issues (e.g., couple in later life, adult children in child-rearing phase with aging parents) pertinent, and how would you make them part of the consultative process?*
5. *What do you see as the choices for this family? How would you explore them in a collaborative manner?*

## CASE 5

*Bill, a highly competent first-year pediatric resident, sought brief therapy complaining of intense feelings of guilt and anger toward his mentally retarded brother and his parents, which had surfaced a few months after starting his residency. During the initial visit he exclaimed, "No matter what I do, I never feel I can do enough to make everyone happy." Bill grew up in a working-class family as the oldest son, and the first of his family with a college education. He was the family "success story." His family situation was compounded by his father's seeing the disabled son as a source of shame. Bill was aware that his choice to become a pediatrician was motivated partly by his deep desire to overcome his feelings of well-sibling survivor guilt by helping other children with chronic disorders.*

1. *Using this vignette as a stimulus, consider your own multigenerational family history regarding illness and loss. Is there an illness story that stands out? How were you involved? How has this experience affected you, in particular your choice to become a health professional? Are there aspects of this experience that are a source of strength? Any that are a source of fear or vulnerability? In what clinical situations do you think this experience might come to the fore, and in what ways?*

# RECOMMENDED READINGS

*Families, Systems, and Health: The Journal of Collaborative Family Health Care* (formerly *Family Systems Medicine*).

This is the only journal that is interdisciplinary and devoted to the area of families and health, with a particular focus on models of collaboration. Topics include family or systems approaches to chronic and life-threatening illness. Formats include review articles, clinical research, theory, commentary, and dialogue. For subscription information contact: Families, Systems and Health, Inc. Subscription Department, P.O. Box 20838, Rochester, NY, 14602-0838.

McDaniel S, Hepworth J, Doherty W (eds): *Medical Family Therapy: A Biopsychosocial Approach to Families with Health Problems.* New York, Basic Books Inc, 1992.

This book does an excellent job of describing the various uses and roles for family consultation and therapy in a variety of healthcare contexts and medical situations.

Rolland JS: *Families, Illness, and Disability: An Integrative Treatment Model.* New York, Basic Books Inc, 1994.

Rich with practical clinical detail, this book provides a much fuller description of the Family Systems-Illness Model outlined in this chapter. Includes separate chapters on assessment and treatment issues for families, couples, and common personal issues and strains for clinicians working with chronic and life-threatening illness. Nominated by American Medical Writers Association as Book of the Year.

# REFERENCES

Antonovsky A: *Health, Stress, and Coping: New Perspectives on Mental and Physical Well-Being.* San Francisco, Jossey–Bass Inc, 1979.
Antonovsky A, Sourani T: Family sense of coherence and family adaptation. *Marriage Fam,* 50:79–92, 1988.
Becker E: *The Denial of Death.* New York, Free Press, 1973.
Boss P: *Ambiguous Loss: Learning to Live with Unresolved Grief.* Cambridge, Mass, Harvard University Press, 1999.
Boszormenyi-Nagy I, Spark G: *Invisible Loyalties: Reciprocity in Intergenerational Family Therapy.* New York, Harper & Row Publishers Inc, 1973.
Bowen M: *Family Therapy in Clinical Practice.* New York, Jason Aronson Inc, 1978.

Campbell TL, Patterson JM: The effectiveness of family interventions in the treatment of physical illness. *J Marital Fam Ther* 21(4):545–583, 1995.

Carter EA, McGoldrick M (eds): *The Evolving Family Life Cycle: Individual, Family, and Social Perspectives*, ed 3. Boston, Allyn & Bacon, 1998.

Combrinck-Graham L: A developmental model for family systems. *Fam Process* 24:139–150, 1985.

Engel GL: The need for a new medical model: A challenge for biomedicine. *Science* 196:129–136, 1977

Engel GL: The clinical application of the biopsychosocial model. *Amer J Psychiatry* 137:535–544, 1980.

Framo JL: *Family-of-Origin Therapy: An Intergeneratonal Approach*. New York, Brunner/Mazel, 1992.

Griffith J, Griffith M: *The Body Speaks*. New York, Basic Books Inc, 1994.

Imber-Black E: *Rituals and the healing process*, in Walsh F, McGoldrick M (eds): *Living Beyond Loss. Death in the Family*. New York, WW Norton & Co, Inc, 1991.

Kleinman AM: *The Illness Narratives: Suffering, Healing, and the Human Condition*. New York, Basic Books Inc, 1988.

Kluckhohn FR: Variations in the basic values of family systems, in Bell NW, Vogel EF (eds): A Modern Introduction to the Family. Glencoe, Ill: The Free Press, 1960.

Kubler-Ross E: *On Death and Dying*. New York, Macmillan Publishing Co, Inc, 1969.

Lefcourt HM: *Locus of Control*, ed 2. Hillsdale, NJ, Lawrence Erlbaum Associates, 1982.

Levinson DJ: A conception of adult development. *Am Psychol*, 41:3–13, 1986.

McDaniel S, Hepworth J, Doherty W (eds): *Medical Family Therapy: A Biopsychosocial Approach to Families with Health Problems*. New York: Basic Books Inc, 1992.

McDaniel S, Hepworth J, Doherty W (eds): *The Shared Experience of Illness: Stories of Patients, Families, and Their Therapists*. New York, Basic Books Inc, 1997.

McGoldrick M, Pearce JK, Giordano J: *Ethnicity and Family Therapy*, ed 2. New York, Guilford Press, 1996.

McGoldrick M, Gerson R, Schellenberger S: *Genograms in Family Assessment*, ed 2. New York, WW Norton & Co, Inc, 1999.

Mechanic D: *Medical Sociology*, ed 2. New York, Free Press, 1978.

Minuchin S, Baker L, Rosman BL, Liebman R, Milman L, Todd T: A conceptual model of psychosomatic illness in children: Family organization and family therapy. *Arch Gen Psychiatry* 32:1031–1038, 1975.

Minuchin S, Rosman BL, Baker L: *Psychosomatic Families: Anorexia Nervosa in Context*. Cambridge, Mass, Harvard University Press, 1978.

Moos R (ed): *Coping with Physical Illness*. 2: *New Perspectives*. New York, Plenum Press, 1984.

Neugarten B: Adaptation and the life cycle. *Couns Psychol* 6:16–20, 1976.

Olkin R: What psychotherapists should know about disability. New York, Guilford Press, 1999.

Penn P: Coalitions and binding interactions in families with chronic illness. *Fam Syst Med* 1(2):16–25, 1983.

Reiss D: *The Family's Construction of Reality*. Cambridge, Mass, Harvard University Press, 1981.

Reiss D, Kaplan De-Nour A: The family and medical team in chronic illness: A transactional and developmental perspective, in Ramsey C Jr (ed): *Family Systems in Medicine*. New York, Guilford Press, 1989.

Rolland JS: Toward a psychosocial typology of chronic and life-threatening illness. *Fam Syst Med* 2:245–263, 1984.

Rolland JS: Chronic illness and the life cycle: A conceptual framework. *Fam Process* 26(2):203–221, 1987a.

Rolland JS: Family illness paradigms: Evolution and significance. *Fam Syst Med* 5(4):467–486, 1987b.

Rolland JS: Anticipatory loss: A family systems developmental framework. *Fam Process* 29(3):229-244, 1990.

Rolland JS: *Families, Illness, and Disability: An Integrative Treatment Model*. New York, Basic Books Inc, 1994a.

Rolland JS: In sickness and in health: The impact of illness on couple's relationship. *J Marital Fam Ther* 20(4):327–347, 1994b.

Rolland JS: Beliefs and collaboration in illness: Evolution over time. *Fam Syst Health* (formerly *Fam Syst Med*) 16(1/2):7–27, 1998.

Rolland JS: Families and parental illness: A conceptual framework. *J Fam Ther* 21(3):242–267, 1999.

Seaburn D, Gunn W, Mauksch L, Gawinski B, Lorenz A: *Models of Collaboration: A Guide for Mental Health Professionals Working with Physicians and Health Care Providers*. New York, Basic Books Inc, 1997.

Sontag S: *Illness as Metaphor*. New York, McGraw–Hill Book Co, 1978.

Sontag S: *AIDS and Its Metaphors*. New York, Farrar, Straus & Giroux Inc, 1988.

Strauss AL: *Chronic Illness and the Quality of Life*. St. Louis, Mo, Mosby, 1975.

Walker G: The pact: The caretaker-parent/ill-child coalition in families with chronic illness. *Fam Syst Med* 1(4):6–29, 1983.

Walsh F: *Normal Family Processes*, ed 2. New York, Guilford Press, 1993.

Walsh F: *Strengthening Family Resilience*. New York, Guilford Press, 1998.

Walsh F (ed): *Spiritual Resources in Family Therapy*. New York, Guilford Press, 1999.

Walsh F, McGoldrick M: *Living beyond Loss: Death in the Family*. New York, WW Norton & Co, Inc, 1991.

Weihs K, Fisher L, Baird M: Families, health, and behavior. Commissioned Report: Institute of Medicine, National Academy of Sciences, 2001.

Wolin SJ, Bennett LA: Family rituals. *Fam Process* 23(3):401–420, 1984.

Wortman C, Silver R: The myths of coping with loss. *J Consult Clin Psychol* 57:349–357, 1989.

Wright LM, Watson WL, Bell JM: *Beliefs: The Heart of Healing in Families and Illness*. New York, Basic Books Inc, 1996.

Wynne LC, Shields C, Sirkin M: Illness, family theory, and family therapy: I. Conceptual issues. *Fam Process* 31:3–18, 1992.

## CHAPTER 15

# Counseling and Behavioral Change

*Larry B. Mauksch*

*Dr. Jacobson entered the room of his patient, Mr. Lawford. During the last 2 years Mr. Lawford gained 20 pounds and had rising blood pressure. Dr. Jacobson was concerned about these changes and wanted to help his patient address them before more serious health problems emerged. Dr. Jacobson expressed curiosity about Mr. Lawford's day-to-day activities. Mr. Lawford described working long hours with burgeoning responsibilities in recent years. He used to exercise at least four times a week and now was lucky to exercise once on the weekend. Neither of his parents exercised and both of them had been overweight. His father worked hard as a plumber, retired 5 years ago, and died 1 year later at 67 of a heart attack. Although Mr. Lawford acknowledged his weight gain, decreased exercise, and stress at work, he was not concerned about his health.*

## EDUCATIONAL OBJECTIVES

By the end of this chapter the learner should be able to:

1. Define the basic attributes of the effective physician-counselor
2. Demonstrate the use of questioning to determine the patient's readiness for change
3. Describe one model of change, namely, Motivational Interviewing
4. Perform reflective listening
5. Demonstrate establishing focus in counseling
6. Define the BATHE model of counseling
7. Describe the components of Problem Solving Therapy
8. Define the contextual factors affecting patient behavior
9. Demonstrate interview skills to assess relationships within the patient's family
10. Describe why physicians and mental health professionals benefit from working together

In Case 15-1 Dr. Jacobson is faced with a challenge. Which skills will be useful in helping his patient? Whose responsibility is it to muster the motivation to change, the physician's or the patient's? Most people go to their physician first for help with mental health and life-style concerns (Regier *et al.*, 1978, 1993; Schurman *et al.*, 1985). Requests for help sometimes come disguised as complaints about physical ails. Physicians who work effectively with these patients are sometimes said to practice "the art of medicine." The use of the term *art* gives the medical trainee a mixed message. This leaves students wondering if they will be fortunate to manifest this innate talent. An alternative view of the "art of medicine" is a *skill-based* perspective.

The skills and knowledge described in this chapter are useful to physicians, irrespective of the setting, medical discipline, or length of time spent with patients. Although psychiatrists and primary care physicians may employ these skills more often than others, all physicians are confronted with patients who resist recommendations or are fearful or simply need support in dealing with health problems. For example, in Case 15-1, Mr. Lawford might present first to a cardiologist with complaints of chest pain or to a gastroenterologist with irritable bowel problems. These and other medical specialists, along with primary care physicians, share the same challenge. In each patient they are confronted with a unique world of ideas and experiences on health and illness. Physicians who master counseling skills have learned to study the world of their patients and create plans that patients support.

Physicians are often reluctant to engage patients in counseling because opening up "the can of worms" takes too much time (Dugdale *et al.*, 1999). However, available research suggests that the opposite is true. One study of primary care physicians and surgeons found that those physicians who picked up on patient clues for emotional problems took less time than physicians who missed or ignored clues (Levinson *et al.*, 2000). In another study the communication patterns of 98 primary care physicians were studied (Roter *et al.*, 1997). Physicians were classified as either biomedical-narrow, biomedical-expanded, biopsychosocial, psychosocial, or consumerist. There were no significant differences in the average length of interviews between groups. Physicians in the two biomedical groups reported lower satisfaction than the other groups, with the psychosocial physicians reporting the highest satisfaction. And physicians in the psychosocial group diagnosed significantly more psychosocial problems than physicians in the other groups! Other research suggests that attending to psychosocial problems decreases complications with the management of chronic illness (Katon, 1998). Engaging in psychosocial discussions with patients is less concrete than pursuing a cure in a biomedical problem. However, when the most important issue in the patient's life is a psychosocial one, this avenue may be more satisfying to you and the patient and need not take more time. This chapter will help you integrate time management microskills with therapeutic interviewing to help you provide better care without taking more time.

Mastering psychosocial skills has practical value beyond enhancing the quality of care and physician satisfaction. At least half of high users of medical services have psychiatric diagnoses (Katon *et al.*, 1992). Neglecting the mental health of these patients usually means spending more dollars on duplicated and overdone medical assessments, unnecessary procedures, and hospital admissions. Frustration in dealing with complicated patients who are high users of medical service can sour medical practice. Physician job satisfaction is compromised by fears of malpractice litigation. Moreover, a strong hedge against malpractice litigation is the formation of a strong physician–patient relationship (Beckman *et al.*, 1994). The integration of counseling skills into the physician's repertoire promotes better care for patients, cost savings, and greater physician job satisfaction.

## BEHAVIORAL CHANGE AND THE PHYSICIAN-COUNSELOR

### CASE 15-1 (continued)

*Dr. Jacobson is confronted with a difficult situation. Mr. Lawford has a paternal history of heart disease and appears to be using his father as a model for his behavior. The weight gain, decreased exercise, rising blood pressure, and increased work stress combined with a family history devoid of health-conscious role models suggest that Mr. Lawford's health is at significant risk. However, he reveals no sign of concern.*

*Dr. Jacobson expressed awareness that things must be stressful for his patient. He then asked what Mr. Lawford's workday was like. Mr. Lawford rarely took time for lunch or other breaks. He "ate on the run" and frequently went to the company store for snacks. In response to Dr. Jacobson's appreciation of the hurried work pace, Mr. Lawford noted that he felt out of control. He had never considered how eating and rushing were linked. Dr. Jacobson shared the idea that his patient's behavior seemed similar to what his father had done. This comparison interested Mr. Lawford, who then pondered the comparison and expressed concern about the long-term implications of continuing this pattern. As time was limited, Dr. Jacobson ended the interview with a request for a follow-up appointment in 2 weeks. He expressed appreciation to Mr. Lawford for talking with him.*

*At their next meeting, Dr. Jacobson asked Mr. Lawford about the good things and less good things of his eating and exercise patterns. Mr. Lawford noted that the major advantage of decreased exercise and missing lunch was increased time for work. After a long pause, he also questioned this advantage. When Dr. Jacobson acknowledged this confusion, Mr. Lawford admitted that he didn't always work in the most creative or efficient fashion. He added that he realized that his behaviors were not healthy. Dr. Jacobson asked for clarification. With obvious sadness, Mr. Lawford admitted that he did not want his life cut short as happened to his father. His father had been gone a lot during his childhood and adolescent years. He expressed grief about the death of his father and fear that he might miss time with his family.*

*At this point Dr. Jacobson summarized their discussion and again expressed appreciation and empathy to Mr. Lawford. Dr. Jacobson asked Mr. Lawford if he wanted help adjusting his lifestyle to promote a healthier and longer life. Mr. Lawford said yes and agreed to return in 2 weeks to make specific plans for change.*

Mental health professionals have their version of the light bulb joke. Namely, how many psychotherapists does it take to change a light bulb? Answer: Only one, but the light bulb must want to change.

To many people around the world, Western physicians have the reputation of being miracle workers. However, it is easy to lose sight of the role patients play in the process of change. While we focus on the dramatic effects of new surgeries or medications, we forget that for each medical success there is a patient who has consented to treatment and followed a prescribed protocol. Transplant surgeons have learned to consult mental health professionals to assess and prepare patients for difficult surgeries (Leedham *et al.*, 1995). They recognize that the patient is an essential part of the team. In less dramatic circumstances the same is true. The best diagnostician and medical therapist is ineffectual without a patient who believes in the treatment and is willing to participate in therapy. Hypertension, often called "the silent killer," is a good example. While it is easy to diagnose and treat most cases of hypertension, only a third of the people treated will follow a physician's advice after 1 year (Clark, 1991; Miller, 1997). Those who aspire to help people make changes in their lives should be on guard for those patients who believe that physicians can do it all. During their training, psychotherapists are taught that the patient's motivation to change should equal or surpass the psychotherapist's desire for change. When physicians believe they "can do it all" they exhaust themselves and eventually resent their patients.

Why do people change? Attempts to answer this question have filled volumes over centuries. While no easy answer exists, we do know that certain ingredients increase the likelihood of change. First, people have to identify a reason to change. Simply doing something different because one is told what to do does not motivate most people to change. To the contrary, telling someone what to do often creates an oppositional response. People who feel more control over their lives are healthier. When physicians help patients articulate reasons to change that are personally meaningful, those patients take more responsibility for their own health (Ryan & Deci, 2000). Reasons to change come in different forms. Sometimes a major life event like marriage, birth, or death alters one's perspective. A major illness affecting an individual or a significant other may prompt change. Sometimes new information, like the connection between smoking and cancer, creates the incentive to change.

Second, people have to believe in their capacity to change. While many people know why they ought to change, they may lack the confidence to proceed. "I think I can, I think I can," the motto of The Little Engine That Could, is an example of one storyteller's appreciation of this principle. Contemplating how to instill confidence in patients desiring to change leads to a third essential ingredient. Change is facilitated by supportive networks of family, friends, and, hopefully, healthcare providers.

Attributes of the effective (physician) counselor are described in texts spanning all of the helping and healthcare professions (Patterson, 1986; Wilson *et al.*, 1991). These attributes help create a relationship in which the patient can feel safe. Interpersonal safety, the sense that one will be cared for and not judged, is an essential prerequisite for the exploration of feelings and ideas about which one feels vulnerable. These attributes include:

- A respectful and nonjudgmental presence
- Accurate empathy (compassion)
- Skillful listening
- A belief in the patient's capacity to change and grow
- Willingness to find a way to like the patient

A professional stance that is helpful to patients but protects providers from becoming overly responsible for creating change is curiosity. It is hard to be curious and authoritarian at the same time. When a physician is genuinely curious, the patient is more likely to feel cared for and willing to be vulnerable. Patients who have curious physicians begin to be curious about themselves, their beliefs and behaviors. Genuine curiosity expressed by the physician, not to be confused with coercion, is unlikely to compromise the patient's sense of autonomy.

Physicians who skillfully counsel their patients have an ability to measure a patient's readiness for change. Offering interventions requiring motivational levels higher than the patient possesses runs the risk of alienating the patient, creating guilt, inadequacy, and even resentment. The physician confronted with a patient who stumbled after being forced down the path to change may be left feeling disappointed and deflated in her attempts to provide assistance.

## ASSESSING READINESS FOR CHANGE AS A GUIDE FOR TREATMENT

The Transtheoretical Model of change describes stages of readiness for people in a variety of clinical situations, including smoking, alcohol abuse, drug abuse, and weight gain (Prochaska *et al.*, 1994). Developed in the early 1980s by Prochaska and DiClemente (Prochaska & DiClemente, 1982), this model has six stages (see Table 15.1).

Rather than thinking of readiness for change as occurring in discrete stages, Miller and Rollnick (1991) suggest it be viewed on a continuum. They have developed a progression of strategic questions. These questions serve two functions. First, they are tools to assess the patient's degree of readiness. Second, they are

**Table 15.1**
The Transtheoretical Model of Change

Precontemplation: Not thinking about behavior change
Contemplation: Considering the possibility and value of change but feeling ambivalence that includes consideration of the disadvantages of change
Preparation: A commitment to change exists and the effort is imminent
Action: A plan to change is implemented
Maintenance: Sustained change, usually lasting longer than 6 months
Relapse: Return to an old behavior pattern, exercise avoidance, safe sex/condom use, and sunscreen use

## DOES THE STAGES OF CHANGE MODEL GENERALIZE?

*The original research describing stages of change (precontemplation, contemplation, preparation, action, maintenance, and relapse) focused mostly on addictive behaviors like cigarette smoking and drug use. Does this model apply to common medical problems? Researchers compared studies of 12 problems across 3860 patients (Prochaska et al., 1994). Problems included counseling about safe sex, sunscreen use, mammography screening, dietary fat reduction, weight control, exercising, smoking cessation, quitting cocaine, adolescent delinquent behaviors, radon gas exposure, and changing physician preventive practice with smokers. Patients and physicians in these studies represent a diverse collection of populations from college students, to intravenous drug users, to prostitutes, to street youth. Some samples were of blue-collar workers while others were from middle class homes and still others were from low-income settings. Findings are similar across 11 of the 12 problems with cocaine users being the exception. Stages of change are evident in all samples. Those in the precontemplation or contemplation stage were characterized by seeing more "cons" than "pros" to change. Those in the action and maintenance phases listed more "pros" than "cons." Today clinicians are applying the stages of change model and related motivational techniques across the broad spectrum of health behaviors including patients with diabetes, those recovering from heart attacks, or people managing HIV medication regimens. When you talk to your next patient who is challenged with making health behavior change, ask yourself, "how ready is this person?" Work with the patient where he or she is, not where you want them to be.*

designed to gently motivate the patient to move to states of greater readiness. They term their approach *motivational interviewing*. The value of these strategies is drawn from five foundational concepts representing a creative synthesis of effective counseling protocols (see Table 15.2). Combined, these general principles promote respectful ways to help people help themselves. Successfully translating this approach into action requires training and practice. Physicians who use this approach become skilled at gauging a patient's readiness for change, adjusting their approach to meet the patient.

What should the physician do when she is concerned about a behavior or relationship such as smoking, sedentary lifestyle, relationship conflict, or drug use? Miller and Rollnick's (1991) menu of questions includes the following approaches demonstrated above by Dr. Jacobson:

**Table 15.2**
General Principles of Motivational Interviewing

1. *Express empathy.* The empathic (compassionate) physician conveys acceptance of the patient, making it easier for the patient to feel safe in experimenting with change.
2. *Develop discrepancy.* Physicians help patients contrast where they are and where they want to be. This process is done in a respectful, curious, and patient fashion. It is the patient who must make the comparisons and acknowledge discrepancies between current patterns and long-term goals. Physicians often make the mistake of setting goals for their patients. This easily creates guilt and alienation.
3. *Avoid argumentation.* Motivational interviewing uses "soft confrontation" through curious, respectful inquiry about the patient's decision to maintain behaviors that compromise health. However, the physician should avoid trying to convince the patient that he or she has a problem. Coercion creates resistance and defensiveness.
4. *Roll with resistance.* Remember that the decision to change is made by the patient. Hesitance is normal and predictable and exists for a reason. Its purpose should be explored and respected. Often the acceptance and examination of resistance reveals a new understanding of the world. This perceptual shift may decrease resistance.
5. *Support self-efficacy.* The physician must believe in the patient's capacity to change. This belief fosters confidence in the patient's ability to cope with the challenges of change. The physician empowers the patient through supportive, encouraging, and tolerant responses.

1. A curious question about how the patient's lifestyle, health, and daily activities involve the unhealthy behavior will offer a glimpse of readiness. "Tell me about your day-to-day activities. How does smoking fit in?"

2. Those who acknowledge ambivalence may be able to compare what Miller and Rollnick call "the good things and the less good things" about the behavior in question. "What are some good things about smoking and some not so good things about smoking?"

3. Patients who can distinguish the benefits from the deficits of a behavior may be ready to receive some information. This should be confirmed first: "Would you like some information about the effect of smoking on health?"

4. For patients who are clearly ready to discuss the problematic aspects of a behavior, ask about their concerns. "What concerns do you have about smoking?"

5. When concerns are expressed, the final step before creating a plan is to ask, "You sound concerned about the effect of smoking on your health. What do you want to do next?" At this point you will hear a commitment to change or hear more ambivalence. Sorting through ambivalence is necessary, predictable, and normal, although time-consuming. The patient who is encouraged to examine goals and values and contrast these with the health implications of current behaviors will fare better than the patient who is simply pressured to change.

The continuing saga of Mr. Lawford in Case 15-1 illustrates several ingredients of successful counseling beginning with curious, empathic, and reflective listening. Dr. Jacobson's pace and choice of questions combined with skillful listening demonstrate his effort to assess the patient's readiness for change. He trusted that helping his patient carefully examine his decisions in the context of their long-term implications would foster a reevaluation of his behaviors. Once Mr. Lawford acknowledged clear concern about the future, a contract for change could be negotiated.

## CASE 15-2

*Dr. Fred Richard entered the room of his next patient, Ms. Laura Thompson.*

DR. R:    *Hello, Laura, how are you doing? How can I help you today?*

MS. T:    *(Looking up briefly, smiles, then eyes drift to the floor) Well ... OK. I want to try to quit. But I'm afraid I'll fail again. (Ms. Thompson had tried to quit smoking on three occasions, each effort lasting at least 6 months but never longer than a year. The most recent relapse occurred a few months ago.)*

DR. R:    *Quitting has been hard for you. (Noting to himself that she seems subdued)*

MS. T:    *Yeah, there is always something that gets in the way.*

DR. R:    *Something that gets in the way ... I'm not sure I understand.*

MS. T:    *Sooner or later something gets to me ... and I get stressed out*

DR. R:    *So something in your life gets hard, and that makes staying away from cigarettes a challenge.*

## COUNSELING SKILLS/REFLECTIVE LISTENING

The most important counseling skill to learn is often simply described in one word—*listening*. If we expand the name of this skill by calling it *reflective listening*, the core listening behaviors become more explicit. The skilled listener incorporates four skills, which can be remembered with the acronym LUCE (listen, understand, clarify, energy).

*Listen.* The skilled practitioner conveys interest and understanding with nonverbal behaviors such as eye contact, head nodding, and a focused body position. Many behaviors are destructive to listening such as looking around the room, standing for long periods of time, folding arms, and clock watching.

*Understand*. Paraphrasing the speaker conveys an understanding of what is heard or perceived, as Dr. R demonstrated in Case 15-2. This is the heart of reflection. True understanding builds compassion. Another benefit of reflection is overlooked. Reflected statements force the speaker to listen to himself. People who seek professional help are frequently stuck in efforts to solve a problem. They go over and over the same ideas, not progressing beyond an invisible barrier. Hearing the sequences of one's own thought forces the speaker to evaluate his reasoning and feelings. The famous "pregnant pause" often occurs after sensitive, accurate reflections. Comfort with silence, lasting 3–5 seconds, is crucial to this process. The patient feels compelled to carry ideas and questions to more evolved states. To beginners, offering reflections and tolerating silence is awkward and slow. Many trainees admit feeling guilty for charging patients for reflective listening. "I didn't do anything" is the frequent novice report.

Two dynamics may interfere with reflective listening, namely, listener disagreement and mixed messages. Efforts to show understanding may be more difficult if the speaker's message conflicts with the listener's beliefs. Remember, understanding is not synonymous with agreement.

The listener should reflect back to the speaker verbal and nonverbal messages. Sometimes verbal and nonverbal messages are incongruent. For example, while frowning, a patient may report feeling "great." Conversely, a patient may describe life as "awful" while wearing a smile. In these situations it is wise to reflect the painful portion of the message. If incongruent messages persist, try reflecting both the verbal and nonverbal messages and then acknowledge confusion. Incongruent communication patterns are often born in families where the honest expression of feelings or ideas is discouraged.

*Clarify*. When the message is unclear or confusing, it is best to ask for clarification. The listener may experience feeling lost, not being able to trace the speaker's progression of reasoning. Confusion may be caused by the speaker switching topics, going on tangents, or lapsing into stories where the meaning is not apparent. Novice physicians will assume that the confusion is the result of a lapse in their own concentration. Most of the time this is not the case. The listener's need for clarification may come from the speaker making a "leap" in reasoning. The novice listener may assume an understanding of the reasoning leap. Whether correct or not, the listener may unwittingly perpetuate dysfunctional thought patterns if clarification is not requested. Whatever the cause, trust yourself. Your confusion is usually diagnostic of confusion within the speaker.

*Energy*. The effective listener puts energy into the relationship. Therapeutic listening is not a passive process. The listener should track the speaker's thought patterns and emotions. Empathy and compassion require energy. It takes energy to monitor one's own emotions, and keep them separate from the experience of the speaker. While listening requires the expenditure of energy, it need not be draining. Experienced healthcare providers regularly leave therapeutic interactions feeling energized. The patient feels an enhanced sense of responsibility and motivation. Helping another person help herself is an honor with its own rewards.

## CASE 15-2 (continued)

*The interview between Dr. Richard and Ms. Thompson, the woman who wants to stop smoking but noted that "sooner or later something gets to me" causing a relapse, continues:*

DR. R: *Something gets to you... ?*
MS. T: *I don't enjoy my work. It's boring and I don't feel valued. I want to get a new job but don't ever seem to do anything about it. The money is too important.*
DR. R: *So your job is not satisfying but it's been hard to look for something else. Anything else?*
MS. T: *My husband and I don't get along. Also, I worry about my daughter. She has a boyfriend who mistreats her.*
DR. R: *You and your husband have some difficulties and you are troubled about your daughter. That sounds like two concerns.*

MS. T:     *Yeah, my husband smokes more than I do.*

DR. R:     *I see. Is this a separate concern from you and your husband not getting along? Or is this part of what makes it hard for the two of you?*

MS. T:     *Well, we fight about other things too. He won't clean up his mess and won't do the laundry. I end up doing too much work.*

DR. R:     *It sounds like you and your husband are having a hard time for several reasons. Outside of your marriage, your concerns at work, and worries about your daughter, does anything else concern you?*

MS. T:     *I wish we made more money, but we get by. It is hard to save and I am tired of living from month to month.*

DR. R:     *I see. Anything else?*

MS. T:     *Not that I can think of.*

DR. R:     *That is a lot of stuff to be thinking about, to have going around and around in your head.*

MS. T:     *Sometimes I just feel worn down and it is just too much.*

DR. R:     *You have begun to separate the areas of stress in your life. These are marital issues such as chores, support for smoking, and how to deal with your daughter's boyfriend. You also mention work and finances. Maybe if you didn't think about them together, but in separate parts, things might be easier to handle. After you chip away at the parts, one at a time, it might be easier to work on stopping the smoking. How does that sound?*

MS. T:     *OK, that makes sense.*

## ESTABLISHING FOCUS (AGENDA SETTING)

Identifying a focus is at the heart of psychological change (Gendlin, 1981). It accomplishes several things. The inability to define discrete, manageable problem areas is characteristic of many who are depressed and anxious. People jump from issue to issue, avoiding a commitment to solving any single problem. This process affects all physician encounters. Not surprisingly, communication experts (Simpson *et al.*, 1991) recommend that successful encounters between physician and patient include agenda setting in the early phase of the interview. If a focus for the interview is *not* overtly established, then one or more problems commonly occur:

1. Physicians and patients pursue mismatched goals because they have not overtly agreed on what problem to work on. This can cause frustration and compromise outcomes
2. More than one problem is addressed at the same time. Such "multitasking" can produce incomplete problem solving ending with plans that are not well thought out and not agreed on by both physician and patient. These interviews often end in a hurry with prescriptions being written and instructions given as physician and patient are walking out of the exam room
3. Agenda items are introduced late in the interview with the dreaded "oh by the way" comments, derailing an organized and thorough problem-solving effort.

In the physician–patient encounter agenda setting occurs in layers. Patients may produce a list of concerns comprised of a series of physical, social, psychological, or behavioral concerns. The first phase of the encounter is devoted to naming and prioritizing the major items on the patient's (and sometimes the physician's) agenda. The second phase of the interview entails identifying a tangible goal related to the problem that is of highest priority. For example, if the initial focus is diabetes, patient and physician must then determine what aspect of diabetes deserves attention first. This might be basic education about sugar metabolism, or learning procedures for testing blood sugar, or discussion about diet or examining the patient's frustration managing a complicated illness. Today's "disease management protocols" recognize that successful outcomes depend on breaking down the healthcare process into parts the patient can readily assimilate. This process applies to common psychosocial problems, too.

Case 15-2 reveals this process. People desiring to change may be paralyzed by multiple, intersecting problems that feel like an undifferentiated glob of pain and confusion. When these problems are dissected and then individually addressed, change will flow more easily. For Ms. Thompson in Case 15-2, finding time to talk about finances and chores with her husband became the focus.

Four useful skills needed to establish focus are:

1. *Make a list.* Before delving into any one problem area, make a list of all concerns you can elicit from the patient. This means never accepting the first answer when inquiring about a patient's concerns. Many people need to be convinced that their physician is genuinely interested in their feelings and concerns. Issues that come out on the second, third, or fourth request ("anything else?") are often associated with more pain and confusion than initially evident. After each request for a new item, wait 2 or 3 seconds. This skill is useful for physicians in all facets of practice.
2. *Avoid premature diving.* After the mention of the first problem, physicians or patients often prematurely dive into asking diagnostic questions (the physician) or telling a story (the patient). This dynamic prevents the creation of a complete list of concerns. Physicians commonly "dive" because they fear long lists will take too much time. As such, it is critical to use some time management strategies. These follow.
3. *Prioritize the list.* Once you are satisfied that the patient has no more concerns to list: (a) review the entire list of concerns; (b) let the patient know that each concern deserves attention and, if the list is too long, determine which issue to address first; (c) suggest follow-up visits for those problems you will not be able to address. *Do not try to do it all in one visit.* In helping patients with chronic illnesses, whether it be diabetes or depression, continuity of care ensures that you and the patient can revisit issues that take time to change.
4. *Negotiate when necessary.* Sometimes you may have a concern that the patient does not list or has placed at a low priority. For example, if your concern is about chest pain, domestic violence, substance abuse, or suicidal thought, you are ethically and legally obliged to pursue these problems. In these situations it is always important to acknowledge the patient's priorities before expressing your concerns. A common mistake is for providers to prioritize this list without patient input. This "provider-centered" approach risks missing the area of greatest concern to the patient. The patient may feel discounted or misunderstood. In such cases, the patient is less likely to follow through with plans that end up feeling imposed.

Once a full list of concerns is created and prioritized, then the visit has focus. The next task is to develop a refined, deeper understanding of the problem. One way of gaining a deeper understanding of the most important problem is to BATHE the patient.

## THE BATHE APPROACH

BATHE (Stuart & Lieberman, 1993) is an acronym developed by psychologist Marion R. Stuart and family physician Joseph A. Lieberman to begin the counseling process. The acronym is a clever mnemonic because it conjures up images of immersing the patient in a cleansing process. The questions included in the BATHE approach may be used to start visits and in response to a patient's request for help. Here we examine what constitutes "BATHEing" a patient.

*B* reminds you to examine the background of the patient. Stuart and Lieberman suggest using the question, "What is going on in your life?" as one way to begin all primary care encounters. This question begins to establish a focus by asking the patient to describe important life events. Gaining insight into current and past life experiences is essential to understanding and placing the patient's response in an appropriate context. If the answer to this question is a list of health concerns, the establishing focus protocol above can help focus the visit.

*A* reminds you to attend to the affect of the patient. Stuart and Lieberman recommend asking, "How do you feel about what is going on?" Helping patients identify and describe feelings is as central to counseling as balance is to riding a bicycle. Left unexpressed, feelings that build up promote anxiety and depression. Stored emotions are eventually expressed in some fashion, but often in a way that is out of control. These out-of-control expressions of emotion can erode self-esteem or damage relationships, worsening the patient's situation.

Many people do not use a "feeling language." Words such as *sad, lonely, scared, inadequate,* and *disappointed* are not evident in the way they describe troubles. Even in response to a direct question about feelings, many will answer with a statement about how they think. Consistently asking "How are you feeling?" or "How is this for you?" will help them learn to identify and express their feelings. Sometimes even asking about specific feelings is necessary because it teaches a vocabulary of feelings. An empathic reflection ("You were sad when your friend left") or an empathic inquiry ("I imagine you were sad when your friend left?") helps patients name their feelings. However, be prepared that your perception of the feeling that the patient experiences may not agree with the patient's. ("No, I wasn't sad, I was lonely.")

*T* reminds you to ask what most troubles the patient. Asking "What about this situation troubles you the most?" will help establish focus. As discussed earlier, it is important to help patients name which problems are of most concern.

*H* reminds you to ask how the patient is handling the problem. "How are you handling the problem?" The answer to this question provides information about what has and has not worked to solve the problem. Common areas of difficulty in "handling" problems include: family relationships, thought patterns, educational issues, and underappreciated strengths and successes. These areas will be discussed in the section below on Problem Solving Therapy.

*E* reminds you that the expression of empathy validates the patient's feelings. Empathy is the oxygen of counseling. If it is not present, the counseling effort will suffocate.

After you BATHE the patient you will have a refined understanding of his or her distress. The next step is to move into creating workable solutions. Problem Solving Therapy (PST) is a counseling approach that embodies elements of Establishing Focus and BATHEing but goes on to help the patient design a plan. It has been taught to primary care physicians and nurse practitioners with consultation from experienced psychotherapists, tested in a series of randomized controlled trials (Mynors-Wallis, 1996, 2000). These studies found PST to be more effective than placebo and as effective as antidepressant medications. Below are the basic steps of PST.

1. *Explanation of the treatment process and its rationale.* The clinician outlines the steps described below.
2. *Clarification and definition of the problems.* This step is the first part of an agenda-setting process that began when you established focus and continued during the BATHE process. Common areas of difficulty include the following.
   - *Family relationships.* Patients may have difficulty in managing relationships. Helping patients learn communication and negotiation skills is helpful. Patients may not recognize that their emotional pain extends from relationship dynamics in nuclear families or families of origin. The patient may be assuming disproportional responsibility for family problems. Others in the family may have unappreciated painful feelings. In these cases, including spouses, parents, and children in counseling is a productive and efficient means of facilitating change (McDaniel *et al.*, 1990).
   - *Thought patterns.* It is prudent to assess the thought patterns of patients. People who experience anxiety or depression often create self-defeating ("I'm not smart enough"), self-deprecating ("I'm not attractive"), and catastrophic ("I'll get fired") thoughts. In a parallel manner, these patients imagine that they are seen in a negative way by others ("He doesn't think I am capable" or "She doesn't care how I feel"). Dysfunctional family patterns are often the source of these negative thoughts. Negative thoughts create emotional pain. Helping patients become aware of their negative thoughts, learn ways to stop creating them, and replace them with self-accepting thoughts decreases emotional pain. This approach, termed *cognitive therapy*, is effective in the treatment of depression and anxiety (Burns, 1980).

- *Educational issues.* Education helps motivated patients who lack the knowledge about how to handle stressful life circumstances. For example, struggling parents, couples with communication difficulties, or those with financial problems can benefit from education

- *Underappreciated strengths and successes.* Patients may not recognize their own strengths and successes. Dwelling on failures and hopelessness can take on a life of its own. Pessimistic views of the world may become self-fulfilling prophecies. In the last 15 years, psychotherapists have emphasized "solution-oriented" approaches (Berg, 1994), and more recently, these have been adapted to use by physicians (Giorlando & Schilling, 1997). In essence, physicians can help patients find "exceptions" to their failures. Examining the characteristics of these unusual successes and expanding their use is the strategy of counseling.

3. *Choice of achievable goals.* In this step, the goal setting is refined. Goals are selected that are discrete and can be realistically accomplished in a reasonable period of time. In Case 15-2 Ms. Thompson may have chosen to work on the relationship with her husband and the first step was to find time to talk about chores, specifically taking out the garbage and loading the dishwasher.

4. *Generation of alternative solutions.* The patient is asked to brainstorm a list of possible solutions. All ideas are included to encourage a creative exploration of options. Ms. Thompson listed several ways to engage her husband: confronting him, leaving him a note, having a neighbor talk to him, not taking out the garbage or emptying the dishwasher, and arranging a time to talk in advance.

5. *Selection of a preferred solution.* The clinician and patient decide on one plan based on feasibility and the direct connection to the initial goal. She settled on asking him for time ahead of time, preferably on the weekend.

6. *Clarification of the necessary steps to implement the solution.* A careful plan is outlined, often rehearsed, and possible obstacles are predicted. Dr. Richard coached Ms. Thompson to practice her approach. They predicted obstacles to success like poor timing, using a critical or demanding tone, or being vague about when to meet.

7. *Evaluation of progress.* The patient reviews the problem-solving effort. Successes are celebrated. Strategies are refined. When failures occur, then reassessment of goals may be indicated. Ms. Thompson returned the following week to report on progress. Her husband was willing to talk and they met over the weekend. After some discussion, he agreed to take out the garbage and fill the dishwasher on the weekdays. She felt better and told him so.

The PST process is designed to address concerns that the patient, not the provider, identifies as most important. The learning of this counseling approach is done best in consultation with experienced psychotherapists.

---

## CASE 15-3

*Mr. Oakly developed a bleeding ulcer. In addition to direct medical management, his physician, Dr. Claren, thought it wise to learn about her patient's world. Mr. Oakly worked as a supervisor in a software company. His job was difficult because it seemed that those he supervised needed to be "checked on constantly." Now, at age 45, Mr. Oakly was in his second marriage, in which he had his third child, 10-year-old Mark, and was the primary parent for his children from the first marriage, 17-year-old Craig and 16-year-old Julie. Julie had struggled through high school, failing a few courses, and had begun experimenting with alcohol. He and his second wife, Tricia, had developed marital problems and blamed their difficulties on Julie. Mr. Oakly admitted that it was hard to trust Tricia as a parent for his children, particularly his daughter. However, he did describe Tricia as a competent, loving person.*

*Mr. Oakly was the oldest child in a family where his father was absent much of the time. His mother was depressed during much of his childhood and drank alcohol excessively. He raised his two younger siblings. As an adult he was married at 24 and divorced at 30. He left his wife, Nancy, who abused alcohol and drugs and did not care for their two children.*

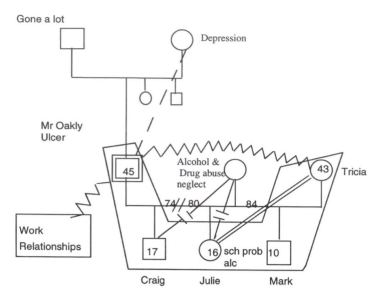

**Figure 15.1.** Oakly family genogram.

*Through asking questions about Mr. Oakly's relationships and life events, Dr. Claren con-structed a genogram (see Fig. 15.1), a map of Mr. Oakly's relational world. In studying his family history, it became apparent to Mr. Oakly that he had difficulty trusting the work of others, par-ticularly women, because of his experiences in his family of origin and his marriage. At work his supervisees felt that he "hovered" too much. Tricia complained about his interference in her relationship with Julie. Julie needed a supportive connection with an adult female. Mr. Oakly agreed to meet with his wife and physician. Dr. Claren helped Mrs. Oakly express her frustration and concerns. During subsequent family meetings that included Julie and then all three children, the family acknowledged their love and concern for Mr. Oakly, but described him as "too controlling." He agreed to "pull back" and be more supportive of his wife's role in the family and more trusting of his children.*

*One year later Mr. Oakly was symptom-free. His daughter was doing better in her last year of high school. Mr. Oakly took his lessons from home into work. He felt relief in pulling back from hovering over his supervisees.*

## UNDERSTANDING PATIENTS IN LARGER CONTEXTS

The biopsychosocial model (Engel, 1980) is a problem-solving method useful for many of the challenges in clinical medicine. This model, based in systems theory, served as the framework for Dr. Claren in helping Mr. Oakly and his family. While it is beyond the scope of this chapter to describe the biopsychosocial model and systems theory in detail, a few applications will be provided:

1. *If 2 + 2 ≠ 4, it is time to examine the patient in her surrounding contexts.* There are two common examples of "things not adding up": (a) when symptoms persist after treatment is administered or (b) when the cause of symptoms is not apparent or does not make sense. Examples of surrounding contexts are: a marital or couple's relationship, the nuclear family, the family of origin, the work setting, the community, the culture. A large proportion, if not all, of human experience and human behavior is influenced by relationships in one of these domains. In Case 15-3, Mr. Oakly's family of origin and marital experience made it difficult for him to rely on women and to trust his supervisees.

2. *Look for circles and tree branches.* A patient's symptom can be seen as (a) part of a circular chain of events that go around and around or (b) created by several, seemingly independent causes converging to

## DOES ETHICAL CARE MEAN BETTER CARE?

*Ethicists argue that respecting patient autonomy is a central principle defining proper care. While this issue is most apparent in decisions around death and dying, the principle holds for all health care encounters. But does ethical care mean better care?*

*In the last 10 to 15 years a branch of research has examined the relationship between providers who are more "autonomy supportive" and healthcare outcomes. The results of these studies show that patients who rank their providers as more supportive of their autonomy have better health outcomes with social and psychological well-being, weight control, diabetes management, and medication adherence (Ryan & Deci, 2000; Williams et al., 2000). A similar finding is evident in the psychotherapy literature where a central predictor of therapeutic success is the therapist and client alliance. A common cause of "alliance ruptures" is when the therapist, without patient input, chooses the therapeutic goal and/or treatment modality (Safran & Muran, 2000). In this chapter all of the approaches presented—motivational interviewing, establishing focus, BATHE, and Problem Solving Therapy—rely heavily on patient involvement in decision making about therapeutic goals.*

*How often are patients involved in clinical decision making? Braddock et al. (1999) analyzed 1057 audiotaped outpatient encounters containing 3552 decisions. They assessed the presence of seven elements of informed decision making. Below is a list of those elements followed by the percentage of interviews in which the element was determined to be present:*

*1. Discussion of the patient's role in decision making* — 5.9%
*2. Discussion of the clinical issue or nature of the decision* — 71%
*3. Discussion of alternatives* — 11.3%
*4. Discussion of pros and cons of alternatives* — 7.8%
*5. Discussion of uncertainties associated with the decision* — 4.1%
*6. Assessment of the patient's understanding* — 1.5%
*7. Exploration of patient preference* — 21%

*The subjects in the Braddock et al. study were primary care physicians and surgeons. No psychotherapists were included and I am not aware of any similar surveys of psychotherapists but suspect the results would be the same. As can be seen, there is a powerful force undergirding physician dominance in the healthcare encounter. How often do you elicit patient involvement in decision making? What are the barriers to doing this? How can you overcome these barriers?*

---

produce symptoms. Mr. Oakly's family contains an example of "circular causation." He interfered with the relationship between his wife and daughter. The absence of a female parent figure contributed to his daughter's behavioral and school problems. Mr. Oakly's effort to solve his daughter's problem created tension between him and his daughter and between him and his wife. Several sources of stress converging to create or inflame a symptom creates a tree branch design. This is known as multicausality. A combination of stresses in Mr. Oakly's life including work difficulties, conflict with his daughter, conflict with his wife, and worry about his daughter contributed to his ulcer symptoms.

3. *Families need effective leadership.* Systems need a hierarchical organization for optimal function. As a cell needs a nucleus, so does a family need effective parents. When parents are ineffective, absent, abusive, or in conflict with one another, children often exhibit behavioral or emotional problems, e.g., school difficulties, fighting, stealing, withdrawal, disobedience, or physical symptoms such as headaches, stomachaches, chronic illness instability. Julie's symptoms are related to insufficient connections to a female parent and to conflict between her parents.

Using systems thinking to solve problems means looking for the interrelatedness of things. Two skills are helpful in making systemic assessments and initiating treatment: (a) asking relationship questions and (b) constructing a genogram.

## RELATIONSHIP QUESTIONS

A relationship question asks the interviewee to think about relationships and begins the process of examining a problem in context. A relationship question is created to test a hypothesis. For example, in knowing of Julie's problems in Case 15-3, Dr. Claren reasoned that relationships in her life may be troublesome. Dr. Claren was also curious about connections between Mr. Oakly's symptoms and his daughter's difficulties. A series of questions designed to assess the Oakly family might include: "Mr. Oakly, how are things between you and your daughter?" and "What is the relationship like between your wife and Julie?" Sometimes it is helpful to compare perspectives on a relationship. Noting differences can stimulate change. "How does Julie feel about Tricia as a stepmother?" "How is it for Tricia to be a stepparent for Julie?" "What has the relationship been like between Julie and her biological mother, Nancy?" The answers to these questions might reveal Julie's need for a female parent figure. It is useful to ask questions that include three parties. For example, "Mr. Oakly, how do you feel about Tricia as a parent for Julie?" Then, "How does Tricia feel when you prevent her from parenting Julie?"

These questions are particularly helpful to physicians who usually see only one person in a family but need to know about the perspectives of others. The use of these questions extends beyond family problems. Family beliefs and support, or lack thereof, have enormous influence on the course of chronic illnesses. For example, after suggesting dietary changes to an overweight man with hypertension, like Mr. Lawford in Case 15-1, it would be wise to ask, "How will it be for your wife to change her cooking?"

In summary, relationship questions are constructed in the following way: (1) They extend from the clinician's curiosity about the connection between interpersonal relationships and physical symptoms. (2) Two or more people are included in each question. The person to whom the question is asked is not always the focus of the question. That is, you may ask one person about the relationship between two or more others. (3) Questions may also be constructed to compare perspectives between people. This is done by first asking for one person's perspective on a relationship and then asking for another person's perspective on the same relationship. Additional information on relationship questions, also called *circular questions*, can be found in Mauksch and Roesler (1990) and Cole-Kelly and Seaburn (1999).

## USING A GENOGRAM

Over the last 15 years the genogram has emerged as a versatile, efficient method for storing family information (McGoldrick *et al.*, 1999). In fact, a genogram, introduced in Chapter 20, is more than just a recordkeeping device. Its maplike format forces the clinician and patient to view problems in context, essentially, to think systemically. Genograms help clinicians develop hypotheses that, in turn, guide treatment efforts.

The genogram is an adaptation of the pedigree or family tree used in genetics. In addition to basic family structure, it includes information about age, marital status, major illnesses, life events, and important relationships.

When familiar with genogram symbols, this format (see Fig. 15.1) conveys a lot of information about Mr. Oakly and his family in Case 15-3. The jagged line between Mr. Oakly and Tricia and between Mr. Oakly and his work describes a conflictual relationship. The dashed line between Mr. Oakly and his mother describes a distant relationship. The lines between Craig, Julie, and their mother denote a "cut-off" relationship. The double line between Julie and Tricia describes a close relationship. The line surrounding Mr. Oakly, the children, and Tricia denotes the people living together with Mr. Oakly. This genogram displays the combination of stresses in the various relationships in Mr. Oakly's world. Imagine knowing nothing about Mr. Oakly before seeing this genogram. If you were told that Mr. Oakly suffered from a stress-related disorder, such as irritable bowel, hypertension, or an ulcer, what would your reaction be? For most of us, possible causes jump off the page on viewing Mr. Oakly in his network of his relationships. (See Chapter 20 for more on genograms.)

Genograms record pregnancies, including history of termination, miscarriage, or stillbirth, overclose relationships, major life events, religious information, and significant relationships with friends. The minimal time necessary to complete a detailed genogram is 12 to 15 minutes and revisions occur during subsequent visits. When physicians construct a genogram, patients feel cared for and understood. While it may not be practical to draw a genogram during every patient visit, there are certain times when it pays to do so. These times include the following situations:

- When symptoms persist despite expected resolution
- When symptoms do not make sense
- When a severe or chronic illness is diagnosed
- When there are psychosocial problems

---

## CASE 15-4

*Dr. Michaels finished performing the fourth termination of pregnancy for his patient, Ms. Stanley. During the procedure she was very tearful. In his office, after the procedure, they talked. In the back of Dr. Michaels's mind were Ms. Stanley's frequent visits to his office. Her life seemed to be in constant chaos. She described feeling overwhelmed in the last 6 months. Dr. Michaels asked if she would consider seeing a counselor. Ms. Stanley was afraid to talk with someone about her problems because she feared "falling apart" and being diagnosed as "crazy." Her family didn't believe in seeing "head doctors." Dr. Michaels explained that he worked with a family counselor, Mr. Phillips. He assured Ms. Stanley that she was not crazy nor would counseling make her crazy. He described the counseling process and the personal characteristics of Mr. Phillips. Ms. Stanley was assured that he (Dr. Michaels) would stay involved in her care. She agreed to meet the counselor. A few minutes later, Mr. Phillips was introduced to Ms. Stanley. Dr. Michaels summarized his concerns about Ms. Stanley to Mr. Phillips while Ms. Stanley listened. They made an initial follow-up appointment.*

*Six months later, Ms. Stanley had seen Mr. Phillips ten times and sorted out many of her issues. Her father had sexualized their relationship. He was gone from the home for long periods of time during her early childhood. When her parents divorced, he rarely saw the children, often not showing up when he promised to visit. As a teenager and young adult, Ms. Stanley had a series of relationships with abusive men. Therapy helped her to build self-esteem and become more selective in choosing men. Medical utilization decreased. Regular communications between Dr. Michaels and Mr. Phillips improved care and saved money. When Ms. Stanley spoke about physical problems to Mr. Phillips, he discussed these with Dr. Michaels, often saving unnecessary tests and visits. Each member of this treatment triangle regularly received input from two others, creating an atmosphere of stability and enhanced quality of care.*

## COLLABORATION BETWEEN NONPSYCHIATRIC PHYSICIANS AND MENTAL HEALTH PROFESSIONALS

There are several reasons why mental health professionals and medical providers should work together. Yet, significant barriers prevent collaboration between these two professional worlds.

Why should mental health providers and medical providers work together? The majority of mental health problems present first in the general medical arena (Regier *et al.*, 1993). The highest healthcare users have a complicated mix of medical and psychosocial problems (Katon *et al.*, 1992). For a variety of reasons, most patients resist referrals "away" from their physician. However, when patients are referred to a mental health provider in the same clinic, referrals are more likely to be accepted. Mental health consultation and treatment improves quality of care and can help control costs (Von Korff *et al.*, 1998). Beyond quality and cost savings, professional rewards are notable. Working in an interdisciplinary team provides a support and educational network.

How can the chasm between mental health and medicine be so great when there are so many reasons to work together? Seventeenth-century Cartesian thought, often described as "mind–body dualism," has persisted in its influence (McDaniel, 1995). Despite what we know about the myriad of interactions between the mind and the body, healthcare systems still function as if these connections did not exist. Insurance benefits for mental health do not equal medical benefits, creating financial barriers to treatment (Glenn, 1987). Members of each profession have maintained derogatory stereotypes of one another. Mental health care has always had stigma attached to it. Patients may not have family support for seeing a psychotherapist. Many patients somatize their psychological pain and reject the notion that psychosocial help is relevant. For these reasons and more it is hard to bring mental health and medicine together.

In the last 15 years a variety of books (Blount, 1998; Cummings *et al.*, 1997; Seaburn *et al.*, 1996), articles, journals (see the journal *Families, Systems and Health*), and conferences have explored collaboration. Primary care training in family medicine, general internal medicine, and pediatrics includes behavioral science curricula. The vast majority of family medicine residencies have behavioral science faculty who help create collaborative practice models in training. The influx of managed care demands that professionals from all healthcare disciplines collaborate. The new catchphrase, "integrated care," expresses the need for professionals to educate one another and to avoid duplication of services. Because the majority of medical visits involve a psychosocial component, integrated care should include mental health professionals. Listed below are a few guidelines for collaboration.

1. Arrange to have interdisciplinary teams working together in the same setting. Working in the same setting ensures a level of communication between professionals that is otherwise impossible to maintain, as demonstrated in Case 15-4. This communication creates better care, saves money, and ensures interdisciplinary education.
2. Let your patients know that you work as a part of a team. Patients appreciate when providers communicate with each other to coordinate care.
3. Work to develop relationships with collaborators. Ongoing collaboration means respectful and open communication. Develop mechanisms that facilitate communication such as shared charts, interdisciplinary conferences, and office designs that create proximity instead of distance.
4. Establish a shared purpose or vision for collaboration. Ask yourself, "Why am I collaborating?" Ask your colleague, "Why is collaboration important to you?" Sharing these reasons strengthens relationships.
5. Be suspicious of your feelings of distrust of another provider. Complicated patients often deal with the world in a black-and-white way. They split relationships into "good guys" and "bad guys." This behavior, which is usually habitual, can create conflict between team members. In these situations it makes sense to communicate directly with other providers and avoid solely communicating through the patient.

## CONCLUSION

In this chapter we have examined counseling and behavioral change. Effective counseling means mastering skills like empathic listening, reflective listening, and intentional curiosity. These are summarized in the acronym LUCE. In the course of helping patients change behavior, it is essential to assess readiness for change. This assessment helps create realistic expectations of the patient, reducing "noncompliance" problems and physician–patient conflicts. Helping patients establish and maintain a focus in any medical visit creates an efficient and productive process. A useful way to organize a counseling approach is via BATHE, wherein reflection, focus, and empathy are core components. Proceeding with a Problem Solving approach has been shown to be very helpful. Respecting individual, family, and cultural beliefs is critical in building respect and creating viable treatment plans. Effective counseling requires an ability to monitor the physician–patient relationship. It is essential to examine the patient in the context of important relationships, including the family of origin, the nuclear family, and the school and work setting. Relationship questioning and genograms are two useful tools for assessing relationships. The physician counselor must become an expert in relationships.

Physicians of the twenty-first century, along with other healthcare providers, will work in interdisciplinary teams. These teams can provide better care, save money, and create work atmospheres that maintain vitality and prevent provider burnout. In this regard, it is important to develop collaborative relationships with mental health professionals to create healthcare systems that mirror the complex and dynamic nature of the patients and families we serve.

# CASES FOR DISCUSSION

## CASE 1

*Mr. Anderson asked his physician, Dr. Maxwell, for help with recurrent sleep difficulties. He finds it hard to get to sleep. Once he falls asleep he stays asleep until 9:00 or 10:00 AM. Mr. Anderson, who is unemployed, spends much of his days sitting around. He naps frequently, watches TV, and rarely goes to bed before midnight. He drinks beer most evenings. His wife works a swing shift.*

*Following a series of questions in an interview directed by Dr. Maxwell, Mr. Anderson is told not to nap during the day and to cut down on his drinking. Three weeks later, Mr. Anderson returns, still complaining about sleep difficulty. He is still drinking most evenings and naps most days. He says, "Doc, it was hard to do those things you suggested."*

1. *What approach would you use in working with this patient?*
2. *What are the disadvantages of being too directive and prescriptive early on in treatment?*
3. *How would you assess this patient's stage of readiness?*
4. *What else might you want to know about the patient's family?*

## CASE 2

*A colleague asks you for some advice. He wants to learn counseling skills and has found a patient with whom he wants to work. However, he feels overwhelmed. During the first visit, his patient, a 35-year-old married mother of two boys, aged 2 and 4, noted the following concerns: parenting difficulties with the 2-year-old, some symptoms of depression including lethargy, sleep disturbance, weight gain, and dysphoria. She also noted a lack of sexual interest from her husband and some questions about her dormant professional life.*

1. *Is this an appropriate patient for your physician colleague to counsel?*
2. *If this patient were to receive counseling in primary care, what advice would you offer in response to your colleague's feelings of being overwhelmed? If not, how should the physician handle the next visit?*

## CASE 3

*Mr. and Ms. Foreman come to you with concerns about their 12-year-old daughter, Rachel. One evening last week, after asking her to help clean the dinner table, she exploded. Loud objections and obscenities shocked the parents. Similar outbursts have occurred four or five times in the last year. Ms. Foreman and her husband appear to disagree about how to handle these situations, but both express concern and some anger about their daughter's behavior. Mr. Foreman notes that when he was a child his parents would never have tolerated such behavior. "I would have felt someone's hand," he said. "That kind of discipline doesn't work," fired back Ms. Foreman.*

*The Foremans are a family of six. The oldest child is a 15-year-old boy. Rachel is the next oldest, with younger sisters aged 9 and 7. Ms. Foreman doesn't work outside of the home, but is very involved in community activities related to their children's interests. Mr. Foreman works long hours as a civil engineer and has to travel frequently. The Foremans report having had similar difficulties with their oldest child when he was about 13.*

1. *Construct a genogram from this description and consider what information is missing.*
2. *What hypotheses can you formulate about this family's difficulties?*
3. *What relationship questions would you want to ask to test your hypotheses?*

## CASE 4

*A 35-year-old patient, Mr. Rosner, has made several visits to you in the last 6 months. He has multiple physical complaints, most of which are unresponsive to your suggested treatments. You know that last year his wife was diagnosed with ovarian cancer. He has been assuming the bulk of family responsibilities, cleaning, paying bills, parenting. On today's visit he tells you about a series of anxiety attacks in the last few weeks. To calm himself down and help him sleep he is drinking one or two glasses of wine each night.*

*In the past you have suggested that Mr. Rosner consider counseling. He has never received this suggestion with much enthusiasm. Since his last visit, your practice has expanded to include a medical family therapist.*

1. *What hypotheses do you have about the cause of Mr. Rosner's symptoms?*
2. *To determine the effect of his behavior on the family, what relationship questions would you construct?*
3. *You decide that it would be helpful to share this case with your new family therapist colleague, but feel leery about suggesting the referral because of Mr. Rosner's prior disinterest in counseling. How would you approach this referral with Mr. Rosner?*
4. *Would you consult with the family therapist first?*

## CASE 5

*You receive a call from Dr. Reed, a local psychologist, about Richard McClure, a 14-year-old patient of yours. A school counselor referred Richard to Dr. Reed for behavior problems and suspicion of drug abuse. Dr. Reed has just completed his first visit with Richard and would like to learn about his family whom you have worked with for 12 years.*

*You know that Mr. McClure, Richard's father, has a history of alcohol abuse. He has had two marital separations and 1 year ago you prescribed an antidepressant for Mrs. McClure. You suspect that there are multiple family problems. Despite having concern about this family, you feel ineffective, indeed powerless, in your efforts to treat or refer them.*

*Now Dr. Reed is on the phone. You have three patients waiting and are 30 minutes behind, but you want to talk about your experience with this family and to learn from Dr. Reed how to help the McClures and others like them.*

1. *What information do you share with Dr. Reed?*
2. *How can you arrange to keep in touch with him to learn about working with multiple-problem families?*
3. *What services can you offer to augment Dr. Reed's treatment effort?*

## REFERENCES

Beckman H, Markakis K, Suchman A, Frankel R: The doctor–patient relationship and malpractice: Lessons from plaintiff depositions. *Arch Intern Med* 154(12):1365–1370, 1994.

Berg I: *Family-Based Services: A Solution Focused Approach.* New York, WW Norton & Co, Inc, 1994.

Blount A: *Integrated Primary Care: The Future of Medical and Mental Health Collaboration.* New York, WW Norton & Co, Inc, 1998.

Braddock CH 3rd, Edwards KA, Hasenberg NM, Laidley TL, Levinson W: Informed decision making in outpatient practice: Time to get back to basics [see comments]. *JAMA* 282:2313–2320, 1999.

Burns D: *Feeling Good: The New Mood Therapy.* New York, Avon Books, 1980.

Clark LT: Improving compliance and increasing control of hypertension: Needs of special hypertensive populations. *Amer Heart J* 121:664–669, 1991.

Cole-Kelly K, Seaburn D: Five areas of questioning to promote a family-oriented approach in primary care. *Fam Syst Health* 17:341–348, 1999.

Cummings NA, Cummings JL, Johnson J-N: *Behavioral Health in Primary Care: A Guide for Clinical Integration.* Madison, Psychological Press, 1997.

Dugdale DC, Epstein R, Pantilat SZ: Time and the patient–physician relationship. *J Gen Intern Med* 14(suppl 1):S34–S40, 1999.

Engel GL: The clinical application of the biopsychosocial model. *Am J Psychiatry* 7:535–544, 1980.

Gendlin ET: *Focusing*. New York, Bantam Books, Inc, 1981.

Giorlando ME, Schilling RJ: On becoming a solution-focused physician: The MED-STAT acronym. *Fam Syst Health* 15:361–373, 1997.

Glenn M: *Collaborative Health Care: A Family Oriented Model*. New York, Praeger Pubs, 1987.

Katon W: The effect of major depression on chronic medical illness. *Semin Clin Neuropsychiatry* 3:82–86, 1998.

Katon W, Von Korff M, Lin E, Bush T, Russo J, Lipscomb P, Wagner E: A randomized trial of psychiatric consultation with distressed high utilizers. *Gen Hosp Psychiatry* 14: 86–98, 1992.

Leedham B, Meyerowitz BE, Muirhead J, Frist WH: Positive expectations predict health after heart transplantation. *Health Psychol* 14(1):74–79, 1995.

Levinson W, Gorawara-Bhat R, Lamb J: A study of patient clues and physician responses in primary care and surgical settings. *JAMA* 284:1021–1027, 2000.

Like R, Steiner P: Medical anthropology and the family physician. *Fam Med* 19(2):87–92, 1986.

Mauksch L, Roesler T: Expanding the context of the patient's explanatory model using circular questioning. *Fam Syst Med* 8(1):3–13, 1990.

McDaniel S: Collaboration between psychologists and family physicians: Implementing the biopsychosocial model. *Prof Psychol Res Pract* 26(2):117–122, 1995.

McDaniel S, Campbell T, Seaburn D: *Family-Oriented Primary Care: A Manual for Medical Providers*. Berlin, Springer-Verlag, 1990.

McGoldrick M, Gerson R, Schellenberger S: *Genograms in Family Assessment*. New York, WW Norton & Co, Inc, 1999.

Miller HN: Compliance with treatment regimens in chronic asymptomatic diseases [Epidemiology and Treatment of Hypercholesterolemia: Where We Are Today]. *Am J Med* 102(2suppl):43–49, 1997.

Miller W, Rollnick S: *Motivational Interviewing: Preparing People to Change Addictive Behavior*. New York, Guilford Press, 1991.

Mynors-Wallis L: Problem-solving treatment: Evidence for effectiveness and feasibility in primary care. *Int J Psychiatry Med* 26: 249–262, 1996.

Mynors-Wallis LM, Gath DH, Baker F: Randomized controlled trial of problem solving treatment, antidepressant medications, and combined treatment for major depression in primary care. *Br Med J* 320:26–30, 2000.

Patterson CH: *Theories of Counseling and Psychotherapy*. New York, Harper & Row Publishers Inc, 1986.

Prochaska JO, DiClemente CC: Transtheoretical therapy: Toward a more integrative model of change. *Psychother Theory Res Pract* 19:276–288, 1982.

Prochaska J, Velicer W, Rossi J, Goldstein M, Marcus B, Radowski W, Fiore C, Harlow L, Redding C, Rosenbloom D, Rossi S: Stages of change and decisional balance for 12 problem behaviors. *Health Psychol* 13(1):39–46, 1994.

Regier DA, Goldberg ID, Taube CA: The de facto US mental health services system: A public health perspective. *Arch Gen Psychiatry* 35:685–693, 1978.

Regier DA, Narrow WE, Rae DS, Manderscheid RW, Locke BZ, Goodwin FK: The de facto US mental and addictive disorders service system. Epidemiologic catchment area prospective 1-year prevalence rates of disorders and services. *Arch Gen Psychiatry* 50:85–94, 1993.

Rollnick S, Mason P, Butler C: *Health Behavior Change*. Edinburgh, Churchill Livingstone, 1999.

Roter DL, Stewart M, Putnam SM, Lipkin M Jr, Stiles W, Inui TS: Communication patterns of primary care physicians. *JAMA* 277: 350–356, 1997.

Ryan RM, Deci EL: Self-determination theory and the facilitation of intrinsic motivation, social development, and well-being. *Amer Psychol* 55(1):68–78, 2000.

Safran J, Muran J: Resolving therapeutic alliance ruptures: Diversity and integration. *J Clin Psychol* 56:233–243, 2000.

Schurman R, Kramer P, Mitchell J: The hidden mental health network: Treatment of mental illness by nonpsychiatrist physicians. *Arch Gen Psychiatry* 42:89–94, 1985.

Seaburn DB, Gawanski BA, Gunn WB, Lorenz A, Mauksch L: *Models of Collaboration: A Guide for Mental Health Professionals Working with Physicians and Health Care Practitioners*. New York, Basic Books Inc, 1996.

Simpson M, Buckman R, Stewart M, Maguire P, Lipkin M, Novack D, Till J: Doctor–patient communication: The Toronto consensus statement. *Br Med J* 303:1385–1387, 1991.

Stuart M, Lieberman J: *The Fifteen Minute Hour: Applied Psychotherapy for the Primary Care Physician*, ed 2. New York, Praeger Publishers, 1993.

Von Korff M, Katon W, Bush T, *et al*: Treatment costs, cost offset, and cost-effectiveness of collaborative management of depression. *Psychosom Med* 60:143–149, 1998.

Williams G, Frankel R, Campbell T, Deci E: Research on relationship-centered care and healthcare outcomes from the Rochester Biopsychosocial Program: A self-determination theory integration. *Fam Syst Health* 18:79–90, 2000.

Wilson J, Braunwald E, Isselbacher K, Petersdorf R, Martin J, Fauci A, Root R (eds): *Harrison's Principles of Internal Medicine*. New York, McGraw-Hill Book Co, 1991.

## CHAPTER 16

# Functional Assessment

*Kathleen R. Farrell*

*Mr. Kim, an 82-year-old man with a history of dementia, hypertension, and osteoarthritis, visited the physician's office because of his wife's concerns that her husband "hadn't been himself" lately. Questioning by the physician revealed that the patient had strained his back 2 weeks earlier while helping his wife move a table. When prompted, the patient complained of back pain, and Mrs. Kim reported that her husband now spent most of his time lying on a couch. His appetite diminished, he slept fitfully, and he had worsening constipation. Mrs. Kim now needed to help her spouse with bathing and dressing. Two days before the visit, she borrowed a neighbor's cane for her husband because he appeared unsteady when walking. Being frail herself, Mrs. Kim worried about her own health and inability to continue caring for her husband. She asked the physician if her husband needed placement in a nursing home.*

*On examination, Mr. Kim had marked kyphosis and point tenderness at the L1 and L2 spine levels. His gait was hesitant and unsteady. He held the borrowed cane incorrectly as he walked, and the physician observed that it was incorrectly adjusted for Mr. Kim's height. A rectal examine showed a large amount of hard stool in the rectal vault. Lumbar spine x-rays revealed diffuse osteopenia with a new compression fracture at L1 and old fractures at T10 and L4.*

*Mr. Kim had become deconditioned and fecally impacted from back pain and inactivity. The physician prescribed scheduled analgesics for the back pain and laxatives for the fecal impaction. A social worker arranged for a home health aide to help Mr. Kim bathe, and a physical therapist organized an exercise program for him. A month later, Mr. Kim had minimal back pain and normal bowel movements. He displayed increased strength, endurance, and appetite. He walked independently with a pistol-grip cane correctly adjusted for his height.*

## EDUCATIONAL OBJECTIVES

1. Contrast the traditional medical model of care with the functional model
2. List five characteristics of geriatric patients that affect function
3. Define and list the components of functional assessment

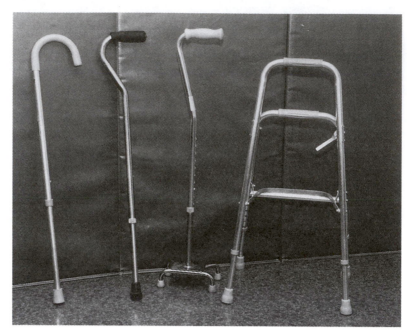

**Figure 16.1.** From left to right: A traditional single-prong cane with curved handle, a single-prong cane with pistol grip, a quadripod cane with pistol grip, and a hemi-walker.

4. List the Activities of Daily Living
5. List the Instrumental Activities of Daily Living
6. Describe the components of mobility
7. Describe the indications for and the correct use of common ambulatory devices
8. Describe how to evaluate gait and balance
9. Define comprehensive geriatric assessment
10. List five benefits of comprehensive geriatric assessment

## INTRODUCTION

Case 16-1 illustrates a common situation that physicians encounter when treating older adults, namely, a patient who presents with multiple—and often ill-defined—problems. Rather than describing specific signs or symptoms, the patient or caregiver describes problems that reflect functional limitations. In Mr. Kim's case, he could no longer bathe, dress, or walk without help.

Many adults find functional limitations that affect their ability to perform previously habitual activities more bothersome than the disease or illness that caused those limitations. Their inability to perform ordinary activities, which they previously took for granted, translates into a loss of function and a loss of independence. Physicians play an important role in helping adults of all ages to adapt and to cope with debilitating conditions.

This chapter will describe how to recognize and successfully treat patients with functional problems. It will also describe instruments and techniques useful for evaluating functional skills, such as self-care and mobility. Although the chapter will focus on older adults, many of the functional principles and instruments it discusses can also apply to younger adults. Everyone has functional concerns and needs.

What is function? In the simplest sense, function is the ability to perform a given activity or role. Patients with normal function can dress and bathe themselves, drive, and use the telephone. Function becomes a concern to people when they lose it. Loss of function can be defined at more than one level (World Health Organization, 1980), as follows:

1. *Diseases*, such as diabetes or hypertension, cause loss of function via pathology at the cellular or molecular level. A person is often unaware of a disease at this stage.
2. *Impairments*, such as renal insufficiency or atherosclerosis, cause loss of function at the organ level. With an impairment, a person may develop signs or symptoms of the disease, but still can perform daily activities.
3. *Disabilities*, also called functional limitations, cause loss of physical function at the person level. With a disability, a person is aware of physical limitations while performing activities. Two examples of disability are a person with hemiplegia from a stroke who can no longer walk or a person with blindness from diabetic retinopathy who can no longer drive. Loss of function in this chapter will generally refer to disabilities, that is, loss of physical function.
4. *Handicaps* cause loss of function at the societal level by preventing a person from fulfilling expected roles. Handicaps are reversible problems if society addresses them. A blind person can travel independently if public signs are printed in Braille. A paraplegic can work if wheelchair access is provided at the workplace.

Loss of function can occur at any or all of these levels, and it is often the first indication of disease or illness in an older patient. Even small changes in function can profoundly affect that person's independence and self-respect. Older people, when asked what they fear most, often respond "loss of independence," which may mean being unable to perform or enjoy everyday activities, needing help from others, or requiring nursing home placement—a common fear of many older adults.

In Case 16-1, Mrs. Kim and her husband shared these concerns. Mr. Kim had a functional decline that caused his wife to assume more of his care. Her presenting complaints focused on her husband's inability to perform physical activities such as bathing and dressing. Pain and deconditioning caused difficulty with self-care (a disability); compression fractures (an impairment) caused pain; osteoporosis (a disease) caused the compression fractures.

The traditional medical model of care focuses on disease, which is presented as a single problem or as a well-defined constellation of signs and symptoms. Signs, such as melenic stools, hypotension, or skin pallor, direct the physician to work up a patient for causes of gastrointestinal blood loss. Symptoms, such as shortness of breath or chest pain, elicit a prompt search for cardiovascular or pulmonary disease. The medical model of disease works well for acute, reversible conditions, such as infections or metabolic abnormalities. It does not always work well for older adults or for younger adults with many disabilities.

Thus, the functional model of care, in addition to diagnosing and treating disease, incorporates *functional assessment* into the evaluation and treatment of a patient's health problems. Functional assessment, the systematic evaluation of a person's abilities, is useful in identifying the causes of functional decline and targeting goals for recovery. The standard history and physical, designed to diagnose disease, provides a general sense of patients' health; but it overlooks function, since patients with long problem lists may be functionally independent while those with short problem lists may be completely dependent on others. Measurement of physical skills complements the history and physical. In its strictest sense, functional assessment evaluates a person's physical abilities, e.g., self-care, household skills, and mobility.

The functional model is particularly useful to physicians caring for older adults, since such patients have unique characteristics and problems. For one, elderly patients often present with *nonspecific complaints*, such as weakness, falling, or "just not feeling well." In Mr. Kim's case, his wife's concern that "he wasn't himself" became more meaningful in the context of his functional decline. Older patients also present with *multiple problems*. Sorting through these lists of problems, especially if complex, poses a challenge to physicians.

On the other hand, some older patients *underreport health problems* because they believe that these problems are a normal part of aging. Many older adults and their families accept without question that forgetfulness, incontinence, and hearing or visual impairment are the inevitable consequences of aging. Physicians are also susceptible to this bias, termed *ageism*, leading them to delete evaluations and treatments that could benefit older patients. *Atypical presentation* of illness is another characteristic of older adults' health problems. For example, a patient with a urinary tract infection may present with confusion or falls instead of the classic dysuria or urinary frequency. Similarly, a patient who presents with weight loss may have an underlying depression rather than cancer. Even when an older patient's problem is well-defined, the problem is likely to have *multiple causes*. An older patient who falls probably has several contributing factors to the falls. Poor vision, side effects from medications, muscle weakness, and a cluttered house could all be cofactors.

Finally, older patients often have *chronic problems*, and these may require more attention than their acute problems. Most older persons have at least one chronic condition and many have several conditions. Of the ten most common chronic conditions reported by adults over age 65, half are problems with physical function: arthritis, hearing impairment, cataracts, visual impairment, and orthopedic impairments (Schick & Schick, 1994). Seeing, hearing, and walking are abilities most people take for granted—until lost.

In an acute model of care, illness occurs episodically, and treatment is cure-driven. Adults of all ages may suffer loss of function after an illness or injury. A person's independence and sense of well-being depend on his or her ability to adapt or cope with loss of function. For older adults or disabled younger adults, where a chronic model of care predominates, illness may be progressive or permanent, and treatment is restorative to whatever extent possible.

## CASE 16-2

*Mrs. Wilson, an 85-year-old widow, slipped on a patch of ice one winter day while getting her mail and fell. A neighbor heard her calls for help and found Mrs. Wilson complaining of right hip and thigh pain. She was taken to a nearby emergency room, diagnosed with a right hip fracture, and taken to surgery that evening to stabilize the fracture. Mrs. Wilson developed a postoperative confusion that slowly cleared. She also developed diarrhea from an antibiotic-associated colitis. Seven days after admission, Mrs. Wilson remained weak and required help with most of her self-care, including bathing, dressing, and toileting. She was also incontinent of urine and walked only with the help of two people.*

*Her physician consulted the rehabilitative services, including physical therapy, occupational therapy, and social work. The physical therapist worked with Mrs. Wilson every day to increase her bed and chair mobility and provided a front-wheel walker for support. The occupational therapist learned that Mrs. Wilson could dress herself when given a reacher to grab her clothes and a long-handled shoehorn to put on her shoes. The social worker contacted a nearby niece who was willing to help her aunt with errands on her return home. A short-term stay at a nearby skilled nursing facility was arranged for Mrs. Wilson to complete her rehabilitation.*

*Three weeks later, Mrs. Wilson returned home. She walked up to 50 feet at a time with a front-wheel walker. Home adaptive equipment, including a tub transfer bench and raised toilet seat, were provided to make bathing and toileting easier for her. Meals-on-Wheels came daily.*

## ASSESSMENT OF PHYSICAL FUNCTION

### Activities of Daily Living

Case 16-2 illustrates another common situation, namely, a patient who suffers a functional decline during hospitalization. Functional assessment allows healthcare providers to recognize loss of function. Elderly

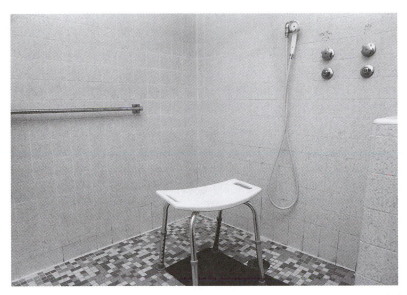

**Figure 16.2.** A shower chair with a hand-held shower head and grab bar.

patients, particularly if frail or lacking social support, may not fully recover from an illness or injury unless prompt interventions are taken to reverse the causes of decline.

Two categories of physical skills have been defined to provide physicians with a broader view of a person's capabilities. The first category, Activities of Daily Living (ADLs), are basic self-care skills that people of all ages and cultures habitually perform: feeding, walking, toileting, dressing, grooming, and bathing. Continence of bowel and bladder, while not functional activities in the same sense, are usually included as ADLs, since social independence requires both. Katz originally defined and measured these abilities after observing that elderly patients on rehabilitation units needed to perform certain physical activities before regaining their independence (Katz *et al.*, 1963). The Katz ADL scale, shown in Table 16.1, remains one of the most commonly used functional assessment instruments.

The Katz ADL scale measures independence in six physical skills: feeding, continence, transfer (the ability to get in and out of bed or chairs), toileting, dressing, and bathing. Independence with each skill usually means that a person can perform it without help from another person. A person who loses function usually loses physical skills in a predictable order: first bathing, then dressing, then toileting, followed by transferring, continence, and feeding. As a person regains function, recovery of those same abilities often occurs in reverse

---

## MEALS-ON-WHEELS

*Loaves and Fishes Centers, Inc., also known as Meals-on-Wheels, is a private, nonprofit, nonsectarian organization that helps older adults to stay independent within a community. Although best known for providing hot meals to adults at senior centers or delivering meals directly to homebound adults, Loaves and Fishes also helps older adults with transportation, shopping, and referrals to other services. Many of this organization's volunteers are themselves older, active adults. Many communities also have local organizations or charities that provide various services to older adults, such as housekeeping, grocery shopping, and transportation. Clinic or hospital social workers can provide information about such resources.*

---

**Table 16.1**
Basic Activities of Daily Living (ADLs)[a]

| Activity | Independent | |
|---|---|---|
| Bathing (sponge bath, tub bath, or shower): receives either no assistance or assistance in bathing only one part of the body | Yes | No |
| Dressing: gets clothes and dresses without any assistance except for tying shoes | Yes | No |
| Toileting: goes to toilet room, uses toilet, arranges clothes, and returns without any assistance (may use cane or walker for support, and may use bedpan or urinal at night) | Yes | No |
| Transferring: moves in and out of bed and chair without assistance (may use cane or walker) | Yes | No |
| Continence: controls bowel and bladder completely by self (without occasional "accidents") | Yes | No |
| Feeding: feeds self without assistance (except for help with cutting meat or buttering bread) | Yes | No |
| Total ADL score = number of "yes" answers, out of possible 6. | | |

[a]Modified from Katz S, Ford AB, Moskowitz RW, Jackson BA, Jaffe MW: Studies of illness in the aged: The index of ADL: a standardized measure of biological and psychosocial function. *JAMA* 185:914–919, 1963. Copyright by the Gerontological Society of America. Reprinted with permission.

order: first feeding, then continence, then transfer, and so on. Katz arranged the elements of the scale to show the typical progression in loss or recovery of these skills. Sociologists have speculated that this sequence of skills parallels the development of self-care skills during childhood—and perhaps their emergence in primitive man (Katz *et al.*, 1963).

The Katz ADL scale has been shown to be valid, reliable, and easy to administer. Its major drawback, as with many assessment instruments, is its inability to detect small changes in function that may over time reflect a large loss of function. The Katz ADL scale nevertheless remains a useful tool for assessing physical function. Other ADL instruments are available (Applegate *et al.*, 1990), which vary in length and in the skills assessed (e.g., walking, climbing stairs, and grooming). Such instruments are clinically useful because they provide a practical way to obtain information about a person's abilities. During her hospitalization, Mrs. Wilson, in Case 16-2, lost several key ADLs, and her functional decline resulted in loss of independence. Addressing these functional deficits was as important to her recovery as treating her medical–surgical problems. A rehabilitative approach was used. *Rehabilitation* is the restoration of function following disease, illness, or injury. Geriatrics emphasizes a rehabilitative approach since maintaining function and preventing its loss are key to an older patient's health and well-being.

## Instrumental Activities of Daily Living

The second category of functional skills, the Instrumental Activities of Daily Living (IADLs), comprise a more complex set of skills: shopping, preparing food, keeping house, using transportation, and handling finances. As with the ADLs, everyone needs IADLs to live independently in a community. The Lawton–Brody IADL scale, shown in Table 16.2, is one of the earliest IADL instruments (Lawton & Brody, 1969). Adults vary in level of independence with IADLs just as with ADLs. Their functional level measured with IADLs often determines whether a person can continue to live in the community. Mrs. Wilson, for instance, would have been unable to return home without help from her niece and community services. Capability versus performance is an issue when assessing ADLs and IADLs. A good rule of thumb is "Say do, can do, do do." That is, patients sometimes *say* they can perform an activity whether they can or not; patients *can* perform an activity but choose not to for whatever reason; and patients may actually *do* the activity that they say they do. Similarly, patients who are in denial about illness or who have cognitive impairment often overestimate their physical abilities, while patients who lack motivation or who are depressed often underestimate them.

Cultural biases also complicate the accurate assessment of IADLs. For example, many older men have never cooked or kept house, but these same men might be able to perform such activities if the need arose. Their lack of actual performance does not necessarily mean they are incapable of those activities.

**Table 16.2**
Instrumental Activities of Daily Living Scale (IADLs)[a]

| | |
|---|---|
| Ability to use telephone | |
|   Operates telephone on own initiative; looks up and dials numbers, etc. | 1 |
|   Dials a few well-known numbers | 1 |
|   Answers telephone but does not dial | 1 |
|   Does not use telephone at all | 0 |
| Shopping | |
|   Takes care of all shopping needs independently | 1 |
|   Shops independently for small purchases | 0 |
|   Needs to be accompanied on any shopping trip | 0 |
|   Completely unable to shop | 0 |
| Food preparation | |
|   Plans, operates, and serves adequate meals independently | 1 |
|   Prepares adequate meals if supplied with ingredients | 0 |
|   Heats and serves prepared meals or prepares meals but does not maintain adequate diet | 0 |
|   Needs to have meals prepared and served | 0 |
| Housekeeping | |
|   Maintains house alone or with occasional assistance (e.g., heavy work, domestic help) | 1 |
|   Performs light daily tasks such as dish washing, bed making | 1 |
|   Performs light daily tasks but cannot maintain acceptable level of cleanliness | 1 |
|   Needs help with all home-maintenance tasks | 1 |
|   Does not participate in any housekeeping tasks | 0 |
| Laundry | |
|   Does personal laundry completely | 1 |
|   Launders small items, rinses stockings, etc. | 1 |
|   All laundry must be done by others | 0 |
| Mode of transportation | |
|   Travels independently on public transportation or drives own car | 1 |
|   Arranges own travel via taxi but does not otherwise use public transportation | 1 |
|   Travels on public transportation when initiated or accompanied by another | 1 |
|   Travel limited to taxi or automobile with assistance of another | 0 |
|   Does not travel at all | 0 |
| Responsibility for own medications | |
|   Is responsible for taking medication in correct dosages at correct time | 1 |
|   Takes responsibility if medication is prepared in advance in separate dosages | 0 |
|   Is not capable of dispensing own medication | 0 |
| Ability to handle finances | |
|   Manages financial matters independently (budgets, writes checks, pays rent and bills, goes to bank), collects and keeps track of income | 1 |
|   Manages day-to-day purchases but needs help with banking, major purchases, etc. | 1 |
|   Incapable of handling money | 0 |

Score = points out of a possible 8

[a]From Lawton MP, Brody EM: Assessment of older people: Self-maintaining and instrumental activities of daily living. *Gerontologist* 9:179–186, 1969. Copyright by the Gerontological Society of America. Reprinted with permission.

Most functional assessments are obtained directly from the patient or from the patient's family or caregivers. While direct observation of a patient's physical performance is the most objective and accurate way to assess a patient, such observations are often impractical, especially with IADLs. Hence, most functional evaluations come from patient or family reports and limited observations. Patients tend to report their own abilities at higher levels than nurses do, while families tend to report patients' abilities at lower levels than nurses do (Rubenstein *et al.*, 1984).

Physicians should routinely ask patients about their function. Ask for a description of their daily routine. Ask how or if the presenting problem affects that routine. Find out what activities are no longer performed compared with a year ago. Ask how the patient performs the stated activity. Sometimes, such open-ended questions yield surprising information. For example, one gentleman, who asserted that he bathed independently, did so only by using his cane as a hook on the bathroom doorknob to get in and out of the tub!

During the interview, observe what the patient does for herself. Does a family member answer questions for the patient? Can the patient state what medications are taken? Is help needed to sit on the examination table? Does the patient have difficulty unbuttoning a shirt or releasing a belt? Questions and observations such as these provide clues about a patient's function.

Two common causes of functional decline in hospitalized patients are *deconditioning* and *iatrogenesis*. Deconditioning refers to the physiological changes that occur with prolonged bed rest or inactivity (Vorhies & Riley, 1993). Such changes can develop quickly, in a matter of days, and affect almost every organ system in the body. Early signs and symptoms of deconditioning include shortness of breath with minimal exertion, a resting heart rate elevated above the patient's baseline, orthostasis, decreased endurance, and decreased muscle strength. Muscle strength may decline as much as 1.3 to 3.0% per day of bed rest in adults of all ages (Hoenig & Rubenstein, 1991). Such losses in an older patient—whose physical reserve is already at a low threshold—may markedly slow the rate of recovery.

Iatrogenesis—complications resulting from medical care—is a serious problem for older hospitalized adults. Iatrogenesis takes many forms: deconditioning from enforced bed rest, pressure ulcers from poor skin care, nosocomial infections, malnutrition, incontinence, and adverse effects from almost any medication. Medications alone account for nearly half of all iatrogenic problems (Gorbien *et al.*, 1992).

Mrs. Wilson suffered both deconditioning and iatrogensis while in the hospital. Her deconditioning, while a natural consequence of a broken hip, might have been lessened by more aggressive postoperative mobilization. Her confusion, a common complication after hip fractures, probably had multiple causes: side effects from medications (anesthetics, analgesics, sedatives), an unfamiliar hospital environment, and an infection (colitis). Her original injury interacted with the subsequent problems to produce a functional decline.

## CASE 16-3 (Part 1)

*Mr. Warren, a 75-year-old retired automobile mechanic, came to the physician's office because of falls. The patient could not recall the details, but Mrs. Warren counted four falls in the previous 3 months. She suspected there had been others as well. Two occurred while her husband was getting up to void at night. After one of those falls, he required treatment in an emergency room for a scalp laceration. Mr. Warren's medications include hydrochlorothiazide and enalapril for hypertension, a nitroglycerin patch for stable angina, and triazolam for insomnia.*

## ASSESSMENT OF MOBILITY

Falls are a classic presentation of functional decline in older adults. At least one-third of all community-dwelling older adults—and one-half of those institutionalized—fall each year (Tinetti & Speechley, 1989). Some falls, for example Mr. Warren's, result in serious injury. Most do not, but even these can have serious consequences. Older patients who have fallen may develop a fear of falling, which leads to decreased activity, followed by deconditioning and eventually immobility.

Falls indicate a problem with mobility, defined as the ability to maneuver throughout the environment. Mobility is an important functional skill that interacts with ADLs and IADLs. Lack of mobility compromises a patient's function and independence and often is the determining factor for nursing home placement. Physicians treating elderly patients therefore should routinely evaluate their mobility. Areas of interest include gait, balance, and range of motion in the upper and lower extremities.

As illustrated in Case 16-3, the first step to successfully evaluating falls is to obtain a description of the event(s). Many older patients do not recall the details surrounding a fall. Therefore, witnesses are invaluable sources for confirming particulars of the event: how the patient fell, whether there was loss of consciousness or continence of bowel or bladder, or whether hazards, such as throw rugs or poor lighting, were present.

Since falls are a common nonspecific presentation of underlying illness, the clinician also should inquire about signs and symptoms of acute illness, e.g., infection or heart disease. The review of systems should focus on potential sensory or neuromuscular deficits that might interfere with mobility. Questions about vision, hearing, joint pain, balance, strength, and sensation provide important information.

Lastly, a careful review of the patient's medications, both prescription and over the counter, is critical. Certain classes of medications, including antihypertensives and sedatives, as well as the total number of medications, increase the risk of falls (Tinetti & Speechley, 1989).

After completing the history, the physical examination should include the musculoskeletal and neurologic systems. The musculoskeletal examination focuses on range of motion in the upper and lower extremities, joint deformities, and pain in these areas. Simple exercises, such as asking patients to put both hands behind their head or to touch their toes with the opposite hand, mimic the types of movements needed when putting on a shirt or shoes. Picking up a pen from the table mimics the use of eating utensils. Simply observing the patient taking off a coat, buttoning it, or reaching for a glass gives almost as much information about range of motion as formal testing.

The standard neurologic examination, originally designed to localize neurologic lesions, is an important part of the examination but provides limited information about function. The abnormalities detected by a neurologic examination do not necessarily correlate with those detected by a mobility evaluation. Tinetti and Ginter (1988) showed that the neuromuscular abnormalities detected on a standard neurologic examination in older patients did not predict who had difficulty getting in and out of a chair.

Assessment of mobility includes analysis of a patient's gait and balance. At least 15% of patients over age 60 have an abnormal gait (Sudarsky, 1990), and gait disturbances are a known risk factor for falls. The normal gait cycle has three phases: stance, swing, and double-limb support. The stance phase, which occupies about 60 to 65% of the gait cycle, begins when the right heel contacts a surface. It ends when the right toe leaves that surface. The swing phase, occupying about 15 to 20% of the cycle, begins when the right toe leaves a surface and lasts until the right heel again contacts that surface. The double-limb support phase, the part of the cycle when both feet are on the ground, is about 20 to 25% of total cycle time (Sudarsky, 1990).

Many diseases produce characteristic gait patterns that physicians can learn to recognize. Cerebellar disease produces a wide-based stance and ataxia (an unsteady and wandering path). Stroke patients often circumduct (swing outward) the affected leg and have minimal flexion at the hip and knee during the swing phase. Patients with dementia may have difficulty initiating steps and shuffle as they walk. Older patients, even in the absence of pathology, develop a characteristic gait pattern. Step length is decreased, stride is broader-based, and velocity is decreased.

## CASE 16-3 (Part 2)

*Mr. Warren was orthostatic on physical examination with a blood pressure of 152/82 mm Hg and a pulse of 78 while sitting and a blood pressure of 128/64 mm Hg and a pulse of 82 after standing 1 minute. He had a mild resting tremor in his right hand and cogwheel rigidity in both arms. It took him three attempts to rise from the chair, and he became unsteady after a few minutes. His step length, step height, and arm swing were decreased symmetrically, and he displayed a flexed posture in the trunk and extremities. Initiation of gait was delayed, but when achieved, his gait speed accelerated. Questioning by the physician revealed that Mr. Warren had had the tremor at least a year, and that it took him longer to dress and bathe.*

*Mr. Warren was diagnosed with Parkinson's disease. His falls were attributed to several causes: orthostasis from medications and from probable underlying autonomic insufficiency (a common problem with Parkinson's patients), deconditioning from chronic immobility, and sedation from the hypnotic triazolam. He received a trial of carbidopa/levodopa, which improved his bradykinesia and ability to dress. Hydrochlorothiazide was discontinued. His blood pressure remained well controlled on enalapril alone. The triazolam was discontinued after the physician reviewed sleep hygiene techniques with him and his wife. Lastly, a physical therapist provided a front-wheel walker and a home exercise program to improve strength and endurance. Mr. Warren's orthostasis improved. Six months later, his wife reported only one fall.*

Assessing Mr. Warren's mobility helped the physician to determine the causes of his falls. His gait provided an important clue for the diagnosis of Parkinson's disease. Gait analysis is easily accomplished, once a clinician recognizes the elements of normal and abnormal gait. The Performance-Oriented Assessment of Mobility, often called the Tinetti Balance and Gait Evaluation, is a standardized clinical instrument used to analyze mobility of older patients (Tinetti, 1986). This instrument, shown in Table 16.3, divides the components of mobility into a detailed list of observations about balance and gait.

To evaluate balance, first observe how patients sit in a chair. Patients with large strokes, for example, often have poor sitting balance and lean toward the affected side. Next, ask the patients to stand without using the hands as support. The need for multiple attempts or for the use of the arms to rise from sitting is typical in patients with lower extremity weakness, osteoarthritis of the hips or knees, or deconditioning. Likewise, falling into the chair when sitting suggests similar problems or poor vision. On standing, observe immediate (first 5 seconds) and delayed (after about 1 minute) standing balance. Unsteadiness could be from orthostasis, cerebellar disease, or weakness. Asking patients to stand with their eyes closed tests dependency on sensory input from proprioception and vision.

Important observations while patients walk include step length and height. Normal step length is at least the length of the patient's foot, and normal step height is 1 to 2 inches above the floor. The heel of the swing foot usually clears the opposite foot by 1 to 2 inches. Observe how quickly a patient initiates walking. Mr. Warren, like many Parkinson patients, had difficulty initiating walking but accelerated once started (called *festination*). An erratic gait path and excessive truncal sway suggest cerebellar dysfunction. The Tinetti Balance and Gait Evaluation takes only a few minutes to complete once the physician is familiar with the tool. Scoring of the instrument has been useful primarily in research settings. Clinicians find the Tinetti Evaluation useful because it teaches them to observe the subtleties of gait and balance and because it provides a practical and objective way to evaluate mobility.

A shorter version of the test, called "the get-up and go test" (Mathias *et al.*, 1986), is a quick screen for gait and balance. To perform the test, instruct the patient to stand up from a chair without using his hands, walk 15 meters, turn around, and return. Before the patient sits down, perform the "nudge test." Ask the patient to close his eyes, then gently but firmly push on the patient's sternum, taking care to guard against a fall. Finally, ask the patient to sit down, again without using the hands. The "nudge test" evaluates a patient's

---

## PARKINSON'S DISEASE

*Parkinson's disease is a progressive neurologic disorder that most commonly occurs in adults over 60 years old. The condition is caused by degeneration of nerve cells and a deficiency of dopamine, a neurotransmitter, within a part of the brain called the basal ganglia. Classic symptoms of Parkinson's disease include a resting tremor, bradykinesia (slow movement), rigidity (stiffness with movement), and gait and balance problems. Several medications, such as carbidopa/levodopa, can improve symptoms by increasing dopamine levels within the brain.*

---

**Table 16.3**
Tinetti Balance and Gait Evaluation[a]

BALANCE

Instructions: Subject is seated in hard, armless chair. The following maneuvers are tests.

| | | |
|---|---|---|
| 1. Sitting balance | Leans or slides in chair | = 0 |
| | Steady, safe | = 1 |
| 2. Arises | Unable without help | = 0 |
| | Able, but uses arms to help | = 1 |
| | Able without use of arms | = 2 |
| 3. Attempts to arise | Unable without help | = 0 |
| | Able, but requires more than one attempt | = 1 |
| | Able to arise with one attempt | = 2 |
| 4. Immediate standing balance (first 5 seconds) | Unsteady (staggers, moves feet, marked trunk away) | = 0 |
| | Steady, but uses walker or cane or grabs other objects for support | = 1 |
| | Steady without walker or cane or other support | = 2 |
| 5. Standing balance | Unsteady | = 0 |
| | Steady, but wide stance (medial heels more than 4 inches apart), or uses cane, walker, or other support | = 1 |
| | Narrow stance without support | = 2 |
| 6. Nudge (subject at maximum position with feet as close together as possible, examiner pushes lightly on subject's sternum with palm of hand three times) | Begins to fall | = 0 |
| | Staggers, grabs, but catches self | = 1 |
| | Steady | = 2 |
| 7. Eyes closed (at maximum position #6) | Unsteady | = 0 |
| | Steady | = 1 |
| 8. Turning 360° | Discontinuous steps | = 0 |
| | Continuous steps | = 1 |
| | Unsteady (grabs, staggers) | = 0 |
| | Steady | = 1 |
| 9. Sitting down | Unsafe (misjudged distance, falls into chair) | = 0 |
| | Uses arms or not a smooth motion | = 1 |
| | Safe, smooth motion | = 2 |

Balance score = _____/16

*continued*

righting reflexes, i.e., the ability to adjust the body's posture to changes in the environment. A patient with a positive "nudge" is unable to correct his posture without falling.

Sometimes even informal observations are helpful in evaluating mobility. When circumstances allow, watch the patient walk in or out of the examination room. At those times, patients are likely to perform in their usual manner. Is there unsteadiness? Does a family member or nurse need to help? Does the patient use an assistive device, such as a cane or walker? Is it used correctly? These observations provide information that is often unavailable in the examination room.

## Ambulatory Devices

Older patients who need ambulatory devices often use them incorrectly. Physicians should know which ambulatory devices help patients with poor mobility. They should also know how to use these devices correctly. The decision about the correct device and its use should be made in conjunction with physical therapists, however, who have expertise in treating mobility problems.

Canes, which can support up to 25% of a person's weight, are a good choice for older adults with unilateral weakness or pain while walking. Stroke patients with normal balance or those with hip osteoarthritis often benefit. When a patient uses a cane, make sure it is correctly adjusted for the patient's height.

**Table 16.3**

*(Continued)*[a]

GAIT

Instruction: Subject stands with examiner, walks down hallway or across room, first at "usual" pace, then back at "rapid, but safe" pace (using using walking aid such as cane, walker).

| | | |
|---|---|---|
| 10. Initiation of gait (immediately after told to "go") | Any hesitancy or multiple attempts to start | = 0 |
| | No hesitancy | = 1 |
| 11. Step length and height<br>    A. Right swing foot | Does not pass left stance foot with step | = 0 |
| | Passes left stance foot | = 1 |
| | Right foot does not clear floor completely with step | = 0 |
| | Right foot completely clears floor | = 1 |
|     B. Left swing foot | Does not pass right stance foot with step | = 0 |
| | Passes right stance foot | = 1 |
| | Left foot does not clear floor completely with step | = 0 |
| | Left foot completely clears floor | = 1 |
| 12. Step symmetry | Right and left step length not equal (estimate) | = 0 |
| | Right and left step length appear equal | = 1 |
| 13. Step continuity | Stopping or discontinuity between steps | = 0 |
| | Steps appear continuous | = 1 |
| 14. Path (estimated in relation to floor tiles, 12 inch diameter. Observe excusion of one foot over about 10 feet of the course.) | Marked deviation | = 0 |
| | Mild/moderate deviation or uses walking aid | = 1 |
| | Straight without walking aid | = 2 |
| 15. Trunk | Marked sway or uses walking aid | = 0 |
| | No sway but flexion or knees or back or spreads arms out while walking | = 1 |
| | No sway, no flexion, no use of arms, and no walking aid | = 2 |
| 16. Walking stance | Heels apart | = 0 |
| | Heels almost touching while walking | = 1 |

Gait score: _____/12

Total score: _____/28

[a]From Tinetti ME: Performance-oriented assessment of mobility problems in elderly patients. *JAGS* 34:119–126, 1986. Permission obtained from author.

Look for a 20 to 30° angle at the elbow. The patient should hold the cane on the unaffected side, which decreases stance time and shifts weight away from the affected side. For example, Mrs. Wilson, who had a right hip fracture, should hold her cane in the left hand. To use it correctly, she should step forward simultaneously with her right leg and the cane in her left hand, then she should step forward with her unaffected left leg.

Walkers, which can support up to 50% of a person's weight, are better for patients with poor balance or general weakness. Demented patients, who have difficulty learning or remembering new information (e.g., how to properly use a cane), may be good candidates for walkers. Pickup walkers are useful to patients with poor endurance, such as those with chronic obstructive pulmonary disease or congestive heart failure. Pickup walkers require adequate balance and upper extremity strength, however. Front-wheel walkers offer more stability to patients with balance deficits, since this type of walker forces the patient's center of gravity forward into the walker. Parkinson patients, like Mr. Warren, tend to be retropulsive, i.e., to fall backward. A standard pickup walker might exaggerate retropulsion and increase Mr. Warren's fall risk, whereas a front-wheel walker would offer more stability.

Wheelchairs provide mobility for patients who need postural support, or who have severe weakness. They provide patients who have progressive diseases, such as multiple sclerosis or amyotrophic lateral sclerosis, with mobility that they would not have otherwise. Safely transferring in and out of the wheelchair is a prerequisite for its use. When prescribing wheelchairs, always collaborate with physical therapists who have the expertise to recommend the right model and to teach its correct use.

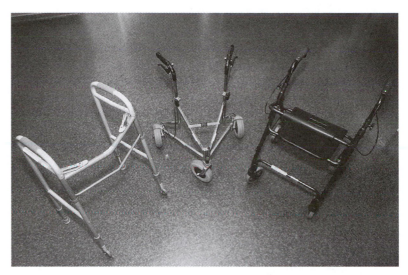

**Figure 16.3.** From left to right: A front-wheeled walker, a three-wheeled walker with hand brakes, and a four-wheeled walker with hand brakes and seat.

Knowing the basics of ambulatory devices, especially canes and walkers, enables physicians to promote mobility and function for their patients.

## CASE 16-4 (Part 1)

*Mrs. Goldendale, a 91-year-old lady, came to the physician's office with her son, Steve, because of weight loss. He had observed a loss of almost 10 pounds over the preceding 8 months; his mother now weighed 78 pounds. She had a remote history of peptic ulcer disease, but denied gastrointestinal complaints. Steve observed that she needed frequent encouragement to eat and that she complained of back and right hip pain, relieved by anti-inflammatory medication. Mrs. Goldendale had been living with her children over the past 3 years because of their concerns about her forgetfulness. Prior physicians attributed the memory loss to "old timer's disease."*

*Steve's brother and sister-in-law were recently frustrated when his mother left a bathroom faucet running, which flooded the upstairs and caused considerable damage. He and his brother worried about their mother's health and disagreed about the need for nursing home placement. Until 2 months ago, Mrs. Goldendale had been independent with all ADLs; she now needed prompting to bathe and dress. Physical examination revealed a petite and cachectic older woman who was disoriented to the date. She nodded to questions and motioned toward her son to answer most of them. Mrs. Goldendale had marked kyphosis and a limp while walking. She became unsteady while turning around; her "nudge test" was positive. The physician recognized that Mrs. Goldendale had many problems: weight loss, forgetfulness, and a functional decline. The physician also wondered if she would need nursing home placement. Since Mrs. Goldendale lived in the area, the physician arranged for an outpatient, multidisciplinary evaluation to sort through her problems.*

## COMPREHENSIVE GERIATRIC ASSESSMENT

When patients like Mrs. Goldendale come to the office, their problems often cover many domains— medical, cognitive, affective, functional, social, economic, and environmental—that interact with one another to affect function. A multidisciplinary evaluation called Comprehensive Geriatric Assessment (CGA) assists healthcare professionals in developing diagnostic and treatment plans that maintain or improve an older adult's function. CGA is useful to patients who have well-defined rehabilitation needs, e.g., strokes, amputations, or hip fractures. It is also useful for frail patients who may have less well defined problems or who have multiple problems, as in Case 16-4.

CGA has been performed in a variety of settings including dedicated inpatient and rehabilitation units, outpatient clinics, and patient homes. A physician, nurse, and social worker usually make up the core team, but other health professionals including physical, occupational, and speech therapists, dietitians, mental health specialists, and pharmacists participate as needed. The multidisciplinary team typically meets after the initial evaluation to discuss and coordinate patient care. Team members may meet thereafter, depending on the patient's progress.

The frail population, meaning those with functional limitations, benefit from such evaluations, since this population is most likely to have complex medical and psychosocial problems. Multiple randomized controlled trials (Stuck *et al.*, 1993; Rubenstein, 1987) have shown that CGA improves diagnostic accuracy, function, and affect, while decreasing mortality and medication use in frail, older adults. CGA has also been shown to reduce nursing home placement, hospital admissions, and healthcare costs. More recent studies focusing on healthier, older adults (Bula *et al.*, 1999; Reuben *et al.*, 1999) have shown that CGA may also prevent functional decline and improve quality of life in this population. Patients most likely to benefit from CGA, whether frail or not, are those with recent functional declines, good social support, and relatively intact cognition. Mrs. Goldendale's physician needed to evaluate more than the weight loss *per se*. Her problems extended into other areas of function that affected her medical condition, including self-care, mobility, cognition, affect, and sensory evaluation.

## CASE 16-4 (Part 2)

*On arriving at the outpatient geriatric assessment clinic, team members evaluated Mrs. Goldendale. The medical workup uncovered an iron-deficiency anemia that was eventually attributed to severe gastritis from nonsteroidal anti-inflammatory drugs. For pain control, the physician prescribed scheduled acetaminophen and a heating pad. They removed impacted cerumen from her ears. Her hearing improved and she began to answer questions rather than simply nod as she'd so frequently done before. An audiologist found Mrs. Goldendale had a moderate hearing loss and recommended hearing aids.*

*The geropsychiatrist interviewed Mrs. Goldendale. She expressed feelings of helplessness and hopelessness. She acknowledged that she had never really gotten over her husband's death 5 years earlier and that while living with her sons was helpful, their interests overshadowed hers. Mental status testing showed intact concentration and mild short-term memory loss. She was diagnosed with clinical depression and eventually with a mild underlying dementia. Her physician began a trial of antidepressant medication.*

*The physical therapist prescribed a front-wheel walker for her unsteadiness along with a home exercise program. The occupational therapist, who performed an in-home safety evaluation, recommended installing grab bars and a tub transfer bench in the shower to help her bathe safely. Lastly, the social worker suggested that Mrs. Goldendale attend a local senior center to increase her socialization. Three years later, Mrs. Goldendale was still living with her children and remained independent with her ADLs.*

Good cognitive and affective function are critical to a patient's health. Normal motor skills and endurance are not enough to ensure normal function. Physicians should routinely screen for cognitive impairment and affective disturbances when evaluating patients with a functional decline.

Patients with cognitive impairment often present with forgetfulness, commonly caused by dementia. Both long-term memory (over years) and short-term memory (over hours or days) can be tested with simple

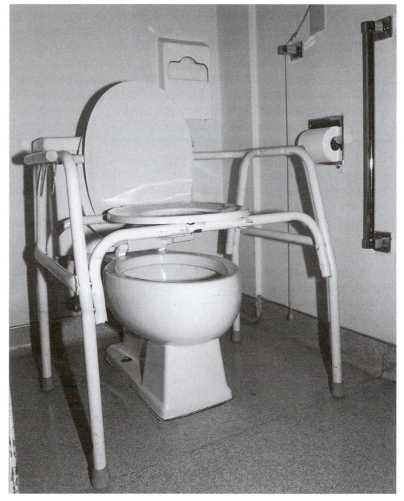

**Figure 16.4.** A raised toilet seat with grab bars and a call light for assistance.

questions. To test long-term memory, ask for a birth date, place of birth, number of children, or date of retirement. Few patients forget these milestones unless cognitive problems are present. Test short-term memory by asking the patient to repeat three common objects immediately, then at 5 minutes. Patients with intact memory should be able to name the objects without prompting. If the person is hesitant to do this, ask less threatening questions. What did they have for breakfast that morning? What is their current address? Can they give directions to their home? An inability to answer these types of questions about everyday life, or vague responses to them, may uncover memory problems.

## ACTIVITIES OF DAILY LIVING

*When interviewing older adults, in addition to taking the standard medical history, remember to ask the patient or family member about function. For example, ask "Have you needed any help recently with your self-care, such as bathing or dressing?" Bathing and dressing are often the first ADL skills lost by an older adult. Other questions might include, "Do you use a cane or walker within your home or when you go outside?" "Have you had difficulty getting to the bathroom on time?" "Have you had accidents with your bowels or bladder recently?" Many adults will not volunteer this information unless asked.*

**Table 16.4**
Mini-Mental State Examination (MMSE)[a]

| Questions | Points |
|---|---|
| 1. What is the: Year? Season? Date? Day? Month? | 5 |
| 2. Where are we: State? County? Town or city? Hospital? Floor? | 5 |
| 3. Name three objects (Apple, Penny, Table), taking one second to say each. Then ask the patient to tell you the three. Repeat the answers until the patient learns all three. | 3 |
| 4. Serial sevens. Subtract 7 from 100. Then subtract 7 from that number, etc. Stop after five answers. Alternative: spell WORLD backward. | 5 |
| 5. Ask for the names of the three objects learned in # 3. | 3 |
| 6. Point to a pencil and watch. Have the patient name them as you point. | 2 |
| 7. Have the patient repeat "No ifs, ands, or buts." | 1 |
| 8. Have the patient follow a three-stage command: "Take the paper in your right hand. Fold the paper in half. Put the paper on the floor." | 3 |
| 9. Have the patient read and obey the following: "CLOSE YOUR EYES." (Write it in large letters.) | 1 |
| 10. Have the patient write a sentence of his or her own choice. | 1 |
| 11. Have the patient copy the following design (overlapping pentagons). | 1 |

Assess level of consciousness along a continuum.
Alert —— Drowsy —— Stupor —— Coma    Total score = _____/30

[a]From Folstein MF, Folstein SE, McHugh PR: Mini-mental state: A practical method for grading the cognitive state of patients for the clinician. *J Psychiatr Res* 12:189–198, 1975. Used with permission of MF Folstein.

The Mini-Mental State Examination (MMSE) is a reliable and easily administered screening test for cognitive impairment (Folstein *et al.*, 1975). It was originally designed to assess the severity of cognitive impairment and to monitor cognitive changes over time. As shown in Table 16.4, the MMSE contains 30 items that test orientation, memory, concentration, and language abilities. Once learned, it takes about 5 to 10 minutes to complete.

When administering the examination, keep several techniques in mind. Some authorities recommend that when asking for the county and floor in the orientation section, the examiner may substitute the county and street, respectively, where the person lives (Tombaugh & McIntyre, 1992). In the registration section, the score is based on the first trial, although it may be necessary for the patient to repeat the three items several times to learn them for later recall. The examiner should confirm that the patient can correctly spell WORLD forward, before asking to spell it backward. Lastly, while WORLD backward and Serial 7s are both tests of concentration, they are not equivalent in difficulty. It is usually best to first ask the patient to spell WORLD backward before performing serial 7s. Count the highest of the two scores. Commonly used cutoff scores for the MMSE are: no cognitive impairment = 24 to 30; mild cognitive impairment = 18 to 23; and severe cognitive impairment = 0 to 17. These scores should always be interpreted with caution. Studies have shown that age, poor fluency in English, and less than an eighth-grade education may produce low scores in patients who do not have true cognitive impairment (Tombaugh & McIntyre, 1992). Nevertheless, the MMSE is a valuable screening tool that can alert physicians to underlying cognitive problems in patients. The physician can subsequently determine the need for further mental status evaluation.

Physicians should also screen for affective or mood disturbances such as depression. Serious depressive symptoms affect more than 10% of older community-dwelling adults. Clinical depression is common in older hospitalized patients (10 to 15%), and even more common in patients with underlying cognitive impairment, e.g., dementia or Parkinson's disease (20 to 40%) (Blazer, 1989). Asking the patient "Do you often feel sad or depressed?" introduces further questions about depression.

The Geriatric Depression Scale (GDS) (Yesavage *et al.*, 1983), a 30-item questionnaire designed to help clinicians detect depressive symptoms in older adults, has been validated in both community-dwelling and hospital populations (Koenig *et al.*, 1988). An example of the GDS is shown in Table 16.5. The GDS can be self-administered or administered by a physician, nurse, or family member. Score one point for each depressed answer. The higher the score, the more likely the patient is depressed. Various cutoff scores have

**Table 16.5**
Geriatric Depression Scale (GDS)[a]

| | | |
|---|---|---|
| Choose the test answer for how you felt this past week: | | |
| * Are you basically satisfied with your life? | Yes | No |
| Have you dropped many of your activities and interests? | Yes | No |
| Do you feel that your life is empty? | Yes | No |
| Do you often get bored? | Yes | No |
| * Are you hopeful for the future? | Yes | No |
| Are you bothered by thoughts you can't get out of your head? | Yes | No |
| * Are you in good spirits most of the time? | Yes | No |
| Are you afraid that something bad is going to happen to you? | Yes | No |
| * Do you feel happy most of the time? | Yes | No |
| Do you often feel helpless? | Yes | No |
| Do you often get restless and fidgety? | Yes | No |
| Do you prefer to stay at home, rather than going out and doing new things? | Yes | No |
| Do you frequently worry about the future? | Yes | No |
| Do you feel you have more problems with memory than most? | Yes | No |
| * Do you think it is wonderful to be alive now? | Yes | No |
| Do you often feel downhearted and blue? | Yes | No |
| Do you feel pretty worthless the way you are now? | Yes | No |
| Do you worry a lot about the past? | Yes | No |
| * Do you find life very exciting? | Yes | No |
| Is it hard for you to get started on new projects? | Yes | No |
| * Do you feel full of energy? | Yes | No |
| Do you think that your situation is hopeless? | Yes | No |
| Do you think that most people are better off than you are? | Yes | No |
| Do you frequently get upset over little things? | Yes | No |
| Do you frequently feel like crying? | Yes | No |
| Do you have trouble concentrating? | Yes | No |
| * Do you enjoy getting up in the morning? | Yes | No |
| Do you prefer to avoid social gatherings? | Yes | No |
| * Is it easy for you to make decisions? | Yes | No |
| * Is your mind as clear as it used to be? | Yes | No |

*Appropriate (nondepressed) answers = yes, all others, no
Score = number of "depressed" answers

[a] From Yesavage JA, Brink TL, Rose RL, Lum O, Huang G, Adey M, Leirer VO: Development and validation of a geriatric depression screening scale: A preliminary report. *J Psychiatr Res* 17:37–49, 1983. Reprinted with permission from JA Yesavage.

been suggested for the GDS. A score of greater than 11 was found to provide a sensitivity of 92% and specificity of 89% in older hospitalized patients (Koenig *et al.*, 1988) and a sensitivity of 84% and specificity of 95% in community-dwelling adults (Yesavage *et al.*, 1983). Many other instruments for assessing cognition and mood disturbances are available (Applegate *et al.*, 1990). These instruments, including the MMSE and the GDS, do not replace a physician's clinical judgment about a patient's condition, but may confirm a diagnosis or catch previously unsuspected cognitive and affective disturbances. Other important functional abilities to screen are hearing and vision (Lachs *et al.*, 1990), since many older adults have trouble with these senses. Their inability to see or hear can profoundly impair function. To screen vision, ask the patient to read the letters of a Snellen chart at 14 inches while wearing corrective lenses. If the chart is unavailable, ask the patient to read a few sentences from a magazine or newspaper.

To screen hearing, use the "whisper test." The physician stands behind the patient, and while covering one of the patient's ears, asks the patient to repeat numbers whispered by the physician. Another screen is the "rub test," performed by rubbing the thumb and index fingers together near one of the patient's ears and asking if the patient heard the sound. One of the most simple but gratifying services a physician can perform for a patient is to remove cerumen occluding the external auditory canals, an easy solution to an often-overlooked problem.

These screening tests do not replace the more detailed examinations of specialists, but they remind physicians that older patients often have vision and hearing impairments. Physicians should have a low threshold for referring patients with these problems.

Mrs. Goldendale had multiple problems, some with multiple causes. Weight loss occurred from gastritis, chronic pain, and depression. Her cognitive impairments occurred from depression, dementia, and hearing loss. These problems were interrelated and produced her functional decline.

## CONCLUSION

Evaluating and treating patients with multiple medical and functional problems challenges even the most experienced physicians. While cures may be impossible, improvement in physical, cognitive, and affective function is often within reach. The Report of the Society of General Internal Medicine Task Force on Health Assessment (Rubenstein *et al.*, 1988) recommends that physicians learn to incorporate a functional approach toward older patients. For all patients over age 65, the task force suggested a targeted clinical interview and examination that focuses on physical function, assessment of the person's IADLs, and a screen for depression. For all patients over age 75 (or over age 65 with clinical indications), the task force also recommended assessing ADLs and cognition. Screening tests, incorporating elements from previously discussed assessment instruments, have been developed to streamline the assessment of older adults (Moore & Siu, 1996). The effectiveness of these tests is currently under evaluation.

Healthcare providers, in all disciplines, are treating larger numbers of older adults. This trend will continue because the percentage of adults over age 65 will almost double from 12.5% to 21% of the total U.S. population by 2030. Furthermore, the oldest old—those over age 85 and even over age 100—are the fastest-growing segments of the population (Schick & Schick, 1994). Levels of disability, rates of hospitalization, and healthcare costs all rise with age. As healthcare providers become increasingly aware of this rapidly growing population, effective models of management that include functional assessment will help physicians to successfully treat older adults as well as younger adults with disabilities.

Adults of all ages may have healthcare needs that do not fit into the traditional medical model of disease. Their concerns often extend to losses of function that require a different approach that complements the traditional model. Physicians who treat these patients can incorporate functional assessment into their daily practice through simple tools and techniques. Assessing ADLs, IADLs, and mobility provides useful information that cannot be obtained from the standard history and physical. Evaluating cognition, affect, and sensory impairments contributes to an even more thorough evaluation. Many patients often need and benefit from the functional approach.

## CASES FOR DISCUSSION

### CASE 1

*Mrs. Morgan, a 69-year-old semiretired teacher with a history of diabetes mellitus, hypertension, and macular degeneration, lived with her spouse and son in their ranch-style home. While preparing breakfast one morning for her family, she developed slurred speech and right-sided weakness. She was taken to a nearby hospital and admitted with a new left cerebrovascular accident. Her neurologic symptoms progressed over the next 24 hours, leaving her with a dense right hemiparalysis.*

*During hospitalization, Mrs. Morgan required many medications for labile hypertension, antibiotics for an aspiration pneumonia, and tube feedings for a severe dysphagia. Twelve days poststroke, Mrs. Morgan showed some signs of neurologic recovery: improved swallowing and increased right-sided motor tone and strength. However, she displayed a moderately severe expressive aphasia, marked right hemiparesis, and urinary incontinence. She appeared to be uncooperative with the staff and required full assistance with all of her ADLs.*

# CEREBRAL VASCULAR ACCIDENTS

*Cerebral vascular accidents, commonly called strokes, are neurologic events caused by a sudden loss of blood supply to part of the brain. The interruption of blood flow most commonly occurs from blood or cholesterol clots (emboli) or from blood vessel rupture (hemorrhage). A person's neurologic deficits and prognosis depend on the size and location of the stroke. Common motor deficits include arm and leg weakness ranging from total paralysis to mild weakness (hemiparesis). Sensory deficits include varying degrees of numbness (paresthesias). Speech disturbances include difficulty thinking of a word (expressive aphasia), difficulty understanding words or phrases (receptive aphasia), or slurred pronunciation (dysarthria). Swallow disturbances are also common. A patient's poststroke prognosis improves with rapid and steady recovery of the neurologic deficits. Some patients, however, may take up to a year to recover the deficits.*

1. List Mrs. Morgan's problems, both medical and functional. What problems would you want to prevent?
2. Which healthcare providers should help with Mrs. Morgan's recovery?
3. Why might Mrs. Morgan be uncooperative with the hospital staff?

## CASE 2

*Pete, a 51-year-old construction foreman, suffered severe crush injuries to both legs after a building collapse. Despite aggressive medical management after his rescue, he eventually required bilateral above-the-knee amputation. You have treated him in the past for hypertension and hyperlipidemia. On several occasions, you've recommended that he stop smoking cigarettes.*

1. What would you predict are Pete's functional limitations? How would you direct his rehabilitation to prevent further disabilities and handicaps?
2. Eight weeks after the accident, Pete remains dependent on caregivers for dressing, transfers, and toileting. How would you evaluate his lack of progress?
3. Pete's wife visits him sporadically. On several occasions, the rehabilitation staff has commented on her reluctance to discuss discharge plans. Which healthcare providers need to be involved at this point? What are their roles?

## CASE 3

*Vera Olson, a 76-year-old retired clerical worker, comes to your office with many concerns: fatigue, dizziness, insomnia, constipation, and back pain. None of these symptoms are new, but she feels that previous physicians have not really "listened" to her. Her medial history includes emphysema, hypertension, osteoporosis, and peptic ulcer disease. Current medications are propranolol, cimetidine, diphenhydramine, conjugated estrogen, calcium supplements, vitamin D, and triamcinolone and albuterol metered-dose inhalers.*

1. How would you approach this patient, who presents with so many complaints?
2. What other information would you want to obtain from Ms. Olson?
3. What instruments would be useful in sorting out Ms. Olson's concerns?

## CASE 4

*You have followed the Brown family in your practice for 12 years. David, 18 years old and the eldest of the four Brown children, is 2 weeks away from high school graduation when he suffers multiple injuries in a motor vehicle accident, including a lacerated spleen, rib fractures, and an incomplete spinal cord injury at the C7 level.*

*After almost 3 weeks in the intensive care unit, David is transferred to the medicine ward. On physical examination, David has resolving ecchymoses around the head and trunk. His abdomen has an intact laparotomy incision that is healing well. A Foley catheter is in place. Neurologically, motor strength in the upper extremities is 3/5 and in the lower extremities 1/5. He has mild flexion contractures of the elbows and wrists. Sensation to pinprick is intact at C7 and inferior.*

*Now that David's condition has stabilized, he and his family wonder what's next. Although David will continue to work with the rehabilitation team, he and his family still consider you his physician. They assume you will continue to follow David throughout his recovery.*

1. *How would you begin to evaluate David's functional abilities? What are his current functional limitations, in terms of diseases, impairments, and disabilities?*
2. *How do David's functional limitations differ from those of an older adult?*
3. *What is your role in David's recovery?*
4. *Before the accident, David had lined up a summer job with plans to enroll that fall at a nearby community college. He now wants to know when he will be "a normal person again." What would you say?*

## CASE 5

*Mrs. Montimore, a 79-year-old widow, is brought to your office by her daughter, Beth, who is worried about her mother. Since her husband's death 2 years ago, Mrs. Montimore has continued to live in her two-story home. Although she denies any falls, Beth is certain several have occurred. One month ago, Beth noticed bruises on her mother's right arm and leg.*

*Beth also feels that her mother's memory is not as sharp as it once was. Mrs. Montimore used to attend a garden club every week, but now rarely leaves her home. On multiple occasions, Beth has observed that her mother is still wearing her pajamas in the late afternoon. Over the past 6 months, Beth has brought over prepared meals regularly and has also cleaned her mother's home to help out. Mrs. Montimore has a history of hypertension, diabetes mellitus, and glaucoma. When you ask what medications she is taking, she replies that she left them at home, but takes them just as the bottles direct her to.*

1. *What further information do you want about Mrs. Montimore's function? How much is she really doing for herself?*
2. *What could be the causes of her functional decline?*
3. *What evaluations would you want to perform?*
4. *Beth is concerned that her mother may be unable to stay in her home much longer. All of her other children live far away, and Beth feels that the burden of care will rest on her. What could you do to help the daughter with her mother's care?*

## RECOMMENDED READINGS

DeLisa JA (ed): *Rehabilitation Medicine, Principles and Practice.* Philadelphia, JB Lippincott Co, 1988.

> This text provides a comprehensive reference for rehabilitation at all ages. It discusses general principles, including functional outcomes, diagnosis and management of common problems (such as contractures and neurogenic bowel and bladder), and specific disorders (such as spinal cord injuries and multiple sclerosis). A busy clinician can look up answers to rehabilitative questions with ease from the detailed index.

Kemp B, Brummel-Smith K, Ramsdell J (eds): *Geriatric Rehabilitation.* Boston, College-Hill Press, 1990.

> This text provides a comprehensive overview of geriatric rehabilitation. It discusses the general aspects of rehabilitation such as functional assessment and organization of rehabilitation programs. It also discusses specific disabling conditions, such as stroke, emphysema, and arthritis. Several chapters delve into the psychosocial aspects of geriatric medicine.

Reuben DB, Yoshikawa TT, Besdine RW (eds): *Geriatrics Review Syllabus.* Dubuque, Kendall/Hunt Publishing Co, 1996.

> Sponsored by the American Geriatrics Society, this text offers a core curriculum in geriatric medicine that provides current, detailed, and practical information on older adult topics.

Whittle MW: *Gait Analysis, An Introduction.* London, Butterworth–Heinemann Ltd, 1991.

> A detailed and readable text about analysis of gait and balance. The book begins with a concise review of the anatomy, physiology, and biomechanics of gait. It then discusses the characteristics of normal and pathological gaits and suggests ways to apply gait analysis to clinical practice. Diagrams provide good visualization of the author's descriptions.

Applegate WB, Blass JP, Williams TF: Instruments for the functional assessment of older patients. *N Engl J Med* 32:1207–1121, 1990.

Blazer D: Depression in the elderly. *N Engl J Med* 320:164–166, 1989.

Brink TL, Yesavage JA, Lum O, et al: Screening tests for geriatric depression. *Clin Gerontol* 1:37–43, 1982.

Bula CJ, et al: Effectiveness of preventive in-home geriatric assessment in well functioning, community-dwelling older people: Secondary analysis of a randomized trial. *J Am Geriatr Soc* 47:389–395, 1999.

Folstein MR, Folstein SE, McHugh PR: Mini-mental state: A practical method for grading the cognitive state of patients for the clinician. *J Psychiatr Res* 12:189–198, 1975.

Gorbien MJ, Bishop J, Beers MH, Norman D, Osterweil D, Rubenstein LZ: Iatrogenic illness in hospitalized elderly people. *J Am Geriatr Soc* 40:1031–1042, 1992.

Hoenig HM, Rubenstein LZ: Hospital-associated deconditioning and dysfunction. *J Am Geriatr Soc* 39:220–222, 1991.

Katz S, Ford AB, Moskowitz RW, Jackson BA, Jaffee W: Studies of illness in the aged: The index of AD: a standardized measure of biological and psychosocial function: *JAMA* 185:914–919, 1963.

Koenig HG, Meador KG, Cohen HG, Blazer DG: Self-rate depression scales and screening for major depression in the older hospitalized patient with medical illness. *J Am Geriatr Soc* 36:699–706, 1988.

Lachs MS, Feinstein AR, Cooney LM, Drickamer MA, Marottoli RA, Pannill FC, Tinetti ME: A simple procedure for general screening for functional disability in elderly patients. *Ann Intern Med* 112:699–706, 1990.

Lawton MP, Brody EM: Assessment of older people: Self-maintaining and instrumental activities of daily living. *Gerontologist* 9:179–186, 1969.

Mathias S, Nayak US, Isaacs B: Balance in elderly patients: The "get-up and go" test. *Arch Phys Med Rehabil* 67:387–389, 1986.

Moore AA, Siu AL: Screening for common problems in ambulatory elderly: Clinical confirmation of a screening instrument. *Am J Med* 100:438–443, 1996.

Reuben DB, et al: A randomized clinical trial of outpatient comprehensive geriatric assessment coupled with an intervention to increase adherence to recommendations. *J Am Geriatr Soc* 47:269–276, 1999.

Rubenstein LV, Calkins DR, Greenfield S, Jette AM, Meenan RF, Nevins MA, Rubenstein LZ, Wasson JH, Williams ME: Health status assessment for elderly patients, Report of the Society of General Internal Medicine Task Force on Health Assessment. *J Am Geriatr Soc* 37:562–569, 1988.

Rubenstein LZ: Geriatric assessment: An overview of its impacts. *Clin Geriatr Med* February, 1987.

Rubenstein LZ, Schairer C, Wieland GD, Kane R: Systematic biases in functional status assessment of elderly adults: Effects of different data sources. *J Gerontol* 39:686–691, 1984.

Schick FL, Schick R (eds): *Statistical Handbook on Aging Americans*. Phoenix, Ariz, Oryx Press, 1994; Table C2-4, p 119; Table A1-9, p 8.

Stuck AE, Diu AL, Wieland GD, Adams J, Rubenstein LZ: Comprehensive geriatric assessment: A meta-analysis of controlled trials. *Lancet* 342:1032–1036, 1993.

Sudarsky L: Geriatrics: Gait disorders in the elderly. *N Engl J Med* 322:1441–1445, 1990.

Tinetti ME: Performance-oriented assessment of mobility problems in elderly patients. *J Am Geriatr* Soc 34:119–126, 1986.

Tinetti ME, Ginter SF: Identifying mobility dysfunctions in elderly patients. Standard neuromuscular examination or direct assessment? *JAMA* 259:1190–1193, 1988.

Tinetti ME, Speechley M: Prevention of falls among the elderly. *N Engl J Med* 320:1055–1059, 1989.

Tombaugh T, McIntyre NJ: The mini-mental state examination: A comprehensive review. *J Am Geriatr Soc* 40:922–935, 1992.

Vorhies, D, Riley B: *Deconditioning Geriatric Rehabilitation , Clinics in Geriatric Medicine*. Philadelphia, WB Saunders Co, 1993, vol 9, No. 4, 745–762.

World Health Organization: *International Classification of Impairments, Disabilities, and Handicaps: A Manual of Classification Relating to the Consequences of Disease*. Geneva, World Health Organization, 1980.

Yesavage JA, Brink TL, Rose RL, Lum O, Huang V, Adey M, Leirer VO: Development and validation of a geriatric depression screening scale: A preliminary report. *J Psychiatr Res* 17:37–49, 1983.

## CHAPTER 17

# Health Promotion and Disease Prevention

*Larry L. Dickey*

*John T. is a 25-year-old patient who is seen by you because of pain in his right hand after bending a finger playing basketball. You diagnose mild soft tissue injury and suggest that he treat it with ice, ibuprofen, and rest. He also brings up that he would like his cholesterol tested because he "wants to live to be 100." Further discussion reveals that he has no medical or family history factors that would put him at risk for coronary artery disease. You have only 5 minutes left before you will need to go to see a patient in the hospital. Rather than order a cholesterol test, you decide to use the time to talk with John and discover that he drinks six beers daily, has had two serious traffic accidents in the last 2 years, and has had unprotected sex with five different partners in the last year. You advise him to not worry about a cholesterol test despite recommendations he has seen on television, but instead to eat a low-fat, low-cholesterol diet, limit his alcohol intake to two drinks a day, wear seat belts, and use condoms with every sexual partner. He declines an HIV test. All of this makes you 5 minutes late getting to the hospital.*

## EDUCATIONAL OBJECTIVES

1. Appreciate the importance of health promotion and disease prevention
2. Describe the basic principles of performing the four types of clinical preventive services: counseling, screening testing and examination, immunization, and chemoprophylaxis
3. Describe how guidelines for clinical preventive medicine are formulated by major authorities
4. Formulate a protocol of preventive medicine procedures for your "own" practice
5. Demonstrate the use of basic office resources for efficiently performing health promotion and disease prevention

Preventive care is no longer as simple as the annual physical, having been replaced by an array of screening tests and other procedures that have different periodicities depending on patient age, sex, and risk factors. Case 17-1 illustrates many of the practical challenges facing clinicians today: how to decide on the most effective health promotion and disease prevention interventions in the context of differing recommendations from major authorities, pressure from a motivated but often poorly informed public, and time and economic constraints.

This chapter will give the student some of the basic knowledge and tools needed to begin coping with these challenges. It should be read with attention to detail while keeping in mind that the content of preventive care, like acute care, will change and grow as the knowledge base increases in future years. As you progress in your future training there will be many factors that may serve to convince you that preventive care isn't important. For the time being at least, suspend judgment on that issue and attempt to understand the sound scientific principles that underpin the field.

You should consider the cases described carefully, because they have been chosen to accurately reflect what you will see in everyday practice, particularly in a primary care field. Preventive care will probably consume a large portion of your future professional life, in some cases as much as 50% or more. Patients like these will enter your office or clinic every day. The pattern of care you begin to develop today will likely persist throughout your career.

## CASE 17-2

*Roger J. is a 53-year-old businessman who was referred to you by his previous physician in his former city of residence. His presenting complaint is "high blood pressure" controlled with medication. You note that he is 50 pounds overweight, and on questioning discover that 50% of the calories in his diet come from fat. You also determine that physical activity for him is limited to bowling one night a week and an occasional walk with the family dog. You prescribe a diet that has only 30% of calories from fat and suggest that he increase his physical activity by briskly walking 2 miles every other night. Over the course of the next 6 months he tries to follow your instructions and loses 20 pounds. His blood pressure decreases and you tell him that if he continues to lose weight and exercise, he may be ready to discontinue his blood pressure medication.*

## THE IMPORTANCE OF PREVENTION

Table 17.1 lists the leading causes of death in the United States for all ages in 1990 (National Center for Health Statistics, 1993). These leading causes are familiar to most health professionals and perhaps would more appropriately be called the proximal causes of death, the diagnoses entered onto death certificates. In reality, the underlying causes of death, the factors that eventually (but not finally) lead to death, may be more important. McGinnis and Foege (1993) published a list of what they called the "actual causes of death in the United States in 1990" (see Table 17.2). Using a complex methodology, they separated out the contributions of various nongenetic ("external") risk factors for mortality. Even when using the most conservative estimates they demonstrated that half of all deaths could be attributed to only nine causes, all of which are modifiable or preventable to some extent.

Most of these "actual causes" are the result of social and personal behaviors, e.g., smoking, substance abuse, unhealthy nutrition, and physical and sexual activity patterns. Although responsibility for their modification resides largely in the realms of personal responsibility and public policy, there is much that providers can do to help stem the tide of preventable and premature death. Clinicians are firsthand witnesses of the destructive effects of unhealthy behaviors and remain a trusted source of health-related information for

**Table 17.1**
Leading Causes of Death, United States, 1990[a]

| Cause | Number |
|---|---|
| Heart disease | 720,000 |
| Cancer | 505,000 |
| Cerebrovascular disease | 144,000 |
| Accidents | 92,000 |
| Chronic obstructive pulmonary disease | 87,000 |
| Pneumonia and influenza | 80,000 |
| Diabetes mellitus | 48,000 |
| Suicide | 31,000 |
| Chronic liver disease and cirrhosis | 26,000 |
| Human immunodeficiency disease | 25,000 |
| | 2,148,000 |

[s]Source: National Center for Health Statistics. *Advance Report of Final Mortality, 1990.* Hyattsville, MD, US Department of Health and Human Services, 1993. Monthly Vital Statistics Report, Vol. 41, No. 7.

most patients. Most Americans see a physician multiple times during each year—the average number of visits to a physician in 1995 was 5.8 (National Center for Health Statistics, 1998)—often when they are ill and most receptive to medical and lifestyle interventions.

The range of preventive interventions that a clinician can deliver can be divided into four basic types:

Counseling
Screening tests and examinations
Immunizations
Chemoprophylaxis

## Counseling

Counseling can take many forms but usually consists of the clinician speaking directly with the patient about a health problem or health-related behavior, as in Case 17-2. Pamphlets and other printed media are

**Table 17.2**
Actual Causes of Death in the United States in 1990[a]

| Cause | Deaths | |
|---|---|---|
| | Estimated no.[b] | % of total deaths |
| Tobacco | 400,000 | 19 |
| Diet/activity patterns | 300,000 | 14 |
| Alcohol | 100,000 | 5 |
| Microbial agents | 90,000 | 4 |
| Toxic agents | 60,000 | 3 |
| Firearms | 35,000 | 2 |
| Sexual behavior | 30,000 | 1 |
| Motor vehicles | 25,000 | 1 |
| Illicit drug use | 20,000 | $\leq 1$ |
| | 1,060,000 | 50 |

[a]Source: McGinnis JM, Foege WH: *JAMA* 270:2207–2212, 1983.
[b]Composite approximation drawn from studies that use different approaches to derive estimates, ranging from actual accounts (e.g., firearms) to population attributable risk calculations (e.g., tobacco). Numbers over 100,000 rounded to the nearest 100,000; over 50,000 rounded to the nearest 10,000; below 50,000 rounded to the nearest 5000.

**Table 17.3**
USPSTF Principles of Patient Education and Counseling[a]

1. Develop a therapeutic alliance
2. Counsel all patients
3. Ensure that patients understand the relationship between behavior and health
4. Work with patients to assess barriers to behavior change
5. Gain commitment from patients to change
6. Involve patients in selecting risk factors to change
7. Use a combination of strategies
8. Design a behavior modification plan
9. Monitor progress through follow-up contact
10. Involve office staff

[a]Source: U.S. Preventive Services Task Force. Recommendations for patient education and counseling, in *Guide to Clinical Preventive Services*. Baltimore: Williams & Wilkins Co, 1989.

useful adjuncts to verbal counseling, but by themselves are generally not sufficient to influence patient behavior significantly (Kottke *et al.*, 1988; Mead *et al.*, 1995). Recently, electronic media, such as interactive video disks, have been developed to help patients share in difficult medical decision-making processes (Kasper *et al.*, 1992). However, such tools are not widely used and in-person counseling remains the most trusted modality.

Patient counseling is an area of medicine that remains almost as much of an art as a science. However, some basic guidelines have been delineated, such as those published by the U.S. Preventive Services Task Force (1989) (see Table 17.3). These principles, while clear and comprehensive, require explanation and expansion. Principle 1, of course, applies to all clinical encounters, not only counseling or preventive interventions. Principle 2 addresses the fact that almost all patients have some health issues for which they could benefit from advice and guidance. Since many patients don't spontaneously volunteer problems and concerns, these must be assessed through actively soliciting information from patients. This can be either in person or through brief written questionnaires. Principle 3 is important because cognitive understanding of the relationship of behavior and health seems to be a necessary, although not usually sufficient, prerequisite to change.

Principles 4 to 6 address the importance of active patient involvement and commitment. Counseling provided to patients in only one form and on only one occasion tends to quickly lose effectiveness. For this reason it is important to use different strategies, Principle 7, and follow-up interventions, Principle 9, to reinforce the message and progress. Many patients can benefit from the concrete reinforcements of behavior modification techniques. Involvement of office staff, Principle 10, can be crucial, since they often have more time and training for counseling and follow-up than do busy clinicians.

Personal experiences teach us that behavior and lifestyle changes are not quick or linear (see Chapter 15, "Counseling and Behavioral Change"). Small improvements are usually followed by relapses, hopefully smaller than the improvements. The work of Prochaska and colleagues has delineated six "stages of change" that are useful for clinicians. These stages are: precontemplation, contemplation, preparation, action, maintenance, and termination (Prochaska *et al.*, 1994a,b). During precontemplation, people are in denial and have not yet recognized the problem behavior. During the contemplation stage they have acknowledged the problem and during the preparation stage have begun to plan concrete steps for dealing with it. During the action stage they actively carry out changes in behavior and during the maintenance stage endeavor to prevent relapses and consolidate gains. In the termination stage the temptation to relapse is no longer present and the problem is no longer active. Progress between stages can take months or years and the entire process a lifetime, with numerous episodes of relapse. Patience and persistence are vital.

Perhaps the most useful contribution of Prochaska's work is the identification of the types of interventions that are likely to be effective at each stage (see Table 17.4). Too much clinician effort is expended

**Table 17.4**
Stages of Change in Which Particular Change Processes Are Most Useful[a,b]

| Precontemplation | Contemplation | Preparation | Action | Maintenance |
|---|---|---|---|---|
| Consciousness-raising ⟶ | | | | |
| Social liberation ———————————————————————————⟶ | | | | |
| | Emotional arousal ——————⟶ | | | |
| | Self-reevaluation ——————⟶ | | | |
| | | Commitment ———————————————————⟶ | | |
| | | | Reward ⟶ | |
| | | | Countering ————————————————⟶ | |
| | | | Environmental control ——————⟶ | |
| | | | Helping relationships ——————⟶ | |

[a]From Prochaska JO, Norcross JC, DiClemente CC: *Changing for Good*. New York, William Morrow & Co, 1994. Used with permission of the publisher. Copyright 1994.
[b]Examples of change processes: consciousness raising—education; social liberation—activities of advocacy groups; emotional arousal—fear, anger, or other strong emotions; self-reevaluation—thoughtful reassessment of personal situation and characteristics; commitment—promise to self and others to change; reward—emotional, material, or health gain from change; countering—substituting a healthy behavior for an unhealthy one; environmental control—changing surroundings to support and maintain change; helping relationships—supprotive friends and family.

providing interventions that are either too advanced or too basic for the patient's stage of change. For example, establishing a behavior modification plan for a patient in the precontemplation or contemplation stages probably will fail; providing consciousness-raising information to a patient in the action stage will be of little use when what is really needed is supportive relationships and concrete rewards.

How effective is patient counseling for behavior change and is it really worth the effort? Data obtained from smoking cessation projects are helpful in answering this question. As a result of counseling by physicians, about 5% of smokers will quit for at least 6 months (Kottke *et al.*, 1988). It has been estimated that if all providers counseled their smoking patients to quit, the national smoking quit rate would almost double (U.S. Public Health Service, 1991). While 5% effectiveness may not seem like much to the individual clinician, for society as a whole and for individuals saved from fatal illnesses, this level of effectiveness may be highly significant. When considering the impact of counseling interventions, it is useful to keep in mind McGinnis and Foege's actual causes of mortality (Table 17.2) and the great burden of suffering ultimately brought on by unhealthy behaviors. From this perspective, counseling interventions may be the most important services clinicians provide.

For many providers the most basic challenge is providing not the most effective counseling, but any counseling at all. A 1994 survey of health plan subscribers in California found that on average only 20% of counseling topics recommended by the U.S. Preventive Services Task Force had been discussed with patients by providers during the preceding 3 years (Schauffler *et al.*, 1996). Low rates of counseling have also been found in studies of patient charts and clinician self-reports, less than 50% for most counseling areas (Lewis, 1988). Although very basic interventions can be effective (such as advising a patient to quit smoking), these are not consistently provided. For counseling interventions perhaps the first rule of practice should be: Above all, say something—regardless of how basic.

## CASE 17-3

*Mrs. Kawasaki is a 55-year-old woman who had a routine screening mammogram in July 1998 that was read as negative for abnormality. In August 1998 she noticed a small lump in her right breast but was not alarmed because of her recent negative mammogram. In October 1998 she saw her physician for treatment of a sprained ankle and mentioned the small lump. He quickly performed a breast examination but wasn't able to feel the lump clearly. He told her that he wasn't concerned because of her recent negative mammogram. He advised her to get another annual mammogram in July 1999. This mammogram clearly revealed breast cancer and a subsequent bone scan revealed widespread metastases.*

## CASE 17-4

*Mr. Jones is a 55-year-old white man who had prostate-specific antigen (PSA) testing at the suggestion of his physician as part of an annual checkup. Mr. Jones was without symptoms of prostate cancer, but very alarmed when his test results were elevated at 5 ng/ml. He had a good friend who died of prostate cancer at the age of 60. He was so distressed, in fact, that he was unable to work for 2 weeks while waiting for an appointment with the urologist. A needle biopsy was performed, the pathology report for which was "benign hypertrophy." Mr. Jones developed a mild prostate infection after the biopsy that was successfully treated with antibiotics. During this treatment he took off another 2 days of work. During the course of his workup and treatment he was passed over for a promotion in favor of a younger employee. Mr. Jones subsequently felt that he had been misled by his physicians since he had not been told that most men of his age and race with a PSA level of 5 ng/ml do not have prostate cancer.*

## Screening Tests and Examinations

Screening tests, such as mammograms and PSA tests, are intended to detect a disease at an early, asymptomatic stage when it can be cured or effectively treated. Several criteria for judging the value of screening tests have been proposed. Those of Frame and Carlson (1975) are presented in Table 17.5. Principles 1 to 4 can be briefly summarized: Screening is not worthwhile (and may cause more harm than good) if the condition cannot be treated more effectively as a result of early detection. Principles 5 and 6 touch on the increasingly important issue of cost, both for the individual patient and for society. In general, screening tests do not save society money, although they do save years of life. For example, mammography has been found to cost $20,000 to $50,000 for each year of life saved. Although this may seem high, it compared favorably with the cost-effectiveness of many treatment interventions, such as the treatment of mild hypertension with medications or the treatment of angina with coronary artery bypass surgery, $32,600 and $62,900, respectively, per year of life saved (Mushlin & Fintor, 1992).

The U.S. Preventive Services Task Force (1989) has employed an additional criterion for judging the worth of a screening test: "The test must be able to detect the target condition... with sufficient accuracy to avoid producing large numbers of false-positive and false-negative results."

To appreciate the importance of this criterion, it is necessary to understand the concepts of sensitivity and specificity, previously addressed in Chapter 9, "Appropriate Use of Laboratory Tests." Recall that sensitivity

**Table 17.5**
Judging the Value of Screening Tests in Medical Practice[a]

1. The condition must have a significant effect on the quality and quantity of life.
2. Acceptable methods of treatment must be available.
3. The condition must have an asymptomatic period during which detection and treatment significantly reduce morbidity and mortality.
4. Treatment in the asymptomatic phase must yield a therapeutic result superior to that obtained by delaying treatment until symptoms appear.
5. Tests that are acceptable to patients must be available, at a reasonable cost, to detect the condition in the asymptomatic period.
6. The incidence of the condition must be sufficient to justify the cost of screening.

[a]From Frame PS, Carlson SJ: A critical review of periodic health screening using specific screening criteria. *J Fam Pract* 2:29–36, 1975. Copyright 1975. Reprinted by permission of Appleton & Lange Inc.

is the ability of a test to detect the presence of the target condition. With a sensitivity of 80%, 20% of patients who have the target condition will not be detected, a false negative. Specificity is the ability of a test to correctly identify those without a condition as not having the condition. Thus, with a specificity of 80%, 20% of patients without the condition will be falsely identified as having the condition, a false positive. As the incidence of a condition in the population declines, the proportion of people screened who do not have the condition will increase and, as a consequence, the proportion of people wrongly identified as having the condition will increase.

Since most routine screening tests have limited sensitivity, usually less than 90%, a negative test result does not ensure that the disease is absent. For example, 10% of breast cancers will not be identified by mammography. Screening tests may thus lead to an unjustified sense of security for both clinicians and patients. Significant symptoms and signs must not be overlooked, as in Case 17-3, despite negative screening test results.

It is important for the clinician and the patient to keep in mind that, because of the low incidence of most diseases targeted for screening and the limited specificity of most screening tests, usually less than 90%, patients identified as having a disease by routine screening often do not have the disease. For example, the specificity of a PSA test with a cutoff of 4 ng/ml is only about 30%. Up to 70% of men, such as Mr. Jones in Case 17-4, identified as positive by PSA screening do not have prostate cancer. Thus, a false-positive screening test can result in unnecessary anxiety, cost, and iatrogenic side effects from procedures performed, e.g., needle biopsy of the prostate, to work up falsely positive test results. When targeting asymptomatic individuals for screening tests and other preventive services, clinicians should keep in mind the ancient precept, "primum non nocere"—above all do no harm.

Cases 17-3 and 17-4 demonstrate the importance of clearly educating patients about the capabilities and limitations of screening tests both before they are performed and after results are returned. Some authorities have even proposed that this education be part of a formalized informed consent process for screening tests (Lee, 1993).

## Immunization

Immunizations are the prototypical clinical preventive service, with a distinguished history spanning from the first use of cowpox vaccine in the 1700s to the first complete eradication of an infectious disease, smallpox, in the 1970s. Immunizations are probably the easiest, most effective type of preventive service to administer, but are often overlooked by clinicians. It is important for clinicians to understand some basic facts about the effectiveness and administration of immunizations.

Immunizations need not totally prevent clinical disease in order to be effective. For example, influenza immunization of the elderly is only 30 to 40% effective at preventing clinical illness in the elderly, but 70 to 90% effective at preventing death from influenza in the elderly. Immunizations also need not confer immunity on 100% of recipients or be given to every member of the population to be effective. In fact, much of the value of immunizations is in the induction of "herd immunity," which protects all members of the population by limiting exposure and transmission. When a clinician immunizes a child against an infectious disease, protection is also provided to other children who have not been immunized or who have not responded to the vaccine.

Adults, like children, need to receive immunizations. This fact is often overlooked. Immunization rates for adults are in the 40% (pneumococcus) to 60% (influenza) range. Conversely, some children and younger adults need immunizations routinely reserved for older adults, i.e., pneumococcus and influenza. In general, patients of any age with chronic respiratory or cardiovascular diseases, diabetes, or immunosuppression need these immunizations. Recipients need not be totally clinically well in order to receive routine vaccinations. Misconceptions regarding this point result in many missed opportunities for immunization. Clinicians should be aware of the true contraindications and relative contraindications for immunizations, especially since one of the main opportunities to immunize patients is when they are seen for treatment of an illness of some type.

## INFORMED CONSENT FOR PROSTATE CANCER SCREENING

*Mr. Johnson is a 55 year-old white male who has come to his primary care provider, Dr. Nelson, for a routine check up. He has no current illness or symptoms. Dr. Nelson raises the issue of prostate cancer.*

DR. NELSON:     *Prostate cancer is the second leading cause of cancer death for men in the United States. About one in six men will get invasive cancer of the prostate during their life time. However, only about one in four men with invasive prostate cancer end up dying of the disease. Because it is slow growing and occurs most frequently in older men, most will not die of it.*

MR. JOHNSON:     *Yes, I've known many friends with this disease—and some have died. Is their anything I can do?*

DR. NELSON:     *Some authorities, such as the American Cancer Society, recommend a blood test yearly beginning at 50 years of age. This test detects prostate specific antigen (PSA) in the blood. An elevated level may indicate the presence of prostate cancer. However, other authorities, such as the National Cancer Institute and the U.S. Preventive Services Task Force, do not recommend this screening test.*

MR. JOHNSON:     *Why not? What could be wrong with detecting cancer early?*

DR. NELSON:     *Detecting cancer early may not be worthwhile if the available treatments do not help prolong life. Thus far, studies have not shown that men who have cancers detected by PSA live longer than those whose cancers are detected by symptoms. This may be because we just haven't done the proper studies yet. However, it is not clear whether treating prostate cancer at an early stage leads to better results than not treating it. Treatments (such as surgery or radiation) may cause side effects, such as impotence or incontinence.*

MR. JOHNSON:     *What's the harm of doing the test? I don't mind having blood drawn.*

DR. NELSON:     *Because of what we call limited "specificity" of the test, approximately two-thirds of men who have an elevated level on the test do not have cancer. This leads to many biopsies which can be painful and lead to considerable anxiety. Also, because of limited "sensitivity" of the test, approximately one in ten cancers will not be detected by the test. This may lead to false reassurance and may cause some patients to later ignore symptoms. Also, the test costs money (approximately $100), which is definitely a factor for some people. You are fortunate since your insurance will pay for it.*

MR. JOHNSON:     *So, you're telling me that the test may give me a jump on a leading cause of cancer but authorities aren't in agreement that it works and it may lead to unnecessary or more painful tests for me. What should I do?*

DR. NELSON:     *I can't really tell you that. It's a matter of personal preference. All authorities recommend that I inform you of these risks and potential benefits in order to help you make up your own mind. I'll be glad to discuss this further and answer any more questions you may have.*

# Chemoprophylaxis

Chemoprophylaxis is the use of a chemical, usually a drug or medication, to prevent the development of disease. Despite numerous theories and trials, there are currently only two chemoprophylactic agents widely endorsed for use with asymptomatic, low-risk populations: fluoride supplementation to prevent dental caries in children living in areas with low amounts of fluoride in the drinking water and folate supplementation for women of childbearing age to help prevent neural tube disorders in their offspring. For adults, the two most widely used agents are aspirin, for the prevention of heart disease in middle-aged men, and estrogen, for the prevention of osteoporosis and heart disease in postmenopausal women. All chemoprophylactic agents have potential side effects that can make their use problematic. Fluoride can lead to mottled teeth, folate supplementation can mask vitamin $B_{12}$ deficiencies, aspirin may cause hemorrhagic stroke and gastrointestinal bleeding, and estrogen may increase the risks for breast cancer and uterine cancer.

Clinicians should carefully weigh the potential benefits and harms of each agent in light of each patient's medical characteristics and personal desires. Because the trade-off of potential benefits against side effects is often close, patient participation in decision-making is vital. For this reason, most major authorities have classified the provision of chemoprophylaxis in the general category of health counseling.

## CASE 17-5

*Dr. T. graduated from a good medical school and a good residency program in internal medicine. On finishing his training he established a successful practice in a medium-sized, Midwest city. Dr. T. liked to approach the preventive care of his patients as he did their acute care, by relying on his excellent clinical judgment. Mr. J. was a 55-year-old man whom Dr. T. saw for a checkup once in 1995. Results of his examination and cholesterol and fecal occult blood tests ordered at this visit were normal. Mr. J. was not seen again until 1999, when he came into Dr. T.'s office complaining of rectal bleeding. Subsequent tests revealed metastatic colon cancer. Dr. T. told Mr. J. that it was too bad that he had not come back to see him earlier, because he might have ordered a fecal occult blood test or screening sigmoidoscopy examination that might have discovered the cancer earlier. Mr. J. said that he did not know that he should have come back earlier because Dr. T. had not told him to and that, in any case, he expected Dr. T. to notify him of any need for preventive care, as does his dentist. Now Mr. J.'s lawyer wants to know what schedule of preventive care Dr. T. follows and what system he has to make sure that patients receive it.*

## CASE 17-6

*Ms. T. is a 25-year-old woman who comes to Dr. J. for a routine checkup. Dr. J. knows that based on her age and gender she will definitely need Pap smears every 1 to 3 years; blood pressure, height, and weight measurements every 1 to 2 years; tetanus–diphtheria immunizations every 10 years; periodic counseling on nutrition, including folate supplementation; and counseling on physical activity. In order to assess her need for other preventive care interventions, Dr. J. asks her about a number of different aspects of her life and history. Based on the following information about Ms. T., he orders additional types of preventive care (in parentheses): she is a Native American who has spent much of her life living on a reservation (plasma glucose and tuberculosis screening), her mother died of heart disease at age 54 (cholesterol screening), she has had moderate asthma for 10 years (influenza and pneumococcal immunization), she works as a pottery maker (lead screening for her children), she is monogamously married with two young children but has had multiple male partners in the past (HIV screening), and drinks about 20 beers per week (alcohol abuse counseling).*

## ESTABLISHING A PREVENTIVE CARE PROTOCOL

One of the most basic tasks facing any primary care clinician is to decide on the types and frequencies of preventive services to be routinely provided to patients. Surprisingly, many clinicians never get around to doing this in any formal fashion. This results in confusion for clinicians, staff, and patients, which in turn probably contributes to poor performance rates. This is unnecessary since a number of major authorities,

# Clinical Preventive Services for Normal-Risk Children

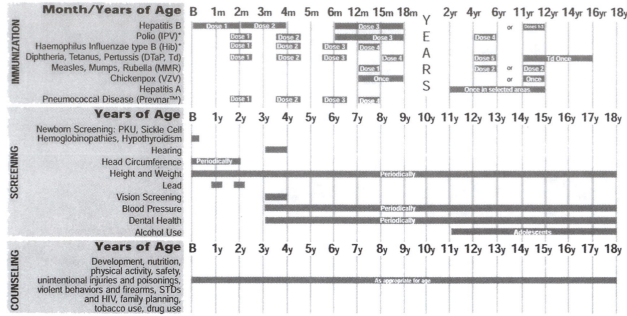

**Figure 17.1.** Child preventive care time line: recommendations of major authorities.

including all four major primary care physician organizations, have issued comprehensive schedules for preventive care that can serve as templates for clinicians to follow (American Academy of Family Physicians, 1997; American Academy of Pediatrics, 1995; American College of Obstetricians and Gynecologists, 1993; Eddy, 1992; American College of Physicians Task Force on Adult Immunization and Infectious Disease Society of America, 1994).

There is a considerable amount of consensus among authorities (see Figs. 17.1 and 17.2 adapted from tables published by the U.S. Public Health Service in the *Clinician's Handbook of Preventive Services, Second Edition*) (U.S. Department of Health and Human Services, 1998). In these charts, dark bars denote preventive services recommended by every major authority for asymptomatic patients, while the light bars denote preventive services recommended by only some major authorities. It is reasonable that every clinician include the preventive services denoted by dark bars in any preventive care protocol for his or her practice.

The next step is to address the preventive services for which there is some disagreement among major authorities (light bars in Figs. 17.1 and 17.2). In order to do this it is useful to have some basic knowledge about the major authorities and how their recommendations for preventive care are formulated. It is also wise to keep in mind that, from a medicolegal standpoint, there are no clear right or wrong answers for these gray areas.

## Assessing the Authorities and the Evidence

The first attempts to bring order to the expanding area of clinical prevention in the United States were made by individual experts, such as Frame and Carlson (1975) and Breslow and Sommers (1977) in the late 1970s. Soon voluntary organizations, such as the American Cancer Society (1980), professional societies,

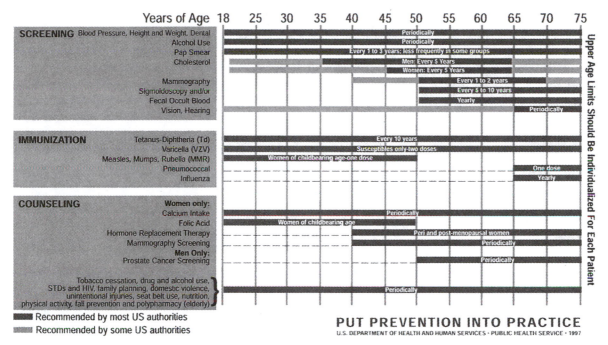

**Figure 17.2.** Adult preventive care time line: recommendations of major authorities.

such as the American College of Physicians (1981), and governmental agencies, such as the National Cancer Institute (1987), became active in the field. All of these authorities used somewhat different methodologies and often reached different conclusions. To help resolve the confusion, in 1984 the U.S. Public Health Service convened the U.S. Preventive Services Task Force (USPSTF). This group was composed of health professionals with expertise in assessing scientific and epidemiologic evidence. The USPSTF's comprehensive recommendations were issued in 1989 and 1996 in the Guide to Clinical Preventive Services (U.S. Preventive Services Task Force, 1989, 1996).

The USPSTF was the first U.S. body to employ a well-defined, explicit methodology for assessing scientific evidence and reporting recommendations. This methodology, which was largely adopted from the Canadian Task Force on the Periodic Health Examination (1979), emphasized carefully grading the quality of scientific evidence (see Table 17.6), with evidence from randomized controlled trials receiving the most weight and that from expert opinions receiving the least. In general, only preventive services supported by evidence in the top two categories, and occasionally reaching down to the third category, were recommended. The USPSTF has also emphasized the importance of actual health outcomes, as opposed to intermediate outcomes, such as service delivery, in formulating its recommendations. As a consequence, the USPSTF recommendations are among the most conservative, but scientifically respected, of any issued by a U.S. group.

The controversy regarding recommendations for mammography screening of women less than 50 years of age demonstrates how the USPSTF methodology differs from that of some other authorities. The American Cancer Society recommends routine mammography for all women beginning at age 40 (American Cancer Society, 1992), a position also supported by the National Cancer Institute. This position is largely based on evidence that mammography can successfully detect cancer at an early stage in women of this age. Large trials, however, have failed to clearly demonstrate that mammography in women younger than 50, unlike that in women 50 or older, leads to a reduction in mortality (Miller *et al.*, 1992; Tabar *et al.*, 1985; Verbeek *et al.*, 1984; Woolf & Dickey, 1999). Lacking data to support this important health outcome, the USPSTF and some other authorities have not recommended beginning routine mammography before age 50. Proponents of early mammography have argued that it is logical that early detection and treatment of breast cancer will lead to improved survival for younger women, as it has for older women, and that studies have failed to detect this effect because of defects in their designs. Proponents also argue that even if mammography does not lead to

**Table 17.6**
USPSTF Rating System for Quality of Scientific Evidence[a]

| | |
|---|---|
| I: | Evidence obtained from at least one properly designed randomized controlled trial |
| II-1: | Evidence obtained from well-designed controlled trials without randomization |
| II-2: | Evidence obtained from well-designed cohort or case–control analytic studies, preferably from more than one center or research group |
| II-3: | Evidence obtained from multiple time series with or without the intervention, or dramatic results in uncontrolled experiments (such as the results of the introduction of penicillin treatment in the 1940s) |
| III: | Opinions of respected authorities, based on clinical experience, descriptive studies, or reports of expert committees |

[a]From U.S. Preventive Services Task Force: Task force ratings, in *Guide to Clinical Preventive Services*. Baltimore: Williams & Wilkins Co, 1989, p. 388.

improved mortality for younger women, it may lead to improved quality of life. Opponents counter that breast cancer may be a biologically different, more aggressive disease in women younger than 50 such that early detection has no effect on mortality and that quality-of-life outcomes cannot be quantitatively assessed.

Large healthcare purchasers and insurers often refuse to provide services that have not been demonstrated in well-designed studies to result in improved health outcomes. As a result, many insurers and healthcare purchasers have endorsed the preventive care recommendations of the USPSTF and other "evidence-based" groups over those based on expert opinion. Because the lack of insurance coverage can be a major barrier to obtaining preventive care, it is reasonable for the clinician to consider the realities of insurance coverage and availability of free or subsidized screening facilities in the community in determining a preventive care protocol for his or her practice.

Primary care clinicians face a dilemma when considering the preventive care recommendations of subspecialty societies. Primary care clinicians frequently defer to the judgment of subspecialists on treatment issues. Should not these same subspecialists also be the most reliable source of information on screening issues as well? Unfortunately, subspecialty training does not usually provide any expertise in epidemiology, public health, cost-effectiveness analysis, or other areas of central importance in determining population-based guidelines. On the contrary, subspecialists may be so invested professionally and financially in studying or treating a particular organ or disease that they don't understand or value these wider issues.

## Considering Risk Factors

Most patients are at increased risk for preventable disease because of factors in one or more of the following categories: ethnic/geographic origin, family history, personal medical history, occupational/recreational history, sexual history, substance abuse history, and social/living situation. The major risk factors for each of these categories that have been described by major authorities, the relevant diseases, and the potentially effective preventive services have been compiled in Table 17.7. In treating large numbers of patients with pertinent risk factors, it may be advisable to include the relevant preventive services in the routine preventive care protocol for all patients. For example, a clinician who treats many migrant farm workers may choose to perform routine tuberculosis screening on all patients.

Information about the risk factor profile of a community or population can be obtained by consulting state and local public health officials. Information about the risk factors of individual patients must, in general, be obtained from the patient. In this task the use of brief questionnaires, either at the first or subsequent visits, can be very valuable. Electronic tools for soliciting and analyzing patient risk factor information have been developed (Roizen *et al.*, 1992). Such tools, although not widely used, can make the complex task of tailoring preventive care to the patient much easier.

## Implementing Health Promotion and Disease Prevention

Having decided on a preventive care protocol, the clinician has taken the first, most essential step toward making health promotion and disease prevention a prominent part of practice. There are, however, many steps left to be taken. The most mundane, but nonetheless critical, is instituting an office system to carry out the protocol.

**Table 17.7**
Summary Table of Risk Factors, Diseases, and Preventive Services[a]

| Risk factor | Disease(s) | Preventive service(s) |
|---|---|---|
| Ethnic and geographic origin | | |
| Asian, African, Mediterranean, Caribbean, Latin American | Hemoglobinopathies | Sickledex text and/or hemoglobin electrophoresis |
| Native American, Hispanic, African American (adults) | Diabetes mellitus | Plasma glucose test |
| Native American, foreign-born from countries with high TB prevalence (i.e., Africa, Asia, Latin America) | Tuberculosis | Tuberculosis skin test |
| African-American (adults ≥ age 40) | Glaucoma | Comprehensive eye exam |
| Family history | | |
| Iron-deficit mother (infant) | Anemia | Hemoglobin/hematocrit test |
| Sibling treated for lead poisoning (child) | Lead poisoning | Lead test |
| Parent cholesterol level ≥240 mg/dl, parent or grandparent ≤55 had myocardial infarction, angina pectoris, peripheral vascular disease, sudden cardiac death, coronary artery bypass or angioplasty (child ≥ age 2) | Hypercholesterolemia | Total cholesterol test |
| Breast cancer in first-degree relative (women ≥ age 35) | Breast cancer | Mammography |
| Colon cancer in first-degree relative | Colon cancer, familial polyposis, cancer family syndrome | Sigmoidoscopy, colonoscopy, or barium enema |
| Prostate cancer (men ≥ age 40) | Prostate cancer | Digital rectal exam, prostate-specific antigen test |
| Skin cancer (adults) | Skin cancer | Skin exam |
| Diabetes mellitus in first-degree relative | Diabetes mellitus | Plasma glucose |
| Personal medical history | | |
| Low birth weight, prematurity (infant) | Anemia | Hemoglobin/hematocrit test |
| | Hearing loss | Hearing testing |
| | Visual loss | Comprehensive eye exam |
| Excessive menstrual flow | Anemia | Hemoglobin/hematocrit test |
| Inflammatory bowel disease, colorectal adenomatous polyps, breast, endometrial, ovarian cancer | Colorectal cancer | Sigmoidoscopy, colonoscopy, or barium enema |
| Blood transfusion between 1978 and 1985 | HIV disease | HIV test |
| Diabetes mellitus | Vision loss | Comprehensive eye exam |
| | Urinary tract infection | Urinalysis test |
| | Influenza | Influenza immunization |
| | Pneumococcal disease | Pneumococcal immunization |
| Chronic pulmonary or respiratory disease | Influenza | Influenza immunization |
| | Pneumococcal disease | Pneumococcal immunization |
| Splenectomy, splenic dysfunction | Pneumococcal disease | Pneumococcal immunization |
| Renal dysfunction | Influenza | Influenza immunization |
| | Pneumococcal disease | Pneumococcal immunization |
| | Hepatitis B (if hemodialysis) | Hepatitis B immunization |
| Cirrhosis | Influenza | Influenza immunization |
| | Pneumococcal disease | Pneumococcal immunization |
| Immunosuppression, including HIV, organ transplantation, medication induced | Influenza | Influenza immunization |
| | Pneumococcal disease | Pneumococcal disease |
| | Tuberculosis | Tuberculosis skin test |
| Lack of immunity to measles and born after 1956 | Measles | MMR immunization |
| Lack of immunity to rubella, especially women of childbearing age | Rubella, congenital rubella syndrome in offspring | Rubella immunization |
| Cryptorchidism, orchiopexy, infertile or atrophic testes, ambiguous genitalia, gonadal dysgensis, Klinefelter's syndrome (men) | Testicular cancer | Testicular exam |

*continued*

**Table 17.7**
*(Continued)*

| Risk factor | Disease(s) | Preventive service(s) |
|---|---|---|
| | Sexual history | |
| Multiple sexual partners | HIV disease and other STDs | HIV testing and counseling, STD testing and counseling |
| | Hepatitis B disease | Hepatitis B immunization |
| Homosexual and bisexual males | HIV disease and other STDs | HIV testing and counseling, STD testing and counseling |
| | Hepatitis B disease | Hepatitis B immunization |
| Sexual partners who have been | | |
|   HIV positive | HIV disease | HIV test |
|   Hepatitis B positive | Hepatitis B disease | Hepatitis B immunization |
| Heterosexually active, do not desire children | Unintended pregnancy | Contraception counseling |
| Prostitution, trading sex for money or drugs | HIV disease | HIV testing and counseling, STD testing and counseling |
| | Hepatitis B disease | Hepatitis B immunization |
| | Substance abuse history | |
| Alcohol abuse | Pneumococcal disease | Pneumococcal immunization |
| | Tuberculosis | Tuberculosis test |
| | Oral cancer | Oral exam |
| | Injuries | Injury prevention counseling, Alcoholism counseling |
| Tobacco use | Oral and lung cancer | Oral exam |
| | Lung and other organ dysfunction | Smoking cessation counseling |
| Illicit drug use | HIV disease | HIV test |
| | Hepatitis B disease | Hepatitis B immunization |
| | Tuberculosis | Tuberculosis test |
| | Social/living situation | |
| Inadequate fluoridation of water supply (<0.3 ppm if < age 6 months, <0.6 ppm if 3 to 16 years of age) | Dental caries | Fluoride prophylaxis |
| Residence in or regular visits to a house built before 1960 with recent, ongoing, or planned renovations or remodeling or peeling or chipping paint (child) | Lead poisoning | Lead test |
| Residence near smelter, battery recycling plant or other industry likely to release lead (child) | Lead poisoning | Lead test |
| Household member being followed or treated for lead poisoning, adult member with hobby or job working with lead (child) | Lead poisoning | Lead test |
| Homelessness | Tuberculosis | Tuberculosis test |
| Institutionalization | | |
|   Criminals, developmentally disabled | Hepatitis B disease | Hepatitis B immunization |
|   Elderly, chronic medical problems | Influenza | Influenza immunization |
|   All | Tuberculosis | Tuberculosis test |
| Firearms in home | Injury and violence | Firearms and injury prevention counseling |
| | Occupational/recreational history | |
| Migrant laborers | Tuberculosis | Tuberculosis test |
| Healthcare workers | | |
|   Contact with blood | Hepatitis B disease | Hepatitis B immunization |
|   Might transmit influenza to persons at increased risk for complications | Influenza | Influenza B immunization |
|   All | Tuberculosis | Tuberculosis test |
| Staff of residential care facilities | Tuberculosis | Tuberculosis test |
| Exposure to increased | | |
|   Sunlight | Skin cancer | Skin exam and protection counseling |
|   Noise | Hearing loss | Hearing test and protection counseling |

[a] Adapted from *Clinician's Handbook of Preventive Services*, 1994. U.S. Government Printing Office.

It should be clear to the reader that modern health promotion and disease prevention practice is very complex, consisting of an array of immunizations, chemoprophylaxis, screening tests, and counseling interventions that need to be tailored to age, sex, and risk factor characteristics of patients. Keeping track of these for any one patient can be a chore; for an entire practice it can be an overwhelming task. To cope with this the assistance of office systems and nursing and office staff is essential.

The most important office system component is a tracking device of some type. Such a device can be as simple as a paper flow sheet/checklist in patient charts, or as sophisticated as a completely electronic medical record. The U.S. Public Health Service has published flow sheet templates as part of the Put Prevention Into Practice campaign (see Fig. 17.3) (Dickey & Kamerow, 1994).

A survey of primary care physicians in 1992 revealed that approximately 75% reported using a paper flow sheet/checklist of some type, while only 15% reported using a computerized tracking system. Only 1% used a computerized tracking system without also using a paper flow sheet/checklist (Dickey & Kamerow, 1996). Of those using a paper flow sheet/checklist, according to other studies, probably fewer than 50% actually enter data onto them consistently (Belcher, 1990; Prislin et al., 1986). The act of having to enter data twice, once onto flow sheets and again into patient progress notes, has undoubtedly been a major burden for many busy practitioners.

Computerized tracking systems have been found to be very effective at promoting the delivery of preventive services (McPhee & Detmer, 1993; Ornstein et al., 1991). It is striking how little delivery of medical care is tracked by computers relative to the delivery of other seemingly less important commodities in our society, such as groceries in supermarkets or packages by delivery services. Several computerized systems for tracking preventive care have been developed and marketed. These systems have been reviewed by an expert panel (American Cancer Society Advisory Group on Preventive Health Care Reminder Systems, 1995). All "stand-alone" tracking systems for preventive care have the same serious drawback as paper flow sheets: they require double data entry. Either the clinician or staff has to take the time to enter data into the computer as well as manually writing it into patient charts.

Clinicians entering practice should seriously consider using a totally electronic patient record that can track all aspects of patient care, including health maintenance services. Initial adoption of a totally electronic patient record will obviate the need to later convert written records into an electronic format. Data entry for electronic systems must now be done by keyboard, either by the physician or staff, but advances in voice recognition technology hold promise for simplifying this task.

The recent ascendance of managed healthcare has resulted in increased pressure on clinicians to provide ongoing accounting of preventive services provided to patients. The Joint Commission on the Accreditation of Healthcare Organizations has recently joined with the National Committee for Quality Assurance, which accredits health maintenance organizations, in requiring reporting on a number of practice parameters as part of the Health Plan Employer Data and Information Set (HEDIS). Several parameters address preventive services (mammography, Pap smears, cholesterol testing, fecal occult blood testing, smoking cessation counseling, and childhood immunizations). Pressure from managed care is beginning to bring clinical accounting methods used by clinicians into the modern information age.

## Using Reminders

Regardless of the tracking system used, it should be capable of generating reminders for the clinician and the patient about health maintenance. A number of studies have demonstrated that reminders both to clinicians and to patients are helpful in the timely delivery of preventive care (McPhee & Detmer, 1993). Reminders can take several forms. Letters generated by staff review of paper records or computer review of electronic records can be mailed to patients to remind them of needed preventive care. Letters or alert notices can also be prepared for clinician use at the time of patient visits. The more specific these reminders are as to each patient's health maintenance needs, the more effective they tend to be. Permanent, practicewide reminders can also be used, such as wall charts of preventive care protocols for examination and waiting rooms for easy patient and clinician reference.

Name

D.O.B.

No.

## Child Preventive Care
## Flow Sheet

**PUT PREVENTION**

**INTO PRACTICE**

**Health Counseling**

| Age | | | | | | | | |
|---|---|---|---|---|---|---|---|---|

**Suggested Topics (Circle if appropriate)**

1. Drugs/Alcohol
2. Dental and Oral Health
3. Nutrition
4. Physical Activity
5. Safety/Injuries/Poisons
6. Sexual Activity
7. STDs/HIV
8. Tobacco
9. UV Exposure
10. Violent Behavior and Firearms
11. _____
12. _____

| | | | | | | | | |
|---|---|---|---|---|---|---|---|---|
| Date / Type(s) | | | | | | | | |
| Date / Type(s) | | | | | | | | |
| Date / Type(s) | | | | | | | | |
| Date / Type(s) | | | | | | | | |
| Date / Type(s) | | | | | | | | |
| Date / Type(s) | | | | | | | | |

**Screening and Tests**

**Suggested Examinations and Tests:***

*EXAMINATIONS AND TESTS MAY INCLUDE:*

| ANEMIA | BLOOD PRESSURE | CHOLESTEROL | DEPRESSION |
|---|---|---|---|
| HEARING | HEIGHT/WEIGHT | LEAD | NEWBORN SCREENING |
| TUBERCULIN SKIN TESTING | URINALYSIS | VISION | |

* Specific preventive protocols should be tailored to the individual and individual's risk factors and based on discussion between the individual and provider

| Examinations and Tests | Schedule | | | | | | | | |
|---|---|---|---|---|---|---|---|---|---|
| | | Date / Result | | | | | | | |
| | | Date / Result | | | | | | | |
| | | Date / Result | | | | | | | |
| | | Date / Result | | | | | | | |
| | | Date / Result | | | | | | | |
| | | Date / Result | | | | | | | |

Suggested Result Codes:   O = Ordered   N = Result Normal   A = Result Abnormal   R = Refused   E = Done Elsewhere

**Immunizations**

| | | | | | | |
|---|---|---|---|---|---|---|
| Polio (OPV) | 2 mos. | 4 mos. | 6–18 mos. Depends on type of vaccination | | 4–6 yrs. | |
| Diphtheria, Tetanus, Pertussis (DTaP/DTP, Td) | 2 mos. DTaP/DTP | 4 mos. DTaP/DTP | 6 mos. DTaP/DTP | 15–18 mos. DTaP/DTP | 4–6 yrs. DTaP/DTP | 11–16 yrs. Td |
| Measles, Mumps, Rubella (MMR) | | | | 12–15 mos. | 4–6 yrs. or 11–12 yrs. | |
| *Haemophilus influenzae* type b (Hib) | 2 mos. | 4 mos. (PRP-OMP once only, age 4–6 months) | 6 mos. | 12–15 mos. | | |
| Hepatitis B (HBV) | Birth–2 mos. | 1–4 mos. | 6–18 mos. | | | |
| Varicella (VZV) | | | | 1–12 yrs. (1 dose) *OR* ≥ 13 yrs. (2 doses) | | |

1/98

**Figure 17.3.** Child preventive care flow sheet.

## COMPUTER REMINDERS

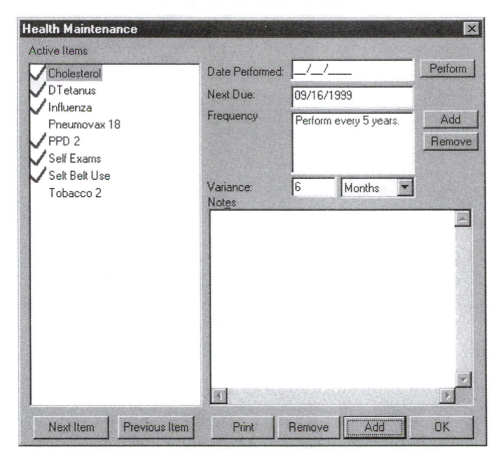

*Figure 17-4 shows the health maintenance tracking page of the SOAPware™ electronic medical record. The checked active items in the left-hand column are the immunizations, tests, or counseling items that the provider has determined the patient needs based on age, sex, and risk factors. In this case, the patient is a female (needs breast self-exams), nonsmoker (does not need tobacco counseling) under the age of 65 years (does not need pneumovax immunization). For the highlighted item (cholesterol), the date when the test is next due (9/16/99) is displayed as well as the designated frequency. This frequency can be individualized for each patient by the provider using a separate "protocol" entry screen.*

*This electronic medical record has the capability of generating printed reminders that can be mailed to the patient as well as printed reminders for the provider. The use of electronic medical records with the capability to actively remind patients and providers has been shown to significantly increase the rate of delivery of preventive services of all types.*

Reminders are necessary because health maintenance, unlike illness care, does not call attention to itself if neglected. Illness symptoms tend to get worse, but the effects of neglected preventive care tend to be silent and insidious. By the time a woman who has not had a screening mammogram develops symptoms from a breast cancer, it may be too advanced to cure.

## Working with Nursing and Office Staff

The responsibility for preventive care must also be shared with nursing and office staff. Some authorities recommend designating a staff member to supervise and maintain the office system and the office milieu promoting the performance of preventive care (Carney *et al.*, 1992). Examples of functions of this person might include: maintaining the tracking system, sending out reminders to providers and patients, keeping educational materials about preventive care current and well stocked, and organizing in-service training sessions. Clinicians are often too busy responding to the acute care needs of the practice to ensure that such important activities occur.

---

## CASE 17-7

*Dr. J. is a family physician who set up practice in a retirement community in the desert Southwest. In the spring of his first year he did a small survey of 100 charts of patients over the age of 65 and was surprised to see that only 30% had received an influenza immunization during the winter, and those were mainly the ones who had been seen for an illness. He called a few patients who hadn't gotten flu shots and asked them why. Some typical answers were, "Those things don't work," "Flu shots give you the flu, so why should I want one?" and "I had a flu shot 2 years ago and thought I didn't need another one for 10 years."*

*It was clear to Dr. J. that his patients had a lot of misconceptions about influenza immunizations. In late summer he prepared a short letter to patients clearly explaining the potential benefits and side effects of influenza immunizations and asking patients to call and schedule an appointment for the immunizations. He also did a short public service message for a local television station in the area. When he repeated the chart survey the next spring, he was pleased to find that 60% of his elderly patients had gotten immunizations. Other physicians in the community reported a slight increase as well and the administrator of the local hospital thought there were fewer hospitalizations for pneumonia than usual.*

---

## INVOLVING AND EDUCATING PATIENTS

Patients have a lot of interest in preventive care. They are, after all, the prime benefactors of good health. This interest can be utilized to help promote not only healthy behaviors but also performance of proper preventive services. All preventive care requires some active patient participation. At a minimum, patients have to come into the office or clinic, hopefully not only when acutely ill, and follow up with the performance of services, such as mammograms or fecal occult blood tests.

For some types of preventive care the lack of knowledge by patients is a major barrier. For example, the two main reasons given by women for never having had a mammogram in a series of National Cancer Institute studies were: they didn't know that they needed one and their physician had never told them to get one (NCI Breast Cancer Screening Consortium, 1990). Proper patient education is essential not only to help identify need, but also to help deal with fear and misunderstanding about services.

Patients can play a proactive role in their own preventive care by prompting their providers or self-referring for their own preventive services, such as mammograms or immunizations. With regard to the latter, influenza vaccinations for the elderly have been widely and successfully provided in community settings, as in Case 17-7. One approach, modeled on the childhood immunization card, is to give patients a protocol and tracking tool for their own preventive care. The Personal Health Guide and Child Health Guide are passport-sized documents recently published by the U.S. Public Health Service for this purpose (Dickey & Kamerow, 1994). Similar patient-held records have been tested and found to be well received by patients and helpful in promoting preventive care (Dickey, 1993).

---

## CONCLUSION

Health promotion and disease prevention are important aspects of modern medical care. As many as half of all deaths may be premature and the result of preventable risk factors. Even modest reductions in these risk factors through counseling and other behavior interventions in the clinical setting can result in a large number of years of life saved.

Clinical preventive services are of four major types: counseling, screening tests, immunizations, and chemoprophylaxis. It is important for the clinician to understand the basic principles underlying each of these types of care. It is also important for the clinician to understand how major authorities make recommendations regarding schedules for these types of care. In particular, the clinician should understand the process of scientific review of evidence.

Clinicians should decide on a protocol of preventive care that is based on science and fits the particular needs of their practice and patients. This protocol should be clearly displayed and explained to staff and patients. Office systems and practice routines should be instituted that aid in the timely delivery of appropriate preventive care. It is important to fully inform and involve patients in decision-making about and prompting of their own preventive care. Good health promotion and disease prevention practice requires teamwork on the part of clinicians, staff, and patients.

# CASES FOR DISCUSSION

## CASE 1

*Jane T. is a 45-year-old white female who has been coming to the clinic intermittently, every 2 to 3 years, for treatment of adult-onset diabetes mellitus, which has been relatively well controlled without insulin. Her medical history is otherwise unremarkable. A review of her family, social, sexual, substance use, and occupational/recreational histories reveals the following risk factors: she works as a nurse's aide in a nursing home and her mother died of breast cancer at age 55.*

1. *What preventive services (don't forget counseling) will she need based on her age and sex? Based on her diabetes mellitus? Based on her other risk factors?*
2. *Given the intermittent nature of her visits, what types of office resources might you use to help ensure that she comes in at more appropriate intervals?*

## CASE 2

*John S. is a 5-year-old boy brought in by his mother for well-child care before starting kindergarten. He is healthy, lives in a modern middle-class neighborhood, and received his last immunizations at age 2 years. His mother states that she would like him to have all of the testing and immunizations recommended by medical authorities and that she will pay for anything that her insurance does not cover.*

1. *List all of the immunizations, screening tests, and counseling interventions that you could provide to him.*
2. *List the preventive services that he may not need.*
3. *What reasons would you give his mother for not providing unnecessary preventive services?*

## CASE 3

*You are the director of a student health service at a state college. The administrator of the college has read about the health consequences of genital chlamydia infections and requests that you study screening all 10,000 female students. You research the issue and find that the prevalence of genital chlamydia infections in similar populations is 5%. The sensitivity of the chlamydia test is 90% and the specificity is also 90%. Each test costs $5 and treatment with antibiotics costs $7 per patient.*

1. *Approximately how many cases of infection will the screening program be expected to detect? How many will the program miss?*
2. *How many false positives will occur during the testing?*
3. *What will be the cost per case of infection properly identified?*
4. *From a cost standpoint, is screening followed by treatment preferable to presumptively treating every female student?*

## CASE 4

*Robert J. is a 35-year-old male who stopped smoking 1 month ago at your urging. He is struggling to avoid starting again.*

1. *According to Prochaska, what "stage of change" is he in? What types of interventions are likely to be most helpful to him? What type least helpful?*
2. *How could you or your office staff be helpful to him between visits?*
3. *What screening examination(s) will he need as a result of his smoking?*

## CASE 5

*Mrs. J. is a 53-year-old white woman who is experiencing menopause. Although she does not have hot flashes or other symptoms, she tells you that she is interested in taking estrogen. You explain to her the potential health advantages and disadvantages of taking estrogen and counsel her that she should probably also take progestin if she elects to take estrogen.*

1. *What diseases will hormone replacement therapy possibly help her avoid?*
2. *What diseases will hormone replacement therapy possibly put her at increased risk for?*
3. *Overall, do you think Mrs. J.'s life span will be increased by taking hormone replacement therapy?*
4. *Overall, do you think the quality of Mrs. J.'s life will be improved by hormone replacement therapy?*

## RECOMMENDED READINGS

Prochaska JO, Norcross J, DiClemente C: *Changing for Good*. New York, William Morrow & Co, 1994.

> Over the last decade the authors of this book have published a large number of excellent scientific articles detailing the stages people progress through in making behavioral and lifestyle changes. Because of their work, assessment of "readiness to change" has become a widely accepted component of counseling by health professionals of many types. This book, written as a self-help guide for the general public, is the first exposition of their model outside of the professional psychology literature. Although leaning a bit too far in the "pop psychology" direction, it is a useful and enjoyable introduction to their work for health professionals.

U.S. Department of Health and Human Services. *Clinician's Handbook of Preventive Services*. Washington, DC, US Department of Health and Human Services, 1998.

> Part of the U.S. Public Health Service's Put Prevention Into Practice campaign, this book was designed as a "how-to" manual to complement the "what-to-do" information of the *Guide to Clinical Preventive Services*. Each type of preventive service recommended by any major U.S. authority is addressed in separate chapters. Five types of information are furnished: the burden of suffering of target conditions; the recommendations of all major U.S. authorities for the frequency of performance based on age, sex, and risk factors; the basics of how to perform the preventive service in simple steps corresponding to their temporal sequence in practice; current information on where to obtain patient and provider educational materials; and scientific references. The handbook was prepared by the U.S. Office of Disease Prevention and Health Promotion with input from every federal health agency and many professional and voluntary health organizations. This is a valuable reference for the busy practitioner and educational tool for health professionals in training. An updated edition was issued in the fall of 1996. It is available from the Superintendent of Documents, Mail Stop: SSOP, Washington, DC 20402-9328 (ISBN 0-16-049227-0). It is also published (Product No. 1980) by the American Academy of Family Physicians (1-800-944-0000) and International Medical Publishing, Inc (1-703-519-0807).

U.S. Department of Health and Human Services. *Put Prevention Into Practice Education and Action Kit*. Washington, DC, US Department of Health and Human Services, 1994.

> In addition to one copy of the *Clinician's Handbook of Preventive Services*, this contains several copies of a variety of paper-based tools for implementing preventive care in the office or clinic. These include: the *Personal Health Guide*, *Child Health Guide*, and Staying Healthy at 50+, passport-sized documents that provide patients and parents with basic information about preventive care and personal records for tracking preventive care; templates of flow sheets for patient charts; a *Prevention Prescription* pad; and posters for examination rooms depicting preventive care for children and adults in time-line formats. The entire kit can be ordered from the AHRQ Publications Clearinghouse, P.O. Box 8547, Silver Spring, MD 20907, 1-800-358-9295. Online versions of some of the materials can be obtained at http://www.ahrq.gov/ppip/pporder.htm.

U.S. Preventive Services Task Force. *Guide to Clinical Preventive Services: Report of the US Preventive Services Task Force, Second Edition Baltimore*, Williams & Wilkins Co, 1996.

> This new edition updated and expanded on the classic report produced by this expert panel in 1989. The scientific evidence

regarding 70 different types of clinical preventive care has been exhaustively researched, evaluated, and clearly summarized for the practitioner, student, or policymaker. Recommendations for and against performance are presented based on patient age, sex, and other risk factors. A third edition is expected to be published by 2002.

# REFERENCES

American Academy of Family Physicians: *Summary of Policy Recommendations for Periodic Health Examination.* Kansas City, Mo: American Academy of Family Physicians, 1997.

American Academy of Pediatrics: Committee on Practice and Ambulatory Care. Recommendations for preventive pediatric health care. *Pediatrics* 96:373–374, 1995.

American Cancer Society: Report on the cancer-related health check-up. *CA* 30:194–240, 1980.

American Cancer Society: *Summary of American Cancer Society Recommendations for Early Detection of Cancer in Asymptomatic People.* Atlanta, American Cancer Society, 1992.

American Cancer Society Advisory Group on Preventive Health Care Reminder Systems: Computerized health maintenance tracking systems: A clinicians guide to necessary and optional features. *J Am Board Fam Pract* 8:221–229, 1995.

American College of Obstetricians and Gynecologists: *The Obstetrician-Gynecologist and Primary Preventive Health Care.* Washington, DC, American College of Obstetricians and Gynecologists, 1993.

American College of Physicians: Periodic health examination: A guide for designing individualized preventive health care in the asymptomatic patient. *Ann Intern Med* 95:729–732, 1981.

American College of Physicians Task Force on Adult Immunization and Infectious Disease Society of America: *Guide for Adult Immunization,* edition 3. Philadelphia, American College of Physicians, 1994.

Belcher DW: Implementing preventive services: Success and failure in an outpatient trial. *Arch Intern Med* 159:2533–2541, 1990.

Breslow L, Somers AR: The lifetime health-monitoring program: A practical approach to preventive medicine. *N Engl J Med* 292:601–608, 1977.

Canadian Task Force on the Periodic Health Examination. The periodic health examination. *Can Med Assoc J* 121:1194–1254, 1979.

Carney PA, Dietrich AJ, Landgraff J, O'Connor GT: Tools, teamwork, and tenacity: An office system for cancer prevention. *J Fam Pract* 35:388–394, 1992.

Dickey LL: Promoting preventive care with patient-held minirecords: A review. *Patient Educ Couns* 20:37–47, 1993.

Dickey LL, Kamerow DB: The put prevention into practice campaign: Office tools and beyond. *J Fam Pract* 39:321–323, 1994.

Dickey LL, Kamerow DB: Primary care providers use of office tools in the provision of preventive care. *Arch Fam Med* 5:399–404, 1996.

Eddy DM: *A Manual for Assessing Health Practices and Designing Practice Policies: The Explicit Approach.* Philadelphia, American College of Physicians, 1992.

Frame PS, Carlson SJ: A critical review of periodic health screening using specific screening criteria. *J Fam Pract* 2:29–36, 1975.

Kasper JF, Mulley AG, Wennberg JE: Developing shared decision-making programs to improve the quality of health care. *Qual Rev Bull,* June 1992, pp 183–190.

Kottke TE, Battista RN, Defriense GH, Brekke ML: Attributes of successful smoking cessation interventions in medical practice: A meta-analysis of 39 controlled trials. *JAMA* 259:2882–2889, 1988.

Lee JM: Screening and informed consent. *N Engl J Med* 328:438–439, 1993.

Lewis CE: Disease prevention and health promotion practices of primary care physicians in the United States, *Am J Prev Med* 4(suppl 1):9–16, 1988.

McGinnis JM, Foege WH: Actual causes of death in the United States. *JAMA* 270:2207–2212, 1993.

McPhee SJ, Detmer WM: Office-based interventions to improve delivery of cancer prevention services by primary care physicians. *Cancer* 72(suppl):1100–1112, 1993.

Mead VP, Rhyne RL, Wiese WH, et al: Impact of environmental patient education on preventive medicine practices. *J Fam Pract* 40:363–369, 1995.

Miller AB, Baines CJ, To T, Wall C: Canadian national breast screening study: 1. Breast cancer detection and death rates among women aged 40 to 49 years. *Can Med Assoc J* 147:1459–1476, 1992.

Mushlin AI, Fintor L: Is screening for breast cancer cost-effective? *Cancer* 69(suppl):1957–1962, 1992.

National Cancer Institute: *Working Guidelines for Early Cancer Detection: Rationale and Supporting Evidence to Decrease Mortality.* Bethesda, National Cancer Institute, 1987.

National Center for Health Statistics: *Advance Report of Final Mortality, 1990.* Hyattsville, Md, US Department of Health and Human Services, 1993. Monthly Vital Statistics Report, 41(7)

National Center for Health Statistics. *Health, United States, 1998 With Socioeconomic Status and Health Chartbook.* Hyattsville, Md, 1998.

NCI Breast Cancer Screening Consortium: Screening mammography: A missed clinical opportunity? *JAMA* 264:54–58, 1990.

Ornstein SM, Garr DR, Jenkins RG, et al: Computer-generated physician and patient reminders: Tools to improve population adherence to selected preventive services. *J Fam Pract* 32:82–90, 1991.

Prislin MD, Vandenbark MS, Clarkson QD: The impact of a health screening flowsheet on the performance and documentation of health screening procedures. *Fam Med* 18:290–292, 1986.

Prochaska JO, Norcross JC, DiClemente CC: *Changing for Good.* New York, William Morrow & Co Inc, 1994a.

Prochaska J, Velicer W, Rossi J, Goldstein M, Marcus B, Radowski W, Fiore C, Harlow L, Redding C, Rosenbloom D, Rossi S: Stages of change and decisional balance for 12 problem behaviors. *Health Psychol* 13(1):39–46, 1994b.

Roizen MF, Coalson D, Hayward RS, *et al*: Can patients use an automated questionnaire to define their current health status? *Med Care* 30:MS74–MS84, 1992.

Schauffler HH, Rodriguez T, Milstein A. Health education and patient satisfaction. *J Fam Pract* 42:62–68, 1996.

Tabar L, Fagerberg CJG, Gad A, *et al*: Reduction in mortality from breast cancer after mass screening with mammography: Randomized trial from the Breast Cancer Screening Working Group of the Swedish National Board of Health and Welfare. *Lancet* 1:829–832, 1985.

US Department of Health and Human Services: *Clinician's Handbook of Preventive Services*. Washington, DC, US Department of Health and Human Services, 1994.

US Department of Health and Human Services: *Clinician's Handbook of Preventive Services, Second Edition*. Washington, DC, US Department of Health and Human Services, 1998.

US Preventive Services Task Force: *Guide to Clinical Preventive Services: An Assessment of the Effectiveness of 169 Interventions*. Baltimore, Williams & Wilkins Co, 1989

US Preventive Services Task Force: *Guide to Clinical Preventive Services, Second Edition*. Baltimore, Williams & Wilkins Co, 1996

US Public Health Service: *Healthy People 2000: National Health Promotion and Disease Prevention Objectives*. US Department of Health and Human Services Publication No. PHS 91-50212, 1991.

Verbeek ALM, Hendricks JHCL, Hollan Tr, *et al*: Reduction of breast cancer mortality through mass screening with modern mammography: First results of the Nijmegen Project, 1975–1981. *Lancet* 1:1222–1224, 1984.

Woolf SH, Dickey LL: Differing perspectives on preventive care guidelines: A new look at the mammography controversy. *Am J Prev Med* 17:260–268, 1999.

## CHAPTER 18

# Keeping Up to Date

*Warren P. Newton*

*At 10:00 PM, the junior medical student on her medicine clerkship learns about her first admission of the night, a 34-year-old man with a history of alcohol abuse who now complains of epigastric pain and an inability to keep any liquids down. On physical examination, he is mildly uncomfortable, with orthostatic changes in pressure and pulse and significant epigastric tenderness. Lab results are normal except for an amylase of 324 mg/dl.*

*After examining the patient, the student is expected to prepare a formal written history and physical examination as well as a short oral presentation at morning rounds. For background information on pancreatitis, she looks in her textbook of medicine. Noting that the textbook was updated 4 years before, she does an online search for a recent evidence-based review.*

*At morning rounds, she briefly summarizes the prognosis and treatment of pancreatitis, recommending i.v. fluids, pain control, and withholding an NG tube in view of his mild course. The patient recovers in 2 days and is discharged to outpatient alcohol rehabilitation.*

## EDUCATIONAL OBJECTIVES

1. Describe three sources of medical information and identify their strengths and weaknesses
2. Identify the principles of effective computer searching and apply them to actual clinical problems
3. Describe the criteria for critically appraising articles on diagnosis, prognosis, treatment, meta-analysis, and causation of disease
4. Apply the principles of critical appraisal to specific articles and clinical situations

## INTRODUCTION

Medical students, residents, and practicing physicians spend a great deal of time obtaining and evaluating medical information, but rarely get practical training in how to do this efficiently and effectively. Over the

## PANCREATITIS

*Pancreatitis is an inflammation of the pancreas, commonly as the result of alcohol abuse or gallstone disease but also as a side effect of medications given by physicians. Symptoms include nausea and abdominal pain associated with elevated serum analysis and lipase. Patients need assessment to exclude other causes of these symptoms and need hospitalization if i.v. fluids or pain medication are necessary. Rarely, patients with pancreatitis can become critically ill. It is important to identify these patients early and treat them aggressively.*

last 30 years, there has been an explosion of medical information available to physicians. Unfortunately, however, there has not been a similar expansion in the hours of the day available for physicians to review this information. As a result, practitioners have become increasingly like the rabbit in Alice in Wonderland, running ever faster to stay in the same place.

To make incorporating new information into practice more feasible, a group of physicians with training in epidemiology at McMaster University developed techniques for "critical appraisal of the literature" (Sackett *et al.*, 1991) and putting evidence into practice. Based on the application of the principles of epidemiology to clinical research, critical appraisal allows physicians to prioritize the information available and systematically to review the quality of the information they receive. Using this approach, searching for appropriate literature is dramatically faster, and evaluation of what is found is substantially more rigorous.

## CASE 18-2

*As part of a didactic seminar in the obstetrics and gynecology clerkship, a medical student is asked to present a 15-minute talk about epidural anesthesia: common techniques, mechanism of action, effectiveness, and adverse consequences. The talk is scheduled to be given in 1 week; the student reviews the relevant sections of his obstetrics text, as well as an anesthesiology text from the library. He also talks with the obstetric anesthesiologist to learn the techniques in use at this hospital and with the hospital business office to learn the current charges for epidurals. The talk goes well; the seminar leader, after praising the student's resourcefulness in learning the charges for epidurals, comments that his search was incomplete, in that his presentation did not address a recent important work including a controversial randomized trial suggesting epidurals increase the rate of cesarean section.*

## RELIEVING THE DISCOMFORT OF LABOR

*Management of discomfort of labor is a perennial clinical challenge. Since the early 1900s, there have been a series of "revolutionary" interventions aimed at this purpose—"twilight sleep" (general anesthesia), nitrous oxide, different formulations of narcotics and saddle blocks—all later being found to have adverse effects for mother and/or baby. The latest attempt is epidural anesthesia, typically placed by an anesthesiologist with the onset of active labor. Epidural anesthesia provides excellent pain relief but may lead to dural puncture headaches, prolonged labor, and increased risk of cesarean section.*

## How Much Time for What Kind of Answer?

Searching for medical information depends on both the time available for the search and the detail of the information needed. In Case 18-1, the student who has just admitted the patient with pancreatitis has overnight to learn the basics of pancreatitis—its differential diagnosis, prognosis, and treatment—prior to her oral presentation in the morning. Time is quite limited, but there is rarely the expectation that the junior medical student will need to know in detail the problems with Ranson's prognostic criteria or recent randomized trials on the management of pancreatitis. By contrast, the task given to the student in Case 18-2 allowed him ample time to search the literature and to review carefully primary research articles. The trade-off between the time available and depth of answer needed continues through residency and into practice. Practicing physicians often turn to *Facts and Comparisons* for a quick question about drug dosage, but may need to do more involved research when it is their turn to do Grand Rounds at their local community hospital or develop their group's practice guideline on a common medical problem.

Whatever the level of training, clinicians face a similar set of possible sources of clinical information. As Slawson and Shaughnessy (Slawson *et al.*, 1994) have described, a helpful way of thinking about sources of information is the usefulness equation:

$$\text{Usefulness} = \frac{\text{Relevance} \times \text{Validity}}{\text{Work}}$$

Clinicians regularly make pragmatic decisions about their sources of information. Within the limits of their task at the moment, they seek to increase the relevance to their patients and the validity of their information, while decreasing the work or time necessary to get the information.

Most accessible and easiest to use are textbooks or recent review articles. Textbooks—in print, online, or on CD — are portable, available wherever and whenever needed, and represent the best opinion of an "expert" in that field; disadvantages are that they are often out of date and they provide overviews that may be too superficial for specific clinical questions. Web-based medical information sources are proliferating rapidly. Like textbooks, they are very convenient but subject to being out of date—just because they are available online instantly does not mean that the information presented is current! Also, like print review articles, many Web sites are dependent on expert advice and in most cases, they have not been written from the perspective of "evidence-based medicine," that is, incorporating an assessment of the strength of the evidence behind specific recommendations (Sackett *et al.*, 2000). Table 18.1 provides a list of noncommercial Web sites that are evidence based. Reviews published in journals possess advantages and disadvantages similar to textbook chapters, but are likely to be more up to date.

A second source of information are local experts, such as a colleague or consultant. Local experts are relatively easy to contact, know local conditions, and provide information more specific to the patient at hand. They may be more up to date than textbooks. However, there may be problems with the information provided by local experts. Most consultants have not been trained in evidence-based medicine, and their clinical

**Table 18.1**
Evidence-Based Web Sites

*www.clinicalevidence.org* (BMJ)
*www.guidelines.gov* (National Guideline Clearinghouse)
*www.update-software.com/ccweb/cochrane/revabstr/mainindex.htm* (Cochrane Collaborative Database)
158.72.20.10/pubs/guidecps (US Guide to Clinical Preventive Services)
cebm.jr2.ox.ac.uk/ (Center for Evidence Based Medicine at Oxford)

experience since training has often been shaped by patients very different from those of the physicians who refer to them. Moreover, consultation may also include a direct monetary cost to the patient.

A third source of information is the primary medical literature, accessed by computer through software facilitating Medline searching. Original research reports, appropriately analyzed, remain the best information on which to base clinical practice. The great advantage of this source is that it is as up to date as possible; this is particularly important when what is at issue is a recently recognized disease or problem, or when recent information is substantially better than what was known before. Another advantage of reviewing the medical literature personally is that the clinician can analyze the evidence directly, without looking through the lens of another reviewer. The major disadvantage of searching the primary medical literature is the time and effort necessary to retrieve, review, and synthesize the individual articles.

Practicing clinicians use all three sources of information regularly, switching from one to the other as the situation and their comfort with their sources vary. An important goal of training in both medical school and residency should be to become facile with the process of searching, including quickly deciding the best strategy for getting specific information, the tactics of searching a particular source, and the synthesis of information from different sources. Regardless of the specific question or search strategy, it is the professional responsibility of the clinician to find the best quality information for patient care.

## Computer Searching of the Literature

Computer searching of the medical literature has become increasingly important for clinicians, and it is important for students to develop good searching skills. The first step is a clear, focused clinical question. As much as possible, it is important to break down general questions into more specific clinically focused questions. For example, rather than searching a very general topic like "knowing about Alzheimer's disease," it is important for the clinician to decide what aspects of its diagnosis, prognosis, or treatment she wants to know about. More specific questions make searching more efficient.

The clinician should also keep in mind what would be the ideal kind of evidence for answering her specific question. As will be discussed later, the ideal study will vary according to the kind of clinical question, but knowing what the ideal study would be greatly speeds the process of sorting "wheat from chaff." For example, for a question about the risks and benefits of treating isolated systolic hypertension, the best possible study will be a randomized clinical trial (RCT) or, possibly, a meta-analysis of randomized trials. Knowing this information means that the search process can focus on finding just RCTs, ignoring the many case series that have been published.

The next step is to consider how many years and what languages the search should include. Again, this decision will depend in part on the topic. For some clinical questions, e.g., the use of AZT in pregnant patients who are seropositive for HIV, it may make sense to limit your search to the last 5 years, but for other questions, e.g., the role of dietary restriction of purines in treatment of gout, searching back to the late 1960s and early 1970s may be more appropriate. For most clinical questions, it is not necessary to search other languages, but such a search may be necessary if the purpose is to prepare a research proposal or write a paper.

---

### WHAT IS THE CLINICAL FOCUS OF ARTICLES IN THE LITERATURE?

*Articles on the medical literature are weighted toward therapy and diagnosis. In a recent study of all articles on pneumonia in a specific year, the majority of articles were case reports and reviews, while therapy accounted for 10% and diagnosis 16%. Articles about prognosis were least common (5%).*

---

Once searching online, the best strategy is to get as many citations as possible initially and then to narrow down. Start with only a disease term or a therapy and use the medical subject headings terms (MeSH) as much as possible. The MeSH headings are the terms used by the National Library of Medicine to code each article as it is entered into the computerized data base. MeSH headings are available in an online thesaurus in many searching programs as well as in books in the library. Some, but not all online searching programs, automatically map to MeSH terms; users should know what their software does. Using MeSH headings will improve retrieval of articles. For example, using our local system, PC OVID, to search 1995–2000 text and key words, *heart attack* yields 44 references, *MI* yields 6317, and the MeSH term *myocardial infarction* yields 11,203 references.

After getting a large pool of citations, the next step is to focus on the best articles for the clinical questions. Major MeSH headings, which select for articles with a major emphasis on the subject, are very useful, as are subheadings, like *drug therapy* or *prevention and control*, as well as the age of subjects or language of publication. Increasingly valuable is searching by publication type such as *meta-analysis* or by methodological terms, such as *randomized controlled trial*. Care must be taken not to weed too vigorously; the searcher should regularly look at the articles in the list to see if they are appropriate.

It is important to keep in mind that computer searching is sometimes insensitive, as medical students learn when they discover a critical article that should have been identified after they have made a presentation or handed in their paper! Even in the best of hands, with an experienced clinician searching along with a librarian, using multiple data bases, a substantial number of references will be missed. The major cause for the insensitivity of searching is the human role in attributing subject headings to articles. With practice, and by using MeSH headings, searching several different ways, and, if necessary, following up the references in articles, the sensitivity of computer searching can be maximized.

## CASE 18-3

*Your family practice preceptors have developed a system for obtaining information from pharmaceutical representatives: In return for the purchase of medical textbooks, your preceptor and his partners have a bag lunch once a month over which they hear the sales pitches of the representatives. Today, the representative is from a company selling a calcium channel blocker. Her goal is to comment on a recent article (Furberg et al., 1995), which attributed a higher mortality rate to calcium channel blockers in routine use. She does not have a copy of the original article to give you, but she does have a public statement by a cardiologist at an academic medical center in the state that the evidence is suspect and that clinical practice should not change at this point, "in view of the obvious effectiveness and safety that these agents have had over the years." The student does a search and retrieves the relevant articles but is still confused after reading studies that report conflicting results.*

## CRITICAL APPRAISAL OF THE LITERATURE

### General Principles

Case 18-3 illustrates the need for critical appraisal of the medical literature. As popularized at McMaster University, critical appraisal is the application of clinical epidemiology to published human research. It has several key principles. First, there is an emphasis on the clinicians' perspective. Whereas traditional epidemiology focuses on the causation of disease, clinical epidemiology recognizes that there are a limited number of fundamental kinds of problems physicians face—diagnosis, prognosis, and treatment—and these problems typically require methodology that is specific to the clinical problem. Second, for each of these kinds of problems, there are some methodologies that are stronger than others, in the sense that they are more likely to

## WHAT IS THE QUALITY OF THE ARTICLES IN THE LITERATURE?

*Despite the attention being paid to methodological rigor, the vast majority of the articles available on Medline are of poor quality. In a recent study of the quality of articles about pneumonia, 38% were case reports. Of 95 articles on treatment, only 4 were methodologically rigorous and applicable to primary care.*

get a valid answer for the patients in the study. Thus, for example, RCTs are in general stronger than cohort studies, which are stronger than case–control studies or case series. The third principle of critical appraisal is that there is little need to review studies that are methodologically weak if stronger studies are available. Time is crucial for busy clinicians, and critical appraisal allows them to focus their attention only on evidence that is worthwhile.

In practical terms, critical appraisal of the literature involves the application of a set of rules derived from epidemiology to specific articles. The particular set of rules will vary according to the kind of clinical question—e.g., diagnosis, prognosis, or treatment—being addressed. In general, the rules will address two different domains, internal validity and external validity or generalizability. Internal validity is the ability of the study to achieve a valid answer for the subjects in the study. Concerns of internal validity revolve around whether the design is randomized, whether the outcomes are appropriate, whether there are confounding effects, and so on. There is general consensus about what kinds of study designs are stronger, so that it is usually relatively easy to rank studies by quality, at least in a general way. Concerns of external validity revolve around the generalizability of the findings to the patient and clinical setting at hand. Are the subjects similar to those of the clinician asking the question? In contrast to the criteria related to internal validity, it is harder to rank studies based on their generalizability to the searcher's clinical context: there is no "scale" for "patients similar to mine"! Nevertheless, both internal and external validity are important, and the clinician should use both kinds of rules to assess the quality of the evidence relating to his or her clinical question.

## CASE 18-4

*An otherwise healthy 23-year-old woman presents with dysuria and urinary frequency for 12 hours, along with a subjective history of chills. Physical examination reveals no fever, costovertebral angle tenderness, vaginal discharge, or cervical motion tenderness; urinalysis shows 0–2 white cells/high-power field and trace leukocyte esterase. The preceptor asks the medical student how sensitive a test urinalysis is for urinary tract infection (UTI). The student finds the information in a text on laboratory medicine (Black et al., 1999), and reports that the sensitivity of urinalysis for UTI is between 60 and 80%—good, but not perfect. The woman is treated for a UTI and improves.*

## DIAGNOSIS

Questions about diagnosis occur frequently in both inpatient and outpatient settings. Typically, physicians are interested in articles evaluating a new diagnostic test or strategy [e.g., urinalysis to diagnose UTI in Case 18-4, prostate-specific antigen (PSA) for prostatic cancer, or the Michigan Alcohol Screening Test (MAST) questionnaire for alcoholism]; occasionally, the "diagnostic test" being evaluated is physician history taking (e.g., a history of angina for coronary artery disease) or physical examination (e.g., calf tenderness as a sign of deep venous thrombosis).

There are many texts available that describe various laboratory tests and list the diseases that can cause abnormalities, but most do not provide information on test performance. An exception is *Diagnostic Strategies for Common Medical Problems*, which provides in-depth discussion of specific clinical questions with data about test performance (Black *et al.*, 1999). Computer searching the literature for diagnostic information can usually be done most efficiently by looking up the disease with a subheading of *diagnosis*; if this yields too many articles to scan, the methodological term *sensitivity and specificity* will select for methodologically stronger studies. Occasionally, meta-analyses of diagnostic tests are performed and can be found by searching by that term. For aspects of the history and physical examination, the recent *JAMA* series on the rational physical examination is an excellent source of information; computer searching should be supplemented by looking for references in textbooks of physical examination, since many of the references are older.

In order to understand how to evaluate articles on diagnosis, it is necessary to review some basic definitions. All diagnostic tests need to be evaluated against a *gold standard*, which is the best single test or combination of tests that is relevant to the particular diagnosis and should be applied to each subject who receives a diagnostic test. Thus, when thinking of exercise tolerance test as a diagnostic test for coronary artery disease, the gold standard would be angiography or autopsy. Gold standards may not be perfect—e.g., chlamydial culture, which is insensitive in clinical practice—and they may be impossible to obtain except under unusual situations such as autopsy. It is a clinical judgment about whether a particular gold standard is the appropriate one.

Articles on diagnostic tests should include the *sensitivity, specificity, positive predictive value*, and *negative predictive value* of the test, as defined in Chapter 9 on laboratory tests. Both sensitivity and specificity are characteristics of the test, and typically do not vary from setting to setting. By contrast, the *positive* and *negative predictive values* vary from setting to setting. It is the predictive value that physicians use when treating for a positive test and reassuring for a negative test. Statistics for a test are usually given in percentages, so that, for example, a 70% sensitivity for a new test for mycoplasma would mean that, on average, the test would read positive for 70% of women who have mycoplasma infections.

The predictive value of a test will depend on the prevalence of the disease in the population. According to the Bayes theorem, for diseases with high prevalence, the positive predictive value will be high; as the prevalence drops, however, the positive predictive value will decrease. The negative predictive value moves in the opposite fashion. In practical terms, given a particular test, if a clinician uses a diagnostic test in a high-prevalence setting, a positive test will be more likely to be truly positive than a positive test in a low-prevalence setting. For example, San Francisco gay males living in the Castro district have an HIV seroprevalence estimated to be at least 80%, while asymptomatic low-risk people from rural North Carolina have a prevalence of disease of <1%. A positive HIV screen in North Carolina is very likely to be a false positive; in a gay San Franciscan, the chances of a true positive are much greater.

Figure 18.1 summarizes the criteria for reading an article about a diagnostic test. The clinician should first decide if the test is one he might use in his clinical setting and whether the gold standard test was used for all subjects. If the answer to both of these questions is yes, the article is worth taking the time to read. Then the clinician should ask what the disease being tested for is. Usually, this is straightforward, but occasionally not, as, for example, when routine urinalysis is done as part of an annual physical examination to screen for infection, renal tumor, glomerular disease, and kidney stones. Next consider the gold standard test. Is it clinically appropriate? If not, the sensitivity and specificity reported by the study may be misleading. Then, review the sensitivity and specificity of the test; how does this test compare with other tests available? Most useful screening tests have sensitivities above 70%, e.g., mammography has a sensitivity of 75 to 85% and HIV testing has a sensitivity of 99%. Finally, compare the prevalence of the disease in the study with your own patients. Keeping the Bayes theorem in mind will allow an estimate of how the test will perform when you use it on your patients.

Is this article worth taking the time to read?

☐ Yes, because I use or might use the test regularly, a "gold standard" test was used on all subjects.

☐ No.

*If yes, answer the following:*

1. What disease is being looked for? What is the diagnostic test?

2. What is the "gold standard" test? Is it reasonable, and what are its limitations?

3. What is the sensitivity, specificity, and predictive value of the test?

4. In terms of prevalence of the disease, are the study subjects similar to your patients? Will the predictive value of the test be the same for your patients?

*UNC Critical Appraisal Group; adapted from materials developed at McMaster University*

**Figure 18.1.** Worksheet for articles about diagnostic tests.

## CASE 18-5

*At a routine home visit 68 hours after delivery, the family physician notices that the baby he delivered is jaundiced in both the arms and the legs. The baby was a full-term product of an uncomplicated labor and delivery, with Apgars of 8 at 1 minute and 9 at 5 minutes. Neonatal course was uncomplicated, and the mother had requested discharge at 6 hours. The mother's first child had breast-fed to 15 months, and the mother has no concerns at this time. Except for the jaundice, results of the*

### HYPERBILIRUBINEMIA AND KERNICTERUS

*High circulating concentrations of bilirubin are toxic to the central nervous system, with the basal ganglia most affected. In the 1950s, an association was noted between elevated hyperbilirubin levels and neurologic disease. That ushered in an era of aggressive treatment with hospitalization and UV lights up to exchange transfusions. In the late 1980s and early 1990s, it began to be recognized that the condition of the child and the etiology of the hyperbilirubinemia were also critical variables, resulting in less aggressive treatment protocols.*

*physical examination were reassuring; the infant was sucking well and was neurologically intact. Review of records shows that the mother is blood type A positive; the cord blood was Coombs negative. Laboratory examination of the newborn reveals a total bilirubin of 12, a normal hematocrit, and no evidence of hemolysis. The family physician asks the medical student accompanying him about the risk of kernicterus from hyperbilirubinemia as well as whether phototherapy is indicated. A computer search with key terms* **jaundice,** **neonatal** *and subheadings* **therapy,** **complications** *and publication type* **practice guidelines** *yields relatively recent practice guidelines (Newman & Maisels, 1992) for the management of neonatal jaundice, as well as a recent reanalysis of a large study of prognosis (Newman & Klebanoff, 1993). Based on their findings from the computer search, the mother and baby are expectantly managed and do well.*

# PROGNOSIS

Questions about prognosis are a common part of the practice of medicine in both inpatient and outpatient settings. Physicians use prognostic information to give patients advice about what symptoms to expect, when to expect them, and what the benefits of treatment are. Unfortunately, there is much less information available in the medical literature on prognosis than on diagnosis and treatment. Textbooks and review articles will sometimes have citations of classic articles; for computer searches, combining the disease term with the subheading *prognosis* or the methodological terms *cohort study* or *prospective study* is the best approach. Also helpful are the control wings of randomized trials, although one has to be careful that the patients enrolled are similar to one's own patients.

A good approach to describing what studies of prognosis ought to include is to describe a clinical question, imagine the best possible study to answer the question, and then extrapolate from this ideal. Regarding the issues raised by Case 18-5, as for many studies of prognosis, a randomized design is not possible, since one cannot usually randomize hazardous exposures like hyperbilirubinemia. As a consequence, the next strongest design would be a cohort study, in which people are identified and followed over years. Identifying the people at the beginning of a disease's course—an *inception cohort*—allows better measurements of exposures and better tracking of the group and is stronger methodologically than identifying a group retrospectively. In the case of neonatal hyperbilirubinemia, it would be important to include patients who were similar to the patients the clinician is most concerned with—full-term babies without evidence of distress or sepsis, who are enrolled at birth rather than referred in, and to follow them for enough years to make sure that the clinically relevant outcomes (neurological abnormalities, school dysfunction, learning problems) have an opportunity to occur, at least 8 years. One would want to have enough numbers of patients to pick up rare outcomes like kernicterus, and keep track of all possible confounding variables, or the other factors that may influence outcomes. For neonatal jaundice, this may require tens of thousands of subjects. Finally, one would want to follow as many patients as possible to the end; if a study does not follow up at least 80% of the patients, the potential bias becomes very large, and the paper is not worth reading.

Obviously, this kind of "ideal study" could only rarely be done, but it does allow us to identify the key criteria for articles on prognosis. As Fig. 18.2 depicts, the cardinal characteristics of studies of prognosis are use of an inception cohort and adequate follow-up. If neither of these features is present, the likelihood of getting valid information is so low that it is usually not worth the time to read the article. As it happens, most articles on prognosis in the medical literature do not meet this standard. Next, assess whether the subjects are similar to yours, both in terms of clinical characteristics required for entry into the trial as well as whether they represent a referral population. Prognosis may vary dramatically with clinical characteristics; patients who are referred to specialists and then followed may have a very different prognosis than other patients who are followed by their primary care physicians. Finally, did the estimates of prognosis take into account the confounding factors? These are factors that may influence outcomes significantly and should be accounted for in the analysis.

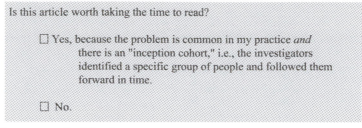

Is this article worth taking the time to read?

☐ Yes, because the problem is common in my practice *and*
there is an "inception cohort," i.e., the investigators
identified a specific group of people and followed them
forward in time.

☐ No.

*If yes, answer the following:*

1.  Were the criteria for entry into the study objective and/or reasonable?

2.  Where did the subjects come from? Was the referral pattern specified?

3.  Were the outcomes assessed objectively and blindly?

4.  Was follow-up of subjects adequate (at least 70-80%)?

5.  Were the patients similar to yours in terms of age, sex, race,
    severity of disease and other factors that might influence
    the course of the disease?

*UNC Critical Appraisal Group; adapted from materials developed at McMaster University*

**Figure 18.2.** Worksheet for articles about prognosis.

## CASE 18-6

*A 33-year-old man presents with a purulent nasal discharge, a temperature of 38.3°C, and right maxillary tenderness. The medical student diagnoses sinusitis and suggests treatment for 10 days with trimethoprim–sulfamethoxazole to the preceptor. The preceptor asks the student if there is any new information in the treatment of sinusitis. The student performs a literature search using the search terms* sinusitis *(exploded) and publication type* randomized controlled trial, *and discovers a randomized trial showing that 3 days of antibiotic treatment has outcomes similar to 10 days (Williams* et al., *1995). The patient is treated with decongestants and 3 days of antibiotics and recovers well.*

## THERAPY

Therapy is any intervention made by a clinician to prevent, cure, or ameliorate disease. Thus, therapy includes not only medication, as in Case 18-6, but also other kinds of interventions as well, such as surgery, an exercise program to lower cholesterol, physician advice about screening mammograms, or over-the-counter medication for allergies.

Textbooks, reviews, and manuals are easily available and give therapeutic recommendations that are relatively applicable; in recent years, textbooks in obstetrics and pediatrics organized solely around the available randomized trials have been published. In situations in which you wish to look at the primary evidence for treating, a good first start for searching the literature is to enter the disease and a subheading, *drug therapy* or *therapy*; the specific drug or therapy can also be used. The publication-type term *randomized controlled trial* has the potential to increase the efficiency of the search dramatically, but not all randomized controlled trials have been given this subject heading, particularly in earlier years.

To illustrate the principles underlying the critical review of articles on therapy, it is valuable to consider a hypothetical case. On a recent trip to Russia, the author visited the Russian National Institute of Physical Therapy, where a physician reported favorably on the therapeutic benefits of a particular type of mud found in the Crimea. She claimed that, when applied hot three to five times a week for up to an hour, this mud was useful for a variety of conditions, including psoriasis, hepatoma, and hypertension.

Consider a trial of the therapeutic benefit of mud for hypertension. Assuming adequate quantities of good-quality mud from the Crimea were available, the most important feature of this trial would be that it was *controlled*—or, in other words, that two groups are compared, one of which gets the new treatment and one of which does not. This sounds basic, but it is surprising how often new technologies or drugs are promoted on the basis of uncontrolled tests. Recent examples include single lung transplants in patients with COPD, diagnostic techniques such as chorionic villus sampling, and the use of buspar for smoking cessation.

Another important feature of a trial would be that the two groups be as similar as possible at the beginning of the trial, except for the therapy. To illustrate, suppose the group getting mud therapy started out with a diastolic blood pressure averaging 91 mm Hg, whereas the control group averaged 106 mm Hg. If blood pressure were measured at the end without making sure the two groups were similar at the beginning, the result might be attributed to the good effect of the mud rather than the fact they started out differently. An actual example of this is the old debate of medical or surgical management of esophageal varices. Early comparisons found that patients getting surgery did better. What was not addressed initially, however, was that, as a group, sicker patients did not go to surgery, so that better outcome was related to being less sick at the beginning of the study rather than the particular treatment.

Randomization is the best way to make the control and intervention groups similar. Why is randomization so powerful? Because it provides the best protection against unequal distribution of factors that may influence the outcomes. In the case of a randomized trial of mud therapy, with a large number of patients, age, race, dietary sodium intake, and other factors that are known to influence blood pressure will be relatively similar in the intervention and control groups. Randomization also protects against the influence of currently unknown factors that may influence outcomes. So, for example, it may be that a future study finds that a particular plasma renin greatly modifies the impact of hypertension therapy. In that case, the integrity of the mud therapy would probably be protected, because randomization would likely have made sure that the average renin level of those getting mud was the same as the average renin for those not getting mud, assuming adequate numbers of patients. An actual example of this is the Lipid Research Clinics Coronary Primary Prevention Trial. This trial was designed to test the hypothesis that lowering serum cholesterol would prevent myocardial infarctions. The two groups in this trial were randomized to receive either cholestyramine or placebo, resulting in a nearly identical distribution of known risk factors for myocardial infarction (e.g., cigarette smoking, hypertension). Now, more than two decades after the CPPT began, new data have suggested that persons who take aspirin are at lower risk for developing myocardial infarctions. Does this mean that the earlier observed results of the CPPT might be related to differences in aspirin consumption in the two groups rather than lowering cholesterol? Probably not, because the earlier study was randomized.

The next step in designing a clinical trial of mud therapy is to decide on which outcomes one wants to measure. The best way to choose outcomes is to apply clinical common sense. With respect to mud therapy for hypertension, blood pressure response is important insofar as it affects incidence of stroke and myocardial function, but other factors are also important, such as the cost in dollars and time and the quality of life of patients receiving the treatment. Frequent mud baths may be relaxing! Also important are side effects, which, in the case of mud therapy, might be burns from mud, time spent in treatment, and skin staining.

Who will measure the outcomes? It would be convenient, but probably not appropriate, to have a mud-room attendant measure blood pressure and other outcomes. Despite the best of intentions, there is a natural human tendency to bias recording to make what one is testing seem better than it is. This is the principle of *blinding* or masking: The people measuring or recording outcomes should not, if possible, know whether the subject was in the treatment or control group.

How long should the trial last? Ideally, of course, it would be nice to run a 20-year trial of the effects of mud therapy on the clinical outcomes of stroke and myocardial infarction, but limited resources dictate more limited durations. Use clinical common sense; in the case of mud therapy for hypertension, 2–4 weeks is probably too short and between 6 and 12 months would be much better. No matter what duration, all subjects should be accounted for at the end of the study. In analyzing the mud trial, it is not appropriate to compare the two groups if a large number of one of the groups dropped out. Subjects who drop out of studies tend to do worse than those who stay in; not paying attention to dropout may lead to the error of assuming that the treatment worked when in fact most of those who got it may have done so poorly that they went elsewhere.

Finally, in considering the results of the trial of mud therapy, it is important to distinguish between statistical and clinical significance. If the trial has 2000 subjects and finds that mud therapy lowers blood pressure by 1 mm Hg and that this finding is statistically significant, this would be nice to know, perhaps, but it would not be clinically useful. A 1 mm Hg change in blood pressure is clinically trivial. Only a trial that is both statistically and clinically significant should influence the clinician to adopt a new therapy. If the trial were negative—that is, if it was unable to show a significant effect of mud therapy on blood pressure—the first question to ask in interpretation of the results is: How large is the study? The *power* of a study is the likelihood that it has of showing a difference between the intervention and control groups; a small study may not have sufficient power to show a difference. In terms of the mud trial, suppose there were four cases treated with mud that showed a 14-mm decline in blood pressure and two placebo-treated subjects in which blood pressure dropped 6 mm. The difference, 8 mm, is clinically significant but, with the small numbers in the trial, may not reach statistical significance. One could imagine that a larger trial might confirm the 8-mm difference and if it did, we would herald a new age in the treatment of hypertension. A negative study might or might not be proof that the particular therapy does not work.

The last section discussed an *efficacy* trial of mud therapy for hypertension—that is, asking the question, "Under the best possible conditions, does mud therapy reduce blood pressure?" The best possible conditions include the best possible mud and physical therapists, physicians who are interested in the projects, subjects who are paid to get the treatments and stay in the trial, and carefully blinded assessment of multiple important clinical outcomes. Practicing clinicians, however, work in settings far removed from the hothouse atmosphere of well-funded clinical trials. Their patients are not homogeneous, they don't pay patients to show up, and high-quality mud may not be available. What they need to guide their actions are *effectiveness* trials, in other words, trials using more realistic conditions. Frequently, effectiveness trials have very different findings from efficacy trials; unfortunately, however, for most new technologies, drugs, and other medical interventions, effectiveness trials are not often done.

In addition to evaluating the methodological strength of studies, it is also necessary to assess the relevance or generalizability of the study to the clinicians' practice. Would the therapy be used or referred for frequently? If not, it is not often worth taking the time to read. Is the drug or therapy available locally? Even if the drug or operation is available locally, it may be used differently than the way it is reported. For example, initial advertising for ciprofloxacin cited a study of the effectiveness of ciprofloxacin in which the average dose was double what the sales representative was recommending. Are the patients similar to yours? Sometimes the patients are of substantially different age, gender, or ethnic background than yours. This is significant if these differences are related to differences in the biology of the disease, health-seeking behavior, or any other factor that will influence the effect of the therapy.

Figure 18.3 lists the criteria for evaluating articles on therapy. The cardinal criteria are: Is the therapy something you would use or refer for, and is the trial randomized? If the answer to either question is no, it is usually not necessary to read the paper unless no other information is available. If the article is worth the time

Is this article worth taking the time to read?

☐ Yes, because I might use or recommend this treatment
in my practice and treatment was randomly allocated
to students.

☐ No.

*If yes, answer the following:*

1.  Were the intervention and control groups similar?

2.  Were all clinically relevant outcomes assessed?

3.  Were all subjects accounted for at the end of the study?
    Were outcomes assessed blindly? Were other factors which
    might influence outcomes accounted for?

4.  Are the results clinically as well as statistically significant? If
    a negative trial, was the power of the study adequate?

5.  Are the patients similar to yours?

*UNC Critical Appraisal Group; adapted from materials developed at McMaster University*

**Figure 18.3.** Worksheet for articles about therapy.

to read, systematically review the paper, looking first at subjects. Are they similar to yours? Did randomization work to divide the subjects into two similar groups? Was there good follow-up? Then look at the outcomes. Were all of the relevant outcomes chosen? Were outcomes assessed in a nonbiased way? Finally, look at the results. Are they clinically as well as statistically significant? Were confounding variables accounted for in the analysis?

## CASE 18-7

*A 53-year-old woman presents for her routine well-woman care. She has begun to develop mild hot flashes and wants to discuss the possibility of estrogen replacement. She tells the family physician that she has heard news reports and wonders whether estrogen causes breast cancer. She does not have a family history of breast cancer, but she is concerned. What does the physician tell her? A computer search with key words* breast cancer, *with subheadings* prevention and control, etiology, *and* estrogen *yields the recent articles that have been in the press (Colditz et al., 1995) as well as a series of conflicting meta-analyses (Brinton & Schairer, 1993; Collaborative Group on Hormonal Factors in Breast Cancer, 1997; Henrich, 1992; Steinberg et al., 1991). The family physician concludes that there is some good evidence that long-term replacement with estrogen increases the risk of breast cancer, and excellent evidence that estrogen reduces complications from osteoporosis and conflicting evidence about the impact of estrogens on cardiac disease. After discussion of risks and benefits, the patient decides to start estrogen replacement. The family physician documents the discussion of risks and benefits in the medical record.*

## CAUSATION

As Case 18-7 illustrates, questions of causation come up frequently when physicians address prevention or give advice about lifestyle or other aspects of personal life, or when patients ask about medical studies reported in the popular press. While common, however, it is rarely as important for physicians to know the fine details of epidemiologic issues around causation, except insofar as they need to know them in order to form an opinion.

Information about causation is readily available but usually superficial in medical textbooks, and effective searching depends on review articles and computer searching. The best strategy is to search for the disease itself, with the subheadings *etiology* or *prevention and control*. Useful methodologic terms are *prospective study, cohort study, case–control study*; the publication term *meta-analysis* is also helpful for topics that have been the focus of a lot of research.

Critical appraisal of issues of causation is more complex than that of diagnosis, prognosis, or treatment, because the number of papers is greater, the study designs are often weaker, and final answers are less common than for many clinical questions. For most causal questions, true experiments are impossible for ethical reasons; for example, it would be impossible to randomly assign some people to smoke cigarettes to see whether lung cancer occurred. Determining causation is thus a judgment, based on a review of all of the evidence. To help with this judgment, epidemiologists have developed a list of criteria that may be used to judge when associations reflect causation. These criteria are listed in Table 18.2.

The most important criteria are temporality, strength of the association, dose response, and consistency. *Temporality* is the requirement that the exposure (smoking) precede the disease (lung cancer). This may seem self-evident, but some study designs like case–series and case–control studies often do not allow the assessment of temporality. The *strength of the association* is determined by the risk ratio or odds ratio; the higher the number, the more likely the association is causal. For smoking and lung cancer, many studies have put the risk ratio at between 4 and 18, whereas for alcohol and breast cancer, the risk ratio is probably less than 2. *Dose response* is the finding that more exposure leads to more of the disease, and *consistency* refers to whether the findings of one study are supported by findings in other populations.

Less helpful are biologic plausibility, specificity, and analogy. *Biologic plausibility* refers to what is known about the pathophysiology of disease; to suggest that a certain mechanism of disease is possible, however, falls well short of proving that it is the mechanism of disease. *Specificity* holds that one cause yields one effect, in the sense that an infectious agent like *M. tuberculosis* causes tuberculosis. This is less important

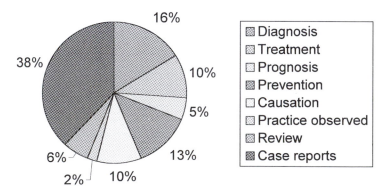

**Figure 18.4.** Major clinical focus of articles.

**Table 18.2**
Criteria for Causation

Temporality
Strength
Dose response
Consistency
Biologic plausibility
Specificity
Analogy

for chronic diseases. Smoking causes COPD and myocardial infarctions as well as lung cancer: The lack of specificity is a weak argument against causality. Finally, *analogy* refers to the existence of a similar disease. The well-known consequences of thalidomide for developing fetuses suggest that other drugs can cause major developmental problems. Like specificity, however, analogy is a weak argument for causation.

Clinicians often have to review a single article that has been reported extensively, and usually incompletely, in the popular press. In this case, many of the principles discussed with other types of articles will hold true. More importantly, how strong was the study design? As noted before, randomized controlled trials are stronger than cohort trials, which are stronger than case–control studies. Beyond this question are the methodological details. Were the measures of exposure and disease appropriate and collected in a blinded fashion? Were other factors that might influence outcome accounted for in the design of the study, the baseline information, and the analysis? Are the risks strong and with evidence of a dose–response curve?

## CASE 18-8

*A 62-year-old woman e-mails her family physician with a concern. A breast cancer survivor, she had received cosmetic silicone breast implants 10 years before. She is pleased with the implants but has become concerned because of reports in the media. Her anxiety is fueled by her daughter, who has done a lot of Internet searching and found numerous reports linking silicone implants to a variety of diseases. Recognizing that an important role for family physicians is to provide authoritative counsel about risk, her family physician suggests she come in for a visit and conducts a literature search. Amidst a swarm of case reports stretching back to the 1990s, the family physician finds a recent meta-analysis (Janowsky et al., 2000) which found no association between silicone implants and any connective tissue disease. At the visit, the family physician discusses with the patient what is known about the risks and benefits of silicone implants and gives her a copy of the article and accompanying editorial in the* New England Journal of Medicine.

## META-ANALYSIS AND SYSTEMATIC REVIEWS

As illustrated by Case 18-8, clinicians often need articles that provide an overview of previous literature. Traditionally, as illustrated in Case 18-1, these take the form of reviews in which the author informally reviews the clinical topic. In the last decade, however, there has been increasing recognition of the value of systematic reviews of previous literature. Systematic reviews differ from traditional reviews in that the process is explicit: Specific questions are defined, the literature search and process of reviewing the literature are detailed, and an attempt is made to summarize the findings of the published literature in an unbiased fashion. The explicit process allows the reader to judge the quality of the review. For some clinical questions, such as that in Case 18-8 about which there have been many small studies, it is possible to go further and do a meta-analysis, or quantitative synthesis, of the previously published articles. Pooling data allows greater numbers of subjects and hence better precision in estimates of the effect of the intervention or exposure.

Most systematic reviews and meta-analyses relate to therapy—e.g. how efficacious is a particular treatment?—but some address diagnosis, prognosis, or causation. Searching for meta-analyses has been made much easier in recent years. The methodological search term *review* is often not useful, since it is typically used for all articles in which there is a review of the literature, including case reports. The search term *meta-analysis* is valuable, although, as with other methodological terms, it is not always used by indexers. The Web sites listed in Table 18.1 provide meta-analyses and information organized around therapeutic questions.

How should meta-analyses be critically appraised? The reader should keep in mind the key questions raised above depending on the kind of clinical question—diagnosis, prognosis, and therapy. In addition, critical appraisal of meta-analyses depends on an assessment of the process of the review. A meta-analysis should begin with a specific clinical question. In Case 18-8, the question is the strength of the relationship between exposure to silicone and autoimmune diseases. The search strategy should be explicit, with a listing of search terms, years, and languages. Thorough search strategies should include the references from all articles found, other review articles, and consultation with experts who may be aware of other studies. The process of review of the prior studies should be explicit; the most rigorous reviews require multiple raters who are unbiased and whose summaries are tested for interrater agreement. The quality of the studies should be rated.

Statistical combination of prior trials depends on whether the trials to be combined are similar, for which there are statistical tests but which is also a matter of judgment. As in the article cited in Case 18-8, the analysis should reveal a pooled effect size with a standard deviation. The final step is a sensitivity analysis. Good meta-analyses should address the impact of a variety of variables of study methodology on the pooled effect size and explore the potential impact of unpublished studies.

# CONCLUSION

This chapter has provided a brief introduction to searching and critically appraising the medical literature. How should one continue to develop one's skills? To some extent, of course, medical students have no choice. At most medical schools, many clinical rotations require searching and interpretation of the literature in some fashion. Beyond medical school, residencies in most specialties have built journal clubs into their training programs. The formats vary greatly, but, typically, journal clubs meet every 1 to 4 weeks to review recent findings from the literature as well as to train skills in critical appraisal. As with any clinical procedure, practice is critical for proficiency, and these required exercises provide a good opportunity to improve skills. Beyond such required practice, however, should be the commitment to taking the time to improve skills. Improving the speed and effectiveness of searching and evaluating the medical literature becomes self-perpetuating, so that the clinician becomes more comfortable seeking out good-quality information.

The ultimate goal of critical appraisal is keeping up to date and in control of one's clinical practices. Practicing clinicians have a responsibility to keep current and to practice as effectively as possible, but changes in the volume of available information have made this increasingly difficult. Adding to the challenge is the format of traditional continuing medical education, in which practicing physicians receive didactic lectures, and which has very little impact on clinical practice.

To remedy the situation, dramatic changes have begun to appear in the way practicing physicians acquire new information. In the decade, most journals have switched over to structured abstracts, which force the authors to name their methods at the beginning and allow clinicians to weed out quickly articles that are weak or not applicable to their practice. The National Library of Medicine has begun to pay more attention to clinical consumers of Medline, which has resulted in more attention to methodological terms as searching tools. Continuing medical education itself is changing, experimenting with formats to allow more inclusion of data from physicians' own practice as well as increased use of evidence-based formats. Finally, the last decade has seen the popularization of practice guidelines published by the federal government, specialty societies, and insurers, some of which are evidence based. Central to all of these efforts is critical appraisal of the literature. Critical appraisal empowers physicians by giving them the tools to cut through the reams of useless data that confront them every day; it facilitates the change of practice because it holds old practice up to the standard of evidence rather than tradition.

## CASES FOR DISCUSSION

### CASE 1

*John Cotton is a 26-year-old man who comes to your office for evaluation of an ankle sprain. It happened in a pickup basketball game the night before. After going up for a rebound, he landed on someone else's foot and inverted his foot. Now there is no ecchymosis, but there is swelling and pain over the top of the foot. He asks you whether he needs an x-ray. In recent years, the Ottawa rules have been promulgated as a guideline for this problem, but you don't remember the details.*

1. *What are the Ottawa rules? Where can you find them?*
2. *How sensitive and specific are they?*
3. *Should you use them routinely? Should Mr. Cotton have an x-ray?*

### CASE 2

*You are seeing Mrs. Walthrop, a 58-year-old woman with hypertension, who is well controlled on a long-acting preparation of diltiazem. An executive for a local software company, she pays close attention to the health information available in the local press and on the radio. At a routine visit, she mentions hearing that calcium channel blockers may lead to increased mortality in some patients. She asks you whether she should change medications. She has no other cardiac risk factors or symptoms and is otherwise healthy except for a sedentary lifestyle.*

1. *How strong is the evidence against calcium channel blockers?*
2. *Should this evidence affect our prescribing for hypertension and angina?*
3. *What do you say to Mrs. Walthrop?*

### CASE 3

*You and your partners are discussing the health education information you will have routinely available to peri-menopausal women considering estrogen replacement therapy (ERT). A key issue is the possible risk regarding ERT and breast cancer, and the consensus of the group is that you need to find or develop some material for patients that explains and assesses the possible risk. You volunteer to do that and you begin by reviewing the literature relating ERT to breast cancer.*

1. *Is there a clinically significant risk of breast cancer with ERT?*
2. *What are the outcomes with the combined regimens now common?*
3. *How should this be expressed in a health education leaflet?*

### CASE 4

*Your staff model HMO is developing a practice guideline around the management of hypertension. Your assignment is to prepare a recommendation for the role of drugs in the management of mild hypertension. You decide to consult the recent JNC guidelines and search for studies of the treatment of mild hypertension.*

1. *Should all patients with mild hypertension be treated?*
2. *What are the benefits, the risks, and the costs of treatment of mild hypertension?*
3. *What is the role of medication as opposed to other therapies in the management of mild hypertension?*

## CASE 5

*Thirty-year-old R. Perrin and his second wife come to your office for contraceptive counseling. Mr. Perrin has two children by his first marriage, which ended in divorce 10 years ago; his current wife has one child by a previous marriage. The couple has been married for 2 years and is emphatic about not wanting to have any more children. They are interested in the possibility of vasectomy and have come to you to discuss it. One of their questions is whether vasectomy causes prostate cancer.*

1. *How strong is the evidence that vasectomy causes prostate cancer?*
2. *How should we incorporate that evidence into contraceptive counseling for our patients?*
3. *Specifically, what words would you use to describe the risk of prostate cancer to Mr. Perrin?*

## RECOMMENDED READINGS

Black ER, *et al.* (eds): *Diagnostic Strategies for Common Medical Problems.* Philadelphia, American College of Physicians, 1999.

This is the best single text on diagnostic tests. It critically evaluates the usefulness of common diagnostic tests.

*Canadian Medical Association Journal.* 1980, 123:499–504, 613–617; 1981, 124:555–558, 703–710, 869–872, 985–990, 1156–1182; 1984, 130:377–381, 1428–1433, 1542–1549.

The best introduction to critical appraisal is this series published in the early 1980s. It is relentlessly clinical, giving practical examples and providing "how to read" approaches for a variety of different questions; it is also very humorous.

*JAMA.* Evidence Based Medicine Working Group. 1992, 268:2420–2425; 1993, 270:2093–2095, 2598–2601; 1994, 271:59–63, 389–391, 703–707, 1815–1819; 1994, 272:234–237, 1367–1371; 1995, 273:1292–1295; 1995, 274:570–574, 1800–1804, 1830–1832; 1996, 275:554–558, 1232, 1435–1439; 1997, 277:1232–1237, 1552–1557, 1802–1806; 1998, 279:545–549; 1999, 282:771–778; 1999, 281:1214–1219, 1836–1843, 2029–2034; 2000, 283:1875–1879, 2829–2836; 2000, 284:79–84, 357–362, 478–482, 869–875, 1290–1296.

In recent years, the Evidence Based Medicine Working Group has published another series of articles. It is not quite as practical for practicing physicians, but it provides an excellent introduction to likelihood ratios, number needed to treat, decision analysis, practice guidelines, and other approaches that are used increasingly frequently.

*JAMA*: The Rational Clinical Examination. 1992, 267:2645–2648; 1993, 270:1242–1246, 2218–2221, 2843–2845; 1994, 271:54–58, 385–388; 1994, 272:1782–1787; 1995, 273:813–817, 1211–1218; 1996, 275:630–634; 1996, 276:1589–1594; 1997, 277:564–571, 1712–1719; 1997, 278:586–591, 1440–1445; 1998, 279:696–701, 1094–1099, 1264, 1614; 1998, 280:328, 1256–1263; 1999, 281:77–82, 1022–1029, 2231–2238; 1999, 282:175–181, 819, 1270–1280; 2000, 283:3110–3117.

This excellent series provides critical reviews about clinical examination.

Shaughnessy AF, Slawson DC, Bennett JS: Becoming an information master: A guidebook to the medical information jungle. *J Fam Pract* 39:489–499, 1994. Slawson DC, Shaughnessy AF, Bennett JS: Becoming an information master: Feeling good about not knowing everything. *J Fam Pract* 38:505–513, 1994.

These articles provide an excellent introduction to Information Mastery, comparing and contrasting different sources of information from the perspective of a busy practitioner.

## REFERENCES

Black ER, *et al* (eds): *Diagnostic Strategics for Common Medical Problems.* Philadelphia, American College of Physicians, 1999.

Brinton LA, Schairer C: Estrogen replacement and breast cancer risk. *Epidemiol Rev* 15:66–79, 1993.

Colditz GA, Hankinson SE, Hunter DJ, Willett WC, Manson JE, Stampfer MJ, Hennekens C, Rosuer B, Speizer FE: The use of estrogens and progestins and the risk of breast cancer in postmenopausal women. *N Engl J Med* 332:1589–1593, 1995.

Collaborative Group on Hormonal Factors in Breast Cancer: *Lancet* 350(9089):1484, 1997.

Furberg CD, Psaty BM, Meyer JV: Nifedipine: Dose related increase in mortality in patients with coronary heart disease *Circulation* 92:1326–1331, 1995.

Henrich JB: The post-menopausal estrogen/breast cancer controversy. *JAMA* 268:1900–1902, 1992.

Janowsky EC, Kupper LL, Hulka BA: Meta-analysis of the relation between silicone breast implants and the risk of connective-tissue diseases. *N Engl J Med* 342:781–790, 2000.

Newman TB, Klebanoff MA: Neonatal hyperbilirubinemia and longterm outcome: Another look at the collaborative perinatal project. *Pediatrics* 92:651–657, 1993.

Newman TB, Maisels MJ: Evaluation and treatment of jaundice in the term newborn: A kinder, gentler approach. *Pediatrics* 89:809–818, 1992.

Sackett DL, Haynes RB, Guyatt GH, Tugwell P: *Clinical Epidemiology: A Basic Science for Clinical Medicine*, ed 2. Boston, Little Brown & Co, 1991.

Sackett DL, *et al* (eds): *Evidence-Based Medicine: How to Practice and Teach EBM*. Edinburgh, Churchill Livingstone, 2000.

Shaughnessy AF, Slawson DC: Becoming an information master: A guidebook to the medical information jungle. *J Fam Pract* 39:489–499, 1994.

Slawson DC, Shaughnessy AF, Bennett JS: Becoming an information master: Feeling good about not knowing everything. *J Fam Pract* 38:505–513, 1994.

Steinberg KK, Thacher SB, Smith SJ, Stroup DF, Zach MM, Flanders WD, Berkelman RL: A meta-analysis of the effect of estrogen replacement therapy on the risk of breast cancer. *JAMA* 266:1358–1360, 1991.

Williams JW, Holleman DR, Samsa GP, Simel DL: Randomized controlled trial of 3 vs 10 days of trimethoprim/sulfamethoxazole for acute maxillary sinusitis. *JAMA* 273:1015–1021, 1995.

# PART III

# Society

The patient–physician relationship is surrounded by a social context. Understanding that context facilitates the growth of the relationship between the patient and the physician, while ignoring it can result in many problems and misunderstandings. The first section on relationships describes the profound effect these societal relationships can have on health and the clinical care of patients. Arising from many perspectives and theoretical models, this research also indicates that if physicians take information about relationships into account when formulating a therapeutic plan with patients, they are more successful in understanding the barriers that promote patient "unhealthiness" and can facilitate the removal of those families.

As technology has expanded the boundaries of care, patient, physician, and societal values are becoming more important in clinical decision-making. An especially difficult dynamic covered in these chapters is the tension between patients who want top-quality, easily accessible, low-cost healthcare, and the fact that resources devoted to medical care are not inhaustible. Another difficult dynamic discussed is that physicians often work to extend patients' lives without regard to cost. However, such extension of life, if it occurs at the expense of quality of life, is not a top priority for many patients. Learning to recognize where the values of the patient and physician differ and then negotiating an effective solution that respects the values of both parties is an important skill. Understanding how to allocate scare medical resources to get the most "bang for the buck" is also essential in this age of cost containment.

The last section of this part of the text deal with societal problems that all physicians will confront. These problems, seemingly intractable, often frustrate physicians into lethargy. However, this section will help physicians in training understand that these problems are not insurmountable and will help them develop appropriate intervention strategies to help their patients cope. Finally it is also hoped that some students will be stimulated to deal with these problems on a larger political level to reduce the toll they bear on our patients and on the fabric of our society.

## CHAPTER 19

# A. Relationships

# The Patient–Physician Relationship

*Ronald M. Epstein*

| CASE 19-1 |
|---|

*Joyce Samuels had chronic joint pains, shortness of breath, difficulty urinating, abdominal pains, and several other illness episodes over the past 8 years about which she was very anxious. Her husband had regarded these as minor concerns. Diagnostic testing revealed no cause, and she felt either that her physicians were not taking her concerns seriously or that they were withholding information. She frequently did not follow through with medical advice. On a routine gynecologic examination, her physician discovered a large pelvic mass that was diagnosed as advanced ovarian cancer. Her prognosis was poor. To her physician's surprise, Mrs. Samuels became much less anxious, and was grateful for having been provided an explanation for her suffering. Her interpersonal relationships with her husband and the medical community became more mutually satisfying.*

## EDUCATIONAL OBJECTIVES

1. List three patient outcomes that are improved by strengthening the patient–physician relationship
2. Distinguish paternalistic, consumerist, patient-centered, and family systems approaches to the patient–physician relationship.
3. Describe five positive and five negative aspects of power in the patient–physician relationship
4. Describe five responsibilities of the physician and five of the patient in the patient–physician relationship
5. Describe major threats to the patient–physician relationship and means for overcoming them

## INTRODUCTION

The patient–physician relationship* is the cornerstone of medical care. Each relationship that a physician forms with a patient is unique, often intimate, and has characteristics, expectations, and means of

---

*For clarity, and to place emphasis on the centrality of the patient, I will use the term *patient–physician relationship* rather than *doctor–patient relationship* or *physician–patient relationship*.

communication different from other social interactions. The patient–physician relationship is not simply bedside manner, or an appendage to technologically competent medical care. The nature of the relationship can have a profound influence on the patient's well-being (Bass *et al.*, 1986a; Stewart *et al.*, 1979), the patient's satisfaction with medical care (Starfield *et al.*, 1981), and the outcomes of diseases as diverse as peptic ulcers (Greenfield *et al.*, 1985), diabetes mellitus (Greenfield *et al.*, 1988), and respiratory infections (Bass *et al.*, 1986b). The fundamental goals of the patient–physician relationship are to assist the patient's own healing powers (McWhinney, 1989b), relieve suffering (Cassell, 1982), and foster healthy behaviors. To do this, the physician needs to understand the patient, the patient needs to understand her illness, and the patient must know that she has been understood.

In this chapter, I will provide general guidelines for a multifaceted appreciation of this complex social relationship. In my experience, most clinicians learn more about the nature of patient–physician relationships from their patients than from teachers and mentors. Rather than starting with abstract principles and providing cases to illustrate them, I will examine stories of actual patient–physician relationships. The "messiness" that inevitably occurs when one examines individual stories is part of what makes medicine a human endeavor (McWhinney, 1989b). I will emphasize the importance of meaningful and respectful human relationships, the family and social context, and the need for physicians to develop the capacity for organized self-reflection.

The relief of suffering is a central goal of medicine, and, therefore, of the patient–physician relationship. Eric Cassell (1982) has defined suffering to include an "injury to the integrity of the person," often associated with perceived disassembling of the patient's world as it has been known and requiring adaptations that may not be desired. Health, on the other hand, includes the ability to grow and adapt to change, to rebuild, and to transcend in response to injury. Suffering is ultimately a very personal experience; only parts of it can be shared, usually with intimates. Healthcare is concerned with disease, an abnormality in the structure or function, as well as illness, the experience of being unwell.

Understanding a patient's suffering involves far more than interpreting specific symptoms related to a disease or illness. The biopsychosocial model (Engel, 1977, 1980) emphasizes that it is crucial to understand each patient as a unique person, including past experiences, bodily and emotional memories, and expectations for the future. Each person has relationships with others (including physicians) within which personal experiences are expressed, redefined, and given meaning. The family usually contains the most important set of interpersonal relationships; its members, in turn, have experiences, roles, and expectations (Baird & Doherty, 1990; Doherty & Campbell, 1988; McDaniel *et al.*, 1990), as well as genetic and historical legacies. Within a particular culture, people are defined by social roles and political power. Aside from beliefs and values, our actions also help to define who we are. All of these factors are involved in suffering, in health, and in the patient–physician relationship.

Suffering can be caused by the illness, the meaning of the illness, the treatment for the illness, or personal and social sequelae of illness. It is difficult to know all of the sources of a patient's suffering without asking the patient.

The significance of the meaning of an illness is illustrated by an important study by Beecher (1959) during the Second World War. While stationed at a bloody battle in which there were many casualties, Beecher studied the meaning of injuries and requests for pain medications among soldiers wounded in combat. He noted that soldiers wounded in battle required substantially less pain medication and experienced less distress when compared with soldiers with similar injuries not sustained in battle. The difference was explained only by the meaning of the injury to the soldier. The injury in battle means that the soldier would be taken out of danger and his life would be saved; for others, a similar injury might mean prolonged disability, decreased income, and loss of a meaningful activity.

As in Beecher's study, the meaning of the illness to the patient described in Case 19-1 played an important part in the experience of and the relief of suffering. Her diagnosis of ovarian cancer validated her suffering and reassured her that she was not crazy. This life-threatening illness carried meanings to the patient and her family that would not have been apparent from casual inquiry. Therefore, it is critical for the physician to understand the illness from the patient's perspective (Stewart *et al.*, 1995) in order to understand the patient's response to illness or disability. Furthermore, physicians, by virtue of our ability to make proclamations about a patient's health, can strongly influence the meaning a patient gives to an illness, and, consequently, the patient's experience of illness. Consider, for example, how differently a patient recently diagnosed with cancer might respond if he were told that he has a 70% chance of cure as opposed to being told that he has a 30% chance of dying within 2 years.

The patient–physician relationship is also dependent on experiences with previous relationships, even if they are from different contexts. The most powerful early socialization experiences are usually with our own families of origin (the family in which each of us grew up) (McDaniel & Landau-Stanton, 1991). These experiences have a powerful effect on the nature of relationships that we form throughout the rest of life, especially intimate and emotionally charged relationships. Thus, some physicians are more formal than others, some feel more comfortable with uncertainty, and some are more comfortable caring for dying patients. Some share decision-making easily, and some find it difficult to care for patients who abuse drugs.

---

## CASE 19-2

*Mario Spola is a 45-year-old, mildly mentally retarded, Italian-born man. He acquired HIV infection at least 5 years ago from one of multiple anonymous same-sex partners. He has had no symptoms of HIV disease other than a mild yeast infection in the mouth. He comes to the office regularly, usually every 3 months, to talk, have a brief physical examination, and have blood tests done. He had several discussions in the past about his sexual behavior with his physician, Dr. Sherrie Newton, but he continued to have sexual relations with men whom he met in public parks and bars. After much encouragement, he began to use condoms, although he was still somewhat reluctant. He had difficulty understanding that, even though he felt healthy, he could transmit a fatal infection to others. He feared being rejected by potential partners if he used condoms; during a frank discussion, he reported that he used condoms only if his partner requested that he do so. He is always cheerful, agreeable, and otherwise follows medical advice. On a recent visit, Dr. Newton told him that his CD4 count, a measure of immune system functioning, has declined further, despite having added a second new combination of three anti-HIV medications. "But I feel great, doc, really great!" he said with pride, making the point that he is healthy enough to work as a machinist, sometimes 10 hours a day, 6 to 7 days a week. His risk of developing complications is now quite high. He has told no one in his family about his HIV disease, including his ex-wife and teenage children. He is certain that he became infected after they separated.*

## MODELS OF THE PATIENT–PHYSICIAN RELATIONSHIP

Case 19-2 illustrates several important features of the patient–physician relationship. The case shows how the sharing of illness stories is the basis of the relationships between patients and their physicians. It also shows that the medical interview is a narrative history involving the transfer of information as well as the development of frames of reference for interpretation of that information. These frames of reference are sometimes shared between physician and patient; often they are not. Therefore, the physician must engage the patient in dialogue to uncover the meaning of his distress. Further, the differing interpretations of a single patient's story points to the fact that a physician, a patient, and relevant family members construct the story of the patient's illness together. This is in contrast to the view that the physician is the disinterested impartial collector and processor of objective information.

It is difficult, and probably undesirable, to define an "ideal" patient–physician relationship. Szasz and Hollender (1956) described three basic models of the patient–physician relationship: the activity/passivity

**Table 19.1**
Models of the Patient–Physician Relationship

| Model | Physician's role | Values and assumptions |
|---|---|---|
| Activity/passivity | Does something to the patient without patient involvement | Physician knows best; patient cannot participate in care |
| Guidance/ cooperation (paternalistic) | Tells patient what to do in order to help patient; uses reassurance rather than explanation | Physician knows how to promote patient's best interest; values are shared between physician and patient |
| Consumer/ informative | Helps patient to help herself. Physician is a technical expert who informs patient of options; patient chooses | Patient bases decisions on her own values, of which she is aware |
| Interpretive | Counsels patient to make decisions in keeping with patient's values | Patient needs help from physician to clarify his values. Physician does not try to change patient's values |
| Deliberative | Engages patient in discussion to develop values; suggests a course of action | Patient values are malleable; physician's duty is to persuade (not coerce) patient to adopt healthy values |
| Contractual/ covenantal | Provides a philanthropic, consensual, negotiated, and mutually beneficial relationship with patient | Values are discussed openly. Moral responsibility is shared between physician and patient in the context of acknowledged power differential |
| Patient-centered | Finds common ground with patient on which to base medical decision-making | Illness must be understood from the patient's perspective as well as the diagnostic perspective. Moral obligation of physician to share power and show a human face |
| Family systems | Cares for patient in context of family unit. Physician helps patient help herself *and* helps family help the patient | Individual and family values are taken into account. Moral responsibility is shared between physician, patient, and family |
| Ethnographic | Discovers, with patient, personal and cultural meanings of illness | Cultural values are embedded in illness and must be addressed comprehensively |

model, the guidance/cooperation model, and the mutual participation model. These, along with more recently described models, are presented in Table 19.1.

The activity/passivity model takes as its assumption that physicians are technicians who perform procedures on patients with little or no input from the latter. Stated in its extreme form, it seems repugnant as a model for patient care in general, yet physicians commonly make decisions on a patient's behalf when there is an immediate, life-threatening illness and when the patient is not capable of communicating. Thus, if a patient without prior advance directives suffers a cardiac arrest with no close friends or family present, a physician uses the activity/passivity model by default. Similarly, physicians frequently have to make decisions for patients who are delirious, demented, psychotic, or comatose, without input from the patient or the family. Also, physicians and parents are empowered to make decisions on behalf of children.

The guidance/cooperation model has been referred to as a parent–child (Szasz & Hollender, 1956), paternalistic (Emanuel & Emanuel, 1992; McKinstry, 1992; Spittle, 1992), or priestly (Veatch, 1972) relationship. The physician assumes sole responsibility for making decisions that benefit the patient, without doing harm (Veatch, 1972). Until recently, this was the predominant model of medical care, and remains so in many parts of the world. For example, in Italy, it is still common for physicians to withhold the diagnosis of cancer from a patient and prescribe treatment without involvement of the patient in therapeutic decisions (Pellegrino, 1992). From a paternalistic viewpoint, the physician's job is to provide reassurance ("Don't worry, I'll take care of everything") rather than information. Underlying assumptions are that the patient's and the physician's values are identical, obviating a need to explore them further, and that the patient will comply with, and not question, the physician's recommendations. In more homogeneous societies, and in those where the range of possible treatments is small, it is reasonable to see how these assumptions could arise. In North American culture, these assumptions are not useful and may be perilous. However, some patients may want to be relieved of the onerous responsibility of making difficult decisions. Older patients may be accustomed to a paternalistic style and may find invitations for their expanded involvement in medical care initially unsettling. When caring for some children or mentally incapacitated adults, or when insurmountable communication barriers are present, physicians must make paternalistic decisions by default. However, respect must be shown for patients' preferences prior to becoming disabled (if known) and for the preferences of family members.

The mutual participation model's central tenets are patient autonomy, respect for the patient's values and experience, and the fundamental equality of all humans (Szasz & Hollender, 1956). According to Szasz, the physician becomes a participant in a partnership rather than telling the patient what to do. There are several different models developed more recently that are subsumed under Szasz's mutual participation model, such as the consumer model (Emanuel & Emanuel, 1992; Lazare *et al.*, 1975), the ethnographic model (Katon & Kleinman, 1981; Kleinman, 1987; Kleinman *et al.*, 1978; Stoeckle & Barsky, 1981), the interpretive model (Emanuel & Emanuel, 1992), the deliberative model (Emanuel & Emanuel, 1992), the contractual/covenantal model (Quill, 1983; Veatch, 1972), and the family systems model (McDaniel *et al.*, 1990). The features of each of these, including the physician's role and responsibilities, are summarized in Table 19.1. All of these models assume that a competent adult has the capacity to synthesize information and to articulate values and preferences. They also assume that the physician has sufficient communication skills to elicit the patient's preferences and sufficient self-awareness to know the difference between the patient's preferences and what the physician imagines or assumes the patient would want (Epstein, 1999; Novack *et al.*, 1997).

As an example, consider a seemingly simple situation (Case 19-3)—and compare the different approaches of four hypothetical physicians.

## CASE 19-3

*John Matthews, a 23-year-old psychology graduate student, has had a productive cough for 5 days. He was well until a week ago when he began to feel fatigued and feverish. He developed an aching sensation in his joints. The cough has worsened, and he is now coughing up green-brown sputum. He has lost his appetite and has stayed home from work and from school. The cough keeps him and his partner up at night. He has had bronchitis in the past and reported that antibiotics have helped; he inquired whether he could be prescribed an antibiotic. He smokes one pack of cigarettes a day. He looked ill and fatigued. On physical examination, there were some crackles in the right lung base, indicating that he has pneumonia.*

Consider the following four alternative ways physicians might handle this situation:

**A paternalistic approach.** Dr. Carol Francis told the patient that this was a "little touch of pneumonia," said not to worry, that the medication would help, and that John should feel better within 3 to 5 days. She wrote prescriptions for amoxicillin and codeine and explained how they were to be used. She advised John to stop smoking and described a method for helping John to quit, including nicotine patches, substitution of noncaloric foods, a smoking cessation group, and follow-up visits. She said that her office would call John in 3 days to see how he was doing and that John should call sooner if he became worse.

**A consumer approach.** Dr. Dennis Graham informed the patient that this was pneumonia and ascertained that the patient had no drug allergies. Dr. Graham explained the common causes of pneumonia in lay language, indicating that smokers have a much higher incidence of respiratory illnesses. He told the patient that continuing to smoke would shorten his life span, but that it would be his choice whether he wished to stop. Dr. Graham presented three options to the patient: (1) if John did nothing, most probably his infection would eventually improve; (2) amoxicillin, which is inexpensive and 90% effective, but must be given three times daily for 10 days; or (3) azithromycin, which is possibly more effective and has few side effects, but is much more expensive than amoxicillin. He asked the patient to make a choice. A similar choice was presented for antitussive medications. After the patient chose amoxicillin and codeine, Dr. Graham asked the patient if his findings and recommendations seemed reasonable. He told the patient to call if there were any further problems.

# BRONCHITIS AND SMOKING

*Many respiratory infections occur in humans. One of those, acute bronchitis, is a direct result of an infectious agent infiltrating the epithelial lining of the bronchi, the tubes that carry air from the throat to the alveoli of the lungs. This inflammation causes symptoms of coughing, sputum production, fever, and malaise. Bronchitis is usually self-limited, but the coughing often so disrupts sleep that the patient becomes fatigued and lethargic.*

*Smoking decreases the body's natural defenses in the lungs, thus predisposing the smoker to an upper respiratory infection. One of these defenses, the ciliated hair cells that line the bronchi, is responsible for trapping infectious agents in the sputum and moving that sputum on the "carpet" of these hair cells out of the lung. Unfortunately, the toxic chemicals in smoking slow the action of cilia initially and then destroy the cilia entirely, resulting in the pooling of these secretions in the lung rather than rapid clearance. Infectious agents flourish in the nutrient-rich sputum trapped in the lung, multiply, and cause infections. Thus, smoking not only causes lung cancer but more frequent lung infections as well.*

*Many controversies surround the diagnosis and treatment of bronchitis in the primary care setting. Many patients with bronchitis want antibiotics. Yet, half of all cases are caused by viruses, and antibiotics kill bacteria, not viruses. Many authorities feel that our overuse of antibiotics in patients with bronchitis and other infections may lead to an emergence of resistant organisms. Additionally, randomized controlled trials have suggested that the one agent that does seem to reduce the duration of bronchitis, inhaled β-agonist, is still not widely prescribed by physicians for this indication.*

*Regardless of these controversies, if a smoker does get bronchitis that visit should be recognized as an opportunity to council the patient regarding smoking cessation in order to reduce the frequency and severity of the patient's bronchitis infections in the future.*

**A patient-centered, deliberative approach**. Dr. Samuel Harris asked John why he thought he had become ill, and John reported being under considerable stress with graduate studies and a full-time job. Dr. Harris told John that he had pneumonia, that he had some understanding of how stressful graduate studies can be, and that rest and antibiotics are usually helpful. They discussed what the most reasonable plan would be. They agreed that it was wise to take time off from work; however, John felt that he had to try to keep up with readings at school. John felt that he could rest in bed some of the time, but would plan to go to the library to keep up with his reading. John felt that he was under too much stress to stop smoking; besides, his father and grandfather smoked heavily and had no adverse consequences. Dr. Harris asked John about what was important in his life right now. John felt that he needed to get more control of his life and needed to take better care of himself. Based on those values, Dr. Harris asked John what he hoped to do to accomplish those goals. John realized that it was probably in his best interest to do his reading at home rather than the library, so he could rest. Further, Dr. Harris strongly encouraged John to set up an appointment in a week to talk about his smoking. He recognized the patient's reluctance, but emphasized that if John stopped smoking he would regain health faster and would be taking better care of himself. John agreed to talk further about his smoking at a follow-up visit, but did not know if he was interested in quitting. Dr. Harris prescribed amoxicillin and offered him a prescription for codeine and asked him if his findings and recommendations seemed reasonable.

**A family systems approach**. Dr. Mary Jacobs asked John how the illness has been affecting his life. John reported being under considerable stress with graduate studies and a full-time job. He felt that he could not afford to take time off, that his life was out of control, and that he wanted to take better care of himself. She told him that he had pneumonia and prescribed amoxicillin and codeine. Although they agreed that it was wise to take time off from work, John felt that he had to try to keep up with readings at school. Dr. Jacobs also asked John if his partner would be able to help at home for the next few days. John replied that he would and that his partner would be pleased if John were not "hacking away" all night. John also mentioned that both he and his partner had tested HIV-negative 2 months previously and were at no current risk for infection. Dr. Jacobs inquired whether his partner smoked. When John indicated that they both smoked, she invited both of them to come in for a follow-up appointment to discuss how they could help each other take better care of themselves.

Although these may seem like simplistic caricatures, the four vignettes following Case 19-3 are based on observations of actual patient–physician encounters, all of which took approximately the same amount of time. These same styles of interaction are equally common in other, more "charged" clinical encounters, such as when a patient is informed she has cancer or when discussing major changes in therapy for chronic illness.

In the first vignette, Dr. Francis was practicing within a paternalistic (Emanuel & Emanuel, 1992; May, 1975; Neighbour, 1992; Spittle, 1992) model, making choices for the patient and instructing the patient on how to comply with the prescribed treatment. Dr. Francis's care was kind and competent; however, she assumed total responsibility for the patient's care: The patient was not informed of any treatment options, the illness was treated out of context of the patient's life, and the patient's values were never explored. Thus, the physician missed an opportunity to address additional concerns of the patient and did not help the patient to participate in his own care.

By contrast, in the second vignette, Dr. Graham completely informed the patient of his treatment options, and, utilizing a consumer model of care (Emanuel & Emanuel, 1992; Lazare *et al.*, 1975), left the choice to the patient. The patient was assumed to have the capacity to synthesize information on his own; conversely, the physician's responsibility was only to provide "value-free" information about the patient's illness. An analogy can be made to the choice of products in a supermarket. The educated consumer reads the well-labeled contents of the product on the side of the box and makes an informed choice about which product to purchase. The patient, willingly or unwillingly, was given total responsibility for his care. This approach, while appropriate for some clinical decisions, often does not address the context of the decision, or the values that the patient brings to the situation, and avoids the positive and negative uses of power in a relationship wherein power is distributed asymmetrically. While giving the illusion of empowering the patient, such an approach is not patient-centered, that is, it places importance only on the diagnosis as defined by the physician's medical frame of reference, rather than including the patient's perspective as well. This approach does not call on the physician to help the patient make an informed choice within the context of the patient's values and does not place the physician in the position of questioning or attempting to influence the values that underlie the patient's choices.

Dr. Harris, in the third vignette, took a more patient-centered (Levenstein *et al.*, 1986; Stewart *et al.*, 1995) approach by exploring the patient's life context, values, and preferences and by offering accurate and appropriate empathy. The physician worked with the patient in a collaborative style and gave the patient meaningful choices. Compared with the consumer approach described above, the range of choices of antibiotic was narrower, and there was less deliberation about issues that the physician imagined might be important to the patient. Instead, by clarifying and interpreting the patient's values, the physician was able to use the time to address important underlying concerns of the patient—that he learn to care for himself better. By taking this approach, Dr. Harris helped the patient to formulate his own solution to a dilemma, a solution John was more likely to follow than had the physician directed the patient to take a similar action. This is in keeping with research that shows that patients who are active participants in their own care have improved medical outcomes and improved satisfaction (Kaplan *et al.*, 1989; Starfield *et al.*, 1981). Dr. Harris went further, by adopting a deliberative (Emanuel & Emanuel, 1992) style of interaction. He did not accept at face value John's reluctance to quit smoking, but rather encouraged (but, importantly, did not coerce) John to adopt a different perspective on the problem. While appearing to have elements in common with a paternalistic approach, this approach was different in several important ways. Dr. Harris took into account the patient's values and life context and engaged in dialogue with the patient as an equal, but the physician retained the obligation to advise and to convince the patient to pursue health-promoting actions. This incorporates elements of a covenantal model (May, 1975), wherein the moral responsibility is shared between physician and patient. It acknowledges that physician and patient have differing expertise and that physician and patient have unequal power in the medical realm.

Dr. Jacobs, in the fourth vignette, incorporated many of the features of a patient-centered, deliberative relationship, but included the patient's family context in the information-gathering, problem list, and potential sources of solutions for the patient's concerns. The family systems model will be discussed in greater detail in Chapter 20. For now, it is important to consider the family as "not limited to ties of blood, marriage, sexual partnership or adoption, [but may include] any group whose bonds are based on trust, mutual support and common destiny" (World Health Organization, 1994). Dr. Jacobs, on hearing that smoking and HIV risk were concerns affecting John and his partner, enlisted the help of a family member to characterize further and manage John's problems, and, in so doing, defined the family as the unit of care. The responsibility for healthcare was shared between physician, patient, and family. By considering it a shared rather than individual effort, John was less reluctant to consider a major lifestyle change.

Finally, an ethnographic approach (Good & Good, 1981; Kleinman, 1983, 1987; Kleinman *et al.*, 1978; Stein & Apprey, 1990) would include inquiry not only into the patient's family, but also into the cultural traditions and values that shape the patient's healthcare-seeking behavior, illness experience, and expectations of the physician. In addition to individual attributions about the nature of illness and treatments, there are strongly held cultural beliefs that influence patients and physicians. For example, a patient from an Asian culture where there is a widely held belief that exposure to wind is harmful, may lose trust in a physician who suggests unbundling an infant with a fever. Care must be taken, however, not to infer individual beliefs solely from ethnicity; there are frequently more variations within an ethnic group than between them. These issues are discussed further in Chapter 24.

## CASE 19-4

*When Sam Walters first met Dr. David Isaacson, Mr. Walters was a 43-year-old, intermittently homeless man with cirrhosis caused by heavy alcohol use, and infection with hepatitis B and C virus, which in turn were acquired through intravenous cocaine use. He was very jaundiced, gaunt, and wasted. Mr. Walters thought that he did not have much time to live. Tests confirmed recurrent hepatitis and that he was not HIV-infected. His liver disease had resulted in a coagulopathy, portal hypertension with splenomegaly, esophageal varices, and thrombocytopenia.*

*Dr. Isaacson asked Mr. Walters what he wanted to do with the time he had remaining. He replied that he wished to reunite with his daughters (whom he had not seen in several years) who were then in foster care. He also wanted to live, and would do "anything" to extend his life. At Dr. Isaacson's suggestion, he stopped drinking and remained abstinent. He was referred to a family therapist, who helped him and his daughters heal the wounds of their difficult relationship. He also expressed remorse about several serious crimes he had committed (he had been arrested but never prosecuted). It was a "secret" that he had never told anyone, but could not live with alone any longer. The nature and details of the crimes were kept in confidence; there was no one was currently endangered.*

*After 2 years, he began having severe recurrent right-sided abdominal pain caused by gallstones. Because of his cirrhosis and portal hypertension, his surgical risk was too high to consider cholecystectomy. He refused narcotics for these episodes for fear of becoming addicted again. He came to the office and the emergency room with frequent recurrences of his pain. He had episodes of encephalopathy and felt progressively worse. He asked if he would likely die of liver failure; Dr. Isaacson's honest affirmative answer changed Mr. Walters's self-concept to that of a dying man.*

*After another 2 years, his episodes of abdominal pain became more severe, and his liver function deteriorated further during those episodes. His right-sided abdominal pain became constant. He began to feel hopeless, began using i.v. cocaine, and again became homeless, living in "crack houses." He was ashamed to have his daughters see him this way. Despite this relapse, he continued to come to the office for regular appointments and assiduously abstained from alcohol. He continued using cocaine, because "there was no purpose in living anyway." He brought up the possibility of liver transplant. At that time, transplant centers were beginning to accept patients with a recent history of drug use. He was put on the transplant list with the proviso that he be tested periodically to document abstinence.*

## HEPATITIS C AND CIRRHOSIS

*Hepatitis C is an RNA virus that attacks the liver. At highest risk for hepatitis C infections are intravenous drug users who share needles and powder cocaine users who share straws. Mother-to-infant spread occurs in approximately 5% of cases with sexual transmission of hepatitis C being rare.*

*While acute hepatitis typically causes symptoms of nausea, fatigue, and jaundice due to elevations in serum bilirubin, chronic hepatitis is usually asymptomatic until the cirrhosis stage is reached. Seventy to eight-five percent of all cases of hepatitis C are chronic, and about 20% of individuals with chronic hepatitis C infections develop cirrhosis. Depending on the degree of cirrhosis, during which the liver becomes fibrotic (scarred), symptoms and effects can include: gastrointestinal bleeding; confusion from encephalopathy; swelling of the abdomen (ascites) and feet (peripheral edema); malnutrition; and, eventually, death. Patients with chronic hepatitis C cirrhosis are predisposed to the development of hepatocellular carcinoma (liver cancer).*

*Current treatments, interferon and ribavirin, are difficult to take due to side effects and often do not prevent the progression to cirrhosis in those with chronic hepatitis C infections. Additionally, many patients with hepatitis C infections have other problems such as HIV, hepatitis B infections or alcoholism, which also worsen liver functioning. Thus, care of patients with hepatitis C, particularly those with cirrhosis, can be quite difficult.*

## ATTRIBUTES OF THE PATIENT–PHYSICIAN RELATIONSHIP

Sam Walters's story in Case 19-4 demonstrates that the patient–physician relationship involves far more than the communication that occurs in a single medical encounter. Relationships develop over time (Stewart *et al.*, 1995). Physician and patient grow through life, have crises, share experiences, and develop trust. The nature of the relationship changes with time. As in this case, physicians can, at different times, act solely as a source of technical competence, make contracts, make judgments, act as agent of change, assume an advocacy role, be charitable, and use power in a variety of ways. These roles are listed in Table 19.2. Also fundamental to the patient–physician relationship is the principle of nonabandonment. According to Quill and Cassel (1995), this is a "continuous caring partnership between physician and patient" that transcends the multiple challenges that the relationship may face.

It is commonly observed that the act of prescribing treatment can be more curative than the pharmacologic value of the medication (Balint, 1957). This may reflect offering hope to the patient in the face of suffering, mutual participation in a treatment plan, and the psychoneuroimmunologic mechanisms that relate psychological states such as hopefulness and feeling supported with biological phenomena such as improved survival in breast cancer patients (Spiegel *et al.*, 1989). Strategies for facilitating healing in the patient–physician relationship include attending to the patient's need for information, negotiating a treatment plan that is concordant with the patient's values, eliciting and responding to the patient's emotions, offering hope, using touch, involving family members, and activating the patient to take part in her medical care (Novack, 1987; Simpson *et al.*, 1991). The patient–physician relationship can be a way for the patient to create meaning in suffering, above and beyond the offering of hope (Cassell, 1982). The patient can be helped to find meaningful

**Table 19.2**
Physician Roles

| | |
|---|---|
| Agent of change | Contractual partner |
| Facilitator of change | Priest/judge |
| Colllaborative partner | Mentor |
| Advocate on patient's behalf | Friend |

connections with medical personnel (Suchman & Matthews, 1988), social support networks, and family members (McDaniel *et al.*, 1990), to help her to reconstruct a world that may seem to have been irreversibly altered by illness (Toombs, 1992). In addition, all of these factors may include the therapeutic aspects of the "placebo effect," which, in part, refers to the use of the patient–physician relationship itself as an important primary therapeutic modality, regardless of whether a drug is prescribed (Brody, 1992).

Physicians are given power by social institutions, by patients, and by their own families (Brody, 1992). Access to knowledge is one of the most potent sources of power (May, 1975). This power is invested in physicians with some direction for its use (see Chapter 26 on ethics), but also with considerable latitude. Some aspects of the power relationship will always be asymmetrical. Physicians have knowledge and skills that, at best, will be shared incompletely with patients.

Physicians can use their power to empower a patient by providing information with which a patient can make an informed choice, exploring the patient's values and preferences, respecting the patient's autonomy, and finding means to help the patient achieve a desired behavior change. This does not involve simply a transfer of power from physician to patient (as would be the case in the consumer model of the patient–physician relationship), but rather a sharing of power to the extent possible to achieve a good outcome as defined by the patient and by the physician. The physician can be active in identifying patients who may feel powerless and providing them with the means to have more control over their medical care. This has important implications for patient outcomes as well. In a series of studies, Greenfield and Kaplan (Kaplan *et al.*, 1989) have showed that "activated patients," that is, those who are naturally more involved in their care or who are taught how to be more involved in their care, have significantly better medical outcomes. This included better control of diabetes mellitus, fewer chemotherapy-associated symptoms in patients with breast cancer, and improved functional status in patients with peptic ulcer disease. These findings were independent of stage of disease and treatment given.

Physicians can act in an advocacy role that directly uses their socially given power. For example, physicians sometimes write letters to the telephone company asking them to provide free telephone service to chronically ill patients who otherwise could not afford a telephone. In some countries, physicians have identified and publicized victims of torture in the hope of preventing future abuses (Mishler E, 1994, personal communication).

Sometimes the physician must use her power to act on the patient's behalf, but contrary to the patient's wishes. Common examples are initiating involuntary psychiatric hospitalization for a suicidal patient, identifying perpetrators of child abuse, or refusing to authorize a renewal of a driver's license for a patient with poorly controlled epilepsy.

Physicians continue to serve judicial and priestly roles. Physicians make judgments on patients' ability to work, and determinations of disability and culpability for injury. There are also more subtle judgments of character that influence the patient–physician relationship. Once a patient is described as "difficult," either verbally or in a written correspondence, this pejorative label is likely to be communicated to future healthcare providers. The "priestly" role also has both positive and negative attributes. Physicians are in a position to use moral persuasion to the patient's benefit, such as the alcoholic who is reluctant to stop drinking. Also, physicians, by virtue of their power, can make performatives (Havens, 1986), that is, statements that transform a situation just by having uttered words. An example in everyday life is when a justice says, "I pronounce you husband and wife." A layperson, uttering the same words, clearly would not have the same effect. Similarly, physicians, by uttering words such as "You have cancer" or "I consider you to be permanently disabled," can also achieve profound (as defined by themselves or by society) changes in patients.

Finally, the patient–physician relationship involves a personal commitment to patients. In long-term caring relationships, as in Case 19-4, feelings and affections form between physician and patient that allow the relationship to withstand tragedy, conflict, and absences. These connections (Branch & Suchman, 1990; Suchman & Matthews, 1988) attend to the spiritual aspect of suffering, which, for many patients, is inseparable from physical or psychological distress. Mutual gift-giving, of objects, time, or attention, often is a manifesta-

## CARING FOR PATIENTS

*The good physician knows his patients through and through, and his knowledge is bought dearly. Time, sympathy, and understanding must be lavishly dispensed, but the reward is to be found in that personal bond which forms the greatest satisfaction in the practice of medicine. One of the essential qualities of the clinician is interest in humanity, for the secret of the care of the patient is caring for the patient. (Peabody, 1927/1984)*

tion of such strong relationships. In this way, patient–physician relationships often involve charity, "giving with love despite the presence or absence of affection for the patient" (McWhinney, 1989a). It is important, however, to emphasize that, in all cases, the patient–physician relationship must first serve the patient's needs, and not primarily the emotional needs of the physician.

## CASE 19-5

*Frank Rowe is a 77-year-old widowed man who formerly ran a newspaper distribution warehouse. Dr. Laura Cobb knew him for 10 years, but took over his care 3 years ago when his primary physician left the practice. She probably knew him better than any of his prior physicians, because he always seemed to get sick when they were out of town and Dr. Cobb was on call. The first time they met, he had an episode of bronchitis. She mentioned that smoking was probably related to his having developed the illness, and he became annoyed. "Why do you doctors keep lecturing me and why don't you just mind your own business?" He would die when his time came, and had filled out living wills and DNAR (do not attempt resuscitation) papers. The next week he had a cardiac arrest in the parking lot of Dr. Cobb's office. The physicians who came to the scene were not aware of his wishes. Dr. Cobb went outside to see what all of the commotion was about, only to discover that he had been "successfully" resuscitated and brought to the hospital. The patient recovered and went home, but voiced resentment at having been resuscitated against his wishes. He was relatively well for 4 years. The next 4 years brought a sequence of increasingly frequent hospitalizations for heart failure, pneumonia, weakness, and syncopal (fainting) episodes. His wife died, and he was increasingly unable to care for himself. He took medications including antidepressants as he felt he needed them. He was often angry and depressed. He would demand to speak to his physicians in the middle of the night when he knew they were at home sleeping. He frequently expressed fear of dying, and often felt that each exacerbation of his disease would be the last. He was offered counseling but was not interested. In the last few months of his life, his congestive heart failure worsened so that he was housebound, on continuous oxygen. He refused nursing home placement, regarding that option as "worse than death." He asked Dr. Cobb if she would prescribe some sleeping pills. She asked him why, and he said, "because I'm too weak to jump off a bridge." They began a discussion about his request, and she offered to discuss it further with him at their next appointment. He died later that week; it was never clear whether the immediate cause of death was the natural progression of his disease, failure to take his medications, or a deliberate suicide.*

## RESPONSIBILITIES OF THE PHYSICIAN AND PATIENT

In Case 19-5, Dr. Cobb had a long and complex relationship with Mr. Rowe; contributing to the complexity were the explicit and implicit responsibilities that physician and patient had toward each other (see Table 19.3). First, physicians are expected to be competent. Competence has been defined by some to consist of a good fund of knowledge, technical skill, clinical judgment, and awareness of limitations

# CHRONIC ILLNESS AND SUICIDE

*In a recent survey of suicidal ideation and suicide attempts, persons with chronic illnesses were found to be at much higher risk. The prevalence of lifetime suicidal ideation among those with a general medical condition was 25.2%, and among those with two medical conditions the numbers rose to 35.0%. The prevalence was 16.3% among the general population, some of whom had medical conditions and some did not. The prevalence of suicide attempts among those with a general medical condition was 8.9% and among those with two medical conditions the prevalence was 16.2%. Among the total respondents, the prevalence of suicide attempts was 5.5%. Patients with cancer or asthma had a four-fold greater chance of a suicide attempt than others, even after controlling for depressive illness and alcohol use. (Source: Druss B, Pincus H: Suicidal ideation and suicide attempts in general medical illness.* Arch Intern Med *160:1522–1526, 2000.)*

(Emanuel & Dubler, 1995). Competence must also include the ability to communicate effectively with patients, their families, and colleagues; to elicit and take into account patients' values and experiences (Engel, 1980); to understand and intervene appropriately with the social aspects of illness; and to be empathic (Rudebeck, 1992; Suchman *et al.*, 1997). These last two features are essential; without understanding the patient's distress, and communicating that understanding to the patient, a physician cannot relieve it. Further, "the doctor's competence is more about accompanying the patient up to her own choice than about giving lots of advice" (Rudebeck, 1992). Part of the competence of a physician is her ability to foster meaningful change.

Moral responsibilities of the physician go beyond the ethical principles of nonmaleficence, beneficence, justice, and autonomy (see Chapter 26 on medical ethics). The physician must not abandon a patient, even when there are difficult decisions to be made and when there are no clear solutions. Mr. Rowe in Case 19-5 would be a demanding patient for most physicians. That made it even more imperative for his physician to listen, to acknowledge Mr. Rowe's requests and needs in a nonjudgmental fashion, and to respect him as a person. At the same time, Dr. Cobb had to make explicit her own limitations. She had to make her values known while respecting his. When mistakes occur, addressing them openly often will win a patient's trust more than trying to hide them. In this case, the "mistake" was a lifesaving one, as the patient expressed resentment at having been resuscitated.

Trust is not implicit in any relationship. It is usually won after having faced a challenge together (O'Rourke, 1993). Physicians' honesty and integrity are usually judged by actions, not only words. When patients are ill and emotions are raised, it is difficult not to promise a good outcome. Consider the following story, reported to me thirdhand, and thus probably better considered a parable.

**Table 19.3**
Physician's Responsibilities toward Patients

Being technically competent
Being with the patient
Providing information
Being truthful/trustworthy
Avoiding conflict of interest
Advocating for the patient
Expressing personal commitment to care
Avoiding harm (nonmaleficence)
Acting in the patient's best interest (beneficence)
Maximizing patient autonomy
Negotiating a treatment plan that is concordant with the patient's values

## CASE 19-6

*Shortly after a young Anglo physician began to work at a clinic on the Navajo reservation, a father brought his daughter into the office. They had traveled a long distance to the clinic. She had had minor upper respiratory symptoms. The physician examined her carefully, shared his findings, prescribed Tylenol for fever, and sent them home.*

*The next day, the father returned with his mother, a chronically ill-appearing woman with poorly controlled diabetes mellitus and a gangrenous foot. The physician then understood that he had brought in his daughter the previous day in order to "check out" the new physician before trusting him with his mother.*

Physicians have the responsibility, in my view, to collaborate with the patient. A collaborative approach to care means taking the patient's perspective on an equal footing with the physician's diagnostic perspective (Brown *et al.*, 1986; Katon & Kleinman, 1981; Levenstein *et al.*, 1986). The patient is recruited as an ally in planning further investigation of a problem and in formulating a treatment plan. Patients are given information that will empower them to make important clinical decisions. Information is shared with relevant family members, important social supports, and other healthcare professionals; maintaining a focus on the patient's values, all of these others may make valuable contributions to the patient's care.

In any healthcare system, there is the possibility of physician conflict of interest in caring for patients (Emanuel & Dubler, 1995). Financial conflict of interest in a fee-for-service system is of concern when patients are referred to for-profit, physician-owned diagnostic or treatment facilities. Conversely, in managed care settings, there may be financial incentives to minimize the use of resources. Conflict of interest can be more subtle, and unavoidable; for example, a patient may receive short shrift if a physician is running late and has an important social engagement. Similarly, bias is prevalent in medical settings. For example, it has been shown that women who have the same percentage of excess body weight as men are more likely to be labeled as obese by their physicians (Franks *et al.*, 1982), that black patients are less likely to be screened for hypercholesterolemia than whites (Naumberg *et al.*, 1993), and that Hispanic patients are less likely to receive adequate pain relief compared with non-Hispanic patients in an emergency room setting (Todd *et al.*, 1993). Recognizing, accommodating to, and correcting conflict of interest and systematic bias are part of the physician's responsibility.

To accomplish these tasks, physicians need to have a means for organized reflection on their behavior (Epstein, 1999; Novack *et al.*, 1999). Commitment to becoming more self-aware will help the physician to reduce miscommunication, recognize the difference between what the patient wishes and what the physician would wish in a similar circumstance, and find more satisfaction with patient care.

Just as physicians have responsibilities in a patient–physician relationship, so do patients. Our notions of what is a "good patient" have changed over the years. Historically, patients have been responsible for accurately reporting symptoms and following physicians' recommendations. A more recent view is that,

## MEDICAL PATERNALISM

*The whole procedure was just what he expected, just what one always encounters. There was the waiting, the doctor's air of importance ... the tapping, the listening, the questions requiring answers that were clearly superfluous since they were foregone conclusions, and the significant look that implied: "Just put yourself in our hands and we'll take care of everything; we know exactly what has to be done—we always use one and the same method for every patient, no matter who." ... The celebrated doctor dealt with him in precisely the manner [that Ivan Ilych, the prosecutor] dealt with men on trial. (Tolstoy, 1886/1981)*

rather than being passive recipients of healthcare, patients should be more active in their care and take more responsibility for health-promoting activities. However, our language often still suggests that the patient take a passive role in healthcare. For example, the term *compliance* implies that the patient will unquestioningly follow the orders of the physician. Perhaps "adherence to a mutually negotiated plan" comes closer to a more balanced locus of responsibility for health. Still, some questions remain that will need to be answered by each physician who cares for patients. For example, whose responsibility is it to remind patients about screening tests? Does a physician have the responsibility to provide a treatment requested by a patient if she does not believe that it will be helpful? Should the physician initiate inquiry into "personal" issues such as sexual behavior or HIV risk, or should the physician wait for the patient to bring these up? What is the physician's responsibility if a patient does not follow through with a treatment plan? There is little consensus among physicians regarding the answers to these questions.

## CASE 19-7

*Dr. Carole Sanchez had taken over the care of Ethel Burke 3 months previously because she was dissatisfied with her prior physician. Ethel is a 66-year-old woman with chronic severe unremitting neurogenic shoulder pain resulting from an automobile accident 4 years previously. She also has an anxiety disorder and mild congestive heart failure. After trying several courses of physical therapy, different medication regimens, anesthetic and steroid injections, chiropractic, psycho-therapy, acupuncture, and electrical stimulation, the only treatment that offered relief was high-dose oral narcotics. She also had taken diazepam at moderate dose for many years for anxiety.*

*Dr. Sanchez expressed willingness to maintain her on these medications as long as she used them as prescribed. Two months after she began caring for Mrs. Burke, the patient requested an urgent refill of her medications 3 days before she was due for a refill. She had gone to the emergency department by ambulance and claimed that the ambulance crew had taken her medication from her and had not returned it. The next month, 2 weeks after having been prescribed a month's supply of medication, she called requesting an urgent refill prescription, claiming that all of her medication was gone. She said that the pharmacy only filled part of her prescription. Dr. Sanchez called the pharmacist, who disconfirmed her allegation. She reported having taken it as prescribed and could not account for the missing medication. She complained of extreme, uncontrolled pain.*

*On a routine prenatal visit, Mrs. Burke's daughter said that she had something important to tell Dr. Sanchez about her mother. She reported that Mrs. Burke was an addict, unable to control her use of medication, and had been receiving prescriptions for narcotics from several physicians simul-taneously.*

*Dr. Sanchez deliberated whether to discharge the patient from the practice for having been dishonest or try to work with her to control her narcotic use. Not discharging the patient would mean working through a time-consuming process of contacting other physicians, contracting with the patient on use of medications, dispensing supplies of narcotics every 3 days rather than monthly, having the patient evaluated by a drug dependency program, and discussing this plan further in a family meeting. Mrs. Burke and her family came into the office. They negotiated a plan to monitor her narcotic use, and they signed a contract to that effect.*

## TOOLS FOR RELATIONSHIP-BUILDING

Case 19-7 illustrates a situation where there were multiple threats to the patient–physician relationship. Caring for Mrs. Burke would be challenging for most experienced physicians. For some physicians, patient dishonesty is a cause for immediate termination of the patient–physician relationship. In my view, direct confrontation about dishonest behavior need not always result in termination of the relationship, but requires careful contracting and rebuilding trust.

Because the patient–physician relationship is a specialized social relationship, no one is born with all of

**Table 19.4**
Tools for Relationship-Building

Demonstrating unconditional positive regard for the patient as a person
Being dependable and consistent
Being caring and charitable
Understanding the patient's perspective on illness
Eliciting and responding to the patient's emotions
Legitimizing the patient's concerns
Demonstrating respect and support
Offering hope
Using touch
Involving family members
Activating the patient to take part in his medical care
Helping the patient find meaning in suffering
Fostering healthy coping
Activating psychoneuroimmunologic mechanisms (the placebo response)
Respecting boundaries
Being committed to becoming more self-aware
Using self-disclosure judiciously

the skills she will need to form effective patient–physician relationships. The noted psychologist Carl Rogers (1961) provided a series of principles for health professionals to consider when forming and developing therapeutic relationships, all of which were useful in caring for Mrs. Burke. These principles are listed in Table 19.4 and are described here:

- Act in such a way that you will be perceived by the patient as trustworthy, dependable, and consistent. The emphasis on action implies that trustworthiness must be demonstrated in a way that is understandable to the patient. Patients' interpretations of physicians' actions may be different than the intent of those actions.
- Communicate clearly and unambiguously. This includes nonverbal as well as verbal communication. It is important to let the patient take the lead, agree on an agenda, avoid use of medical jargon until you are sure the patient understands, summarize periodically, and check with the patient to make sure you have understood him, and that he has understood you (Epstein *et al.*, 1993). When there is hope, let the patient know.
- In all situations, learn to experience and communicate some positive attitudes toward the patient. In situations when the patient's life resembles your own, this may be easy. However, it is crucial, in order to sustain a long-term patient–physician relationship, to develop an unconditional positive regard for the patient (Rogers, 1961). This does not mean condoning unacceptable behavior, as in Case 19-7, but does mean being capable of understanding the patient's behavior from the patient's perspective. This may involve viewing unacceptable behavior as a cry for help or a misguided attempt at healing. It is important to acknowledge and articulate respect for patients' attempts at problem-solving, even if not successful.
- Enter as fully as possible into the patient's experience of suffering and personal meanings to see these as he does. Then, communicate your understanding to the patient. Empathy is the basis for therapeutic human relationships, and involves taking a perspective other than our own (Bellet & Maloney, 1991). Physical touch can communicate empathy as well. Once having taken the patient's perspective, it is important to let the patient know that you understand his perspective. Reflection ("You clearly were in

---

## SYMPTOMS AS SIGNALS

*Doctors never meet symptoms adjusted to suit their knowledge, [rather] they meet human beings who try through their symptom presentations to communicate signals from within their own bodies (Rudebeck, 1992).*

pain") and legitimation ("It is only natural to feel this way facing this situation") are techniques for communicating empathy (Bird & Cohen-Cole, 1990).

- Be sure to separate your needs from those of the patient. Conflict of interest can be financial, emotional, and logistical. Some emotional needs may not be within the physician's awareness. Because this is a thorny issue, there will be a detailed discussion of boundaries in the next section. When such conflicts do arise, organized self-reflection or a neutral third party can be helpful in resolving them.

- Act in such a way that the patient does not perceive you as a threat. An anxious or frightened patient will not be able to listen well or will not feel empowered to change. If a patient feels that she is being blamed for her illness or humiliated in the course of medical care (Lazare, 1987), she will be less likely to share information and participate in her care. By taking a nonjudgmental stance, you will help the patient trust you and help her participate in her care. Mrs. Burke and her family in Case 19-7 were well aware that she might be stigmatized for having a narcotics addiction; only when she and her family felt that Dr. Sanchez would treat her with respect were they able to disclose the extent of her problem.

- Inquire into and utilize the strengths in the patient's family and cultural background. Patients' families are intimately involved in the interpretation of symptoms, provision of medical care, and relationships between the identified patient and the healthcare system (Doherty & Baird, 1983; Epstein *et al.*, 1993; McDaniel *et al.*, 1990). In Case 19-7, Mrs. Burke's family proved invaluable in providing necessary information to understand the patient's problem, developing a therapeutic plan, monitoring her pain control, and driving to the pharmacy every 3 days so that she had lower potential for abusing narcotic medications. Even when the family is not present, inquiry into strengths and attributes of family members is often fruitful. Asking a patient to solicit the assistance of a family member who successfully quit smoking, for example, may reinforce a patient's efforts to quit. Similarly, culture influences significantly the way symptoms are presented to physicians, patients' expectations of care, and patients' explanatory models of illness (Kleinman *et al.*, 1978). These are crucial factors and will be discussed in more detail in Chapters 20 and 25.

- Demonstrate that you can work together in a partnership. Make explicit your wish to work on a problem together. Be clear about what you can and cannot do. Follow through with your promises. Don't make promises that you cannot deliver. Describe, and then demonstrate a relationship based on collaboration. With Mrs. Burke, it was critical for Dr. Sanchez to indicate that she would continue to care for her, but would not tolerate her unrestricted use of narcotics.

- Advocate for the patient in gaining access to healthcare services, social services, and justice. You can offer support ("I will be here with you no matter what happens," or "Mr. Z, the social worker, can help you with that problem; I will give him a call") that is realistic and perceived as helpful by the patient. Also, you can facilitate access to a variety of services that would otherwise be inaccessible to the patient.

- Communicate your own experience to the patient in a way that will be helpful and meaningful to her. Be aware of your own experiences, emotional reactions, and prejudices and their sources (Epstein, 1999; Mengel, 1987; Novack *et al.*, 1997; Weinberg & Mauksch, 1991). With Mrs. Burke, it was helpful to the patient and family to know that Dr. Sanchez had treated patients successfully who had similar difficulties. Judicious use of physician self-disclosure can sometimes be helpful to patients. Take care, however, that disclosure is for the benefit of the patient and not the physician.

## CASE 19-8

*Dr. Peter Blank lives next door to the Dwyer family. The Dwyers' 3-year-old daughter is ill with a temperature of 102°F, cough, and nasal congestion. It is Sunday of a 3-day holiday weekend. Mrs. Dwyer calls to see if Dr. Blank will take a look in her daughter's ears to make sure that she does not have an infection. Dr. Blank is not their usual physician; however, as a family physician, he would be competent to diagnose and treat an ear infection. He is not on call, but does have an otoscope at home. He feels somewhat uncomfortable about this because he does not know the child's prior medical history nor would he be able to follow up, but he examines the child, makes a diagnosis of otitis media, and prescribes an antibiotic. He suggests follow-up with the child's family physician.*

## OTITIS MEDIA

*Otitis media is an infection of the middle ear, usually in children, that typically presents with symptoms of fever, ear pain, and loss of hearing; very young children will often only present with fever. A diagnosis is made by looking at the tympanic membrane with an otoscope to see if the membrane is red and bulging due to infected fluid in the middle ear pushing out the tympanic membrane into the ear canal. Usually the infection is caused by one of three bacteria:* Streptococcus pneumoniae, Haemophilus influenzae, *and* Moraxella catarrhalis.*

*Antibiotics are usually used for treatment, although some studies suggest that most children with otitis media will undergo symptom resolution in 1 to 7 days even without antibiotics. A recent guideline published by the Agency for Healthcare Research and Quality* (http://www.ahrq.gov/clinic/otitisum.htm) *suggests that treatment will speed resolution. Most authorities feel that 5 days of antibiotics is sufficient, although some feel that in children under 2 a full 10-day course is necessary.*

*Like most diagnoses relying on clinician observation, otitis media is a difficult diagnosis to make with confidence. A squirming, crying child will often have a red tympanic membrane from agitation alone and many parents will not leave the physician's office satisfied unless they bear a prescription for an antibiotic. While many authorities recommend insufflating the ear canal through the otoscope, judging tympanic membrane motion in a squirming child is difficult. Thus, even among experienced clinicians, the diagnosis of acute otitis media is often fraught with uncertainty and ambiguity, particularly in children.*

## BOUNDARIES OF THE PATIENT–PHYSICIAN RELATIONSHIP

Although diverse, in order to meet complex human needs, the patient–physician relationship is governed by explicit legal regulations, ethical principles, and complex social conventions. The boundaries of the patient–physician relationship protect both physician and patient (Linklater & MacDougall, 1993) so that they can maintain a professional helping relationship that meets the patient's needs. Boundaries define expected and accepted physical, social, and emotional interactions between physicians and patients.

Some examples of blatant boundary violations by physicians include sexual misconduct, abuse of confidential disclosures, inappropriate disclosure of personal information, accepting expensive gifts, and seeing patients for medical problems at unusual times and places (Gabbard & Nadelson, 1995). Such violations are common. For example, in a variety of settings, 3–12% of male physicians report having had sexual relations with a patient (Gabbard & Nadelson, 1995). Usually, boundary violations such as these involve misuse of the physician's power, place the physician's interest ahead of the patient's, put patients in a double bind where clinical care depends on continued violations, and involve secrecy (Linklater & MacDougall, 1993).

Patients can also test and violate boundaries. Requesting frequent or "special" appointments, wearing seductive clothing, giving large gifts, sexually harassing the physician (Phillips & Schneider, 1993), being dishonest, and exhibiting threatening or demanding behaviors can all test the integrity of the patient–physician relationship. Family members can test boundaries by requesting access to confidential information about a patient, and third parties can demand information about a patient as a condition of providing benefits.

There are more subtle boundary issues that physicians face on a daily basis. Despite the complexities raised when physicians treat or offer medical advice to family members or friends, as in Case 19-8 (Epstein, 1994; La Puma *et al.*, 1991), sometimes it is unavoidable, such as in the case of physicians in rural areas, or desirable, such as when the physician is the most qualified person to treat the problem. Often physicians seek colleagues whom they know professionally or personally for their own healthcare. The most conservative approach is to avoid such "dual relationships"; however, in certain situations, they can work well if approached with caution. A patient may feel comfortable approaching a physician-friend (or relative) about routine problems, but would not feel comfortable talking about a sexually transmitted disease, diagnosis of terminal illness, or psychiatric problems. Usually, it is best to discuss with the patient-friend how to deal with such situations before they occur. The physician must first reflect on whether she would be able to probe the patient's intimate history, bear bad news, be objective enough to give appropriate care, and recruit the patient-friend's cooperation with care plans. The same questions also should be directed toward the patient. If the friendship is unable to support a therapeutic relationship, then parts or all of the care of the patient should be transferred to another physician (Rourke *et al.*, 1993).

Some rituals help to protect the sanctity of the patient–physician relationship. Physicians use more formal speech and less small talk than used in typical social conversation. They also use professional attire and the office setting to set therapeutic encounters apart from other social interactions. This context often helps the patient feel safe enough to trust the physician with personal and intimate information. Deviations from established personal practice norms require self-reflection. Even though a patient might offer to come to a physician's home for treatment rather than the physician making a home visit, this is rarely acceptable. Medical consultations should not take place in the supermarket, if physician and patient happen to meet there.

## CASE 19-9

*Dr. Reuben Marks was caring for Carol Wang, a 71-year-old retired librarian who had multiple medical complaints. Typically, the patient would come into the office having recently seen a television program or read a newspaper article about a new technology or screening procedure. Despite Dr. Marks's explanations that the procedure was not appropriate or necessary, the patient would appear dissatisfied. Sometimes she would seek another physician who would be willing to perform the procedure. Dr. Marks found himself dreading Mrs. Wang's visits, and would feel very frustrated and angry at the end of them.*

*At one point, Dr. Marks realized that he had never ordered a screening colonoscopy, even though he knew Mrs. Wang had two first-degree relatives who died of colon cancer. This realization was startling to Dr. Marks, who otherwise was a careful and thoughtful physician. On reflection, he realized that, in many ways, Mrs. Wang's behavior reminded him of his grandmother, who played a prominent part in his childhood. She was never satisfied with anything that he did, was relentlessly demanding, and belittled his accomplishments. Dr. Marks's response was to avoid contact with his grandmother; he recognized this same pattern of behavior with Mrs. Wang. Having realized that connection, Dr. Marks found it easier to understand his own anger and could become more patient with and attentive to Mrs. Wang's needs, while providing appropriate medical care.*

## DIFFICULT RELATIONSHIPS

Medical care is emotionally demanding and intense for physicians, patients, and their families. Physicians have a responsibility to care for all patients, regardless of race, sex, personality, and personal values. Physicians face their own limitations when caring for patients with incurable illnesses, ambiguous or vague symptoms, or unsolvable social problems. Environmental barriers, disabilities, cognitive impairment, language barriers, and cultural factors make some relationships intrinsically more difficult (Klein *et al.*, 1982). Also, the stress of illness may bring out more "primitive" or maladaptive aspects of a patient's personality in an attempt to deal with unfamiliar and overwhelming situations. This may result in the patient acting in a hostile or abrasive manner, becoming passive and dependent, appearing manipulative, presenting symptoms in a dramatic way, or avoiding medical care (Groves, 1978). Some patients are dishonest and falsify prescriptions for controlled substances, lie about their drug use, and feign injury to claim disability payments.

When there are difficulties in a patient–physician relationship, most often, it is a combination of factors contribute to the difficulty. Some of these are listed in Table 19.5.

**Table 19.5**
Difficult Patient–Physician Relationships

Characteristics of difficult situations
Problems perceived as unsolvable
   Incurable diseases
   Ambiguous, vague symptoms
   Terminal illness
Conditions for which patient is perceived as culpable
Physician feeling helpless or inadequate
Patient behavior that threatens physician authority
Violation of physician's personal norms
Perception of personal risk to physician (e.g., contagion of HIV)
Specific diagnoses
   Psychopathology—moderate to severe
   Substance abuse
   Obesity
   Chronic pain
   Sexual behavior-related conditions—patient perceived as culpable
   Hypochondriasis
   "Symptom amplification"
Personality characteristics and behaviors of patients that may predispose to difficulties
   Expression of anger, hostility, or frustration
   Addiction to or seeking of drugs
   Not following physician's advice
   Expression of seemingly endless needs (overdependency)
   Expression of entitlement for special attention
   Attempts to manipulate the physician
   Rejection of help while continuing to complain of symptoms
   Self-destructive behavior
Personality characteristics of physicians that may predispose to difficulties
   Enjoyment of problem-solving and sense of closure
   Satisfaction in being able to help
   Belief in self-sacrifice, stoicism, and hard work
   Belief that science can solve human suffering
   Aversion to risk
   Expectation that patients will share these values

Just as strong patient–physician relationships have the potential to enhance outcomes, difficulties can lead to patient and physician dissatisfaction because of uncommunicated needs, unmet expectations, and failure of the physician to respond empathically to the patient's suffering (Schwenk & Romano, 1992). There is also a strong relationship between communication failure, increased healthcare utilization (Lin *et al.*, 1991), and more requests for specialty consultation. Breakdown of the patient–physician relationship was identified as a reason for malpractice litigation in 71% of depositions reviewed in a study by Beckman and colleagues (Beckman *et al.*, 1994); specific issues identified by the plaintiffs included being abandoned by the physician, failing to acknowledge the patient's or family's concerns, delivering information poorly, and failing to understand the patient's or family's perspective.

Case 19-9 illustrates some of the effects that a physician's prior experiences can have on his behavior that was outside of his moment-to-moment awareness. Dr. Marks found Mrs. Wang annoying, without quite knowing why, and these feelings affected the quality of care that Mrs. Wang received. In other situations, physician and patient may have difficulty reaching agreement on treatment, physicians can make mistakes (Dimsdale, 1984), or a patient may not take medication as prescribed, without knowing why. Part of understanding these difficulties lies in understanding the concepts of transference, countertransference, and projection.

Transference refers to the unconscious reactions that patients have to physicians who, in some way, remind them of another important person in their past (usually a close family member). Countertransference is the corresponding phenomenon in physicians; as much as physicians may want to consider their relationships with patients "professional," the intimate nature of medical care makes it common for some patients to provoke powerful positive or negative emotions in physicians as in Case 19-9. Projection refers to assigning one's own unconscious or conscious feelings or beliefs to another person, often in emotionally charged situations. Case 19-1 is a good example of a situation wherein projection might occur; the physician expected that the patient would become more anxious and afraid based on the meaning that he assigned to the illness. Sometimes transference/countertransference and family-of-origin issues can impair a physician's ability to provide optimal medical care (Epstein, 1999; Mengel, 1987).

Mindfulness, on the other hand, is a moment-to-moment awareness of one's own thoughts, emotions, and actions that permits the clinician to observe and "be with" the patient without being judgmental (Epstein, 1999). Mindfulness allows the physician also to distinguish the patient's thoughts and feelings from her own. If the physician can become aware of and utilize her own background, experiences, feelings, and values, she can be more effective in helping patients through difficult times and can reinforce rather than erode therapeutic relationships (Epstein *et al.*, 1993; McDaniel & Landau-Stanton, 1991; Novack *et al.*, 1997).

While physicians are a diverse population, there are some common personality characteristics among physicians that can contribute to difficulties in the patient–physician relationship and that may be connected to their choice of career. Physicians describe themselves, and are described, as being hard-working, self-sacrificing, and averse to taking risks (Gerber, 1985; Schwenk *et al.*, 1989). Physicians generally like to solve problems, like a sense of closure, and like to help. Further, physicians expect that their patients will share these values. It is inevitable that some patients may have behaviors or belief systems that violate physicians' personal norms. Consider the physician from a conservative religious and cultural background caring for a patient who acquired AIDS through male prostitution, the patient who arrives late for appointments to a physician who values punctuality, and a patient who continues to abuse drugs seeing a physician who values self-control. Other common situations that physicians find frustrating are listed in Table 19.5.

Difficulties in the patient–physician relationship can also involve family members, friends, social contacts, and social agencies. For example, a patient may come into the office reluctantly on the insistence of a spouse, or a patient may become angry because his HMO has denied payment to a psychotherapist whom he has been seeing for a year. A patient may want validation for his symptoms to receive attention and care from family members. Even if the other person or agency is not physically present in the office, the influence is clearly felt. Particularly challenging is when triangulation (McDaniel *et al.*, 1989) occurs. In these situations, the physician is invited to take sides in a two-way dispute, often between family members. Consider a situation where the spouse of a diabetic woman reports to a physician that the patient is not as careful with her diet as she reports. On the surface, this may seem like useful information, until the physician looks at the dynamics of the relationship further. The diabetic woman has been criticized by her spouse at home. She insists that she is doing a good enough job of managing her diabetes; she wants the physician to validate this. The spouse wants the physician to make the patient more careful with her diet. Consider what would happen if the physician took either partner's side in the dispute. If the physician were to criticize the patient for her noncompliance, the physician might imperil the relationship with the patient and unknowingly discourage the patient from returning. On the other hand, excluding the spouse from the discussion might escalate his unhelpful criticism at home. In either case, the physician would create a dysfunctional compensatory alliance (Hahn *et al.*, 1988).

When difficulties arise, it is even more important to attend to the principles of mindfulness and relationship-building listed in the previous section. Anxiety tends to make difficult situations more difficult. It is therefore important for the physician to put himself at ease, to attend to his own feelings, and to inquire, in an open-ended way, into the sources of the patient's frustrations. Recognition that there is a problem is usually helpful, along with an offer of help (e.g., "It seems that I haven't addressed all of your concerns. Could you tell me how I could help?"). It is helpful to explore the meaning of the illness with the patient in a nonjudgmental way, letting the patient know that his needs have been understood and legitimizing the patient's concerns no matter how trivial they may seem to you. Communicating clearly what you can and cannot do for the patient avoids the problem of promising what cannot be delivered. When the patient's demands are excessive, the physician can set clear boundaries and be consistent. When a patient has been dishonest, a written behavioral contract is helpful (Quill, 1983). The contract should list specific unacceptable behaviors in observable terms. It should also be spelled out that violations of the contract would initiate a series of measures that might result in termination of the relationship. When problems seem mysterious, expanding the focus of the inquiry, and including relevant family members and important social contacts can help. In family meetings, everyone's perspective should be articulated and heard; even though the physician may agree more with some perspectives than others, he or she must avoid the temptation to take sides. Often, the physician's job is to facilitate the resolution of conflict by the family, not to provide a solution. Most importantly, physicians should recognize their own needs. Not every patient will appreciate the physician's hard work, but a colleague might. For practicing physicians, calling on medical consultants and psychotherapists can be very helpful in providing reassurance and support (Epstein, 1995). Similarly, medical students should be encouraged to make use of mentors, peers, and faculty to discuss cases that are emotionally difficult, and to explore the reasons why. Support groups are another means of dealing with difficult situations, and are increasingly used in medical training (Quill & Williamson, 1990).

Sometimes differences between physicians and patients are irreconcilable. Patients may expect that the physician will be available at all times, prescribe desired medications, order desired laboratory tests, validate disability, or spend exceptional amounts of time in caring for the patient. Often these differences can be negotiated after respectful inquiry and principled discussion about the disagreement. The next step is to inform the patient clearly of the reasons for not complying with her request(s), along with a willingness to work together despite the disagreement (Quill, 1989). When the conflict escalates, and when the issues affect clinical care of the patient, the physician should relinquish care of the patient rather than capitulate to the patient's demands for inappropriate care.

Secrets deserve special mention (Karpel & Strauss, 1983; Newman, 1993). There is a difference between information that is private and information that is secret. Private information has little or no power to harm third parties, and requires little psychological energy to sustain. Secrets, on the other hand, have the potential to be destructive to the patient or to others if disclosed or if not disclosed. It can be especially destructive if the physician is asked to compromise his integrity in order to keep a secret. Bearing private information is part of the burden and privilege of being a physician. Some confidential information must be disclosed if the physician feels that a life is in danger. Suicidal and homicidal intent, child abuse, and elder abuse require prompt evaluation, even if promises of confidentiality have been made. There are many other situations, where there is not universal agreement among the involved parties, when the physician must reflect on his own values and communicate them unambiguously to the patient. Consultation with a trusted colleague can be invaluable in untangling some of these difficult situations. These issues are discussed further in Chapter 26.

## CONCLUSION

The patient–physician relationship is a complex professional relationship with the goals of relieving suffering, promoting healing, and preventing illness. It is a personal relationship and a social contract that needs to be flexible enough to accommodate to a wide variety of situations, but well defined enough to maintain the primacy of the patient's interest.

The philosophical basis for the patient–physician relationship evolved considerably during the twentieth century from a predominantly paternalistic model to models that promote patient autonomy. It is critical, though, that the emphasis on patient autonomy not relieve physicians of the obligation to make therapeutic recommendations and to foster behavior modifications in patients who may be reluctant to change. Physicians' wise use of their intimate connections with patients and their socially given power can make them strong advocates for patient well-being.

Earning trust, nonabandonment, continuity, being empathic, and taking a nonjudgmental stance are critical to the development and maintenance of a strong patient–physician relationship. Families and culture have a powerful influence on patient well-being and patient–physician relationships; it is essential to take a family and social perspective on all illness episodes, regardless of whether family members are actually present at the visit.

No aspect of human suffering is excluded from the physician's office. It is a burden and a privilege to bear witness to patients' suffering and to intervene on patients' behalf. Physicians can have a profound impact on a patient's life when they are willing to listen respectfully and courageous enough to accompany her in her suffering. Each patient has a personal language through which she expresses her distress; the task of a physician will be to help the patient interpret her symptoms, to find meaning, and to establish a common purpose. Just as there is a distinction between illness and disease, there is a distinction between curing, caring, and healing. Curing can sometimes be a purely technical matter. Caring involves developing a personal bond with a patient. The physician can only become a healer when the patient knows that her suffering has been understood.

## CASES FOR DISCUSSION

### CASE 1

*Veronica Jones was a 37-year-old woman with advanced AIDS on renal dialysis for HIV-related kidney failure. She was admitted to hospital with respiratory failure and was put on a ventilator in the intensive care unit. Her prognosis was very poor. Dr. John Graham, with whom she had a strong relationship, was out of town; his mother had died suddenly of a stroke. Despite many attempts to discuss end-of-life issues, she would change the topic and make statements that she would later retract. She believed that her family did not know that she had AIDS.*

*Dr. Tom Rubin was covering for Dr. Graham and knew the patient and her family from a prior hospitalization. Ms. Jones was lethargic and confused. At times she would become more lucid. On one occasion, while on the ventilator, she expressed a wish to die and be disconnected from the ventilator. Dr. Rubin contacted her niece, who was the patient's healthcare proxy listed on an advance directive. However, she could not make decisions on the patient's behalf unless she knew the patient's diagnosis and prognosis.*

*During a time when Ms. Jones was more lucid, Dr. Rubin strongly advocated that he be permitted to disclose the diagnosis to Ms. Jones's niece, so that she could help make decisions on the patient's behalf. She gave permission; the niece indicated that she was already aware of the AIDS diagnosis, as was most of the family.*

*Despite the patient's wishes, the niece refused to consider a do-not-resuscitate order. To everyone's surprise, Ms. Jones came off the ventilator and became more lucid. Later in the hospitalization, the patient learned that the niece had been stealing money from her bank account. Dr. Rubin convened a family meeting, to discuss end-of-life care. The discussion provoked heated family conflict, and no resolution was reached.*

*Dr. Graham returned to town. It was clear to him, and all physicians involved, that the patient, although improved, would likely die in the next few weeks. She required morphine for pain, and she was intermittently sedated and lucid. Ms. Jones asked to go home, but home services could not be arranged because no family member would be available to take 24-hour responsibility for her. During a dialysis session, she asked that the dialysis be stopped. She refused dialysis the next day, consented the following day, but again stopped halfway through the treatment. Dr. Graham asked her if she would like another dialysis treatment, and Ms. Jones replied, "I've had enough." She would not answer whether she would want to be resuscitated in case of now imminent cardiac arrest. Dr. Graham made a decision that resuscitation would be futile, and wrote a DNAR order. The patient remained comfortable on morphine and died quietly 2 days later.*

1. *What were the physician's responsibilities in this situation?*
2. *Using your knowledge of models of patient–physician relationships, what approaches were used? Which would you have used in this situation?*
3. *Who should have responsibility for making decisions about the do-not-resuscitate order for this patient?*
4. *What is the physician's role in facing family conflict of this magnitude?*

### CASE 2

*Joanne Williams is a mentally retarded 48-year-old woman who lives alone in an apartment complex for people with disabilities. She comes to the office frequently for a variety of medical concerns. Many of these concerns are chronic, such as back pain that does not interfere with her activity, or self-limited, such as colds. It is very difficult to keep office visits to their allotted time—the patient continues to ask for more time, and always has additional concerns. Each time that she needs a medication refill for her antiseizure medications, she calls at least three times within an afternoon to make sure that it has been called into the pharmacy. She is on the phone to the office daily with a variety of concerns. She has written many letters to her physician, Dr. Beverly Price, describing how difficult her life has been and how lonely she feels. The patient is on an insurance plan that provides Dr. Price with minimal reimbursement. Dr. Price feels burdened by the patient's unrelenting needs.*

1. *What is the responsibility of the physician in this situation?*
2. *What are the boundaries to this relationship?*
3. *How can the physician care for this patient without becoming overwhelmed?*
4. *What feelings would you have caring for this patient? How would you approach this relationship?*

## CASE 3

*Mr. Ray Kapsberger is a patient whom Dr. Glenda Lee has seen for many visits for right ankle pain. He fractured his ankle several years ago while intoxicated and recalls nothing of the event. Since then, he has reinjured his ankle on several occasions, mostly while intoxicated. He has a long history of alcoholism, and has been in many alcohol rehabilitation programs, with only a few weeks of abstinence at a time. Mr. Kapsberger frequently comes in complaining of ankle pain. Dr. Lee has referred him to a surgeon who recommended an ankle fusion operation. This is complex surgery that requires a long rehabilitation including physical therapy for 3–4 months following the procedure. The surgeon refuses to operate unless the patient is sober for at least 3 months, as reinjury would be very dangerous during the recuperation period. Also, Dr. Lee is reluctant to prescribe the patient with narcotic pain relievers, given his heavy intermittent binge drinking. The pain pills take the edge off the pain, but don't get rid of it completely. Mr. Kapsberger is angry. He has several demands: that he be referred to a surgeon who will do the operation regardless, that Dr. Lee fill out a form indicating that he is unable to work, and that he get some narcotics for pain.*

1. *How should Dr. Lee deal with Mr. Kapsberger's demands?*
2. *What can Dr. Lee do to create a more satisfactory patient–physician relationship?*
3. *How can Dr. Lee help the patient to become more active in his care?*
4. *How would you feel taking care of this patient?*

## CASE 4

*Charles Johnson is a 78-year-old man, a retired professor of psychology. For several weeks he had not been feeling well, with decreased appetite and some mild upper abdominal pain. After several visits to Dr. Sam Green, he had a CT scan and found out that he has unresectable metastatic pancreatic cancer. Since the diagnosis 3 weeks ago, he has consulted a medical oncologist, a surgeon, and a radiologist for the consideration of palliative procedures, including surgery, percutaneous insertion of a stent, and radiation. None of these are possible, as there is too much tumor surrounding the bile ducts. Mr. Johnson was given a prognosis of 4 to 8 weeks at the time of diagnosis. It has now been 4 weeks. He has been getting weaker by the day. He has some upper abdominal pain but does not like to complain about it, especially to his daughter Denise, whom he views as overconcerned and very intrusive. He would like to spend his last days at home in peace and quiet without many visitors. He approaches death with grace but still harbors some fears about what the end will be like, especially as the tumor spreads. Mr. Johnson's wife, Sarah, has been extremely involved and supportive during this time. She has made many calls to the children to update them on his condition, and has passed along his instructions to have them not come to visit.*

*Because Mr. Johnson previously had been healthy, he has seen Dr. Green rarely until recently. Mr. Johnson is aware that some physicians have prescribed medications for terminally ill patients who wish to end their lives with dignity. While his wife is out one day, Mr. Johnson calls Dr. Green to ask him if he would be willing to prescribe some medicine to end his life before things become intolerable.*

1. *How would you approach this patient's request?*
2. *What models of the patient–physician relationship would be appropriate?*
3. *What are your own feelings about assisted suicide?*
4. *How would those feelings affect your care of Mr. Johnson?*
5. *Would you involve Mr. Johnson's family? How?*

## CASE 5

*Frank Roth is a 75-year-old retired schoolteacher in generally good health. Many of his close friends have died, and his two brothers are chronically ill and live far away. He comes into the office to see Dr. Beth Green frequently for concerns that seemed minor to Dr. Green. Once, Mr. Roth had a blood pressure check at a shopping mall screening program; his pressure was 142/88, and he made an appointment to discuss this further. He would call several times a week with mild respiratory symptoms, muscle aches, and other concerns; he would take a long time to describe his symptoms in great detail. He would be easily reassured, and he did not seem to have hypochondriacal preoccupations. The frequent contacts with the office were a social outlet for a patient who led a very lonely life. The patient was not otherwise depressed.*

1. *How would you approach caring for this patient?*
2. *What goals would you have for his care?*
3. *How would you feel about not being able to meet all of Mr. Roth's needs?*
4. *How could you still remain patient-centered but set appropriate limits?*

## CASE 6

*Muriel Bristol is a 46-year-old woman who has visited Dr. Reginald Bruce occasionally for seasonal allergies and irritable bowel syndrome. Among other concerns at her annual physical examination, she indicated that she would like a series of laboratory tests to check micronutrient levels, immune function, viral titers, and allergy to a wide variety of substances. Although she had generally felt well, she had been advised by an alternative health practitioner that she may have chronic candida syndrome. She presented the physician with articles from the lay press suggesting that a wide variety of symptoms may result from candida, and that intensive nutritional and pharmacologic treatment should be used to eradicate it. Dr. Bruce offered to discuss the patient's concerns, while explaining that these tests are very expensive, often inconclusive, and would likely yield no benefit. Ms. Bristol insisted on testing and accused the physician of being too narrow-minded.*

1. *Would you be able to care for this patient?*
2. *How would you maintain a relationship with her given her demands?*
3. *At what point would you refer her to another physician?*
4. *What would you do if you did not know a physician who shared her health beliefs?*

## CASE 7

*On a routine physical examination visit, Dr. Carla Long asked Mr. Tom Garcia about sexual risk behaviors for HIV infection. After an uncomfortable silence, Mr. Garcia reported that, while on business trips, he would occasionally have sexual encounters with men. Often he would meet the men at a bar or health club, and have sex afterwards. None of these encounters has resulted in a long-term relationship. He reported always using condoms for oral sex; he does not engage in anal sex. Mr. Garcia is married and has three teenage children. He reports that his marriage has been generally good, and feels that disclosure of his bisexuality to his wife would be devastating. The results of an HIV test a year ago at the county health department were negative. His wife has not been tested, as far as Dr. Long knows. His wife is also a patient of Dr. Long. Dr. Long felt uncomfortable harboring this secret from the patient's wife, even though her risk for HIV is very low. On the other hand, she would not tell the patient's wife without Mr. Garcia's permission. Dr. Long found this situation very troubling also because of her own religious beliefs: As a fundamentalist Christian, she believed that homosexuality was an abomination and that Mr. Garcia should abandon his current sexual practices.*

1. *Should Dr. Long care for Mr. Garcia?*
2. *What principles should she use in approaching his care?*
3. *How would you advise her to deal with her own feelings about Mr. Garcia's sexual orientation and behaviors?*
4. *How should Dr. Long handle the secret that Mr. Garcia is keeping from his wife?*

**Acknowledgments.** I have learned the most about patient–physician relationships from my patients, to whom I am greatly indebted. Drs. Cecile Carson, Dan Duffy, George Engel, Leston Havens, Ian McWhinney, Susan McDaniel, Tim Quill, Peter Reich, and Charles Solky provided guidance and inspiration at critical points. My children, Eli and Malka, taught me how to listen with both ears.

# RECOMMENDED READINGS

Cassell EJ: The nature of suffering and the goals of medicine. *N Engl J Med* 306:639–645, 1982.

> This is an eloquent exposition of the need for physicians to understand the totality of patients' experiences and to communicate empathy. It provides guidelines on a clinical approach based on understanding the patient as person.

Emanuel EJ, Emanuel LL: Four models of the physician-patient relationship. *JAMA* 267:2221–2226, 1992; May WF: Code, covenant, contract, or philanthropy? *Hastings Cent Rep* 5:29–38, 1975; Szasz TS, Hollender MH: The basic models of the doctor–patient relationship. *Arch Intern Med* 97:585–592, 1956.

> These three articles are all excellent descriptions of models of the patient–physician relationship. Each takes a different perspective on patient autonomy and the role of the physician.

Epstein RM: Mindful practice. *JAMA* 282: 833–839, 1999.

> In this article, I propose a model for self-awareness, reflection, and presence that informs technical, interpersonal, and cognitive aspects of medical care.

Stewart M, Brown JB, Weston WW, McWhinney IR, McWilliam CL, Freeman TR: *Patient-Centered Medicine: Transforming the Clinical Method.* Thousand Oaks, Calif, Sage Publications Inc, 1995.

> This book examines the practice of medicine, from theoretical models to the provision of care, from a patient-centered perspective that takes the patient's experience of illness on equal ground with the physician's diagnostic perspective.

# REFERENCES

Anonymous: December 1, 1994—World AIDS Day. *JAMA* 272:1568, 1994.

Baird MA, Doherty WJ: Risks and benefits of a family systems approach to medical care. *Fam Med* 22:396–403, 1990.

Balint M: *The Doctor, His Patient, and the Illness.* New York, International Universities Press Inc, 1957.

Bass MJ, Buck C, Turner L: Predictors of outcome in headache patients presenting to family physicians—A one year prospective study. *Headache* 26:285–294, 1986a.

Bass MJ, Buck C, Turner L: The physician's actions and the outcome of illness. *J Fam Pract* 23:43–47, 1986b.

Beckman HB, Markakis KM, Suchman AL, Frankel RM: The doctor–patient relationship and malpractice. Lessons from plaintiff depositions. *Arch Intern Med* 154:1365–1370, 1994.

Beecher HK: *Measurement of Subjective Responses.* New York, Oxford University Press, 1959.

Bellet PS, Maloney MJ: The importance of empathy as an interviewing skill in medicine. *JAMA* 266:1831–1832, 1991.

Bird J, Cohen-Cole SA: The three function model of the medical interview: An educational device, in Hale MS (ed): *Methods in Teaching Consultation-Liaison Psychiatry.* Basel, Karger, 1990, pp 65–88.

Branch WT, Suchman A: Meaningful experiences in medicine. *Am J Med* 88:56–59, 1990.

Brody H: *The Healer's Power.* New Haven, Yale University Press, 1992.

Brown J, Stewart M, McCracken EC: The patient centered clinical method. II. Definition and application. *Fam Pract* 3(2):75–79, 1986.

Cassell EJ: The nature of suffering and the goals of medicine. *N Engl J Med* 306:639–645, 1982.

Dimsdale JE: Delays and slips in medical diagnosis. *Perspect Biol Med* 27:213–220, 1984.

Doherty WA, Campbell TL: *Families and Health.* Beverly Hills, Calif, Sage Press, 1988.

Doherty WJ, Baird MA: *Family Therapy and Family Medicine: Toward the Primary Care of Families.* New York, Guilford Press, 1983.

Emanuel EJ, Dubler NN: Preserving the physician–patient relationship in the era of managed care. *JAMA* 273:323–335, 1995.

Emanuel EJ, Emanuel LL: Four models of the physician–patient relationship. *JAMA* 267:2221–2226, 1992.

Engel GL: The need for a new medical model: A challenge for biomedicine. *Science* 196:129–136, 1977.

Engel GL: The clinical application of the biopsychosocial model. *Am J Psychiatry* 137:535–544, 1980.

Epstein R: Taking care of. *Arch Fam Med* 3:9–10, 1994.

Epstein RM: Communication between primary care physicians and consultants [see comments]. *Arch Fam Med* 4:403–409, 1995.

Epstein RM: Mindful practice. *JAMA* 282:833–839, 1999.

Epstein RM, Campbell TL, Cohen-Cole SA, McWhinney IR, Smilkstein G: Perspectives on patient–doctor communication. *J Fam Pract* 37:377–388, 1993.

Franks P, Culpepper L, Dickinson J: Psychosocial bias in the diagnosis of obesity. *J Fam Pract* 14:745–750, 1982.

Gabbard GO, Nadelson, C: Professional boundaries in the physician–patient relationship. *JAMA* 273:1445–1449, 1995.

Gerber LA: Career and family dilemmas in doctor's lives. *Fam Med* 17:109–112, 1985.

Good BJ, Good MD: The meaning of symptoms: A cultural hermeneutic model for clinical practice, in Eisenberg L, Kleinman A (eds): *The Relevance of Social Science for Medicine.* Dordrecht, Reidel, 1981, pp 165–196.

Greenfield S, Kaplan S, Ware JE Jr: Expanding patient involvement in care. Effects on patient outcomes. *Ann Intern Med* 102:520–528, 1985.

Greenfield S, Kaplan SH, Ware JE, Jr, Yano EM, Frank HJ: Patients' participation in medical care: Effects on blood sugar control and quality of life in diabetes. *J Gen Intern Med* 3:448–457, 1988.

Groves JE: Taking care of the hateful patient. *N Engl J Med* 298:883–887, 1978.

Hahn SR, Feiner JS, Bellin EH: The doctor–patient–family relationship: A compensatory alliance. *Ann Intern Med* 109(1):884–889, 1988.

Havens L: *Making Contact*. Cambridge, Mass, Harvard University Press, 1986.

Kaplan SH, Greenfield S, Ware JE Jr: Assessing the effects of physician–patient interactions on the outcomes of chronic disease [published erratum appears in *Med Care* 27(7):679, 1989]. *Med Care* 27:S110–S127, 1989.

Karpel MA, Strauss ES: Family secrets, in Karpel MA, Strauss ES (eds): *Family Evaluation*. New York, Gardner Press, 1983, pp 245–263.

Katon W, Kleinman A: Doctor–patient negotiation and other social science strategies in patient care, in Eisenberg L, Kleinman A (eds): *The Relevance of Social Science for Medicine*. Dordrecht, Reidel, 1981, pp 253–279.

Klein D, Najman J, Kohrman AF, Munro C: Patient characteristics that elicit negative responses from family physicians. *J Fam Pract* 14:881–888, 1982.

Kleinman A: The cultural meanings and social uses of illness. *J Fam Pract* 16:539–545, 1983.

Kleinman AM: *The Illness Narratives: Suffering, Healing, and the Human Condition*. New York, Basic Books Inc, 1987.

Kleinman A, Eisenberg L, Good B: Culture, illness, and care: Clinical lessons from anthropologic and cross-cultural research. *Ann Intern Med* 88:251–258, 1978.

La Puma J, Stocking CB, La Voie D, Darling CA: When physicians treat members of their own families. Practices in a community hospital. *N Engl J Med* 325:1290–1294, 1991.

Lazare A: Shame and humiliation in the medical encounter. *Arch Intern Med* 147:1653–1658, 1987.

Lazare A, Eisenthal S, Wasserman L: The customer approach to patienthood. Attending to patient requests in a walk-in clinic. *Arch Gen Psychiatry* 32:553–558, 1975.

Levenstein JH, McCracken EC, McWhinney IR: The patient centered clinical method I. A model for the doctor patient interaction in family medicine. *Fam Pract* 1:24–30, 1986.

Lin EH, Katon W, Von Korff M, Bush T, Lipscomb P, Russo J, Wagner E: Frustrating patients: Physician and patient perspectives among distressed high users of medical services. *J Gen Intern Med* 6:241–246, 1991.

Linklater D, MacDougall S: Boundary issues. What do they mean for family physicians? *Can Fam Physician* 39:2569–2573, 1993.

May WF: Code, covenant, contract, or philanthropy? *Hastings Cent Rep* 5:29–38, 1975.

McDaniel SH, Landau-Stanton J: Family-of-origin work and family therapy skills training: Both-and. *Fam Process* 30:459–471, 1991.

McDaniel SH, Campbell TL, Seaburn D: Managing personal and professional boundaries: How to make the physician's own issues a resource in patient care. *Fam Syst Med* 7:1–12, 1989.

McDaniel SH, Campbell TL, Seaburn DB: *Family-Oriented Primary Care: A Manual for Medical Providers*. Berlin, Springer-Verlag, 1990.

McKinstry B: Paternalism and the doctor–patient relationship in general practice. *Br J Gen Pract* 42:340–342, 1992.

McWhinney IR: Illness, suffering, and healing, in McWhinney IR (ed*): A Textbook of Family Medicine*. London, Oxford University Press, 1989a, pp 73–86.

McWhinney IR: 'An acquaintance with particulars …'. *Fam Med* 21:296–298, 1989b.

Mengel M: Physician ineffectiveness due to family of origin issues. *Fam Syst Med* 5(2):176–190, 1987.

Naumberg E, Franks P, Bell B, Gold M, Engerman J: Racial differentials in the identification of hypercholesterolemia. *J Fam Pract* 36:425–430, 1993.

Neighbour R: Paternalism or autonomy? *Practitioner* 236:860–864, 1992.

Newman NK: Family secrets: A challenge for family physicians. *J Fam Pract* 36:494–496, 1993.

Novack DH: Therapeutic aspects of the clinical encounter. *J Gen Intern Med* 2:346–354, 1987.

Novack DH, Suchman AL, Clark W, Epstein RM, Najberg E, Kaplan C: Calibrating the physician: Personal awareness and effective patient care. *JAMA* 278:502–509, 1997.

Novack DH, Epstein RM, Paulsen RH: Toward creating physician-healers: Fostering medical students' self-awareness, personal growth, and well-being. *Acad Med* 74:516–520, 1999.

O'Rourke K: Trust and the patient–physician relationship. *Am J Kidney Dis* 21:684–685, 1993.

Peabody FW: Landmark article March 19, 1927: The care of the patient. By Francis W. Peabody. *JAMA* 252:813–818, 1984.

Pellegrino ED: Is truth telling to the patient a cultural artifact? *JAMA* 268:1734–1735, 1992.

Phillips SP, Schneider MS: Sexual harassment of female doctors by patients. *N Engl J Med* 329:1936–1939, 1993.

Quill TE: Partnerships in patient care: A contractual approach. *Ann Intern Med* 98:228–234, 1983.

Quill TE: Recognizing and adjusting to barriers in doctor–patient communication. *Ann Intern Med* 111:51–57, 1989.

Quill TE, Cassel CK: Nonabandonment: A central obligation for physicians. *Ann Intern Med* 122:368–374, 1995.

Quill TE, Williamson PR: Healthy approaches to physician stress. *Arch Intern Med* 150:1857–1861, 1990.

Rogers CR: The characteristics of a helping relationship, in Rogers CR (ed): *On Becoming a Person: A Therapist's View of Psychotherapy*. Boston, Houghton Mifflin, 1961, pp 39–58.

Rourke JT, Smith LF, Brown JB: Patients, friends, and relationship boundaries. *Can Fam Physician* 39:2557–2564, 1993.

Rudebeck CE: General practice and the dialogue of clinical practice: On symptoms, symptom presentations, and bodily empathy. *Scand J Primary Health Care Suppl*, 1992, pp 1–87.

Schwenk TL, Romano SE: Managing the difficult physician–patient relationship. *Am Fam Physician* 46:1503–1509, 1992.

Schwenk TL, Marquez JT, Lefever RD, Cohen M: Physician and patient determinants of difficult physician–patient relationships. *J Fam Pract* 28:59–63, 1989.

Simpson M, Buckman R, Stewart M, Maguire P, Lipkin M, Novack D: Doctor–patient communication: The Toronto consensus statement. *Br Med J* 303:1385–1387, 1991.

Spiegel D, Kraemer H, Bloom J, Gottheil E: Effect of psychosocial treatment on survival of patients with metastatic breast cancer. *Lancet* (ii):888–891, 1989.

Spittle B: Paternalistic interventions with the gravely disabled. *Aust NZ J Psychiatry* 26:107–110, 1992.

Starfield B, Wray C, Hess K, Gross R, Birk PS, D'Lugoff BC: The influence of patient–practitioner agreement on outcome of care. *Am J Public Health* 71:127–131, 1981.

Stein HF, Apprey M: *Clinical Stories and Their Translations*. Charlottesville, University of Virginia Press, 1990.

Stewart MA, McWhinney IR, Buck CW: The doctor/patient relationship and its effect upon outcome. *J R Coll Gen Pract* 29:77–82, 1979.

Stewart M, Brown JB, Weston WW, McWhinney IR, McWilliam CL, Freeman TR: *Patient-Centered Medicine: Transforming the Clinical Method*. Thousand Oaks, Calif, Sage Publications, Inc, 1995.

Stoeckle JD, Barsky AJ: Attributions: Uses of social science knowledge in the 'doctoring' of primary care, in Eisenberg L, Kleinman A (eds): *The Relevance of Social Science for Medicine*. Dordrecht, Reidel, 1981, pp 223–240.

Suchman AL, Matthews DA: What makes the patient–doctor relationship therapeutic? Exploring the connexional dimension of medical care. *Ann Intern Med* 108(1):125–130, 1988.

Suchman AL, Markakis K, Beckman HB, Frankel R: A model of empathic communication in the medical interview. *JAMA* 277:678–682, 1997.

Szasz TS, Hollender MH: The basic models of the doctor–patient relationship. *Arch Intern Med* 97:585–592, 1956.

Todd KH, Samaroo N, Hoffman JR: Ethnicity as a risk factor for inadequate emergency department analgesia. *JAMA* 269:1537–1539, 1993.

Tolstoy L: *The Death of Ivan Illyich*. Toronto, Bantam Books Inc, 1981.

Toombs K: *The Experience of Illness*. Boston, Kluwer Academic Publishing, 1992.

Veatch RM: Models for ethical medicine in a revolutionary age. What physician–patient roles foster the most ethical relationship? *Hastings Cent Rep* 2:5–7, 1972.

Weinberg RB, Mauksch LB: Examining family of origin influences in life at work. *J Marital Fam Ther* 17(3):233–242, 1991.

World Health Organization: World AIDS Day. *JAMA* 272:1568, 1994.

## CHAPTER 20

# The Family System

*Thomas L. Campbell, Susan H. McDaniel, and David B. Seaburn*

## CASE 20-1

*When Bill Guyer, a 52-year-old accountant, arrived at the emergency room, it was obvious to the staff that he was having a heart attack. Pale and sweating, he looked terrified as he clutched his chest. He was accompanied by his new wife Cathy, a 38-year-old nurse whom he had married shortly after his divorce, 1 year ago. Distressed, Cathy shouted continually at the ambulance and ER staff that they were doing something wrong or not working quickly enough. Finally, two of the nurses were able to escort her into the ER waiting room, while her husband was being treated.*

*Several minutes later, Bill's ex-wife Martha arrived in the waiting room demanding to know what had happened. Apparently, Bill had developed chest pain in the midst of a heated argument with their 17-year-old daughter Jane after she returned home drunk at 2 AM. When the ambulance took Bill to the hospital Cathy, her stepmother, had not allowed Jane to come. Jane then called her mother and explained that she had caused her father's heart attack.*

## EDUCATIONAL OBJECTIVES

1. Understand the importance of the family in health and illness: how families can influence health and how health affects families
2. Know how to implement a family-oriented approach in clinical practice and particularly in the treatment of chronic illnesses
3. Know how to obtain and utilize a family tree or genogram
4. Understand the concept of the "therapeutic triangle" and how to maintain alliances with all family members without taking sides
5. Know when to meet with family members or convene a family conference, and when to refer to a mental health professional
6. Understand how the physician's own family-of-origin issues can influence clinical practice

The family remains the most important social unit in our culture and plays an essential role in all aspects of health, illness, and medical care. As illustrated in Case 20-1, family relationships have a powerful impact on health, and illness strongly influences the family (Campbell, 1986; Doherty & Campbell, 1988). In clinical practice, family members may act as informants, customers for treatment, part of the problem, or members of the treatment team (McDaniel *et al.*, 1990). Whether in primary care or a subspecialty, the physician must have some understanding of the patient's family system and how the family context influences the patient's health and vice versa.

This chapter will present a basic approach to understanding and working with the family in medical practice. Using examples and research data, we will demonstrate how the family is an important source of stress, social support, health beliefs, and health behaviors. We will discuss the basic principles of a family systems approach to healthcare, including how to understand the family context of presenting symptoms, the use of genograms, the value of meeting with families and convening family conferences, and the importance of working collaboratively with mental health professionals.

## THE FAMILY SYSTEM

### Definition

Despite rapid changes in the demographics of U.S. families, most Americans live with other family members. The traditional or stereotypical U.S. family, however, which included father as breadwinner, mother as homemaker, and one or more children, has become a shrinking minority of U.S. households. Today, families are couples, two parents and children, blended families, single-parent households, and nonfamily households. As the U.S. family evolves, we need to adapt our understanding and definitions of family to capture its diversity. We define "family" as "any group of people related either biologically, emotionally, or legally" (McDaniel *et al.*, 1990). The World Health Organization has a broader definition:

> The concept of family need not be limited to ties of blood, marriage, sexual partnership or adoption. Any group whose bonds are based upon trust, mutual support and a common destiny may be regarded as family. (World Health Organization, 1994)

The relevant family context may include family members who live a distance from the patient, although physicians are most often involved with family members who live in the same household. In caring for Bill Guyer in Case 20-1, the relevant family included three generations of this remarried and blended family.

A biopsychosocial approach to healthcare is central to working effectively with families. The biopsycho-

## EMOTIONS AND HEART DISEASE

*Several lines of research have demonstrated a strong relationship between psychological factors and heart disease. Initial studies found a relationship between Type A personality and coronary artery disease. The Type A individual was characterized as competitive, impatient, and aggressive (Rosenman, 1990). More recent studies have clearly shown that it is the hostility component of Type A personality that is a risk factor of CHD. In multiple prospective studies, both anger and hostility, measured by several different methods, have predicted the development of angina and myocardial infarction (Friedman, 1992). Other studies have found that interpersonal conflict, particularly within the family, is a powerful risk factor for CHD (Sanders et al., 1991).*

social model, first described by George Engel (Engel, 1977), is more than the addition of psychosocial data to biomedical data. It is based on a systems approach to healthcare that emphasizes the interdependency and interplay among the different levels of any system, whether it is the cardiovascular system, the individual, family members, or the community. In Case 20-1, Bill Guyer's health is affected not only by the complex interrelationships of his organ systems, particularly his cardiovascular and nervous systems, but also by the complex relationships within his own extended family system. The Guyer family system is in turn influenced by larger community and social forces, such as the changing roles of women in society, increasing rates of divorce, and drug and alcohol problems in our schools and communities.

The family is a system, like the cardiovascular system, in which the whole is greater than the sum of its parts, and its component parts (family members) reciprocally influence each other. The relationships between family members are as important as individual characteristics of family members. One useful analogy to the family system is the solar system, in which one cannot understand the behavior or movements of a single planet without considering the movements and gravitational influence of other planets. Thus, we cannot fully understand a patient's behavior or health without considering the influence of the family and other larger systems, including work, community, and culture.

## The Family's Impact on Health

Numerous studies have shown that an individual's physical health and longevity are influenced by the quality and quantity of her social relationships, especially within the family (Doherty & Campbell, 1988). In a review of the research on social relationships and health, sociologist James House concludes:

> The evidence regarding social relationships and health increasingly approximates the evidence in the 1964 Surgeon General's report that established cigarette smoking as a cause or risk factor for mortality and morbidity from a range of diseases. The age-adjusted relative risk ratios are stronger than the relative risks for all cause mortality for cigarette smoking. (House *et al.*, 1988)

The marital relationship seems to have a particularly strong influence on health. Men and women who are in unhappy marriages have been shown to have poorer health status and immune functioning (Kiecolt-Glaser *et al.*, 1987). The adverse effects of the two most stressful life events, the death of a spouse and divorce, are well documented (Campbell, 1986; Doherty & Campbell, 1988). The family is the primary social context in which health promotion and disease prevention takes place. The World Health Organization has characterized the family as the "primary social agent in the promotion of health and well-being" (World Health Organization, 1976). A healthy lifestyle is usually developed, maintained, or changed within the family setting. Behavioral risk factors tend to cluster within families, as family members share similar diets, physical activities, and tobacco and alcohol use. In a 1985 Gallup survey of health-related behaviors, over 1000 adults reported that their spouse or significant other was more likely to influence their health habits than anyone else, including their family physician (Gallup Poll, 1985).

A number of studies have demonstrated the effectiveness of couple and family interventions for physical health problems (Campbell & Patterson, 1995). Family-oriented cardiovascular risk reduction programs are more effective and cost-effective than individually oriented programs. Couples-based weight reduction

---

## CARDIOVASCULAR RISK FACTORS WITHIN FAMILIES

*The Framingham Heart Study found a higher than expected concordance between spouses for blood pressure, cholesterol, triglycerides, blood sugar, smoking, and lung function. Parent–child blood pressure, body fat, and cholesterol were also significantly correlated (Sackett et al., 1975). Several family-focused cardiac risk factor trials have resulted in healthier lifestyles for the entire family (Anonymous, 1994).*

# PSYCHOSOMATIC FAMILIES

*To determine how family interactions affect chronic illness, Minuchin and his colleagues (1978) at the Philadelphia Child Guidance Center studied the physiologic responses of poorly controlled diabetic children to stressful family interviews. They observed a specific pattern of family interaction in some of these children, characterized by enmeshment (emotional overinvolvement), overprotectiveness, rigidity, and conflict avoidance. During the family interview, the diabetic children from these psychosomatic families had a rapid rise in their free fatty acids (a precursor to diabetic ketoacidosis). Minuchin hypothesized that in psychosomatic families, parental conflict is detoured or defused by the chronically ill child, and the resulting stress leads to exacerbations of the illness.*

programs result in greater maintenance of weight loss (Black *et al.*, 1990). Family therapy and psychoeducation for childhood illnesses seem to be particularly effective. Interventions for family caregivers of dementia and stroke patients reduce caregiver burden and depression and can delay institutionalization of these patients (Mittelman *et al.*, 1996).

## CASE 20-1 continued

*As their family physician, Dr. C. knew the Guyer family quite well. He had delivered their second child, Mike, who was now 14 and had insulin-dependent diabetes mellitus. He had treated Martha for depression, which developed at the time of their stormy divorce. He had rarely seen Bill in the office, despite years of efforts by Martha and more recently Cathy encouraging him to visit their physician. Dr. C. knew that Bill was overweight and smoked, despite having a strong family history of heart disease. The few times Dr. C. saw Bill, he was fatalistic about his health, stating that if heart disease was in his genes, there was nothing he could do about it. Dr. C. also knew that his daughter Jane was having serious problems at school and had been suspended several times over the past year. In addition, he was the physician for Martha's father, who had moderately severe Alzheimer's disease and had moved into the family's home 2 years before. With all of these issues occurring over the past several years, Dr. C. knew that this illness episode would be a challenge.*

# THE BIOPSYCHOSOCIAL APPROACH

To implement a family systems approach, the physician must not split biomedical from psychosocial issues during patient care. Using an integrated, biopsychosocial approach is a challenging task: Our culture and medical training encourage diagnosing problems as either physical or emotional and often focuses exclusively on one aspect of the problem. This mind–body split causes particular difficulties when caring for patients who present with physical symptoms for which no biomedical cause can be found or for which the psychosocial factors are significant. The challenge for physicians is to evaluate the biomedical and psychosocial aspects of the problem simultaneously and to decide at which level of the biopsychosocial model one should intervene. Occasionally, when faced with urgent problems or emergency medical problems, as in this case, the biomedical issues must be addressed first, followed by the psychosocial issues as soon as possible.

Because Dr. C. has a longstanding relationship with the Guyer family in Case 20-1, he has a good understanding of the family context and some hypotheses about what family stresses may have contributed to the patient's heart disease. However, initially Dr. C. needed to address the family's urgent need for information and reassurance and begin to assess the circumstances surrounding the onset of symptoms.

## FAMILY INFLUENCE ON IMMUNE FUNCTION

*Kiecolt-Glaser and her colleagues (1987, 1988a,b, 1991) at Ohio State University have studied the effects of marital conflict and family stress on immune functioning. In a series of studies, she found that divorced men and women had poorer cellular immunity (T-cell functioning) than married couples, and that individuals who were unhappy in their marriages had poorer immunity than those who were happily married. She also found that distressed family caregivers of Alzheimer's disease patients had poorer immune function than matched controls.*

### CASE 20-1 (continued)

*Shortly after Bill stabilized in the intensive care unit, Dr. C. met with Bill's wife Cathy, explained what had happened and the treatment her husband was receiving, and reassured her about his prognosis. Then, he gathered more history of the events surrounding his heart attack.*

*Dr. C. learned that Cathy had been concerned about Bill's health ever since they had met 2 years earlier. As a nurse, she knew he was at high risk for heart disease, because of his family history, smoking, poor nutrition, and lack of exercise. Since being married, she had completely changed his diet, serving him only low-fat meals. However, she knew that he went regularly to McDonald's for lunch and brought home pints of Ben and Jerry's ice cream for late-night snacks. She occasionally fought with him about his smoking and would hide or throw out any cigarettes she could find. He refused to join her aerobics classes at the local YMCA. Cathy thought he had episodes of angina over the past few months, but he always denied it and refused to see a physician.*

*Cathy also described the increasingly conflictual relationship between Bill and his daughter Jane. Jane blamed her father for the divorce and had become openly rebellious. She was failing in high school, drinking alcohol regularly, and dating a college junior whom neither Bill nor Cathy liked or trusted. They were also worried that she was using drugs.*

## The Family Context of the Presenting Problem

Most illnesses either influence the family or are influenced by the family, so it is helpful for the physician to have some understanding of the family context of every presenting problem. This may involve knowing who is in the household, what treatments other family members have recommended, or who is the primary caretaker of the patient. Patients often present with physical symptoms that are related to family stress or family problems. These somatic symptoms may represent a stress-related illness, an exacerbation of an underlying chronic illness, or some type of somatization for which no physiological abnormalities can be found. Physicians should be aware of "red flags" that alert them that a more complete exploration of the context is indicated. These "red flags" may include stress-related symptoms, such as chronic headaches, unexplained or inconsistent physical symptoms, abnormal mood, or who accompanies the patient to the visit (Doherty & Baird, 1983). In these situations, more detailed information about the family should be obtained. In Case 20-1, the history of Bill's presenting complaint makes it obvious that family stresses and conflict are contributing to his health problems. The arrival of both his wife and ex-wife to the emergency room suggests that there may be more complex issues.

A few simple questions can be used to assess the family context quickly (Cole-Kelly & Seaburn, 1999). Asking "Who is at home?" provides information about the family structure. Knowing the ages of family members allows one to hypothesize what developmental issues the family may be handling at the moment. Other useful questions include:

- How has this problem affected you and your family?
- Has anyone else in your family ever had this problem?
- Who knows about this problem?
- What does your family think about the problem you are having?
- What suggestions has your family made?
- Have there been any recent changes or stresses at home that you have had to deal with?

A family systems approach provides a way to understand the patient and his problem in a larger context of meaningful relationships. It does not mean the physician meets with the family at every visit. Most of the time, physicians meet with individual patients. But by being alert to "red flags" and asking a few routine family questions, the physician can make an initial assessment of the family context as it relates to the presenting problem. If that initial assessment suggests that family issues play an important role in the patient's health problem, more detailed information about the family needs to be obtained.

## CASE 20-1 (continued)

*Dr. C. reviewed the genogram that he had constructed over many visits with different members of the Guyer family (Fig. 20.1). He had been very involved in the care of the son, Mike, who developed insulin-dependent diabetes mellitus at the age of 10. During the first few years of his illness, Mike was in and out of the hospital with frequent episodes of diabetic ketoacidosis. Mike's illness had been very stressful on his parents and their relationship. Bill felt that Martha "smothered" their son and was overprotective, not letting him become as involved in sports as Bill felt he could. Though Mike's illness stabilized, the conflict between his parents had escalated.*

*Dr. C. knew that Mike's father, Bill, was an only child and that Bill's parents had divorced when he was 16. A few years after the divorce, Bill's father died suddenly of a heart attack. Bill's father had*

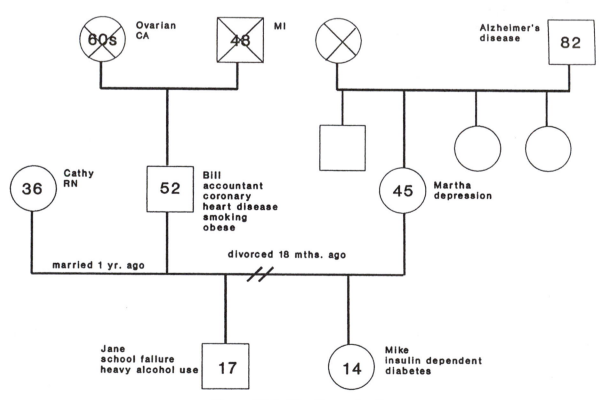

**Figure 20.1.** The Guyer family.

*been an alcoholic and his relationship with Bill had been conflictual. Bill did not have any contact with his father after his parent's divorce and refused to attend his father's funeral. On the other hand, Bill remained close to his mother until she died of ovarian cancer in her late 60s.*

## Use of the Genogram for Family Assessment

The family tree or genogram is one of the most basic and useful family systems tools. It allows the physician to obtain and record basic family information and provides a visual record of the family (McGoldrick *et al.*, 1999). With recent advances in human genetics, obtaining a genogram is essential for understanding genetic risk factors that occur in the family (Rose *et al.*, 1999). While obtaining information about genetic and other medical disorders in the family, information about family structure, developmental issues, relationship patterns, life cycle stages, and stressful life events can also be elicited. By reviewing the Guyer genogram (Fig. 20.1) before seeing Bill, Dr. C. has a snapshot of the family context and is alerted to the relevant individual and family issues.

During a patient's initial visit or physical examination, a brief, skeletal genogram can be obtained in less than 5 minutes as part of the family and social history. Patients are usually comfortable helping to construct the family tree. The genogram communicates to the patient that the physician is interested in all aspects of the patient's life. When the genogram is obtained in a nonthreatening manner, as a part of routine practice, patients are more likely to reveal sensitive and important family issues, such as substance abuse or domestic violence.

The genogram is particularly important when caring for divorced, remarried, or blended families, such as the Guyer family. In these families, adults and children often have different last names. It is essential to know which children belong to which parents, and who lives in which household. For example, if one falsely assumed that Cathy Guyer was Jane's mother and that Jane lived full-time in their household, it would have caused major difficulties in treatment. With a genogram, the physician can recognize immediately the relationships between family members.

When the physician cares for more than one member of a family, as with the Guyer family, it is also helpful to organize these individual charts into a family folder (Farley, 1990). The family's genogram can be included in the folder and added to during any family members' visits. With a family folder, the provider has access to other family members' charts during a patient's visit.

---

### CASE 20-1 (continued)

*Dr. C. was aware that the Guyer family was facing numerous developmental stresses. The most immediate concern was Bill's health and whether he would recover completely and be able to return to work. Bill and Martha's bitter divorce and Bill's remarriage was the greatest challenge that the family had confronted. Occurring at a time when their daughter Jane was beginning plans for college and leaving home, she was having the most difficulty coping with the divorce. Protective of her mother, she blamed her father and rarely visited him since he remarried. Her grades in school plummeted, and her prospects for college looked poor. Martha was essentially a single parent while also caring for her demented father. She had been forced to quit her job, which she enjoyed, to be home with her father. Over the past year, she had entered early menopause and began treatment for her depression.*

## The Family Life Cycle

By knowing the ages of the family members and examining the genogram, the physician can identify developmental issues affecting the family and whether these normative stresses are affecting the presenting health concerns. The family life cycle is a useful conceptual framework for understanding family development (Carter & McGoldrick, 1998) (see Chapter 2). Similar to the individual life cycle, the family life cycle assumes that families go through different stages for which there are specific developmental tasks to be accomplished. Families who do not accomplish these developmental tasks at one stage may develop difficulties with subsequent family development.

Many normative family life transitions can be very stressful and can precipitate or exacerbate health problems. Many women, like Martha Guyer, and some men in their 40s are faced with the demands of caring for elderly and disabled parents while they are simultaneously raising young children. As in the Guyer family, an increasing number of families are coping with the stress of divorce. Since one-half of all couples will eventually divorce, divorce and remarriage is a common developmental stressor for many families (Carter & McGoldrick, 1998). Today's physicians care for higher numbers of divorced and remarried families than ever before. These physicians are often asked by family members to choose sides; it takes a skillful clinician to avoid being pulled into such family conflicts.

## CASE 20-1 (continued)

*Dr. C. realized that the stress of Bill's heart attack and the circumstances around which it developed were contributing to the problems and conflicts that already existed in the family. Shortly after Bill's admission to the MICU, Dr. C. met briefly with Cathy and Martha together in the waiting room. After answering their questions about Bill, he asked how they were both doing. Cathy expressed her fears about Bill and Martha talked about her worries about Jane, who felt responsible for what had happened. This provoked an argument between Cathy and Martha, which Dr. C. quickly interrupted.*

*Dr. C.: "Excuse me. I need to interrupt this discussion. I realize that some of your family's relationships have become quite conflictual since the divorce and that Bill's illness has only added to the enormous stress that both of you are experiencing right now. I really think some of the problems will need to be dealt with, but not now. While Bill is in the hospital, it is very important for his health and for the kids' well-being that both of you put aside your conflicts as much as possible and help Bill recover and the kids to cope with their father's illness. Do you think you can do that?"*

## The Therapeutic Triangle

Another principle of a family systems approach is that medical visits are not just between physician and patient but involve the family, even when they are not in the examination room. Doherty and Baird (1987) have called this physician–patient–family interaction the therapeutic triangle in medicine (Fig. 20.2). The triangle emphasizes the important role of the family in every encounter and how the family affects the patient and vice versa, as well as how family members can influence the physician–patient relationship. By giving their opinions about the care the patient is receiving, family members can undermine or support the physician–patient relationship. When there is a poor medical outcome, the family often decides whether the physician was at fault and should be sued.

Whenever two people are in conflict, one person is likely to involve or triangulate a third person into the relationship to reduce the tension, anxiety, and seek an ally. Most people prefer to complain to a third person about their problems with a spouse, friend, or co-worker than to confront the offending person directly about the problem. When a patient complains to the physician about an interpersonal problem, he will often try to get the physician to take his side. Depressed or anxious patients may complain to the physician about another family member, such as "My husband drinks too much," "I think my wife is having an affair," or "Our son won't listen to us anymore." Physicians will often support and empathize with the patient, inadvertently taking sides in the conflict.

The difficult task for the physician is to develop and maintain a positive relationship with each family

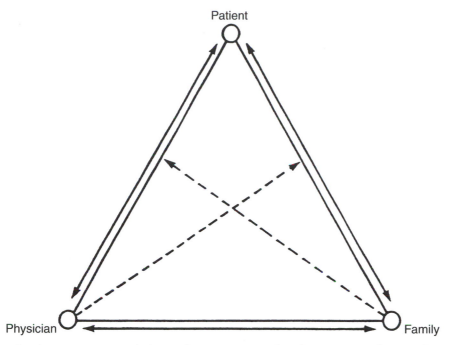

**Figure 20.2.** The therapeutic triangle in medicine. Reprinted with permission from Doherty and Baird (1983).

member and avoid blaming or taking sides in any conflict. To listen repeatedly to a patient complain about another family member is similar to only prescribing pain medication for a peptic ulcer: It may make the patient feel better acutely while the underlying problem gets worse.

In Case 20-1, there are multiple triangles into which Dr. C. may be pulled, being pressured to take sides. The most obvious and conflictual is between the divorced parents. In conflictual divorced families, parents and stepparents may try to get the physician to take sides with them, particularly with regard to the children. For example, one parent may bring his child for an acute visit to a physician and try to get the physician to agree that the health problem is somehow the result of what the ex-wife did, sometimes without even letting the physician know that the parents are divorced. In extreme cases, warring parents may take their children to different physicians and then try to pull these physicians into the divorce conflict.

The conflict between Jane and her parents is another common situation into which physicians can be pulled. One parent may try to get the physician to convince their teenager not to be sexually active or not to smoke. In another triangle, Cathy might ask Dr. C. to reinforce her message that Bill should eat better and exercise. While the physician will always advocate for a healthy lifestyle, if she takes sides in family conflicts, she usually loses effectiveness in working with the family member who is being sided against. When there is family conflict, the challenge is to remain allied with each member of the conflict and not take sides, while still being clear about what good healthcare warrants. Often, this can be done most effectively by meeting with the entire family.

## CASE 20-1 (continued)

*On the day prior to discharge from the hospital, Dr. C. met with Bill, Cathy, and the children. During the hospitalization, Cathy had agreed to participate in Bill's cardiac rehabilitation program and had attended informational classes on exercise and nutrition. She was relieved to see how much exercise he was allowed to do prior to his discharge. Dr. C. met separately with Bill and Cathy to discuss medication and resumption of sexual activity.*

*During the family meeting, Dr. C. reviewed Bill's hospital course and the plans for rehabilitation as an outpatient. He answered several of the children's questions about what had caused their father's heart attack and in what activities he could participate. He asked all of them how they felt about what had happened and what fears they had.*

# The Family Conference

Although a family systems approach can be used with individual patients, meeting with the family is frequently useful and sometimes necessary. Physicians often meet other family members at regular office visits, during hospital rounds, or for more extended family conferences. Family members often accompany patients to the physician's office and may be invited in from the waiting room. One study of primary care practices found that another family member was present in 32% of all visits (Medalie *et al.*, 1998). In another study, 39% of patients came to a family medicine center with a family member or friend, and two-thirds of these accompanied the patient into the examination room (Botelho *et al.*, 1997). These family members serve various roles for the patient, including helping to communicate the patient's concerns to the physician, helping patients remember the physician's recommendations, and assisting the patient in making decisions. Examination and consultation rooms should have a second chair for family members, so that they do not have to stand alone or sit on the examination table. Seeing elderly couples together for joint appointments acknowledges their interdependency, especially about health concerns.

A family meeting or conference can be particularly helpful in certain circumstances (McDaniel *et al.*, 1990). It is generally useful to meet with the family at least twice during a hospitalization, at the time of admission and shortly before discharge. Family members always want information about the patient's medical condition and often provide valuable information about events leading up to the admission. At the time of hospital discharge the family usually takes over the care of the patient. Before discharge, the physician should meet with the family to review the hospital course and ongoing treatment plans and elicit any family concerns about the patient returning home. Patients should receive "bad news" when they have the support of their families. In a family meeting, the physician can assess how well the family is coping with the illness and how to assist them.

It is particularly important to meet with the family when the diagnosis of a terminal illness is made or when a patient dies. Family members may be in a state of shock or denial. They may need empathy and support. They may need assistance in communicating with each other. Or, they may need information. Oftentimes physicians view death as a failure and feel guilty about it. This guilt may result in the physician avoiding the family when it is most important for both parties to meet

Family members are usually willing to accompany the patient to a physician's appointment or a family meeting. However, if there are serious family conflicts such as in the Guyer family, some family members may be reluctant to attend, fearing they will be blamed for the problem.

---

## CASE 20-1 (continued)

*In discussing their fears, both children said they were worried that a family argument might precipitate another heart attack. Dr. C. explained that Bill's heart attack was not caused by the argument with Jane prior to his admission. His heart disease resulted from a combination of genetics, poor diet and exercise, and smoking. Dr. C. added that he would be working with Bill to help him deal with family stresses in a healthier manner, and that the family needed to find better ways of resolving their conflicts.*

*This comment led to a broader discussion by the family of some of their conflicts. Dr. C. mostly listened, occasionally interrupting when arguments seemed to be escalating. Collectively, the family agreed that for the sake of Bill's health, they needed to work together to resolve their difficulties.*

## LEVELS OF WORKING WITH FAMILIES

When using a family systems approach, it is important to assess continuously what level of involvement the physician wishes to have with the families in her practice. As with other areas in medicine, she needs to decide what level of skills and knowledge she has or wishes to have in a particular area. For example, when treating cardiac patients, she must decide whether she has the skills to treat complicated post-MI patients in the intensive care unit, or refer them to a cardiologist.

Based on the physician's knowledge, personal development, and skills, Doherty and Baird (1987) have outlined five levels of physicians' involvement with families (Table 20.1). They developed these levels to emphasize that all physicians work with families at some level and that some problems require the expertise of a trained family therapist. Some physicians only deal with families when it is necessary for medical–legal reasons, Level One.

Most physicians usually work at Level Two, providing ongoing medical information and advice to families. For the Guyer family, this involved assembling the family before hospital discharge and providing detailed information about the illness and treatment plans. If this kind of information is only provided to the individual patient, it can create confusion and conflict as the family tries to decide what activities are safe for the patient.

Working at Level Three involves eliciting feelings and providing support to families and can be very therapeutic for patients and families. Many families never share their worries and fears about a family member's illness unless encouraged to do so in a family meeting. These families often have the belief that expressing their feelings will upset the patient and worsen his illness. Level Three requires the physician to be comfortable eliciting, attending to, and normalizing strong emotions. As in the Guyer family, simply asking how they are feeling about the illness or what has happened usually elicits family members' feelings.

Level Four, Systematic Assessment and Planned Intervention, requires additional training in family systems theory and its application. At this level, physicians provide brief and focused family counseling for uncomplicated family problems. This involves getting family members to talk with each other, intervening to change communication patterns, but not engaging in therapy to address ongoing relationship problems. More complex and chronic family problems need family therapy, Level Five, a specialty service that requires 3 to 5 years of postgraduate training and supervision and is beyond the interest and training of most physicians. Since physicians often see these types of problems in their practice, they need to work collaboratively with family therapists so effective referrals can occur.

---

### CASE 20-1 (continued)

*Because Dr. C. had a longstanding relationship with the family and they trusted him, they asked him if he would help them with some of their conflicts. Although flattered and initially tempted to take on the challenge, Dr. C. recognized that he was over his head and that the Guyers' difficulties were beyond the training in family counseling that he had received in residency.*

*Dr. C. expressed his desire to help the family with these problems, but said they needed and deserved a specialist who has special expertise dealing with family problems. He made the analogy to Bill's need to see a cardiologist to do a cardiac catheterization and help decide on further*

**Table 20.1**
Levels of Physician Involvement with Families

| Level One: Minimal Emphasis on Family | Level Two: Ongoing Medical Information and Advice | Level Three: Feelings and Support | Level Four: Systematic Assessment and Planned Intervention | Level Five: Family Therapy |
|---|---|---|---|---|
| This baseline level of involvement consists of dealing with families only as necessary for practical and medical legal reasons, but not viewing communicating with families as integral to the physician's role or as involving skills for the physician to develop. This level presumably characterizes most medical school training where biomedical issues are the sole conscious focus of patient care. | **Knowledge Base:** Primarily medical plus awareness of the triangular dimension of the physician–patient relationship.<br><br>**Personal Development:** Openness to engage patients and families in a collaborative way.<br><br>**Skills:**<br>1. Regularly and clearly communicating medical findings and treatment options to family members.<br>2. Asking family members questions that elicit relevant diagnostic and treatment information.<br>3. Attentively listening to family members' questions and concerns.<br>4. Advising families about how to handle the medical and rehabilitation needs of the patient.<br>5. For large or demanding families, knowing how to channel communication through one or two key members.<br>6. Identifying gross family dysfunction that interferes with medical treatment and referring the family to a therapist. | **Knowledge Base:** Normal family development and reactions to stress.<br><br>**Personal Development:** Awareness of one's own feelings in relationship to the patient and family.<br><br>**Skills:**<br>1. Asking questions that elicit family members' expressions of concerns and feelings related to the patient's condition and its effect on the family.<br>2. Empathetically listening to family members' concerns and feelings and normalizing them where appropriate.<br>3. Forming a preliminary assessment of the family's level of functioning as it relates to the patient's problem.<br>4. Encouraging family members in their efforts to cope as a family with their situation.<br>5. Tailoring medical advice to the unique needs, concerns, and feelings of the family.<br>6. Identifying family dysfunction and fitting a referral recommendation to the unique situation of the family. | **Knowledge Base:** Family systems.<br><br>**Personal Development:** Awareness of one's own participation in systems, including the therapeutic triangle, the medical system, one's own family system, and larger community systems.<br><br>**Skills:**<br>1. Engaging family members, including reluctant ones, in a planned family conference or a series of conferences.<br>2. Structuring a conference with even a poorly communicating family in such a way that all members have a chance to express themselves.<br>3. Systematically assessing the family's level of functioning.<br>4. Supporting individual members while avoiding coalitions.<br>5. Reframing the family's definition of their problem in a way that makes problem solving more achievable.<br>6. Helping the family members view their difficulty as requiring new forms of collaborative efforts.<br>7. Helping family members generate alternative, mutually acceptable ways to cope with their difficulty.<br>8. Helping the family balance their coping efforts by calibrating their various roles in a way that allows support without sacrificing anyone's autonomy.<br>9. Identifying family dysfunction that lies beyond primary care treatment and orchestrating a referral by educating the family and the therapist about what to expect from one another. | **Knowledge Base:** Family systems and patterns whereby dysfunctional families interact with professionals and other health-care systems.<br><br>**Personal Development:** Ability to handle intense emotions in families and self and to maintain neutrality in the face of strong pressure from family members or other professionals.<br><br>**Skills:**<br>The following is not an exhaustive list of family therapy skills but rather a list of several key skills that distinguish Level Five involvement from primary care involvement with families:<br>1. Interviewing families or family members who are quite difficult to engage.<br>2. Efficiently generating and testing hypotheses about the family's difficulties and interaction patterns.<br>3. Escalating conflict in the family in order to break a family impasse.<br>4. Temporarily siding with one family member against another.<br>5. Constructively dealing with a family's strong resistance to change.<br>6. Negotiating collaborative relationships with other professionals and other systems who are working with the family, even when these groups are at odds with one another. |

*treatment. Dr. C. explained that he would remain involved in their care and work closely with the family therapist he recommended. Dr. C. recommended that they contact Dr. M., a family therapist with whom he has worked closely. He agreed to join the family at the first visit with Dr. M.*

## COLLABORATION WITH A MENTAL HEALTH PROVIDER

Using a biopsychosocial and family systems approach to medical care requires the physician to assess problems at multiple levels and to decide at what level or levels to intervene. In Case 20-1, it was important to intervene at the cardiovascular system level (cardiac catheterization and medication), the individual level (change in diet, exercise, and smoking), and the family system (family therapy). However, it is crucial for the physician to know what the limits of his expertise and skills are and when to consult or refer to a specialist. Most physicians have learned to do this quite skillfully for medical problems.

Many psychosocial problems can be handled by primary care family counseling (Level Four) by physicians who have the time, interest, and skill to do such counseling. Table 20.2 lists the common types of problems amenable to family counseling, as well as those that usually need referral to a mental health provider. Factors that influence whether a problem should be referred to a therapist include the severity of the problem, its chronicity, and previous attempts to treat the problem. The more severe and chronic problems that have failed previous treatments require referral. Sometimes the patient or family may request a referral to a mental health provider, either because they recognize the severity of the problem or because they prefer to discuss a sensitive topic with someone other than their physician who they see regularly (McDaniel *et al.*, 1992). Finally, the physician may decide that the issues that the family is dealing with are too close to unresolved issues in the physician's own life.

### CASE 20-1 (continued)

*Dr. C. had recently gone through his own painful and sometimes conflictual divorce. He knew how important it was to buffer the children from the effects of the divorce by keeping them out of conflicts between ex-spouses, by reducing these conflicts, and by developing as smooth a working relationship as possible. He also knew that his divorce was still fresh and that he had not yet resolved many of his own issues. As a result, he was very cautious about advising or counseling the family on how they should deal with their postdivorce conflicts. He was tempted to suggest the best custody arrangements and how to communicate between ex-spouses, but realized that part of his desire resulted from his need to convince himself that what he had done was the best approach (see Chapter 19, "projection"). Dr. C. also had some struggles with his teenage son, who was at a rebellious stage. He used his own experience to empathize with Bill about the difficulties of raising teenagers but realized that he did not have any expertise in how to deal with these problems.*

**Table 20.2**
When to Treat and When to Refer Problems Seen in Primary Care[a]

| Problems commonly seen in primary care counseling | Problems commonly referred on to a mental health specialist |
| --- | --- |
| Adjustment to the diagnosis of a new illness | Suicidal or homicidal ideation, intent, or behavior |
| Other adjustment or situational disorders | Psychotic behavior |
| Crises of limited severity or duration | Sexual or physical abuse |
| Behavior problems | Substance abuse |
| Mild depressive reactions | Somatic fixation |
| Mild anxiety reactions | Moderate-severe marital and sexual problems |
| Uncomplicated grief reactions | Multi-problem family situations |
| | Problems resistant to change in primary care counseling |

[a]Reprinted with permission from McDaniel *et al.* (1990).

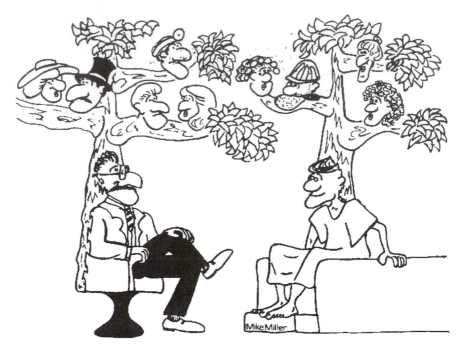

**Figure 20.3.** Family influences on the physician and patient.

## PHYSICIAN SELF-AWARENESS AND FAMILY OF ORIGIN

A physician's past and current personal issues can be either a major resource or a profound hindrance in the patient–physician relationship. All physicians carry with them influences from the family that they grew up in (see Fig. 20.3). Styles of caretaking and authority as well as tolerance for affect (emotions) are all learned in our families of origin. Many physicians are able to use their past experiences to enhance their empathy and their credibility with patients. However, current problems or unresolved struggles from the past can cloud or distort our perceptions of patients and their families. For example, medical students or practicing physicians who grew up with family members with serious alcohol problems may have difficulty dealing with alcoholic patients, either getting angry at them or "giving up" on them. Difficult or "problem" patients often elicit strong reactions in their physicians and may result in "stuck" interactions where the physician is spending a great deal of time with little change in the patient or relationship. These problematic relationships often result from experiences in the physician's own family of origin (Mengel, 1986). The patient's family may mirror some of the same relationships or issues in the physician's own family. A physician who grew up with very authoritarian parents may find it very difficult to treat demanding or entitled patients (see Chapter 19, "transference" and "countertransference").

Utilizing personal issues as a resource depends on being able to recognize these issues when they occur in our work (Novack *et al.*, 1997). When the physician recognizes that a patient or family is stimulating an important personal issue, the physician then has the opportunity to decide whether to treat, collaborate with a colleague, or refer. Physicians can benefit their own practice by regularly consulting with colleagues, such as in a Balint group (Balint, 1964) or, in some instances, seeking personal psychotherapy.

### CASE 20-1 (continued)

*The Guyer family met with the family therapist, Dr. M., for 10 visits over the following 6 months. Dr. C. joined the family for the first session and shared his concerns about the conflict in the family and how it was affecting each family member. He stressed how he thought Dr. M. could be helpful to the family.*

*Dr. M. met with the entire family for several sessions and helped them address the conflicts and loyalties that had developed because of the divorce. Bill, Martha, and Cathy met separately with Dr. M. to address parenting issues and how to help and support their daughter Jane. Dr. M. also held separate sessions for Bill and Cathy to deal with stresses that had developed in their marriage and the impact of Bill's MI, and with Martha to help her decide what to do about her demented father.*

## CONCLUSION: COLLABORATIVE FAMILY HEALTH CARE

Because of the complex nature of patients' problems, the increasing age of the general population, and the growing emphasis of primary care, it will be important for physicians to develop effective partnerships with families and mental health professionals (Seaburn *et al.*, 1996). Applying a family systems approach to healthcare provides helpful information for diagnosis and opens new options for treatment of patients and their families. This approach is based on the biopsychosocial model, but puts special emphasis on the role of the family in health care. It can be implemented in daily practice by considering the family context of all presenting health problems, including the developmental phase of patients and their families, through the regular use of genograms. It does not require seeing family members at every visit.

In addition, some physicians may obtain additional training in order to counsel families in their practices (Level Four). However, many family problems will require referral to a mental health professional, usually a family therapist (McDaniel *et al.*, 1992; Seaburn *et al.*, 1996). Collaborative family healthcare, working collaboratively with families and mental health providers, helps physicians practice a fully integrated bio-psychosocial approach and provides comprehensive and effective care for a broad spectrum of health problems (Dym, 1994).

## CASES FOR DISCUSSION

### CASE 1

*J. P. is a 35-year-old woman who has a partner of 6 years and a daughter, aged 4. This medical visit is the second one regarding low back pain, leg pain, and headaches. The patient is very anxious about these symptoms: They have persisted for many years but have worsened in the last 3 months. The patient has not been able to work for over a month. She presents her symptoms in an anxious manner, moving quickly from one symptom to the next. Unknown to the physician, the patient's mother had similar problems. The mother feels that her daughter has "something serious," maybe cancer.*

*The patient's partner is unconcerned and not supportive. He has a drinking problem. The patient is worried about their relationship. Her father has told her to leave him. The patient's daughter worries about her and tries to take care of her. As a child the patient was sexually abused by an uncle. She is seeing a therapist about this, but the physician is unaware of the abuse or the therapy.*

1. *How might the patient's family be influencing her presenting symptoms? What role might her history of sexual abuse play in her current problems?*
2. *How would you involve this patient's family in her care? How would you work with her partner, daughter, and parents?*
3. *How would you work with the therapist who is seeing the patient?*

### CASE 2

*M. S. is a 65-year-old mother of 10 who presented to the hospital 3 days after a myocardial infarction. She had experienced chest pain and shortness of breath at home where she lived with her son, but refused to go to the hospital or to see a physician. When her children finally prevailed on her to go to the hospital, she was very argumentative with the residents on the floor. It took several days to convince her to have the appropriate tests and begin medical treatment for her cardiac disease. The patient felt frustrated that her children were "smothering me," and the adult children were upset that their mother was not receiving the care she needed.*

1. *Why do you think the patient is not seeking timely medical care for her health problems? How might her family be affecting her behavior?*
2. *How would you help this patient and her family? How might a family meeting be helpful? What additional information would you want to obtain from the patient and her family?*

## CASE 3

*H. M. is a 48-year-old businessman who rarely seeks medical care. The morning before his scheduled routine physical examination, his wife calls the office to tell you that he has a serious drinking problem and asks, "Could you talk with him about it?"*

1. *What do you tell the wife on the telephone? How would you address her concerns? If you ask the wife to join him at his visit and she refuses, what do you say?*
2. *How would you deal with this information when you see the husband, if his wife comes, and if she doesn't come?*

## CASE 4

*G. R. is a 70-year-old man with a long smoking history who is brought to your office by his daughter who is his primary caretaker. He has had some difficulty urinating and has passed some blood. On rectal examination, you feel a hard nodule in his prostate. You order blood work and refer him to a urologist for a biopsy.*

*As they are leaving the office, his daughter pulls you aside and says that if he has cancer, she does not want him to be told. She says that she knows her father very well, that he has always been terrified of cancer, and that he cannot deal with the diagnosis.*

1. *How do you respond to her request? What further information would you want from her?*
2. *The nodule is malignant, and you decide to meet with the patient and his daughter. How would you deal with his new diagnosis and his daughter's concerns?*

## RECOMMENDED READINGS

Campbell TL: *Family's Impact on Health: A Critical Review and Annotated Bibliography*. NIMH Series DN, No. 6, DHHS Publ. No. (ADM) 86-1461, 1986. Also published in *Fam Syst Med* 4(2&3):135–328, 1986.

This monograph and special issue of *Family Systems Medicine* review the research literature on how family factors, especially family relationships, influence health. It also includes an annotated bibliography of the reviewed studies.

Doherty WJ, Baird MA: *Family Therapy and Family Medicine*. New York, Guilford Press, 1983.

This landmark book outlines the theory and practice of a family systems approach to healthcare. It has excellent chapters on how to assess, refer, and counsel families in primary care.

Doherty WJ, Baird MA (eds): *Family-Centered Medical Care: A Clinical Casebook*. New York, Guilford Press, 1987.

Family physicians and collaborating therapists describe 71 cases of working with families in clinical practice. The cases are organized around the editors' Levels of Working with Families and include commentaries by the editors.

Doherty WJ, Campbell TL: *Families and Health*. Beverly Hills, Calif, Sage Publications, 1988.

This book is part of the Sage Family Studies literature and is written for family professionals as well as medical providers. It reviews the literature on families and health and its implications for health professionals. It is organized around the Family Health and Illness Cycle.

McDaniel SH, Campbell TL, Seaburn DB: *Family-Oriented Primary Care: A Manual for Medical Providers*. New York, Springer-Verlag, 1990.

This practical guide to implementing a family-oriented approach in primary care has chapters on how to convene a family conference, conduct a family interview, and specific practical guidelines for dealing with numerous life-cycle and health-related issues.

Anonymous: Randomised controlled trial evaluating cardiovascular screening and intervention in general practice: Principal results of British family heart study. Family Heart Study Group. *BMJ* 308:313–320, 1994.

Balint M: *The Doctor, His Patient, and the Illness*. London, Pitman, 1964.

Black DR, Gleser LJ, Kooyers KJ: A meta-analytic evaluation of couples weight loss programs. *Health Psychol* 9:330–347, 1990.

Botelho RJ, Lue BH, Fiscella K: Family involvement in routine health care: A survey of patients' behaviors and preferences. *J Fam Pract* 42(6):572–576, 1997.

Campbell TL: *Family's Impact on Health: A Critical Review and Annotated Bibliography*. NIMH Series DN, No. 6, DHHS Publication No. (ADM) 86-1461, 1986. Also published in *Fam Syst Med* 4(2&3):135–328, 1986.

Campbell TL, Patterson J: The effectiveness of family interventions in the treatment of physical illness. *J Marital Fam Ther* 21(4):545–583, 1995.

Carter B, McGoldrick M (eds): *The Expanded Family Life Cycle: Individual, Family and Social Perspectives*, ed 3. Boston, Allyn & Bacon, 1998.

Cole-Kelly K, Seaburn D: Five areas of questioning to promote a family-oriented approach to primary care. *Fam Syst Health* 17(3):341–348, 1999.

Doherty WJ, Baird MA: *Family Therapy and Family Medicine: Toward the Primary Care of Families*. New York, Guilford Press, 1983.

Doherty WJ, Baird MA (eds): *Family-Centered Medical Care: A Clinical Casebook*. New York, Guilford Press, 1987.

Doherty WJ, Campbell TL: *Families and Health*. Beverly Hills, Calif, Sage Publications, 1988.

Dym B (ed): *Working Together: The Newsletter of the Collaborative Family Health Care Coalition*. 1(1), 1994.

Engel GL: The need for a new medical model: A challenge for biomedicine. *Science* 196:129–136, 1977.

Farley ES Jr: Is it worthwhile to file by family folders in family practice: An affirmative view. *J Fam Pract* 30:697–700, 1990.

Friedman HS: *Hostility, Coping & Health*. Washington, DC, APA Press, 1992.

Gallup Poll (1985) as quoted in Public Health Service: *Healthy People 2000: National Health Promotion and Disease Prevention Objectives*. Washington, DC, 1990, p 258.

House JS, Landis KR, Umberson D: Social relationships and health. *Science* 241:540–545, 1988.

Kiecolt-Glaser JK, Fisher LD, Ogrocki P, Stout JC, Speicher CE, Glaser R: Marital quality, marital disruption, and immune function. *Psychosom Med* 49:13–34, 1987.

Kiecolt-Glaser JK, Dyer CS, Shuttleworth EC: Upsetting social interactions and distress among Alzheimer's disease family care-givers: A replication and extension. *Am J Comm Psychol* 16:825–837, 1988a.

Kiecolt-Glaser JK, Kennedy S, Malkoff S, Fisher L, Speicher CE, Glaser R: Marital discord and immunity in males. *Psychosom Med* 50:213–229, 1988b.

Kiecolt-Glaser JK, Glaser R: Caregiving, mental health, and immune function, in Light E, Lebowitz B (eds): *Alzheimer's Disease Treatment and Family Stress: Direction for Research*. Rockville, Md, NIMH, 1991.

McDaniel SH, Campbell TL, Seaburn D: *Family-Oriented Primary Care: A Manual for Medical Providers*. New York, Springer-Verlag, 1990.

McDaniel SH, Hepworth J, Doherty W: *Medical Family Therapy*. New York, Basic Books Inc, 1992.

McGoldrick M, Gerson R, Shellenberger S: *Genograms: Assessment and Interventions*, ed 2. New York, WW Norton & Co Inc, 1999.

Medalie JH, Zyzanski SJ, Langa D, Stange KC: The family in family practice: Is it a reality? *J Fam Pract* 46(5):390–396, 1998.

Mengel M: Physician ineffectiveness due to family of origin issues. *Fam Syst Med* 5(2):176–190, 1986.

Minuchin S, Rosman BL, Baker L: *Psychosomatic Families*. Cambridge, Mass, Harvard University Press, 1978.

Mittelman MS, Ferris SH, Shulman E, Steinberg G, Levin B: A family intervention to delay nursing home placement of patients with Alzheimer disease. A randomized controlled trial. *JAMA* 276:1725–1731, 1996.

Novack DH, Suchman AL, Clark W, Epstein RM, Najberg E, Kaplan C: Calibrating the physician. Personal awareness and effective patient care. *JAMA* 278(6):502–509, 1997.

Rose P, Humm E, Hey K, Jones L, Huson SM: Family history taking and genetic counseling in primary care. *Fam Pract* 16:78–83, 1999.

Rosenman RH: Type A behavior pattern: A personal overview. Special Issue: Type A behavior. *J Soc Behav Pers* 5:1–24, 1990.

Sackett DL, Anderson GD, Milner R, *et al*: Concordance for coronary risk factors among spouses. *Circulation* 52:589–593, 1975.

Sanders JD, Smith TW, Alexander JF: Type A behavior and marital interaction: Hostile-dominant responses during conflict. *J Behav Med* 14:567–580, 1991.

Seaburn D, Lorenz A, Gunn B, Mauksch L, Gawinski B: *Models of Collaborative Health Care*. New York, Basic Books Inc, 1996.

World Health Organization. Statistical Indices of Family Health 1976, No. 589:17.

World Health Organization. World AIDS Day. *JAMA* 272:1568, 1994.

## CHAPTER 21

# The Community

*Laura B. Frankenstein and Elisabeth D. Babcock*

*Mrs. Josephs was an 81-year-old woman living on her own in a third-floor tenement apartment in a crowded urban area. She had no family and was in very frail health. Despite repeated urging by her regular physician, she had refused to enter a nursing home.*

*During a 3-day period of 90-degree weather, Mrs. Joseph's home health aide found her hyperthermic and dehydrated. The aide called an ambulance and Mrs. Josephs was rushed to the local emergency room.*

*At the hospital, Mrs. Joseph's physician in conjunction with the hospital social worker stressed to her that she could not continue living at home without greater support. They suggested she either enter a nursing home or join a new managed care program designed to provide extensive support to frail elders who wished to remain in their homes.*

## EDUCATIONAL OBJECTIVES

1. Recognize how poverty, language, culture, transportation barriers, and other aspects of a community affect a patient's health
2. Understand how shortages of primary care physicians affect communities
3. Identify resources within the community for improving patient care and be effective in sharing this information with patients
4. Recognize the limitations of treating one person at a time in the office setting, and utilize Healthy People 2010 to evaluate health promotion and disease prevention
5. Develop a community project to address a public health problem

## INTRODUCTION

Just as it is impossible to understand and treat patients without understanding the dynamics of the families in which they live, it is equally important to understand their communities. The community will often

449

## PHYSICIANS CAN INTERACT
## WITH THEIR COMMUNITIES IN FOUR WAYS

*1. Informed and appropriate use of community health resources*
*2. Sociocultural awareness in the care of patients*
*3. Identifying and intervening in health promotion and disease prevention activities in the*
   *community in collaboration with other concerned individuals*
*4. Community participation on committees, as board members, as speakers, by writing in*
   *the lay press or perhaps involvement in politics*

(Source: Pathman, 1998)

house clues to the causes of patients' diseases as well as the resources with which to treat them. A recent study by the Province of Ontario, Canada, Department of Public Health, showed that the entire healthcare system of Ontario accounted for only 11% of the total variation in patient outcome; the balance of 89% was controlled by factors outside of the healthcare system such as level of education, poverty, housing, and ethnicity (Society for Ambulatory Care Professionals, 1993).

Carefully defining the factors within a community that create barriers to good health as well as barriers to care, and then seeking to remedy those barriers, can often yield far-reaching and cost-effective improvements in patient outcome. This approach to understanding and caring for patients through understanding and caring for their communities is called community-oriented primary care (COPC). COPC gives the clinician tools for more rapid diagnosis of patients, better mechanisms for devising treatment plans, and the opportunity to provide new programs of care within communities to benefit not only patients the clinician treats directly, but also patients the clinician might never see.

As Case 21-1 demonstrates, patients often present with a host of obstacles to receiving good care within the limitations of the traditional medical system. To adequately treat such patients, the clinician may have to devise new programs to bridge barriers to care. The patient in Case 21-1 was fortunate that she could participate in a new program of managed care for the frail elderly within her community called PACE (Program of All-inclusive Care for the Elderly). Physicians and other caregivers had observed many of the frail elderly of the community going into nursing homes because of lack of resources to care for them in their homes. Many of these patients did not wish to be admitted to the nursing home and once admitted had significant diminution in health status including mental decompensation and death.

To address this problem, the clinic joined with the local elder services agency to seek ways to provide better supports for frail elders to remain in their homes. They successfully applied for a Robert Wood Johnson Program grant to begin a PACE program in their community. The program provided special capitation rates from Medicaid and Medicare that paid the clinic a monthly stipend in place of the traditional system of billing for medical services rendered. Under this new PACE program, funds paid by Medicaid and Medicare could be used for anything that clinicians determined would lead to healthy patient outcomes and prevent unwanted nursing home admissions. In addition to inpatient and outpatient medical care, medications, and transportation to an adult day health site and to any necessary medical visits to specialists, this money was used for group activities, social work, and meals at the site. Therefore, instead of entering a nursing home, the patient

## HEAT-RELATED DEATHS

*Nearly 70% of all heat-related deaths occur among the poor, urban elders in our communities.*

## HOW TO TELL WHEN A PERSON IS HYPERTHERMIC AND DEHYDRATED

1. *Confusion, irritability, lethargy, or loss of consciousness*
2. *Intense thirst*
3. *Weakness*
4. *Orthostatic dizziness (blood pressure drops when a person stands up)*
5. *Dry mucous membranes (mouth and tongue)*
6. *Increase in skin turgor (when you pinch the skin on the hand or arm it "tents" or stays in that shape much longer than it does normally)*
7. *Hot to the touch*
8. *Tachycardia and tachypnea (rapid heart and respiratory rates)*

in Case 21-1 received an air conditioner from her PACE program. She enjoyed coming to the PACE site 5 days a week, and saw her physician and nurse practitioner there between bingo, group exercises, and health lunches. She thus remained happily in her own apartment and her health status was restored. Needless to say, the air conditioner cost much less than a nursing home admission and Mrs. Josephs retained her independence and dignity. By looking at patient needs within the context of the community and devising community-based solutions, the physician was able to provide Mrs. Josephs a better outcome while adding a new cost-effective tool for patient care to her clinical armamentarium.

This chapter offers clinicians a framework for learning about their patients' communities and ideas as to how such knowledge can improve the diagnosis and treatment of patients as well as the development of new resources for patient care.

## CASE 21-2

*Dr. Jenkins was the medical director of a 230-bed hospital that served the population of an aging factory town. Over the years, as the factories closed and jobs had been lost, the old corps of general practitioners who had provided most of the town's primary care had retired and Dr. Jenkins had found it increasingly difficult to attract new physicians to the community.*

*During this period, Dr. Jenkins also began to observe significant increases in the numbers of patients seeking emergency care at the hospital for diabetes mellitus, asthma, and bacterial pneumonia. He wondered what conditions in the community might be contributing to the sharp increase in the incidence of these diseases and what he could do to prevent their occurrence.*

## HOW TO PREVENT ELDERS FROM BECOMING DEHYDRATED

1. *Many elderly drink little more than a few cups of coffee or tea, sometimes a fair amount of alcohol. Encourage them to drink fluids, especially water, every day.*
2. *Elderly individuals should avoid going outside and should stay in an air-conditioned building when temperatures are extremely hot.*
3. *Many older individuals habitually keep their thermostats very high and bundle themselves in multiple layers of clothing. Encourage them to avoid these habits in warm weather.*
4. *Share information about local programs that provide fans and air conditioners to elders.*

## HOW TO BECOME A COMMUNITY-ORIENTED PHYSICIAN

*1. Consider the types of patients you see whose health is not helped significantly by office-based clinical care alone; e.g.,*
   *a. Obese patients*
   *b. Partners of HIV patients*
   *c. Teenagers*
   *d. Homebound elders*
*2. Consider alternative ways you can help each population; e.g.,*
   *a. Obese patients: form a fitness support group, create a flier of healthy alternatives to fast food.*
   *b. Partners of HIV patients: provide information about confidential, free testing and counseling locations and support groups for patients and their partners; invite patients to bring their partners to their next visit.*
   *c. Teenagers: encourage the use of or the development of school-based health centers, volunteer as a team physician or offer to give talks in the schools to expose teens to healthcare, support programs that help teens deal with the issues of substance use, pregnancy prevention, and safety.*
   *d. Homebound elders: work with visiting nurses and local homecare agencies that provide meals and other services, make home visits, and support their caregivers.*
*3. Recruit other health professionals to join you in these activities.*

## PRIMARY CARE SHORTAGES

The U.S. healthcare system is specialty dominated. Unlike many European countries, which have at least two primary care physicians for each specialty physician, the United States has almost the exact opposite: two specialists for every one generalist (Council on Graduate Medical Education, 1992). There are 2.07 active generalist physicians per 1000 U.S. citizens; ratios should be twice that number per thousand (Whitcomb, 1995). When health insurance was predominantly indemnity-based and patients could freely gain access to specialists, this specialty-dominated model did not pose a barrier to access. Now that fewer than 5% of patients are insured by indemnity plans and the rest must seek the care of a primary care physician who in turn controls access to specialty physicians, many areas of the nation are experiencing shortages of primary care physicians (Bindman *et al.*, 1995).

These shortages are especially severe in areas of the country where there are high concentrations of the most vulnerable patients, such as communities of urban or rural poor. Competition for primary care physicians is so extreme that most physicians settle in the more affluent communities where salaries and benefits are highest. Communities with high numbers of uninsured or publicly insured residents are often unable to attract and keep the physicians they need to maintain basic health. Such communities are termed *medically underserved.*

## THE IMPACT OF THE NATIONAL HEALTH SERVICE CORPS

*There are currently 2400 NHSC clinicians in the 50 states, the District of Columbia, Puerto Rico, the Virgin Islands, and the Pacific Basin.*

*They serve in community and migrant health centers, private practices, the Indian Health Service, the Bureau of Prisons, and in State, County, and local health departments.*

*More than 21,000 health professionals have served with NHSC since 1972 and many remain after their required commitment is over.*

The Bureau of Primary Health Care defines health profession shortage areas and medically underserved populations based on a composite of seven variables that reflect the need for and access to primary care services (*Federal Register*, 1998).

1. *Population-to-primary care practitioner ratio*. A ratio of 1250 persons per primary care practitioner is considered to be the lower end of the acceptable range. This definition includes obstetricians, gynecologists, nurse practitioners, physician assistants, and certified nurse midwives. Historically this has been accepted as the primary indicator of shortages.

2. *Percentage of population with income below 200% of the poverty level*. This variable represents the economic access barrier faced by many underserved populations, including not only Medicaid-eligibles but also many uninsured or underinsured working poor not eligible for Medicaid. The poverty level is set by federal officials, although individual states determine at what percentage of poverty children and adults qualify for Medicaid. Community Health Centers are required to provide a sliding fee scale to patients with incomes below 200% of the poverty level.

3. *Infant mortality (deaths per 1000 live births) and low birth weight rates (percentage of live births less than 2500 grams)*. The normal accepted rates are based on the Healthy People 2000 targets of no more than 7 infant deaths for every 1000 live births and no more than 5% low-weight live births. The low birth weight is a more helpful indicator because the event occurs more often than infant mortality. Access to primary care has been shown to lower the incidence of low-birth-weight infants.

4. *Percentage of the population that is a racial minority*. Like the rest of these variables, this one is based on census data which include African-Americans, Asian and Pacific Islanders, Native Americans, and other nonwhites in the definition of racial minority. This indicator is included because independent of income, some minority groups have a higher prevalence of certain diseases than the general population and poorer health. In addition, cultural barriers and discrimination can create access barriers to healthcare.

5. *Percentage of the population of Hispanic ethnicity*. Many individuals of Hispanic ethnicity experience negative health status effects and discriminatory and cultural barriers, independent of their income level, in the same way as the racial minorities described above. This group is considered separately because the census does not include persons of Hispanic origin in the "racial minority" group unless individuals identify themselves as "nonwhite."

6. *Percentage of the population that is linguistically isolated*. This is defined as the percentage of persons in households where no one over the age of 14 speaks English well. This is used as a direct measure of those persons with a severe language barrier. A person who cannot speak English will have difficulty calling a physician for advice, accessing emergency care, trying to explain his or her symptoms, or trying to comprehend the physician's instructions.

7. *Low population density*. This is a proxy for the long distances and travel times people in rural communities face. Even if the ratio of primary care practitioner to population approaches an acceptable level, people who have to travel an hour or more to reach a medical provider are at a distinct disadvantage.

Like Dr. Jenkins in Case 21-2, clinicians may first suspect that they are serving a medically underserved community when they find themselves delivering care to patients who they feel should have received earlier intervention. Often patients in such communities are able to access physicians only when they are ill or in the later stages of disease. Patients may lack a history of preventive care such as good immunization compliance or regular care for chronic diseases such as congestive heart disease. There may be significant discontinuity of care such as problems with coordination of medications or posthospitalization follow-up. There may also be difficulties in obtaining accurate patient histories; patients in medically underserved communities often do not know the name of their previous physician or their instructions for care. Providing care to patients in such communities is often frustrating and substandard. Although clinicians in such communities may attempt to provide good care, the dynamics of provider availability will often undermine the best-laid treatment plans.

The best long-term treatment plan may be to treat the underlying problem of physician shortages. Areas of the country federally designated as Medically Underserved Areas (MUA) qualify for special programs to expand physician availability.

The federal Public Health Service within the Department of Health and Human Services provides two loan repayment programs for clinicians who are willing to locate within an MUA. The first program is the National Health Service Corps (NHSC) Scholarship Program. Under this program, students pursuing medical degrees agree to place within an underserved area at the completion of their training. In exchange for this commitment, the federal government pays most or all of the cost of their training. Students are given a limited number of choices as to where they can practice.

In the 1980s, over 6000 medical graduates per year were NHSC scholars, but in recent years, because of funding cuts and high default rates by the scholars, the number of annual graduates has dropped significantly. Reducing the default rate and restoring this program to earlier levels of funding would help alleviate the current shortage of primary care physicians.

The federal government recently developed a second program called the National Health Services Corps Loan Repayment Program, which has greater flexibility than the first program and less financial benefit. Under this program, healthcare organizations located within an MUA may apply to be designated as eligible to hire an NHSC Loan Repayment Clinician. The federal government then assumes the debts incurred for previous medical training of the new clinician. The normal maximum obligation of the program is repayment of $25,000 in school debts per year of service for 3 years.

The NHSC program allows clinicians to match with any site that is deemed eligible for loan repayment and therefore provides a wider range of placement opportunities than the NHSC Scholarship Program. The wide selection of placement opportunities has made the NHSC Loan Repayment Program much more successful; its default rates are practically zero.

Many states and some local governments also offer various loan repayment and education incentives to attract providers to underserved areas. These programs range from formal programs such as grants to medical and nursing schools that provide care in underserved areas and state loan repayment programs, to less formal initiatives such as local community sponsorship of an individual clinician's training. Most physicians who choose to work in medically underserved areas find the experience challenging, rewarding, and meaningful while having a huge impact on the health and quality of life for people in the community that they serve.

## CASE 21-3

*Maria Contreras had come with her parents and four siblings to the United States from her native Dominican Republic in search of a better life. What the 17-year-old woman had found was that with no high school education and only limited ability to speak English, she and most of the other members of her family could not find work. Because of this, they all shared a two-bedroom apartment with an aunt and uncle who cleaned office buildings for a living.*

*When Maria became pregnant, she would not consider having an abortion or giving the child up for adoption. She had her baby and she then qualified for welfare, but the waiting list for permanent housing was so long that she had no hope of getting her own apartment for at least 2 years. Her medical providers had strongly urged Maria to breast-feed her child, but the infant was fussy and Maria gave up trying to nurse because she was exhausted from trying to keep the baby quiet in the overcrowded apartment and a girlfriend had told her that the baby would sleep better on formula. However, Maria had no space to refrigerate or store all of her baby's bottles. Her child had repeated problems with the formula and started to lose weight. The infant did not sleep and neither did other household members.*

## SEEING PATIENTS AND THEIR FAMILIES
## IN THEIR COMMUNITY CONTEXT

*As Salvador Minuchin (1984) has written in* Family Kaleidoscope, *"Looking at the family apart from its social context is like studying the dynamics of swimming by examining a fish in a frying pan. The result is intervention without perspective." We cannot always see patients in their communities, but we can infer from their stories what their homes, schools, churches, and other institutions are like, and when we do this, our effectiveness increases greatly.*

*On the sporadic visits when Maria brought her child to a clinic, the child was not well dressed for cold weather and had upper respiratory and ear infections, as well as symptoms of failure to thrive. Maria was usually exhausted and seemed totally unable to cope.*

## POVERTY

In 1999, 12.7% of all Americans were living below the poverty level. Racial disparities are noteworthy: 10.5% of whites lived below the poverty level while 26.1% of blacks and 25.6% of Hispanics lived below the poverty level in 1999. The data for children 6 years old and younger are dismal: 16.8% of white children live below the poverty level—a high number for an affluent country. More alarming is the fact that 39.6% of black children and 35.8% of Hispanic children 6 years old and under live below the poverty level. Unfortunately, Maria and her child are not alone.

The poverty level is defined as $17,050 for a family of four (*Federal Register*, 2000). When treating patients with such a lack of resources, even the simplest treatment plan may be virtually impossible for a patient to follow. Paying for food, housing, heat, electricity, day care for those trying to work, and transportation are among the expenses competing for the very scarce dollars in these homes.

In Case 21-3, we see the results of poverty: overcrowding, limited education, and stress on the provision of basic care to a newborn. In these circumstances, the provider would certainly advise the patient to move into her own apartment where she could get more sleep and where her baby would not be exposed to so many infections, if this were feasible. She would also be advised to pay more attention to her diet and that of her child. She obviously needs help with her parenting skills.

Patients such as Maria have needs that extend far beyond the capacity of the medical system to satisfy. There is no simple prescription for this patient. The thoughtful clinician will often have to seek resources beyond the healthcare system to care adequately for patients such as Maria and her child.

## BREAST-FEEDING VERSUS BOTTLE-FEEDING

*Breast-fed infants and their mothers benefit in many ways;*
- *Fewer infant infections because of maternal antibodies*
- *No formula intolerance (digestive problems, rashes)*
- *Less costly*
- *Easier for mother (no bottles to prepare)*
- *Mother often loses weight more readily*
- *Many feel it promotes closer bonding*

Indicators of extensive poverty within communities include significant numbers of people living below the federal poverty line, high infant mortality rates, higher than average unemployment rates, unaffordable housing, extreme overcrowding of living conditions, high rates of crime, and high rates of people without health insurance.

Clinicians who provide care in impoverished communities will often encounter patients who have histories of episodic illness and care, and who often delay seeking care until they are in the advanced stages of an illness.

The lack of financial resources will also cause patients not to follow through on recommended treatment plans including the purchase of necessary medications. Patients with chronic conditions such as hypertension and diabetes mellitus who could remain very healthy with appropriate use of medications will often be unable to afford those medications or, if they can occasionally afford them, will take them only when their budgets permit. They may take the medications at only half the recommended dosages or intervals. Similarly, when told to reduce work levels, or to change dressings regularly, poor patients may fail to comply because they simply cannot afford to do so.

The overcrowded living circumstances of patients in these communities often lead to high rates of infectious diseases such as tuberculosis, hepatitis, and upper respiratory infections. Such living conditions and the poverty that causes them also lead to increased stress, higher rates of domestic violence, and mental health problems. Finally, clinicians like those who treated Maria in Case 21-3 will often find higher rates of malnutrition and failure to thrive in poor communities.

Obviously clinicians cannot cure all of the social ills that cause their patients' disease, but many communities do have social supports that may benefit patients living in poverty. Community Action Programs (the so-called CAP Agencies) help patients obtain subsidized housing, temporary shelter, fuel assistance, and day care. Early Intervention Programs and Head Start are federally and state-supported programs that provide early stimulation and education to children at risk. They also occasionally provide training in parenting skills.

Children from low-income families qualify for federally and state-financed Medicaid Early Periodic Screening and Treatment of Disease (EPSTD) care. Such care guarantees payment to clinicians providing primary care and specialty services such as hearing and vision screening; occupational, physical, and speech therapy; and mental health treatment, when any of the aforementioned care is necessary for normal development of children and readiness to learn in school.

The Women, Infants, and Children (WIC) Program of the federal government provides nutritional counseling and food supplementation to women and children living below 185% of the federal poverty limit ($31,542 for a family of four) (Massachusetts Department of Public Health, 2000). This federal program, which began during the War on Poverty era of the Johnson Administration, provides pregnant and breast-feeding women and their children up to the age of 5 with vouchers for food "prescribed" by a nutritionist. Prescribed food items are those that will provide the greatest health outcome and cannot be substituted for others. Pregnant and breast-feeding mothers are given food vouchers for milk and other high-protein items;

---

## WIC

*WIC services are provided in the community where women can find them:*
- *County health departments*
- *Hospitals*
- *Mobile clinics (vans)*
- *Schools*
- *Public housing sites*
- *Migrant health centers and camps*
- *Indian Health Service facilities*

# BREAST-FEEDING

*The Healthy People 2000 goal for breast-feeding initiation is "to increase to at least 75 percent, the proportion of mothers who breast-feed their babies in the early postpartum period." If the "early postpartum period" is interpreted as the time of hospital discharge, the comparable percentage for WIC mothers is 45%. More than one-half of WIC mothers initiate breast-feeding. At the time of hospital discharge, less than one-half of all WIC mothers were still breast-feeding.*

*The breast-feeding duration goal in the Healthy People 2000 report is that at least 50% of infants are to be breast-fed until 5–6 months of age. Thirty-one percent of WIC mothers currently initiate breast-feeding, and only 16% of all WIC mothers continue breast-feeding until their infant is 5 months old.*

*Women who are less likely to breast-feed and who are most likely to quit if they try to breast-feed:*

- *Younger women*
- *African-American women (Hispanic women are more likely to breast-feed than either white or African-American women)*
- *Those born and raised in the United States*
- *Those who did not complete high school*
- *Those who were not encouraged by their physician to breast-feed*
- *Women who supplement breast milk with bottle-feeding*
- *Women who are discouraged by their own mothers*

infants whose mothers are not breast-feeding will have an appropriate formula prescribed. Clients in the program have their weights and hematocrits checked regularly to ensure good outcomes. The federal government estimates that for every dollar spent on WIC, three dollars is saved in medical costs as a result of prevention of premature birth, failure to thrive, and other health complications (Massachusetts Department of Public Health, 1995c).

It is very important for a clinician who is caring for poor patients to also know the services provided by the various public agencies run by that state. Most states will have local welfare, social service, youth service, public health, mental health, and public housing departments that provide an array of services helpful to the impoverished patient. Although it is often difficult to know exactly which services are provided by such public agencies, many social service departments of hospitals will have printed lists of agencies with a guide to the services they provide.

Although the services of the agencies mentioned here may help ameliorate the environmental conditions in which a patient lives, they usually do not improve the problems the poor and uninsured patient encounters when trying to obtain care within the medical system. It can be very difficult if not impossible to get patients the care they require when they are poor and uninsured. When trying to obtain emergency care for uninsured patients, providers may refer them to Hill–Burton-funded emergency rooms, which under federal law are required to treat any patient with a life-threatening condition and to provide care until the patient is stable. The Hill–Burton program was a federally funded program providing funds for the construction of hospitals under the proviso that the hospitals would agree to provide emergency services regardless of ability to pay. Increasingly, the offices of the attorneys general of many states are also producing guidelines of the community services required to be rendered by nonprofit hospitals. Nonprofit hospitals are exempt as charities from state and federal taxes and are therefore required to provide charitable services in exchange for this exemption. State guidelines for the services provided by the hospital usually include, at a minimum, free emergency care for patients with life-threatening illnesses. A description of the other services required of nonprofit hospitals to their communities may usually be found at the attorney general's office of each state.

An estimated 44.3 million people in the United States, or 16.3% of the population, had no health insurance in 1998, an increase of about 1 million people since 1997 (Bureau of the Census, 1998). In 1989, only

## UTILIZING COMMUNITY RESOURCES

*Sometimes all we need to do to improve a patient's health is to be aware of effective community resources and to help connect the patient with the resource.*

*Ways to increase your awareness:*

1. *Read the local newspapers, listen to radio and television paying attention to possible resources.*
2. *Listen to your patients when they tell you about resources that they have benefited from, perhaps a support group, a sliding scale membership at the YMCA, or a particularly helpful AA group in town.*
3. *Use the Internet.*
4. *Talk to other healthcare providers who care for patients similar to yours.*
5. *Stay in touch with your local health department.*

14.3% were uninsured (Employee Benefit Research Institute, 1995). Because of this alarming rate, and because the federal government has failed to institute any program to deal with it, many states have formulated their own programs for the uninsured. These programs range from virtual statewide entitlement to care in such states as Hawaii and Oregon, to pilot programs such as the free-car pools of Massachusetts and Florida. Many states have liberalized the eligibility requirements for Medicaid beyond those promulgated by the federal government. Providers should familiarize themselves with the programs that provide a "safety net" to the uninsured in their states.

The only federal program that provides primary care services to the uninsured is the Community Health Center Program (defined under Sections 329, 330, and 340 of the Public Health Service Act). Community Health Centers (CHCs) are outpatient primary care organizations specifically designed to provide care to undeserved communities. CHCs were started in 1965 by the Office of Economic Opportunity of the federal government to provide care for patients who lacked access to providers because of poverty or living in an underserved area. CHCs are supported by federal, state, and local grants as well as patient revenues and provide the single largest source of care to underserved patients in MUAs.

CHCs must provide care to patients without regard to their ability to pay or insurance status. These centers are designed to treat patients with barriers to care in the traditional medical system and frequently have bilingual staff, special transportation programs, and health education and disease prevention programs tailored to their communities. Most CHCs are independent charitable organizations run by community-based boards of directors and are therefore very familiar with the needs of the communities they serve. Over 850 CHCs provide care from more than 2000 locations to 8.8 million patients per year (National Association of Community Health Centers, 1995). They are essential resources for communities with high numbers of uninsured citizens.

## CASE 21-4

*A Bus Stop in Every Differential*

*—by Laura Frankenstein, M.D.*

**It left as we watched
Muddy, defaced, wounded by
Bullets
But it was ours, and had been for decades.
Abducted on a flatbed truck,
Yanked from the hard earth so near**

*Our door*
*Without notice, without alternative.*
*Now, if they came, they descended*
*Bus stops six blocks from our clinic's chaos.*
*Unfamiliar*
*Scary blocks, wet, cold, or searing hot, often dark blocks.*
*Inside the clinic we continued to care for people.*
*Or did we? Why did he miss his visit? Why did she*
*Stay at home*
*With her febrile infant's swollen red eyelid?*
*The day they took it*
*They said it was a mistake, changed the route,*
*"Forgot"*
*The stop served a clinic for the medically indigent.*
*Didn't mean to abandon the elderly, the frail, the addicted,*
*The wounded, the ill, the newborn of all colors, really.*
*But*
*Can't change a route for a year. "Takes that long."*
*"Takes that long" to alter a bus route, but*
*At least it might happen before a generation slips by.*
*How long*
*Before we value people, especially those unlike ourselves?*
*Together we scrambled, using mighty phone and*
*Pen, tried a few connections, and waited*
*Longer*
*Than a full-term pregnancy.*
*They heard our noise about the bus stop, but not our*
*Outrage about insidious sanctions that allow poverty to fester,*
*To flourish,*
*That makes it OK to shove away the undesirables.*
*We were students, residents, patients, members of staff*
*And board, determined to be heard.*
*We got it*
*Back, just outside our rusty door, and people came again.*

*(Reprinted with permission from the* **Journal of Family Practice***)*

## TRANSPORTATION BARRIERS

The above poem was written by a physician at a CHC after learning a lesson that had been omitted from her medical school residency training. Many patients are logistically barred from a regular source of primary care, and as Case 21-4 indicates, the lack of transportation can be an enormous barrier to effective patient care.

When patients live in a high-poverty area and there is no regular source of affordable public transportation or the average travel time to an affordable source of primary care exceeds 30 minutes, clinicians will begin to observe the effects of logistical barriers to care. These effects will usually include increased patient "no-show" rates for appointments and difficulties with patient compliance with follow-up treatment plans such as referrals, pediatric prevention visits and immunizations, as well as failure of some patients to obtain prescribed medications.

As Case 21-4 suggests, sometimes the provider needs to advocate for transportation necessary for adequate patient care. Other options open to the provider include working with Medicaid to provide transportation vouchers for deserving patients. Transportation programs also are occasionally provided by certain philanthropic organizations. For example, local chapters of the American Cancer Society often provide

## EASY WAYS TO SHARE INFORMATION WITH YOUR PATIENTS

*1. Provide pamphlets for commonly used resources such as the Women, Infant and Children's Nutrition Program (WIC), local AA and NA meetings, and domestic violence hotline numbers.*

*2. Offer credible Internet site addresses.*

*3. Place posters in your waiting or examination rooms.*

*4. Write your suggestion on your prescription pad to emphasize how much you value it.*

*5. Make an introductory phone call to an organization such as Hospice or to a Visiting Nurses Association.*

volunteers who will drive patients for visits necessary for diagnosis and treatment of cancer. Also, CHCs, which receive funding from the federal government, are required to provide funding for transportation of their patients to necessary medical services.

If a clinician suspects that a patient may not receive necessary medical treatment because of the lack of transportation, the provider should broach the subject of transportation problems with the patient and recommend one of the alternatives just mentioned.

## CASE 21-5

*Mr. and Mrs. Ieng had resided in the United States only 18 months when Mrs. Ieng discovered she was pregnant. They spoke no English and worked in a Cambodian market. Mrs. Ieng had very little knowledge of our medical system and did not seek any prenatal healthcare. She went to her local hospital when she realized that she was in labor. She felt very frightened because she guessed that her baby was coming too soon and because she did not know anyone at the hospital and none of the hospital staff spoke Khmer. Mrs. Ieng soon gave birth to twin sons who weighed 3 pounds each and had to be transferred to a tertiary care facility at the next largest city more than 30 miles away. When Mrs. Ieng was discharged, she was told by the telephone translation service used by the local hospital that her babies had been sent to another hospital, but she was never told the hospital address or that she was allowed to visit her babies. She was given the hospital address and visiting hours written in Khmer on a printed sheet that the hospital used for directing patients to the tertiary care facility. However, like many Cambodian patients, the Iengs were not literate in Khmer and therefore could not read the directions. Days went by, and when the parents of the twins did not attempt to visit them in the tertiary care hospital, the hospital social workers tried to contact the Iengs, but they had no telephone. As the twins improved, the social workers moved to have the children placed in foster care, feeling that the parents had abandoned them. It was only when, in a final effort to contact the parents, they called the CHC in the Iengs' hometown that they were finally able to reach the Iengs. As luck would have it, the Iengs had received their immigration physicals at the CHC and were known to one of the Cambodian caseworkers there. The caseworker went to the Iengs' market and found them totally distraught, having thought, when no one returned their children, that their babies had died or were severely ill.*

*Without the help of the health center staff who assisted the Iengs at the custody hearing for their children, the children would have been placed in foster care.*

## ———— LANGUAGE, LITERACY, AND CULTURAL BARRIERS

As Case 21-5 illustrates, language and cultural barriers, coupled with illiteracy, can have tragic consequences. The family in that case almost lost their children as a result of the inability of the medical system to cope with those barriers.

Over 1.1 million individuals immigrated to the United States in 1993; 700,000 permanent residents, 100,000–150,000 refugees, and 300,000 undocumented immigrants (U.S. Department of Justice, 1994). Many of them are not even literate in their own first languages. Often these newcomers have little or no knowledge of Western medicine and bring their own deeply ingrained beliefs and methods of healing.

To provide adequate care to patients from communities where there are significant numbers of residents who are not native to the United States, do not speak English, or who cannot read, it is extremely important to know the degree to which these problems exist. Information about your community that will help you provide effective care includes: the percentage of students in bilingual classes, the percentage of people who are non-English speaking, the percentage of residents with a high school education, and the availability of English as a second language classes for adults. Your local schools have most of this information. Community agencies that serve immigrant and refugee populations are aware of both the extent of the problem for those they serve as well as available resources.

When conditions such as the above prevail, patients will often have difficulty with written instructions, even when those instructions are written in their own language. Many times, patients will not readily admit that they cannot read and the clinician will have to reiterate instructions verbally and have patients repeat them back to ensure understanding. Videotapes in a patient's native language can be culturally and linguistically effective.

With patients who are newcomers to this country, there may be higher rates of atypical infectious microbial and parasitic diseases, and higher rates of preexisting conditions. One CHC with considerable numbers of newcomers diagnosed within a 6-month span both preexisting tumors in one child who had lived close to the Chernobyl nuclear plant and tuberculosis of the bone in a Hispanic child. These conditions would be highly unusual in children native to the United States.

Newcomer populations may have strongly held healing traditions native to their own countries and very limited knowledge of or appreciation for Western medicine. They may distrust providers who do not know or respect their cultural roots. To be effective, physicians should learn about the culture and religion of the patient populations they treat (see Chapters 24 and 29 for additional information). Without such knowledge, treatment can be impossible.

For example, if a clinician is treating a primarily Chinese-born population and decides to give the clinic a touch-up coat of paint, she might be very surprised when no prenatal patients come to the clinic. One might think that a simple "Caution! Wet Paint" sign would suffice to make patients comfortable. However, many Chinese people believe that if a pregnant woman inhales paint fumes, her baby will have birthmarks. Such unique beliefs can be found in all cultures, and must be known as well as respected if the provider is to forge a bond of mutual trust with newcomer patients.

Providing care to newcomer populations obviously poses some unique problems. Local cultural organizations can provide great resources in training caregivers about prevailing customs and perspectives on disease and treatment. Such in-service training is not only helpful to the clinic staff, but also sends a signal to the community that the providers are trying to understand and respect the beliefs and customs of their patients.

Language barriers are also difficult for the provider. Failure to bridge such language barriers can have drastic consequences, including impaired information flow from physician to patient that may result in inaccurate assessment of symptoms and misdiagnosis, increased dependency on testing with resulting increased inconvenience to patients, higher costs of care, and higher risks of false-positive results, problems with informed consent for procedures, and decreased medical compliance (Woloshin *et al.*, 1995).

Although translation services provided by the telephone company for a fee exist in most areas and are available in most languages, such services provide a very poor alternative to communicating directly with the patient in the patient's own language. Hiring bilingual office and medical assisting staff is a very good intermediate step to this problem. Where bilingual education programs exist, courses in the patient's native tongue are also often available. Many Community Action Programs, public schools, and colleges offer such foreign language programs. Also, large teaching hospitals in areas of high concentrations of foreign-born patients often offer medical foreign language programs. These programs are usually available at little or no cost.

If the clinician is consistently seeing patients who speak a language other than English, it is surprising how relatively little training in a foreign language is necessary to become proficient in basic communication with patients. Clearly one should not rely on limited foreign language skills alone when treating patients, but as a bridge between the patient and translation of some kind, even limited language skills are greatly appreciated by patients and help gain their trust.

Occasionally state or local philanthropic grants are available to organizations trying to hire bilingual staff, training existing staff, or in other ways make themselves more accessible to non-English-speaking minorities. Additionally, areas that have CHCs have fine resources for multilingual, culturally competent care, because CHCs specialize in providing such services to linguistically and culturally barred populations.

## CASE 21-6

*Joseph Connolly was a 45-year-old postal worker who had been employed 10 years in the city where he was born. He liked the work because it gave him a chance to exercise regularly and to be outside daily. Over the years, Joe found himself very short of breath when he hiked around his route. He also started getting sharp pains down both legs and he became increasingly worried that there was something seriously wrong with his health. However, even though his symptoms persisted and even worsened over the course of several months, his diagnosis of severe hypertension and sciatica was not made until Joe was forced to see a physician to obtain a premarital blood test.*

## PROVIDER DISCRIMINATION

It may well be a puzzle that the patient in Case 21-6 had worked around the corner from a large group practice and even though he had insurance and had worried about his symptoms, he had not sought medical care. However, the physician he sought for his blood test gradually uncovered a previous history of severe alcoholism that had left the patient destitute, without family, and living on the streets. In the past, when he had sought care, he had been so shabbily treated by his medical providers that he had decided to never seek care again unless absolutely necessary. Treating patients who are substance abusers, seriously mentally ill,

## SILENT KILLERS

*Hypertension is a chronic illness that is silent until it has caused significant damage. The only way to detect it is to check an individual's blood pressure with a blood pressure cuff. Once diagnosed, diet, weight loss, smoking cessation, and medications are used as treatments. Untreated, hypertension can eventually cause heart disease, strokes, renal failure, and peripheral vascular disease that can lead to amputations. The patient in Case 21-6 was experiencing shortness of breath, a symptom of congestive heart failure, due to his heart having to pump against significant resistance for many years. If he smokes or has high cholesterol or diabetes, his risks of complications are much greater. Without medical care the high cholesterol and diabetes will go undetected and treatment will be unnecessarily delayed. Sometimes people who are reluctant or cannot seek medical care, do have their blood pressure, even glucose and cholesterol levels checked at a health fair at a church or a shopping mall. This can be a less threatening place for some people and where they can be encouraged to connect with a physician.*

## SCIATICA

*Sciatica is an extremely painful acute or chronic condition that is caused by pressure on the sciatic nerve. This nerve is the size of your thumb, the largest of the body, running from the lumbar area of your spine to the legs and feet. Most often a vertebral disk protrudes from the spine putting pressure on the nerve, causing pain to run down one or both legs. Sciatica often prevents people from working. Treatments include heat, massage, rest (not bedrest as was once advised), physical therapy, judicious use of nonsteroidal anti-inflammatory medication (like ibuprofen) and muscle relaxants, and infrequently surgery. To prevent recurrences, patients should be taught how to exercise appropriately and to walk regularly. Smoking cessation has been shown to decrease the incidence and recurrence of back pain.*

homeless, or have personal beliefs that differ strongly from the caregiver's can be quite challenging. Discrimination against such patients, however, prevents adequate caregiving and can cause patients to refuse to seek or accept treatment. For these reasons, providers who work in communities with high numbers of complex and vulnerable patients need to be aware of the problems that exist within their communities and aware of the resources available to help such vulnerable patients. Characteristics of communities with high concentrations of patients with complex needs include:

- Total reported violent crime greater than 746 per 100,000 population (U.S. FBI, 1994)
- Drug arrest rates higher than 400 per 100,000 (U.S. FBI, 1994)
- Driving while intoxicated arrest rates greater than 120 per 100,000 (U.S. FBI, 1994)
- Alcohol- or drug-related hospital discharge rates higher than 600 per 100,000 (Massachusetts Department of Public Health, 1995a)
- HIV positivity rates greater than 4 per 1000 (Massachusetts Department of Public Health, 1995b)
- AIDS rates greater than 1.8 per 1000 (Massachusetts Department of Public Health, 1995b)

When a provider is working in a community with significant problems such as those listed above, caregiving can become complicated. Often patients in such communities display the lack of trust shown by the mail carrier in Case 21-6. They may also have difficulty providing an adequate history of past treatment because of discontinuity of care or memory lapses.

Patients with alcoholism, substance abuse, or mental health problems may have multiple primary diagnoses coupled with their history of poor prior treatment. They may also show considerable lack of willingness to work with the provider to treat underlying medical problems and may integrate into the medical system only as long as it takes to alleviate the symptoms that brought the patient to the provider in the first place. Providers of complex patients such as these may feel "used," thinking that the patient is only trying to "get something from them" and that they can't trust the reliability of their patients' reporting. The important thing is to render the best care that one can in a nonjudgmental way, thus leaving the door open to future patient contact should the patient desire it.

Most areas have free substance abuse treatment programs supported by the federal government. These federal Office of Substance Abuse Prevention (OSAP) programs provide outpatient as well as inpatient treatment for patients with substance abuse problems. Sometimes the waiting lists for such programs are long. However, there are no waiting lists for 12-step programs such as Alcoholics Anonymous or Narcotics Anonymous available in most communities. Although the 12-step programs do not take the place of comprehensive OSAP programs, they can help maintain patients' sobriety and provide a supportive environment for patients.

Additionally, many states offer mental health programs through Medicaid, disability and general relief status, or through Departments of Mental and Public Health, which provide clinical support to those with

## UNLIKELY COMMUNITY RESOURCES

1. Building managers and landlords *often know elders without family or friends better than anyone else. They may contact you when they have concerns about a patient falling, wandering, or acting strangely. With the patient's permission they can help relay information to a patient without a phone or continue to keep you up-to-date the way a family member might.*

2. *An alcoholic, schizophrenic man, who had severe asthma and was a heavy smoker living alone in a boarding house room without a phone, couldn't use a nebulizer on his own. Fortunately the convenience store he frequented many times a day took an interest in him. They encouraged him to cut back on the cigarettes he purchased and smoked, hooked up and supervised his nebulizer treatments T.I.D., and gave him messages when the physician's assistant caring for him needed to reach him. He eventually quit smoking and rarely was hospitalized for asthma exacerbations.*

3. *An elderly man became depressed, ate irregularly, and stopped taking his medications for hypertension a year after the death of his wife. His physician wrote a prescription for him to enroll in a volunteer program at a local school where he began reading stories to second graders. A nurse referred him to an animal shelter where he adopted a beagle puppy. The depression began to lift, nutrition improved, and the man began taking his medications again.*

substance abuse or mental health problems. Once a patient has a mental health provider, that provider can often bypass waiting lists for programs such as OSAP and can get patients much-needed treatment more efficiently.

### CASE 21-7

*Anne is a family physician who has been in practice 7 years. By now she knows not only her patients' medical problems, she also knows a lot about their social, economic, occupational, and family situations. Maybe because she knows her patients so well and cares about them, she gets frustrated when she cannot prevent progression of disabling chronic illnesses such as diabetes, hypertension, and heart disease. Florence is a 62-year-old high school mathematics teacher. Although Anne has treated her for hypertension, hypercholesterolemia, and obesity, she has a stroke that leaves her paralyzed on one side and unable to speak clearly. Without family nearby who can care for her she has to go to a nursing home. Florence is depressed and angry about her situation. Anne is saddened and discouraged. She had helped Florence stop smoking and had met with her every 3 months to adjust her medications: what else could she do to prevent such tragedies?*

## HEALTHY PEOPLE 2010

Anne is not alone. It can seem futile when physicians do everything they can to counsel and treat patients effectively and yet patients still have bad outcomes. In this case Anne felt that she and her patient had a good relationship, that the patient was doing everything she could, and that they were making progress treating her illnesses. Unfortunately, Florence, like many of Anne's patients, had been heavy most of her life and had trouble keeping fit. The more Anne thought about it, the more she admitted to herself that she was not very effective at helping people lose weight. Was it her inadequacy as a physician, or was it something more pervasive?

# HEALTHY PEOPLE 2010

*Healthy People 2010 is firmly dedicated to the principle that—regardless of age, gender, race, ethnicity, income, education, geographic location, disability, and sexual orientation—every person in every community in the United States deserves equal access to comprehensive, culturally competent, community-based healthcare systems that are committed to serving the needs of the individual and promoting community health.*

*Healthy People 2010 recognizes that communities, states, and national organizations will need to take a multidisciplinary approach to achieving health equity that involves improving health, education, housing, labor, justice, transportation, agriculture, and the environment.*

Anne starts to do some research and comes across Healthy People 2010 on the Internet (U.S. Department of Health and Human Services, 2000). She finds it well organized and quite powerful. She finds herself drawn into reading about more than treatments for obesity. She discovers that Healthy People 2010 represents the ideas and expertise of a diverse range of individuals and organizations concerned about the nation's health. The Healthy People Consortium—an alliance of more than 350 national organizations and 250 state public health, mental health, substance abuse, and environmental agencies—conducted three national meetings on the development of Healthy People 2010. In addition, many individuals and organizations gave testimony about health priorities at five Healthy People 2010 regional meetings held in late 1998.

On two occasions—in 1997 and 1998—the U.S. public was even given the opportunity to share its thoughts and ideas. More than 11,000 comments on draft materials were received by mail or via the Internet from individuals in every State, the District of Columbia, and Puerto Rico. The final Healthy People 2010 objectives were developed by teams of experts from a variety of federal agencies under the direction of Health and Human Services Secretary Donna Shalala, Assistant Secretary for Health and Surgeon General David Satcher, and former Assistant Secretaries for Health. The process was coordinated by the Office of Disease Prevention and Health Promotion, U.S. Department of Health and Human Services.

Healthy People 2010 is designed to achieve two general goals. The first is to increase quality and years of healthy life, and the second is to eliminate health disparities among different segments of the population. These include differences that occur by gender, race or ethnicity, education or income, disability, living in rural localities, or sexual orientation.

These goals serve as a guide for developing a set of objectives that will actually measure progress within a specified amount of time. The objectives focus on the determinants of health, which encompass the

# THE COST OF OBESITY

*Fifty-five percent of adults in the United States are overweight or obese. Over two decades, the number of cases of obesity alone has increased more than 50%—from 14.5% of the adult population to 22.5%. Approximately 25% of adult women and 20% of adult men in the United States are obese. Many diseases are associated with overweight and obesity: high blood pressure, type II diabetes, coronary heart disease, stroke, gallbladder disease, osteoarthritis, sleep apnea, respiratory problems, and some types of cancer. The health outcomes related to these diseases, however, often can be improved through weight loss or, at a minimum, no further weight gain. Total costs (medical costs and lost productivity) attributable to obesity alone amounted to an estimated $99 billion in 1995 (U.S. Department of Health and Human Services, 2000, Healthy People, 2010).*

## BODY MASS INDEX

*Body mass index (BMI) is a measure of obesity. It is calculated by dividing weight (in kilograms) by the square of the height (in meters). A BMI >27 is equivalent to being more than 20% overweight and is associated with increased health risk. To make this a more useful tool in the office setting, physicians often carry a small chart that lists the BMI for weights in pounds and heights in inches.*

combined effects of individual and community physical and social environments and the policies and interventions used to promote health, prevent disease, and ensure access to quality healthcare. The ultimate measure of success in any health improvement effort is the health status of the target population. The nation's progress in achieving the two goals of Healthy People 2010 will be monitored through 467 objectives in 28 focus areas. Many objectives focus on interventions designed to reduce or eliminate illness, disability, and premature death among individuals and communities. Others focus on broader issues, such as improving access to quality healthcare, strengthening public health services, and improving the availability and dissemination of health-related information. Each objective has a target for specific improvements to be achieved by the year 2010.

One of the most compelling and encouraging lessons learned from the past decade's work, the Healthy People 2000 initiative, is that we, as a nation, can make dramatic progress in improving the nation's health in a relatively short period of time (U.S. Department of Health and Human Services, 1990). For example, during the last decade, we achieved significant reductions in infant mortality. Childhood vaccinations are at the highest levels ever recorded in the United States. Fewer teenagers are becoming parents. Overall, alcohol, tobacco, and illicit drug use is leveling off. Death rates for coronary heart disease and stroke have declined. Significant advances have been made in the diagnosis and treatment of cancer and in reducing unintentional injuries.

There are other devastating areas yet to be addressed successfully. Of note to Anne, obesity in adults has increased 50% over the past two decades. Nearly 40% of adults engage in no leisure time physical activity.

Healthy People 2010 emphasizes the key role of community partnerships particularly when they reach out to nontraditional partners to improve health in communities. Anne felt less alone when she read of cooperation between the federal government, states, local governments, communities, businesses, civic, professional, and religious organizations. These types of groups have been inspired by previous Healthy People objectives to print immunization reminders, set up hotlines, change cafeteria menus, begin community recycling, establish worksite fitness programs, assess school health education curriculums, sponsor health fairs, and engage in myriad other activities. Opportunities for reducing health disparities include empowering individuals to make informed healthcare decisions and promoting communitywide safety, education, and access to healthcare.

A great deal of data will be gathered during the next decade to determine how much progress is made. The leading health indicators reflect the major public health concerns in the United States and were chosen based on their ability to motivate action, the availability of data to measure their progress, and their relevance as broad public health issues. These indicators illuminate individual behaviors, physical and social environmental factors, and important health system issues that affect the health of individuals and communities. Underlying each of these indicators is the significant influence of income and education. These indicators are:

- Physical Activity & Fitness
- Nutrition & Obesity
- Tobacco Use
- Substance Abuse
- Responsible Sexual Behavior

- Mental Health
- Injury and Violence
- Environmental Quality
- Immunization
- Access to Health Care

Turning her attention to 2 of the 28 focus areas in Healthy People 2010, those of Nutrition & Obesity and Physical Activity & Fitness, Anne discovers that the sections include background information and ample references. Disparities in health status indicators and risk factors for diet-related disease are evident in many segments of the population based on gender, age, race and ethnicity, and income. For example, overweight and obesity are observed in all population groups, but obesity is particularly common among Hispanic, African-American, Native American, and Pacific Islander women.

She concentrates on the opportunities sections, which describe efforts that many segments of society can make together to improve this growing problem. She reads all of the objectives for these areas. One objective is to increase the proportion of adults who are at a healthy weight. The target by 2010 is that 60% of adults aged 20 and older will be at a healthy weight [defined as a body mass index (BMI) equal to or greater than 18.5 and less than 25]. In 1988–1994 only 42% of adults met this criterion. She realizes she needs to concentrate more on children to prevent obesity and more on helping people of every age increase their physical activity. She considers doing the following herself:

1. Check with the schools in her town to see if nutrition education is in the curriculum since research suggests that parents who understand proper nutrition can help preschoolers choose healthful foods, but they have less influence on the choices of school-aged children. She has learned that a survey done in 1994 showed that only 69% of states and 80% of school districts required nutrition education for students in at least some grades from kindergarten through 12th grade.
2. At the same time check with the schools about the nutritional content of meals and find out how much time they have each week for physical activity.
3. Based on the objectives in Healthy People 2010 she can discuss her concerns with the schools or write an editorial to the newspaper emphasizing the importance of these issues.
4. She will add to her waiting room literature that is easy to read, in the languages her patients speak, and will include a list of resources for patients of all ages with local opportunities for exercising.
5. She may purchase interesting, well-researched nutrition and fitness videotapes for her waiting room. If she or her staff can't find any, especially in languages other than English, perhaps the local college communications department would like to take this on as a project.
6. When she gets a chance she could call the closest YMCA for sliding fee information and see if they would like to cosponsor a promotional event with her hospital to promote healthy eating and exercise.
7. She will ask the medical student who will join her next week to consider doing a community project that addresses these issues, based on his interests. She knows he was on the track team in college; perhaps he has some ideas.

---

*Go in search of people.*
*Begin with what they know.*
*Build on what they have.*
—Chinese proverb

*People find us in our offices and hospitals. Sometimes directing them to useful community resources is as simple as reinforcing an opportunity familiar to them. An elderly grieving widow I care for this year was suffering alone until I encouraged her to talk with her priest and seek out the comfort of women she knew from church. She discovered a bereavement support group and since then I have been able to refer another family to the same church. The patients are healthier, they spend less time and money in my office, and the priest likes the fact that I am giving him some business.*

---

## WHY BOTHER WITH COMMUNITY HEALTH PROMOTION? DON'T WE HAVE ENOUGH TO DO ALREADY?

*1. We can increase our effectiveness by linking patients to resources.*
*2. We can reduce our own frustration and burnout.*
*3. Working with others on a board of directors or a committee can be fun and helps reduce the isolation we can feel working in an office setting.*
*4. It may remind us of the reasons we became physicians in the first place.*

---

8. As soon as she sees one of the nutritionists in the hospital when she is rounding, she will check to see what initiatives she knows about and what materials she can share.
9. She will pay closer attention to opportunities she has for participating in health fairs, perhaps speaking to community groups or supporting a proposal for a bike path in her area.

Anne returns to her practice knowing she will continue to face this problem daily with individuals and families, but she feels a little less frustrated, is glad to have some effective interventions, and is relieved that others in many other fields and segments of society are making this a national priority.

---

# CONCLUSION

Patients come into their caregivers' offices encumbered with many and varied obstacles to care related to their environments and social circumstances. Adequate treatment of patients depends on the ability of the provider to diagnose not only the patient, but also the community from which the patient comes. Only then will the provider have the correct context in which to make assumptions about the likely diagnosis and prognosis of the patient's disease; only then will the provider know the treatment plan most likely to effect a satisfactory outcome; only then will the provider know the most efficient and effective resources to bring to bear on the patient's problem.

When patients repeatedly seek care for the same problem and obstacles to effective treatment exist in the community, the most efficient and comprehensive treatment plan the provider can effectuate may be a change within the environment itself. We have seen that when environmental resources fall short in the treatment of disease, sometimes the caring provider can help create them. At a minimum, he can make others aware of the barriers to care that exist within the community and, through advocacy, can remove them.

---

# CASES FOR DISCUSSION

## CASE 1

*The local elder service agency has called you to make a home visit to assess the status of an 81-year-old woman who is allegedly a victim of abuse by her daughter and son-in-law with whom she lives. On reviewing her records from the VNA, you find that she is status-post two hip fractures and has Parkinson's disease, chronic obstructive pulmonary disease, and a seizure disorder. Your examination reveals that she has severe rheumatoid arthritis and angina pectoris, as well as failure to thrive. You suspect that both the daughter and the son-in-law with whom she lives are schizophrenic and labile. You also suspect that they may be substance-dependent and may be stealing your patient's Social Security checks.*
*The patient is reluctant to leave the home because she is very attached to her two granddaughters, aged 7 and 13, who also live with her.*

*1. How do you best stabilize and treat this patient?*

2. *What are the implications of supporting the elder service agency's recommendation to file a protective court order which would have her removed from the home and placed in a safe environment?*
3. *Are there other options for the protection and care of this patient?*

## CASE 2

*Your patient is a Hispanic woman with advanced AIDS (CD4 count = 15). Even though you had told her many times to call you if she had any problems, one night when she couldn't breathe, had a temperature of 102°F, and was very frightened, she drove herself to the nearest emergency room and was admitted with a diagnosis of histoplasmosis. You did not have staff privileges at the hospital where she was admitted, and that hospital was not used to treating patients with AIDS.*

*Her care during her hospitalization was uncoordinated. Even though you discussed her case over the telephone with her attending physician, an open lung biopsy was performed instead of the bronchoscopy you recommended. Staff at the hospital shared her AIDS diagnosis with family members without the patient's permission.*

1. *How can you best help your patient under these circumstances?*
2. *The Hispanic social worker from your clinic is very concerned about the patient's two children who are staying with an aunt. The social worker says that the aunt cannot care for the children much longer and they will be placed in foster care if something is not done.*
3. *Finally the patient is stable and discharged. You want to prevent this type of occurrence again, but you realize that the hospital where she was admitted is the closest one to her home. What should you do to help your patient in future care?*

## CASE 3

*The triage nurse in your clinic asks you to see a walk-in patient who has never been treated at your clinic. The patient is highly agitated, disheveled, and confused. She tells you that she thinks she has "bugs" and that her dog has them too, whereupon she opens a large shoulder bag she is carrying and her dog scampers out into your examination room. She says that she can't take the itching anymore and that she will kill herself if you can't help her. She states that she has already "chopped" her own hair and she will chop herself next.*

1. *How should you begin to assess this patient? She has no self-reported history of primary care or mental health treatment. In fact, she says that physicians "give her the creeps."*
2. *Should you attempt to begin a primary care relationship with this patient, and if so, how do you do so?*
3. *The patient tells you that she wants you to help her dog and her boyfriend too because she knows that they have the "bugs too" and she'll just get them back. How do you respond to her?*

## CASE 4

*A 19-month-old child is brought to your clinic with a temperature of 102°F and tugging at his ear. You quickly diagnose otitis media, but on reading his chart you realize that he is long overdue for a history and physical examination. His last immunizations were at 6 months of age.*

1. *How do you best care for the child?*
2. *When you ask the mother why she has missed so many appointments, she states that she "just forgot" and that she also has changed addresses twice since the last visit and she has no car. How do you help her and reinforce the importance of the child's regular primary care?*

## CASE 5

*A 50-year-old black Haitian-American man who speaks only French Creole comes to your office with his wife. His wife speaks enough English to serve as the translator and when you request the patient's chief complaint, the patient seems to gesture and say that he has chest pains. His wife adds that the chest pains come from an evil spirit placed on the husband because he had an affair with the woman next door. She states that the only way the husband will get any better is if he goes to her French Pentecostal church, confesses his sin, and is exorcised. The wife appears to you to be attending the patient's appointment grudgingly and with great hostility. You are not convinced that she is providing a word-for-word translation of your dialogue with the patient.*

1. *What is the best way to begin to treat this patient?*
2. *Should you continue to use his wife as the translator for his care?*
3. *You have in your office a young nursing student who is fluent in French and says that she understands some Creole. Should you use her as a translator instead?*

## CASE 6

*You work in a clinic in an impoverished inner-city area. The wait for an appointment for a physical examination of a new patient is 12 weeks, and a regular patient of the clinic must wait at least 8 weeks. Your patients call all the time needing immediate physical examinations for entry into school, Head Start, summer camp, or to get jobs. Without these examinations, you know that your patients will suffer.*

1. *How do you handle your patients' requests?*
2. *In the long run, how should you begin to deal with this problem?*

# RECOMMENDED READINGS

Aday LA: *At Risk in America. The Health and Health Care Needs of Vulnerable Populations in the United States.* San Francisco, Jossey–Bass, 1993.

> A comprehensive examination of vulnerable patient populations as well as a description of approaches to their care.

Birrer RB: *Urban Family Medicine.* New York, Springer-Verlag, 1987.

> A practical guide to physician practice within the community.

Nutting PA: *Community Oriented Primary Care: From Principle to Practice.* Albuquerque, University of New Mexico Press, 1990.

> A thorough examination of the COPC approach to defining and then preventing and treating disease within a community.

Pathman DE: The four community dimensions of primary care practice. *J Fam Pract* 46(4), 1998.

> A description of the practical ways physicians can incorporate community experience in their practice. Based on a study supporting the hypothesis that the community plays a role in the work of physicians.

Sardell A: *The U.S. Experiment in Social Medicine. The Community Health Center Program, 1965–1986.* Pittsburgh, University of Pittsburgh Press, 1988.

> An interesting exploration of the history of community health centers and the role they play in today's medical system.

U.S. Department of Health and Human Service: Healthy People 2010: Objectives for Improving Health. Washington, DC, Government Printing Office, 2000. *www.health.gov/healthypeople/.*

> Setting the nation's health agenda for the next decade, this comprehensive document combines the efforts of experts in many fields to set goals to improve the health status of all Americans. Full of background data and references, it motivates us to work within communities to promote health.

# REFERENCES

Bindman A, *et al*: Preventable hospitalization and health care access. *JAMA* 274:305–311, 1995.

Bureau of the Census: *Statistical Abstract of the United States.* Washington, DC, Department of Commerce, 1998.

Council on Graduate Medical Education (COGME): *Improving Access to Health through Physician Workforce Reform: Dimensions for the Twenty-first Century.* Washington, DC, Health Resource Services Administration, 1992.

Employee Benefit Research Institute: *Sources of Health Insurance and Characteristics of the Uninsured.* Special Report: Issue Brief 158, 1995.

*Federal Register*: Designation of Medically Underserved Areas 63(169):46541–46542, 1998.

*Federal Register*: Poverty Income Guidelines 60(27):7772, 2000.

Massachusetts Department of Public Health: *CHNA 14 Report.* Boston, Massachusetts Department of Public Health, 1995a.

Massachusetts Department of Public Health: *HIV/AIDS Surveillance Monthly Update.* Boston, Massachusetts Department of Public Health, 1995b.

Massachusetts Department of Public Health: *WIC Program Coordination and Outreach Manual*. Boston, Massachusetts Department of Public Health, 1995c.

Massachusetts Department of Public Health: *WIC Program Coordination and Outreach Manual*. Boston, Massachusetts Department of Public Health, 2000.

Minuchin S: *Family Kaleidoscope*. Cambridge, Mass, Harvard University Press, 1984.

National Association of Community Health Centers (NACHC): *America's Health Centers*. Washington, DC, National Association of Community Health Centers, 1995.

Pathman DE: The four community dimensions of primary care practice. *J Fam Pract* 46(4), 1998.

Society for Ambulatory Care Professionals (SACP): Community health centers in Ontario: A paper presented by Ms. Wendy Muckle, Executive Director of the Ontario Community Health Center, 1993.

U.S. Department of Health and Human Services: Healthy People 2000: Objectives for Improving Health. Washington, DC, Government Printing Office, 1990.

U.S. Department of Health and Human Services: Healthy People 2010: Objectives for Improving Health. Washington, DC, Government Printing Office, 2000. *www.health.gov/healthypeople/*

U.S. Department of Justice: *Immigration and Naturalization Service Fact Book: Summary of Recent Immigration Data*. Washington, DC, Department of Justice, U.S. Immigration and Naturalization Service Statistics Division, 1994.

U.S. Federal Bureau of Investigation: *Crime in the US, 1993*. Washington, DC, Federal Bureau of Investigation, 1994.

Whitcomb ME: A cross-national comparison of generalist physician workforce data: Evidence for US supply adequacy. *JAMA* 274: 692–695, 1995.

Woloshin S, *et al*: Language barriers in medicine in the United States. *JAMA* 273:724–728, 1995.

## CHAPTER 22

# The Workplace

*Annette M. David and Mark R. Cullen*

There are many things that a doctor, on his first visit to a patient, ought to find out either from the patient or from those present. For so runs the oracle of our inspired teacher: "When you come into a patient's house, you should ask him what sort of pains he has, what caused them, how many days he has been ill, whether his bowels are working, and what sort of food he eats." ... I may venture to add one more question: What occupation does he follow?

Bernardino Ramazzini
De Morbis Artificum (Diseases of Workers), 1713

## CASE 22-1

*Mr. A. K. is a 43-year-old man who was seen at the Primary Care Clinic with a chief complaint of "fatigue." He stated that he had been feeling "crummy" for over a month and was concerned about his health. The physician was unable to elicit a coherent history of any illness. However, the review of systems indicated numerous nonspecific symptoms such as joint aches and several episodes of crampy abdominal pain, which Mr. A. K. attributed to "dyspepsia." The results of the physical examination were unremarkable.*

*At this point, the physician began to suspect a nonorganic etiology for Mr. A. K.'s symptoms. Still, because the patient insisted on it, blood was drawn for a CBC. This revealed a low hemoglobin and hematocrit, results that surprised the clinician. Red blood cell indices were indicative of a normocytic, normochromic anemia. He called Mr. A. K. back for a follow-up visit, during which a second blood draw was done for a reticulocyte count, which proved to be elevated.*

*Called back for his third clinic visit, Mr. A. K. was questioned extensively about a family history of hemolytic anemia, which he denied. There was no previous history of sickle cell trait, G6PD deficiency, or the presence of an intravascular prosthesis. However, Mr. A. K. did mention that his symptoms began shortly after he started restoration work on a 150-year-old farmhouse. Intrigued, the physician asked Mr. A. K. what his job entailed. "I'm a painter," replied Mr. A. K. Properly enlightened, the physician did a third blood draw, which indicated a marked elevation in blood lead level and zinc protoporphyrin. The diagnosis: acute lead poisoning.*

1. Appreciate the impact of workplace exposures on health
2. Recognize the different types of clinical encounters that may involve workplace issues
3. Understand the factors that lead to ethical dilemmas when dealing with work-related illness
4. Apply the principles of occupational medicine when analyzing clinical cases resulting from potential workplace exposures

## INTRODUCTION

The Bureau of Labor Statistics of the U.S. Department of Labor estimates that in November 1999 134.1 million people were employed in private industry. Not included in that figure are the self-employed or the employees of federal and state agencies. Altogether, the total number of workers in the United States comprises the majority of the adult population.

Physicians and public health officials are becoming more cognizant of the impact of the workplace on the health of workers. On the one hand, the workplace is being targeted for interventions to promote health and to prevent disease. On the other hand, we continue to discover many potentially damaging effects of workplace exposures. Clearly, the workplace is an arena that must be of interest to all practitioners of medicine caring for adults.

Most working men and women obtain their healthcare not from occupational or worksite-based clinics but from primary care providers: internists, family practitioners, physician's assistants, and nurse practitioners. Mr. A. K. in Case 8-1, for example, sought help from a physician at a primary care clinic. Whether they are conscious of it, these clinicians are engaged in the practice of occupational medicine and should be knowledgeable about the basic principles of occupational disease.

Unfortunately, occupational medicine training remains outside the mainstream of U.S. medical education and training. For instance, in 1985, a survey showed that only 50% of U.S. medical schools included occupational and environmental health in their curricula; the average time spent on occupational medicine during 4 years was 4 hours (Levy, 1985). By 1992, not much improvement was noted, with 66% of schools devoting an average of 6 hours to occupational and environmental medicine (Burstein & Levy, 1994). Residency training in the primary care specialties offers little as well (Cullen & Rosenstock, 1988).

## Work-Related Medical Visits

How many medical encounters involve work-related problems? Definitive data to answer this question do not exist. In the inpatient setting, one study found that occupational factors were implicated in over 10% of all admissions to a general medicine ward (Gannart *et al.*, 1991). A more recent survey done in Israel revealed that more than 40% of patients hospitalized on general medicine wards believed that occupational risk factors contributed significantly to the development of their current illness, but in none of the medical records was the exposure documented by the attending physicians.

Few studies have focused on outpatient medical visits. However, experienced primary care providers would agree that a significant portion of their patient encounters are generated by health concerns that are directly related to workplace issues. There are straightforward "industrial medicine" visits that require healthcare providers to evaluate individuals for work fitness. Preplacement physicals and respiratory fitness evaluations are good examples. In addition, many corporations are downsizing their medical departments for economic reasons and utilizing community primary care facilities to do urgent care for their employees who suffer from on-the-job accidents and injuries. Because of recent federal mandates on drug and alcohol testing in the workplace, physicians are being asked to serve as medical review officers by both government and private sector companies.

## WORLDWIDE, TWO PEOPLE DIE EACH MINUTE FROM OCCUPATIONALLY RELATED CAUSES

*Each year, work-related injuries and illnesses kill an estimated 1.1 million people. Annually, approximately 160 million new cases of work-related diseases occur. These figures are almost certainly based on underestimates.*

*WHO, 1999*

Increasingly, third-party payers are expecting primary care practitioners to provide information regarding disability and work restrictions. Such requests also come from lawyers involved in workers' compensation cases or class action suits related to workplace exposures. Patients themselves may present to their healthcare providers for a variety of reasons. Some may request an evaluation and a letter to excuse themselves from absence at work because of an illness—the sickness excuse. Others have illnesses that they suspect may be attributed to their work. A survey in 1991 determined that 17% of patients seen in a primary care clinic thought their health problems were work-related (Schwartz *et al.*, 1991). Most importantly, patients with symptoms that were not initially ascribed to a workplace exposure may turn out to have an occupational disease. The case of Mr. A. K. presented at the beginning of this chapter is a good example.

## Work and Disease Causation

Where does the workplace fit in disease causation? Medicine has traditionally focused on the infectious disease model that emphasizes the host–agent interaction, almost to the exclusion of the environment within which this interaction occurs and of the patient's activities in that setting. Occupational medicine broadens that view, with agent, environment, and activity all assuming major roles in disease causation. Most working people spend an average of 8 hours at work per day, which translates into at least a quarter of one's entire life spent at the workplace. It should be apparent that the work environment may have a substantial impact on an individual's state of health. A good physician must spend some time understanding what the work environment entails to better understand the nature of the work-related health problem.

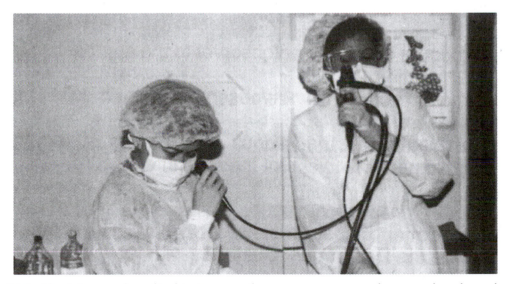

**Figure 22.1.** Physicians and medical trainees perform numerous procedures, such as bronchoscopy, that put them at risk for exposure to airborne pathogens like *Mycobacterium tuberculosis*. Photo courtesy of the Pulmonary Division, Department of Medicine, Philippine General Hospital.

In the infectious disease model, the infectious agent and the host assume paramount importance. Measures to prevent or control disease can be targeted toward either the agent causing disease or the susceptible host. For example, if the virus causing an infection can be identified, an antiviral agent can be developed against that virus. Antibiotics can be manufactured to combat specific bacteria. The host can be immunized or prevented from coming into contact with agents of disease. Occupational health extends this concept one step further by taking the broader workplace environment as a third potential target for interventions designed to prevent or cure disease. Thus, engineering and administrative controls can be instituted to reduce harmful exposures. Work processes can be changed to alter their impact on disease. And when necessary, protective devices can be used to further control risks. How can work cause disease? There are certain health hazards that exist because of harmful agents in an individual's work. The miner exposed to silica, the firefighter exposed to carbon monoxide, the medical intern exposed to *Mycobacterium tuberculosis*, the pathology technician who uses formalin (formalin can contain up to 50% formaldehyde by weight), and the house painter exposed to lead in paint are good examples.

In other cases, the work itself is the hazard. The movie stuntman is constantly at risk of losing life and limb. A data entry clerk who uses a keyboard 8 hours a day can eventually develop cumulative trauma to her wrists and hands. Outdoor workers must contend with markedly enhanced ultraviolet radiation exposure and hazards associated with the elements.

Preexisting health conditions can be aggravated by work. The asthmatic laborer in a dusty factory and the diabetic with neuropathy who works with solvents are both at risk of worsening their preexisting health problems.

Psychological and social stresses at work can also affect an individual's health and sense of well-being. In today's economic climate, the constant threat of unemployment is a real fear for many people. In addition, in this technological age, workers have to grapple with uncertainty about the future as automation replaces skilled craftsworkers and laborers. Persons employed in factory lines and large office pools have to come to terms with the drudgery of their work. For the sake of efficiency, their workplaces have been dehumanized, and their tasks reduced to often meaningless, repetitive motions. An increasing number of working adults no longer obtain a sense of satisfaction and personal identity from what they do. Instead, work to them is a chore, something that must be done in order to survive, nothing more than a distasteful necessity to be gotten over with each day as quickly as possible. The anxiety and resentment that this situation generates can contribute to ill health. In fact, work-related stress has been found to be strongly associated with sleep disturbance and depression, as well as with elevated risks of cardiovascular diseases, particularly hypertension. In addition, work-related tensions often spill over into the personal lives of these individuals. Indeed, the complex interplay of work, health, and personal and family life is a reality that healthcare providers need to recognize, assess, and be able to address.

## Work and Health

While acknowledging that the work environment is an integral component of disease causation, an experienced physician also recognizes the positive effects of work on health. Work can be defined as any activity that is expended to support the basic needs of the individual and of society. From an individual perspective, work is the means by which people procure the ability to provide for their desires and needs. By working, one also makes a contribution to society and establishes a social identity. A successful worker is a successful person. Work achievement becomes a measure of adult functional capacity and is therefore an affirmation of health (Deubner, 1987b). Occupational medicine is as committed to supporting well-being and excellent function in the healthy worker as it is to uncovering work-related illness and preventing disease *per se*.

*In the United States, healthcare expenditures are nearly 50% greater for workers who report high levels of stress at work.*

*WHO, 1999*

# Ethical Dilemmas in the Occupational Medicine Encounter

By its nature, dealing with occupational health problems often gives rise to ethical dilemmas. When the referral source is other than the individual patient, the issue of loyalty or allegiance arises. Can the healthcare provider function in an unbiased, objective manner toward the worker when the paycheck comes from the company or third-party payer? On the other hand, will the provider be fair to the employer when the individual worker or his labor union is footing the bill? Where should the provider's loyalty lie? Another area of conflict in the occupational setting is that of patient confidentiality. To what extent do employers and third-party payers have a right to know about individual employees' health histories? If a provider is aware of a condition in an individual worker that could pose a potential risk to that individual, his co-workers, or that segment of the public whom he serves (e.g., a school bus driver who has a substance abuse problem), can the provider break confidentiality? Sometimes, a provider's health concerns may be in direct conflict with the patient's economic security. When removal from a workplace exposure is the safest means to control an occupational illness, what do you do when the patient has no other source of income? Although ethical guidelines exist, there is no consensus as to how to respond to these dilemmas. The primary care provider must be sensitized to these issues and should have a sound ethical framework within which to resolve the ethical dilemmas she may encounter (Deubner, 1987a; Rest & Patterson, 1986).

The following sections of this chapter revolve around some of the key issues in the practice of occupational medicine. Special considerations in the diagnosis and management of work-related disease are emphasized. The last few pages introduce the reader to the concepts pertinent to disability and impairment evaluation and to the federal agencies involved in workplace regulation.

## CASE 22-2

*A previously healthy 40-year-old Hispanic man presented to the emergency room of a tertiary care teaching hospital with chief complaints of headache, abdominal pain, and nausea. He reported that his symptoms appeared shortly after he began work as a machine operator coating fabrics with a plastic compound. On further questioning, he stated that other co-workers suffered similar symptoms. Liver function tests showed an elevated aspartate aminotransferase level with normal alkaline phosphatase and bilirubin levels, consistent with hepatocellular injury. Results of the hepatitis screen were negative. There was no history of alcohol or drug abuse, or of previous blood transfusions. The emergency room physician, suspecting a possible occupational cause of the man's hepatitis, consulted the occupational medicine specialist. The man was temporarily removed from work.*

*In the meantime, the occupational medicine physician consulted an industrial hygienist. Together, they went to the man's workplace and evaluated the potential exposures. They noted the presence of numerous solvents that were mixed into the polyurethane compound used to coat fabrics; a number of these were known or suspected hepatotoxins. The index patient's co-workers were evaluated for subclinical liver disease; several of them turned out to have abnormal elevations in their liver transaminases. An epidemiological investigation pointed toward one particular hepatotoxic solvent, dimethylformamide, as the most likely culprit. The employers, aware of the possible legal and health consequences of the problem, stopped production and installed an improved ventilation system. The company substituted a less toxic agent for the dimethylformamide and returned to full production. The index patient eventually recovered normal liver function. At the urging of the labor union, a medical screening program was instituted for the workers. Those employees who chose to leave the company were referred to an experienced social worker for counseling and assistance with job placement (Redlich et al., 1988).*

## THE FIELD OF OCCUPATIONAL MEDICINE

Unlike other medical specialties that delineate themselves on the basis of organ systems (e.g., cardiology, neurology) or medical procedures and technology (e.g., nuclear medicine, radiology, or surgery), occupational medicine is defined by the environment in which work-related health and illness occur. The workplace is usually an easily identifiable entity and in many cases its structure is conducive to developing a healthcare delivery system specific to it. The design of an occupational medicine healthcare delivery system and the players involved differ from the more traditional medical specialties.

Occupational medicine is an established specialty of medicine that seeks to identify, treat, and prevent disorders related to hazards and exposures in the workplace as well as to institute measures designed to promote the health and fitness of workers. The practice of occupational medicine goes beyond the care of the individual patient; public health and prevention are of paramount importance. Diagnostic and therapeutic interventions are targeted toward the work environment as well as toward the individual patient. Finally, social, legal, and economic factors are incorporated into the occupational health provider's decision-making strategies to a much larger extent than in other fields of clinical medicine. It is a dynamic, rapidly evolving medical specialty that requires energy, ingenuity, and the ability to grasp intuitively the "big picture."

Although several models of occupational medicine practice exist, the composition of the occupational health team always requires certain key components. The primary provider is a physician, nurse practitioner, or physician's assistant who is well grounded in the principles of general medicine and in addition has specialized knowledge about work requirements, workplace hazards, and legal issues relating to the workplace. This individual is responsible for the diagnosis, treatment, and determination of the work-relatedness of illness or injury in the working population being served. The primary provider works in coordination with an industrial hygienist whose role is to evaluate the workplace for chemical, physical, and biological hazards and to recommend measures designed to minimize or control them. Ideally, the primary provider also has access to a social worker or counselor who is well versed in social and legal issues affecting the workplace. Patients often need such assistance if work disability occurs, when considering a job change for health reasons, or when negotiating the tangled path of workers' compensation. These professionals form the core of the occupational health team.

Case 22-2 demonstrates the "team approach" that is so crucial to the successful resolution of work-related problems. The physician of first contact in the emergency room, suspecting an occupational cause for the patient's problem, called in an internist who was trained in occupational medicine. She, in turn, consulted with an industrial hygienist during the process of evaluating the worksite. While the occupational medicine physician managed the medical problems of the patient and his affected co-workers and the industrial

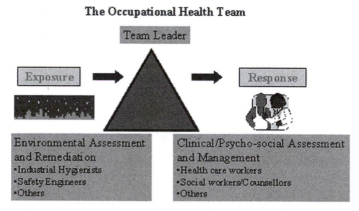

**Figure 22.2.** In occupational medicine, exposures in the work environment can result in disease in worker-patients. To be effective, measures to assess and control work-related illness must focus simultaneously on the environment (where exposures occur) and on the worker-patient(s) (where disease manifests). A team approach is necessary, with some members knowledgeable in environmental science and others with clinical expertise. The team leader, often an occupational health professional, plays a pivotal role in directing the efforts of these various professionals.

hygienist addressed the engineering requirements of the workplace, the social dilemmas were resolved with the assistance of a social worker. An occupational physician working alone would not have been able to address the various facets of this case so thoroughly.

In general medicine, the therapeutic relationship used to have only two parties, the provider and the patient. Increasingly, "payers" are becoming third parties to be coped with. Unique to occupational medicine is the addition of yet other parties to the therapeutic relationship, including employers, labor unions, and lawyers. A significant proportion of patient referrals to occupational medicine providers may come from these parties. The special interests of these groups may parallel or conflict with those of the patient. Although the actual diagnosis and assessment of workplace risk remains unchanged, the provider needs to be aware of the forces that motivate each party. In Case 22-2, for example, the employers wanted to avoid legal repercussions while maintaining productivity. The labor union wanted to ensure the safety of all of its members by securing adequate medical care and surveillance as well as engineering controls such as improved ventilation. The individual workers were anxious to keep their jobs but were concerned about their personal health at the same time. The different agendas of these parties and of the patient can affect access to information and can limit the range of therapeutic options available. While the provider needs to maintain her objectivity, she must also constantly attempt to see the situation in its entirety to make effective diagnoses and therapeutic recommendations. This is one aspect of the field that constantly challenges physicians dealing with occupational health problems. It is a good reason for consulting an occupational medicine specialist.

## CASE 22-3

*Mrs. G. B., a 48-year-old previously healthy nonsmoker, consulted her family physician because of periodic shortness of breath. About 2 months ago, she started having dyspnea at night, accompanied by wheezing. She experienced no chest pain, orthopnea, paroxysmal nocturnal dyspnea, or symptoms of gastroesophageal reflux. On further questioning, she recognized that her symptoms seemed to be worse during midweek. In the past 2 months, the only time she was asymptomatic was when she went on vacation to Bermuda. Results of her physical examination were unremarkable. Spirometry revealed a pattern of mild airway obstruction.*

*Asthma was diagnosed, but the physician could not find the trigger factor. She then reviewed the original screening questionnaire that Mrs. G. B. filled out during her first clinic visit 6 months ago. On that questionnaire, she noted that her patient was a furniture maker who had just started working with western red cedar. She did a Medline search and discovered that western red cedar is a known precipitant of occupational asthma and that the pattern of airway dysfunction may be of the delayed type, that is, symptoms may occur several hours after exposure, consistent with Mrs. G. B.'s nocturnal episodes. Mrs. G. B.'s symptoms were relatively well controlled by standard bronchodilator therapy, but only after she stopped using western red cedar did the symptoms abate completely.*

## HAZARDS IN THE WORKPLACE

Every healthcare provider will encounter cases in his practice that involve unfamiliar hazards or activities, leading to difficulty in recognizing and diagnosing occupational disease. General principles that can be applied to all work-induced disorders exist. These principles can provide a conceptual framework to aid providers in approaching work-related illness, especially when specific knowledge of toxicity is limited (Rosenstock & Cullen, 1994).

*Principle No. 1: The clinical and pathologic expressions of most occupational diseases are indistinguishable from those of nonoccupational diseases.* To be diagnosed, occupational disease must first be recognized. Many healthcare providers imagine that the patterns of illness produced by hazards in the workplace are somehow unique and that the clinical presentation of occupational diseases will distinguish them from non-

**Table 22.1**
Principles of Occupational Disease[a]

1. The clinical and pathologic expressions of most occupational diseases are indistinguishable from those of nonoccupational diseases
2. More often than not, it is the history of the illness that will provide clues pointing toward a work-related cause
3. Nonoccupational factors can contribute to the development of work-related disease
4. There is a biologically predictable latency period between occupational exposure and overt disease
5. A dose–response relationship typically holds true for occupational exposures
6. Individuals vary in their clinical response to workplace hazards

[a]Modified from Rosenstock & Cullen (1994).

work-related disorders. In reality, occupational diseases present in much the same way as common disorders of nonoccupational origin. Usually, there is nothing in the clinical presentation of a disease that will indicate a work-related etiology.

Consider Mrs. G. B. in Case 22-3. Although she was ultimately diagnosed with occupational asthma, her presenting symptoms were indistinguishable from those of "garden-variety" asthma that is unrelated to workplace exposures.

*Principle No. 2: More often than not, it is the history of the illness in relation to work activities and exposures that will provide clues pointing toward a work-related cause.* The occupational health history is fundamental to the assessment of the work-relatedness of a health problem. It must be incorporated into the routine health history obtained from every patient. This point cannot be overemphasized.

The occupational history has several purposes. These include increasing patient awareness of occupational and environmental factors, making accurate diagnoses, preventing the development of occupational disease, preventing the aggravation of underlying medical conditions by workplace factors, identifying potential workplace hazards, detecting new associations between exposure and disease, and establishing the basis for compensation of work-related disease.

The two major components of the occupational history are the work and exposure history and the general health history. In the work and exposure history, information about current and previous jobs and other nonoccupational environmental exposures should be obtained. This portion of the history should include not only the patient's job title but also information regarding the nature of her work and a description of the actual tasks performed. The job title alone often is insufficient to provide clues as to what the significant exposures are. For example, a painter involved in new construction does not have the same risk of lead exposure as Mr. A. K. in Case 22-1, who had to scrape and burn lead-based paint on the 150-year-old farmhouse that he was refurbishing.

Potential work exposures should be sought and enumerated. If the worker is well informed about his specific workplace exposures, the information that he provides may be sufficient. By law, employers must make exposure information available to their workers in the form of Manufacturers' Safety Data Sheets

## THREE ESSENTIAL QUESTIONS
## IN THE OCCUPATIONAL HISTORY

- *Please describe your job.*
- *Have you ever worked with any health hazard, such as asbestos, chemicals, noise, or repetitive motion?*
- *Do you have any health problems that you believe may be related to work?*
  *Source: Textbook of Clinical Occupational and Environmental Medicine,*
  *Rosenstock & Cullen (1994)*

(MSDSs). MSDSs can be a rich source of data; the worker has the right of access to them and should be encouraged to exercise this right. Occasionally, hazardous exposures are identified during an industrial hygienist's worksite evaluation, which is what happened in the case of the solvent-exposed factory worker in Case 22-2.

Nonoccupational exposures need to be pinpointed. The physician should ask about hobbies, recreational activities, and the home environment. Some extremely toxic chemicals are available for home use, e.g., caustic substances in household cleaners and pesticides for use in gardening. Tobacco and alcohol use should be investigated, since these environmental exposures may interact with or aggravate occupational exposures. If the factory worker in Case 22-2 also happened to be an alcoholic, the extent of his liver injury would probably have been much worse because of the combined hepatotoxicity of dimethylformamide and alcohol. Had Mrs. G. B. in Case 22-3 been a heavy smoker, her asthmatic reaction to western red cedar would likely have been more severe.

An inquiry about habits as they relate to hygiene at work should be made. In Case 22-1, the house painter's body burden of lead would have increased significantly from hand-to-mouth contact if he ate or smoked in the workplace.

Information regarding health problems and symptoms as they relate to work should be elicited in the general health history. The temporal relationship of these symptoms with the work day or work shift may be crucial to the diagnosis and should not be overlooked. Some work-related conditions will have a strong relationship to time spent at work. Airway irritation with cough and bronchial spasm from high levels of formaldehyde occurs within a short time of exposure and resolves within hours to days from cessation of exposure. Occupational asthma from red cedar, on the other hand, is of the delayed-onset type, with nocturnal wheezing as the first manifestation. Hence, the timing of Mrs. G. B.'s wheezing and dyspnea together with her workplace exposure were crucial in making the diagnosis in Case 22-3. Finally, a number of chronic work-related conditions may exhibit no particular variation with work exposure; most conditions with long latency have this character.

Information can be obtained by interview or by a self-administered questionnaire. Studies affirmed the validity of self-reported data for occupational and environmental exposures (Rosenstock *et al.*, 1984). Of course, whenever possible, other sources of supplemental information should be sought. These include prior medical records of the affected worker, exposure information from the employer (e.g., MSDSs), results of prior inspections of the workplace by a regulatory agency such as the Occupational Safety and Health Administration (OSHA) or the local Department of Health, and direct exposure assessment from a site visit. Substantial amounts of information, often of good quality, can sometimes be obtained from labor unions and community groups concerned about potentially hazardous exposures.

*Principle No. 3: Nonoccupational factors can contribute to the development of work-related disease.* Most occupational illnesses have a multifactorial etiology. For example, the risk of developing lung cancer is much higher in asbestos workers who also smoke. Clinicians must recognize that identifying a nonoccupational cause of a disease does not eliminate the possibility of a second work-related factor. Even if Mrs. G. B. in Case 23-3 were a heavy smoker, the occupational exposure to western red cedar remains the primary etiologic agent of her asthma. The potential role of a workplace hazard should not be overlooked just because another nonoccupational hazard exists.

*Principle No. 4: There is a biologically predictable latency period between occupational exposure and overt disease.* This fact is crucial in correctly attributing a disease to an occupational exposure. Certain illnesses may manifest long after the original exposure. Mesothelioma, for example, has a mean latency period of about 35 years from the initial asbestos exposure. On the other hand, a number of irritants and toxins are unlikely to cause delayed reactions. For example, acute upper airway irritation cannot be ascribed to an ammonia exposure that occurred uneventfully 5 weeks earlier (Beckett, 2000).

*Principle No. 5: The dose–response relationships are important for the diagnosis of occupational diseases.* The dose of an exposure to a workplace hazard is a strong predictor of the type and intensity of the

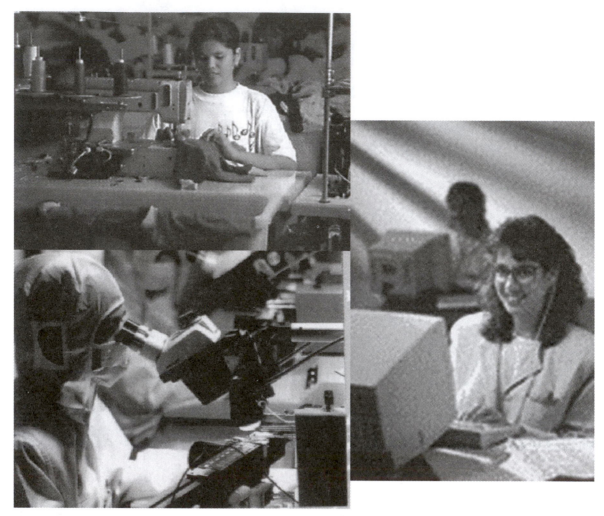

**Figures 22.3, 22.4, and 22.5.** While occupations and work-related hazards can be extremely diverse, knowledge of the basic principles of occupational medicine can help healthcare providers understand the interplay of environmental exposures and disease causation. Source: Clark Development Corporation, Philippines photo files, with permission.

response (Greenberg, 1997). For example, acute silicosis, an aggressive disease characterized histologically by alveolar proteinosis, is unlikely unless an overwhelming exposure to freshly fractured silica occurred. On the other hand, once sensitized, even a very small exposure to western red cedar can trigger an asthmatic attack in someone like Mrs. G. B. from Case 22-3. The clinician's ability to make a reasonably accurate assessment of previous and current exposure dose will determine to a large extent the successful evaluation and management of a patient suspected of having an occupational disease.

*Principle No. 6: Individuals vary in their clinical response to workplace hazards.* Persons respond differently to the same type of exposure. In Case 22-3, for example, there were three other furniture makers who were not susceptible to the sensitizing effects of western red cedar and who never developed respiratory symptoms. The response to solvent exposure in Case 22-2 ranged from no response to subclinical liver enzyme abnormalities to overt hepatitis. This variation may cause a provider to underestimate the relationship between a workplace hazard and a disease. Astute clinicians will acknowledge that this variability in response may be a function of variability between individuals and not necessarily proof that the occupational exposure is unrelated to the health outcome.

# Evaluating the Worksite

If, after evaluating the patient with a thorough history and physical examination, the possibility of an occupational disease is seriously considered, the ideal next step is to do an assessment of the workplace.

The usual concept of "the workplace" is that of a physical entity that is geographically defined. A factory in the suburbs, a city office, and a mine in West Virginia are good examples. However, there may be instances when "the workplace" is not confined to one location. Consider Mr. A. K., the painter in Case 22-1. His workplace, rightfully defined, is wherever he is currently working. It could be a bridge, an old building, or a construction site. It could be one construction site today and a different one tomorrow. Some workplaces may not conform with the conventional image of a worksite. Think of the airline pilot. A housekeeper's place

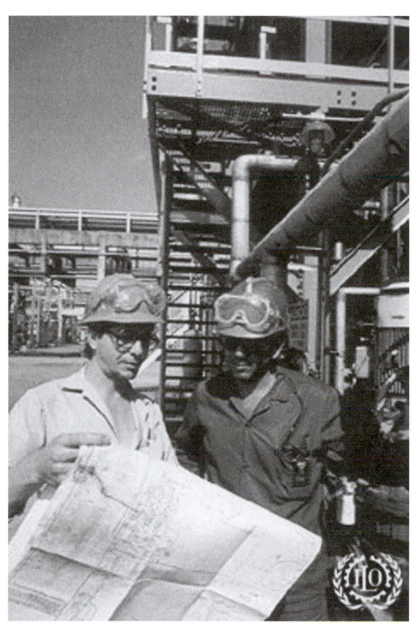

**Figure 22.6.** Safety engineers at an alcohol producing plant in São Paulo, Brazil. Source: ILO Photo Files, *www.ilo.org* (photographer: J. Maillard).

of work is another person's home. With the advent of computer technology, more and more people are opting to work in their own homes. The point is that "the workplace" is not always defined by structure.

An essential prerequisite to a worksite evaluation is familiarity with the work itself. By knowing what a specific job entails, what materials are handled, what processes/tasks are carried out, and what products are generated, hazard recognition is facilitated. In Case 22-3, for example, knowing that Mrs. G. B. was a furniture maker who worked with western red cedar was crucial in establishing the deleterious exposure. Although patients may not know much about specific chemicals, they can almost always provide good information about the major products and materials and the kinds of activities that they and others do.

## Diagnostic Decision-Making

The principles of medical diagnostic decision-making also apply to occupational disease (Rosenstock & Cullen, 1986). The clinical presentation should be consistent with the nature of the illness. The interval between onset of disease and exposure should conform to the known latency of the suspected causal agent. The intensity of the exposure should be appropriate for the magnitude of the disease, given the known dose–response characteristic of the suspected workplace hazard. The hazard itself should be verified and the dose range established to the fullest extent possible. Supplemental information should be obtained from other sources, such as employers, labor unions, other physicians, manufacturers, and even regulatory agencies if required. The final step is processing all of this information and deciding the likelihood that the disease is work-related.

In practice, the information available to the healthcare provider will often be insufficient to establish with absolute certainty that a disease is occupational. Commonly, the decision regarding the work-relatedness of a disease will require a judgment. Such a decision merits careful thought because, unlike general medicine, the consequences of that decision go beyond medical concerns. There are economic, social, and legal ramifications in making the diagnosis of an occupational disease and dreadful personal and public health consequences of not making the diagnosis. All of these factors must be taken into consideration so that the probable outcome is in the patient's best interest. For example, from a purely medical perspective, Mrs. G. B. in Case 22-3 should have been removed from further exposure to western red cedar. However, quitting her job would have a considerable impact on her life, especially since she is a widow with two young children. Fortunately, her employer assigned her to work with less allergenic hardwoods and provided her with the appropriate respirator. On the other hand, if the diagnosis was missed and the exposure to western red cedar continued, Mrs. G. B.'s asthma very likely would have progressed, perhaps to the point of incapacitating her.

## Managing a Work-Related Illness

Once a diagnosis is established, the clinician can then proceed to formulate a treatment plan. Depending on the circumstances, this plan can operate on two levels: The first is tailored toward the individual patient, and the second addresses the public health dimension of the problem.

The portion of the treatment plan that concerns itself with the individual patient needs to take into account not only medical concerns but also the various economic, social, and legal factors that may be pertinent to the case. One text puts this succinctly: "Although one choice or another may seem preferable from a strictly medical perspective, it cannot be presumed that this choice satisfies the needs of the patient, or that it is included among the options offered by the employer or other relevant parties" (Rosenstock & Cullen, 1994). This is the point in the encounter when a thoughtful consideration of the various agendas of the patient and other parties is crucial. Options need to be explored and alternatives considered, with the main goal of optimizing benefit for the patient. It is also at this point that the services of a social worker may be required.

Responsibility may not end with the conclusion of care of the individual patient. When a workplace hazard is identified and other workers may be at risk of exposure, the provider should consider acting on the public health implications of the situation. At the very least, the opinion that others may be at risk should be documented and reported to local health authorities. In some instances, hazardous workplaces will be recognized about which little can be done, though often employers will respond directly to such concerns. The clinician may have additional recourse through a regulatory agency such as OSHA or through a labor union so that employees may be informed of their potential risk. In addition, it is vital that the employer or whoever has ultimate responsibility for the workplace be made aware whenever safety concerns have been raised.

## CASE 22-4

*Mr. D. L. is a right-handed 27-year-old mechanic who was working on a car engine when an accident occurred. The rod holding the car's hood open buckled and the car hood came down on his left hand. His left thumb had to be amputated from the metacarpophalangeal joint. He was evaluated to have a 100% loss of the left thumb, which translated into a 40% impairment of the upper extremity. With appropriate occupational rehabilitation, he was able to return to his job in 3 months.*

## CASE 22-5

*Ms. M. F. is a 53-year-old data entry clerk for a large corporation. She joined the company in 1980 and has been doing data entry for 15 years. Over the past year, she noticed the onset of bilateral forearm pain. The pain progressively worsened over time. Eventually, she was unable to perform activities of daily living because of the severe pain. Results of repeated physical examinations including neurologic testing were inconsistent with carpal tunnel syndrome or other well-characterized clinical entities. She underwent various radiographic and electrophysiologic tests under the supervision of a hand surgeon. Although a mild nerve conduction abnormality was noted bilaterally, it was insufficient to explain her degree of dysfunction. A psychiatric evaluation was not helpful. She was diagnosed with repetitive stress disorder. Despite physical therapy and active participation in a pain management program, she was unable to regain function in both arms. Although impairment could not be documented, she was awarded permanent partial disability after a year of treatment, but she was never able to return to her job and suffered enormous economic and personal loss.*

# EVALUATING DISABILITY, IMPAIRMENT, AND WORK-RELATEDNESS

Disability problems are the most common reasons that persons with work-induced illnesses are evaluated by primary care providers. Often the referral source is a third party, usually an employer or insurance agency. The task for the provider is to determine the extent and permanency of functional loss, what residual work capacity is left, what work restrictions should apply, and what degree of impairment or disability should be awarded for purposes of workers' compensation or disability benefit allocation.

Certain terms need to be defined. Impairment, as defined in the American Medical Association's *Guides to the Evaluation of Permanent Impairment*, is "an alteration of an individual's health status that is assessed by medical means" (American Medical Association, 1988). It refers to the objective loss of the function of an organ or part of the body relative to a preexisting baseline. Because it is an objective finding, it can generally be demonstrated by clinical maneuvers and quantified. It is independent of the patient's functional status.

Disability, on the other hand, is defined as "an alteration of an individual's capacity to meet personal, social, or occupational demands, or to meet statutory or regulatory requirements" (American Medical Association, 1988). Disability is assessed by nonmedical means; the patient's functional status and occupational and social circumstances need to be taken into account. Disability may be temporary or permanent.

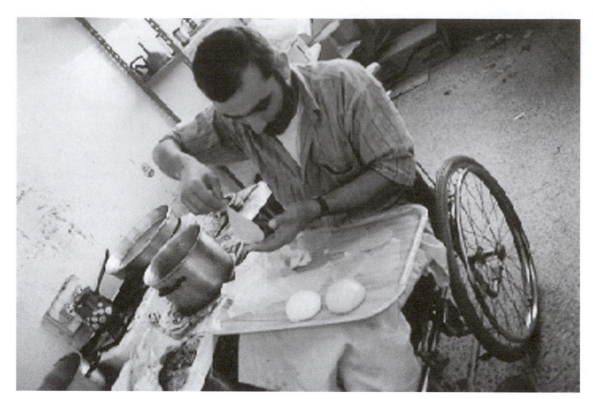

**Figure 22.7** Physical impairment and functional disability are different. This paraplegic worker earns a living by crafting candles. Source: ILO Photo Files, *www.ilo.org* (photographer: J. Maillard).

Permanent disability is usually determined after a period during which maximum medical improvement can be expected to occur. Note that an impaired individual is not necessarily disabled. The mechanic in Case 22-4 is impaired because he lost his left thumb. However, he was able to return to his job after a period of rehabilitation; hence, he is not, by definition, disabled. In contrast, the woman in Case 22-5 exhibits significant disability in the absence of measurable impairment.

A component of most disability evaluations is the determination of the work-relatedness of an injury or illness. Simply put, an injury or illness is work-related if it resulted from some activity or exposure at work. Although the work-related nature of most on-the-job accidents is evident, the situation with chronic illnesses is more complicated. Because of the multifactorial nature of most chronic diseases, it is often difficult to ascertain the cause of a particular disorder with certainty. The legal standard is less rigorous than the medical one, and benefits are based on the legal standard. Therefore, it is the more important one for this decision, a fact that makes many physicians uneasy. Cause is established from a legal perspective if it is more likely than not that a workplace exposure caused or aggravated the disease. In numerical terms, if the probability that an occupational factor resulted in disease is greater than 50%, then sufficient cause exists.

A more detailed discussion of this topic is beyond the scope of this chapter. Because it puts a different slant to the traditional role of the provider as patient advocate, however, certain guidelines need to be mentioned.

First, to be effective, the provider who is doing the evaluation needs to distance herself from personal feelings regarding the appropriateness of the benefit system. For example, a provider may believe on a personal level that any person who seeks disability insurance is "out to milk the system." If she is unable to prevent that personal belief from influencing her professional judgment, she will not be able to make a reliable assessment. To do a credible job, the provider as evaluator must be unbiased. Second, both provider and patient need to understand that the traditional clinician–patient relationship is modified when disability is being evaluated. If the provider is doing an evaluation on an individual who also happens to be a patient whose medical care she oversees, then she needs to be able to distinguish her role as evaluator from that of medical caregiver. It may be appropriate in this situation to refer the patient to another provider, a social worker or some other professional who can take over the role of patient advocate. Third, if the provider is uncertain about the disability and its cause, she should consider obtaining a second opinion early on during the course of the evaluation. The evaluator's opinion should always be communicated in an unequivocal fashion to the patient as well as to the referral source in writing. Finally, the decision to remove a patient from his job should be done only after a thoughtful consideration of the consequences, both financial and psychological, that such an action could have.

## Workers' Compensation

A significant number of disability and work-relatedness evaluations are performed for worker's compensation purposes. Workers' compensation is a system defined by a set of federal and state laws instituted to provide income replacement, medical expense benefits, and rehabilitation services to workers disabled by work-related injury or illness. In essence, it is a form of insurance against occupational disease or injury that is paid for by the employer. In return, it operates on a "no-fault" assumption that precludes the worker from suing the employer. Any injury or illness that fulfills the legal standard for work-relatedness is compensable regardless of who was at fault. The worker bears the burden of proof of the work-relatedness of his health condition. Claims are paid for either directly by the employer or indirectly by an insurance company contracted by the employer. Claims have to be filed in a timely manner with the state agency that administers the worker's compensation system. Claimants do not become eligible for benefits until after a waiting period in which claims can be, and often are, contested. When this happens, they undergo review by either an administrative or a judicial agency.

The benefits received by a disabled worker from the workers' compensation fund may be insufficient to meet his needs. There are other sources of benefits available to him. Social Security Disability Insurance (SSDI) supplements worker's compensation with monthly benefits for qualified workers. Income from SSDI is paid in coordination with workers' compensation provided the sum of the combined benefits does not exceed 80% of the worker's current average earnings. The Social Security benefits would be reduced, not the workers' compensation, in order to meet the 80% limit.

To qualify for Social Security disability benefits, the injured worker must meet several criteria. First, he must be totally disabled; that is, he must be unable to do any substantial gainful work. Second, the disability must be expected to last for at least 12 months or result in premature death. Finally, the worker must have worked long enough and recently enough and paid the required number of quarters into Social Security to be insured. SSDI begins to provide benefits to the worker 6 months after the onset of total disability (Division of Worker Education, Workers' Compensation Commission, 1989).

A worker, however, may be ineligible for SSDI benefits because he has not worked long enough to qualify. This individual can apply for benefits under the Supplemental Security Income (SSI) program. SSI is designed to assist the disabled with limited income and few resources. Unlike SSDI, a person does not need to have worked to qualify. Economic need is the basis for determining SSI eligibility. Monthly payments begin once eligibility criteria are met. Although workers' compensation pays for all medical bills from an on-the-job injury or illness, a disabled worker who is unemployed or waiting for worker's compensation may need some basic health insurance. If this individual qualified for Social Security disability (SSDI) benefits and has been receiving these for 2 consecutive years, then she is eligible for Medicare Part A coverage. On the other hand, a worker who did not qualify for SSDI but who instead obtained SSI benefits is covered by Medicaid. Medicaid is a state-administered public assistance program for persons who cannot meet the cost of the medical care that they need. Individuals who receive SSI benefits are automatically entitled to Medicaid since they have already proved disability and economic need (Goldenson *et al.*, 1978).

The physician's role in worker's compensation, SSDI, and SSI centers on the determination of impairment, disability, and work-relatedness. Medical certification of the extent of disability is required to establish eligibility for these benefits (Herrington & Morse, 1995). To do a credible job, clinicians need to be knowledgeable about the different benefits systems and the various medical, social, and legal issues involved.

---

## CASE 22-6

*When E. L., a 34-year-old factory worker, was diagnosed with noise-induced hearing loss, his physician suspected an occupational cause. E. L. had no other risk factors such as the use of guns or noisy equipment at home, and he disliked loud music. E. L. told his physician that the grinder he operated at work seemed excessively noisy. E. L. further stated that hearing protection was not provided by his employer. As far as he knew, noise levels had never been monitored at the factory.*

*Concerned, the physician called E. L.'s employers. He explained the problem and offered to do a workplace evaluation together with an industrial hygienist. The factory owners refused. Several other attempts to obtain their consent were unsuccessful. Frustrated by his employers' lack of cooperation, E. L. called the nearest OSHA office and explained the problem. An OSHA inspector appeared at the factory 2 weeks later for an inspection. The factory noise levels were found to be in excess of the noise standard. The factory owners were cited and fined a considerable sum. They were required to institute a hearing protection program for their employees. During the initial screening, four other cases of noise-induced hearing loss were identified.*

---

## REGULATION IN THE WORKPLACE

Case 22-6 illustrates the important role that government agencies such as OSHA play in regulating workplace safety. Sometimes, the efforts of the individual worker and her private physician may be insufficient to generate the necessary action to improve the conditions at a particular worksite. Knowledge about the various entities involved in workplace regulation and knowledge of the various laws enacted to safeguard worker safety is helpful to clinicians who encounter work-related problems in their medical practice.

In 1970, the Occupational Health and Safety Act was passed with the objective of reducing the risk of injury and illness to workers in the workplace. It mandated the creation of OSHA, housed under the Department of Labor. The legislation envisioned controlling workplace hazards by promulgating safety standards that are enforceable by safety inspectors. Compliance with these standards is monitored by complaint, by set priorities, by random inspections, or after a major disaster. Written into the Act was the option for individual states to take over part or all of the role of federal OSHA if they proved to be as effective as the federal agency. Standards relate to plant operations and physical setups. Inspections are conducted either according to priority or in response to complaints by employees, healthcare providers, labor representatives, or other concerned parties. Citations are issued for failure to maintain specific standards. Violators are fined and violations must be corrected within a stipulated time period.

The National Institute for Occupational Safety and Health (NIOSH) is a component of the Centers for Disease Control (CDC). Its major tasks are to support education and research in the field of occupational health and to establish new workplace standards. NIOSH has a branch that conducts Health Hazard Evaluations (HHEs) at the request of private industry, labor unions, or other employee groups. Unlike OSHA inspections, which focus primarily on the industrial hygiene aspects of a workplace, HHEs include health evaluations in their investigations. NIOSH is not limited to evaluating only those substances for which standards already exist. However, it has no capacity to enforce its recommendations.

Other laws exist for specific industries in the United States. The Mine Safety and Health Act; the Clean Air Act; the Clean Water and Safe Drinking Water Acts; the Federal Insecticide, Fungicide and Rodenticide Act; and the Federal Food, Drug and Cosmetic Act are examples of legislation that affects the safety of the workplace. The Mine Safety and Health Act, for example, created the Mine Safety and Health Administration

(MSHA) in the Department of Labor to deal with health and safety risks to all surface and underground miners. The Federal Insecticide, Fungicide and Rodenticide Act gave authority to the Environmental Protection Agency (EPA) to protect both consumers and workers who handle pesticides.

Despite their number, these laws remain insufficient to guarantee workplace safety for every worker. At best, they provide standards to reduce risk at work. The regulatory process traditionally is slow to react to crises in the workplace. Economic interests often conflict with safety concerns, further complicating the picture. Vigilance and commitment to the highest level of worker safety will therefore remain the responsibility of employers, workers, and the healthcare providers of workers.

> Not only in antiquity but in our own times also laws have been passed in well-ordered cities to secure good conditions for the workers; so it is only right that the art of medicine should contribute its portion for the benefit and relief of those for whom the law has shown such foresight; indeed we ought to show peculiar zeal, though so far we have neglected to do so, in taking precautions for their safety, so that as far as possible they may work at their chosen calling without loss of health.
>
> Bernardino Ramazzini
> De Morbis Artificum (Diseases of Workers), 1713

## CONCLUSION

This chapter has focused on some of the issues that pertain to health and the workplace that are important for practitioners of medicine. Occupational factors play a role in numerous general medical encounters. Because there are no clinical markers to distinguish occupational disease from non-work-related disorders, it is imperative that a good occupational history be included in any health evaluation. Providers need to be sensitized to the various issues involved in work-related illness. An environmental perspective and coordination with other professionals involved in workplace issues is crucial to the successful control of work-related medical problems.

Clinicians should use the general principles in the diagnosis of occupational disease presented in this chapter as guidelines when confronted with a potentially work-related clinical problem. Concurrent diagnostic evaluation of the workplace, a key difference from the traditional medical encounter, and familiarity with the work itself are necessary components of a thorough occupational evaluation. Management of occupational disease requires a careful consideration of the medical, social, legal, psychological, and economic consequences of each therapeutic option. Care does not end with the resolution of the individual patient's problem; prevention of further disease in other workers and the protection of the general public from potential environmental hazards must be considered.

A brief discussion of the issues related to the evaluation of impairment, disability, and work-relatedness is provided since this type of evaluation is commonly encountered in a primary care practice. The chapter ends with an overview of the various government agencies and legislation that seek to regulate the workplace. However, these are inadequate to safeguard the safety of every worker. Clinicians have the responsibility to advocate for safety in the workplace for as long as they continue to provide services to the working population.

## CASES FOR DISCUSSION

### CASE 1

*Mr. E. F. is a 52-year-old firefighter. During a fire, he was noted to be pale and clammy by his colleagues, who measured his blood pressure at 200/110 mm Hg. A physician diagnosed his problem as new-onset hypertension. E. F.'s father, who died of a heart attack at the age of 42, also had hypertension. The insurance carrier for the Firemen's Disability Board referred Mr. E. F. to you. During the initial interview, you discover that Mr. E. F.'s favorite snack food is salted peanuts. Physical examination revealed a 28-lb excess over ideal body weight. The fundi were normal.*

*1. Is Mr. E. F.'s hypertension job-related? Why or why not?*

*2. What, if any, work restrictions would you recommend?*

*3. What do you think was the underlying agenda of the insurance carrier in referring Mr. E. F. to you? Mr. E. F.'s supervisor strongly encouraged him to keep the appointment with you. What could his agenda be? What of Mr. E. F. himself? How do you take all of these different agendas into account when making your recommendations?*

## CASE 2

*S. D., a 26-year-old secretary, comes to your office because she needs a letter from you excusing her from the previous week's absence from work. She tells you that she had a "stomach virus" and was too sick to work. Results of her physical examination are completely normal.*

*1. Do you accede to her request?*

*2. What ethical guidelines can you think of to help you whenever you are confronted with a similar situation?*

## CASE 3

*The director of human resources of a large company refers one of their employees to your medical practice for a health evaluation because of recurrent absenteeism. During your encounter with the patient, you learn that he is in the midst of divorce proceedings. To help cope, he has started smoking again, after having quit for 3 years, and is consuming an average of six to eight alcoholic drinks daily. His appearance is unkempt, he has trouble sleeping, and his appetite is poor. He works as a forklift operator.*

*1. What ethical dilemmas can you identify? How would you address them?*

*2. How much information do you provide the human resources director who referred the patient to you?*

*3. What recommendations would you give the patient? Would you refer him to anyone else?*

*4. Would you remove him from his job? If yes, how would this potentially affect your patient's situation?*

## CASE 4

*You work at an urgent care clinic. A 30-year-old woman is brought in for evaluation. She had fainted while at work. Shortly after she is brought into your clinic, she wakes up. She describes feeling dizzy and nauseous just before passing out. She works in a company that manufactures formica cabinets. In the past month, four other co-workers were brought into your clinic with similar complaints. Unfortunately, the patient doesn't know the names of the chemicals she is using.*

*1. Could your patient's fainting spell be work-related? How would you go about investigating the possible work-relatedness of the problem?*

*2. You decide to call the factory owner to obtain additional information. He tells you to mind your own business. What other options do you have to learn more about the workplace?*

*3. The employees finally complain to OSHA. During the inspection, the air levels of a number of organic solvents were found to exceed the Permissible Exposure Limits (PELs). The factory owner is fined and given 3 months to install a ventilation system capable of reducing the solvent air levels. Two weeks later, you receive a phone call from attorney X. He wants to know if the young lady with the fainting spell, whom he now represents, had acute solvent intoxication, because if so, she will be filing a worker's compensation case. In the meantime, the results of the beta-HCG test that you did when the patient came to your clinic come back positive; your patient is pregnant. What is your opinion now? Does the case meet the legal standard for causation? Does it meet the medical standard with the same degree of certainty? If you feel there is a conflict here, how do you resolve it?*

## CASE 5

*D. V., a 60-year-old plumber, is referred to you by the local plumber's union for a screening evaluation. D. V. tells you that he started working as an apprentice plumber at the age of 17. He intends to retire in 5 years. During your review of systems, you elicit a history of exertional dyspnea that started about 3 years ago. Results of the physical examination were unremarkable. However, the chest x-ray showed extensive pleural disease from asbestos exposure and a suspicious-looking nodule in the right upper lung zone. After a diagnostic workup, adenocarcinoma is diagnosed. D. V. is a heavy smoker with a 75-pack per year smoking history. His father and uncle, both heavy smokers, also died of lung cancer.*

1. *What questions would you ask in the occupational history to help you assess the amount of asbestos exposure of this patient?*
2. *Is D. V.'s lung cancer work-related? What elements in the history would support a diagnosis of asbestos-related lung cancer?*
3. *How would you explain the role of D. V.'s smoking and family history? Do they go against the diagnosis of a work-related cancer?*
4. *D. V.'s lawyer contacts you and asks if you believe the legal standard is met for a diagnosis of asbestos-related lung cancer, because if so, D. V. will apply for worker's compensation benefits. What is your reply? How do you feel about becoming involved in the process of applying for compensation?*

## RECOMMENDED READINGS

Fallon LF Jr. Ethics in the practice of occupational medicine. *Occup Med* 16(3):517–24, v. Review, 2001.

Goldman RH, Peters JM: The occupational and environmental health history. *JAMA* 246:2831–2836, 1981.

> In this journal article, the authors discuss the elements of good history-taking in the occupational setting. Key points in eliciting a thorough exposure history are stressed.

Greaves WW, Pearson DO (eds): Occupational medicine: A primary care perspective. *Patient Care* 30(3), 1996.

> A special issue with a pragmatic discussion of the issues surrounding the practice of occupational medicine from the perspective of primary care.

Hadler NM: Occupational illness: The issue of causality. *J Occup Med* 26:587–593, 1984.

> This article focuses on the legal issues surrounding causality as it applies to disability benefits and worker's compensation claims.

Harber P, et al. Frequency of occupational health concerns in general clinics. *J Occup Environ Med* 43(11):939–45, 2001.

Rest KM, Patterson WB: Ethics and moral reasoning in occupational health. *Semin Occup Med* 1:49–57, 1986.

> A thoughtful, well-written essay that explores the ethical dilemmas often encountered in the practice of occupational health.

Rosenstock L, Cullen MR: *Clinical Occupational Medicine.* Philadelphia, WB Saunders Co, 1986.

> Paper-cover volume that provides the essential information that general practitioners and occupational health providers require when faced with patients with possible work-related illness.

Rosenstock L, Cullen MR: *Textbook of Clinical Occupational and Environmental Medicine.* Philadelphia, WB Saunders Co, 1994.

> A reference textbook that covers the entire range of occupational medicine issues with depth and clarity.

World Health Organization. Global strategy on occupational health for all: a way to health at work. *Recommendation of the Second Meeting of the WHO Collaborating Centres in Occupational Health, 11–14 October 1994, Beijing, China.* Geneva: World Health Organization, 1995.

## REFERENCES

Beckett WS. Occupational respiratory disease. *NEJM* 342:406–413, 2000.

Goldman RH, Peters JM. The occupational and environmental health history. *JAMA* 246:2831–2836, 1981.

Greaves WW, Pearson DO, eds. Occupational medicine: A primary care perspective. *Patient Care* 30(3), 1996.

Greenberg MI, Hamilton RJ, Phillips SD. *Occupational, Industrial and Environmental Toxicology.* St. Louis, Mo, Mosby-Year Book, Inc, 1997.

Hadler NM. Occupational illness: The issue of causality. *J Occup Med* 26:587–593, 1984.

Rest KM, Patterson WB. Ethics and moral reasoning in occupational health. *Semin Occup Med* 1:49–57, 1986.

Rosenstock L, Cullen MR. *Clinical Occupational Medicine.* Philadelphia, WB Saunders Co, 1986.

Rosenstock L, Cullen MR. *Textbook of Clinical Occupational and Environmental Medicine.* Philadelphia, WB Saunders Co, 1994.

World Health Organization. Occupational health: ethically correct, economically sound, Fact sheet no. 84 (revised). Geneva, World Health Organization, 1999.

## CHAPTER 23

# Public Health and the Environment

*James N. Hyde and Barry S. Levy*

## CASE 23-1

*Bill Small had a successful and growing primary care practice in a medium-sized city of 100,000 in the Midwest. Among the things he enjoyed most was the new role he had begun as physician consultant to the city's largest nursing home facility. He looked forward to his regular visits to the facility both for the opportunity to visit his own patients as well as the chance to talk to a wide variety of others. This nursing home facility was modern, well run, and provided excellent care.*

*Dr. Small was surprised, therefore, when he arrived at the nursing home one day and learned that two of his six patients were seriously ill with diarrhea and severe gastrointestinal symptoms. He started both immediately on symptomatic medication and ordered appropriate tests. He was relieved to find that his other patients apparently were not sick.*

*In discussions with the nursing staff, however, Dr. Small learned to his dismay that several other patients at the nursing home were experiencing similar symptoms, suggesting the possibility of a common-source outbreak of diarrheal illness.*

*As a precaution, Dr. Small ordered that stool samples be taken on all patients, that they be carefully monitored for GI symptoms, and that the staff be reminded about the critical importance of maintaining a high level of sanitation. He also advised the nursing home administrator that he intended to report a probable outbreak of diarrheal illness to the chief epidemiologist at the state health department. While concerned about the prospects of potentially adverse publicity, the administrator was well aware of the mandate under the state's licensure laws to report the existence of a potential disease outbreak. The chief epidemiologist expressed gratitude to Dr. Small when he called to report on the situation. She concurred with the steps that had been initiated but on a hunch requested that all stool samples be sent to the state laboratory for analysis.*

*A few days later the report came back from the state laboratory indicating that 10 of the 12 patients with symptoms were positive for* **Cryptosporidium parvum.** *In reporting this finding to Dr. Small, the state epidemiologist explained that* **C. parvum** *has been recognized as a serious human pathogen only since 1976 (CDC, 1995). Prior to the AIDS epidemic, it was reported only sporadically and then only in cases of persons who were immunocompromised. With the development of more sophisticated laboratory techniques, the organism can now be identified among immunocompetent individuals as well, particularly the elderly.*

*The epidemiologist went on to explain that* Cryptosporidium *is a protozoan parasite that is transmitted by the ingestion of oocysts excreted by infected animals or humans. Transmission can take place through person-to-person contact, animal-to-person contact, or the ingestion of fecally contaminated food or water. Of particular concern is the potential for waterborne spread. The oocyst is present, at least periodically, in 65–97% of all surface waters tested in the United States. Conventional chlorine disinfection does not inactivate the organism. Filtration methods used at most water treatment plants are inadequate to remove all oocysts, and some localities do not filter their water.*

*Particularly troublesome, she said, was the potential for waterborne outbreaks, several of which had occurred in the United States since 1984. The most serious was in Milwaukee, Wisconsin, in 1993, involving an estimated 400,000 people, 4000 of whom required hospitalization (MacKenzie et al., 1994). Equally worrisome was the fact that all of these outbreaks occurred in municipalities that either met or exceeded state and federal drinking water quality standards (CDC, 1995).*

*The search was on for the source of the infection.*

## EDUCATIONAL OBJECTIVES

1. Provide examples of the wide range of environmental exposures that adversely affect human health
2. Explain the concept of natural history of disease and how it affects the prevention and control of disease
3. Explain the concept of the multifactorial nature of disease and how it affects disease prevention programs
4. Discuss the concept of the primary care physician as sentinel reporter
5. Describe the steps a physician should take when presented with a case of environmentally induced illness

## INTRODUCTION

We live in a world of increasing complexity with the constant threat of a myriad of unanticipated environmental exposures. Among such exposures are: infectious agents as in Case 23-1, pesticides and other toxic substances, microcontaminants, ionizing and nonionizing radiation, ambient air pollutants, noise, and indoor air contaminants.

Consider the following clinical scenarios:

*A 45-year-old fisherman is diagnosed by his primary care physician with malignant melanoma. Does his cancer result from degradation of the ozone layer or an excess exposure to UV light as a result of his occupation? What might a physician do to prevent this event? Counsel on the use of sunscreen? Fight for the elimination of fluorocarbon propellants? Advocate for the establishment of education programs for all commercial fishermen?*

*A young mother, one of whose children has leukemia, calls her primary care physician's office after the neighbors next door contract with a lawn service company to care for their yard. She is concerned that her neighbor's desire for a green lawn may expose her family to toxic chemicals. As her physician, how would you counsel her about the risks? What is the role of the state, county, and local regulatory agencies to ensure that the agents used are "safe" and that those applying them have been trained in their proper application and disposal?*

*A 30-year-old father of two young children calls for your advice on whether to buy an otherwise perfect house that he and his wife have found after a lengthy search. His concern is that the house is located within 100 yards of a cellular telephone tower. He has heard about the possible association of radiofrequency emissions from cell phones as a cancer risk. How does the physician help his patient place this risk in perspective? How can a father's concerns and worries be channeled into positive or constructive directions?*

**495**

**EPIDEMIOLOGY AND PUBLIC HEALTH PRACTICE**

Case 23-1 and these vignettes illustrate the range of environmental concerns confronting physicians today. The effective management of these situations requires developing and maintaining a particular set of clinical skills: taking an exposure history, conducting a thorough physical examination, educating about risk, reporting to public health authorities. It also requires a willingness to take on and play a larger role as an advocate for patients and the community at large.

While medical education tends to emphasize one-on-one clinical skills, the training and skills required to equip physicians to serve as population physicians receive far less attention. It is critical for the practicing clinician to be aware of the basic principles and concepts that underlie the science and practice of public health. The purpose of this chapter is to acquaint readers with these principles and concepts and to illustrate and explore some of the conflicts and dilemmas they pose.

## CASE 23-2

*Late in January, 21-year-old Hortensia Valasquez was taken by ambulance to the hospital emergency department 1 hour after being found unconscious in her apartment by a neighbor. She had been intubated by EMTs at the scene and had received 100% oxygen while en route to the hospital. Hortensia's husband, Carlos, was also found at the scene and brought to the hospital. Although disoriented, he was lucid at the time of arrival at the emergency department.*

*From the history given it was determined that the couple's furnace had broken. They were using a portable propane construction heater to heat their unventilated home. Carlos also revealed that his wife was pregnant.*

*Dr. Katherine Woolesy, their primary care physician, happened to be in the hospital at the time of admission. During her physical examination she noted that the patient was combative and confused, her carboxyhemoglobin level was 7%, and abdominal examination results were consistent with a 28-week intrauterine pregnancy, although no fetal movement could be detected. The patient was being treated with oxygen continuously.*

*On the second day following admission, Hortensia went into labor spontaneously and delivered an 1100-g stillborn female fetus of approximately 27 weeks gestation. The gross autopsy findings were unremarkable except for bright red discoloration of the skin and visceral organs.*

*Hortensia continued to recover slowly postdelivery and was discharged on the ninth day postadmission. Dr. Woolesy and her colleagues agreed that the loss of the Valasquez child was almost certainly the result of carbon monoxide exposure from the use of a propane construction heater in an unventilated mobile home (Adapted from: Farrow et al., 1990).*

## EPIDEMIOLOGY AND PUBLIC HEALTH PRACTICE

Epidemiology is the basic science of public health. Although there are many good definitions of epidemiology, we would propose the following: *Epidemiology is the study of the patterns, distribution,*

*Of the 2.3 million deaths reported in the United States in 1997, 146,400 were due to injuries. Of these 65% (95,644) were due to "accidents," 21% (30,535) suicides, 14% (19,846) homicides, and 3% (3043) other causes. In that same year carbon monoxide poisoning accounted for fewer than 150 deaths. (National Vital Statistics Reports, Vol 47, No. 19, June 1999, p.11.)*

*antecedents, and determinants of illness and health-related events in human populations and the application of that study to the prevention and control of disease.* There are several important conceptual notions inherent in this definition that have a bearing on how epidemiologists and public health practitioners function and how they view the world.

The first is that epidemiology is an applied science. It is concerned with the prevention and control of disease and not with the acquisition of knowledge for its own sake. Efforts to study HCV infection, Legionnaires' disease, breast cancer, traffic fatalities, and carbon monoxide poisoning are all predicated on the desire to reduce the incidence of morbidity and mortality from these events, not to study them for the sake of satisfying idle intellectual curiosity.

Second, epidemiology is concerned with understanding etiology. While it is not always necessary to understand the etiologic mechanism of disease to reduce its incidence, understanding causes is usually an important step in devising plans that ultimately lead to their elimination. Conversely, it should be noted that understanding causes is not always synonymous with prevention of morbidity and mortality. Case 23-2 illustrates this quite dramatically.

Third, epidemiology is concerned with understanding the patterns and distribution of disease in human populations. Most often this is addressed in terms of trying to identify common characteristics of the individuals who are affected. The epidemiologist looks for common characteristics of the *persons* affected, e.g., their age, sex, occupation, education. Also of interest is the *place* where these events have occurred, e.g., on one floor of a nursing home (Case 23-1) or in one part of the city. Finally, the epidemiologist checks to see if there are certain patterns or characteristics in the *timing* of these events. Figure 23.1, which shows deaths in the United States from carbon monoxide poisoning over a 10-year interval, illustrates this point.

A knowledge and understanding of the characteristics and antecedent events associated with an outbreak are often essential ingredients in constructing a strategy of prevention and control. The figure shows clearly that carbon monoxide poisoning is most prominent during late fall and winter, not surprising since these seasons are often associated with incomplete or unventilated combustion. What these temporal data do not show is that carbon monoxide poisoning is most prevalent among people in lower socioeconomic settings where the costs of central heating are prohibitively expensive, forcing them to use gas heaters, stoves, or even barbecue grills. Understanding the characteristics of CO poisoning victims leads quite naturally to certain conclusions about how to target educational or regulatory efforts.

Fourth, epidemiology seeks knowledge of antecedent events and/or the characteristics of those affected, since such information may provide clues to causes or may allow the development of profiles of people who are at greatest risk of developing a given illness.

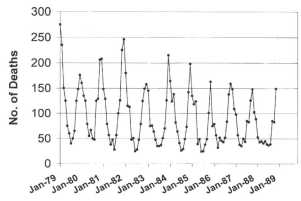

**Figure 23.1.** Deaths by month from carbon monoxide poisoning for the United States 1979–1989. Adapted from: Cobb N, Etzel RA: Unintentional carbon monoxide-related deaths in the United States, 1979 through 1988. *JAMA* 266:659–663, 1991.

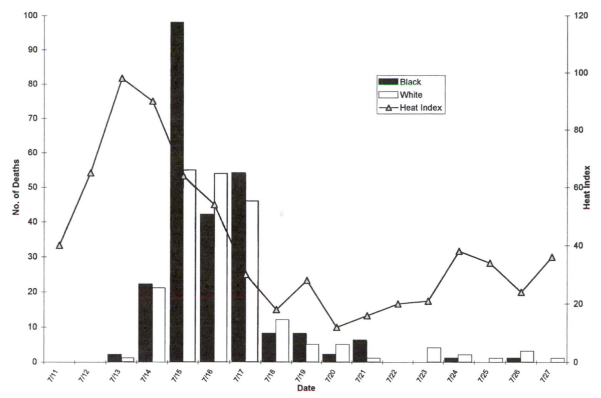

**Figure 23.2.** Number of heat-related deaths by date of occurrence and race of decedent, and heat index by date (Chicago July 11–29 1995). From: U.S. Centers for Disease Control and Prevention. *MMWR*, August 11, 1995, p. 578.

For example, data from the Cook County Medical Examiner's Office of heat-related deaths that took place in the last 2 weeks of July 1995 in Chicago showed that blacks, males, and the elderly were most susceptible. Blacks comprise 26% of the population yet account for the majority of heat-related deaths. In addition, the data in Fig. 23.2 indicate that the incidence of heat-related deaths is likely to remain high for several days after the heat wave peaks. This suggests that educational outreach, public warnings, and clinical vigilance need to continue for some time after the heat wave has subsided.

One important concept that underlies the epidemiologist's view of the world but is not explicitly contained in the definition given is the concept of the natural history of disease. Figure 23.3 provides a schematic representation of what is meant by natural history.

Every clinician knows that in treating otitis media, Type II diabetes mellitus, or a urinary tract infection, the progression of events will generally fall into a definite pattern. In public health, the epidemiologist sees these same patterns, with each disease having a unique signature in the absence of any outside intervention. The stages or phases through which disease is seen to progress include preexposure, a period of susceptibility, the exposure phase, biologic onset, a symptomatic phase, and then certain end points—either cure, a chronic phase, or death.

A critical feature of the natural history is the length of time between onset of exposure and the manifestaton of disease. The longer this period, the better are the prospects for prevention. In the case of infectious diseases this period can be is very short, i.e., days or weeks. In the case of chronic disease, such as coronary heart disease and cancer, this period may be quite long. A characteristic of environmentally induced illnesses is that this latent period can be either very lengthy, e.g., UV exposure and melanoma, or incredibly short, as was the outcome in the case of Hortensia Valasquez's stillborn child or the deaths associated with Chicago's heat wave of the summer of 1995.

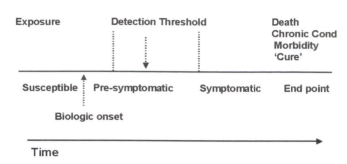

**Figure 23.3.** Phases in the natural history of disease and illness.

## CASE 23-3

*Six adults and three children present to the emergency department of a hospital in a small town in the South. All complain of fever, nausea and vomiting, abdominal pain, and other symptoms. Each of them ate the day before at a church picnic catered by a local restaurant in town. There are indirect reports that other people have been similarly affected.*

*The local health officer closes the restaurant as a precaution and asks local physicians and community residents to report any additional cases. She asks local physicians to also advise their affected patients about precautions to prevent secondary spread of this likely infectious disease within households. She finally asks for assistance from the state health department in investigating the outbreak.*

*The state epidemiologist, with the assistance of local public health nurses and sanitarians, conducts a questionnaire survey of people who had eaten at the church picnic, specifically focusing on which food items they had eaten and which symptoms they had that might be related to the outbreak. Local physicians report 46 additional cases suspected to be part of the outbreak. The team inspects the restaurant's food preparation area, interviews food service workers about symptoms before and during the outbreak, and obtains stool samples from several of those affected as well as all food handlers.*

*The investigators develop a working definition of illness in this outbreak. Analysis of question-naire data involves calculating attack rates of illness for those who had eaten each food item. This analysis reveals that those affected had eaten potato salad more frequently (**p < 0.05**).* **Salmonella typhimurium** *bacteria are grown in cultures of stool from several of those affected and one of the food handlers as well. Further investigation finds opportunities where this food handler may have contaminated the potato salad during its preparation. In addition, it is found that the potato salad had been kept at room temperature overnight (for 12 hours), allowing* **Salmonella** *bacteria in it to multiply.*

*After training food handlers at the restaurant in safe food handling techniques and removing the infected food handler from work (until his stool cultures became negative), the restaurant is allowed to reopen. Those who became ill during the outbreak all recover within 1 week.*

---

*Salmonella comprises more than 2000 serotypes of bacteria that are spread to humans by ingestion of organisms in food from infected animals or contaminated by feces of an infected animal or person. Some domestic and wild animals, such as chickens, are often reservoirs of infection. Salmonella infection can be asymptomatic, or cause a range of symptoms of gastroenteritis, including nausea, vomiting, diarrhea, fever, and sometimes dehydration, especially in the elderly and infants and young children. Prevention is achieved largely through careful practices of food handling, preparation, and storage; public awareness and education; and treating those who are infected.*

---

The outbreak in Case 23-3 is typical of the approximately 500 foodborne disease outbreaks reported each year in the United States. However, these reported outbreaks are just the tip of the iceberg. Were it not for the fact that all of those affected in this particular outbreak had eaten a catered meal, the outbreak might not have been detected or reported.

Foodborne illness accounts for much of the morbidity and some mortality in the United States and abroad. Many types of agents account for these disorders (see Table 23.1).

Large-scale, centralized food production and processing and substantial imports of fresh produce and other food items from other countries may be increasing the risk of foodborne illnesses in the United States today.

Prevention of foodborne illness depends on epidemiologic and laboratory surveillance of gastrointestinal illness and pathogenic organisms responsible for foodborne disease, investigation of outbreaks, the institution of control measures, education of food service workers, inspection of food service establishments, and other measures. Costs of preventive measures like these are substantially lower than the costs of foodborne illness.

Clinicians play important roles in diagnosing, treating, and reporting to public health authorities cases of suspected foodborne disease. In addition to alerting public health authorities to the possible existence of an outbreak such as in Cases 23-1 and 23-3, physicians may be asked to cooperate in an investigation of a disease outbreak or to participate in the screening of food handlers. It is important, therefore, to have some understanding of how these investigations are conducted. While the example we have chosen relates to a foodborne illness, the steps followed in the investigation are quite similar to those that might be followed in the field investigation of any type of exposure.

Basic steps in an epidemiologic investigation:

1. *Collect information*. The first step in undertaking the investigation of any disease outbreak is to collect all available data about the cases of interest. Basic descriptive epidemiologic measures are used to characterize those affected, and those not affected, in terms of person, place, and time. This involves interviewing persons who are ill as well as those who may have recovered, collecting data on the time of onset and duration of illness, gathering information on demographics, and other important antecedent events. As an essential part of this process, it is critical to develop a good "working" case definition. Without a good operational definition of what constitutes a "case," it is not possible to mount a thorough and rigorous investigation. One might decide to employ a strict case definition, in which event only the most severely affected individuals would be included. Alternatively, a loose case definition would include more cases, but might, as a consequence, include some individuals without the illness under investigation.

**Table 23.1**
Classification of Foodborne Disease, with Illustrative Examples[a]

| Category | Examples |
| --- | --- |
| Bacterial infection | *Salmonella* and *Clostridium perfringens* infections |
| Bacterial poison | Staphylococcal and botulinal toxins |
| Viral infection | Hepatitis A |
| Parasitic infection | Trichinosis |
| Chemical poison | Poisoning caused by salts and oxides of arsenic, antimony, copper, and lead |
| Plant or fungal poison | Mushroom poisoning |
| Animal (including marine) | Ciguatera and scombroid poisoning |
| Radionuclide | Strontium-90 poisoning |

[a]Adapted from Werner SB: Food poisoning, in Last JM, Wallace RB (eds): *Maxcy–Rosenau–Last Public Health & Preventive Medicine*, ed 13. Norwalk, Conn, Appleton & Lange, 1992, p 193.

2. *Formulate a hypothesis.* At this stage investigators often develop a working hypothesis based on data gathered in the field, e.g., the culprit is the potato salad, the mayonnaise, or the baked ham. The working hypothesis is tested in a subsequent analytic study.

3. *Choose an appropriate study design.* Most often the investigation of an outbreak will employ a retrospective case–control methodology. Persons who are ill will be identified and are matched with persons who are not ill but have similar demographic characteristics. Data collection will focus on possible exposures. In the case of a foodborne illness, information about the types of food, frequency, and amount consumed are gathered for both cases and controls.

4. *Case identification.* Ascertain all of the cases possible that meet the case definition during a pre-scribed time interval and area. Failure to ascertain all cases during an illness investigation may bias the outcome of the investigation.

5. *Instrument construction.* Develop and, if possible, pretest, refine, and retest instruments (question-naires, interview instruments, data-abstracting forms) in order to gather data on subject characteristics, e.g., person, place, and time, symptoms, and exposure history. The single weakest link in field epidemiologic investigations is often the quality of the data that are gathered. There can be weaknesses in relying on self-reported information. The epidemiologist tries to obtain information from multiple sources wherever possible, in addition to self-reported data such as medical records and employment records. Using alternative sources to augment self-reports often provides a mechanism for validating the data collected in the field.

6. *Analyze the data.* The analytic approach in examining the results of a case-control study proceeds from the premise that a putative causal exposure will be reported more frequently among the cases than among the controls. Hence, the investigator looks for a higher proportion of potato salad-eaters among the cases than the controls. The term that epidemiologists use in describing the association between an exposure and an outcome is *relative risk*. Crudely stated, the relative risk is simply an expression of how much more likely an outcome is, given a particular exposure. For example, given that one eats a portion of potato salad, one has a 4.0-fold greater chance of reporting gastrointestinal illness. (These concepts have been simplified for the purposes of this discussion. In fact, in a case–control study, one often must estimate the relative risk using another measure called an *odds ratio*.)

In addition to sloppiness and carelessness in the design and execution of any investigation, sampling variability and chance are always possible explanations for the results that are observed. An estimate of relative risk of 4.0 for potato salad-eaters versus noneaters could well be a chance finding and not reflect a valid association. To determine whether an association is a chance finding, the epidemiologist employs the tools of inferential statistics. Statistical procedures permit the epidemiologist to assess the likelihood that chance accounts for a particular finding. It is these procedures, called *statistical tests*, that produce the much discussed "*p* value." The *p* value is merely a statement of the probability that chance accounts for the finding observed. Hence, in Case 23-3, the statement that "those affected had eaten potato salad more frequently ($p < 0.05$)" may be interpreted as meaning that there is a less than 5 in 100 (5%) chance that the observed association between potato salad and the illness occurred by chance alone. In the language of the statistician we say that the finding is statistically significant at the 0.05 level. Conversely, there is always a chance, less than 5 in 100, that we are wrong in making such an assertion. The power and promise of inferential statistics is that it allows the epidemiologist/researcher to make inferences from samples of subjects when it is impractical or impossible to study everyone.

---

*When presented with a statistically significant finding, e.g.* $p < 0.05$, *an investigator must always consider the possibility that the finding occurred by chance. The* p *value provides an estimate of the likelihood that chance accounts for the results observed from a given sample.*

---

7. *Examine the results in the light of consistency with previous studies and biologic plausibility.* Epidemiology is a fusion of many different disciplines: the basic biological sciences, clinical medicine, laboratory sciences, and the science of statistics. It is always more impressive in examining the results of an epidemiologic investigation to find that the results observed are not only unlikely due to chance but are also consistent with what we know and what previous investigators have observed and reported. The epidemiologist usually looks for indirect support of a hypothesis before arriving at a conclusion.

8. *Formulate a conclusion.* The conclusion of this analytic process is often an action that will likely have an important programmatic or policy impact, e.g., closing a restaurant (Case 23-3), closing a reservoir (Case 23-1), or regulating the use of space heaters (Case 23-2). Such conclusions are often the last act of the process, but because these conclusions may have sweeping implications, they must be carefully considered by the epidemiologist, the public health official, and the government policymaker.

---

## CASE 23-4

*Maria is a 3-year-old who has just been brought into the community health center. She is accompanied by her mother, Dorothy (aged 28), and two other children, Kenneth (7) and Susan (5). Maria's father, Frank (29), had been working at various jobs in rural Maine until 6 months ago, when the family moved to the city. He found part-time employment with West Bridge Construction Company, where he has been working on the maintenance and reconstruction of highway bridges across the state. The family has no source of health insurance, since Frank's company only provides insurance for full-time employees. The family is currently living on the top floor of a three-family "triple-decker" where they pay $1250 a month for rent.*

*Maria's mother reports that the child was in generally good health until a few weeks ago when she began to notice a loss of appetite. Dorothy described Maria as an easygoing child although recently she has become more and more irritable and difficult to control. She decided to bring Maria to the health center after Maria stopped eating. The other two children appear to be in good health although Kenneth has been having behavioral problems at school. Dorothy thinks that it is because Kenneth is having difficulty adjusting to a new school and finding new friends. Dorothy is very concerned about how she is going to be able to afford the cost of the health center visit.*

*The physical examination revealed that Maria was of normal height although she was below the 5th percentile for weight, perhaps as a result of her loss of appetite. Her vital signs were all within normal limits. She had a hematocrit of 31% and a blood lead level of 28 µg/dl.*

## THE MULTIFACTORIAL NATURE OF DISEASE

The adverse health effects of high levels of lead exposure have been known since Roman times, although only in the past 20 years have the adverse effects of low-level lead exposure been well understood (DHHS, 1991). Lead affects virtually every system of the body, causing among other effects, encephalopathy, nephropathy, and even death at levels around 100 µg/dl.

Subtler neurological effects, such as slowed nerve conduction and subtle developmental effects at levels of 10–20 µg/dl, exact a terrible toll on our nation's children. Those at highest risk are children living in pre-1970's housing, which was built before lead had been banned as a color stabilizer in paint, and adults working in industries or occupations that use some form of lead (see Table 23.2).

As the more subtle neurological, behavioral, and developmental effects of lead have become increasingly well understood, expert groups ranging from the American Academy of Pediatrics to the U.S. Centers for Disease Control and Prevention (CDC) have continued to lower the criteria for blood lead levels that

**Table 23.2**
Sources of Lead Exposure[a]

| Occupational | Environmental | Hobbies and related activities | Substance use |
|---|---|---|---|
| Plumbers, pipefitters | Lead-containing paint | Glazed pottery making | Folk remedies |
| Lead miners | Soil/dust near lead industries, | Target shooting at firing ranges | "Health foods" |
| Auto repairers | roadways, lead-painted homes | Lead soldering (e.g., electronics) | Cosmetics |
| Glass manufacturers | Plumbing leachate | Painting | Moonshine whiskey |
| Shipbuilders | Ceramicware | Preparing lead shot, fishing sinkers | Gasoline sniffing |
| Printers | Leaded gasoline[b] | Stained-glass making | |
| Plastic manufacturers | | Car or boat repair | |
| Lead smelters and refiners | | Home remodeling | |
| Police officers | | | |
| Steel welders or cutters | | | |
| Construction workers | | | |
| Rubber product | | | |
| manufacturers | | | |
| Battery manufacturers | | | |
| Bridge reconstruction workers | | | |
| Firing range instructors | | | |

[a]Adapted from Needleman HL (ed): Case studies in environmental medicine: Lead toxicity, in *Environmental Medicine*, U.S. Department of Health and Human Services, Public Health Service, Agency for Toxic Substances and Disease Registry, Institute of Medicine. Washington, DC, National Academy Press, 1995, p 415.
[b]In countries where lead is not banned in gasoline.

require immediate action. The CDC currently recommends that children with blood lead levels greater than 10 μg/dl be retested and closely monitored (see Fig. 23.4).

With the knowledge that blood lead levels once considered "safe" may indeed constitute a threat to a child's normal growth and development, a greater and greater appreciation of the diversity of sources of lead in the environment and the importance of a multiplicity of different exposure routes has also developed. While flaking and peeling paint chips and dust generated by home improvement activities constitute the principal source of exposure for children, it is clear that lead in soils, in drinking water from soldered pipes, and from work environments (e.g., bridge maintenance and construction) also constitute important sources of exposure.

Lead has been used without restriction for many generations in paint as a color enhancer, in industrial manufacturing (solder, car batteries), as an additive (tetraethyl lead in gasoline banned in 1976 in the United States), in construction (flashing, pipes), by hobbyists (in some pottery glazes), and in recreation (fishing weights and lures). Pathways or sources of childhood exposure are varied and include paint, dust, soil,

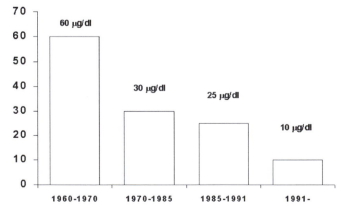

**Figure 23.4.** Steady decline of the CDC's action level for blood lead in children.

drinking water, air, and food. Because lead is extremely stable and persistent, millions of tons of lead that are already in the environment will not soon disappear and will remain a threat to human health whenever it is dislodged or disturbed.

In many ways lead presents a paradigm for many of the environmental exposures that society faces: It is pervasive, it is persistent, and its effects range from subtle neurological and developmental effects, which are nonspecific and often easily confused with other exposures, at low levels, to life-threatening effects at the higher levels of exposure.

Case 23-4 presents the physician with multiple challenges: (1) the need to manage the patient's clinical care; (2) the need to follow up the other two children, making certain they are screened and treated if necessary; (3) the need to explore other possible sources of lead exposure, e.g., through Frank's employment and through dirt in the children's playground; (4) the need to alert the appropriate authorities so that an environmental assessment can be conducted; and (5) the need to advise the landlord so that remedial action can be taken to protect the family from further exposure and insult. Each of these steps should be done without threatening Frank's employment status, without creating higher exposure levels than already exist, i.e., such as by having the family de-lead their apartment themselves, and without adequate medical insurance coverage. Maria's physician also has a responsibility to the families and children who live in the two other units in their "triple-decker" and to the other children and families in the city for whom protection from this environmental exposure is vital to their health and well-being. (See "Role of Physician as Citizen," p. 507.)

Were the clinical management of Maria's low-level lead exposure the only goal of clinical practice, the next steps would be reasonably straightforward: Identify the source of lead, erect barriers to it or protect Maria from it, monitor her blood lead levels carefully, assess her nutritional status, and monitor her neurological and developmental milestones frequently to ensure that they were not compromised in any way. However, managing the physician's larger role is not as simple. Where does one intervene? What are the factors that will likely affect the problem? Which individuals, agencies, and businesses should be contacted? It is in this context that the basic tools and science of epidemiology are so valuable.

Epidemiology, as has been seen, focuses in part on studying the patterns and distribution of health and illness in human populations. One of the critical insights gained through the use of these analytic methods is that causes of morbidity and mortality are multifactorial. There are indeed few, if any, instances in public health in which there exists a single cause and a simple cure. People who develop public policy, e.g., how to prevent and control substance abuse in the population, understand and are often frustrated by the lack of simple "silver bullet" solutions to large-scale intractable problems. Many models have been proposed to explain the determinants of disease and disability and in turn define appropriate intervention strategies. For example, there is the classic agent–host–environment model (Mausner & Kramer, 1985) in which the determinants of morbidity and mortality are seen as resulting from the confluence of factors associated with the individual (host), exposure to some chemical, biological, or physical factor (agent), all taking place within an environmental context, e.g., the workplace, home, school (environment). Although an often cited framework, this model is not terribly helpful to the clinician or public health practitioner who may need to consider other aspects of the problem, for example, what is the potential contribution of the organization and delivery of health services in creating or solving the problem?

In 1974, the Canadian Government published the LaLonde Report, a pivotal document in the evolution of thinking about public health as public policy. Entitled *A New Perspective on the Health of Canadians*, it suggested that there were four categories of factors that had to be considered in developing effective prevention and control strategies (Government of Canada, 1974):

1. Biological factors. These factors include those that are unalterable, such as age, gender, ethnic background, family history, and those that can be altered, such as immune status, cholesterol level, blood pressure.
2. Environmental factors. Included are elements of the physical environment such as chemicals, noise, air and water pollution, tobacco smoke. However, the LaLonde Report also speaks more broadly of

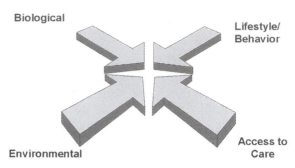

**Figure 23.5.** Determinants of health status.

the political, social, and cultural environment in which people live and work as a source of concern, such as the tolerance for violence as a means of resolving disputes and attitudes about sexual behavior.

3. Lifestyle/behavioral factors. One of the conceptual breakthroughs reflected in this report is the inclusion of individual behavior as one of the critical determinants of health. The framework reminds us of something every practicing physician knows, namely, that individual behaviors are as important determinants of health status as pharmacologic and other therapeutic interventions. Choices that people make about diet, exercise, use of licit and illicit substances, seat belts, helmets, and other protective devices are all critical factors in moderating or eliminating the risk of adverse health outcomes.

4. Access to medical care. One of the fundamental insights of the LaLonde model is that it underscores the importance of the organization, financing, and availability of medical care as an instrument for the prevention of disease and the protection of the public. Timely, appropriate, affordable, and accessible care, while the cornerstone of clinical practice, must also be seen as a major axis for crafting population-based intervention strategies.

Implicit in the LaLonde approach is a population-based perspective essential to the clinician designing an effective management plan for diseases with a known environmental etiology. Using this framework can help the physician craft a management plan responsive to the needs of the patient, the extended family, and the community. Viewing problems in terms of the four categories of the framework enables the physician to consider how interventions can be identified that will address each of these contributing groups of factors. The inescapable conclusion that one reaches in this process is that preventing and controlling environmentally induced illness requires a multifactorial approach and hence the coordinated action of an interdisciplinary group of professionals.

The physician must consider all of Maria's family members at risk. For example, Kenneth may already be showing signs of low-level lead exposure; Maria's mother is at risk of becoming pregnant again and may as a consequence place her unborn fetus at risk; and Frank, Maria's father, may be both occupationally exposed and the source of lead exposure for his family. At the next level, quite literally, are the families who live in the same building who may unknowingly also be exposed to high lead levels in the environment and who also may require medical care. Finally, there is the responsibility to protect others in the community.

While we have already addressed the physician's responsibility to act on behalf of others, she cannot possibly hope to manage this complex situation without the active involvement of others. Just as the physician treating a child with a chronic long-term condition such as asthma requires the assistance of a broad range of helping professionals, so too the physician managing the acute and chronic effects of an environmental exposure must rely on the expertise, advice, and action of other health professionals. This requires alerting state, local, and sometimes federal officials depending on the nature of the exposure and requires working with health and allied health professionals whose roles and responsibilities are sometimes foreign to those who have worked all of their lives in clinical settings. In the worst case, management of these problems

**Table 23.3**
Steps to Take in Addressing Lead Poisoning and Other Environmental Health Problems

1. Screen all children in the nuclear and extended family who may be at risk.
   (Determine if there are any other children potentially at risk.)
2. Conduct appropriate diagnostic tests and initiate treatment where indicated.
3. Educate parents about ways to reduce exposure levels.
4. Educate children about avoiding exposures, if age and developmental level are appropriate.
5. Alert local public health authorities.
6. Make certain that you, or a designated health professional, coordinate and manage the various aspects of the case.
7. Ensure that all poisoned children are followed up and receive appropriate care.
8. If needed, advocate for changes in policy at the state, local, and national levels.

can sometimes lead to a "circus-type" atmosphere in which a huge cast of characters swirl around the child and family and everybody's business becomes nobody's responsibility.

In dealing with a well-recognized problem such as lead poisoning, physicians will often discover a large cadre of helping professionals from both public and private sectors who are available, experienced, and share concern for the best interests of the family and child. Over time physicians learn which aspects or components of the problem they feel competent to address and which aspects are best left to others. Physicians develop a better understanding and appreciation for contributions and competencies of others while at the same time fulfilling their responsibility to serve as an advocate for both their patients and their community.

Table 23.3 provides a summary of the basic steps physicians should follow in crafting management plans to assist in the clinical management of lead poisoning as well as other environmentally induced illnesses. Following these steps will not only assist in clinical management but will also help the family and protect the larger community of families living in the area.

## CASE 23-5

*Amanda Stuart has been in practice for just 3 years. She and her husband, who is also a physician, decided to join the same staff model HMO, he with a general primary care practice and she with a subspecialty in pulmonary medicine. As part of her staff role and responsibilities, she works a half day each week in the HMO's employee health service department providing both primary care and specialty consultation in pulmonary medicine.*

*During the course of the last 6 weeks she has seen a total of seven employees each with similar nonspecific complaints including eyes watering, wheezing, coughing, headache, and nausea. A thorough workup including, history, physical examination, and laboratory tests, revealed no basic underlying etiology for the complaints. Furthermore, there was no common work or exposure history that might explain the symptoms other than the fact that they all worked in the same building.*

*The clustering of these symptoms bothered her since, though nonspecific, they appeared so striking in their presentation. After thinking about them for several days, she attributed them to coincidence and her lack of experience and went about her routine as before.*

## THE ROLE OF PHYSICIAN AS SENTINEL REPORTER

Because of their background and training in science and the scientific method and because of their close contact with individual patients and their families, physicians are in a unique position to provide an early warning of the adverse effects of environmental exposures. While surveillance systems exist at both state and federal levels to alert officials of the existence of threats to the public's health, physicians in practice are the ones most likely to supply these data. The alert clinician who sees seven cases of upper respiratory discomfort in seven patients all of whom work in the same facility (Case 23-5) should consider, as did Dr. Stuart, the possibility that these are not isolated random events. Do these cases have anything in common? Do the patients work in the same setting? Are they neighbors? Are they using the same water supply?

The basic principle that underlies the functioning and operation of any of the state or national reporting systems is that, taken alone, seven cases do not mean very much. By aggregating data over a broad geographic or temporal expanse, one can begin to look for patterns or common characteristics in the distribution of cases. Once identified, such patterns may well provide clues either to the etiology of the illness or disease or to methods for its prevention. Often, many reported cases are needed before these patterns become apparent. Unless an outbreak is a massive and geographically restricted event, e.g., the Legionnaires' disease outbreak in Philadelphia in 1976, it is quite likely that it may go unrecognized for a long time. Advances in communications technology and the use of computers to aggregate and manage data have shortened the time it takes to identify new manifestations of disease or illness and the patterns that are inherent within them.

There are times when the savvy and observant clinician is in the position to serve as an observer and reporter of patterns and trends in health events. As physicians develop their observational skills as part of clinical practice, they also need to remain highly alert to the possibility of unusual patterns or distributions in the events that they observe. Depending on the type of data and situation, physicians need to be aware of the different reporting systems that exist at the state health department level. A discussion of a cluster of cases with an epidemiologist or other expert in the field will help determine whether a more thorough investigation is warranted.

## CASE 23-6

*Dr. Frank Fulton had lived and practiced medicine in Jefferson township for over 15 years. His two children had grown up in the community; attended elementary, junior high, and high school; and were now a sophomore and senior in the high school. Jefferson was an economically struggling community in the southeastern United States, having lost its last remaining textile mill to foreign competition 5 years ago. Notwithstanding these realities, Dr. Fulton had a good practice and had achieved a high level of prominence in the community.*

*Recently, a wave of optimism and euphoria had swept through Jefferson when it was announced that the community had secured a contract with a huge waste management company to build a massive waste management facility at an abandoned mill site a mile and a half from the center of town. Part of the site would be used to construct and operate a high-temperature waste disposal incinerator to handle nonradioactive medical and infectious waste from regional hospitals and medical providers. While acknowledging that special care would be needed to handle infectious waste and contaminants contained in the residual ash from this facility, the company had convinced city, county, and state officials that the state-of-the-art facility posed no health risks to the community.*

*Dr. Fulton was not so sure. He had read about studies in which dioxin and other potent carcinogens had been identified in the breast milk of women living in proximity to waste incinerators.*

*In deciding to report an environmental exposure, ask yourself:*
*1. Is it hazardous or potentially hazardous?*
*2. Are people exposed or potentially exposed?*
*3. Are people experiencing adverse health effects?*

*He also had concerns about possible contaminants from stack emissions since the regulations for waste incinerators had been loosened considerably in recent years. He was concerned for his patients, his family, and his community and he knew that he had sufficient credibility in Jefferson such that his voice would be heard. What concerned him the most was the impact on his practice, his family, and the economic well-being of his community if he raised his voice too high.*

## THE ROLE OF PHYSICIAN AS CITIZEN

Implicit in the notion of the physician as sentinel reporter is that of the physician's responsibility as a citizen of a broader community, a theme evident in all cases we have examined thus far. Because physicians have background and training in the basic and clinical sciences, they are often afforded wide-ranging credibility on a variety of issues that may exceed their training and knowledge. It is not unusual for community-based physicians to be asked to comment on or interpret information from diverse technical and scientific sources. While there is always the danger of misrepresenting one's expertise, it is equally tempting to avoid involvement due to the controversial nature of many local issues, such as a large company that may be endangering the health of its employees and the community, as described in Case 23-6.

In addition to being providers of healthcare services in a community, physicians and their families are also members of that community, a fact that often complicates the physician's role. There are no easy rules or guidelines for assessing which actions to take when presented with public health problems. Threats to one's professional standing and influence, the potential for civil liability, the fiscal integrity of one's practice, and the effects on one's own personal life and family have to be weighed against the moral imperative to act to protect the health both of patients and of the community. The availability of federal, state, and local agencies, whose responsibilities include protection of all citizens, will not necessarily make these choices any easier.

---

### CASE 23-7

*Cynthia Burdick is a 13-year-old who was diagnosed with asthma at the age of 10 by her family's physician, Dr. Herbert Robinson. Her condition has been generally well managed by her mother, who lives with Cynthia and her brother, Brian, aged 8. Cynthia's mother has struggled to make a living on the farm that she inherited from her husband when he died in an automobile accident 6 years ago. Both children attend school 6 miles away. Brian has been actively involved in school sports, but Cynthia has been unable to compete in athletics, her first love, because of her asthma. Recently, Cynthia has become moody and temperamental and has had two recent asthmatic attacks, one of which required hospitalization.*

*Adding to the stress in the household, Mrs. Burdick's brother Edwin, his wife, and their 1-year-old are staying with the family while they look for a place of their own. Edwin and his wife both smoke a pack and a half of cigarettes a day. Although Mrs. Burdick has asked them not to smoke in the house, they continue to do so.*

## ENVIRONMENTAL EXPOSURES: IMPLICATIONS FOR CLINICAL PRACTICE

Asthma affects approximately 17.3 million people in the United States, 4.8 million of whom are children, making it the most common chronic disease of childhood (Committee on the Assessment of Asthma and Indoor Air, 2000). Asthma hospitalization rates for children 14 years of age and under were 338 per 100,000 in 1997, a 20% increase from the baseline year of 1987. Asthma remains the most frequent admitting diagnosis in children's hospitals across the country. In terms of economic costs, it was estimated that by 2000, asthma-related costs would exceed $14.5 billion (*Healthy People 2000 Review*, National Center for Health Statistics, 1999). As is the case with so many chronic diseases, asthmatic death rates for blacks are higher than for whites (DHHS, 1995). Among Puerto Rican children residing in the United States, the prevalence of asthma is higher than in the non-Hispanic or black communities. Epidemiologic evidence suggests that race/ethnicity may serve as a proxy for socioeconomic status, which is itself another known risk factor for asthma. Additionally, urban dwelling clearly poses its own risks, with dust, pollution, ozone, and other ambient air factors contributing to asthma development. In summary, asthma provides a convenient paradigm for examining the synergistic and potentiating effects of race/ethnicity, poverty, housing, and geography on the natural history of a chronic disease.

Aggressive medical management of the asthmatic child with bronchodilators and anti-inflammatory agents along with careful monitoring using peak flow meters are most often the bases for therapy. Of critical importance to the success of this therapeutic approach is the provision of careful instruction and training for both the child and parents so that they will be able to deal quickly and effectively with an asthmatic episode. In fact, several studies have demonstrated that increasing parental knowledge of asthma is effective in decreasing the subsequent use of healthcare services (Brook *et al.*, 1993; Clark *et al.*, 1986).

Strangely, there is little discussion in the clinical literature of the role of in-home management of pollutants and/or the role of pollution prevention in the home environment as a critical component of asthma management practice. For people who spend much time indoors, as is the case for many urban dwellers, the concentrations of many indoor air pollutants can exceed those found in ambient air. Development or exacerbation of asthmatic episodes has been associated with dust, dander (from cats and dogs), cigarette smoke, mold spores, and vapor and mists from chemicals and cosmetics.

Anyone with children understands how difficult it is to implement aggressive in-home pollution control measures. While it may be possible to control the myriad indoor factors likely to precipitate or exacerbate an asthmatic episode for a short period of time, it takes an extraordinary commitment to engage in such behaviors over long periods of time. If one couples this with the difficulties attendant with various sources of pollution likely to be found in certain other venues, e.g., living on a farm, the scope of the problem becomes enormous.

While anxiety and stress are a part of Mrs. Burdick's life in Case 23-7 and also a factor in the clinical management of Cynthia's asthma, these factors are not often easy to eliminate. Similarly, occupational exposures in a farm environment from dust, pollens and other allergens, and the like cannot be easily eliminated from the family's life without a change of venue. The primary care physician does have a role to play in counseling family members about ways to reduce exposure to these factors through the use of barrier techniques, such as a dust mask, or through anticipatory guidance, such as having Cynthia perform chores less likely to expose her to environmental factors that will exacerbate her condition.

There are, however, exposures such as environmental tobacco smoke (ETS) that pose a very real threat to the health and well-being of the asthmatic child or adult but that are far more easily preventable or avoidable. The U.S. Environmental Protection Agency (U.S. EPA), in its Scientific Advisory Committee Report on Environmental Tobacco Smoke, stopped short of identifying ETS as a "cause" of asthma but it did conclude that "ETS is a known cause of exacerbation of asthma in persons known to have the disease" (U.S. EPA, 1993). While it may not be possible for Mrs. Burdick to refuse her brother and his family a place to stay, it is critically important for Cynthia's physician to emphasize the importance of Cynthia's avoiding any unnecessary exposure to ETS. The evidence implicating ETS in the etiology of a range of chronic and acute conditions is mounting rapidly. ETS exposure has been linked to lung cancer, asthma, lower respiratory tract infections, otitis media, and, most recently, SIDS, and coronary heart disease (Glantz & Parmley, 1995; Klonoff-Cohen *et al.*, 1995; National Cancer Institute, 1999; U.S. EPA, 1993).

Recognizing the adverse health effects of ETS exposure and fearing potential liability, several well-known restaurant chains that cater to children have banned all smoking in their establishments. Similarly, large businesses and employers are increasingly moving in the direction of restricting or banning smoking altogether. Although a volatile subject for discussion, Edwin Burdick's smoking behavior in Case 23-7 requires careful attention. Dr. Robinson should explain to Edwin the likely negative effect of his behavior not only on his niece but also on his own child, citing the data on otitis media, lower respiratory tract infections, and SIDS. While Edwin and his wife certainly should be encouraged to stop smoking, failing that, a reasonable goal would be to have them agree only to smoke outside and away from Cynthia and her family. Research shows that even among smokers there is an acknowledgment of the need to keep children from initiating the behavior as well as the need to avoid their involuntary exposure to tobacco smoke. A little judicious counseling can go a long way toward eliminating this risk factor.

As with lead and other environmental exposures, Dr. Robinson and his colleagues should become involved in efforts to control involuntary exposure to ETS. He should consider joining with local and county public health officials working on the development of ETS regulations and curbing youth access to tobacco. Similarly, large employers and insurers in the area should be approached about reducing involuntary exposure to ETS and other pollutants. Because so many sources of pollution are inaccessible to the average consumer and provider, it is essential to act when the opportunity presents itself.

Asthma, along with other diseases having important environmental cofactors, poses many dilemmas for the clinician. While effective pharmacologic agents exist to help in the clinical management of the disease, long-term success requires a threefold approach:

1. It is essential that the patient receive clear and precise instructions concerning when, where, and how to use the standard medications that you prescribe. To assist in this effort, several excellent materials have been developed to help with patient education and instruction (see the Asthma Prevention Program of the National Center for Environmental Health, U.S. Centers for Disease Control and Prevention, www.cdc.gov/nech/programs/asthma).
2. It is essential that the patient and family have access to clinical care when needed to manage any exacerbations that may occur. Since asthmatic attacks can be life-threatening, it is essential that patients and their families have easy access to emergency care when needed.
3. It is essential that families receive assistance evaluating the sources of environmental exposure in their living spaces as well as assistance in taking steps to reduce these factors to the lowest possible threshold levels. Pollution prevention and pollution control are as important in the environmental management of the asthmatic child as they are in the larger environment.

# CONCLUSION

In this chapter we have emphasized four points of critical importance to the primary care physician faced with the clinical management of a problem having an environmental etiology:

1. Practicing physicians must be vigilant for situations involving disease and illness that may have an underlying environmental etiology. This implies paying special attention to exposures peculiar to the geographic location of the physician's practice. It also requires special care and attention when obtaining a history to cover areas of possible environmental exposure.
2. Physicians in primary care practice have an important responsibility to serve as sentinel reporters of adverse health events that may be associated with environmental exposures. This requires that physicians be familiar with the various state and local agencies having responsibility for receiving and analyzing reports of environmental disease and illness.
3. Primary care physicians have important roles to play as "risk communicators" sharing information with the communities in which they live, and their patients and patient families about the relative importance of various environmental exposures and methods of avoiding them.
4. The physician faced with environmentally induced illness must look beyond the individual patient and consider the population health consequences of environmental exposures. The effective management of environmentally induced disease forces the physician to assume both roles of medical doctor and public health physician.

While these various roles are important, traditional medical education does not prepare the primary care physician to assume these roles. Thus, many physicians shy away from problems with a suspected environmental etiology. Attention to the basic principles outlined in this chapter should make that experience both rewarding and meaningful.

## CASES FOR DISCUSSION

### CASE 1

*A young male office worker comes to your clinic with a chief complaint of a rash on his hands and wrists that appeared 5 days ago. The company he works for is the largest employer in your community and is just beginning to recover from a dramatic series of "downsizing" layoffs triggered by cutbacks in the defense industry.*

*He has just relocated to an older building that has been totally remodeled. Private offices were replaced with cubicles and a large open work environment, new carpeting was laid throughout the work area, and the walls were finished with new wallboard and painted.*

*Many of his co-workers also have reported a wide range of symptoms from fatigue, lightheadedness, watery eyes, and an assortment of GI symptoms. He reports that to his knowledge he is the only one who has developed a rash, although most other employees attribute their symptoms to the new work environment.*

*1. What areas would you want to cover in taking a history?*
*2. What other possible non-work-related exposures might account for these symptoms?*
*3. What obligations do you have to validate the reports of other affected employees?*
*4. To whom would you turn at the state and local level to assist you in unraveling the etiology of this illness episode?*

### CASE 2

*For years residents of the Fairview neighborhood have been complaining about the foul odors emanating from the abandoned landfill adjacent to the nearby river. The state Department of Environmental Management closed the landfill 5 years ago, installed vents to bleed off methane from beneath the landfill, and instituted a monitoring program to sample groundwater for volatile organic compounds. A nearby elementary school is adjacent to the landfill.*

*Articles have recently appeared in the local paper suggesting that an "abnormal number of cancer deaths" have occurred in the Fairview neighborhood among longtime residents of the area. The mayor has notified the county health department and has asked you to represent the medical community on an advisory board he is establishing to investigate these allegations.*

*1. How would you determine whether this constitutes an environmentally induced cluster of cases or is a "natural cluster" due to chance?*
*2. How would you define a "case"?*
*3. What type of investigation should be conducted? Who should be interviewed? What about those who have left the area?*
*4. How would you define the exposure? How would you measure it?*
*5. What would you tell your patients who live in the area or whose children attend the elementary school about the risks?*

### CASE 3

*A mother with two young children calls your office in a near state of hysteria having just seen a report on national television on the association between leukemia and electromagnetic fields. She and her family live two blocks from a major power substation just like one of those implicated in the television documentary. She wonders what she can do to protect her children while she contemplates putting her house on the market. You admit to her that you are not totally familiar with the recent research on electromagnetic fields and human cancer but that you will get back to her once you have done some research and made some inquiries of your own.*

1. *Where would you look for information about an exposure with which you were unfamiliar? What state and local agencies might you contact for additional information?*
2. *Does common sense provide any clues as to what steps this mother ought to take?*
3. *Assuming the data you gathered were equivocal, as they often are, what would you tell this mother about the risks? Should she sell her house?*

## CASE 4

*Over 40 hours, 19 patients have come to your clinic complaining of feverishness, abdominal cramps, and diarrhea. Nine of these patients are women and ten are men. They range in age from 6 to 71.*

1. *How would you go about determining if this was a foodborne or waterborne outbreak with a common source of infection?*
2. *When and to whom would you report this outbreak?*
3. *How would you determine if there were additional cases in your community that might be part of this outbreak?*
4. *Without yet knowing the cause and the source of this outbreak of illness, how would you advise your patients about minimizing the spread of this illness?*

## CASE 5

*You have just treated the second case in a month of a child with persistent upper respiratory symptoms. The only unusual aspect to the two cases was that the parents reported that the symptoms appeared after the purchase and use of an ultrasonic humidifier. After seeing the second case, you asked both sets of parents to stop using the humidifier in their children's rooms. In both instances the parents reported that the symptoms abated and disappeared a few days after discontinuing use of the room humidifier.*

1. *Is there a cause-and-effect relationship between humidifier use and the children's symptoms?*
2. *What subsequent steps, if any, might you take to alert other parents and families?*
3. *How might an epidemiologic investigation be undertaken to investigate the relationship between humidifier use and symptoms of upper respiratory infections?*

# RECOMMENDED READINGS

Blumenthal DS, Ruttenber AJ: *Introduction to Environmental Health*. New York, Springer Publishing Co, 1995.

> A good overview of principles and practice of environmental health. The book contains chapters on epidemiology, environmental health law, occupational health, and an overview of pathways of exposure.

Christoffel T, Gallagher SS: *Injury Prevention and Public Health Practical Knowledge, Skills and Strategies*. Gaithersburg, Aspen Publishers, Inc, 1999.

> This is an excellent comprehensive book on injury and public health practice. It provides a thorough discussion of the epidemiology of injuries and approaches to injury prevention and control.

Goldman L: Environmental health and its relationship to occupational health, in Levy BS, Wegman DH (eds): *Occupational Health: Recognizing and Preventing Work-Related Disease and Injury*, ed 4. Philadelphia, Lippincott, Williams & Wilkins, 2000.

Hennekens CH, Buring JE: *Epidemiology in Medicine*. Boston, Little Brown & Co, 1987.

> One of the best and most widely used texts on epidemiology, this book provides an excellent starting point in the theory and practice of epidemiology.

Levy BS, Wegman DH (eds): *Occupational Health: Recognizing and Preventing Work-Related Disease and Injury*, ed 4. Philadelphia, Lippincott, Williams & Wilkins, 2000.

> This textbook provides a comprehensive introduction to the field of occupational health.

Pope AM, Rall DP (eds): *Environmental Medicine: Integrating a Missing Element into Medical Education*. Washington, DC, National Academy Press, 1995.

> An excellent case book and resource guide for developing and implementing environmental health teaching in medical school and residency training settings. The book contains many case studies complete with questions for study, references, and review questions.

Rom WN (ed): *Environmental and Occupational Medicine*, ed 3. Philadelphia, Lippincott–Raven, 1998.

> A well-written, comprehensive, and authoritative book on environmental and occupational medicine.

Wallace RB (ed): *Maxcy–Rosenau–Last Public Health & Preventive Medicine*, ed 14. Stamford, Conn, Appleton & Lange, 1998.

> This classic one-volume text of almost 2000 pages covers the principles and practice of public health. The text, which is in its 14th edition, covers epidemiology, environmental health, infectious disease, and the organization and structure of public health in the United States. If one were to purchase only a single book on public health theory and practice, this would be the one to choose.

# REFERENCES

Asthma Prevention Program of the National Center for Environmental Health, U.S. Centers for Disease Control and Prevention. www.cdc.gov/nech/programs/asthma

Brook U, Mendelberg A, Heim M: Increasing parental knowledge of asthma decreases hospitalization of the child: A pilot study. *J Asthma* 30(1):45–49, 1993.

Clark NM, Feldman CH, Evans D, Levison MJ, Wasilewski Y, Mellins RB: The impact of health education on the frequency and cost of health care use by low income children with asthma. *J Allergy Clin Immunol* 78(1):108–114, 1986.

Cobb N, Etzel RA: Unintentional carbon monoxide-related deaths in the United States, 1979 through 1988. *JAMA* 266:659–663, 1991.

Committee on the Assessment of Asthma and Indoor Air: *Clearing the Air—Asthma and Indoor Air Exposures.* Washington, DC, Institute of Medicine, National Academy of Sciences, 2000.

Department of Health and Human Services, Public Health Service, Centers for Disease Control and Prevention: Asthma—United States 1980–1987. *Morbidity Mortality Weekly Rep* 39:493–497, 1990.

Department of Health and Human Services, Public Health Service, Centers for Disease Control and Prevention: *Preventing Lead Poisoning in Young Children: A Statement by the Centers for Disease Control*, October 1991.

Department of Health and Human Services, Public Health Service, Centers for Disease Control and Prevention: Asthma—United States 1982-1992. *Morbidity Mortality Weekly Rep* 44:952–955, 1995.

Farrow JR, Davis GJ, Roy TM, McCloud LC, Nichols, GR: Fetal death due to nonlethal carbon monoxide poisoning. *J Forensic Sci* 35(6):1448–1452,1990.

Glantz S, Parmley W: Passive smoking and heart disease. Mechanisms and risk. *JAMA* 273(13):1047–1053, 1995.

Government of Canada, Ministry of Health and Welfare: *A New Perspective on the Health of Canadians. A Working Document.* Ottawa, Ministry of Health and Welfare, Government of Canada, 1974.

*Healthy People 2000 Review*, National Center for Health Statistics, 1999.

Klonoff-Cohen H, Edelstein S, Lefkowitz E, Srinivassan I, Kaegi D, Chang JC, Wiley KJ: The effect of passive smoking and tobacco exposure through breast milk on sudden infant death syndrome. *JAMA* 271:795–798, 1995.

MacKenzie WR, Hoxie MS, Proctor MA, Gradus MA, Blair KA, Peterson DE, Kazmierczak JJ, Addiss DG, Fox KR, Rose JB, Davis JP: A massive outbreak in Milwaukee of Cryptosporidium infection transmitted through the public water supply. *N Engl J Med* 331: 161–167, 1994.

Mausner JS, Kramer S: *Epidemiology: An Introductory Text.* Philadelphia, WB Saunders & Co, 1985, p 28.

National Cancer Institute: Health Effects of Exposure to Environmental Tobacco Smoke: The Report of the California Environmental Protection Agency. Smoking and Tobacco Control Monograph No. 10. Bethesda, Md, U.S. Department of Health and Human Services, National Institutes of Health, National Cancer Institute, NIH Publication No. 99-4645, 1999.

Needleman HL (ed): Case studies in environmental medicine: Lead toxicity, in *Environmental Medicine*, U.S. Department of Health and Human Services, Public Health Service, Agency for Toxic Substances and Disease Registry, Institute of Medicine. Washington, DC, National Academy Press, 1995, p 415.

U.S. Centers for Disease Control and Prevention: *Morbidity Mortality Weekly Rep*, August 11, 1995, p 578.

U.S. Environmental Protection Agency. The respiratory health effects of passive smoking: Lung cancer and other disorders. Washington, DC, Office of Health and Environmental Assessment, Office of Research and Development, U.S. Environmental Protection Agency. Publication No. EPA/600/6-90/006F, 1993, pp 7–51.

Werner SB: Food poisoning, in Last JM, Wallace RB (eds): *Maxcy–Rosenau–Last Public Health & Preventive Medicine*, ed 13. Norwalk, Conn, Appleton & Lange, 1992, p 193.

## CHAPTER 24

# The Cultural Role of the Patient

*Howard F. Stein*

---

## CASE 24-1

*The patient, a 63-year-old white man being hospitalized for rehabilitation following a myocardial infarction, suddenly stopped eating, refusing all food and drink. The nurse carefully noted this in the patient's chart, and the attending physician, wanting to rule out depression, asked for a liaison psychiatric consult. As it turned out, the psychiatrist quickly discovered that the refusal to eat occurred on Yom Kippur (the Day of Atonement), a religious fast day, and that the patient was an Orthodox Jew. "Things" in medicine are often not what they seem: "refusal to eat" can have different significances, different consequences, in different frameworks (medical, religious, ethnic).*

## EDUCATIONAL OBJECTIVES

1. To equip the medical student to think and act culturally in patient care
2. To distinguish between cultural stereotype and cultural description
3. To improve physician–patient communication through cultural negotiation
4. To understand ethnic, workplace, and popular cultural facets of patients' health beliefs and practices.

## INTRODUCTION

People live in groups, from small, nuclear to large, extended family groups, from face-to-face village-based societies to complex, urban, nation-based societies cemented by electronic communications media. Even in small, bounded societies such as aboriginal hunting-gathering bands, people are never members of only a single group. Even there, they move in and out of several microcultures, although the differences between them are not as dramatic as those in our industrial society. It is in such groups that people become ill, are defined as ill, receive treatment, recover or decline, and eventually die.

Unlike small-scale, face-to-face, closed, kin-based preliterate societies, in our complex, secularized, urbanized, and pluralistic society, practitioner and patient often come from different cultural groups. Their

513

values, beliefs, rules, roles, attitudes, expectations, and world-views may differ markedly. To further complicate matters, the clinician will have undergone years of socialization in a professional culture that is supposed to supersede all those earlier ones from childhood that bear the mark of being "lay."

Case 24-1 illustrates problems that can arise if the patient and the physician come from different cultures. Had the team taken a rudimentary social history, been more familiar with the cultural and religious tradition of the patient population, or simply asked the patient why he refused to eat, a psychiatric consultation would have been unnecessary.

This chapter explores the cultural world of the patient and its consequences for sickness and treatment. Following a number of conceptual topics, four types of cultural settings will be discussed: ethnic or nation of ancestry, religious, occupational, and popular. The reader should understand, however, that such a classification is at some level heuristic and arbitrary, that all of these overlap, and that culture is a fluid, not a static, process.

As author of this chapter, I wish to serve as the reader's guide on a journey into cultural awareness that did not come easy to me—nor does it now after 25 years of practice. Let me say at the outset that I cannot provide some answers the reader wishes—and that I, too, wish I could provide—even though "answers," "quick answers," "simple answers," and "definitive answers" are what we in the United States are taught to expect of experts. The reader will look in vain for ethnic or denominational formulas that generalize, say, to "all Vietnamese" or "all Southern Baptists." Behind every ethnic or religious label is much diversity, even among seemingly homogeneous tribal groups. Groups change, too, over history, over differing experiences. Twenty years ago, during the Black Power era, I served on the faculty at Meharry Medical College in Nashville, Tennessee. I can still remember the astonishment and disbelief on the faces of medical students who had grown up in New York City as they heard their ethnic brothers and sisters from New Orleans speak of how they left their homes and cars unlocked at night. Ideologically, they thought themselves to be "the same." In experience, they discovered much unwelcomed difference.

No outsider's cultural formulary or "recipe book" can substitute for the physician's painstaking, time-consuming, but rewarding familiarity with the lives of patients and the communities from which they come. This does not make my chapter somehow "too advanced" for medical students—as though a more elementary text should offer ethnic pablum that falsifies the cultural reality the reader will soon see every day in practice. In a real sense, the reader needs to be equipped to be a better clinical anthropologist than I am, because long after the reader has forgotten this chapter, he or she will have to be making difficult cultural assessments about patients' beliefs, values, attitudes, expectations, feelings, and roles. Behind the myriad of facts and vignettes in this chapter is *a method for learning about culture.*

In my 30 years of medical teaching, many medical students and residents have protested to me during their training that "cultural stuff" is interesting but not "real medicine." "If I had the time, I'd find out about patients' culture, but who has the time?" The trouble is: culture is never mere "background." It is as much foreground as is any tissue or organ system. It may lurk behind the very disease etiology we seek to explain and that we wish to cure. Culture is part of every one of those key words we use everyday in biomedicine: diagnosis, symptom, outcome, satisfaction (the physician's as well as the patient's), compliance, prevention, wellness, and yes, litigation. Culture is not extrinsic to medicine or on the periphery. The challenge for busy medical practitioners is to be attentive enough to take culture seriously, while attending to everything else as well. And I know that is never easy.

## CASE 24-2

*The Vietnamese-American parents of a 4-year-old boy brought him to a primary care physician for persistent cough, sore throat, fever, diarrhea, upper respiratory distress, and poor appetite that had lasted a week. On physical examination, the physician found six symmetrical ovoid bruises (ecchymoses) on the boy's back and two on the front of his neck. He immediately suspected child abuse, especially since the child seemed so quiet, docile, and compliant. He wanted immediately to contact child protective services and have a social worker begin an investigation of the boy's home situation.*

## APPROACHES TO THE CONCEPT OF CULTURE

What is culture? How can physicians look and listen for culture? How can physicians recognize and work clinically with culture—that of their patients, themselves, and their clinical colleagues? Let me offer several perspectives, like a surveyor trying to assess a landscape. A crucial distinction that must be made is between the view of culture offered by a member of that group (insider) and a view of that "same" culture by someone external to that group (outsider), such as a physician. We need to correct the deficiencies and blind spots of each group.

At its most basic—and contrary to a widespread view among social scientists—culture does not consist primarily of trait lists of, say, values, language, attitudes, beliefs, expectations, all of which somehow add up to influence health beliefs and behavior. Rather, *culture is first and foremost that sense of "us," "we," "our way,"* the contents of which can and do change over time. Central to the concept of culture is that of group boundary and group identity: what is inside and what is outside.

Culture is the social unit, or often one among many units, to which the sense of belonging and loyalty are attached, the unit associated with one's social boundary. It is as if to say: "This is who and what I am; this is who and what we are; this is what we do." Or: "That is not who and what I am; that is what we do not do." Cultural content here serves to define what is "me" and what is "not me." For example, many male members of the "cowboy culture" of the North American Great Plains associate cowboy boots as an intrinsic part of the self and of one's masculinity. Other forms of footwear are viewed as alien, feminine, if not downright wrong. If a cowboy injures his foot, the prospect of not being able to wear cowboy boots is experienced as a threat to the self. Of course, group boundaries are permeable. At any given moment, and over a lifetime, one can have multiple "group" identities and affiliations—all of which affect health beliefs and behavior.

As a "design for living," culture is a normative system, with both prescriptive and proscriptive rules, values, attitudes, roles, expectations, and the like (Parry, 1984; Spiegel, 1971)—much like physicians' *prescriptions* to patients. It is full of "Thou shalt's" and "Thou shalt not's." Understood this way, culture consists of patterned, preferred solutions to common problems, solutions that often lead to standardized, stereotyped responses to these problems. For instance, among many Irish Catholics the lively sense of sin and guilt leads them to believe that if a medicine is truly beneficial, then it must taste bad or hurt when applied to the body: "Good [powerful] medicine tastes bad."

When we describe people's cultures (our own or others'), we often think only in terms of the "object" we are describing rather than also in terms of the "subject" doing the describing. In many ways, physicians and anthropologists are in the same boat, as they try to understand and work with people whose cultures differ from their own. Here, culture is an abstraction constructed by outside observers and interpreters, an abstraction that may be welcomed or condemned by those whom we are describing. Our own cultural lens as healthcare professionals may help us to see better, or distort our vision.

One virtue of an outsider's viewpoint for biomedicine is that an outsider, say, a physician, might detect a pattern that members of the patient culture or community do not notice or simply take for granted. Further, what people claim about their way of life often differs from what an outsider sees or hears them actually do (Stein & Hill, 1977). An observant physician has access to both kinds of "data sets." A physician can describe a culture statistically, in terms of population characteristics, then interpret it not only to an individual patient, but also to the wider community (from county medical society meetings to newspaper articles). Through careful study of medical records of one-patient-seen-at-a-time, broader community patterns may emerge. At one clinic where I work, for example, "like clockwork" in the middle of March there will be several three-

and four-wheeler vehicle [all-terrain vehicle (ATV)] accident victims, mostly teenagers, in the hospital. With the first sign of a break in the winter weather, young people will take their restless energy to daredevil courses on the clay mounds and in the fields.

No culture stands still over time. Cultures change as their ability to fulfill human functions diminishes. People create and change culture in order to meet needs, whether these needs be rational, reality oriented, or irrational. For instance, once the Spanish and their horses had arrived in North America, Native Americans' hunting and raiding by foot on the Great Plains was succeeded and replaced by equestrian hunting and warfare. But initially this was done only among some groups: Others ate the horses as meat. To turn to a medical example: until the 1950s, entire children's hospitals in North America were filled with iron lung machines for patients with polio. The revolutionary vaccination developed by Jonas Salk was quickly accepted, and by now the massive iron lungs (Drinker respirator) have virtually disappeared. At the same time, the equally revolutionary antiseptic procedure of washing one's hands with chlorinated lime, developed in nineteenth-century Vienna by Ignaz Phillip Semmelweis, was met with fierce and persistent opposition by Western professional culture. As we try to understand the history of Western biomedicine, like the history of all culture, we must realize that, on the one hand, even cultural ideas to which people are committed do change. But on the other hand, the abundance of counterrevolutionary movements over history attests to the fear of change, resistance to change, and the threat of loss of whole ways of life.

Not only do all cultures undergo change over time (often more at the surface than at the core), but all cultures also have some degree of intracultural variation. This internal differentiation is more pronounced and more tolerated in complex, secularized, urban society. In complex society, people move in and out of numerous subcultures, whereas in more primitive, small-scale society, these would tend to merge or at least greatly overlap. The more complex the society, the less homogeneity and the more heterogeneity is found. For instance, in a hunting-gathering band, one's kin group is also one's occupational group and one's religious congregation.

Those of us in healthcare professions need to be able to distinguish between scientific *generalizations* about culture and *stereotypes* we might indulge in about others. It is often difficult to know which form of "discrimination" we are making. (And remember that a good differential list marks the beginning of that crucial form of clinical discrimination called diagnosis!) In theory at least, scientific thinking is open-minded, and theories can therefore be modified, while no amount of new evidence can loosen a stereotype, which people use to defend themselves against thoughts and feelings. However, healthcare practitioners are not the only ones who have stereotypes. All cultures have their stereotypes about themselves and about others (Henry, 1963). That is what ethnocentrism is all about: It says, "*We* are the real human beings; *you* are the dirtballs." Such stereotypes feel and ring true because they perform vital functions of preserving self-esteem and cohesiveness.

But the price of stereotypes is that they distort reality. Groups cannot learn when they feel that they cannot afford to perceive the world differently. For instance, cultural groups that are rife with suspicion and mistrust, and that abound in malevolent supernatural beings who inflict disease and death, will be unlikely candidates for easy acceptance of the more neutral and impersonal biomedical disease model. Similarly, one can only wonder what the effect of the competitive battle among HMOs and their allied physicians for patients will be on physician collegiality in the future culture of U.S. medicine.

To summarize: to say that culture is a *system*, and not a mere collection of elements or traits, is to say that culture is an *organizing principle* of people's lives. This can be taken too far as much as it can be overlooked. Physicians, mental health practitioners, social scientists, and public policymakers frequently use cultural formulations to "pigeonhole" people, to adopt cultural profiles as cookbooks, to turn description, inquiry, and interpretation into stereotypes that oversimplify and distort rather than illumine. Especially in a complex, pluralistic society, a listing of a person's ancestral ethnicity, a label about one's personal or parental religion, a classification of one's job, or a statement that one largely self-medicates based on popular U.S. folk culture should not be construed to be the whole story. It should be the beginning of a conversation, not the end.

There can be no substitute for the painstaking and time-consuming elicitation of the patient's story, including the patient's family and wider intimate network, a fact that is no less true in the era of corporate medicine and managed care than it was in the prior era of fee-for-service practice (Stein & Apprey, 1987). To know that a person is African-American, Ashkenazic Jewish, Latin Rite Catholic, Vietnamese Buddhist, Guatemalan Catholic, Great Plains wheat farmer, or avid reader of *Reader's Digest* and *The National Enquirer* or the Internet as sources for medical advice is rightfully to generate a set of hypotheses that may help to understand and culturally calibrate the *individual* (Hill *et al.*, 1990). On the other hand, uncritical extrapolation from a mere cultural label or stereotype is an indulgence that reveals more the projections of the observer than the cultural worlds inhabited by the one ostensibly under observation.

For example, in Case 24-2, consultation with a behavioral science faculty member and subsequent inquiry of the parents revealed a picture different from that initially supposed by the physician about the Vietnamese-American boy's ecchymoses. The parents practiced an ethnomedical treatment regimen that they widely shared with coastal Vietnamese peoples. Many diseases are believed to be caused by "bad winds" that enter the body and cause an imbalance. "Winds" are believed to be one of the major elements of the universe. This Vietnamese theory of disease is a local variant on a balance theory widespread throughout the Buddhist/ Confucian-influenced Orient. To help the child, the parents resorted to custom to try to help restore the body's natural balance. They took a highly polished coin and rubbed it with an ointment (lubricant) at several places on their son's back and neck until these places bruised, thereby creating openings for the "bad winds" to escape from entrapment in the body, thus enabling the boy's body to restore its natural balance. This procedure is called *Cao gio* ("scratch away the wind": *cao* = scratch away, *gio* = wind) (Primosch & Young, 1980).

The boy and his parents alike described the practice as soothing, a little like a massage, and that the warm ointment felt good being rubbed. The boy insisted that "it didn't hurt." The parents became concerned when their efforts did not result in the boy's rapid return to health. With this explanation, the physician was persuaded that he did not need to pursue a child abuse investigation. It turned out that the boy had an especially virulent form of the flu, one that typically lasted around 10 days; the parents likewise felt reassured on hearing this.

In biomedicine at least most of the time, we do not so much ask the wrong questions as we ask our own cultural, professional questions, e.g., What do you have (disease, acute or chronic; visible lesion; disability)? We need also to ask those kinds of questions—and listen for that kind of information—that address their lives, e.g., Who are you? What is it like to be you? What is it like for you to have (name of disease, disability, accident)? Although we might not ask these questions directly, if we think rather of the type of information they seek, we will be on our way to obtaining personal, and therefore culturally useful, data. What is more, the act of thinking and speaking in this way toward patients makes us more of a person as well. Finally, the approach I am suggesting here is not so much a matter of literally asking (more and more) questions, as of listening and caring to listen to others as persons. The "asking" comes out of the process of "listening" in the broadest sense. The listening, in turn, is a product of a willingness to imagine the disease or the problem as being a part of a life—and of lives (marriage, family, workplace)—that is, to consider the possibility that the patient or family member is coming from a different frame of reference.

Physicians should keep in mind that patients' and families' cultural beliefs, meanings, and practices may well influence any and all aspects of health-related decision-making. Even where patients might accept the naturalistic, mechanistic, diseased entity-oriented biomedical model for certain aspects of their disease and its treatment, they may well harbor more personalistic (Foster, 1976) ideas of why they are sick *now*, why *they* and not another have fallen ill, *what* they might have done in their relations with other people or with God that might have resulted in their "susceptibility" to disease or accident, and what to *do* about it now. Often patients, families, and physicians come to an impasse over how and whether to talk about these issues.

Patients and physicians often think that the other only wants to talk about the "strictly medical" matters; or patients may feel afraid to bring up religious beliefs for fear of looking foolish or superstitious in the physician's eyes. On the other hand, patients may compartmentalize their medical care, allocating the

## DOES READING ABOUT CULTURAL "NONCOMPLIANCE" MAKE YOU ANGRY? SOME SOLUTIONS

1. *Suck it up. This is a common response in biomedical culture. Just memorize, pass the test, and move on.*
2. *Ask yourself some questions. If a particular case makes you angry:*
   - *At whom or what am I angry?*
   - *Is there some cultural issue that the anger is protecting me from knowing or feeling?*
   - *Which types of patients and diseases do I dislike the most? Why?*
   - *What is different about cultural material in comparison with other kinds of medical information?*
3. *Try this chapter on for size in your own life*
   - *Recall an illness episode in your family and how people decided what to treat, what not to treat, what language to use to describe the situation, whom to consult, when to have the situation addressed, and so on.*
   - *Recall an illness or accident of your own and how your cultural values influenced the way you handled it.*

corporeal "why" and biomedical treatment to the physician, while allocating the spiritual or psychological "why" and its restoration to their folk healer or pastor. What physicians construe to be medical "noncompliance" may often in fact constitute a different understanding of the situation, differing agendas or priorities.

### CASE 24-3

*The scene is a rural North Carolina primary care clinic. During an office visit in which the presenting complaint was a "bad cold," a physician also diagnosed his 35-year-old African-American patient as having hypertension. He gave her some samples from the clinic cabinet of a diuretic medication, recommended a low-sodium diet, and exercise. As he concluded the interview, he asked her whether she understood what he had explained and whether she had any questions. She averted looking directly into his eyes, and quietly said she had no questions. He asked her to schedule a return visit in 2 weeks; he wanted to monitor her blood pressure. She left the waiting room without rescheduling. When she arrived home, she said with obvious frustration in her voice to her mother with whom she and her husband and children lived: "I don't understand why this doctor gives me these pills for high blood. How's that supposed to thin out my blood? It doesn't make sense to me." Trying to reassure her daughter, her mother said to her: "I'll get you some pickle juice, and tonight when you sleep, sit up a little so the thick blood can drain down easier. That'll be better than these pills—although it was nice that he didn't give you a prescription you'd have to pay for." The patient felt better now that she thought she understood what was going on with her.*

## PATIENTS' INFORMAL CARE NETWORKS, ROLES, AND TREATMENT CHOICE

Most people's illnesses are totally treated outside the formal healthcare system (see White *et al.*, 1961). Even when this system becomes involved, it is usually after a number of assessments and interventions by the *patient's own personal network*. Indeed, it is helpful for the physician to see the act of "going to the doctor" as an act of including the physician's world within the patient's expanding cultural world, and to ask "What is the patient seeking in doing so?" Chrisman (1977) has identified five steps that characterize the health-seeking process: (1) symptom definition, (2) illness-related shifts in role behavior, (3) lay consultation and referral, (4) treatment actions, and (5) adherence.

People consult with and seek treatment from a variety of others in the popular (lay) folk (e.g., root-worker, medicine man) and professional sectors (Foster & Anderson, 1978). This can be sequential or concurrent. For instance, a person might consult an aunt, a local pharmacist, a chiropractor, and a physician for different facets of the same illness episode, as described in Case 24-3. Or the person might seek help from them in some sequence, as a result of the progression or nonresolution of symptoms. Whether a practitioner is defined as "folk" or "professional" also depends on who is doing the defining: consider only the controversy over chiropractors among biomedical physicians! Johnson and Kleinman (1984) note that

> Most illness episodes are dealt with in the context of the family, regardless of ethnic background. This may involve special diets, foods, herbs, massage, exercise, religious treatment, and prescribed or nonprescribed medications. [They] also may consult with folk practitioners such as *curanderos* among Hispanics, root-workers and spiritualist ministers among blacks, herb doctors and acupuncturists among East Asians, voodoo specialists among Haitians, and medicine men among Native Americans. It is common for patients to engage in lay healing practices and to consult traditional practitioners while simultaneously seeking health care from physicians. (pp. 279–280)

In 1978, Kleinman introduced a useful conceptual distinction between disease and illness, defining "disease" as "malfunctioning and maladaptation of biological and/or psychological processes" (p. 428), and defining "illness" as "the personal and social significance of and life problems created by the experience of perceived disease" (p. 428). Disease is the conceptual domain and chief interest of the medical professional, while illness is the conceptual domain and chief interest of the patient. The degree of congruence between the physician's and patient's cultural models of the illness episode and expectations for treatment deeply affect the clinical relationship and the degree to which a mutually satisfying treatment plan can be developed (Chrisman & Maretzki, 1982; Eisenberg & Kleinman, 1981; Kleinman, 1982). Lack of congruence between the physician and patient in this important area often leads to nonadherence, as in Case 24-3.

Even differences in preferred style of interaction can create clinical conflict. For instance, the physician who identifies with the strictly scientific role might prefer to keep aloof, detached, "objective," while the patient might wish for a physician who is more charismatic. In its powerful expressiveness, the aura and drama of Pentecostal faith healers closely resembles shamanistic healing among North American Native Americans, shamans whose very name means "power man" or "mysterious man" (Hultkrantz, 1992, p. 18). Patients from Evangelical Protestant traditions might expect a physician to be more personally involved than an "objective" medical scientist. To understand the patient's culturally based "explanatory model" of the illness episode, one must observe carefully, listen actively, and ask evocative questions.

All patients have a rationale for their medical actions. This rationale might not be organized into an Aristotelian explanatory system, nor might it follow the same rules of evidence that biomedical decision-making at least officially strives to follow. While many ethnomedical practices might contain irrational elements or aspects (Boyer, 1983), it is prejudicial automatically to infer that simply because a practice is different from one's own, or from one's official medical model, it is ipso facto inferior, wrong, crazy, or dangerous. On the other hand, it is dangerous to romanticize folk or popular medical practices. It is important to become intimately familiar with patients' various cultures, so that one might know what types of questions to ask the patient.

In the late 1980s I presented Case 24-2 about the Vietnamese-American boy to a group of family medicine residents; the topic was patients' and physicians' explanatory models. Their response was far from enthusiastic; one resident said monotonously, "We saw this kind of stuff at the Mecca [teaching hospital]." I then sought to draw a parallel between this "exotic" and "alien" cultural presentation and something perhaps more within their orbit. I said that the Vietnamese model is one among many "balance" theories of sickness, treatment, and health. I continued:

# QUESTIONS TO ASK PATIENTS

*The following questions are helpful in eliciting the patient's culturally-based "explanatory model" of the illness episode:*

*1. What do you call your problem?*
*2. What do you think has caused your problem(s)?*
*3. Why do you think it started when it did?*
*4. What does this sickness do to you? How does it work?*
*5. How serious is this illness? How long will it last?*
*6. What kind of treatment is best for this illness?*
*7. What results do you expect from treatment?*
*8. What are the chief problems your illness has caused you?*
*9. What worries you most about being sick?*

*(from Johnson & Kleinman, 1984, p. 282; Kleinman, 1980; Kleinman et al., 1978).*

---

Many of us in this room probably grew up with some degree of humoral folk medicine. Did your mother ever tell you that, when you finish a hot shower or bath, to be sure to run some cold water on yourself to be sure your pores closed? Otherwise, if you went outside or walked on the cold floor, you could catch a draft and get the flu or a cold.

The group brightened, joking about some of the stories they remembered from their childhoods 20 years earlier. Suddenly, the Vietnamese theory of ill winds gained some experiential plausibility. It was not simply silly and foreign. Rather, we all found aspects of our own lives that could be used to identify with those of a different culture.

Questions about explanatory models that a physician might ask can only go so far in data gathering and in building rapport—whether in the medical history or in a social history. Questions that the physician might consider appropriate might be experienced as intrusive, embarrassing, or judgmental to the patient. Careful listening, attentiveness to a patient's changed emotion, tone of voice, eye movements, or gestures can all provide important cues. We Americans ask many direct questions as a standard mode of communication. In many other cultures, indirectness and modesty are greater virtues. Physicians need to gather information; at the same time, physicians need also to be aware both of the meaning particular questions might have to patients and that questioning itself as a mode of communication may have entirely different meanings to the physician and to the patient.

Sickness and healer *roles*, together with the definition of what qualifies as legitimate illness, are inseparably bound up with shared notions about the self and its boundaries. This collective self-image, together with the range of deviation allowed within the cultural category of "normal," is not only a social fact, but also an important value. In the United States, for instance, disease conceptualization and treatment are embedded in the value system of self-reliance, rugged individualism, independence, pragmatism, empiricism, atomism, privatism, emotional minimalism, and a mechanistic conception of the body and its "repair" (Kluckhohn & Strodtbeck, 1961; Ohnuki-Tierney, 1984). The horror of dependency (the conscious expression of a repudiated wish) is a powerful fuel that influences and confers authority on the biomedical conceptual, diagnostic, and treatment system. Hocking (1987) writes that

> Because the sick are dependent, sickness is seen as deviant behavior, undesirable, and only to be legitimated on certain terms ([Talcott] Parsons sick role concept). Legitimation of sickness has become the prerogative of the medical profession which uses the biomedical concept of disease as its yardstick. (1987, p. 526)

In U.S. culture, the biomedical conceptualization of disease has been welcomed and widely adopted precisely because it fits so well with the image of the self as a physical thing that can be broken but easily repaired.

## TAKE A TOUR OF YOUR OWN CULTURE'S HEALTH BELIEFS: DID YOU GROW UP HEARING ANY OF THESE? DO YOU STILL PRACTICE ANY OF THESE?

- *Finish off a shower with cold water to close your pores.*
- *Stay out of the "night air."*
- *Drink a hot toddy for a bad cold.*
- *Crying is a sign of weakness.*
- *No pain, no gain—if the medicine tastes bad, it's good medicine.*
- *Bottle-feeding is more sanitary than breast-feeding.*
- *If you hold a baby too much, you'll spoil him.*

## ILLNESS-RELATED WORDS AND THEIR MEANINGS

Language is a common area of misunderstanding and ill will between physician and patient (Dirckx, 1982). Physicians often discount irrational-*seeming* patient folk expressions. However, some of the worst impasses occur when the words physicians and patients say *seem* to be the same, but carry divergent meanings. Many African-American patients, for example, visualize illness in terms of blood imbalance. Physicians talk about high and low blood *pressure*, where many lower-socioeconomic-class blacks talk about high and low *blood* (and parallel terms *thick/thin* and *sweet/bitter blood*) (Hill & Mathews, 1981; Snow, 1974, 1983), as in Case 24-3.

According to this classification, the terms *high* and *low blood* "may refer to either the amount of blood in the body or a shift in its location, that is, 'high blood' may be too *much* blood or it may be that a normal amount of blood is present in the body but has suddenly shot up into the head. Changes in blood volume and shifts in location can result from improper dietary practices or emotional shock or both" (Snow, 1983, p. 824). Foods considered as too rich or red in color are included in the etiology of "high blood": among these are red meat (especially pork), beets, red wine, carrots, and grape juice. Blackouts, especially in males, are often regarded as a symptom of high blood. Lack of energy, fainting spells, and constipation are common signs of low blood. Diet modification, herbal remedies, and family counseling to deal with interpersonal relations related to stress are among the treatments for these illnesses (Hill & Mathews, 1981, p. 316).

Typical remedies for high, sweet, thick blood are substances believed to help thin down the blood: bitter herbs, epsom salts, vinegar, garlic, peach leaf, horehound, snake root, and pickle juice (Hill & Mathews, 1981, p. 317). Many of these ingredients increase the patient's sodium intake and are thus anathema from a biomedical viewpoint. In lowering "high blood," the goal is to try to sweat the excess out through the pores, to try to eliminate it through the bowels, or, in women, through menstruation (Snow, 1983, p. 824). In part, conditions of "high" and "low" blood are related to gravity. Elderly black patients who diagnose themselves as suffering from "high blood" might drink pickle brine to *dilute* their blood and might *sleep sitting upright* in bed (propped up with boxes and pillows) so that their thinned blood could run down from their head and redistribute itself in the rest of the body.

Many Americans believe the diagnosis "hypertension" to mean that they are hypertense, anxious, nervous, irritable, high-strung, and that the logical cure is relaxation (Blumhagen, 1982). In such a scheme, drastic diet management, exercise, and medication for life often makes little sense. Also within U.S. popular culture, the heart is a deeply metaphoric subject; one has only to think of its association with Valentine's Day (love, intimacy), sadness and depression (having "a heavy heart"), pride ("a stout heart"), and so on. Americans are attentive to cardiovascular imagery akin to the French and Latin focus on the liver, and the Japanese on the stomach (*hara*). These metaphorical meanings may cause misunderstandings between physician and patient, since physicians are often looking for a mechanical malfunction whereas patients might be referring to a different, personal meaning.

For another example, many Anglo-Americans (narrowly defined, Americans of English ancestry; more broadly, Americans of Protestant, north European ancestry) might feel emotionally "close" to their families and friends, maintaining contact by telephone and travel, yet actually live thousands of miles from them. Mexican-Americans (Keefe, 1984) feel deeply close to their families, but such closeness has a markedly different meaning. "Mexican Americans value the physical presence of family members while Anglo Americans are satisfied with intermittent meetings with kin supplemented by telephone calls and letters" (p. 68). For Mexican-Americans, close familialism is associated with geographic stability and face-to-face interaction, whereas for Anglos, it is associated with considerable social and geographic mobility.

When patients use familiar-sounding words, it is important to find out from them their own meanings. By doing so, say, with respect to the term *close* family, the physician can assess the extent to which closeness corresponds to his or her expectation, or is functional or pathological (as, for instance, in "enmeshed" families). Such inquiry can clarify the extent to which the family can realistically function as support system, and which member(s) the physician can rely on or contact during a sickness episode.

Consider, further, the range of cultural meanings of the seemingly self-evident term *togetherness*, and of the clinical misunderstandings between patient (or family) and physician when the physician assumes that his or her meaning is the same as that of the patient or family. From clinical experience and research, Nguyen Nga (1988), a psychiatrist, has discovered that, while many Americans associate "family togetherness" with the notion of spending the weekend together at the lake or going on a picnic, the Vietnamese-American meaning is that of "us versus them," "our family united against other families and against the world." While the mainstream U.S. connotation is inclusive and expansive, the Vietnamese connotation is exclusive and protectively encapsulating. A clinician would miss crucial information if he or she did not elicit the boundary aspect of Vietnamese family togetherness. For example, in Case 24-2, a physician treating this Vietnamese family should consider the possibility that he or she would have to expend additional effort at building rapport (the therapeutic alliance), since the medical system was not yet incorporated into the trusted world of "us."

A further distinction lies in the fact that when many Americans speak of togetherness, they mean a collection of distinct selves, each with a personal identity. Traditional Vietnamese, on the other hand, regard themselves more in terms of a shared "family identity" from which each member sees him- or herself as inseparable. This family identity encompasses deceased ancestors for whom the living must perform rites so that their souls do not wander aimlessly forever. Thus, something as seemingly elemental and universal as the definition and the experience of the self is influenced by the culture in which one grows up and in which one participates.

In Japan, Korea, and traditional China, the family is also experienced as identical and coextensive with the self. In Confucianism, whose "moral principles...supported the legitimacy of [the Japanese] family and state" (De Vos, 1980, p. 121), there is

> no place for individualistic concepts of the person. There are no individuals as such—only family members whose roles change through the life cycle. At no time is the person regarded as separate from his family and social roles, and maturation is a deepening of understanding of one's place in a system, that is, part of a yet larger social unit. One's ultimate duty, as one's ultimate psychological security, is to be found in family or group continuity, not in the continuity of the self.
> Tensions experienced through a conflict of occupational expectations or family role versus disruptive private feelings are most frequently resolved in Japan by directing the individual back toward the family. The goal of attempts to alleviate psychiatric problems are therefore defined in terms of family or occupational integration. (pp. 121–122)

In such families, duty to the family and wider cultural unit predominates over duty to an individual self, a value organization that may make it difficult for the patient from such cultures to "follow doctor's orders" when they conflict with obligations to one's family role. Obligations to one's kinship network often supersede obligations to strangers such as the physician. U.S. individualism and the tightly bounded physician–patient relationship might differ markedly from the value system and expectations of such patients. As Parry (1984) notes,

Seeking help for oneself may be a threat in cultures in which the family or other social networks are more important than the individuals. A set of behaviors that threatens to change a role in a family would be viewed as displaying selfishness, disloyalty, or even hostility. (p. 930)

Thus, for Americans and a number of families of Asian heritage, to speak of birth, adolescence, marriage, and death as "family events" may carry vastly different cultural meanings and burdens.

---

### CASE 24-4

*A behavioral scientist was working with a married, female family medicine resident who was irate about a pregnant Chinese-American woman. This patient refused to take the prescribed iron-enriched vitamins and seemed otherwise noncompliant (that is, obstinate) and uninterested in her own pregnancy. The patient had evidently not wanted to become pregnant and wanted to have her baby and be over with it (abortion was out of the question). A consultant was brought in to mediate the conflict. The consultant spoke with the patient in Chinese, and learned that in her culture, pregnant women do not take vitamins because it is felt they will throw the body out of balance. The consultant discovered, however, that within the patient's framework, seaweed figured prominently in her diet. Then the consultant and the resident successfully reached agreement with the patient to increase her intake of seaweed to give her the necessary iron supplement. The resident was relieved that her patient was getting the iron albeit in a culturally acceptable form.*

---

I cannot conclude this section without at least some reference to medical terms and abbreviations (often acronyms) that *physicians* often use, but that are ripe for misunderstanding by *patients*. What a physician says or writes is not necessarily identical with what a patient hears or reads. For instance: a dyspneic patient suffering from chronic obstructive pulmonary disease was mortified to read in her medical chart that "Pt. SOB," a common abbreviation. She thought that her physician was calling her a humiliating sobriquet! In another instance, a physician informed a patient with chronic bowel disease that the patient suffered from "terminal ileitis." The patient went home and tearfully notified her family that she was about to die! Thus, even well-intended, scientific medical terms can be misunderstood and become sources of embarrassment and trouble to physicians.

## ETHNICITY AND HEALTH BEHAVIOR

Within the United States, the terms *ethnic* and *ethnicity* denote a major *social typology* according to which people are classified by others, and classify themselves, in terms of nation or tribe of origin: for instance, Poles, Irish, Slovaks, Vietnamese, Cambodians, English, German, Navahos, Hispanics, Latinos, Iroquois, Jews, and so forth. As has been discussed at length elsewhere, the term *ethnicity* is complex (see Committee on International Relations, 1987; De Vos & Romanucci-Ross, 1975; Glazer & Moynihan, 1975; Stein, 1987d; Stein & Hill, 1977). Jews, for example, are sometimes regarded, and sometimes regard themselves, as a nation, as an ethnic group, as a race, and as a religion.

Until the civil rights and Black Power movements of the 1960s, large numbers of U.S. blacks regarded themselves, and were regarded by the larger society, as a race (and anthropologists were quick to point out that the U.S. folk notions about "race" should not be confused with the concept as is used in scientific biology). Since the mid-1960s, many blacks have renounced the racial classification and have strongly identified themselves as Afro-Americans, that is, in terms of their continent of origin. Not only has the black/white/yellow/red U.S. "racial" classification distorted the deep cultural diversity *within* each ostensibly homogeneous racial category, but "race" has often been used as an "ethnic" category. Moreover, groups that now qualify as whites, e.g., Serbians, Poles, Ukrainians, Italians, Spaniards, Greeks, were, earlier in the twentieth century, regarded as inferior, darker races, by those "whites" who feared that the North European, Protestant culture of *their* United States would be defiled.

# PREGNANT WOMAN NEARING DELIVERY

*Big-bellied, rose cheeked,*
*Her eyes—full of life as her uterus—*
*Met mine as she lumbered out*
*The clinic door. She smiled*
*With the knowing gleam*
*Of one who gladly*
*Tells her secret.*
*She deserves better*
*Than for us to call her*
*An "OB."*

*Howard Stein, in* Evocations, *Pittsburgh, Dorrance Publishing, 1997, p. 33. Reprinted with permission of the publisher.*

The important point to keep in mind in all aspects of medical care is that *anything* can have group-shared, symbolic significance that bears consequences for clinical outcome. Consider food, whose symbolic weight is at least as great as its objective, nutritional value. One immigrant Italian-American male in his 60s was recovering postsurgically in the hospital. His physicians and nursing staff were becoming alarmed that he was hardly eating anything from his well-stocked hospital tray. Finally, an Italian-speaking social worker was brought in to find out what was wrong. It turned out that the soft-spoken patient objected to the way the food was served: it was so unappetizing that he could not bring himself to eat it. Yet to regain strength from the surgery he had to eat. He protested: "Couldn't they make the same meat into a nice patty or meat ball and put some garlic and spicy tomato sauce on it?"

For another example: In his last years, my father, a retired, Jewish widower in his late 80s, lived in his longtime apartment in a largely Catholic and Protestant town. Some years ago he contacted the local hospital-based "Meals on Wheels" organization to bring his lunch and dinner meals 5 days per week. Although he was unable to keep a strictly Kosher diet (that is, one in complete accord with Orthodox Jewish dietary law), he was able to arrange that the Meals on Wheels kitchen send him sandwiches and hot meals without pork products (the meat of the pig was perhaps the most forbidden). Through this arrangement, Meals on Wheels could provide him with nutritionally high-quality food that at the same time met his sense of religious obligations.

The *form*, rather than the *substance*, of prescribed medication may become a source of conflict, as illustrated in Case 24-4. Many traditional Hispanic-Americans prefer to have their medicine in the form of a "shot" (which is more masculine) than in the form of a "pill" (which is more sissifying). A 73-year-old Irish-Catholic patient once told me, "Good medicine tastes bad. If it don't hurt going down, it mustn't be very strong." For him and many of his religious/ethnic culture, "taking your medicine" is as much a form of punishment as it is a form of treatment. To soothe the conscience as well as to perform its biomedical function, medicine that is acceptable must inflict some physical pain.

Many traditional Hispanic-American patients (Mexican-American, Puerto Rican) adhere to the Hippocratic, humoral theory-derived "hot–cold" (*caliente–frio*) model of disease (Harwood, 1971, 1981). According to this system, certain diseases are classified as hot, cold, and "cool" (an intermediate category). "Cold-classified illnesses are treated with hot medication and foods, while hot illnesses are treated with cool substances" (Harwood, 1971, pp. 1153–1154). Hispanic women on diuretics might discontinue such physician-prescribed potassium sources as bananas, oranges, or raisins during menstruation (a cold condition, and these foods are likewise regarded as cold or cool). The physician could prescribe potassium in the culturally acceptable form of vitamins (which are "hot"), together with "hot" foods such as coffee and cocoa, which are rich in potassium (p. 1155). Or, consider pregnancy, a "hot" condition during which "many women will not take hot iron supplements or vitamins. These patients might be encouraged to take these prescriptions with fruit juice or an herb tea [both of which are cool] to 'neutralize' them" (p. 1157).

I continue with another example drawn from Hispanic-American culture to illustrate a central issue in physician–patient relationships: attitudes toward authority. Many patients from Central American countries have a tall, hierarchical view of religious and secular authority, ranging from the Roman Catholic priest to the "strong man" leader or *caudillo*, who will protect them from marauding outsiders. Like these other authorities, the physician, especially a male physician in this patriarchal culture area, is to be respected, deferred to, and never questioned, at least in face-to-face behavior. Position or place is important in regulating all relationships. The modern-trained physician who cultivates patient autonomy and informed consent is likely to be frustrated by traditionalist Mexican, Guatemalan, or Honduran patients who live more according to an older "paternalistic" model of care wherein the physician is less concerned with seeking thoroughgoing "informed consent" than with directing the patient to follow the proper course of care. Here, a "You decide from a menu of options" collides with "You're my physician in whom I put my trust; you tell me what I need to do." Moreover, to many Hispanic patients, physician–patient relationships fall into the category of patron–client relationships (as in godparenthood throughout Catholic Europe and Central/South America) in which each person has a personal obligation to the other. An impersonal, professionalized, almost mechanized view of the clinical relationship and of treatment is foreign to such a hierarchical, intimate view and expectation.

In fact, the appearance of respect and conformity with authority's judgment is often far more important than carrying out the "doctor's orders." Hispanic patients, not that unlike, say, many Great Plains whites, African Americans, or Marshall Islanders from Micronesia, are practical, pragmatic, instrumental in medically related decision-making. They wish to avoid open conflict, confrontation, and ridicule. As a consequence, saying "Yes" in the presence of the physician may well mean a later "No" that could never be said directly. Behind the scenes, privately, or with a different "public," with their own family, neighbors, or co-workers, they will compare the physician's prescription with that of their inner and interpersonal standards, and they may decide to "comply" with family rather than with the physician.

East European Jews tend to be as concerned about the meaning of pains as with their immediate alleviation through analgesics. Although U.S. physicians of various ethnicities perceive both Jews and Italians to be vociferous about their pains, they often fail to perceive that the purpose or function of the complaint differs between the groups. Anglo-American patients, like Jews, tend to be health-conscious, but attach very different significance to the search for health. Jews have been depicted as generally worried that something profoundly terrible might be wrong, whereas Anglo-Americans might be seen as viewing the body in a machinelike utilitarian way: When something seems broken, one is obligated to take care of oneself and bring one's body to the physician to be fixed (Zborowski, 1969). Jews may see in the most minor symptom the harbinger or symbol of tragedy; Italians may primarily want to feel better and place less emphasis on the entire prescribed medical regimen; Irish patients might ignore their symptoms as long as possible, report only a few, and avoid the sense of sin that goes with too much preoccupation with the body; and WASP patients might believe that rationality, hard work, control, and "pulling yourself up by your bootstraps" should suffice, in the treatment of disease as with the rest of life.

Ethnic symbolism often appears in what is to us in biomedicine some of the most unexpected places. For example, in a study of diabetes and diabetes management on the Devil's Lake Sioux Reservation in North Dakota, Gretchen Chesley Lang (1985) found that "food preferences, expense, and lack of time in a large household were the most frequently given reasons for lack of compliance" (p. 252) with the diabetes program. As is true in many other ethnic groups as well, for many contemporary Dakota people bigness and heaviness means well-being and health. Three widespread Dakota perceptions about diabetes are that (1) diabetes afflicts the Dakota because their way of life is out of balance; (2) diabetes is the most recent among diseases spread by the white man to destroy Indian society; (3) because few medicine men have the power to treat it, diabetes may not necessarily be treated by traditional Dakota means. As among many other peoples, Dakota people highly regard traditional food and medicinal plants, and eating marks social occasions (p. 255). Further, many Dakota believe the presence of diabetes itself signifies the white man's destruction of their society, that is, that the source of the disease is outside rather than inside their group. Low compliance with medically prescribed diets often serves the purpose of cultural resistance (pp. 255–256). Thus, not only are there cultural and religious aspects to food and diabetes, but *political* ones as well. The presence of a disease, and the way a group responds to that presence, may be used to affirm that group's identity and boundary. Thus, at a very practical level, for one to choose to become more healthy may endanger his or her inner sense of Dakota-ness, and become a source of alienation in others' perceptions as well.

A recent study by Frank *et al.* (1998) contrasts principle-based biomedical ethics and ethnically based decision-making. The authors focus on end-of-life decision-making with a 79-year-old Korean-American woman as an exemplar of Korean-American attitudes. They contrast the abstract "Georgetown mantra" (principles of autonomy, beneficence, nonmalfeasance, justice) with understanding how families decide about end-of-life healthcare. "Although Korean Americans reported extremely negative attitudes about the use of life-sustaining technology (LST) for themselves, they were extremely positive about its use generally. Mrs. Kim explains this paradox: Although she did not want to be kept alive by LST, she believed that it is her children's duty to make the decision for her [filial piety versus individual autonomy]. In her view, family members are obligated to protect patients from learning that their illnesses are life threatening and must strive to keep patients alive 'even one more day' " (p. 406). Here, claims of intimacy clash with claims of legality. The authors urge that in medicine, "a discourse on relationships should supplement the discourse on individual rights" (p. 415). Biomedical ethics needs to engage in dialogue with culture. Notions of "informed consent" are thus far from self-evident or universal.

The study of ethnic (from tribal to national) cultures has long been a productive focus of attention in medicine. The studies of Loudell Snow (1974, 1983) among blacks, of Alan Harwood (1981) among Hispanics, and of Mark Zborowski (1969) among Anglo-Americans, Jews, Irish Catholics, and Italians, have become classics. In my work among Slavic-Americans (Stein, 1976; Stein & Hill, 1977), I have also contributed to this literature. Most recently in this genre, Anne Fadiman has written a popular book entitled *The Spirit Catches You and You Fall Down* (1997), an account of the conflict-ridden encounter between a Hmong family in California and the U.S. biomedical system. The clash in the treatment of a child is over diagnosis, treatment, beliefs, expectations, values, and roles. The difference between a diagnosis of epilepsy and spirit possession becomes a failure of meeting between human worlds. But, for all its poignancy, this account is hardly a new one. Nor is culture-in-medicine to be relegated to the *exotic-seeming* instances, such as the newest waves of immigrants to North American shores. Conspicuous difference in appearance, language, and dress should not be the defining feature for qualifying as "cultural," and hence of clinical interest.

Further, although each ethnic group has distinctive practices and beliefs, one cannot fail to recognize overall similarities in conflicts and in patterns of adaptation between groups that vary widely in space and time in the United States. The *kinds* of physician–patient communication problems, and the *kinds* of intergenerational change and conflict, experienced by, say, Vietnamese, Cambodian, Guatemalans, and Hmong in the late twentieth century are remarkably similar to those faced a century ago by Poles, Italians, Greeks, and Slovaks (e.g., obligation to family versus individual autonomy).

Just as cultural *differences* between patient and physician can make for misunderstandings and conflict, so—surprisingly, perhaps—can *similarities*. In a paper on physicians' "cultural blind spots" with regard to

---

## A PERSONAL EXAMPLE OF SHARED-DECISION-MAKING

*When I was a baby, I was scrawny, underweight. As I was later told, my parents' pediatrician recommended that I be fed bacon to help fatten me up. Since my parents were Conservative Jews, pork was out of the question. Some physicians might have labeled my parents as "noncompliant" and washed their hands of the situation. Fortunately, my physician and parents negotiated a culturally suitable substitute, what then was called "beef fry" or fried corn beef. And the medically sought consequence was accomplished! —HS*

patients, Elizabeth Hiok-Boon Lin (1983), a Western-trained Chinese physician, challenges the popular assumption that similarities in cultural background between patient and physician invariably enhance clinical communication and outcomes. A common cultural heritage does not rule out intraethnic variation influenced by age, sex, personality, political orientation, socioeconomic class, rural/urban background, region of origin, dialect spoken, religion, occupation, education, family structure, or extent of acculturation (e.g., American-ization). Especially when the physician identifies him- or herself as belonging to the same ethnic group as the patient, "cultural stereotyping results in superficial generalizations that are often misleading in the case of individual patients" (p. 92). Lin's caution extends beyond ethnicity or nationality of origin to religion, occupation, and common popular cultural participation. The clinical error in all of these is the assumption that "You are the same as I," a psychological merging that prevents the physician from taking notice of potentially important differences between him- or herself and the patient. The reverse is also possible, where the patient tries to persuade the physician that they are the same. Both of these can be seen to be a variation on physician countertransference/patient transference issues. When one wants to see the patient as the same as oneself, the question to ask is: "What am I trying not to see in the patient?" (Devereux, 1980; Stein & Apprey, 1985).

## CASE 24-5

*"Tinker syndrome": For 6 years (1979–1985) I coordinated behavioral science teaching at the family medicine residency program in Shawnee, Oklahoma, a clinic where many workers from Tinker Air Force Base sought their primary care. Over the years, several residents came to formulate what they wryly referred to as the "Tinker syndrome." The syndrome was characterized by feelings of job dissatisfaction, low productivity, punching the clock, and collecting a paycheck. Many workers came to the clinic intermittently through the year, acknowledging depression or with multiple organic complaints. Toward early spring (March, April), the family medicine residents noticed that many of these workers would come into the clinic with symptoms they would relate to stress (anxiety, can't sleep, nervousness).*

*Early spring was the time of an annual site visit and major review of the air force base, when supervisors were expected to show efficiency and productivity, and units were evaluated for their performance. Suddenly, the base became self-consciously more active and busy. The physicians sur-mised that many of their patients were situationally anxious or suffering from vague guilt and fear of being judged and found inadequate, which they expressed in a wide spectrum of physical symptoms. During this "Tinker syndrome" influx, there were biomedically bona fide physical complaints as well. Some workers would literally strain themselves by trying to cram 12 months of physical labor into 2 to 3 weeks prior to the annual site visit. Unaccustomed to regular strenuous physical labor, some workers injured themselves when they attempted to perform intensive physical labor on their jobs.*

*Apart from this latter group, a visit to the physician usually resulted in reassurance that no severe disease process was taking place. The workers were able to ventilate about their variously frustrating and bureaucratic governmental jobs and confess some anxiety, guilt, and shame for their lack of enthusiasm at an unrewarding job. Through their symptoms they received some degree of punishment for their lackluster attitude toward work and received assurance that neither their body nor their spirit was in that terrible a shape, only to return to the base to commence the cycle anew. It required rather sophisticated cultural thinking on the part of these residents (1) to recognize an epi-demiological pattern rather than think exclusively of patients on a one-by-one basis and (2) to inter-pret a plethora of physical complaints as a metaphor for a disorder related to the culture of the work-place. (Gratitude is expressed to James Michael Pontious, M.D., for his collaboration on this case.)*

## OCCUPATIONAL CULTURE AND HEALTH BEHAVIOR

The culture of the workplace is yet another source of health behavior-related norms. These are often learned not via intergenerational socialization of the young (as is more characteristic of long-term ethnic and religious cultures) but through learning as a participant in one's work culture (an exception, discussed below, is the culture of family farming). One is subject to similar external stresses and expectations. One negotiates common meanings and interpretations of events from day to day interaction with superiors, co-workers, and subordinates.

Although the family farm, the family grocery store, the hospital, and the corporation, for instance, can all be labeled "occupational cultures," one must keep in mind that they differ markedly in the process of recruitment. Family farms and family businesses recruit from within, through procreation and socialization of the next, succeeding generation. However, "Organizations [such as hospitals and corporations] are not self-renewing but must replace their memberships from the outside society" (Grieco, 1988, p. 85). Those recruited from without are already culture-bearers, albeit those whose values are congruent with those of the organization and who are most easily socialized.

As the Tinker syndrome illustrates in Case 24-5, a major element in the healthcare process is timing: When does the patient (in league with relatives, co-workers, drinking partners, and so on) decide to come in for medical care? Physician and patient often become embroiled in conflict from the start, because the physician's sense of timing does not correspond to that of the patient. Consider this issue from the viewpoint of the culture of Great Plains wheat farming families, a regional cultural group congealed over the generations from immigrants and their descendants from western and central Europe, Great Britain, and Ireland. A typical farmer's presenting complaint at the emergency room or in the clinic is frequently a variation of the following:

> My wife made me come. She's been on my back for 2 weeks now. I've had just a little pain in my chest, nothing that working out in the yard or on the tractor won't cure in time. But the only way I could get her off my back is to come in and prove it's nothin'.

Moreover, it is often difficult if not impossible to elicit a "complete history" from the taciturn, terse farmer (who keeps words to a minimum, wants to avoid stirring a fuss over nothing, and serves up plenty of *Yup*'s and *Nope*'s); therefore, it becomes the role of the wife to provide the history of the symptoms. She is the person from whom the explanatory model can often be elicited. As described elsewhere in detail (Stein, 1987a,b), the pre-harvest months and harvest proper are times when only a seriously ill infant or child will be brought to the physician; similarly, during holiday times of family togetherness (Thanksgiving, Christmas) trips to the physician will be postponed (Stein, 1987a,b).

---

## CASE 24-6

*Many rural "white" farming families, like countless of their urban counterparts in the mainstream United States, routinely take sodium bicarbonate (baking soda) frequently for a wide variety of gastric discomforts. Baking soda thus occupies the same place in popular culture as, say, Vicks once did. Also, these farming families usually do not consider baking soda to be a "medicine" or "drug." Thus, when a physician inquires "What medications are your currently taking?", baking soda (like birth control pills, aspirin, and vitamins) is likely to be omitted from the list. The frequent use of sodium bicarbonate could complicate, or at least compromise, the course and medical treatment of hypertension and related cardiovascular diseases, since it increases rather than decreases the sodium in the body.*

## POPULAR CULTURE AND HEALTH BEHAVIOR

In many ways, of the four cultural regions covered in this chapter, this section may be the most difficult for the reader to "stomach" precisely because it comes closest to home. It may feel too personal. For many readers it may be more tolerable to read about ethnic groups, religious groups, and occupational groups that seem sufficiently alien to be safely distant from one's own. But when we examine popular U.S. culture and its link to health beliefs and health behavior, the reader is likely to rear up, as it were, and say: "Wait a minute, buddy, you're talking about *me*!"

There is safety in scrutinizing, even compassionately criticizing, something or someone who seems "foreign," but we are quick to muster our defenses to protect our boundaries when we feel scrutinized ourselves. Yet unfair scrutiny is not my intention; nor do I wish to make any group more foreign-seeming than another. If anything, my goal all along in this chapter is to help make the familiar a little more unfamiliar, to make it a little more remote, and to make the more unfamiliar feel closer to ourselves. I raise the question: How do we in biomedicine think compassionately yet critically about the many links between our own professional culture and national culture? Can we be at once loyal while sometimes critical? If in describing popular U.S. culture, I come uncomfortably close to the home of the reader, I am likewise looking at my own cultural household!

The culture most difficult to gain distance from, and then to be carefully critical of, is one's own. It is much easier to be leery of "their" health practices than of "ours." Don't we all assume that "our" practices (of any kind—food, clothing, gesture, speech—not only medical) are human, natural, while "their" practices are "cultural" if not suspect? When we think of language, do we ever imagine *ourselves* to have an "accent"? Certainly not. Only those who "talk differently" from us have "accents"—but then to them, we have an accent, too! For the sake of patient care, we deserve to increase our own tolerance of anxiety about "difference" and place our own popular culture health beliefs and practices under the same microscope and "macroscope" we do to understand the foundations of others' health values and behaviors.

Powerful folk medical currents exist within mainstream U.S. popular culture (and not only isolated religious sects and newly arrived ethnic groups), currents that flow into official professional culture as well. Over the past decade, popular interest has grown in what has come to be called *alternative medicine* (Fuller, 1992; Murray & Rubel, 1992; O'Connor, 1995) (e.g., herbal teas, crystals, chiropractic, therapeutic touch, meditation, acupuncture, magnets). As the reader has no doubt already discovered throughout this chapter, the designation of cultures and their health-related practices as "professional," "popular," "ethnic," "occupational," "alternative" is ultimately contextual if not arbitrary. A healthy sense of medical history is required to realize that what in one decade is marginal, if not anathema, might in another decade be incorporated into the biomedical "armamentarium" (biofeedback, acupuncture, family therapy)—and vice versa (psycho-analytic theory and therapy in psychiatry, now almost entirely supplanted by psychopharmacology). A century ago, allopathic medicine was itself culturally "alternative" in the United States.

In one family medicine residency setting I have known intimately for over two decades, allopathic and osteopathic physicians (M.D.s and D.O.s) train together. Busy M.D.s with neck and back strains often quietly ask their D.O. colleagues to take them into a nearby examination room and "manipulate" them back into shape so that they will be without pain and able immediately to resume allopathic patient care! Still, the anxious "D.O. jokes" persist. Years ago, an especially perceptive allopathic physician-colleague said to me: "Isn't it strange that we are so hard on chiropractors, but then we turn around and send patients to physical therapists in the hospital?"

We take for granted elements of U.S. popular medical culture, although they become evident as soon as they are pointed out. Over-the-counter, patent medicines available at pharmacies and supermarkets are part of this popular, folk-American culture. The wide-swinging deification and vilification of physicians (who can do nothing wrong and who can do nothing right) is intrinsic to popular culture. The common preference for medication in pill (oral) form, together with the search for a pill-for-every-ailment, "magic bullets," are popular ethnomedicine. Similarly, much of the impetus for high-technology solutions to human suffering comes from this cultural "grass roots." Television commercials (from prime time to soap operas), newspaper and magazine ads, and articles in the popular press are rich treasure troves of fantasies and ideologies and practices within U.S. popular medicine.

Consider the term *germs*. The term blurs fantasy and reality. As science, germs refer to viral and bacterial entities and their adaptation to human hosts; as a folk category they have (like cancer) assumed mythic, malevolent proportions. They are akin to the nuclear mutagenic aliens who threatened to overtake us in films from the 1950s. Every housewife (and now, househusband) is taught by TV commercials to dread the presence of even a single "germ" in the kitchen or bathroom—or on the floor anywhere. With the threat of AIDS and hepatitis B, the return of the nearly banished tuberculosis, and the emergence of drug-resistant *Streptococcus*,

*Time* magazine even featured a cover story in 1994, titled "Revenge of the Killer Microbes—Are we losing the war against infectious diseases?" The listing in the table of contents continues the imagery of assault: "The Microbes Strike Back" and later "Counterattack" (p. 3; note of course the widespread military metaphor in biomedicine).

A strong theme within U.S. popular culture is that of *germ phobia*, a long-term preoccupation of Americans, into which the growing list of sexually transmitted diseases (especially HIV/AIDS and chlamydia) and tuberculosis now fits grimly well. In popular culture, much of the painstaking, scientific method that officially characterizes the ideal self-image of biomedicine is replaced by abundant magical thinking, of which supernaturalized, menacing "germs" are the result. The popular medical cult of cleanliness is obsessed with the ritual purification of the body, both inside and outside. We cleanse and purge ourselves with folk remedies ranging from laxatives through laundry detergents (as in the Ivory Snow commercial's slogan, "99 and 44/100% pure"). The popular image of the physician—conqueror, warrior, doer, teacher, wise caretaker, and master of high technology—holds that the physician is the one in whom the hope rests for the secularized purification of the body for life here on earth. The combination of high (if not magical) expectation and rage at failed expectation leads to frequent lawsuits against those seen as secular priests of perfect health.

The deep embeddedness of biomedicine in the U.S. imagination can be immediately attested to by the consistent popularity of medical programs on television: e.g., *Marcus Welby, M.D.*, *Ben Casey*, *Medical Center*, *MASH*, *After-MASH*, *Trapper John, M.D.*, and most recently, *E.R.*, *Chicago Hope*, *L.A. Doctors*, and *Providence*; the daytime soap operas, such as *General Hospital*, and countless local call-in physician talk shows. Moreover, medical "miracles" and "breakthroughs" are featured on local and national "news" on radio and television, in the newspaper and in national magazines. Pharmaceutical companies now advertise regularly in magazines and market directly to patients-as-consumers. Finally, thanks to the popularity of the personal computer, the Internet is a virtually infinite source of medical information, opinion, and popular demand. One obtains personal medical information through one's own online literature searches and in "chat rooms." To be so worthy of prominence in the media genres of "news" and "entertainment," medicine must tap deeply into the dominant meanings and fantasies of our time.

Professional culture is never far removed from popular U.S. culture. An example is the prevalence of "management" imagery, language, and organization within biomedicine. In the 1910s, the movement led by Frederick Winslow Taylor (1911) introduced principles of "scientific management" into industry and organizational settings. Four decades later, Peter Drucker's (1954) rationalist approach called "management by objective" became widely accepted throughout American business culture. Work was conceived to be a strictly and narrowly linear, impersonal enterprise, having expected outcomes and precise ways of reaching them; and measuring productivity along the path toward that outcome. One might say that this managerial world-view was a decontextualized one or rather one in which the only contexts to be considered were those regarded by the managers as important (e.g., specifically, variables that were supposed to be incentives for greater worker productivity).

This management ethos rapidly diffused throughout various cultural institutions, medicine among them. Common expressions are "medical management," "case management," "pain management," "management conference," "It is a clinical management problem," and so forth. Not only the language, but also the way of imaging or conceptualizing medical problems, the way of treating them, and the way of relating to other medical colleagues in the treatment process are all consequences of the popular culturally managerial style of thinking. Clinically and elsewhere in life, people act toward themselves and toward others in terms of how and what they think of themselves. In medicine as in life, metaphors often become destinies.

In a powerful interpretive passage, Scheper-Hughes and Lock (1987) show how professional and medical cultures collude in the production of the obsession with anorexic fitness and ascetic wellness. In a sinister way, hypochondriasis is transformed from disease into cure!

> In our own increasingly "healthist" and body-conscious culture, the politically correct body for both sexes is the lean, strong, androgynous, and physically "fit" form through which the core cultural values of autonomy, toughness, competitiveness, youth, and self-control are readily manifest (Pollitt 1982). Health is increasingly viewed in the United States as an achieved rather than an ascribed status,

and each individual is expected to "work hard" at being strong, fit, and healthy. Conversely, ill health is no longer viewed as accidental, a mere quirk of nature, but rather is attributed to the individual's failure to live right, to eat well, to exercise, etc. We might ask what it is our society "wants" from this kind of body. DeMause (1984) has speculated that the fitness/toughness craze is a reflection of an international preparation for war. A hardening and toughening of the national fiber corresponds to a toughening of individual bodies. In attitude and ideology the self-help and fitness movements articulate both a militarist and a Social Darwinist ethos: the fast and fit win; the fat and flabby lose and drop out of the human race (Scheper-Hughes and Stein, 1987). Crawford (1985) has interpreted the eating disorders and distortions in body image expressed in obsessional jogging, anorexia, and bulimia as a symbolic mediation of the contradictory demands of postindustrial American society. The double-binding injunction to be self-controlled, fit, and productive workers, and to be at the same time self-indulgent, pleasure-seeking consumers is especially destructive to the self-image of the "modern," "liberated" American woman. Expected to be fun-loving and sensual, she must also remain thin, lovely, and self-disciplined. Since one cannot be hedonistic and controlled simultaneously, one can alternate phases of binge eating, drinking, and drugging with phases of jogging, purging, and vomiting. Out of this cyclical resolution of the injunction to consume and to conserve is born, according to Crawford, the current epidemic of eating disorders (especially bulimia) among young women, some of whom literally eat and diet to death. (pp. 25–26)

At individual, family, workplace, and larger cultural levels, these U.S. eating disorders condense the dread of death, the quest for immortality and the preservation of youthfulness, preoccupation with and intense ambivalence about sexuality, an obsession with elusive perfection and control, and the unreliability of people in the face of plentiful food.

Family medicine and sports medicine physician and faculty colleague James R. Barrett (1994) described a syndrome of "exercise addiction," complete with the triad of dependence, tolerance, and withdrawal symptoms. As often happens in all human culture's attempt to solve life's problems by vicious cycles of anxiety and defense, one day's solutions often become the next day's burdens. Alas, the recent history of medicine's linkage of "wellness" and "fitness" with preventive medicine may be one such triumph and casualty. At its extremes, "wellness" could be considered a culturally acceptable expression of hypochondriasis.

A powerful link between professional biomedical and popular national U.S. cultures is "illness somatization [that] has become a dominant metaphor for expressing individual and social complaint" (Scheper-Hughes & Lock, 1987, p. 27). Physician, health care system, third-party payers, patients, families, and society jointly collude in the diversion of attention from affect (emotion), conscious and unconscious meaning, and the experience of social injustice. Paradoxically, by defining virtually all problems and issues somatically, patients and families inadvertently surrender to physician control much of the autonomy and self-responsibility for which the medical consumerist movement of the 1970s fought so strenuously. Scheper-Hughes and Lock point ironically to "the usefulness to the body politic of filtering more and more human unrest, dissatisfaction, longing, and protest into the idiom of sickness, which can then be safely managed by doctor-agents" (p. 27). In a now-classic article on premenstrual syndrome as a Western culture-specific disorder, Johnson (1987) underscores this very point. An ever-expanding host of syndromes, diseases, and presenting complaints can be included in this process: among them, low-back pain, chronic fatigue, dizziness, pelvic inflammatory disease, carpal tunnel syndrome. Used pejoratively, the concept of "secondary gain" denies the extent of suffering and the location of its cause.

Yet another link between health beliefs in professional biomedical and popular U.S. cultures is an alternate model of alcoholism that diverges from the official disease model endorsed by many physicians and by Alcoholics Anonymous to whom physicians often refer patients. Its essence is captured by patients, spouses of patients, friends, and co-workers of patients who often say, for instance:

"I'm just a different person when I drink"; "I'm not myself when I drink"; "She's not herself when she drinks"; "I just don't know what gets into him when he's drinking"; "It's not him talking, it's the liquor"; "I don't know what overcame me to get into that fight last night—I'm really a quiet person; it must have been all those beers I had at the [football] game."

Within what explanatory frame(s) of reference do statements like these make sense? We Americans have long prided ourselves on our hard-bitten realism, our practicality (pragmatism), our rationality, our goal of objectivity. One could even claim that "medical science" is one of our chief contemporary religions, at least with respect to the salvation and preservation of the youthfulness of the body.

Yet, from research I have conducted over the course of medical teaching (Stein, 1982, 1985a, 1987c, 1993), a widespread model of alcoholism departs markedly from how we prefer to view ourselves. Alcohol is not only *substance* but also *symbol* (Stein, 1993). This symbol serves as a collective excuse for individuals, family members, co-workers, friends, to do and condone for others to do what we secretly wish to do, but which also violates our conscious values, feelings, and roles. Our model of alcohol and alcoholism is the compromise. Foreign as it may seem to the reader, I have come to the conclusion that an implicit popular cultural theory of "possession" underlies the official, professional pharmacological biomedical theory of alcoholism and drug abuse in the United States (Stein, 1982, 1985a, 1987c, 1993).

In this folk model, alcoholism and chemical dependency constitute a form of what I have called *secular possession*. In arguing so, I am quite aware that I am suggesting that we, too, even though we have gone to the moon and returned, are also "primitive" in many ways! In imbibing the spirits, one incorporates the impersonal anima or "spirit" that has been bottled or canned, and is soon possessed by it. Just as religious knowledge is said to come from the outside in, by divine "inspiration" or "revelation," likewise does drunkenness or drug-induced highs. All one need do to confirm this is to consult our cultural semantics, vividly illustrated by the above clinical example.

Everyday language offers clues about the meaning alcohol has for us. We say one becomes "in-toxicated" or "in-ebriated" after consuming alcoholic beverages. We speak of someone being "under the influence" of alcohol or "driving under the influence" (or "while intoxicated"). The term has even made it into the legal vocabulary ("DUI" or "DWI"). Alcohol is associated with being "influenced by" the profane, with badness, with poison that enters the body and does its evil work (e.g., spirits, demon rum). Not unexpectedly, the initial part of our cultural ritual cure for alcoholics is a form of exorcism: *detoxification* to expunge the poisons (toxins) from the body, often performed in special inpatient hospital wards or mental health units. Since possession by the debasing, alien agent of ethanol caused the intoxication in the first place, detoxification will expel the noxious substance from the body. But expulsion is never complete ("Once an alcoholic, always an alcoholic," we Americans also often say.). Alcoholics, even after the exorcism (similar to drug abusers following chemical detoxification), remain vulnerable to being possessed once again by the vile, but fascinating, substance.

We realist Americans scorn as mere superstition the notion of spirit possession. Yet we also practice what we claim not to believe. Scientific theory can serve as a scarcely veiled supernatural, animistic possession in an acceptable cultural form ("It's the booze talking, not him!"). Two cultural models of alcoholism, one official (scientific, disease, naturalistic) and the other unofficial (folk, possession), can coexist alongside each other in the same people's minds. One or both can be used to divert the attention of patient, family, physician, healthcare institution, and the wider culture away from the system of meanings, conscious and unconscious, of which alcoholism or drug abuse are only "the tip of the iceberg."

Sadly, much of human culture—not only U.S. popular health culture—serves precisely the function of allaying anxiety, guilt, shame, and other dysphoric feelings by directing our attention only to the tip of that iceberg. Unfortunately, culture can have both adaptive and maladaptive sides.

## CULTURE, MEDICINE, AND DISASTER

This chapter is written in Oklahoma City, where the author has lived and practiced as a clinically applied medical anthropologist since 1978. The April 19, 1995 bombing of the Murrah Federal Building, and the deadly tornadoes that devastated central Oklahoma the night of May 3, 1999, have made issues of disaster planning, emergency preparedness, and trauma mastery far more ordinary in both medical and wider cultural consciousness than before. The April 20, 1999 massacre at Columbine High School in Littleton, Colorado—a bordering, "sister" state—adds to the haunting sense of catastrophe. With the threat of biological and chemical terrorism, medical conferences on emergency community medical preparedness are increasing. In this section, I want briefly to address some central questions and issues that emerge from these disasters (see Oliver-Smith, 1992). They crosscut all of the topics and categories already discussed in this chapter. I shall focus on matters directly applicable to physicians and medical care. (For a broader discussion of medical and psychological adaptations to the 1995 bombing, see Stein, 1997, 1999.)

There are some basic questions that should be asked, that can help us to understand how people experience disaster, and how they act: What do people do when something catastrophic happens to them? How do they perceive, experience, even define the catastrophic? What is the relationship between the event itself (the "stimulus") and the meaning of the event? How do people "respond" to a disaster, and how do people incorporate its reality into their lives? What is the interplay between many cultural systems: family, neighborhood, community, professional, ethnic, regional, national? What brings communities together, and for how long? What explanatory models compete with one another to help account for the catastrophe (the false dichotomy between "natural disaster" and "man-made disaster")? What "heals" following a disaster? Which models or methods vie with each other for repairing lives and communities following a disaster? What are the cultural timetables for restoration after a disaster? What circumstances do people adapt to; and what do they adapt with? What are the categories of people in disasters (e.g., victims, survivors, rescuers, caregivers), and what are the consequences of this taxonomy for people who are noticed and for those who are overlooked? Who all is "at risk"?

A few answers, all culture-laden, are available: Firefighters are more publicly acknowledged than police, largely because of their mythical compartmentalization into hero/villain, respectively. Short-term, emergency, acute care is the cultural rule among professional and popular cultures alike. Long-term offering of physical and medical relief, let alone of mental health service, is rare in a culture where one is expected to "get a life," to "get your life together and go on down the road." Widespread "communal" response is intense and short-lived; the ultimate and ideal social unit remains the autonomous individual family. Large numbers of people who suffered from the presence of the bombing, or of the tornado, are not regarded as victims or casualties worthy of medical or mental health care because they were not "directly" (physically or residentially) affected.

Disaster "preparedness" takes multiple dimensions, some of which might be counterintuitive. On the one hand, the overwhelming public response to the bombing and to the tornado build culturally on voluntary mutual aid that traces to European-American home rebuilding and barn raising following destructive fires. On the other hand, experience from massive destruction by tornado and recovery from it (e.g., Wichita Falls, Texas, 1979) helped prepare Oklahomans for the bombing, since the *type* of cataclysm was largely similar, e.g., shrapnel. On yet a "third" hand, despite the medical and physical preparation, there was an utter lack of emotional preparation for the bombing because, in contrast to a tornado, it was culturally unimaginable (and hence unanticipatable). This is what makes the experience "traumatic." Into this void we pour such models as "posttraumatic stress disorder" (PTSD) and "critical incident stress management" (CISM), cultural diagnoses and emergency treatment strategies that attempt to control experiences that are utterly out of control. One is led to wonder what clinical realities these approaches omit and cannot hear in their attempt to offer clear-cut explanations and solutions (Young, 1997).

## CONCLUSION

This chapter has introduced the reader to the cultural world of the patient, and perhaps has *re*introduced the reader to the cultural worlds he or she inhabits. In all clinical communication, the practitioner gains access to realms of the patient's experience, values, beliefs, expectations, explanations, feelings, meanings, and conflicts, by having free access to those realms within oneself. The self of the clinician remains one of the finest instruments of observation, assessment, and treatment available. Physicians, no less than patients, are creators and bearers of culture, and suffer the consequences from unexamined assumptions about others' cultures.

All of us in U.S. medicine wish to make the work of medical practice more simple, more efficient, more "cost-effective." Physicians conduct thorough physical examinations, "take" thorough histories, order numerous tests, all to try to obtain a definitive diagnosis and proceed with a decisive treatment plan so that they succeed rather than fail (two culturally loaded words in biomedical culture). But often the more we know biomedically, the more complicated clinical knowledge and decision-making become. It is no different with the culture of the patient: despite our wish for simple cultural answers, the more we know of a patient's, a family's, a physician's culture(s), the more complicated the clinical picture becomes (that is to say, the more real). Just as I wish it were different on the organic side of medicine, so I also wish it were different from the cultural side. But it is not.

*Interest* in the patient's culture, however, can lead to some surprising turns in the physician–patient–family relationship, and to wisdom about people outside the ethnic group or tribe one is currently thinking about. Consider, for example, the widespread practice among Jews of circumcising newborn males on the eighth day, or the widespread practice among Muslims of female circumcision—or, for that matter, the belief among many U.S. physicians that males should be routinely circumcised at birth, and further that such procedures do not require pain control, or much pain control, because infants supposedly do not feel pain or presumably will not remember it in later life anyway. Or consider the question of whether Muslim women should be routinely assigned a female physician to conduct the physical examination. For one thing, there is considerable intragroup variation, which is often to say controversy, among Jews, Muslims, and physicians as to what is culturally acceptable.

Any group's health-related practices (including our own as Americans, as physicians) should be open to further inquiry as to their personal and family meaning. To say simply: "Custom A is practiced in Group B means we should uncritically and automatically abide by it" is to suspend the very judgment we regard as critical in areas we call "clinical." On the other hand, sensitivity to cultural *questions* (e.g., physical examinations, pelvic examinations with female Muslim patients) can be a cue for physicians to ask key questions about gender, modesty, sexuality, exposure of the body, expectation, and the like, of any female patient: for instance, "Are you comfortable having a male physician examine you? Doing a pelvic? Would you like anyone else in the room with you during the examination?", and so on. Often, too, a physician must infer a patient's comfort from nonverbal messages such as facial expression, because many patients would feel it to be disrespectful to ask something, let alone to tell a physician not to do something. Just as physicians often fear retaliation from patients (e.g., lawsuits), patients—especially from newly immigrant families and countries—often fear rejection if not retaliation from their physicians if they are too outspoken or demanding. Cultural issues, alas, far from being mere "background" or "academic" in the medical encounter, may turn out to be among the most intellectually, emotionally, and ethically demanding facets of medicine.

In this chapter, after several approaches to the concept of culture were discussed, two aspects of culture were portrayed: (1) patients' informal care networks and (2) illness-related words and concepts, together with their meanings. Four cultural domains that affect patients' health behavior were then explored: (1) ethnicity, (2) religion, (3) occupation, and (4) popular U.S. culture. It is tempting for the practitioner to memorize lists of cultural traits, just as in medical school the student must memorize thousands of anatomical parts, biochemical terms, physiological processes, and pharmacological actions. The result, however, would be less an intimate understanding of a real other person and family than the imposition of a stereotype and the mistaking of that stereotype for the patient's reality. It is admittedly more difficult, yet at the same time more rewarding, for the physician (or other healthcare provider) to take an interest in the patient as a person, an interest that will quite naturally lead to inquiry into the universes of meaning the patient inhabits, and in turn to a more satisfactory, productive, clinical relationship.

## CASES FOR DISCUSSION

## CASE 1

*The following case is based on Macquire (1978) and Hocking (1987, p. 527). It highlights the fact that (1) pathology occurs in workplace culture and (2) work-culture pathologies occur not only in individuals one at a time but also in groups where persons identify with one another as members of groups. In many U.S. communities, family physicians and general internists have long served as the "company doc" for oil refineries and factories. More recently, in large industries and corporations, or in "outsourced" health facilities, occupational medicine physicians, PAs, nurses, and industrial hygienists, among others, serve in this capacity. Although the case below occurred in England, it easily could have occurred in the United States:*

> *An outbreak of skin disorders took place in a ceramics factory. Those affected consisted of eight female employees who worked in one room, and two male porters. Subsequently, one woman was diagnosed with angioneurotic edema with cholinergic urticaria with impetigo complicating self-inflicted excoriation. The other seven women described that after seeing this woman, they themselves developed transient rashes on exposed surfaces. The two porters had winter eczema. Following an extensive investigation the plant was temporarily closed, the employees were given clear assurance, and the rashes disappeared. Only the first employee had sought medical help. There was consensus among employees that factory management was responsible for the illnesses and that management was likewise responsible for the cure. Employees believed they had lost their sense of individuality and that the factory now consisted only of a system of variously sized, impersonal work-groups. Somatization was the only acceptable way the grievance and protest could take place. The rash was a way to express powerlessness, to exert a small degree of power, and to help the group of employees to redefine themselves as a group. (Hocking, 1987, p. 527)*

*When practitioners and educators in biomedicine speak of "infectious disease," we usually refer to viral and bacterial infection. In this case, one might think of a kind of metaphoric infection based on identification. What is symbolically "infectious" here is discontent based on a sense of group isolation and mistreatment. The organizational culture had changed, making it a far more emotionally sterile place to work. The astute clinician of any specialty needs to inquire into the* kind *of "infection" that is affecting an organization and its* timing *(why now?) as well. A number of questions emerge from this case:*

1. *As a physician in a community or corporate group, how do you learn to think in terms of epidemiological or cultural patterns in addition to thinking clinically, biomedically, one patient at a time?*
2. *As the physician for a corporation or plant, for whom do you work (that is, individual employee, the employee's supervisor, the management, the union)? What role conflicts might you expect in the setting of an industrial or corporate culture?*
3. *Discuss this case in terms of Kleinman's distinction between "disease" and "illness."*
4. *If somatizing responses are corporately and culturally safe, how would you help employees to discuss feelings and grievances if these could be construed by management as threat or rebellion?*
5. *How would you clinically or administratively deal with the issues of female employees' low pay and relative powerlessness—factors over which you as a physician have no control and which management would likely tell you is "off limits" as a medical issue?*

## CASE 2

*(Adapted from Stein, 1987a, pp. 170–171): Mary Tinsley, a woman in her mid-60s, presents at the office of her family physician with a complaint of mid- and low-back pain. It is late September, and her annual visit(s) are like clockwork. Her ritual has been going on for some 30 years. She alleges that years ago she had some back injury but no vertebral fractures or compressions can be detected. Recent workups confirm the present physician's conviction that the problem is psychosomatic. The present physician is one in a distinguished line of family physicians, general practitioners, and orthopedic surgeons, all of whom were able to "find nothing."*

*Every year during the September planting season, John Tinsley, her husband, a man in his late 60s, spends nearly 2 weeks away from the house, working in the field. Mary feels isolated, abandoned. She felt this way even when their young children were living with them, when they lived in a house on the farm. She feels the same, now that she and her husband have moved from the farm to a nearby town. Thirty years ago, her back pain was so bad that she had to move about in a wheelchair, and her irate husband and children had to take care of her. Over the years, she has admirably run the household, reared the children. During the rest of the year, she is not sick a day. But come September and planting, her low-back pain is as predictable as is the change of season. The annual onset of symptoms coincides with John's departure. By the time plowing is finished, she has become veritably incapacitated (while continuing to perform domestic duties to a fault), and seeks medical relief. The physician prescribes meperidine HCl (a narcotic pain medicine) or flurazepam HCl (a tranquilizer) to alleviate the pain.*

*Mary reports that her husband berates her as "excess baggage," accusing her of not holding her own in her responsibilities around the house. As they both have grown older, Mary has apparently "aged" more than John—who even now cannot seem to work enough. John wants the freedom to work his farm, to come and go as he pleases, to be accountable to no one, and to not be tied to home or wife. Over time John's expectations have not at all diminished, while Mary resents being saddled with these expectations, feeling unappreciated for her role, and abandoned and ridiculed as "excess baggage."*

1. *Explain the timing of the wife's symptoms.*
2. *Speculate on the role of her symptoms in her marriage.*
3. *How would you as a physician go about inquiring into the meaning and function of her physical symptoms?*
4. *How would you avoid the temptation to do a "million-dollar workup" on a patient of this kind—who is "presenting" somatically?*
5. *How would you introduce "psychosocial" issues to a patient whose familial–cultural–religious beliefs militate against such an interpretation?*

## CASE 3

*(From Stein, 1985b, pp. 87–88): A farmer in his early 50s was scheduled for gallbladder surgery. Hospitalized, he was being prepped for surgery, his family gathering in the waiting area. As the anesthesiologist approached the patient, he developed supraventricular tachycardia, whereupon she stepped back and waited for him to calm down. She tried this unsuccessfully several times. Finally, she decided to postpone the surgery until a later time—one in which the patient would presumably be less nervous.*

*In the waiting area, the family wondered why it took so long for him to be readied for surgery. First, the anesthesiologist attempted to explain the problem by saying that the patient had developed supraventricular tachycardia; she explained anatomically all that was involved; she even drew an elementary diagram. The family didn't understand, standing around puzzled, wondering whether something undiscovered was wrong. The surgeon then attempted to redeem the situation, going basically through the same explanation as had the anesthesiologist—with similar success.*

*Down the hall walked a family physician who overheard the vain attempts to explain to the family through recourse to anatomy and physiology. He put his arm around the shoulder of one of the members of the family, and said: "Your father's heart is shimmying like the front end of an old Chevy pickup." The family said, with one voice, "Oh!"—finally feeling that they understood what was wrong. Satisfied, they were ready to leave until the next attempt could be made.*

1. *How would you have tried to explain the patient's cardiac reaction to the patient and family?*
2. *How do you think you would have responded (feeling, behavior) to the patient's and family's incomprehension of an accurate, elegant biomedical explanation you had just offered to them?*
3. *What cues would "tell" you that you need to talk with them in a different language?*
4. *Why do you think that the family practitioner's explanation succeeded, since a heart is not the same as the front end of a pickup truck?*
5. *Had this been an emergency situation, how would you have proceeded medically?*

## CASE 4

*Internist and family physician Robert E. Pieroni, M.D. (1981), reported the following case of hypokalemia, here paraphrased: He was asked to evaluate a 42-year-old black woman with a dangerously low serum potassium level. She was 8 months pregnant and had been admitted to the hospital because of weakness and marked hypertension. She reported no significant vomiting, diarrhea, or use of drugs that could have contributed to her considerable loss of potassium. He then questioned her about pica (an abnormal craving), which was frequently found in their area (the deep South). She reported that she had not eaten starch, dirt, or clay, but when directly questioned she did state that she had used chewing tobacco to ease her morning sickness. Such a practice is not uncommon in the deep South and has probably been handed down from generation to generation. Many brands of chewing tobacco, including the brand his patient was using, contained licorice, which not only can deplete the body of potassium but can also cause marked hypertension, weakness, and swelling. Fortunately, her potassium was corrected before further harm was done, and she went on to deliver a healthy baby. She now spreads the word that chewing tobacco is not a panacea for morning sickness (1981, p. 7).*

1. *Describe the two cultural explanatory models (professional and ethnic or folk) that were in conflict.*
2. *How do you decide whether to try to work within a patient's cultural framework or to persuade a patient to change it?*

3. *When you as a physician are unfamiliar with a patient's cultural practices, how would you go about inquiring into them so as to lead—for example—to thinking about licorice?*

# RECOMMENDED READINGS

Abel TM, Metraux R, Roll S: *Psychotherapy and Culture.* Albuquerque, University of New Mexico, 1987.

> The authors offer a view of the therapeutic process based on a psychodynamic model of human relationships and meanings.

Chrisman NJ, Maretzki TW (eds): *Clinically Applied Anthropology.* Dordrecht, Reidel, 1982.

> This edited volume describes the clinical contributions of applied anthropologists who conduct research and teach in health science settings.

Fadiman A: *The Spirit Catches You and You Fall Down: A Hmong Child, Her American Doctors, and the Collision of Two Cultures.* New York, Farrar, Straus & Giroux, 1997.

> This is a gripping narrative study in cross-cultural medicine. It traces the disparity in diagnosis and treatment between "epilepsy" and "soul loss" in a Hmong child and family from Laos. It is a tragic account of differences in understanding that became labeled as noncompliance.

Harwood A (ed): *Ethnicity and Medical Care.* Cambridge, Mass, Harvard University Press, 1981.

> This edited volume offers rich accounts of the role of cultural values, attitudes, expectations, language, and beliefs in a wide array of ethnic groups' members' health behaviors.

Henry J: *Culture Against Man.* New York, Random House, 1963.

> Henry critically examines family, education, values, political ideologies, attitudes toward aging, and much more in this classic work on U.S. culture.

Johnson T, Sargent C (eds): *Medical Anthropology,* ed 2. Westport, Conn, Greenwood Press, 1995.

> This encyclopedic volume represents a state-of-the-art review of the conceptual, methodological, and clinical issues in culture and medicine, including a focus on gender and health and HIV disease.

Stein HF: *American Medicine as Culture.* Boulder, Colo, Westview Press, 1993.

> Stein presents a description and interpretation of U.S. biomedicine as an occupational culture. Topics include values, metaphors, control, group dynamics in clinical decision-making, money and medicine, the process of becoming a physician, and the self of the physician.

Stein HF, Apprey M: *From Metaphor to Meaning: Papers in Psychoanalytic Anthropology.* Charlottesville, University Press of Virginia, 1987.

> Stein and Apprey offer interpretations of the intrapsychic story that is simultaneously represented and veiled by culture. They demonstrate how deceptively simple personal, familial, clinical, and larger cultural symbols condense complex ideas and feelings.

# REFERENCES

Barrett JR. Exercise addiction, in Mellion MB (ed): *Sports Medicine Secrets.* Philadelphia, Hanley & Belfus, 1994, pp 141–144.

Blumhagen D: The meaning of hypertension, in Chrisman N, Maretzki TW (eds): *Clinically Applied Anthropology.* Dordrecht, Reidel, 1982, pp 297–323.

Boyer LB: Approaching cross-cultural psychotherapy. *J Psychoanal Anthropol* 6:237–245, 1983.

Chrisman NJ: The health seeking process: An approach to the natural history of illness. *Culture Med Psychiatry* 1:351–377, 1977.

Chrisman NJ, Maretzki TW (eds): *Clinically Applied Anthropology.* Dordrecht, Reidel, 1982.

Committee on International Relations, Stein HF: *Us and Them: The Psychology of Ethnonationalism.* Group for the Advancement of Psychiatry, Report No. 123. New York, Brunner/Mazel, 1987.

Crawford R: Healthism and the medicalization of everyday life. *Int J Health Serv* 10:365–388, 1980.

Crawford R: A cultural account of health: Self control, release, and the social body, in McKinlay J (ed): *Issues in the Political Economy of Health Care.* London, Tavistock, 1985.

deMause L: *Reagan's America.* New York, Creative Roots, 1984.

Devereux G: *Basic Problems of Ethno-psychiatry,* Gulati BM, Devereux G (trans). Chicago, University of Chicago Press, 1980.

De Vos GA: Afterword, in Reynolds DK: *The Quiet Therapies: Japanese Pathways to Personal Growth.* Honolulu, University of Hawaii Press, 1980.

De Vos GA, Romanucci-Ross, L (eds): *Ethnic Identity: Cultural Continuities and Change.* Palo Alto, Calif, Mayfield Publishing Co, 1975.

Dirckx JH: Speaking of illness. *Pharos* 45:22–26, 1982.

Drucker PF: *The Practice of Management.* New York, Harper, 1954.

Eisenberg L, Kleinman AM (eds): *The Relevance of Social Science for Medicine.* Dordrecht, Reidel, 1981.

Fadiman A: *The Spirit Catches You and You Fall Down: A Hmong Child, Her American Doctors, and the Collision of Two Cultures*. New York, Farrar, Straus & Giroux, 1997.

Foster G: Disease etiologies in non-Western medical systems. *Am Anthropol* 78:773–782, 1976.

Foster GM, Anderson BG: *Medical Anthropology*. New York, John Wiley & Sons Inc, 1978.

Frank G, Blackhall LJ, Michel V, Murphy ST, Azen SP, Park K: A discourse of relationships in bioethics: Patient autonomy and end-of-life decision making among elderly Korean Americans. *Med Anthropol Q* 12(4):403–423, 1998.

Fuller RC: The turn to alternative medicine. *Second Opinion* 18(1): 11–31, 1992.

Glazer N, Moynihan DP (eds): *Ethnicity: Theory and Experience*. Cambridge, Mass, Harvard University Press, 1975.

Grieco MS: Birth-marked? A critical view on analyzing organizational culture. *Hum Org* 47:84–87, 1988.

Harwood A: The hot–cold theory of disease: Implications for treatment of Puerto Rican patients. *JAMA* 216:1153–1158, 1971.

Harwood A: *Ethnicity and Medical Care*. Cambridge, Mass, Harvard University Press, 1981.

Henry J: *Culture against Man*. New York, Random House, 1963.

Hill CE, Mathews H: Traditional health beliefs and practices among southern rural blacks: A complement to biomedicine, in Black M, Reed JS (eds): *Social Science Perspectives on the South*. New York, Gordon & Breach Science Publishers, 1981, pp 307–322.

Hill RF, Fortenberry JD, Stein HF: Culture in clinical medicine. *South Med J* 83(9):1071–1080, 1990.

Hocking B: Anthropologic aspects of occupational illness epidemics. *J Occup Med* 29:526–530, 1987.

Hultkrantz A: *Shamanic Healing and Ritual Drama: Health and Medicine in Native North American Religious Traditions*. New York, Crossroads, for the Lutheran General Health System, 1992.

Johnson TM: Premenstrual syndrome as a Western culture-specific disorder. *Culture Med Psychiatry* 11(3):337–356, 1987.

Johnson TM, Kleinman A: Cultural concerns in consultation psychiatry, in Guggenheim FG, Weiner MF (eds): *Manual of Psychiatric Consultation and Emergency Care*. New York, Jason Aronson, 1984, pp 275–284.

Keefe SE: Real and ideal extended familism among Mexican Americans and Anglo Americans: On the meaning of "close" family ties. *Hum Org* 43:65–70, 1984.

Kleinman AM: Clinical relevance of anthropological and cross-cultural research: Concepts and strategies. *Am J Psychiatry* 135:427–431, 1978.

Kleinman AM: *Patients and Healers in the Context of Culture: An Exploration of the Borderland between Anthropology, Medicine, and Psychiatry*. Los Angeles, University of California Press, 1980.

Kleinman AM: The teaching of clinically applied medical anthropology on a psychiatric consultation-liaison service, in Chrisman NJ, Maretzki TW (eds): *Clinically Applied Anthropology: Anthropologists in Health Science Settings*. Dordrecht, Reidel, 1982, pp 83-115.

Kleinman AM, Eisenberg L, Good B: Culture, illness, and care: Clinical lessons from anthropologic and cross-cultural research. *Ann Intern Med* 88:251–258, 1978.

Kluckhohn F, Strodtbeck F: *Variations in Value Orientations*. Evanston, Ill, Row Peterson, 1961.

Lang GC: Diabetes and health care in a Sioux community. *Hum Org* 44:251–260, 1985.

Lin EH-B: Intraethnic characteristics and the patient–physician interaction. *J Fam Pract* 16:91–98, 1983.

Macquire A: Psychic possession among industrial workers. *Lancet* 2:376–378, 1978.

Murray RH, Rubel AJ: Physicians and healers—Unwitting partners in health care. *N Engl J Med* 326:61–64, 1992.

Nga NA: Vietnamese relocation. Department of Family Medicine Grand Rounds, University of Oklahoma Health Sciences Center, Oklahoma City, 23 February 1988.

O'Connor BB: *Healing Traditions: Alternative Medicine and the Health Professions*. Philadelphia, University of Pennsylvania Press, 1995.

Ohnuki-Tierney E: *Illness and Culture in Contemporary Japan*. New York, Cambridge University Press, 1984.

Oliver-Smith A: *The Martyred City: Death and Rebirth in the Andes*. Prospect Heights, Ill, Waveland Press, 1992.

Parry KK: Concepts from medical anthropology for clinicians. *Phys Ther* 64:929–933, 1984.

Pieroni RE: Folk medicine of the black elderly. *Quarterly Contact* [National Caucus and Center on Black Aged, Inc.] 4:7, 1981.

Pollitt K: The politically correct body. *Mother Jones*, May 1982, pp 66–67.

Primosch R, Young S: Pseudo battering of Vietnamese children (Cao gio). *J Am Dent Assoc* 101:47–48, 1980.

Scheper-Hughes N, Lock MM: The mindful body: A prolegomenon to future work in medical anthropology. *Med Anthropol Q* 1:6–41, 1987.

Scheper-Hughes N, Stein HF: Child-abuse and the unconscious, in Scheper-Hughes N (ed): *Child Survival: Anthropological Approaches to the Treatment and Maltreatment of Children*. Dordrecht, Reidel, 1987.

Snow LF: Folk medical beliefs and implications for care of patients. *An Intern Med* 81:82–96, 1974.

Snow LF: Traditional health beliefs and practices among lower class black Americans. *West J Med* 139:820–828, 1983.

Spiegel J: *Transactions: The Interplay between Individual, Family, and Society*. New York, Science House, 1971.

Stein HF: Ethanol and its discontents: Paradoxes of inebriation and sobriety in American culture. *J Psychoanal Anthropol* 5:355–377, 1982.

Stein HF: Alcoholism as metaphor in American culture: Ritual desecration as social integration. *Ethos* 13:195–235, 1985a.

Stein HF: An argument for more inclusive context in clinical intervention: The case of family medicine, in Stein HF, Apprey M: *Context and Dynamics in Clinical Knowledge*. Charlottesville, University Press of Virginia, 1985b, pp 78–91.

Stein HF: The annual cycle and the cultural nexus of health care behavior among Oklahoma wheat farming families, in Stein HF, Apprey M: *From Metaphor to Meaning: Papers in Psychoanalytic Anthropology*. Charlottesville, University Press of Virginia, 1987a, pp 156–177.

Stein HF: Farmer and cowboy: The duality of the Midwestern male ethos—A study in ethnicity, regionalism, and national identity, in Stein HF, Apprey M: *From Metaphor to Meaning: Papers in Psychoanalytic Anthropology*. Charlottesville, University Press of Virginia, 1987b, pp 178–227.

Stein HF: In what systems do alcohol/chemical addictions make sense? Clinical ideologies and practices as cultural metaphors. Invited presentation for panel "Toward a Critical Clinical Anthropology," for the 86th Annual Meeting of the American Anthropological Association, Chicago, 1987c [later published in *Soc Sci Med* 30(9):987–1000, 1990].

Stein HF: Review of Koenigsberg RA, The psychoanalysis of racism, revolution and nationalism (New York: The Library of Social Science, 1977/1986). *Can Rev Stud Nationalism* 14:345–347, 1987d.

Stein HF: Substance and symbol, in Galanter M (ed): *Recent Developments in Alcoholism, Volume 11: Ten Years of Progress*. New York, Plenum Press, 1993, pp 153–164.

Stein HF: Trauma revisited: Mourning and the unconscious in the Oklahoma City bombing. *J Psychoanal Culture Soc* 2(1):17–37, 1997.

Stein HF: A bombing in April: Culture and disaster in the Oklahoma City bombing. *Illness, Crisis and Loss* 7(1):17–36, 1999.

Stein HF, Apprey M: *Context and Dynamics in Clinical Knowledge*. Charlottesville, University Press of Virginia, 1985.

Stein HF, Apprey M: *From Metaphor to Meaning: Papers in Psychoanalytic Anthropology*. Charlottesville, University Press of Virginia, 1987.

Stein HF, Hill RF: *The Ethnic Imperative: Examining the New White Ethnic Movement*. University Park, Pennsylvania State University Press, 1977.

Stein, HF: A dialectical model of health and illness attitudes and behavior among Slovak-Americans. *Int J Mental Health* 5(2):117–137, 1976.

Taylor FW: *The Principles of Scientific Management*. New York, Harper & Brothers, 1911.

*Time* magazine. Cover story: Revenge of the killer microbes—Are we losing the war against infectious diseases? 24 September 1994, pp 62–69.

White KL, Williams TF, Greenberg BG: The ecology of medical care. *N Engl J Med* 265:885–892, 1961.

Young A: *The Harmony of Illusions: Inventing Post Traumatic Stress Disorder*. Princeton, NJ, Princeton University Press, 1997.

Zborowski M: *People in Pain*. San Francisco, Jossey–Bass Inc, Publishers, 1969.

# The Healthcare System

*James W. Mold\**

*Dr. S. was a member of the medical staff of a comprehensive rehabilitation hospital. He was particularly interested in geriatric rehabilitation, the most frequent admitter of older patients to the facility. With the encouragement of the Chief of Staff and administrator of the hospital he began having meetings with the staff to discuss ways to improve the care of older rehabilitation patients. One of the ideas he proposed to the group made up of physicians, nurses, speech pathologists, occupational therapists, physical therapists, recreational therapists, social workers, case managers, and dietitians was to develop a unified, coordinated assessment process. The advantages would include less duplication of effort, better organization of essential information, and better coordination of care. Each member of the team would contribute his or her unique set of information to a single unified assessment and a set of goals for the hospitalization that all would agree to and sign.*

*Dr. S. was surprised at the resistance to this idea. The physicians were reluctant to trust anyone else's history and examination. The nurses were using a separate chart altogether, had put a great deal of effort into developing it, and saw no reason to change their system. Besides, they argued, their accrediting body would not allow them to reduce the content of their assessment. Some of the therapists were enthusiastic about the idea but were concerned about who would be involved in determining the rehabilitation goals, specifically wondering whether the physicians would control the process. They also stated that their assessments took more time to complete and could not be completed within the time frame that was proposed.*

## EDUCATIONAL OBJECTIVES

1. The roles, settings, training, and certification of the various healthcare professions, both traditional and alternative

*With the assistance of Barbara Barrett, D.P.M.; F. Tohgi, D.C., L.Ac., Ph.D.; Dan Gentry, P.T.; Andre F. Fountain, R.N.; Kevin T. Avery, D.M.D.; Julia Eyer, Ph.D., CCC-SP; David Thompson, LPT, M.P.H.; Don Lanquist, RRT; Carol McCoy, Ph.D., MT (ASCP), CLS; Earl Schmitt, O.D., Ed.D.; Jacqueline Cook, M.S.W./P; Gary Sharp, P.A.; Bob Shahan, R.T.; Carole A. Sullivan, M.Ed., R.T.(R)T, FASRT; Cynthia Omoto, M.S.W.; Shirley Wunder, R.N.; Paul Preslar, D.O.

2. How to consult with and refer to each of these professionals
3. How to build multidisciplinary healthcare teams, and how to overcome the most common obstacles in building such teams

# INTRODUCTION

Although typically considered to be the principal providers of healthcare, physicians represent only one of a large number of healthcare professionals that make up the healthcare system. Many of the other healthcare disciplines are comparatively new (post World War II), reflecting the increasing complexity of modern healthcare. Table 25.1 is a partial list of "traditional" healthcare practitioners. In addition to these, a variety of "alternative" or "complementary" healthcare practitioners have gained recognition in recent years (Table 25.2).

For such a large and complex system to be maximally effective and efficient, a certain amount of teamwork is required. Unfortunately, the training received by the practitioners in each discipline is predominantly discipline specific, with surprisingly little integration with the training programs of the other disciplines. As a result, the conceptual approaches to healthcare and even the languages used by providers from the various disciplines differ considerably. In addition, because of differences in responsibilities and rewards and some overlap of competencies, there is a natural tendency for the various groups to be suspicious and envious of each other, a tendency that, at its worst, leads to what is commonly called protecting one's turf, illustrated in Case 25-1.

When the contributions of the various disciplines are recognized and valued, the healthcare system can function in a truly interdisciplinary way. Cooperation results in improved coordination of healthcare with less duplication of efforts. More overall energy can be applied to patient care.

**Table 25.1**
Characteristics of "Traditional" Healthcare Professionals[a]

| Discipline | Year and Number of Practitioners in U.S. | | Length of Training | Degree |
|---|---|---|---|---|
| Physicians | | | | |
|   Allopathic | 1998 | 777,859 | 5–11 years | M.D. |
|   Osteopathic | 1999 | 44,000 | 7 years | D.O. |
|   Podiatric | 1998 | 7,510 | 5–10 years | D.P.M. |
| Psychologists | 1998 | 84,380 | 5–8 years | Ph.D. |
| Social workers | 1998 | 365,600 | 4–8 years | B.A., M.S.W., Ph.D. |
| Speech pathologists/audiologists | 1998 | 88,390 | 4–6 years | CCC-SP; CCC-A; CCC-SP/A |
| Pharmacists | 1998 | 178,110 | 5–6 years | Pharm.D. |
| Physician assistants | 1998 | 62,000 | 2–4 years | P.A. |
| Dental practitioners | 1998 | 81,510 | 4 years | D.D.S. |
| Nurses | | | | |
|   Registered nurses | 1998 | 2,027,830 | 2–4 years | R.N. |
|   Licensed practical nurses | 1998 | 673,790 | 1 year | L.P.N. |
| Optometrists | 1998 | 23,500 | 4 years | O.D. |
| Dietitians/nutritionists | 1998 | 44,840 | 4–5 years | R.D./L.D. |
| Medical/clinical technologists | 1998 | 151,100 | 3–5 years | |
| Occupational therapists | 1998 | 64,730 | 4–8 years | O.T.R. |
| Recreational therapists | 1998 | 23,300 | 4 years | |
| Physical therapists | 1998 | 111,480 | 4–5 years | P.T. |
| Respiratory therapists | 1988 | 84,730 | 2–5 years | RRT/CRTT |
| Radiology technologists | 1998 | 157,480 | 2–4 years | RTR/RT(N)/RRT; RT(US)/RT(CT) |

[a]Information for this table was obtained from the U.S. Government Bureau of Labor & Statistics Occupational Employment and Wage Data online: http//stats.bls.gov/oes/oes_data.htm

**Table 25.2**
Partial List of Alternative Healthcare Disciplines and Practices

| | | |
|---|---|---|
| Acupuncture | Herbal medicine | Massage |
| Aromatherapy | Homeopathy | Meditation |
| Art therapy | Hypnosis | Naturopathy |
| Ayurveda | Imagery/visualization | Orthomolecular medicine |
| Chelation therapy | Iridology | Reflexology |
| Chiropractic | Macrobiotics | Rolfing |

# PHYSICIANS

Practitioners from several different disciplines use the title "physician" and/or "doctor." These include allopathic physicians, osteopathic physicians, doctors of podiatric medicine, doctors of optometry, chiropractic physicians, and homeopathic and naturopathic physicians. At present, allopathic and osteopathic physicians are most similar in terms of training, credentialing, practice activities, and status. For this reason, after a brief review of their philosophical origins, they will be discussed together while the other groups will be discussed individually later in the chapter.

## Allopathic Physicians

The terms *allopathy* and *allopathic medicine* were coined by Hahnemann around 1849 to distinguish "ordinary" medical practice from the emerging field of homeopathy. *Allopathy* implies an active approach to the treatment of disease using medications and surgery to do what the body is unable to do for itself. Allopathic physicians are currently the predominant physicians in the United States. Their education involves an undergraduate college degree including a variety of prerequisites—mainly math and science, 4 years of medical education leading to the medical doctor (M.D.) degree, and from 1 to 10 years of residency training.

## Osteopathic Physicians

Osteopathy was founded by Andrew Still in 1874 on the following principles, which he felt to be sufficiently distinct from those of allopathic medicine at that time (Jones, 1978).

1. The body is an integral unit, a whole. The structure of the body and its functions work together, interdependently.
2. The body systems have built-in repair processes, which are self-regulating and self-healing in the face of disease.
3. The circulatory system or distributing channels of the body, along with the nervous system, provide the integrating functions for the rest of the body.
4. The contribution of the musculoskeletal system to a person's health is much more than providing framework and support.
5. While disease may be manifested in specific parts of the body, other body parts may contribute to a restoration or correction of the disease.

His original intent was not to create a new discipline but rather to strengthen the existing one (Lesho, 1999).

Dr. Still was fascinated with the musculoskeletal system, spending large amounts of time studying it in great detail. At the same time he opposed many of the pharmaceutical remedies that were in vogue at the time, and was therefore interested in nonpharmacological treatments for disease that could enhance the body's natural repair mechanisms. He became convinced that manipulation of the musculoskeletal system could affect beneficial changes in all other systems, particularly the circulatory and nervous systems, which he believed were critical to the body's natural reparative mechanisms. Musculoskeletal manipulation is now a relatively small but still important part of most osteopathic physicians' practice.

Currently osteopathic physicians receive essentially the same quantity and quality of training as allopathic physicians, with only minor differences in philosophy and emphasis. Their terminal degree is the doctor of osteopathy (D.O.) degree. Although barriers and philosophical distinctions between the two physician groups are diminishing, there are no obvious signs that the two professional bodies intend to unite in the near future.

Osteopaths have always been trained as generalists first and foremost, and although specialty training is available in all of the traditional areas, a larger percentage of osteopaths choose general practice than do allopathic physicians. Osteopathic physicians have also been more likely to practice in rural settings than their allopathic counterparts. An osteopath can choose to do either an osteopathic or an allopathic residency program in primary care or a subspecialty after medical school.

## Physicians and the Healthcare System

Physicians have generally occupied the highest leadership roles in the healthcare system, due to their extensive training and revered position in society. State and national physician organizations, such as state medical societies and the American Medical Association, exert a powerful influence on legislators. Although administrators are now taking away some of the authority and responsibility that has traditionally belonged to physicians, among healthcare providers it is still physicians who most frequently give the orders that other healthcare providers are expected to follow. And it is physicians who bear the greatest liability when something goes wrong. Many physicians still believe that other healthcare professionals should only be involved in patient care by direct order of and under the close supervision of a physician.

Because of the current level of acceptance of a biomedical model of health and illness, physicians, as the most highly trained applied biomedical scientists, are logically the most powerful members of the healthcare team. Other health professionals are often forced, then, to function in supporting roles. There is some reason to believe, however, that the current biomedical model may soon undergo a transformation that may alter this traditional hierarchy. The pressure for such a paradigm shift comes from consumers and, more recently, payors (e.g., employers) who have become increasingly dissatisfied with the current technical, physician-dominated approach, which they view as impersonal, mechanistic, and expensive (Freymann, 1989).

While historically physicians have been predominantly male and other healthcare disciplines predominantly female, since 1967, the percentage of female physicians has increased substantially. Differentials in income undoubtedly reflect differences in training and responsibility but perhaps also a measure of sexism. As more women choose to become physicians and more men become nurses and allied health professionals, these differences may become less significant.

### CASE 25-2

*Mrs. M. was a 78-year-old widow who lived alone. Because of frequent falls and increasing forgetfulness, she had become essentially homebound by choice. She came to the attention of Dr. S., a general internist, on referral from a social worker from Adult Protective Services (APS) who requested a medical evaluation of her falls, forgetfulness, and the recent onset of a blood discharge from one of her breasts. The APS became involved because of the neighbors' concerns that Mrs. M. was in need of assistance.*

*Dr. S., after careful evaluation, concluded that there was a possibility of significant heart disease as well as a breast nodule, bilateral cataracts, and mild dementia. He referred her to a general surgeon for breast biopsy, an ophthalmologist for evaluation of the cataracts, and arranged for her to have some cardiac studies, an echocardiogram, and a 24-hour Holter monitor.*

*The breast nodule was biopsied and proved to be malignant. The consulting surgeon suggested a modified radical mastectomy. The ophthalmologist confirmed the presence of cataracts but was not*

*convinced that removing them would prevent further falls. The results of the cardiac studies were
normal.*

*Mrs. M. was admitted to the hospital for breast surgery. Dr. S. visited her in the hospital and met
with nurses to develop a plan of care that would prevent falls and minimize the confusion he
anticipated might result from the unfamiliar hospital environment. He asked that the surgeon
request a physical therapy consult to help with the evaluation of the falls and to ensure that Mrs. M.
remained as active as possible during the hospitalization. The surgery was a success, no complications occurred, and Mrs. M. was discharged to her home. Dr. S. then scheduled a house call and
invited the social worker from Adult Protective Services to be present for a discussion of further
healthcare needs.*

## Generalists and Subspecialists

As medicine has become more complex, physicians have become increasingly subspecialized. Table
25.3 lists the major medical and surgical subspecialties. Generalist physicians still provide most of the
primary care, managing 80–90% of patients' problems and coordinating the care of other professionals as in
Case 25-2. Many of the same kinds of turf issues that occur between healthcare disciplines also occur to a
somewhat lesser degree between subspecialties of medicine for similar reasons. Subspecialized physicians
tend to have greater status and higher incomes than generalists. This is in contrast to most corporations in
which individuals with the most specialized training head divisions, whereas corporate leaders are of
necessity generalists. Part of the income differential between subspecialists and generalists is the result of
third-party reimbursement practices.

Despite their higher incomes and status, subspecialists are dependent on generalists for consultations and
referrals. Thus, there is some pressure on subspecialists to be gracious and to return patients to the consulting/
referring physicians as promptly as possible. These courtesies often break down within medical centers and
other large organizations in which, for a variety of reasons, subspecialists are less dependent on, or less aware
of their dependency on, primary care physician referrals.

Patients interested in obtaining the best possible medical care are faced with the choice of either seeing
the appropriate subspecialists for each of their health problems, or seeing a generalist (family physician,
internist, or pediatrician), whom they must trust to refer them to subspecialists when appropriate. Studies
indicate that family physicians can adequately manage 85–95% of the healthcare problems that their patients
present to them without consultation or referral (AAFP, 1991). Because of their familiarity with subspecialist
colleagues and the local healthcare system, generalist physicians are in a good position to advise their patients
when consultation with other providers is necessary and which subspecialists would provide them with the
best service in specific situations.

However, generalists are less likely to recognize and diagnose unusual problems as quickly and
accurately as subspecialists. They are therefore susceptible to *errors of omission*. They are also less likely than
subspecialists to follow clinical practice guidelines for individual diseases, being more concerned about the
patient as a whole, and more easily distracted by competing problems. Subspecialists, on the other hand, often

**Table 25.3**
Major Medical and Surgical Subspecialties

| | | |
|---|---|---|
| Allergy and immunology | Neurology | Physical medicine and rehabilitation |
| Anesthesiology | Nuclear medicine | Plastic surgery |
| Colon and rectal surgery | Obstetrics and gynecology | Psychiatry and neurology |
| Dermatology | Ophthalmology | Radiology |
| Emergency medicine | Orthopedic surgery | Surgery |
| Family practice | Otolaryngology | Thoracic surgery |
| Preventive medicine | Pathology | Urology |
| Internal medicine | Pediatrics | |

have less familiarity with the patient, are less able to view health problems in context, are expected not to make errors of omission, and have more technology at their fingertips, making them more susceptible to *errors of commission* (doing too much).

Errors of omission are more obvious than errors of commission, but they are not necessarily more harmful. Increasingly aggressive attempts through testing and other interventions to reduce uncertainty may result in an avalanche of unwanted consequences. This phenomenon has been called the *cascade effect* (Mold & Stein, 1986). Clinical cascades may be catastrophic but are often unrecognized.

## CASE 25-3

*Mrs. F. was a 68-year-old woman who had coronary artery bypass surgery 6 years earlier and now was experiencing recurrent angina pectoris related to severe coronary artery disease, uncontrolled by medications. Her physician, Dr. J., requested a cardiologist's opinion regarding the risks and benefits to Mrs. F. of another coronary artery bypass operation. The cardiologist, after evaluating Mrs. F., agreed that surgery was a possible option and requested the additional input of a cardiothoracic surgeon. The surgeon, after reviewing the cardiac catheterization results, recommended against surgery because of the high operative mortality risk for this particular patient (approximately 20%).*

*However, Dr. J. felt that his questions had not been properly answered. He already knew that the risk associated with a second cardiac surgery would be high, but he believed his patient might be willing to take a substantial risk because of the persistence of her chest pain, which was limiting her to a bed-to-chair existence. What Dr. J. really needed to know were the probability of benefit and the possible likelihoods of the various nonfatal adverse outcomes associated with surgery so that he could help Mrs. F. make the best possible decision, taking into account her own values and preferences.*

### Consultation and Referral

Integral to the professional relationship between physicians is the consultation and referral process. Classically, a physician asks a consultant on behalf of his patient for advice regarding the diagnosis or treatment of a particular health problem. At times it is necessary and appropriate for one physician to refer a patient to another physician for ongoing management of one or more problems. Such requests may be communicated by phone, letter, or by the patient. The more effectively the request is communicated, the more likely the consultant is to be helpful. Once the consultant has reached an opinion, he or she communicates it to the patient and primary physician, generally by phone and/or mail and returns the patient to the care of the consulting physician unless requested to do otherwise (McWhinney, 1989). Obviously, good communication between physicians is essential to the consultative process, but, unfortunately, it doesn't always occur.

A proper consultation request should specify the questions being asked of the consultant and the extent of involvement requested of the consultant in the evaluation and management of the patient. The physician requesting the consultation may, for example, request that the consultant render an opinion regarding diagnosis or treatment but not assume responsibility for implementation of the recommended treatment. Alternatively, the request may be for the physician to assume complete responsibility for the management of a specific problem.

Although the opinion of the consultant should be given a great deal of consideration, it is not binding. Neither the physician requesting the consultation nor the patient is under any ethical or legal obligation to follow the advice of the consultant. It should be remembered that although the consultant brings specialized knowledge and skills to bear on the problem in question, the consulting physician and patient have equally important information that must be considered before a final decision can be made. Under no circumstances should a consultant send the patient to a second consultant without the authorization and approval of the primary physician, as was done in Case 25-3.

## CHOOSING A SPECIALTY

*Several methods have been proposed to help medical students select the medical or surgical field for which they will be best suited. Those who choose primary care tend to be more comfortable with uncertainty and less concerned about money and prestige than those who become subspecialists. Personality inventories such as the Myers Briggs Type Indicator suggest, for example, that students who are "introverted, intuitive, feeling, perceptives" (INFP) tend to choose and be happy in psychiatry while those who are "extroverted, sensing, thinking, judgers" (ESTJ) tend to choose careers in surgery. An alternative conceptualization suggests that medical career choice can be guided by one's level of enjoyment of three categories of activities: need for sensation or excitement, relationships with people, and use of technologies.*

## Physician Associates/Assistants

Once called *physician extenders*, physician associates (PA's) are healthcare professionals who provide services to patients under the supervision of physicians. Physician associates take medical histories, perform physical examinations, order laboratory tests, make diagnoses, and prescribe treatments including medications. They practice in private physicians' offices, health maintenance organizations, nursing homes, student health services, urban and rural clinics, correctional institutions, and industry. In addition, physician associates are involved in medical education, health administration, and research.

Physician associates are trained in programs accredited by the Committee on Allied Health Education and Accreditation (CAHEA), which is sponsored by the American Medical Association. The first phase of the 2-year curriculum includes classroom and laboratory instruction in the basic medical sciences. The second phase consists of structured clinical rotations providing the students with direct patient contact. These rotations are intensive hands-on learning experiences in private and institutional medical settings that emphasize training in primary care (family practice, internal medicine, and pediatrics) but also include experience in obstetrics and gynecology, surgery, and emergency medicine.

Degrees awarded vary, depending on the institution offering the program and the educational background of the student. Most programs offer a baccalaureate degree. A few master's degree and residency programs are available either within the core PA curricula or for postgraduate specialization in such areas as occupational medicine, surgery, and pediatrics.

Physician associates, working with other members of the healthcare team, improve the overall distribution of healthcare services and access to care, particularly in rural areas and underserved communities. They also increase the efficiency of ambulatory care practices, reduce patient waiting time, and allow physicians more time for difficult cases. By stressing preventive health and periodic screening, they may help reduce excess morbidity and mortality (Jones & Crawley, 1994).

### CASE 25-4

*A 40-year-old insulin-dependent diabetic, E.W., who had previously achieved excellent diabetic control, had recently begun to have blood glucose levels in the 200 to 300 mg/dl (normal ≤ 100 mg/dl) range for reasons that were unclear to him. His physician was also puzzled. Because of some gum swelling and irritation, he saw his dentist. The dentist discovered an abscess under one of E.W.'s teeth, which he treated with antibiotics and surgical drainage. One week later, E.W.'s diabetes once again came under good control. No communication occurred between the physician and dentist before or after the event.*

## DENTAL ABSCESS

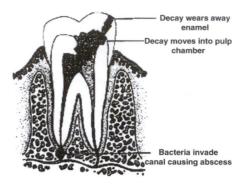

Decay wears away
enamel

Decay moves into pulp
chamber

Bacteria invade
canal causing abscess

Periapical Abscess

*A collection of infected material (pus) resulting from bacterial infection of the center (pulp) of a tooth.*

## DENTISTS

Approximately 85% of dental practitioners in the United States are generalists. Only one state (Delaware) requires a year of residency training. Most states require National Board exams and/or practical clinical exams. The American Dental Association (ADA) recognizes eight dental subspecialties: orthodontics, oral surgery, oral pathology, endodontics, pediatric dentistry, dental public health, periodontics, and prosthodontics, all of which require several years of additional training beyond dental school.

Dentists provide a wide range of services including prevention, diagnosis, and treatment of dental caries; medical and surgical treatment of gingival and periodontal disease; prosthedontic and surgical treatment of malocclusion, temporomandibular joint dysharmony, and cosmetic problems; and treatment of various benign and malignant soft tissue diseases. The dental caries rate in the U.S. population has been substantially reduced by water fluoridation. As a result, the rate of dental loss has been substantially reduced, and many more people are at risk for periodontal disease. The profile of services that dentists provide has therefore shifted to include fewer fillings and extractions and more endodontics, periodontics, and cosmetic restorations (Ring, 1985). Part of this shift is also related to new technology and to patient expectations. People now expect to keep their natural teeth over a lifetime and are demanding treatment approaches that will help them to do so. In 1988 the U.S. population spent more than $37 billion on dental care. Half of that amount came directly from patients, almost half from third parties, and very little from the government.

Physicians and dentists working together could better educate their patients, identify problems early, and make appropriate referrals, in contrast to what more commonly happens, illustrated in Case 25-4. Most dental diseases are either preventable or are much easier and less costly to treat in the incipient stages. Particularly critical to oral health are episodes of severe physical illness when resistance is compromised and oral hygiene is likely to be less adequate. Physicians must be particularly alert to the potential need for dental evaluation and treatment during or following such episodes.

## CASE 25-5

*Mrs. R., a 60-year-old woman with longstanding diabetes mellitus associated with visual impairment, neuropathy, and peripheral vascular disease, was admitted to the hospital with gangrene of several toes on her left foot. After a forefoot amputation, she was discharged home to be followed closely by*

## WHAT IS GANGRENE?

*Gangrene is defined as the destruction of living tissue due to obstruction of the blood and oxygen supply.*

### Dry Gangrene

*Dry gangrene is caused by the gradual loss of blood. Dry gangrene often comes about as a result of diabetes, arteriosclerosis, or severe frostbite. The skin becomes painful and then dark, the dead skin eventually drying and dropping off. This form of gangrene is not life threatening because healing usually takes place naturally at the junction between the living and dead tissue.*

### Moist Gangrene

*A more serious condition, known as moist gangrene, is caused by the loss of blood supply. Some cells may stay alive while surrounding cells begin to quickly die and to leak fluid, causing the affected tissues to become moist. Bacteria flourish in the moist environment. At first, the skin becomes swollen and blisterous, and then foul smelling. This type of gangrene can spread rather quickly and can be fatal.*

### Gas Gangrene

*The most deadly form of gangrene is gas gangrene. It occurs in wounds infected with bacteria that live in low oxygen environments, which release gas and poisons into the body. The symptoms of gas gangrene are high fever, brown pus, and gas bubbles on the skin. This form of gangrene spreads very quickly, and causes a rapid death.*

*her primary care physician and a home health agency. The agency sent a registered nurse to her home to teach her how to change dressings, to monitor her blood sugars and blood pressures (her medications and dosages had been changed), and to measure correctly and administer her insulin. Physical and occupational therapists made home visits as well to help her to modify her home and to learn to care for herself after the amputation. The agency staff communicated with Mrs. R.'s primary care physician by mail, phone, and during monthly luncheon meetings at the physician's office.*

## NURSES

Florence Nightingale described a nurse's role as "putting the patient in the best condition for nature to act upon him." In 1980, the American Nurses' Association redefined nursing as "the diagnosis and treatment of human responses to actual or potential health problems," reflecting a somewhat more expansive concept of the involvement of nurses in patient care (Friedman, 1990). In most clinical settings, nurses spend a greater amount of time working directly with patients than any other healthcare professionals. Their impact on outcomes is often underestimated. Studies of postoperative mortality rates between hospitals have consistently pointed to the experience and qualifications of the nursing staff as one of the major variables determining outcome.

Collaboration between physicians and nurses, though vitally important for optimal patient care, is often suboptimal (Fagin, 1992; Friedman, 1990; Stein *et al.*, 1990). Physicians frequently regard nurses as subordinates whose major responsibility is to carry out their orders. Nurses, on the other hand, consider themselves to be healthcare professionals with roles equally as important as and distinct from those of physicians. Although nurse practice acts vary from state to state, several legal opinions have held nurses responsible for failing to take timely and responsive action, such as failing to communicate patient condition changes to the physician and failure to discover conditions not found by the physician.

Like medicine, nursing has developed a subspecialty structure, allowing nurses to develop greater expertise in more limited areas. This should result in increased status, income, and decision-making responsibility. Nursing specialties have, for the most part, been organized around medical subspecialties, but with a clearer differentiation between ambulatory and hospital-based practice. Subspecialty-trained, master's degree nurses in hospital practice are called clinical nurse specialists, whereas those in ambulatory settings are more often educationally prepared as nurse practitioners or nurse midwives (Kassirer, 1994; Maule, 1994). Their training differs reflecting different roles and responsibilities.

In an era of reduced hospital stays, nurses have become invaluable in the management of patients in their homes as in Case 25-5.

## CASE 25-6

*O.L. was a 79-year-old man admitted to the hospital because of intractable pain and decreased mobility resulting from a vertebral compression fracture. His physician pursued a diagnostic evaluation and ordered narcotics for the pain. He consulted a physical therapist for advice regarding pain management and mobilization. The physical therapist recommended that O.L. see an orthotist to be fitted with a thoracolumbar extension brace and she taught him to use a transcutaneous nerve stimulation unit. She also taught him to do specific bed exercises and provided him with a walker for trips to the bathroom.*

*In several days, although he was much more comfortable, O.L. felt that he would benefit by a short nursing-home stay before returning to his home to care for himself. The hospital social worker helped him make the necessary arrangements and discussed home care options in case he should need them once he returned home. He also mentioned to O.L. that an occupational therapist might be able to suggest some home modifications and adaptive equipment that might allow O.L. to return home more quickly.*

## ALLIED HEALTH PROFESSIONALS

The major allied health professions are listed in Table 25.4. During this century, the development of the allied health disciplines has been one of the most dramatic developments in the healthcare delivery system, reflecting both the increasing complexity of patient care and an increased emphasis on rehabilitative strategies.

The relationships among the various allied health professional associations, the American Medical Association, and the certifying and licensing bodies governing each discipline are complicated, at times strained, and subject to fairly frequent modifications. An additional complicating factor in recent years has

**Table 25.4**
Allied Health Professionals

| | | |
|---|---|---|
| Audiologists | Physical therapists | Recreational therapists |
| Dietitians | Radiologic technologists | Activities therapists |
| Laboratory professionals | CT/MRI technologists | Art therapists |
|   Cytotechnologists | Mammographers | Dance therapists |
|   Histological technicians | Nuclear medicine technologists | Music therapists |
|   Medical laboratory technicians | Radiation therapists | Play therapists |
|   Medical technologists | Ultrasonographers | Respiratory therapists |
| Occupational therapists and OT assistants | | Social workers |
| | | Speech pathologists and audiologists |

been the tension between the federal government (Medicare, Medicaid), state governments (Medicaid), and the private sector created by efforts to contain costs while assuring quality.

## Physical Therapists

Physical therapists are mobility experts. Through neuromusculoskeletal evaluation and the use of a variety of treatment modalities they help patients to maintain or improve their ability to move about. Physical therapists practice in a variety of settings, providing inpatient, outpatient, and community-based services. Unique settings include community health centers, public schools, private practices, athletic centers, and specialty medical clinics as well as hospital, rehabilitation centers, and nursing homes.

Opportunities for specialization following entry-level education are increasing. The American Physical Therapy Association (APTA)-sponsored American Board of Physical Therapy Specialties presently offers board certification in six specialty areas: pediatric physical therapy, orthopedic physical therapy, sports physical therapy, clinical electrophysiology physical therapy, cardiopulmonary physical therapy, and neurological physical therapy.

A physical therapy assessment may include determination of motion, strength, and endurance abilities of the patient; evaluation of balance, coordination, and postural (static and dynamic) abilities; establishment of quantitative and qualitative profiles of movement abilities; development of a profile of the cardiopulmonary abilities of the patient; and definition of electrophysiological responses to various electrical modalities. Therapeutic regimens consist of a wide range of interventions from the application of specific modalities, heat, ice, ultrasound, diathermy, and so on, to exercise, musculoskeletal rehabilitation, and the reeducation of various functions. Many physical therapists provide definitive treatments for wounds such as pressure sores and diabetic ulcers. In addition to treatment of physical impairments, physical therapists provide a wide range of consulting services in areas such as health promotion and fitness, prevention of athletic injuries, and prevention of work-related injuries and trauma.

## Occupational Therapists

Occupational therapists use selected educational, vocational, and rehabilitative activities to help individuals reach the highest functional levels possible, become self-reliant, and build a balanced lifestyle of work and leisure. In partnership with their clients, they frequently work with other members of the healthcare team and with community agencies not only to treat patients with disabilities but also attempt to prevent disabilities from occurring. Whereas physical therapists focus on mobility, strength, and endurance, occupational therapists address activities of daily living such as bathing, dressing, cooking, money management, use of the telephone, and driving (see Case 25-6). Recent randomized controlled trials have documented that occupational therapy provided to homebound elders can improve functional abilities and quality of life (Clark *et al.*, 1997; Walker *et al.*, 1999) and can reduce falls (Cummings *et al.*, 1999).

Occupational therapists work in hospitals, clinics, schools, rehabilitation centers, home care programs, private practice, community health centers, nursing homes, day-care centers, and psychiatric facilities. A registered occupational therapist (OTR) carries professional and administrative responsibilities for occupational therapy programs and services and is responsible for evaluating clients, deciding on program goals, working with clients to implement those goals, and evaluating progress. In addition, OTRs educate students entering the field and may be involved in research.

Certified occupational therapy assistants (COTA) work under the supervision of an OTR. They are high school graduates or the equivalent who complete an associate degree program in an accredited university or community college or a 1-year certificate program in an accredited educational institution. A minimum of 2 months of supervised field work is also included. Graduates are eligible for certification as a COTA on passage of a national certification examination.

# Recreational Therapists

Recreational therapists constitute a diverse group of professionals. Some areas of interest and expertise of recreational therapists are (1) self-esteem/confidence building, (2) independent living/self-reliance development, (3) self-expression/enrichment of life, (4) group acceptance/development of interpersonal skills, (5) hospital and play therapy/fear reduction, (6) art and music therapy/self-expression and fulfillment, and (7) physical activities/physical condition and stress reduction. They are employed in a variety of settings including hospitals, rehabilitation centers, nursing homes, mental health centers, community parks and recreation departments, schools, sheltered workshops, and correctional centers.

Recreational therapists must complete an approved associate's degree program. Certification is awarded by the National Council for Therapeutic Recreational Certification after satisfactory completion of a certifying exam. Licensure or registration is also required in many states, often through the state's Board of Medical Examiners.

# Respiratory Therapists

On successful completion of the registry exam of the National Board for Respiratory Therapy, respiratory therapists become registered respiratory therapists (RRT). Under the direction of a physician, respiratory therapists are responsible for the administration of therapeutic gases (e.g., oxygen, carbon dioxide–oxygen mixtures); aerosols and humidity, bronchodilators, corticosteroids, aerosolized water; assisted ventilation, respirators; positive airway pressure, and chest physical therapy to mobilize secretions and stimulate cough, breathing exercises, and the like. They perform blood gas sampling and pulmonary function testing, and they provide individualized patient education and follow-up.

# Speech–Language Pathologists and Audiologists

Speech–language pathologists and audiologists are health professionals who deal with the normal and developmental aspects of human communication, communication disorders, and clinical techniques for evaluation and management of these disorders. Their training involves a minimum of 300 hours of supervised clinical experience and a 9-month clinical fellowship in a variety of settings including hospitals, rehabilitation facilities, and public and private outpatient settings. They often work closely with otorhinolaryngologists, neurologists, psychiatrists, dentists, and plastic surgeons. Much of their work involves children with congenital and development disorders, and the elderly who have acquired disabilities such as deafness and aphasia.

Audiologists are concerned with diagnosis and remediation of hearing loss. Responsibilities include prescription and fitting of hearing amplification devices. They are accountable for provision of auditory, speech, and reading training. Speech and language pathologists diagnose and remediate speech disorders (e.g., problems of fluency, voice, and articulation) and language disorders (e.g., aphasia, reading disorders, and delayed language development). Many are also involved in the evaluation and treatment of eating and swallowing problems, augmentative communication devices, and alternate forms of communication such as sign language and esophageal speech.

# Clinical Dietitians

Nutritional status is a very important component of health and disease. The evaluation of current nutritional status, calculation of adjustments needed to achieve nutritional well-being, development and implementation of a plan to meet those goals, and education of the patient and other caregivers are all important and expected responsibilities of clinical dietitians.

Most accredited hospitals and rehabilitation facilities require that nutrition support be provided by a *registered* or *licensed* dietitian. These titles denote a level of expertise acquired through an American Dietetics Association (ADA)-regulated combination of didactic and clinical learning. Many facilities require ADA registration, which documents passage of a professional exam and monitored maintenance of continuing education hours in compliance with ADA regulations. Some states have also implemented a licensing procedure through state medical licensure boards, which protects the consumer from persons practicing under false credentials and guards against inappropriate practice behavior of its members. The initials R.D. or L.D. will appear with the person's signature if these higher levels of certification have been achieved. The term *nutritionist* has been used by many to imply professional expertise in the area of human nutrition. However, this title is not protected from misuse by persons with questionable educational background and sometimes inaccurate or unethical presentation of information to the consumer.

## CASE 25-7

*A.R. was an 8-year-old girl brought to the emergency room by her parents for evaluation of recurrent leg pains occurring at night, preventing her from sleeping. The episodes had been occurring occasionally for 4 months but more frequently for the past 2 weeks. Dr. Y. was working in the emergency room on the night that A.R. came in. The results of his examination of her were completely unremarkable. However, he ordered a complete blood count (CBC) with a differential count and an erythrocyte sedimentation rate (ESR) as a precaution. The machine-run CBC results showed normal parameters. The medical technologist who reviewed the differential white blood cell count detected several immature white blood cells. To further investigate the possibility of acute leukemia, a bone marrow biopsy was performed. After results of the special stains performed and review of the bone marrow aspirate by the pathologist, the diagnosis was confirmed. A.R. was expected to have a good prognosis because her disease was diagnosed at such an early stage.*

## Medical Technologists/Cytotechnologists

Laboratory professionals represent the single largest group of allied health professionals. This reflects the heavy reliance of modern patient care on analytical laboratory testing and procedures for diagnosis, treatment, and monitoring. There are several categories of laboratory professionals. Educational requirements differ based on scope of practice.

*Medical technologists* perform analytical testing, evaluate the validity of the results, and report the results to the physicians who requested the tests, as illustrated in Case 25-7. If there is a question regarding the clinical correlation of the results and the patient's condition, a clinical pathologist provides the consultation.

Medical technologists are able to work in any of the clinical laboratory specialties, i.e., blood bank, chemistry, toxicology, microbiology, and hematology. They are employed in hospital and independent laboratories as well as medical and industrial research laboratories. Some obtain specialty certifications after the medical technology certification. Many supervisors and managers hold master's degrees.

A *cytotechnologist* screens slides for the presence of cancer and other disease states. Any diagnosis of malignancy is confirmed by an anatomic pathologist. The largest portion of the work performed by a cytotechnologist is in the screening of Pap smears. Cytotechnologists also screen many nongynecological specimens such as bronchial washing and fine-needle aspirations of masses for the presence of cancer cells. Some take additional training and are employed in cytogenetics laboratories.

*Histological technicians* prepare tissue specimens for viewing by a pathologist. The histology laboratory has recently expanded its diagnostic capabilities via special types of stains, e.g., immunochemistry.

## Radiologic Technologists

Radiologic technologists can be subdivided into four major groups: radiographers, nuclear medicine technologists, radiation therapists, and diagnostic medical sonographers. Members of the first three groups, who are involved in the use of radiation of various types for either diagnostic or therapeutic purposes, are different in several other ways from diagnostic medical ultrasonographers, who are involved in the use of high-frequency sound waves. Diagnostic medical sonographers are credentialed by the American Registry of Medical Sonographers, whereas the others receive their credentialing through the American Registry of Radiologic Technologists.

*Radiographers* [R.T.(R)s] are responsible for obtaining radiographs (x-rays) as requested by a physician to be interpreted by a radiologist. This involves working closely with patients and with a variety of sophisticated equipment. They must know how to properly position the patient, set the proper radiation exposure levels, protect the patient from unnecessary radiation exposure, and determine whether adequate images have been obtained. With the development of computed tomography, magnetic resonance imaging, and mammography, special training and certification are now required to operate these instruments.

*Nuclear medical technologists* [R.T.(N)s] administer radiopharmaceuticals to patients and operate a variety of scanning instruments that produce radiographic images of various parts of the body for diagnostic purposes. Brain, bone, liver, and thyroid scans as well as dynamic cardiac and pulmonary scans are examples of the tests they routinely perform.

*Radiation therapists* are involved in the administration of ionizing radiation primarily to cancer patients for therapeutic purposes. Because of the nature of cancer, and since treatments are generally given repetitively over a period of time, radiation therapy technologists often develop close relationships with patients and their families and are therefore called on to function as members of interdisciplinary teams.

Although most radiologic technologists work in hospital settings or in large clinics, *diagnostic medical ultrasonographers* work in a variety of settings. Cardiologists, obstetricians and gynecologists, and occasionally general surgeons and primary care physicians may employ ultrasonographers to assist them in the evaluation of common problems such as valvular heart disease and congestive heart failure, pelvic masses, pregnancy dating, gallstones, and peripheral vascular diseases.

# Pharmacists

Pharmacy is the third largest health profession after nurses and physicians. Almost 90% of active pharmacists are practicing in clinical settings. Another 10% are involved in the development, production, or distribution of medications, teaching, research, legal and regulatory activities regarding pharmaceutical practice, public health activities, association work, and journalism. The clinical work of pharmacists includes community pharmacy, hospital pharmacy, drug information centers, poison control centers, and supervision of dispensing practices in long-term care facilities such as nursing homes. An increasing number of residencies and fellowships are available for academic and clinical pharmacists in specialized areas such as psychiatry, geriatrics, internal medicine, pediatrics, pharmacokinetics, family medicine, and others.

Pharmacists are involved in many clinical activities: verification of prescriptions for accuracy, legality, and physical and chemical compatibility; advice to patients and other healthcare providers regarding proper administration, potential side effects, and potential drug–drug and drug–nutrient interactions of prescription drugs; advice to patients and other healthcare providers regarding proper use and choice of OTC medications; advice to patients regarding personal health habits, smoking, drug abuse, and so on; referral of patients to other health professionals; instruction of patients and other healthcare providers regarding proper use of medical or surgical appliances, inhalers, colostomy bags, splints, and bandages; participation in mass screening programs, stool occult blood testing, hypertension screening, and the like; and participation in utilization review, medical audits, and other medical care evaluations in hospitals, nursing homes, and so on. Other services of a more innovative and advanced nature include pharmacokinetic and nutrition consultations and primary care of patients with special emphasis on hypertension, diabetes mellitus, and hyperlipidemia. Advanced trained pharmacists are also now able to conduct drug research with human subjects provided that a physician is part of the study team (Schultz & Brushwood, 1991).

Pharmacists may be the nation's most accessible healthcare professionals. However, in retail community pharmacy practice, an important factor that limits the ability of pharmacists to provide good care is their lack of access to complete patient-related information. Pharmacists, more than any other healthcare professionals, are often relatively isolated from other professionals. Patients would benefit greatly from improved communication between physicians and pharmacists.

## Optometrists

Optometrists evaluate, diagnose, and manage a variety of pathological ocular conditions. Binocular and refractive conditions, along with accommodative and convergence relationships that can influence reading, learning, and other visual tasks, are major professional concerns. As is the case with other primary healthcare professions, the scope of optometric practice is governed by individual state laws. Optometrists may prescribe topical diagnostic pharmaceuticals throughout the nation and may administer a wider selection of therapeutic agents in half the states.

Optometric training leading to the O.D. (doctor of optometry) degree requires 4 years in an accredited school or college of optometry. Preadmission and undergraduate optometric requirements are parallel to those of other major health professions and include basic science courses such as biology, physics, advanced mathematics, organic chemistry, and microbiology. Postdoctoral residency programs are widely available. To obtain licensure, the optometric graduate must pass a board exam administered by the state in which he or she would practice.

Demarcations are sometimes indistinct between the professional roles of optometry and ophthalmology. Matters of serious ocular pathology and surgical intervention clearly require the expertise of an ophthalmologist, as well as systemic therapy, as might be suitable to remedy ocular pathologies and related disorders at a secondary or tertiary level of referral. Otherwise, in primary ophthalmic healthcare, the clinical activities of the two professions are very similar. Optometrists are employed as members of HMOs, in group practices, as industrial and sports vision consultants, in research capacities by ophthalmic companies, and in academic institutions.

## Social Workers

Social work practice focuses on the relationship between individuals and their environment and is directed toward defining and resolving problems that develop in this relationship. Social workers are therefore trained to evaluate the psychosocial aspects of an individual's situation. They are often able to provide supportive counseling to individuals and families and act as their advocates in situations where environmental changes would be helpful, as in Case 25-5. They are especially well trained to locate community resources that may enhance the quality of life of an individual or family. A majority of practicing social workers have a master's degree (M.S.W.). Social workers who have received special training in mental healthcare such as individual or family therapy are called *psychiatric social workers*.

The specific activities of a social worker depend somewhat on the occupational setting in which the social worker practices and the amount and type of training she or he has received. Common practice settings include medical and psychiatric hospitals and clinics, schools, nursing homes, special shelters, government agencies, the workplace, family service agencies, churches, and private practice. Social workers often function as case managers in settings in which interdisciplinary teamwork is practiced.

## Podiatrists

Podiatrists are clinicians trained to manage health-related conditions of the feet and ankles. Their 4-year training program, often supplemented with one or more years of residency, prepares them to utilize all of the same diagnostic and treatment approaches employed by allopathic and osteopathic physicians including the prescription of medications and various kinds of adaptive equipment (e.g., special footwear, orthotic devices, casts and splints), and performance of surgery. Many have hospital and operating room privileges.

Most work out of private offices while others are employed by various healthcare facilities. Certification as a doctor of podiatric medicine (D.P.M.) requires a case study preparation and final exam by the American Board of Foot Surgery and successful completion of the National Board Examination. All states require state licensure as well.

# Mental Health Professionals

The emergence of new theoretical perspectives on mental health, an accumulating empirical data base, demonstrations of effective and generalizable clinical procedures and programs, and broader social acceptance of mental health concerns have all contributed to the growth of the mental health professions (Richardson, 1988). The development of the biopsychosocial (Engel, 1977) and multisystem (Tapp & Warner, 1985) theories of health and illness along with theories of stress and coping (Lazarus, 1966; Selye, 1976) have blurred the distinctions between physical and mental health and resulted in the development of the fields of behavioral medicine (Schwartz & Weiss, 1978) and health psychology (Millon *et al.*, 1982). These developments have resulted in a diverse array of distinct yet overlapping mental health professions including psychiatry, psychology, counseling, marital and family therapy, social work, and psychiatric nursing.

## Psychiatry

Psychiatrists are physicians who specialize by completing a 3-year psychiatric residency during which they receive training and experience in the diagnosis and treatment of major mental illness. They may further subspecialize in order to work primarily with adults, children, or other identified groups.

Most contemporary U.S. psychiatrists have a strong biological orientation and are highly trained in the diagnosis and pharmacological treatment of major mental illness. Depending on training and interest, psychiatrists may also be skilled in psychotherapy and other forms of psychosocial treatment. As physicians, psychiatrists are licensed to practice medicine by each state and, after completion of an approved residency and comprehensive exam, are certified by the American Board of Psychiatry.

## Psychology

Psychologists are doctoral-level behavioral scientists, typically holding doctor of philosophy (Ph.D.), doctor of psychology (Psy.D.), or doctor of education (Ed.D.) degrees. The American Psychological Association recognizes four professional specialties within psychology: clinical psychology, counseling psychology, school psychology, and industrial-organizational psychology (American Psychological Association, 1981). Three additional professional specialty areas are emerging: neuropsychology, health psychology, and forensic psychology. Diplomate status granted by the American Board of Professional Psychology requires at least 4 years of postdoctoral experience in the specialty area, a written exam, and direct peer review of clinical skills. Professional psychologists are licensed for independent practice by all states.

*Clinical and counseling psychology* have evolved out of different historical contexts (Tipton, 1983; Whitley, 1984). Clinical psychology has traditionally had a greater emphasis on the diagnosis and treatment of children, severe psychopathology in all ages, and services delivered in inpatient mental health settings, whereas counseling psychology has had a greater focus on assessment and treatment in rehabilitation settings, vocational, educational, and family counseling agencies, and with persons experiencing adjustment problems and other less severe forms of psychopathology. Despite these differences, it has been estimated that these two specialties have 80–90% overlap in training skills, work settings, and professional roles (Watkins *et al.*, 1986). Clinical and counseling psychologists are employed in many settings, including private practice, medical schools, hospitals, universities, mental health centers, other human service agencies, and research foundations. Their training includes basic and clinical coursework, a doctoral dissertation, and a 1-year clinical internship.

*School psychologists* specialize in the learning and mental health needs of children in educational settings. They are usually employed in school systems or academic research institutions. *Industrial-*

*organizational psychologists* specialize in the study and design of organizational settings with regard to human performance and interpersonal relationships and are usually employed by large corporations and public institutions or in academic research settings. *Neuropsychologists* are typically clinical or counseling psychologists who complete special pre- and postdoctoral training in neuropsychology. Neuropsychologists conduct neuropsychological evaluations and contribute to diagnosis and treatment planning of patients with a variety of neurological injuries and rehabilitation concerns. They are typically employed in medical and rehabilitation settings but may also work with school systems and in academic research capacities. *Health psychologists* are also trained as clinical or counseling psychologists but specialize through pre- and postdoctoral work in preventive health and the psychological needs of general medical and surgical patients. Health psychologists work in a variety of hospital and medical settings. *Forensic psychologists* are clinical or counseling psychologists who further specialize in forensic issues and typically work in penal, law enforcement, or psychiatric hospital settings. Individuals trained at the master's level in psychology may be identified as psychological assistants or associates and are licensed by many states to provide limited psychological services under the supervision of a licensed doctoral-level psychologist.

## Other Mental Health Professions

*Counselor*, *therapist*, and *family therapist* are generic terms and have only recently begun to be defined and licensed by states. Typically a *counselor* or family therapist has a master's degree in counseling or family therapy from an accredited college or university and has received a minimum of 6 months to 1 year of supervised clinical experience on at least a half-time basis. A limited number of practicing counselors and family therapists hold doctoral degrees.

Counselors are usually affiliated with the American Association of Counseling and Development. They may specialize through graduate study and work experience in a variety of areas such as mental health counseling, counseling of children, marriage and family counseling, school counseling, or rehabilitation counseling. Counselors who work with persons experiencing mental health problems should be further certified by the National Academy of Certified Clinical Mental Health Counselors. Certified Clinical Mental Health Counselors are licensed for independent practice in 28 states (Weikel & Palmo, 1989).

*Family therapists* are usually affiliated with and should be certified by the American Association of Marriage and Family Therapy (Nichols, 1984). Often counselors and family therapists belong to both organizations but may prefer to refer to their work as either counseling or family therapy. Counselors and family therapists are employed in a variety of settings including mental health centers, guidance and counseling agencies, schools, and increasingly in private practice.

As previously discussed, social workers are also major providers of mental health services. Social workers often have unique skills and training qualifying them for roles as case managers within mental health organizations (Richardson, 1988). They may also be trained as psychotherapists or counselors. Psychiatric nurses are also important providers of mental health services. Nursing training is heterogeneous, and as a result there are multiple levels of training that may qualify a nurse to provide psychiatric services. The term *psychiatric clinical nurse specialist* has been suggested as designating an R.N. with a master's degree in psychiatric services. Such qualified nursing personnel may play an increasing role in the delivery and coordination of mental health services, especially in hospital settings (Richardson, 1988).

# Pastoral Care

Ministers with additional training in either pastoral counseling or pastoral care also provide counseling services. *Pastoral counselors* are individuals who usually have an M.Div. (master of divinity) degree and have completed an additional 3–5 years of residency training in pastoral counseling. Some go on to obtain a D.Min. (doctor of ministry) degree as well. They typically work in outpatient counseling centers, clinics, and through churches, and provide both psychological and spiritual counseling services. They are credentialed by the American Association of Pastoral Counselors.

## MENTAL HEALTH:
## A REPORT OF THE SURGEON GENERAL (1999)

*1. Mental health is fundamental to overall health. Mental disorders are real health conditions that have an immense impact on individuals and families.*

*2. The efficacy of mental health treatments is well documented. A range of treatment exists for most mental disorders. Two broad types of intervention include psychosocial treatments, e.g. psychotherapy or counseling, and psychopharmacologic treatments; these often are most effective when combined.*

*3. About 10% of the U.S. adult population use mental health services in the health sector in any year, with another 5% seeking such services from social service agencies, schools, or religious or self-help groups. Yet critical gaps exist between those who need service and those who receive service. Gaps also exist between optimally effective treatments and what many individuals receive in actual practice settings.*

Hospital chaplains who provide pastoral care receive from 1 to 2 years of residency training after their 3-year M.Div. degree program. They are trained to provide pastoral care to people in crisis, and work primarily in institutional settings such as hospitals, mental health facilities, or hospices. The training is provided by the Association for Clinical Pastoral Education (ACPE), the College of Pastoral Supervision and Psychotherapy (CPSP), and/or the National Association of Catholic Chaplains (NACC). Certification for Chaplaincy is by the College of Chaplains or the NACC. Many chaplains go on to obtain their D.Min. degree.

## CASE 25-8

*Frances Tuttle was a 57-year-old stenographer who had for the last year been experiencing migratory muscle and joint pains. She had seen several allopathic physicians who had diagnosed a nonspecific inflammatory condition and prescribed various nonsteroidal anti-inflammatory medications all of which upset her stomach and caused her blood pressure to go up and her ankles to swell. On the advice of a church friend, she decided to see a naturopath. She was pleased that he did not prescribe any medications other than some vitamins and herbs, and that after his treatments, which included dietary changes and regular exercise, she actually began to feel a great deal better.*

## NONTRADITIONAL HEALTHCARE PRACTICES

In addition to the methods employed by the traditional healthcare disciplines, a variety of alternative approaches to health maximization, maintenance, and restoration exist, some of which are listed in Table 25.2. These alternatives to traditional healthcare are becoming increasingly popular in the United States, particularly in the last decade. Many of these practices are based on entirely different conceptual models of health and illness, and most have not been subjected to the same level of scientific scrutiny as the conventional methods. It should be acknowledged, however, that the effectiveness of many conventional practices has not been clearly established either. While these approaches are considered to be "nontraditional, alternative, or unconventional" in the United States, up to 70% of the world's population rely on nonallopathic systems of healing (Krippner, 1995).

Interest in alternative forms of healthcare has been growing rapidly in the United States primarily among upper-middle-class, well-educated, non-African-American people. In a population survey reported by Druss (1999), 8.3% of respondents reported using at least one unconventional therapy in the past year, of whom 80%

## WHO USES ALTERNATIVE MODALITIES? CONDUCT YOUR OWN SURVEY

*Ask 10 neighbors, friends, relatives, or classmates if they have ever:*

- *Visited a chiropractor, osteopath, homeopath, or naturopath*
- *Visited a* curandero, *Chinese healer, Ayurvedic healer, or other traditional or Asian healer*
- *Visited a sweat lodge*
- *Visited a massage therapist, rolfer, or reflexologist*
- *Been treated with acupuncture, biofeedback, magnets, herbal medicines, dietary supplements, chelation, or aromatherapy*
- *Tried meditation, imagery, or other relaxation technique*
- *Tried tai chi or yoga*
- *Prayed for healing*
- *Attended a support group for a particular illness or disorder*

*Based on this sample, what would you say about the prevalence of "alternative" medicine? Do you consider these modalities alternative, complementary, or mainstream?*

also sought help from a medical doctor. In fact, dissatisfaction with traditional medical care was not predictive of use of alternative approaches in another survey (Astin, 1998). However, many patients who use unconventional methods do not inform their medical doctors that they are doing so. This may be because physicians have been particularly critical of many of these practices or are unable to answer patients' questions about them. Other studies suggest that from 10 to 50% of cancer patients and more than 50% of Alzheimer's victims use some form of alternative therapy (Burstein *et al.*, 1999; Coleman *et al.*, 1995; McGinnis, 1991). Interestingly, the American Medical Association revised its code of ethics in 1980, giving physicians permission to consult with, take referrals from, and make referrals to practitioners "without orthodox medical training" (Krippner, 1995). Recently an Office of Alternative Medicine has been established at the National Institutes of Health to direct research involving nontraditional therapies. Alternative forms of medical treatment can be loosely divided into the following categories: alternative medical systems, bodywork, mind/body treatment approaches, and dietary supplements.

## Alternative Medical Systems

These are comprehensive therapeutic approaches based on conceptualizations of health and disease that differ from those of Western biomedicine. The most popular examples in the United States are chiropractic, traditional Chinese medicine, Ayurveda, naturopathy, homeopathy, and chelation.

### Chiropractic

Doctors of chiropractic (DCs) could be considered either traditional or nontraditional healthcare providers depending on the definitions one chooses. Licensed in all 50 states, they are approved for reimbursement under Medicare, Medicaid, and the Vocational Rehabilitation program. They are authorized providers under Workers' Compensation statutes. The U.S. Public Health Services classifies doctors of chiropractic among "medical specialists and practitioners," includes them in its *Health Manpower Sourcebook*, and includes a chapter on chiropractics in its *Health Resources Statistics*. However, it is still relatively uncommon for chiropractors to work collaboratively with the other traditional healthcare professionals, and while chiropractic physicians regard themselves as primary healthcare providers, they are rarely mentioned in federal and state policymaking discussions regarding primary care manpower. And while the fundamental principles on which chiropractic is based are compatible with the traditional Western biomedical paradigm, the theories derived from those principles and their application have not been particularly well accepted by physicians including osteopaths.

Chiropractic, from the Greek words *cheir* and *praktikos* meaning "done by hand," is based on the beliefs that disease processes may be caused or exacerbated by disturbances of the nervous system and that disturbances of the nervous system are often the result of derangements of the musculoskeletal system. In particular, subluxations of vertebrae in the back or neck are thought to commonly impinge on nerve roots resulting in alterations of function in the tissues innervated by those nerves. After a diagnostic evaluation that commonly includes a history, physical examination, and x-rays, chiropractors utilize spinal and apendicular adjustment and manipulation, physical modalities, traction, diathermy, ultrasound, massage, heat, cold, and so on, nutritional counseling, and adaptive and supportive equipment to maintain or restore the structural and biomechanical integrity in order to prevent or ameliorate a variety of health problems. While the vast majority of patient encounters involve treatment of "neuromusculoskeletal conditions," nearly 15% involve the treatment of conditions involving other organ systems thought to have been caused or exacerbated by neuromusculoskeletal imbalances (*Chiropractic: State of the Art, 1994–1995*). It is their treatment of these latter conditions that most disturbs physicians. Concerns have also been expressed regarding whether chiropractors are qualified to obtain and interpret radiographs and to provide nutritional and psychological counseling.

A number of randomized controlled trials have demonstrated that spinal manipulation can result in more rapid resolution of acute neck and lower back pain and is associated with less analgesic use than traditional medical management. There is also some reasonably good evidence to support its effectiveness for headache, including migraine, and possibly dysmenorrhea, but little evidence that it has any effect on any other health problems (Vickers & Zollman, 1999).

To obtain a doctor of chiropractic degree, one must have a minimum of 2 years of college including certain prerequisite science courses, and then complete 4 years at a chiropractic college. The chiropractic curriculum includes many of the same basic science courses taken by medical students—human anatomy, biochemistry, physiology, human behavior—as well as a variety of clinical rotations. State chiropractic examining boards generally require graduation from an accredited chiropractic college and successful completion of a certifying examination.

## Traditional Chinese Medicine

Traditional Chinese medicine has probably been practiced for more than 23 centuries in the Orient. It is a comprehensive form of healthcare that views the human body as an ecosystem and employs a language based on metaphors from nature. Health is considered "the ability of the organism to respond appropriately to a wide variety of challenges while maintaining equilibrium, integrity, and coherence" (Beinfield & Korngold, 1995). The human body is believed to be the result of the fusion of shen (psyche) and essence (soma), and to be made up of qi (*chee*, energy), moisture (body fluids), and blood (tissue). Disease is thought to result when there has been depletion or congestion of these substances. Qi is believed to flow along distinct paths called *meridians* which can be evaluated and manipulated. Therapeutic modalities include acupuncture, herbal medicine, exercise, and massage (including energy techniques).

### CASE 25-9

*Olive Andrews, a 38-year-old woman with chronic shoulder pain resistant to oral medications, physical therapy, and local corticosteroid injections, decided to try acupuncture therapy. The practitioner, a physician trained in traditional Oriental medicine and acupuncture in Japan and subsequently in chiropractic medicine in this country, used physical clues (palpation of wrist pulses) and electronic equipment designed to detect energy generation from the skin to determine where to place eight acupuncture needles that he then attached to a source of electrical current. Mrs. Andrews received three 30-minute treatments per week for 5 weeks. Following the course of treatment she reported nearly complete resolution of her shoulder pain and full mobility.*

## Acupuncture

Acupuncture is a form of treatment that has been practiced in the Orient for at least 4000 years. It is an attempt to affect the quality and mobility of the life force, Qi Chee, which, it is believed, flows in channels or meridians within each of us and is the primary determinant of health and illness. Very fine needles, usually 8–10, are inserted just beneath the surface of the skin in specific locations dictated by the specific problem being treated. These needles are then manipulated manually, or attached to a source of electrical current. Occasionally the needles are heated with a burning herb stick or cone called *moxa*. For treatment of chronic conditions, a minimum of 10 treatments is usually required as in Case 25-9.

A 1997 National Institutes of Health consensus conference on acupuncture concluded that

> ... promising results have emerged, for example, showing efficacy of acupuncture in adult postoperative and chemotherapy nausea and vomiting and postoperative dental pain. There are other situations such as addiction, stroke rehabilitation, headache, menstrual cramps, tennis elbow, fibromyalgia, myofascial pain, osteoarthritis, low back pain, carpal tunnel syndrome, and asthma in which acupuncture may be useful as an adjunct treatment or an acceptable alternative or be included in a comprehensive management program. Further research is likely to uncover other areas where acupuncture interventions will be useful. (p. 2)

Practitioners of acupuncture can receive their training in an Asian medical school or in one of more than two dozen 3- to 4-year training programs that have been started in the United States and in other parts of the world since 1970 when James Reston, a *New York Times* columnist on assignment in China, underwent an appendectomy with acupuncture needles as the only anesthetic and focused attention on this form of treatment. In the United States, practitioners of acupuncture are often chiropractic, osteopathic, or allopathic physicians, or veterinarians who have received additional training in this method. Length of study varies considerably. Licensure is also quite variable between states, but frequently involves passing both written and skills tests.

## Chinese Herbal Medicine

In traditional Chinese medicine, herbs are generally directed to specific body parts rather than to movement of qi. There are five categories of Chinese herbal remedies: pungent, sour, sweet, bitter, and salty. The flavors are thought to correspond to specific therapeutic effects that are the result of the "energetic" properties of the herbs. These substances, which may actually come from plant, mineral, or animal extracts, are used in complex formulations for specific conditions. In a recent randomized placebo controlled trial, a standard formulation of Chinese herbs was shown to be effective for relief of the symptoms of irritable bowel syndrome (Bensoussan *et al.*, 1998).

In other published clinical trials, various Chinese herbal preparations have shown efficacy for the treatment of a broad spectrum of medical conditions including herpes zoster, retinal vein occlusion, diabetic nephropathy, chronic hepatitis C, bronchiolitis, nonulcer dyspepsia, atopic eczema, and hyperlipidemia.

## Ayurveda

Ayurvedic medicine is a 5000-year-old healing method that originated in India. Literally translated, Ayurveda means *life science*, *life knowledge*, or *longevity knowledge*. Its practitioners believe that optimal health requires a balance both within and between the external and internal environments. Individual human beings are viewed as smaller units of the whole/universe inseparable from the earth that sustains us. Illnesses are believed to be the result of imbalances and disharmonies which can often be eliminated by some combination of dietary changes, daily or seasonal routines, herbal and nutritional therapies, a 2-week rejuvenation program and/or a detoxification program (panchakarma), breathing exercises (e.g., alternate nostril breathing), and specific physical exercises (e.g., yoga). Ayurvedic medicine is typically embraced by those who perceive physical and spiritual health to be inextricably linked.

## Naturopathic Medicine

Naturopathy as a distinct healthcare profession began in the United States about 100 years ago. Its founders, Dr. Benedict Lust and Robert Foster, were concerned that conventional medical practice had become reductionistic and overly reliant on drugs and surgery. They advocated the use of "natural healing methods" designed to assist the body's own healing processes. Modern naturopathy is based on six fundamental principles: the healing power of nature; identification and treatment of the cause of the problem, not just its symptoms; first, do no harm; treat the whole person; the physician as teacher; and prevention. Naturopaths are primary healthcare practitioners whose therapeutic armamentarium includes clinical nutrition, physical modalities, homeopathic strategies, botanical medicine, natural childbirth, traditional Oriental medicine techniques, counseling, and minor surgery as illustrated by Case 25-9.

Naturopathy enjoyed great success during the first quarter of this century but experienced a decline in the 1940s and 1950s. There is now only one college of naturopathic medicine in the United States. Located in Portland, Oregon, its curriculum includes courses in the traditional basic and clinical sciences as well as the areas mentioned above. A 4-year course of study leads to the doctor of naturopathic medicine (N.D.) degree. Licensure is currently required in six states. Scope of practice is specifically defined in the practice acts in the various states that license or regulate naturopathic medicine.

## CASE 25-10

*Frances Gordon was 28 years old and pregnant with her second child. She had had tremendous problems with nausea and vomiting with her first pregnancy and now at 12 weeks gestation was beginning to experience similar problems with her second pregnancy. Remembering the fear that she experienced when taking physician-prescribed medications during her first pregnancy, she decided to consult a homeopath for advice. She was given instructions to take homeopathic doses of ipecac which she was assured would not harm the baby. She found that the treatment seemed to help.*

## Homeopathy

Homeopathy is a healthcare practice based upon the principle that "like treats like." Its practitioners and advocates believe that symptoms are the body's attempt to heal itself, and that they therefore should not be suppressed, but rather promoted. To accomplish this, homeopathic physicians prescribe extremely diluted solutions of substances that in larger amounts would cause the same symptoms as the problem being treated. Their prescription is based on both the type of problem and the patient's reaction to it, that is, the patient's personality style.

In Case 25-10, for example, ipecac when given in pharmacologic doses *causes* nausea and vomiting, but in minute doses it is used by homeopaths to relieve it. Ipecac was chosen for Ms. Gordon because of the pattern, severity of the nausea, and certain characteristics of her personality (Ullman, 1988). Most homeopathic remedies can be purchased without prescription in health-food stores or in a rapidly increasing number of pharmacies. Self-care has been facilitated by the increased availability in pharmacies of homeopathic mixtures containing several of the substances commonly prescribed for particular problems (Debrovner, 1993).

The principles of homeopathy were developed in the early 1800s by Samuel Hahnemann, a German physician and pharmacist. By 1900 there were 22 homeopathic medical schools in the United States alone.

However, with the discovery of antibiotics and other advances in allopathic medicine, the practice fell out of favor in the 1940s (National Center for Homeopathy, 1995). In the last 5–10 years, homeopathy seems once again to be gaining in popularity. The number of pharmacies selling homeopathic products in the United States has increased tenfold in the last 5 years, and the popularity of homeopathy has far outgrown the number of homeopathic practitioners. Patients must largely depend on their own knowledge or the advice of pharmacists and health-food store owners. Many homeopathy "study groups" have been formed, and the National Center for Homeopathy offers short courses for laypeople.

Since 1995, a number of randomized controlled trials comparing homeopathic remedies with placebo or conventional therapies have been conducted, primarily in England and Germany. Homeopathic approaches may be as effective as conventional therapies for a few conditions including allergic rhinitis (Weiser *et al.*, 1999) and vertigo (Weiser *et al.*, 1998), and may have some immunomodulatory effects (Melchart *et al.*, 1995; Rastogi *et al.*, 1999). However, no significant effects were seen in patients with migraine (Whitmarsh *et al.*, 1997), tinnitus (Simpson *et al.*, 1998), warts (Kainz *et al.*, 1996; Smolle *et al.*, 1998), pain following surgery (Hart *et al.*, 1997; Lokken *et al.*, 1995), or pain following exercise (Vickers *et al.*, 1997, 1998).

Individual states regulate the practice of homeopathy. Usually it can be practiced legally by licensed medical practitioners including allopathic physicians, osteopathic physicians, dentists, and veterinarians. In some states, chiropractors and naturopaths may be licensed to prescribe homeopathic remedies. The National Center for Homeopathy lists approximately 800 practitioners throughout the United States. A majority of these have become educated through participation in multiple short courses and workshops and through self-directed reading. There is no certification examination.

# Bodywork

"Bodywork" techniques include rolfing, massage, postural therapies, and therapeutic touch.

---

## CASE 25-11

*Andy Raddisan was a 63-year-old businessman who, when not at work, enjoyed a variety of outdoor activities including jogging and cross-country skiing. However, over a 3- to 5-year period, he developed discomfort and stiffness in his right hip such that it became increasingly difficult to raise his leg to put on his pants. He also had to change his jogging stride to accommodate the impairment, and his ability to ski became more and more limited because of pain. He saw his family physician who prescribed a nonsteroidal anti-inflammatory medication for suspected osteoarthritis. He also referred him to a physical therapist who taught him to follow exercise with appropriate periods of rest, and prescribed joint protection strategies and mobilization exercises. He followed this advice but did not see much improvement. A business associate suggested that he see his rolfer.*

## Rolfing

Rolfing is a system for maximizing human physical structure and function using connective tissue manipulations. The method, developed by Dr. Ida Rolf during the first half of this century, involves the use of the practitioner's hands, knuckles, and elbows to stretch the connective tissues surrounding muscles and joints in an attempt to improve alignment and mobility. The theory is that therapies delivered to purely somatic structures can affect the structure and functions of internal organs (Nansel & Szlazak, 1995). Unlike massage, the manipulations involve static pressure applied to specific structures for periods of time. There tends to be some discomfort involved. Rolfers believe that stress-related chemicals may become trapped within contracted segments of muscle, and that when they are released through rolfing these chemicals enter the circulatory system, sometimes triggering emotional reactions including memories of past traumas. Therefore, rolfers must be prepared to provide supportive counseling.

# ROLFING

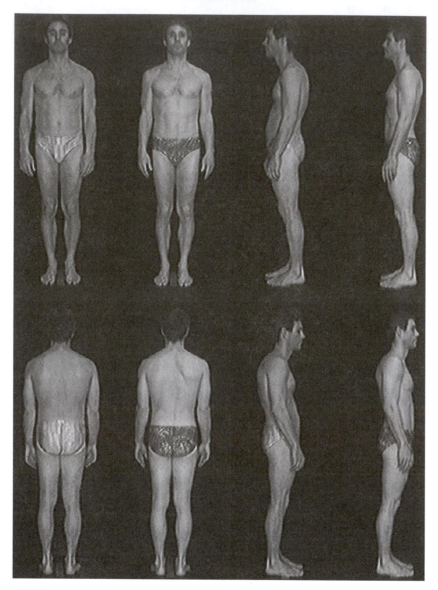

*Rolfing structural integration realigns a person's body and posture. The client is shown after the first and tenth Rolfing sessions. (Source: The Rolf Institute)*

A fundamental assumption of rolfing is that connective tissue disturbances in one part of the body cause compensatory disturbances in other areas. Therefore, a whole-body approach to treatment is necessary. A whole-body realignment is called the *ten series* because it generally requires ten 1-hour sessions to complete. However, depending on the client's needs, a rolfer may choose to use a more focused approach.

There are at least four rolfing institutes in the world that have trained about 800 rolfers. To qualify for admission to one of these institutes one must complete prerequisite courses in anatomy, physiology, kinesiology, and psychology; write a prescribed research paper; and undergo a series of rolfing treatments. Once admitted to an institute, one must complete required course and clinical work that can take from 1½ to 5 years. On graduation, certification is awarded. There are no licensure requirements at this time. A high percentage of rolfers have advanced degrees in another health science, e.g., M.D., R.N., M.S.W.

*Mr. Raddisan saw the rolfer and informed him that he had had a complicated appendectomy many years earlier with perforation and subsequent intra-abdominal adhesion formation. He underwent 20 weekly 1-hour treatments involving the ten series plus efforts focused at stretching and mobilizing contracted and adhered connective tissue in and about the abdomen and right hip. By the end of this series of treatments he had 95% normal painless range of motion in the right hip, was able to jog normally, and had gone cross-country skiing with minimal discomfort. He agreed to monthly maintenance treatments for 6 months followed by less frequent treatments for an undetermined period of time. Mr. Raddisan's health insurance company did not reimburse him for the cost of the sessions.*

## Therapeutic Massage

Massage as a therapeutic modality is practiced by a wide variety of health professionals, both traditional and nontraditional. Its roots go back to the dawn of history. There are four basic types of therapeutic massage with many variations within types: Oriental, athletic, energy, and psychotherapeutic. The major differences between modalities are the intent of the therapist, the amount of pressure used, and the speed of application. All types of massage are noninvasive, nonpainful, and palliative, not curative. The mechanisms of action may include relaxation, stress reduction, mobilization of extracellular fluid, and muscle relaxation (Field, 1998).

Certification as a massage therapist can require anywhere from 20 to 3000 hours, but it usually requires about 500 hours of training. There is no national standard. Currently 17 states have licensure requirements and many cities have ordinances to control prostitution which has been associated with so-called "massage parlors."

## Reflexology

Reflexology involves the manipulation of the hands and feet in an effort to influence the function of other parts of the body. The theory is that there are "reflex areas" on the feet and hands that correspond to every other organ and tissue in the body and that the application of a specific kind of pressure to those areas can positively influence the physiology of those organs and tissues. In some ways this conceptualization resembles the theory underlying acupuncture. This technique, which has been practiced in Europe for several decades, has been used medically primarily in postoperative settings to enhance the rate of recovery. There is, however, little research evidence at this point to support this practice.

# Mind–Body Treatment Approaches

A variety of treatment approaches involve the connection between mental processes and physical disturbances. Some of these include imagery, hypnosis, biofeedback, meditation, and a variety of relaxed techniques.

## Hypnosis

In the eighteenth century, Frantz Anton Mesmer (mesmerize) first used hypnosis to treat a variety of psychological disorders. However, the technique probably dates back at least as far as ancient Greece (*hypnos*, meaning sleep). Today this therapeutic strategy is used to ameliorate a variety of health problems.

Hypnosis is a form of focused concentration. It involves an absorption in the words and/or visualizations described by the therapist, dissociation from internal, rational criticism, and responsiveness to suggestions that are in accordance with their own wishes. The salubrious effects of hypnosis include muscle relaxation, reduced sympathetic nervous system activity, and pain modulation. Dentists and obstetricians have used hypnosis effectively for procedures, labor, and delivery associated with pain and anxiety. It has been promoted for the treatment of obesity and cigarette educational though the evidence to support its effectiveness for these challenging problems is fairly weak (Allison & Faith, 1996). Patients can learn self-hypnosis that can be helpful as a means of stress/anxiety relief.

## Meditation

Meditation is a mental state different from hypnosis in which the mind is empty of extraneous thoughts of past and future and is completely focused on the present. At one level this may involve a clear and intense awareness of present sensations and mood or, at a deeper level, of the inner workings of the mind. In some ways it is the opposite of hypnosis in that hypnosis is an attempt to hide or escape from feelings (e.g., cravings for food or cigarettes) while meditation is an attempt to fully appreciate the origins of those feelings. Like any other mind–body technique, meditation requires a great deal of training and practice. Many variations of meditation exist within the various religious traditions, but it is particularly emphasized in Zen and Tibetan Buddhism. The technique most often used in Western medical settings is transcendental meditation which has been used in the management of pain, anxiety, depression, and addictions to alcohol and cigarettes. There is randomized controlled trial evidence of its effectiveness as an adjunct in the management of psoriasis (Kabat-Zinn *et al.*, 1998), hypertension (Schneider, 1995; Wenneberg *et al.*, 1997), and fibromyalgia (Kaplan *et al.*, 1993). It was also shown to reduce anxiety and psychological distress and increase the empathy scores of medical students (Shapiro *et al.*, 1998).

## Biofeedback

Biofeedback includes any technique that provides continuous feedback regarding the effects of purposeful actions. As such, it is an effective method for learning such things as relaxation or contraction of specific muscle groups and even control over autonomic functions such as pulse rate and blood pressure. Randomized controlled trials have demonstrated the effectiveness of biofeedback techniques in the treatment of fecal and urinary incontinence (Fynes *et al.*, 1999; McDowell *et al.*, 1999), constipation, (Cox *et al.*, 1998; Heymen *et al.*, 1999), headache (Kroner-Herwig *et al.*, 1998), fibromyalgia (Buckelew *et al.*, 1998), hypertension (Henderson *et al.*, 1998), congestive heart failure (Moser *et al.*, 1997), and chronic obstructive pulmonary disease (Esteve *et al.*, 1996).

## Imagery/Visualization

Imagery is a technique in which the patient is asked to create a mental image of a pleasurable event or setting or a desired outcome. This technique can be used to achieve a state of relaxation or to attempt to influence the body's natural defenses. For example, a cancer patient might create a mental image of the cancer melting away or of white blood cells rushing to attack the cancer. The hope is that the mind can encourage and direct the immune system to accomplish the desired task. Because it is relatively easy to do and teach, and has few if any side effects, and because of some data to suggest that it may sometimes make a difference (Burish *et al.*, 1991; Post-White, 1993), imagery has become popular in the treatment of a variety of health conditions. It is prescribed by physicians, nurses, mental health professionals, and many others, but is still considered by most to be nontraditional therapy.

# Dietary Supplements, Herbs, Etc.

## Herbal Medicine

The various parts of plants have been used for medicinal purposes for centuries. At least 25% of modern prescription medicines today are derived from higher plants. As the pharmaceutical industry has become more successful in designing more effective and less toxic medicines, many of the herbal remedies of the past have gone by the wayside. However, in the midst of the most recent trend toward "natural" healing methods, more and more people have once again become enamored with herbal remedies. The variety of herbal products sold in health-food stores and increasingly in pharmacies is large and regulations governing product labeling are loose enough that manufacturers are able to make claims about these products that are often misleading or completely baseless.

There is no question that some herbal products have physiologic effects. In fact, the pharmaceutical industry is actively studying a variety of traditional herbal remedies in hopes of discovering new pharmaceuticals. However, the magnitude of the effects, the doses required to achieve them, their potential toxicity, and potential interactions with other medicines or food products have often not been well studied. The quantities of biologically active ingredients in many, if not most, of the OTC preparations available in the United States are insufficient to cause either benefit (beyond the placebo effect) or harm.

## Orthomolecular Medicine

Based, in part, on the work of Nobel laureate Linus Pauling, the presumption of orthomolecular (*ortho* meaning proper) medicine is that the Recommended Daily Allowances (RDAs) for many vitamins and minerals are far too low, based as they are on the quantities required to prevent overt deficiency states. Advocates of orthomolecular medicine often argue that, over time, essential minerals have been leached out of the soil, and that modern diets and food preparation methods have removed many of the essential vitamins as well. Thus, they argue that large (often huge) doses of a variety of vitamins and minerals taken as supplements can have beneficial health effects. Megadoses of vitamin C (up to 500 times the RDA) have been advocated for the prevention and treatment of viral infections, cancer, and atherosclerosis. Various concoctions of trace minerals have been widely promoted as the antidotes to the degenerative diseases associated with aging. More recently, there have been suggestions that large doses of antioxidants such as vitamin E, beta-carotene, and selenium may prevent cancer and coronary artery disease. While epidemiological data have often been promising, to date, with rare exceptions, randomized controlled trials are either lacking or have failed to demonstrate the purported benefits of these practices.

## Chelation

Chelation involves the intravenous injection of chelating substances such as sodium EDTA in order to bind and ultimately remove from the body substances thought to be responsible for various health problems. It is commonly used, for example, to treat atherosclerosis on the premise that calcium can be removed from the plaques that line the obstructed blood vessels. Other purported benefits include improved lipid profiles, increased effectiveness of hydroxyl-radical scavengers, inhibition of platelet aggregation, and restoration of electromagnetic potential across cell membranes (Chappell, 1995). Diagnostic blood and tissue tests are done to determine the levels of various toxic substances in the body as well as the quantities of various essential vitamins and minerals. Based on the results of these tests and the nature of the presenting problem, a chelating solution is prepared that may include the chelating agent plus supplemental vitamins. Recent randomized controlled trials have found that chelation was no better than placebo for treating patients with symptomatic peripheral arterial occlusive disease (Ernst, 1998). Chelation is generally performed by physicians. Training usually consists of attendance at workshops and short courses.

# INTERDISCIPLINARY TEAMWORK

Patients like Mrs. M. in Case 25-2 require the services of a variety of health professionals simultaneously. How should these services by coordinated? In the above case, Dr. S. took it on himself to coordinate Mrs. M.'s care. Even though his efforts appeared to have been successful, at no time were more than two professionals able to engage in a discussion of Mrs. M.'s situation at the same time, and there were several professionals who were excluded from even those discussions, e.g., the hospital pharmacist, the hospital social worker, the cardiologist who read the cardiac studies, and the anesthesiologist.

As modern healthcare has become more complex because of broader definitions of health, increased medical knowledge, technological advances, and changes in the spectrum of illnesses, so too has the healthcare system become increasingly complex. One aspect of this complexity is the dramatic increase over the last half century in the number of healthcare disciplines and in the degree of specialization within each discipline, particularly medicine, nursing, and dentistry. For such a complicated system to function effectively and efficiently to the benefit of individual patients, teamwork is required.

Interdisciplinary teamwork in healthcare as a concept has been described and advocated for at least 30 years. Enthusiasm was particularly high in the 1960s, when several large demonstration projects were funded. Unfortunately, because of the difficulties involved in implementation and a relative shortage of convincing data proving increased efficacy, the movement lost momentum. However, as health professionals find that they are caring for increasing numbers of chronically ill and disabled patients, there has been a resurgence of interest in interdisciplinary approaches to healthcare. Interdisciplinary teams are now the rule in rehabilitation (Rothberg, 1981), home healthcare, and geriatrics (Rubenstein, 1983), where there is now some reasonably good evidence that interdisciplinary team care is superior to traditional multidisciplinary care (Williams & Williams, 1986).

Of course, any setting in which professionals from more than one discipline work side by side could be considered interdisciplinary teamwork, and that is probably true to a degree. Outpatient clinics, operating rooms, and hospital wards all require interdisciplinary collaboration. However, teamwork in these settings generally means that physicians give orders to the other professionals on the team, who dutifully carry them out. There is very little collaborative decision making.

What are the barriers to true interdisciplinary teamwork? Several have already been mentioned. Professionals from the different disciplines are trained separately in their own specialized fields with little chance to learn about or even interact with professionals from other disciplines until after they graduate. By that time, "turf" boundaries are well established. Specialization tends to emphasize differences more than similarities between professionals (French, 1979). Issues of power, prestige, financial compensation, sexism, and racism also contribute to defensive and distancing behaviors. Attitudes that develop within a group become firmly entrenched through social support and affiliation (French, 1979).

Physicians in particular are trained to be action-oriented, self-contained, autonomous decision makers. Thus, they are systemically educated to be poor team players (Goldstein, 1989). If being a member of an interdisciplinary team means being responsible to other team members, then physicians, whether by selection or training, are often unwilling and ill prepared to do so (Charns, 1976). In addition, teamwork results in significant loss of power and control, items valued highly by many physicians, particularly in today's liability-conscious society.

Effective interdisciplinary teamwork requires that professionals from the various healthcare disciplines understand and respect each other, that there be a common language and method of communication between them, and that the goals of treatment and the roles played by each team member can be agreed on by all. To become an effective team member, a healthcare professional must learn his own discipline well and feel comfortable within its boundaries. In addition, he must learn enough about each of the other disciplines to allow colleague-to-colleague communication, consultation, and referral. The consultative process must be mastered. In situations requiring particularly close and frequent interdisciplinary collaboration, such as geriatrics and rehabilitation, group process skills must also be learned.

Perhaps the most important obstacle to a team approach is the traditional departmental organizational structure that exists in nearly all healthcare institutions. Hospitals, for instance, usually have separate departments of nursing, social work, occupational therapy, physical therapy, radiology, laboratory, and pathology. That type of departmental model puts a client in the middle, making him a victim of territorial struggles for power, control, status, and financial resources. As a result, the staff members serving those same clients do not know one another and cannot communicate, plan together, or support each other. Garner describes teams and departments as being like oil and water (Garner, 1988).

The basic requirements for interdisciplinary teamwork are mutual respect and an understanding of the potential contributions of team members from other disciplines, communication through use of a commonly understood language, and an interdisciplinary decision-making process that facilitates the formation of mutually agreed-on goals and strategies. Teamwork also requires training and practice; it does not occur automatically. For interdisciplinary healthcare to become a universal reality, more and better interaction must occur between disciplines at every stage of training, and administrators must recognize the need to reorganize healthcare systems into interdisciplinary teams rather than discipline-specific departments. The time required for team meetings must be reimbursed by third-party payers. Liability issues must be explored and addressed. If physicians are to function as leaders of interdisciplinary healthcare teams, strategies will need to be developed at both the selection and training stages that will foster appropriate attitudes and skills.

## CONCLUSION

Our modern healthcare system is complex. The number and variety of healthcare practitioners, both traditional and nontraditional, provides patients a great many options. It also presents a formidable challenge. Despite the explosion of health-related information available to the public, most people still know very little about the roles of the various healthcare disciplines. In fact, healthcare professionals often know surprisingly little about other professionals outside their own discipline. It is hoped that this chapter has begun to address this portion of the problem.

Important changes are occurring in the healthcare system. Driven largely by rising costs, a predominantly medical subspecialty-oriented system is evolving into one in which generalists occupy a more important role. Administrators are becoming more powerful as are the other health professions such as nursing. As people in our society have become healthier and better informed, we nevertheless have become increasingly dissatisfied with our health, and particularly with our healthcare system. Interest in nontraditional healthcare methods has grown exponentially in the past two decades. Healthcare reform remains near the top of the political agenda.

Regardless of the changes that occur, there is no question that such a complex system can only run effectively and efficiently when the various providers of care can coordinate their efforts toward the best interests of patients. This requires teamwork, and true interdisciplinary teamwork requires more than good intentions. A critical ingredient is understanding and respect for the skills of others. The consultation and referral process is also essential, but even better methods of communication and coordination are required. Administrative structures may need to be changed, liability issues explored, and record systems revamped. Most importantly, health professionals must be trained to function as members of teams.

## CASES FOR DISCUSSION

### CASE 1

*K.S., a 42-year-old man who had no regular physician, saw a plastic surgeon to have a large lipoma removed from his back. Because of the size of the lesion, which would have required a fairly large dose of local anesthetic, the surgeon ordered an ECG to reassure himself that no heart disease was present. The ECG report was equivocal, showing some minor ST-T wave changes possibly caused by ischemia. He recommended and made arrangements for a consultation with a cardiologist.*

*The cardiologist took a more complete cardiac history and learned that the patient had had a long history of occasional episodes of palpitations never severe enough to require treatment. In fact, he had never before mentioned them to a physician. The cardiologist ordered some blood tests and recommended an exercise tolerance test and a 24-hour Holter monitor study. The results of the blood work were normal except for a fasting serum cholesterol of 250 mg/dl. The exercise test was equivocal with 1.5-mm ST depressions at maximal exercise. He recommended that K.S. begin a low-cholesterol and low-saturated-fat diet.*

*Before the Holter tracing could be done, K.S. had to be seen in the emergency room with the worst episode of palpitations that he had ever had. A rhythm strip showed paroxysmal supraventricular tachycardia. He was converted using digoxin and carotid massage and was sent home only to return several days later with another episode, which was converted similarly. He was then told to continue to take digoxin indefinitely. The Holter monitor was canceled.*

*The cardiologist then requested an echocardiogram to look for valvular disease and chamber enlargement and an exercise nuclear ventriculogram to further evaluate the possibility of ischemia. These studies demonstrated no chamber enlargement, normal valves, but a borderline low left ventricular ejection fraction of 50% (normal 60% or greater) and no real evidence for ischemia. However, because of the low ejection fraction and atrial arrhythmia as well as the elevated serum cholesterol, the cardiologist suggested going ahead with a cardiac catheterization, which demonstrated clean coronary arteries and again a borderline low ejection fraction.*

*One year later, K.S. now follows a low-cholesterol, low-saturated-fat diet to which his wife compulsively forces him to adhere, niacin three times daily to further lower his cholesterol, which remained elevated despite the diet, once-daily digoxin, and once-daily baby aspirin. He has had two more episodes of palpitations requiring emergency room conversions, and he anxiously awaits the results of his follow-up nuclear ventriculogram to see if his "idiopathic cardiomyopathy" has worsened. His lipoma remains intact.*

1. *What happened? In which ways is K.D. better off for having had the cardiac evaluation? In what ways is he worse off? What do you suspect the impact has been on his family?*
2. *At what points in this clinical cascade could it have been stopped? Who could have stopped it most effectively?*
3. *Can too much information ever be harmful? If so, how can we decide how much is enough?*
4. *What do you suspect would happen if K.S. now developed postprandial epigastric pain?*

## CASE 2

*Dr. F.L. requested a consultation from an endocrinologist for his longtime patient, T.Y., whose blood pressure was difficult to control and his serum calcium level was borderline high. Nine months later Dr. L. was fit to be tied when he learned that the endocrinology consultation had led to a pulmonary consultation for a chronic cough, which Dr. L. knew to be allergic in nature and of long standing, and an orthopedic consultation for evaluation of low back pain, which Dr. L. had previously evaluated and found to be associated with marital and job-related stress. Neither of the secondary consultants sent the results of their evaluations to Dr. L., since they were unaware that he was the primary physician. Furthermore, the endocrinologist who had handled the blood pressure and calcium questions with the patient had not communicated with Dr. L.*

1. *Why did the endocrinologist probably act in this way? What kind of trouble did it cause?*
2. *What do you think Dr. L. should do about it?*
3. *Why didn't T.Y. keep it from happening?*

## CASE 3

*When Dr. D.W. decided to admit R.P. to the intensive care unit of the county hospital to rule out an acute myocardial infarction, he was told that he would have to speak with the charge nurse in the ICU. When he was informed by the charge nurse that although there was one open bed, there were not enough nurses available to properly care for any additional patients, and she therefore could not authorize the admission, he was livid. How dare a nurse tell him whether or not he could admit a patient to the ICU. He called the intensivist in charge of the ICU but to his surprise was informed that the nurse's decision was correct and would be upheld.*

1. *Should nurses be making this kind of decision? Was the nurse's decision in this case an appropriate one?*
2. *Why was Dr. W. so angry?*

## CASE 4

*A 46-year-old woman suffered a left hemispheric stroke. After a brief hospitalization, she was referred to an inpatient rehabilitation facility. There she was found to have a right hemiparesis, moderately elevated blood pressure, and blood glucose.*

1. *Which healthcare professionals should be involved in this patient's care? What would each be expected to contribute to her management?*
2. *Who should be the coordinator of the rehabilitation team? Suggest a method of care that would allow interdisciplinary teamwork.*

## CASE 5

S.R., a pharmacist, called Dr. G. to clarify a prescription that Dr. G. had written for D.D. for a potassium-sparing diuretic. He wanted to make Dr. G. aware of the fact that Mr. D. was also taking a potassium supplement and an ACE inhibitor and had just bought a box of Lite Salt, all of which, in combination with the diuretic, might be expected to increase D.D.'s risk of hyperkalemia. He was not terribly surprised when Dr. G. seemed somewhat annoyed and told him in essence to quit practicing medicine. Dr. G. added that he had told Mr. D. not to take any more of the potassium supplement. However, when S.R. had asked D.D. earlier, he had not remembered that advice.

1. What should the pharmacist's role be on the healthcare team? What, if anything, should the pharmacist have done differently in this case?
2. Which obstacles, if any, exist that prevent pharmacists from taking a more active role in patient care?

## CASE 6

G.C. was 71 years old when he came to see Dr. H. for a checkup at the insistence of his daughter. G.C. had had a heart attack 2 years earlier. Now he was having some mild stable angina, but wasn't taking any medication for it, and had had one episode of sudden vision loss in his right eye lasting about 5 minutes. After recommending several tests and a medication, G.C.'s daughter revealed that her father had been receiving chelation therapy weekly for the last 6 months.

1. Could the chelation therapy be contributing to G.C.'s symptoms?
2. What would you say to G.C. and his daughter about chelation therapy?
3. What kind of practitioners generally perform chelation therapy? What is involved in this kind of treatment?
4. What are its purported benefits?

## CASE 7

D.T., on discharge from the hospital after the birth of her second child, when asked to bring the child in for a 2-week checkup, disclosed to you that she would be taking the child to the same chiropractor who had been providing well-child care to her other child for the past 2 years. She said that she was well pleased with his care, which included regular spinal manipulations and dietary advice, but apparently no immunizations.

1. What are your feelings about chiropractors' providing well-child care?
2. What besides immunizations might the child not be getting that would ordinarily be part of traditional well-child care?
3. What advice, if any, would you give to this mother?

# RECOMMENDED READINGS

Jacobs J (ed): *The Encyclopedia of Alternative Medicine: A Complete Family Guide to Complementary Therapies*. Boston, Journey Editions, 1996.

> This text summarizes the principles and practices of a broad range of complementary therapies, as well as questions patients should ask, pictures of the procedures used, and references to other information. It is evidence-based but provides a useful overview.

Lecca PJ, McNiel JD (eds.): *Interdisciplinary Team Practice: Issues and Trends*. New York, Praeger, 1985.

> This text is an excellent state-of-the art review of interdisciplinary team practice, including rationale for development of such an approach, models, and projections for the future. Specific chapters describe various types of team care, including rehabilitation, mental health, and hospice care.

Williams SJ, Torrens RR (eds.): *Introduction to Health Services*, ed 3. New York, John Wiley & Sons Inc, 1988.

> This text describes the major features of the U.S. healthcare system from a macro level and thus serves as a nice complement to this chapter's microview. It also addresses several economic issues, such as health manpower and the evaluation and regulation of healthcare programs, and concludes with a discussion on health policy.

AAFP: *Facts about Family Practice*. Kansas City, KS, American Academy of Family Physicians, 1991.

Acupuncture. *NIH Consensus Statement* 15(5):1–34, November 3–5, 1977.

Allison DB, Faith MS: Hypnosis as an adjunct to cognitive–behavioral psychotherapy for obesity: A meta-analytic reappraisal. *J Consult Clin Psychol* 64(3):513–516, 1996.

American Psychological Association: *Specialty guidelines for the delivery of services in clinical psychology, counseling psychology, industrial/organizational psychology, and school psychology*. Washington, DC, American Psychological Association Committees on Professional Standards, 1981.

Astin JA: Why patients use alternative medicine. *JAMA* 279(19):1548–1553, 1998.

Beinfield H, Korngold E: Chinese traditional medicine: An introductory overview. *Altern Ther* 1(1):44–52, 1995.

Bensoussan A, Talley NJ, Hing M, Menzies R, Guo A, Ngu M: Treatment of irritable bowel syndrome with Chinese herbal medicine: A randomized controlled trial. *JAMA* 280(18):1585–1589, 1998.

Buckelew SP, Conway R, Parker J, Deuser WE, Read J, Witty TE, Hewett JE, Minor M, Johnson JC, Van Male L, McIntosh MJ, Nigh M, Kay DR: Biofeedback/relaxation training and exercise interventions for fibromyalgia: A prospective trial. *Arthritis Care Res* 11(3):196–209, 1998.

Burish TG, Snyder SL, Jenkins RA: Preparation of patients for cancer chemotherapy: Effect of coping preparation and relaxation interventions. *J Consult Clin Psychol* 59(4):518–525, 1991.

Burstein HJ, Gelber S, Guadagnoli E, Weeks JC: Use of alternative medicine by women with early-stage breast cancer. *N Engl J Med* 340(22):1733–1739, 1999.

Chappell LT: EDTA chelation therapy should be more commonly used in the treatment of vascular disease. *Altern Ther* 1(2):53–57, 1995.

Charns M: Breaking the tradition barrier: Managing integration in healthcare facilities. *Health Care Manage Rev* 1:55–67, 1976.

*Chiropractic: State of the Art 1994–1995*. American Chiropractic Association, 1994.

*The Chiropractic Profession: Myths & Facts*. Palmerton, Pa, PracticeMakers Products, Inc, 1993.

Clark F, Azen SP, Zemke R, Jackson J, Carlson M, Mandel D, Hay J, Josephson K, Cherry B, Hessel C, Palmer J, Lipson L: Occupational therapy for independent-living older adults. A randomized controlled trial. *JAMA* 278(16):1321–1326, 1997.

Coleman LM, Fowler LL, Williams ME: Use of unproven therapies by people with Alzheimer's disease. *J Am Geriatr Soc* 43:747–750, 1995.

Cox DJ, Sutphen J, Borowitz S, Kovatchev B, Ling W: Contribution of behavior therapy and biofeedback to laxative therapy in the treatment of pediatric encopresis. *Ann Behav Med* 20(2):70–76, 1998.

Cummings RG, Thomas M, Szonyi G, Salkeld G, O'Neill E, Westbury C, Frampton G: Home visits by an occupational therapist for assessment and modification of environmental hazards: A randomized trial of falls prevention. *J Am Geriatr Soc* 47:1397–1402, 1999.

Debrovner D: Micro medicine. *Am Drug* 208(1):36–41, 1993.

Druss BG, Rosenheck RA: Association between use of unconventional therapies and conventional medical services. *JAMA* 282(7):651–656, 1999.

Engel GL. The need for a new medical model: A challenge for biomedicine. *Science* 196:129–136, 1977.

Ernst E: Review: Chelation therapy is ineffective for peripheral arterial occlusive disease. *ACP Journal Club* March/April 1998, p 38.

Esteve F, Blanc-Gras N, Gallego J, Benchetrit G: The effects of breathing pattern training on ventilatory function in patients with COPD. *Biofeedback Self Regul* 21(4):311–321, 1996.

Fagin CM: Collaboration between nurses and physicians no longer a choice. *Acad Med* 67(5):295–303, 1992.

Field TM: Massage therapy effects. *Am Psychol* 53(12):1270–1281, 1998.

French RM: Interpersonal relations, in *Dynamics of Health Care*, ed 3. New York, McGraw-Hill, 1979, pp 141–143.

Freymann JG: The public's health care paradigm is shifting: Medicine must swing with it. *J Gen Intern Med* 44:313–319, 1989.

Friedman E: Troubled past of "invisible" profession. *JAMA* 264(22):2851–2858, 1990.

Fynes MM, Marshall K, Cassidy M, Behan M, Walsh D, O'Connell PR, O'Herlihy C: A prospective, randomized study comparing the effect of augmented biofeedback with sensory biofeedback alone on fecal incontinence after obstetric trauma. *Dis Colon Rectum* 42(6):753–758, 1999.

Garner HG: *Helping Others through Teamwork*. Washington, DC, Child Welfare League of America, 1988.

Goldstein MK: Physicians and teams, in Ham R (ed): *Geriatric Medicine Annual 1989*. Oradell, NJ, Medical Economics, 1989, pp 265–275.

Hart O, Mullee MA, Lewith G, Miller J: Double-blind, placebo-controlled, randomized clinical trial of homeopathic arnica C30 for pain and infection after total abdominal hysterectomy. *J R Soc Med* 90(2):73–78, 1997.

Henderson RJ, Hart MG, Lal SK, Hunyor SN: The effect of home training with direct blood pressure biofeedback of hypertensives: A placebo-controlled study. *J Hypertens* 16(6):771–778, 1998.

Heymen S, Wexner SD, Vickers D, Nogueras JJ, Weiss EG, Pikarsky AJ: Prospective randomized trial comparing four biofeedback techniques for patients with constipation. *Dis Colon Rectum* 42(11):1388–1393, 1999.

Jones BE: *The Difference a D.O. Makes*. Oklahoma City, Times Journal Publishing Co, 1978.

Jones PE, Crawley JF: Physician assistants and health system reform. *JAMA* 271(16):1266–1272, 1994.

Kabat-Zinn J, Wheeler E, Light T, Skillings A, Scharf MJ, Cropley TG, Hosmer D, Bernhard JD: Influence of a mindfulness meditation-based stress reduction intervention on rates of skin clearing in patients with moderate to severe psoriasis undergoing phototherapy (UVB) and photochemotherapy (PUVA). *Psychosom Med* 60(5):625–632, 1998.

Kainz JT, Kozel G, Haidvogl M, Smolle J: Homoeopathic versus placebo therapy of children with warts on the hands: A randomized, double-blind clinical trial. *Dermatology* 193(4):318–320, 1996.

Kaplan KH, Goldenberg DL, Galvin-Nadeau M: The impact of a meditation-based stress reduction program on fibromyalgia. *Gen Hosp Psychiatry* 15(5):284–289, 1993.

Kassirer JP: What role for nurse practitioners in primary care? *N Engl J Med* 330(3):204–205, 1994.

Krippner S: A cross-cultural comparison of four healing models. *Altern Ther* 1(1):21–29, 1995.

Kroner-Herwig B, Mohn U, Pothmann R: Comparison of biofeedback and relaxation in the treatment of pediatric headache and the influence of parent involvement on outcome. *Appl Psychophysiol Biofeedback* 23(3):143–157, 1998.

Lazarus RS: *Psychological Stress and the Coping Process*. New York, McGraw-Hill, 1966.

Lesho EP: An overview of osteopathic medicine. *Arch Fam Med* 8:477–486, 1999.

Lokken P, Straumsheim PA, Tveiten D, Skjelbred P, Borchgrevink CF: Effect of homeopathy on pain and other events after acute trauma: Placebo controlled trial with bilateral oral surgery. *BMJ* 210(6992):1439–1442, 1995.

Margolis S: Chelation therapy is ineffective for the treatment of peripheral vascular disease. *Altern Ther* 1(2):53–57, 1995.

Maule WF: Screening for colorectal cancer by nurse endoscopists. *N Engl J Med* 330(3):204–205, 1994.

McDowell BJ, Engberg S, Sereika S, Donovan N, Jubeck ME, Weber E, Engberg R: Effectiveness of behavioral therapy to treat incontinence in homebound older adults. *J Am Geriatr Soc* 47(3):309–318, 1999.

McGinnis LS: Alternative therapies. *Cancer* 67(6 suppl):1788–1792, 1991.

McWhinney IR: *A Textbook of Family Medicine*. London, Oxford University Press, 1989.

Melchart D, Linde K, Worku F, Sarkady L, Holzmann M, Jurcic K, Wagner H: Results of five randomized studies on the immunomodulatory activity of preparations of echninacea. *J Altern Complement Med* 1(2):145–160, 1995.

Millon T, Green C, Meagher R (eds): *Handbook of Clinical Health Psychology*. New York, Plenum Press, 1982.

Mold JW, Stein HF: The cascade effect in the clinical care of patients. *N Engl J Med* 314(8):512–514, 1986.

Moser DK, Dracup K, Woo MA, Stevenson LW: Voluntary control of vascular tone by using skin-temperature biofeedback-relaxation in patients with advanced heart failure. *Altern Ther Health Med* 3(1):51–59, 1997.

Nansel D, Szlazak M: Somatic dysfunction and the phenomenon of visceral disease simulation: A probable explanation for the apparent effectiveness of somatic therapy in patients presumed to be suffering from true visceral disease. *J Manipulative Physiol Ther* 18(6):379–397, 1995.

*National Center for Homeopathy Directory: Practitioners, Study Groups, Pharmacies, Resources*. Alexandria VA, National Center for Homeopathy, 1995.

Nichols MJ: *Family Therapy: Concepts and Methods*. New York, Gardner Press, 1984.

Post-White J: The effects of imagery on emotions, immune functions, and cancer outcome. *Mainlines* 14(1):18–20, 1993.

Rastogi DP, Singh VP, Singh V, Dey SK, Rao K: Homeopathy in HIV infection: A trial report of double-blind placebo controlled study. *Br Homeopath J* 88(2):49–57, 1999.

Richardson M: Mental health services: Growth and development of a system, in Williams SJ, Torrens PR (eds): *Introduction to Health Services*, ed 3. New York, John Wiley & Sons, 1988, pp 255–277.

Ring ME: *Dentistry. An Illumined History*. New York, Harry N. Abrams, 1985.

Rothberg JS: The rehabilitation team: Future direction. *Arch Phys Med Rehabil* 62:407–410, 1981.

Rubenstein L: The clinical effectiveness of multidimensional geriatric assessment. *J Am Geriatr Soc* 31(12):758–761, 1983.

Schneider RH, Staggers F, Alexander CN, Sheppard W, Rainforth M, Kondwani K, Smith S, King CG: A randomised controlled trial of stress reduction for hypertension in older African Americans. *Hypertension* 26:820–827, 1995.

Schultz RM, Brushwood DB: The pharmacist's role in patient care. *Hastings Cent Rep*, January–February 1991, pp 12–17.

Schwartz GE, Weiss SM: Yale conference on behavioral medicine: A proposed definition and statement of goals. *J Behav Med* 1:3–12, 1978.

Selye H: *The Stress of Life*. New York, McGraw-Hill, 1976 revised edition.

Shapiro SL, Schwartz GE, Bonner G: Effects of mindfulness-based stress reduction on medical and premedical students. *J Behav Med* 21(6):581–599, 1998.

Simpson JJ, Donaldson I, Davies WE: Use of homeopathy in the treatment of tinnitus. *Br J Audiol* 32(4):227–233, 1998.

Smolle J, Prause G, Kerl H: A double-blind, controlled clinical trial of homeopathy and an analysis of lunar phases and postoperative outcome. *Arch Dermatol* 134(11):1368–1370, 1998.

Stein LI, Watts DT, Howell T: Sounding board: The doctor–nurse game revisited. *N Engl J Med* 322(8):546–549, 1990.

Tapp JT, Warner RW: The multisystems view of health and disease, in Schneiderman N, Tapp JT (eds): *Behavioral Medicine: The Biopsychosocial Approach*. Hillsdale, NJ, Lawrence Erlbaum Associates, 1985.

Tipton RM: Clinical and counseling psychology: A study of rules and functions. *Prof Psychol* 14:837–846, 1983.

Ullman D: A brief history of homeopathy and its legal status in the U.S. *Homeopathy Medicine for the 21st Century*. Berkeley, Calif, North Atlantic Books, 1988, pp 80–81.

Vickers A, Zollman C: The manipulative therapies: Osteopathy and chiropractic. *BMJ* 319:1176–1179, 1999.

Vickers AJ, Fisher P, Smith C, Wyllie SE, Lewith GT: Homeopathy for delayed onset muscle soreness: A randomised double blind placebo controlled trial. *Br J Sports Med* 31(4):304–307, 1997.

Vickers AJ, Fisher P, Smith C, Wyllie SE, Rees R: Homeopathic arnica 30x is ineffective for muscle soreness after long-distance running: A randomized, double-blind, placebo-controlled trial. *Clin J Pain* 14(3):227–231, 1998.

Walker MF, Gladman JR, Lincoln NB, Siemonsma P, Whiteley T: Occupational therapy for stroke patients not admitted to hospital: A randomised controlled trial. *Lancet* 354(9175):278–280, 1999.

Watkins CE, Lopez FG, Campbell VL, Himmell CD: Counseling psychology and clinical psychology: Some preliminary comparative data. *Am Psychol* 41(6):581–582, 1986.

Weikel WJ, Palmo AJ: The evolution and practice of mental health counseling. *J Men Health Counseling* 11(1):7–25, 1989.

Weiser M, Strosser W, Klein P: Homoeopathic vs conventional treatment of vertigo: A randomized double-blind controlled clinical study. *Arch Otolaryngol Head Neck Surg* 124(8):879–885, 1998.

Weiser M, Gegenheimer LH, Klein P: A randomized equivalence trial comparing the efficacy and safety of Luffa comp.-Heel nasal spray with cromolyn sodium spray in the treatment of seasonal allergic rhinitis. *Forsch Komplementarmed* 6(3):142–148, 1999.

Wenneberg SR, Schneider RH, Walton KG, Maclean CR, Levitsky DK, Salerno JW, Wallace RK, Mandarino JV, Rainforth MV, Waziri R: A controlled study of the effects of the Transcendental Meditation program on cardiovascular reactivity and ambulatory blood pressure. *Int J Neurosci* 89(1–2):15–28, 1997.

Whitley JM: Counseling psychology: A historical perspective. *Counseling Psychol* 12:3–109, 1984.

Whitmarsh TE, Coleston-Shields DM, Steiner TJ: Double-blind randomized placebo-controlled study of homeopathic prophylaxis of migraine. *Cephalalgia* 17(5):600–604, 1997.

Williams ME, Williams TF: Evaluation of older persons in the ambulatory setting. *J Am Geriatr Soc* 34:37–43, 1986.

## CHAPTER 26

# B. Values

# Medical Ethics

*Warren L. Holleman*

*Kimetre is a fourth-year medical student doing an oncology elective. At team meeting the first day, she learns about Ms. Little, a patient with apparent breast cancer who is scheduled for surgery the next day. The surgeons plan to obtain a frozen biopsy and, depending on the extensiveness of the cancer, to go ahead and perform a lumpectomy or mastectomy. Later that morning Kimetre visits Ms. Little and discovers she has serious misperceptions about the nature of her illness and the surgery to be performed. She has no inkling that she has breast cancer, that her disease is life-threatening, or that the surgery might significantly disfigure her. She believes she merely has "a cyst."*

*Kimetre wants to believe that too, and wonders momentarily if she misunderstood the discussion earlier that morning. After reflecting, reviewing her notes, and checking with another member of the team, Kimetre confirms that the oncologist is certain the patient has breast cancer.*

*Kimetre then wonders if Ms. Little might be in a state of denial. Perhaps she knows intellectually the nature of her illness and of tomorrow's surgery, but she is hoping against hope that the physicians have made an error in judgment. So Kimetre spends a little extra time with Ms. Little to evaluate her competence, her level of anxiety, and her level of denial. Kimetre finds her lucid and, although she is not as curious about her condition as others might be, it is clear to Kimetre that the team has not informed her truthfully about her illness and the surgery.*

*Now Kimetre is in a difficult position. She is the lone medical student on a team of experienced faculty, fellows, and residents. It is her first day on the service. One of her patients—well, not exactly Kimetre's patient, she's just a medical student—is about to be wheeled into surgery, apparently unaware of the disease that threatens her life or that, on awakening, some or all of her breast may be missing.*

*Kimetre asks the intern whether the patient knows what's going on. "She might. Patients often know more about their condition than we do." "Has anyone told her?" Intern: "Probably not." "Well," Kimetre asks, "don't you think someone ought to tell her?" The intern seems distracted and avoids her question: "You need to check the prostate in 614. He's had catheter problems. Maybe you could be useful THERE." Kimetre wants to be useful here, but she doesn't want to be too pushy. "I'll check on Mr. Shackleton in 614 but first I'm going to talk to Ms. Little." Intern: "Don't do that." "Why not?" Kimetre asks. Intern: "Because I said so. She's an old lady. Trust me, I'm a doctor." He walks away as he says this. Then, halfway down the hallway, he stops, turns, and flashes a knowing grin. The grin could be interpreted any number of ways: a clumsy attempt at understanding, a seductive overture, or a conceited way of saying "I'm in charge here." Kimetre thinks it's probably a little of each.*

*In any other context his smile would have won her over, but here Kimetre finds herself confused, angry, and scared. The patient is 65 years old, the same age as Kimetre's mother. She reflects: "My mother doesn't seem that old, and I know she wouldn't want to be treated like this."*

*Kimetre then helps the gentleman with the catheter problem and someone else's pain problem but she can't get Ms. Little off her mind. In the politest voice she can muster Kimetre asks the fellow to "help" her with her problem. The problem, of course, is that Kimetre doesn't understand why Ms. Little hasn't been told the truth, why she's being wheeled off to surgery without giving an informed consent, and why confidential information is being discussed with her daughter. The fellow begins with a familiar response: "She's an old lady, and we don't want to upset her." Still trying to maintain a courteous pose, Kimetre acknowledges his concern but wonders whether Ms. Little might also be upset at being lied to or at waking up and discovering her breasts mutilated. The fellow says that since she's an old lady, and since this is the best treatment for her, she probably won't be too upset. Trying not to become too upset herself, Kimetre asks, "How can you speak for her? How do you know what she wants?" The fellow's response: "We're working closely with her daughter, and that's what her daughter says. Her daughter is a nurse herself. We're trusting her judgment."*

*The fellow gives Kimetre a friendly discourse on how things are done in his home country, where the oldest child routinely handles all medical decision-making. Cancer, prognosis, and death are never discussed with patients: "It's taboo." Attempting to avoid sounding culturally insensitive, Kimetre points out that, until recently, such behavior was considered taboo in many parts of the United States as well. Then Kimetre realizes that maybe it still is.*

*Kimetre signed up for this elective because of the outstanding reputation of the oncologist and this cancer treatment center. Now, just a few hours into the rotation, she is disillusioned with both.*

## EDUCATIONAL OBJECTIVES

1. Identify the most common ethical issues facing medical students and physicians
2. Understand ethical standards of care regarding confidentiality, truth telling, informed consent, death and dying, and third-party payers
3. Identify factors affecting physician compliance with ethical standards of care
4. Apply ethical standards of care to common clinical situations in both the outpatient and clinical settings

## INTRODUCTION

Case 26-1 is troubling for a number of reasons, not the least of which is that it is true. It happened recently, and at one of the leading cancer treatment facilities in the United States.

Fortunately, this story has a happy ending. Kimetre confronted the oncologist, who responded by admitting his fault, apologizing to the patient, and disclosing truthfully to the patient. The oncologist even thanked the student for her courage and concern. He explained that he generally abided by ethical standards of treatment but that in this case his judgment had been impaired by the fact that the patient's daughter was a nurse, not just any nurse but an oncology nurse, and not just any oncology nurse but *his* nurse! Once the charade ended he breathed a sigh of relief, saying that it was much harder to cover secrets, tell lies, and bend rules than simply to do the right thing, even though in this case that meant telling a patient bad news.

577

FACTORS AFFECTING
PHYSICIAN
COMPLIANCE WITH
ETHICAL STANDARDS
OF CARE

The medical ethics movement of the past quarter-century has made much progress in establishing standards of treatment requiring truthfulness, informed consent, and confidentiality within the physician–patient relationship. Incidents such as the one described in Case 26-1 are becoming less common in the United States. As the foregoing case illustrates, however, deception does happen and for a variety of reasons, including paternalism toward patients, cynicism regarding morality, denial of death, medical hubris, and clumsiness in balancing conflicts of interest.

## FACTORS AFFECTING PHYSICIAN COMPLIANCE WITH ETHICAL STANDARDS OF CARE

Paternalism is often fueled by a desire to protect the patient, but without a fundamental respect for the patient the "helpful" physician becomes coercive, dishonest, and untrustworthy. The attending physician in Case 26-1 may have honestly believed he was doing what was best for his patient, but his judgment had been clouded by his relationship with her daughter. The patient would soon go home, but the physician would continue to work side by side with the daughter. The physician became confused regarding the primacy of the conflicting loyalties and blurred the boundaries between personal, collegial, and professional responsibilities. In so doing he forgot to show a fundamental respect for the autonomy and integrity of the patient.

Cynicism is common in academic medical centers, often fostered by fatigue, stress, peer pressure, and poor mentoring. While psychological, sociological, and institutional factors influence attitudes and behavior, they do not justify them. Those who feel cynical about the moral enterprise should search their souls to consider basic motivations for pursuing a medical vocation. They should also recognize that many standards of medical ethics have been codified into law. Violators have more than a guilty conscience to deal with: They may face fines, imprisonment, malpractice suits, and probation or loss of their medical license.

Those who have difficulty discussing death, disability, and disease with their patients should recognize that this feeling is normal. It is usually rooted in fear and insecurity regarding one's own mortality or in feeling impotent to fix a bad situation. For some students it takes considerable willpower to resist the temptation to flee the bedside of the dying, disabled, or disfigured patient. One rule of thumb I try to follow is: *If I feel the urge to leave, stay. If I find myself staying away from a difficult situation, that's the very place I need to go—right now.* When I get there and feel the urge to leave, I imagine myself on a rambunctious horse and I tell myself to stay in the saddle—that's the only way to learn to ride the tough ones. Similarly, when I feel the urge to leaf through the chart or to carry on small talk with the family, I have another rule: *Don't just do something, stand there.* Or better: sit there. Let the patient comfort you. Then you can begin to care for the patient.

---

## WHAT WOULD YOU DO?

*I'm a fourth-year medical student doing my rural preceptorship in Montana. I've been here 4 weeks working side by side with the only doctor in the entire county. The closest hospital is 80 miles away. My preceptor treats a number of seriously ill patients with little access to the technology we use in the medical center where I train. We've seen every type of injury you can imagine: a man kicked in the head by his horse, a teenager who shredded his arm in an auger, a woman bit by a rattlesnake, a man shot in the foot when he tripped over a rock chasing a pack of coyotes. It's been exciting; just what I hoped for.*

*This afternoon the preceptor told me that, as this is the last week of my rotation, he's going to let me run the clinic for a day. He wants to go hunting tomorrow and this is his only chance to get away. He says I've done a good job and he trusts me. He says if I get in trouble to ask the nurse; she'll know what to do. He says he'll leave before sunrise and be back late. What should I do?*

---

Medical hubris is an occupational disease found among those medical students and physicians who believe that modern medicine can cure every ailment. I have found chronically ill and disabled patients the best teachers in helping rid one of this misconception.

With so many competing interests these days—patients, families, third-party payers, employers, hospital administrations, pharmaceutical companies—it is little wonder that physicians have difficulty weighing the legitimate interests of each party (Morreim, 1991). A thoughtful consideration of ethical foundations and ethical standards of care can go a long way, however, in helping one avoid the most common pitfalls and in learning to juggle multiple competing interests more adroitly.

## CHAPTER OVERVIEW

Although the chapter will touch on controversial areas such as euthanasia, abortion, and access to care, the main focus will be the areas in which some consensus has been reached in hopes that this basic knowledge will enable the student to be more competent and confident on clinical rotations. Case 26-1 illustrates many of the areas covered by the chapter.

First, confidentiality vis-à-vis the patient's family and other third parties: Under what circumstances should the physician discuss diagnosis, prognosis, and treatment options with family members or with other individuals not involved in the patient's care? Second, truth telling: Does the fiduciary nature of the physician–patient relationship require that physicians and patients be honest with one another, and are there any circumstances in which the physician or patient might legitimately withhold information or deceive one another? Third, informed consent: What constitutes a free, informed consent, what types of information should the physician provide the patient, and under what circumstances should a physician seek the consent of a proxy decision-maker rather than the patient?

To appreciate the significance of respect for confidentiality, truth telling, and informed consent to treatment, it is important first to understand the foundations on which these ethical standards are based. The next section will examine these foundations.

## CASE 26-2

*Carlos, a 24-year-old police officer, presented to his primary care physician with a broken nose, an injury sustained 3 months previously while playing soccer. The examination revealed a deviated septum that partially closed the air pathway. Carlos reported mild to moderate difficulty in breathing and sinus allergies and discomforts. The physician, who himself had had a deviated septum for many years and who received a salary bonus at the end of the year for keeping tests, procedures, referrals, and hospitalizations under a certain limit, suggested doing nothing: "No one ever died of a deviated septum, but the other options carry risks." When Carlos asked about those options the physician responded by saying, "There are medicines you could take but they'd probably make you feel worse than you do now. Mother nature is the best healer. If I were you I wouldn't worry."*

*Soon thereafter Carlos's employer switched to a new health plan and Carlos visited a new physician, who referred Carlos immediately to a head and neck surgeon. After a brief examination the specialist told Carlos he ought to have surgery to repair the deviated septum: "Not only will it open the pathway and improve your breathing, but also the girls will like your new nose." After calculating the cost of meeting his deductible and the 20% copayment, Carlos decided he could not afford the surgical procedure at this time. Six months later Carlos presented once again to the primary care physician with sinus headaches and sinusitis. The physician scolded him for not having the surgery and prescribed antibiotics. The problem resolved temporarily but when it recurred Carlos—feeling shamed by the physician's comments—delayed returning to the physician until the headaches became unbearable. This pattern repeated itself several times over the next year, with the physician prescribing an antibiotic but making Carlos feel the blame for his illness.*

*Then Carlos's employer switched healthcare plans once again. The new primary care physician, concerned about the frequency of the recurrences and of Carlos's absences from work, took a complete history, reviewed with Carlos the pros and cons of nontreatment and surgery, and suggested a third option, nasal decongestants, to open the nasal pathway. Carlos agreed to try the medication. When he returned 6 months later for a follow-up examination, Carlos said he felt like his old self again. He reported only occasional mild headaches and no bothersome side effects of the medication.*

## ETHICAL FOUNDATIONS

In every patient encounter, physicians ought to ask themselves four basic ethical questions (Beauchamp & Childress, 1989; McCullough & Ashton, 1994; Pellegrino & Thomasma, 1993). These questions apply whether the patient has a deviated septum or a deviated spine, a cold or cancer. These questions concern whether the patient will be benefited by the treatment (*beneficence*), whether the patient might be harmed by the treatment or the risks, discomforts, and side effects might outweigh the benefits (*nonmaleficence*), whether the patient participates in the decision process (*autonomy*), whether the physician considers the impact of the treatment on other patients, on the patient's family, on caregivers, and on the rest of society (*justice*), and whether the physician's motives reflect personal and professional values and ideals (*virtue*).

The first question to ask is, *What medical benefits can I offer this patient, and what harms are also possible?* In Case 26-2, the medical benefits that can be offered to Carlos are to open his nasal pathway, improve his breathing, reduce his discomfort, and reduce his sinus allergies. These benefits can be achieved by one of two means: surgery and medication. The surgery would permanently correct the problem but would involve considerable expense, 1 week of missed work and postoperative pain and discomfort, and the remote possibility of disfigurement as a result of infection or death as a reaction to the anesthesia. Nasal decongestants usually engender moderate improvement with little risk or cost in the short run. Long-run costs will be much higher, however, and some patients will experience mild to moderate discomfort as a result of insomnia and feeling "wired." Additional factors to consider when comparing the cost of surgery vis-à-vis medication include the patient's life expectancy and which treatments are covered by the patient's health insurance plan. From a medical and societal perspective, the decision becomes even more complicated when the patient's health insurance reimburses the less desirable or more expensive option.

One reason Carlos received suboptimal care is that the first three physicians failed to spell out the entire array of legitimate treatment options. Each was comfortable with one particular option and tried to force Carlos to accept it, without exploring alternatives and without exploring benefits, harms, and costs. As a result, Carlos was sick much longer than he had to be. When the fourth physician took the time to review each treatment option, physician and patient quickly found a mutually satisfactory solution.

Because each patient will weigh benefits and harms differently, it is important to ask a second question: *What are the patient's values and preferences?* For some patients, such as Carlos, the cost of surgery will be prohibitive. Even those patients who could afford the procedure might prefer to spend the money on some other good, such as a downpayment on a car. If the nasal blockage is minor, the patient will probably prefer conservative treatment or no treatment at all, as in the case of the first physician in deciding about his own treatment. What that physician failed to recognize, however, is that the severity of the problem and the tolerance for discomfort vary from patient to patient; he should have assessed Carlos's severity and discomfort more carefully.

For patients whose threshold for risk is low, the risk of anesthesia will seem excessive for an elective procedure. One can imagine, for example, parents of young children deferring the procedure until the children are older. If the discomfort of the nasal blockage and the side effects of decongestants are having a significant impact on one's lifestyle, work, or parenting abilities, then the risk of anesthesia may seem reasonable.

Because values, preferences, and thresholds for risk vary from person to person, it is important for the physician to inform the patient of the risks, benefits, side effects, and costs of the various legitimate treatments—and of nontreatment—so that the patient can make an informed and individually appropriate decision.

Respect for the patient's autonomy includes respect for the patient's right to choose among each of the legitimate treatment options, or to refuse treatment completely. Patients have the right to refuse treatment regardless of whether the treatment is an elective procedure, such as rhinoplasty, or a lifesaving procedure or medication, such as cardiac bypass surgery or chemotherapy. It is quite common, for example, for patients dying of cancer or AIDS to refuse antibiotics for opportunistic infections, even though the antibiotic could prolong their life.

Respect for the patient's autonomy does not mean that physicians are obligated to provide *whatever* treatment the patient requests. If the patient requests a treatment that is outside the standard of care, such as sleeping pills for chronic insomnia, the physician is not obligated to comply. In fact, the principle of nonmaleficence would suggest that the physician is obligated *not* to comply.

More controversial is the patient's request for assistance in suicide or abortion. For many physicians these medical procedures violate personal and professional values. For these physicians there is no legal or professional obligation to comply with the patient's request, even though abortions or medically assisted suicides may be legal or at least permissible in their jurisdictions. Physicians who refuse to do procedures they consider unethical are protected in most states by conscience clauses. Conscience clauses do not apply to emergency abortions in which the mother's life is in danger and do not exempt physicians from the obligation to provide their patients with appropriate referrals.

The third question to consider is, *What is fair in this situation?* Medical decisions have an impact not only on the patient but also on family, caregivers, other patients, and the rest of society. A concern for justice demands that physicians and patients bear this in mind when making decisions about which tests to order and which treatments to pursue. For example, if the deviation of a patient's septum is minor and the benefits of surgery are marginal, the physician should not recommend surgery even if the procedure is covered by insurance. Wasting scarce resources on marginally beneficial treatments is unfair to others in the insurance plan and, in the case of Medicare, to taxpayers in general. In the case of patients who are dying and for whom curative treatments are deemed futile, the physician not only should ask whether the patient wants the treatment and has the ability to pay, but also should consider the cost to other patients in terms of allocation of beds, equipment, and supplies. The physician should also consider the financial, emotional, and physical cost to family and caregivers in providing round-the-clock care: Many spouses become so exhausted in caring for their loved ones that the health of the caregiver becomes a more pressing concern than that of the identified patient.

A concern for justice also demands that nations make primary medical care available to all citizens regardless of ability to pay. Physicians ought to be leading this effort. Unfortunately, too many U.S. physicians are preoccupied with maximizing their incomes or the power and prestige of their specialty.

In light of the tendency to place self-interest above professional service and social responsibility, it is important always to bear in mind a fourth question: *Am I remaining faithful to my values and ideals, and to those of my profession?* One such value is honesty: being truthful with patients, colleagues, and administrators, and on medical records and insurance forms. On some occasions third parties may demand information to which the physician believes they have no right. In some cases other concerns, such as protection of patient confidentiality, must be weighed with the moral demand to be truthful.

Another value is compassion, which means "to suffer with" or "to experience with," along with the inclination to do something to ameliorate the suffering. Fundamental to compassion is empathy, the ability to understand the thoughts and share the feelings of another, without being overwhelmed by those feelings (Reich, 1989). Compassion and empathy improve the competence of the clinician, enabling her to better assess the needs, values, and preferences of the patient. Compassion and empathy are themselves means of healing. Patients who feel known, understood, and cared for can focus on the healing process rather than worrying whether the physician knows what she's doing or being angry that nobody cares. The physician who fails to feel the pain of her patients not only deprives herself of a powerful diagnostic and therapeutic tool, but also denies her own humanity and runs a higher risk of burnout and job dissatisfaction.

Two other values are courage and humility. Courage enables a physician to face a scary situation, make sound judgments, and perform adroit procedures. Humility enables a physician to recognize when she has reached the limitations of her expertise and needs to ask for help. Humility also enables a physician to recognize the limitations of medical science and medical technology so as to avoid hubris. In Carlos's case, the first physician, who had too high an opinion of his ability to take care of Carlos, lacked humility. The second physician, who referred too quickly, lacked courage.

Finally, integrity is the virtue that encompasses all of the other virtues. Integrity is what Polonius had in mind when he advised his son Laertes, "This above all, to thine own self be true" (*Hamlet* I,3). For the physician, integrity requires being faithful to one's own values and to the values of the profession. In addition to the moral values of honesty, compassion, humility, and courage, there are essential medical values to which every physician must ascribe: enhancing health, preventing illness and disability, preserving life, preserving quality of life, and palliating pain and discomfort. These medical values will sometimes conflict and physicians will differ as to the priority given each of them, but professional integrity requires a conscientious effort to be faithful to each of these values. The physician who, for financial gain, told Carlos not to treat his problem was not acting with integrity. He should have disclosed his financial conflict of interest and he should have given Carlos sound medical advice and excellent care.

---

**CASE 26-3**

*Annie Dillon presented to Dr. Lambert with fever, chills, and congestion of the lungs. Dr. Lambert treated her appropriately and, at her request, wrote a note to her employer to indicate that her absence from work was medically justified. The note read as follows: "Annie Dillon was seen in my office today. She was unable to work today because of pneumonia."*

## CONFIDENTIALITY

Most discussions of confidentiality begin with a more dramatic case involving AIDS; alcoholism; a teenager who doesn't want her parents to know that she smokes marijuana or sleeps with her boyfriend; a schoolteacher who is secretly homosexual; a student who is depressed and suicidal; or a husband who goes to a convention, cheats on his wife, and discovers he has a sexually transmitted disease (STD) *after* he has infected his wife. I have intentionally begun this section with a more routine case to make a point: Confidentiality is important in every facet of the practice of medicine, not just the sexy, scary, or scandalous areas.

At first glance, it appears that the physician in Case 26-3 has provided excellent medical care. She did a careful history and physical, ordered the appropriate diagnostic tests, prescribed the right medications, and advised the patient properly regarding rest, diet, and not exposing others to the illness. She judged properly that she was not able to work and was correct in agreeing to write a sickness excuse for her. But she made a serious error in revealing to the employer the nature of the patient's illness.

### The Patient's Employer

Employers have a right to know whether their employees' absences are legitimate. Thus, the physician could have written, "She was unable to work today because of illness." But the precise nature of the illness is a private matter. The reasons for this are obvious in cases of "embarrassing" or taboo illnesses, such as schizophrenia, AIDS, and STDs. Many careers and reputations have been destroyed by the illegitimate release of such information. The movie *Philadelphia* documents one such incident in which a man lost his position with a law firm after it was revealed that he was a homosexual and that he had the AIDS virus. A similar scenario played out in Houston: After discovering that an employee had been infected by the human immunodeficiency virus (HIV), a music company changed its health insurance policy to reduce coverage for HIV from $1 million to $5000 (Holleman *et al.*, 1994). AIDS is not the only taboo: In 1972 Thomas Eagleton was forced off the Democratic presidential ticket after it was revealed that many years previously he had seen a psychiatrist for depression.

At this point the reader may be thinking, "This is all well and good, but certainly none of these disasters could befall Ms. Dillon since, after all, her illness is neither expensive nor socially stigmatic. In fact, by being informed of the precise nature of her illness, and because of the fact that her symptoms are not vague but rather are verifiable, the employer will be assured that she is truly sick and is not malingering. So it is in Ms. Dillon's interest that the physician reveal this information to her employer." This reasoning is specious for several reasons. One is that the employer will become accustomed to being informed of the nature of the illness and when that information is absent will suspect that the employee has an expensive or embarrassing illness (Holleman & Holleman, 1988). Another is that, since pneumonia is a common complication of HIV, even pneumonia could be viewed by a xenophobic employer as a justification for firing or discriminating against an employee.

## The Patient's Family

Another area in which confidentiality must be guarded delicately is in relation to families of patients. Sometimes families want to know what's going on but don't want the patient to know what's going on. Sometimes they don't want the patient to know that they know. If the physician isn't careful to protect boundaries, the diffusion of information can get out-of-hand, more like a soap opera than a textbook case.

In the case of severely ill patients, physicians often prefer to talk with family members: The families may be more lucid and the physician doesn't have to face the angst of the patient. While such an approach may be expedient in terms of time and emotional energy, it is inappropriate as long as the patient is able to communicate with the physician. In some cases, often as a result of cultural traditions, the patient may request that the physician deal directly with a particular family member. Such an approach should not be encouraged and, if adopted, every effort should be made to ensure that the patient was not coerced. The patient's waiver of confidentiality should be expressed in writing and included in the chart.

Patients presenting with STDs often request that their spouses or partners not be informed of the nature of their illnesses. Adolescents seeking treatment related to pregnancy, abortion, STDs, and drugs often make similar requests regarding their parents. The first situation is problematic because the partners are often at risk and the second because the child is still dependent on the parents and the parents are usually footing the bill. Judgments in these cases are often based on the seriousness of the disease, the risk of transmission, the legal reporting requirements, the attitude of the patients, and the degree of trust between physician and patient. Usually the physician will encourage the patient to discuss the matter with the third party, but when persuasive efforts and goodwill fail, the physician is faced with a difficult decision.

Many of these problems can be alleviated by conscientious attention to "preventive ethics" (Mc-Cullough & Ashton, 1994). With regard to adolescents, for example, physicians ought to establish policies of meeting alone with the patient at each visit, as well as meeting with the parent and child together. By following this process in all cases, the parent does not become suspicious when the physician unexpectedly asks the parent to leave the room. Physicians and parents also ought to establish an agreement for treating adolescents whereby the parents allow the adolescent to see the physician privately without requiring patient or physician to report to them. It has become a custom for physicians to treat adolescents for sexual and substance-related problems without insisting on notification of the parents, but an up-front agreement could help prevent many problems caused by secrecy, cover-ups, and the threat of disclosure.

Privacy is particularly important for teenagers. Many will not seek treatment if confidentiality cannot be guaranteed. Many are too embarrassed to reveal their lifestyles to their parents. In many cases embarrassment is but the tip of the iceberg. Many fear physical violence in retaliation for breaking their parents' rules.

For many pregnant teenagers, the father of the child is, well, the father of the child. Or, the stepfather, uncle, a friend of the father's, or some other adult man. A colleague once told me of a case in which a young physician refused to prescribe birth control for a 12-year-old patient, insisting that the girl was too young for sex. Soon thereafter she became pregnant and asked for an abortion. The physician refused to discuss abortion with her and advised her once again to practice abstinence. After the girl delivered the baby she asked once again for birth control. The physician refused and, as before, did not offer a referral. The next time the girl presented to the clinic the physician, a family practice resident, was on another rotation and the girl was assigned a different resident physician. Instead of refusing to discuss sex with the girl outside the presence of her parents, the physician listened and discovered the girl's father to be the father of the baby. As a result of this discovery, the girl's primary physician was placed on probation by the residency program.

As this tragic case illustrates, one purpose of confidentiality is to create a space in which patients feel safe, comfortable, able to be vulnerable, and able to trust their physicians. Only in such an atmosphere will patients reveal embarrassing symptoms, family problems, lifestyle preferences, and other information essential to good medical care.

## Confidentiality as a Cornerstone of the Physician–Patient Relationship

Respect for the patient's privacy is among the oldest and most time-honored traditions in the practice of medicine. The Hippocratic oath regarded medical information as "holy secrets" (Reiser, 1977). More recently, the American Medical Association's Code of Ethics has forbidden the physician from revealing "the confidences entrusted to him in the course of medical attendance, or the deficiencies he may observe in the character of patients, unless he is required to do so by law or unless it becomes necessary in order to protect the welfare of the individual or of the community" (American Medical Association, 1957). As these documents indicate, confidentiality is not simply a "good idea" or "a nice thing we do for our patients." Confidentiality is the cornerstone of the physician-patient relationship. Without it, often there would be no meaningful exchange of information and no effective therapeutic relationship.

## Exceptions

Even so, there may be times when the responsibility to protect the patient's confidentiality must be weighed against other responsibilities. I have already discussed the responsibility of the physician to protect the public's health, as in the case of certain infectious diseases. There may be an ethical obligation, for example, for physicians to notify persons exposed to TB, syphilis, and HIV (Brennan, 1989; Dickens, 1988). The physician's minimum legal obligation is to report the information to the local health department, which in turn notifies endangered parties. The parties are not told the source of their exposure although they often are able to deduce the source.

## WHAT WOULD YOU DO?

*Help! I'm a third-year resident moonlighting at a Doc-in-the-Box in a small town 30 miles from the medical center. A middle-aged man is visiting the clinic for a bad case of athlete's foot. Of greater concern to me, however, is the fact that he's drunk. He has apparently driven himself to the clinic and plans to drive home after the visit. What should I do?*

The famous *Tarasoff* decision (*Tarasoff v. Regents of the University of California*, 1976) dealt with another type of exception, that of a patient who threatens to murder a particular individual. In this case a distraught young man killed his ex-girlfriend after disclosing to his psychiatrist his intention to do so. The psychiatrist had contacted the police but not the young woman. The courts ruled that the psychiatrist had a duty to warn the woman directly. Not every state has made such a strong ruling, and the legal requirements outside California are not yet clear. There does seem to be a consensus among ethicists, however, that in cases where the patient's homicidal threat is specific and there is a reasonable likelihood that the patient will follow through, the physician's ethical obligation to respect the patient's confidentiality is superseded by an ethical obligation to protect the lives of endangered human beings (Cooper, 1982). Thus, notifying both the police and the endangered individual or individuals is in order in such cases.

Of course one problem with notifying potential victims is that they may initiate a preemptive strike and commit a crime themselves. States vary as to the reporting requirements of physicians in this situation, so for legal guidance the medical student is advised to examine his state's laws. For ethical guidance, physicians must rely on their knowledge of the persons involved and on the counsel of colleagues and law enforcement officials. My own experience is that lawyers will advise you to do the minimum legal obligation in order to avoid litigation, but will not advise you regarding the ethically responsible action.

One other area in which traditional views of confidentiality need rethinking is in the large medical center, where the "dyadic" physician–patient relationship is replaced by the patient being cared for by a team of physicians, nurses, and other medical personnel (Holleman *et al.*, 1994; Siegler, 1982). In this atmosphere the patient's medical chart may be read by dozens, even hundreds, of individuals. In academic teaching centers where medical students train, the patient may be examined by a plethora of medical students and the patient's case is often discussed in the hallway, on elevators, and at large conferences. To protect patients and avoid misunderstandings in such situations, the primary physician should inform the patient of the nature of the facility, and should ask the patient's permission for various members of the team, various medical students, and other trainees to examine the patient and to discuss the case.

For their part, medical personnel should refrain from discussing the case in hallways and elevators in a way that others can identify the patient. Persons attending case conferences should be reminded that the anonymity of the patient must be protected outside the confines of the conference room. If presenters or discussants plan to reveal the identity of the patient, pharmaceutical representatives and other persons without professional licenses and fiduciary obligations to protect confidentiality should be asked to leave the conference room before the case discussion begins.

## CASE 26-4

*Blake is a college freshman who presented to the student health center complaining of headaches, a cough, and malaise. The physician, Dr. Aaron, told Blake that it's probably "just a cold" and prescribes fluids, rest, aspirin, and a cough suppressant at bedtime. When Blake returned 1 week later without any improvement and appeared distressed and dejected, Dr. Aaron noted that Blake was facing his first college midterms and took a few minutes to ask Blake about the stressors in his life. Blake refused his offer of a referral to a psychiatrist but returned for weekly follow-up visits. Blake appreciated Dr. Aaron's warm, fatherly manner but the symptoms continued.*

*On the seventh week Blake asked Dr. Aaron for a referral to a specialist and for a sickness excuse to allow him to take incompletes on two of his courses. Dr. Aaron appeared shocked that the "cold" caused Blake to miss so many classes. He signed the sickness excuse but recommended a thorough workup before opting for a referral. The cold agglutinin test was positive, indicating that Blake had mycoplasma pneumonia. Dr. Aaron seemed embarrassed to have missed the diagnosis but told Blake that he had an "atypical presentation" of "a rather rare illness" which is "extremely difficult to diagnose." He prescribed erythromycin and in 3 days the symptoms resolved completely.*

*Meanwhile, two of Blake's roommates have gone home for the winter holidays with "colds" and seen their local physicians, each of whom quickly diagnoses the problem as mycoplasma pneumonia.*

## TRUTH-TELLING

Until recently, physicians routinely withheld the truth from their patients in a number of areas, such as a diagnosis of cancer, a poor prognosis, and any risks and side effects of treatment that might scare the patient from taking the treatment. Many physicians also hid their mistakes from their patients. Physicians believed that patients did not have the mental or emotional wherewithal to "take" the truth—at least when the truth hurt. In reality, it was the physician who felt uncomfortable with truth, particularly if the truth meant that the patient was dying or that the physician had failed the patient.

In Case 26-4, the physician makes a mistake that hampers a young student's college career. Dr. Aaron then makes a second mistake: He lies to the patient in an effort to cover the first mistake. Dr. Aaron's justification for the lie is that he does not want Blake, the patient, to lose confidence in his abilities. After all, confidence is an important ingredient in healing. The real reason, however, is that he feels guilty for the harm he caused Blake and too embarrassed to reveal his shortcomings as a physician. He also fears that Blake might become angry and that his parents might sue.

Now that Blake and his family know that Dr. Aaron has lied, Blake might indeed sue. After all, Dr. Aaron missed a diagnosis that most would have made, this mistake harmed the patient, and then Dr. Aaron lied to cover his mistake. Lying to clients and patients is clearly a violation of the professional's fiduciary obligations. Like many physicians, Dr. Aaron underestimated the ability of his patients to accept his shortcomings, to forgive his mistakes, and to recognize that physicians are, after all, mere mortals. He underestimated his patient's ability to uncover the truth. He had a good relationship with Blake yet, like many physicians and attorneys, underestimated the influence of that relationship in preventing litigation (Garr & Marsh, 1986).

And even if Blake's parents had sued, which they have every right to do, this would not in any way change the fact that the only morally decent thing to do is to disclose one's error to one's patient, to apologize, and, if possible, to make restitution (Peterson & Brennan, 1990). There may be exceptions, such as when the errors are minor or when the errors cause the patient no harm. When the errors are serious, patients have a right to know and physicians have an ethical obligation to tell them. Many attorneys will counsel otherwise, but their job is to tell you your minimal legal obligations, not to tell you the right or even the minimally decent thing to do. Nor is it their job to tell you how to be a good person or a virtuous physician. Most ethicists, and most everyone else, would agree that the minimally decent thing to *be* is to be honest.

### Trust and Confidence

An essential component of an effective physician–patient relationship—or of any successful relationship, for that matter—is trust. Relationships, both personal and professional, are built on the faith that the other can be trusted to tell the truth, to keep promises, to abide by agreed-on ways of doing things.

In the physician–patient relationship, honesty is essential. If the physician cannot trust the patient to tell the truth about symptoms, habits, and lifestyle, as well as willingness to follow the physician's recommenda-

## WHAT WOULD YOU DO?

*Help! I'm a second-year pediatrics resident doing a rural elective in south Texas. I'm 3 days into the rotation and this morning my attending reviewed my charts and told me I'm not prescribing enough medications. "Mothers like to go out of here with a prescription or sample in hand. That way they feel we're doing something for them. If we don't do something for them, they'll find another doctor who will." My impression after 3 days is that these children take far too many medications. Now I'm seeing an 8-year-old girl who is sad and has a tummy ache because her kitten just died. The attending wants me to prescribe antidepressants and antacids. What should I do?*

tions and the side effects of treatment, the physician's best efforts will be stymied. If the patient cannot trust the physician to tell the truth about the nature of the illness or the risks and side effects of treatment, the patient will be less likely to follow the physician's recommendations. Also, an effective placebo will be wasted, as the patient will not place confidence in the healing powers of the physician (Brody, 1980).

Interestingly enough, the terms *confidence* and *confide* stem from the same root, *fidere*, which means trust or faith. To have confidence in a particular physician or healer, one must feel willing and able to confide in that healer. Patients are not likely to confide in persons they cannot trust, in persons they do not deem trust*worthy*. Healthcare professionals earn that confidence and trust through accumulating a steady track record of being honest with their patients. This requires resisting the temptation to avoid telling patients bad news. It requires resisting the temptation to mislead the patient by watering down the bad news.

## Combining Truth with Empathy

It also requires, however, the art of telling the patient bad news in such a way that the patient does not abandon all hope. Physicians and healers who care deeply about their patients not only will want patients to understand the nature and severity of their illness but also will want them to sense that their physicians will not abandon them, that they will receive the best care possible, and that, although "hope" and "good outcome" may need to be redefined, there is always a basis for hope (Kubler-Ross, 1970). Good physicians recognize that patients need to hear the truth and that this might make them depressed. But the best physicians will assist the patients through the depression in such a way as to prevent their reaching a state of utter despair. The best physicians do not shirk from their responsibility to tell their patients the truth, nor do they blast out the bad news, leave the room, and leave the patients devastated by the truth. When the truth is told in a sensitive manner, the physician's voice can be an agent of healing even while the words themselves bring unpleasant news.

Combining truth with empathy is important for all types of physician–patient communications. If a patient with metastatic cancer asks you if she is going to die, you could simply say "yes" and fulfill your obligation to tell your patients the truth. But you would be shirking other responsibilities, such as the responsibility to be a healer and to ease suffering. Here's a better response: "I hope you live a long time, and I'm going to do what I can to help that happen. But I think you ought to know that most patients in your condition live for a shorter time, a few months. Either way, I'm going to be here to help. To help you live as long as you can and, when that's no longer in the cards, to help you be as comfortable as possible." For many patients, the fear of being abandoned is as great as the fear of dying. If the patient feels she can't trust her physician to tell her the truth, then she is unlikely to trust her to be there when she needs her.

Patients with diabetes mellitus, heart disease, and other chronic illnesses often become frustrated with the inconveniences, discomforts, and disabilities caused by their illness. A common defense mechanism is to deny the illness exists and to quit taking medications, or to take them sporadically. Physicians must be frank with these patients in pointing out that their illness is hidden but real and in confronting them regarding the outcome of not taking their medications. Even so, such bad news can be told in a caring manner. Begin by acknowledging their suffering: "I can't imagine the pain, the discomfort, the expense, the inconvenience, and the frustration of living with this disease." Continue by joining with them in their denial: "If I were in your situation I think I'd do just what you're doing. I'd try my damnedest to wish it away." Or: "As your physician and friend, I wish to goodness I could wave a wand and make this illness, this curse, go away. I've seen how it hurts my patients and I wish I could do more to help." Pause to listen to the patient's response. And truly listen: Don't pretend to listen while composing your next lines. In an indirect way, you've already addressed the patient's denial, and this may be sufficient to help the patient work through the denial. But a direct confrontation will often be necessary. "You're not going to like hearing this, but as your physician it's my responsibility to remind you that you've got a serious disease and it's going to kill you if you don't take your medications."

Sometimes physicians are reticent to discuss bad news because they aren't sure how extensively the patient wants to talk about "it." What commonly happens in these situations is that physicians, nurses, patients, and families do a very clumsy dance, dancing around "it." Nobody wants to give "it" a name. One way to break the ice is simply to acknowledge what is happening: "We could go on and on dancing around the truth, talking about 'it,' smoothing things over, or we could just come on out and say what we're thinking. My experience has been that, even though it's painful at first, most patients prefer to get things out in the open. They don't want me hiding things from them. I assume that this is how you feel too, is it?" Most studies show that physicians, not patients, are the ones who feel uncomfortable talking about death, cancer, and all the other "its" and who project this anxiety onto their patients (Edinger & Smucker, 1992). My experience has been that, despite the sting, patients feel relieved to finally know the truth so they can begin dealing with it.

Many medical students feel uncomfortable talking with patients who have terminal illnesses or disabling injuries, or with parents whose children are found to have serious illness, mental retardation, or physical disability. A good way to break the ice is to greet the patient by naming the "it": "Good afternoon, Mrs. Shah. How is the cancer treating you today?" Another technique is to disclose the discomfort: "I feel uncomfortable asking you these questions so soon after you've heard some very disappointing news, but there are a few things we have to talk about if we are to provide the best care possible for your child."

## When the Patient Is in Denial

Sometimes the problem will not be that the physician has withheld the truth from the patient, but that the patient has not heard it. A common defense mechanism for dealing with devastating information is denial. This is a natural, healthy way to avert shock, to allow for time to process the information gradually (Weisman, 1972).

Except in emergency situations in which decisions must be made immediately, patient and family should be given time to absorb the information, to ask questions, and to get used to this new state of affairs. Treatment decisions can usually be delayed a few days, even weeks. During this time the patient might quite rationally seek a second opinion or a repeat of the diagnostic test. Physicians in this situation often feel that their expertise is being questioned or their authority undermined. Such a feeling reflects the physician's failure to recognize that cognitive denial is a normal, healthy reaction. Denial is a means of avoiding shock and reflects the patient's desire to maintain health and independence. It is also quite rational: X-rays do get switched from time to time, physicians have been known to misread EKGs and EEGs, and many tests commonly produce false positives.

Rather than becoming angry with such patients or attempting to bludgeon them with the truth by insisting that the diagnosis is correct and that they must "take or leave" the recommended treatment, the physician should encourage the patient to seek a second opinion or, in some cases, a repeat of the test. Verifying the diagnosis is the first step toward accepting the reality of the illness and what must be done to treat it.

---

### CASE 26-5

*Mr. Martin Salgo presented to a surgeon, Dr. Frank Gerbode, appearing older than his 55 years and reporting leg cramps, hip pain, and pain in the lower right quadrant while walking and exercising.*

*Dr. Gerbode concluded that Mr. Salgo had "probable occlusion of the abdominal aorta which had impaired blood supply to the legs and other areas and advanced arteriosclerosis." Dr. Gerbode recommended x-rays of the GI tract and aortic angiography, the injection of a radiopaque dye into the aorta to visualize the plaque formation and confirm the diagnosis. Dr. Gerbode told Mr. Salgo that the procedure would be done under general anesthesia, but did not explain the possible complications of anesthesia or aortography. Mr. Salgo consented to the procedure. The day following the procedure Mr. Salgo awoke paralyzed in his lower extremities. The paralysis, caused by a hematoma pressing against the spine, proved to be permanent (Salgo v. Leland Stanford, Jr. University Board of Trustees, 1957).*

## INFORMED CONSENT

When people get sick, they commonly experience a loss of control and feel that their privacy and personal integrity have been violated. This vulnerability is related to a number of factors, including the patient's weakness, the nature of hospitals and of medical and surgical tests and treatments, and the insensitivity of some caregivers. As students begin their medical training, it is important for them to appreciate the vulnerability of patients and the need to protect their right to self-determination as expressed through the principle of autonomy and guaranteed by the practice of informed consent to treatment.

For an informed consent to be valid the patient or his proxy must give consent. Yet there are times when the physician, for whatever reason, fails to obtain that consent. In Case 26-1, Ms. Little's oncologist and surgeon conspired with her daughter to have her breast amputated without her knowledge or consent. In past years some obstetricians tied the Fallopian tubes of indigent or mentally ill women without their consent, permanently sterilizing them. Sometimes burn patients have painful treatments forced on them (*Please Let Me Die*, 1974). Sometimes busy physicians *tell* their patients what they're going to do to them rather than offering their recommendation and awaiting the patient's consent before initiating treatment. Such actions are wrong, both legally and ethically, as indicated by a landmark ruling in 1914 by the New York Supreme Court: "Every human being of adult years and of sound mind has the right to determine what shall be done with his own body, and a surgeon who performs an operation without his patient's consent commits an assault for which he is liable in damages" (*Schloendorff v. Society of New York Hospital*, 1914).

In Case 26-5, Mr. Salgo clearly gave his consent, a point that Dr. Gerbode's attorneys felt sufficient to meet the legal requirements. Yet the jury awarded Mr. Salgo a large sum of money, ruling the consent invalid because Dr. Gerbode had failed to warn the patient of the risk of paralysis. Perhaps Dr. Gerbode considered the risk too minimal to mention. Perhaps he feared that Mr. Salgo might be frightened from going through with the procedure. Or perhaps Dr. Gerbode simply didn't feel he had any obligation to share this information with the patient. There certainly had been no legal precedent for doing so, at least not until then. The jury in this case established an important legal precedent in claiming that the physician must not only get the patient's consent but also that the consent must be an *informed* decision:

> A physician violates his duty to his patient and subjects himself to liability if he withholds any facts which are necessary to form the basis of an intelligent consent by the patients to the proposed treatment. Likewise the physician may not minimize the known dangers of a procedure or operation in order to induce his patient's consent (*Salgo v. Leland Stanford, Jr. University Board of Trustees*, 1957).

## Elements of Informed Consent

For the consent to be truly *informed*, what information should be given the patient? First, the patient should be told the nature of his condition. Is it life-threatening? How will it affect his work, his lifestyle, his future? What pain, suffering, disability, or disfigurement might possibly result from this disease or injury? Second, the physician should describe the major recommended treatments for the patient's condition. What are the benefits of each treatment? What are the risks? What are the discomforts and other possible side effects? What are the costs? Third, the physician should describe the likely benefits, risks, discomforts, and

**Table 26.1**
Elements of Informed Consent

| The nature of the patient's condition | Recommended treatment(s) | Nontreatment |
|---|---|---|
| Whether the condition is life-threatening | Benefits | Benefits |
| Anticipated pain, disability, disfigurement | Risks, discomfort, and other side effects | Risks, discomfort, and other side effects |
| | Costs | Potential costs |

side effects of nontreatment. A patient who refuses a Pap smear, for example, should be informed of her risk of cervical cancer and of the seriousness of that disease (*Truman v. Thomas*, 1980). These three elements are presented in Table 26.1.

## Exceptions

There are, of course, a few exceptional situations in which the obligation to initiate a test or treatment supersedes the obligation to obtain informed consent. In medical emergencies in which the patient's life or health is in danger and consent cannot be obtained from the patient or next of kin in a timely fashion, the physician should presume that the patient wishes to be treated aggressively. In situations in which children are in distress as a result of an injury or illness and the parents cannot be reached in a timely fashion, the physician should presume that the parents would want the condition treated in accordance with the standard of care rather than prolonging the suffering of the child. During public health emergencies, vaccines and quarantines may be required by law.

In some cases a patient may choose to waive her right to make an informed decision, turning the decision over to a relative or to her physician. Physicians should discourage this practice and should evaluate and address the underlying cause of the patient's unwillingness to decide for herself. The potential for abuse by paternalistic physicians and coercive family members makes this situation an ethical and legal quagmire. Physicians whose patients waive this right despite counseling should ask the patient to document the waiver in writing or should ask a colleague to witness the verbal waiver.

In the past some physicians have withheld information from patients by invoking the so-called therapeutic privilege. In these cases the physician believes the very attempt to gain informed consent will have serious health-related consequences for the patient. A commonly cited example involves a patient who is depressed, suicidal, and is found to have cancer. Oftentimes the issue is less a fear of suicide than fear that the patient will not choose the therapy the physician thinks the patient needs. The consensus among ethicists is that physicians should seldom, if ever, invoke therapeutic privilege, particularly if for paternalistic fears that the patient will not select the physician's recommendation. The reluctance to gain an informed consent usually reflects the physician's insecurity rather than the patient's and perhaps also unwillingness or incompetence to treat an underlying depression. Even in rare cases where, despite psychiatric treatment, the patient truly is at serious risk of suicide, the testing or treatment often can be delayed a few days or weeks until the patient is able to make an informed decision. In cases where the patient is incompetent to make an informed decision and unlikely to become competent in the near future, the physician should gain an informed consent from the patient's designated agent or next of kin (Faden & Beauchamp, 1986).

## Common Mistakes

Despite the wide ethical and legal acceptance of the patient's right to informed consent for tests and treatments, physicians often fail to respect this right. One of the most common mistakes is that the physician bypasses the competent patient and talks instead with the family. She may do this because she feels uncomfortable being with seriously ill or dying patients. Others lack the patience to communicate with feeble or confused patients who speak softly and slowly, or who may need to have information repeated several times.

Sometimes physicians fail to get a truly informed consent because they fail to explain the information in a way the patient can understand. Medical students can be particularly guilty of this mistake, as they are in the process of mastering a new vocabulary and forget that patients do not know the same jargon, nor do they have the same understanding of disease processes or treatment regimens. I advise students to imagine that the patient is a brother or grandfather or someone else whom one knows well, and to try to communicate the information to him in a way he'll understand. It is also best to ask the patient to explain to you, in his own words, what he hears you saying: what the options are, what the risks and benefits are, and what he wants to do to treat his illness.

Some physicians are guilty of "leading the witness." This occurs when a physician presents a biased version of the information that the patient will use to make her decision. For example, the physician omits or minimizes the risks of Treatment A and omits or minimizes the benefits of Treatment B. Or, the physician may include the pertinent information but may insinuate by voice inflection, word choice, or body language that the risks of Treatment B are more dangerous than the risks of Treatment A, when actually this is not the case: "Mrs. Honda, if you go with Treatment A, the only thing you have to worry about is a myocardial infarction, which most of our patients don't even get, but [lowering voice, speaking slower, and adopting a somber expression] if you choose Treatment B, I'm afraid there is a very real chance you'd develop AN IRREGU-LAR HEARTBEAT. During the first 2 weeks of treatment you might also break out with SOME VERY UNSIGHTLY PINK AND WHITE SPLOTCHES ON YOUR FACE." The physician in this case should have explained the term *myocardial infarction* or used a familiar term, such as *heart attack*. The physician also should have given a more accurate impression of the relative odds and seriousness of each risk.

Some physicians are diligent in getting the patient's consent for the most invasive procedures but forget that every medication and every diagnostic test involves discomforts and risks that ought to be explained to the patient. Some physicians mistakenly believe that getting the patient's signature on an informed consent form is all that is required. Actually, informed consent is a verbal communication between physician and patient. The patient's signature on the form is merely a legal record that the physician discussed the pertinent information with the patient, the patient understood it, and the patient freely decided to accept or refuse recommended tests or treatments.

Some physicians fail to inform patients of costs of recommended tests or treatments. Many prescriptions are never filled for this reason. Physicians often accuse these patients of being "noncompliant," but the real issue is that the patient was never given the opportunity to make an informed consent to treatment. Some physicians err by failing to inform patients of legitimate alternative treatments. For example, a patient with a back problem should be informed not only of the allopathic medical standards of care, but also of the legitimate chiropractic alternatives. Some physicians fail to inform their patients of the risks and benefits of

---

## WHAT WOULD YOU DO?

*Help! I'm a second-year student on my medicine rotation at the public hospital. This afternoon I was about to enter the room of my patient to take a history, when I overheard the following conversation inside:*

*"We're not going to kill you! I promise we won't kill you! Just sign the form. We need your signature on the form."*

*—"I don't know. What are you going to do?"*

*"We're not going to do anything but take a biopsy. But you've gotta sign."*

*—"Let me get my daughter. She'll be here this afternoon."*

*"I just told you it's nothing. You think were going to kill you. We're not going to kill you. We're just going to take a little biopsy. I've gotta get your signature now, because I need to get outta here and go home."*

*As it turned out, it was not my patient but my patient's roommate. The doctor was an intern on the 16th hour of his call. What should I do?*

nontreatment. For many years, Dr. Thomas recommended that Mrs. Cobbs have a Pap smear test. Each time she refused. After Mrs. Cobbs died of cervical cancer, her children sued, and won. The court ruled that the patient must be informed of "the risks of a decision *not* to undergo treatment" as well as the "risks inherent in the procedure ... and the probability of a successful outcome of the treatment" (*Truman v. Thomas*, 1980). Having dealt with Pap smears every day, Dr. Thomas assumed incorrectly that most patients knew what they were and how they helped prevent deaths caused by cancer.

## Competence

Physicians often falsely label certain types of patients as incompetent. We have already discussed one such type: the weak, feeble patient who talks slowly, barely audibly, and who may need to have information repeated two or three times before understanding it. Another type of patient often incorrectly labeled as incompetent is the person with disabilities. This is the result of the physician's inexperience with and prejudice toward persons who are blind, deaf and dumb, mildly retarded, or severely physically disabled.

Other patients often treated as incompetent include those who speak a foreign language or come from a culture with which the physician is unfamiliar. I recall one incident in which our medical team entered the room of a 95-year-old patient who had just been admitted from a local nursing home, heard him speaking "gibberish," and therefore assumed him to be incompetent to make medical decisions. Thus, the team did not attempt to inform him of the nature of his condition and the risks, benefits, and costs of treatment. Nor did they obtain his consent for treatment. Later the team learned that the patient was a Jewish immigrant from Russia. They also learned from a psychology consultant that in times of crisis patients often seek strength in the language of their youth or the language that bears religious significance for them. This patient may have been speaking Russian, Hebrew, Yiddish, or all three. Rather than the "gibberish" being an indication of incompetence, it may have indicated just the opposite: the patient's intelligence, his facility for many languages, and his ability, unlike that of the medical team, to have functioned throughout his life in multicultural settings and also to engage the religious as well as the medical meaning of suffering.

Physicians should presume that their patients are competent unless there is strong evidence to suggest otherwise. Patients who cannot communicate, who cannot understand basic facts, who cannot reason consistent with a personal value, who because of depression or anxiety cannot bring themselves to make any decisions, or who cannot stick with a decision are the types who may legitimately be viewed as incompetent. It should be emphasized that the definition of being unable to communicate is a narrow one: If a paralyzed patient can move her eyeballs once to indicate "yes" and twice to indicate "no," then she should not be considered unable to communicate. It should also be emphasized that patients who make decisions based on deeply held personal values should not be judged incompetent even if the physician dislikes those values. For example, a patient who refuses chemotherapy because he believes "the Lord will heal me" is not incompetent, nor is a patient who states that he believes in the healing power of "a strict macrobiotic diet." Even the patient who refuses chemotherapy because he doesn't want his hair to fall out may be deciding on the basis of a deeply held personal value.

On the other hand, the patient who refuses chemotherapy because he believes "the Viet Cong have poisoned all the medicines" is basing his decision on a psychotic delusion, not on a deeply held personal value, and such a patient should not be viewed as competent to make an informed decision. For such patients a proxy decision-maker should be identified. If the patient did not designate such a decision-maker prior to losing competence, then his spouse or partner, parents, adult children, siblings, or closest friends should be consulted.

### CASE 26-6

*Jackie Thomas, a 26-year-old teacher's aide at a children's day care center, presented to her family physician with lower abdominal pain. She had suffered this pain intermittently throughout her adult life and began seeing Dr. Amin 1 year ago to address the problem. During that time Dr.*

*Amin performed a complete gastrointestinal workup, with no medical findings, and became con-vinced that the pain related to the molestation Jackie suffered as a child. It had taken Jackie most of that year to gather the courage to tell Dr. Amin about the sexual abuse; he was the first person she had ever told.*

*Dr. Amin told Jackie that her pain could be healed through psychotherapy. Jackie agreed and said she was ready to do the work. He asked Jackie to call the number on the back of her health plan card. Jackie called the number, explained the general nature of her problem, and was told she would need to wait 2–3 months and would then be assigned a psychotherapist, allowed six visits, and that her copayment would be $40 rather than the $10 for medical visits. With an income of $23,000 per year and two children to raise alone, the copayment presented a formidable barrier for Jackie. Jackie had anticipated being given a choice of psychotherapists; she did not feel comfortable telling her story to just anybody. And, Jackie worried that six visits might just be long enough to reopen her wounds. Jackie had selected this plan because it included mental health coverage. Now that she realized the limitations of the coverage, she became frustrated, hopeless, and depressed. She decided to keep seeing Dr. Amin and to treat her pain with medication.*

*One month later Jackie learned that her employer was in the process of switching managed care plans. Dr. Amin called and discovered that in 3 months Jackie would no longer be able to see him. Dr. Amin called to request that the new provider add him to their list of approved providers, but was told they were currently full.*

*Faced with the prospect of starting over with a new physician, Jackie's depression worsened and she missed several days of work. She was fired by her employer, lost her health insurance, lost her apartment, and moved into a shelter for homeless, battered, and abused women.*

## MANAGED CARE

Events such as those described in Case 26-6 have occurred much too often in recent years: a physician works to gain the trust of a patient; the patient begins to respond; then all that work goes down the drain when they discover the needed therapy is not covered or the patient must switch to another physician. Such a situation can be extremely frustrating for the physician. He spends more time on the phone and filling out forms than seeing patients. He is unable to establish long-term relationships with patients and follow them from womb to tomb. He is powerless to get his patients the help they need. He wonders what attracted him to medicine, and begins to think about switching professions.

Such a situation is even more devastating for the patient. She needs continuity of care to address a chronic condition, but is forced to treat her problem with episodic acute care. When she started her new job 1 year ago and signed up for a health plan, she made a personal commitment to address her chronic problem. She felt safe with Dr. Amin and began to believe she was on the road to recovery. Now she feels the rug pulled out from under her and does not know when she will dare to hope and trust again.

The best situations in life are "win–win." This one, unfortunately, is a "lose–lose," not only for physician and patient, but also for society as a whole. Most of the progress made over the past year has been squandered, and now Jackie is unemployed, homeless, and depressed. Even if Jackie recovered her courage and got a new job and a new apartment, she must start over with a new physician, logging many hours in a physician's office while he or she repeats the work Dr. Amin already completed. She may never get the counseling she needs to address her underlying problem. Clearly, the cost of *not* providing psychotherapy and continuity of care is but a fraction of the cost deferred to society. Yet it is not in the interest of Jackie's original health plan to address chronic problems: the board and stockholders know that their patients will be in another plan before any savings will be realized, so they pass these costs on to society.

It is tempting to frame managed care as the villain of this disastrous scenario. After all, the managed care plan is failing to provide the patient what she needs to be healed and is causing iatrogenic harm by pushing her and her physicians through revolving doors of bureaucracy and denial of care. Yet many of the problems described in this scenario existed in the fee-for-service system as well, and may have been created by the fee-for-service system (Holleman *et al.*, 1997).

First, in the fee-for-service system, poor patients were routinely denied care because they could not afford insurance and lacked an ability to pay. Managed care has attempted to make healthcare more affordable for the working poor. We may disagree with the areas they have chosen to cut costs, but must acknowledge that managed care is attempting to address the injustices of the fee-for-service system by making healthcare more affordable.

Second, some critics will charge that under managed systems the physician's fiduciary obligations to the patient are compromised by competing obligations to business managers and payment policies. This is true, but under the fee-for-service system such obligations did not exist since many physicians simply refused to treat poor patients. They chose to accept no obligations at all to poor patients. Most would agree that, for those unable to afford healthcare under the fee-for-service system, a situation of competing obligations is morally superior to a situation of no obligations at all.

Third, many managed systems give physicians financial incentives to keep costs down. Some charge that physicians who participate in such plans have compromised their integrity by accepting financial incentives to undertreat their patients. Lest we forget, in the fee-for-service system physicians benefited from financial incentives to overtreat their patients. The costs of medical care skyrocketed, creating a privileged class of wealthy physicians and a disenfranchised class of working Americans who could not afford healthcare. This created the public demand for more affordable healthcare.

Fourth, some critics point to cases such as Jackie's to illustrate how managed care and employment-based health coverage have failed to provide continuity of care to patients with chronic conditions. The constant changes in managed systems and in our employment environment are indeed problems that need to be addressed by making coverage more portable, and significant progress is being made in this area. But lest we forget, if continuous and comprehensive care were such important values in U.S. medicine, why did we allow to develop "a specialist-dominated fee-for-service system in which so many patients lacked a primary-care physician?" (Holleman *et al.*, 1997).

In weighing their responsibilities to patients like Jackie, physicians should consider four questions. The first involves harms and benefits. Switching physicians in midstream constitutes a harm, particularly for patients with chronic or sensitive conditions. For patients suffering pain, depression, anxiety, relational difficulties, and other effects of sexual trauma, psychotherapy is clearly a benefit.

The second involves the patient's values and preferences, often referred to as *patient autonomy*. In this case the patient made a conscious choice: to discover and address the underlying cause of her symptoms; to work with Dr. Amin as her primary care physician and coordinator of her care; and to seek the additional help of a psychotherapist for healing of the trauma of sexual abuse. These choices seem reasonable enough, yet Jackie's health plan does not allow her to make these choices.

The third involves fairness. To expect a health plan to cover expensive treatments of marginal or questionable value is unfair to others paying into the system. But to expect a health plan to cover appropriate, reasonably priced treatments with a high likelihood of benefit seems fair indeed. Not to cover such benefits, while deferring the cost to future health plans and to society, and causing harm to the patient, seems unfair.

The fourth area involves the physician's personal and professional values. One such value is honesty. In the past some managed plans forbade their physicians from telling patients about treatments not covered under their plan. Gag orders are now illegal in most states (Miller, 1997), but at the time Dr. Amin was struggling with this case he faced a difficult decision: whether to tell Jackie that what she needed was psychotherapy and that she ought to find a health plan that included psychotherapy, or whether to treat her with psychotropic medications alone. From an ethical perspective, the obligation to tell the truth to one's patients outweighs the obligation to protect the self-interest of the managed care company, particularly when the benefits to the patient are clear and when corporate profits are high (Holleman *et al.*, 2000). Other relevant values include compassion and courage. Physicians should feel sympathy for their patient's condition and have the desire to do what they can to heal it. In their role as advocates, they should have the courage to challenge unfair or irrational policies that prevent her from getting the care she needs.

Based on these four ethical considerations, it is clear that physicians faced with patients such as Jackie should make every reasonable effort to provide continuity of care and access to psychotherapy. In his role as patient advocate, Dr. Amin should pursue the matter up the chain of command to the medical director of the managed plan. If efforts by phone fail, a letter presenting the four points specified above can help document the case and encourage the health managers to reconsider the rationality, prudence, and medical and ethical justification of their decision to deny coverage of psychotherapy. With Jackie's permission, a letter to her employer identifying her major needs—continuity of care and psychotherapy—might also be in order.

If efforts to provide continuity of care and psychotherapy through Jackie's managed plan and her employer fail, her physician still has at least three remaining obligations. The first is to find some form of affordable counseling for Jackie. Some agencies offer free or sliding scale counseling services. Many ministers are trained in pastoral counseling. Some women's shelters and other organizations provide group therapy for sexually traumatized women. Most communities offer support groups and 12-step groups that are free of charge.

Dr. Amin's second obligation is to ease Jackie's transition from one primary care physician to another. He can help her identify a physician with whom she would feel comfortable and who would have the knowledge and skills to address her problem effectively. With Jackie's permission, Dr. Amin can call the physician and/or write a letter reviewing the course of her care and specifying her needs as a patient. He can send the new physician a copy of her medical records and offer to be available by phone if any questions arise.

Third, physicians working in managed care plans have a moral obligation to address the systemic cause of problems affecting their patients. They can work within professional organizations and political structures to reform the injustices affecting their patients. They can challenge gag orders and rationing by exhaustion. In this case, Dr. Amin can lobby for reasonable mental health coverage and portability of care.

There is no guarantee that these additional efforts would prevent Jackie's depression, unemployment, and homelessness, but failure to make these efforts makes her physician partially responsible for the disastrous turn of events in Jackie's life.

---

## WHAT WOULD YOU DO?

*I'm a third-year medical student doing my family practice rotation. One of the requirements is to do a home visit and write a home visit report. I was asked to visit Ms. Sparrowhawk, a 55-year-old woman with diabetes whose foot wounds have not healed since surgery 9 weeks ago. She is in danger of losing the foot. I visited her yesterday afternoon.*

*At first she was pleasant but vague about her medical problems. Then when I asked her about her family situation she broke down and sobbed for 5 minutes. She said she had felt confused ever since her husband died a year ago. She told me she hasn't filled any of the prescriptions since she left the hospital. Nor had she been monitoring her glucose or eating properly. She could not recall the name of her physician. She said she saw a different one every time she went to the medical center, and they all looked like they were still wet behind the ears. What should I do?*

*Tom Edwards, a 78-year-old man with advanced Alzheimer's disease, presented to Dr. Wycliff, his longtime physician, with cough, sore throat, and pneumonia. Dr. Wycliff treated Mr. Edwards with fluids and cough syrup but, in accordance with the wishes expressed by Mr. Edwards prior to becoming demented, did not prescribe antibiotics. Dr. Wycliff then called a family conference at the nursing home where Mr. Edwards lived.*

*Mr. Edwards's oldest son demanded that his father be given antibiotics and admitted to the local hospital where he could be placed in an ICU and receive "the best care possible." Dr. Wycliff explained that Mr. Edwards had asked to be allowed to die when his Alzheimer's reached an advanced stage. When the son continued to object, Dr. Wycliff showed him a copy of his father's Living Will and explained that as a physician he was legally bound to comply with this request. He explained that Mr. Edwards no longer remembered who he was and that his condition was irreversible. Dr. Wycliff also explained that Mr. Edwards had been concerned not to spend his wife and children's inheritance. Mrs. Edwards affirmed that this had been her husband's wish and that she was ready to "let him go."*

*The second son said it was a disgrace that their father, who had once been such a friendly, outgoing member of the community, should be spending the last days of his life in an institutional setting. "Let's bring him home. If it's too much for mom to handle, we sons can rotate shifts to care for him 'round the clock." Dr. Wycliff acknowledged that many patients prefer to die at home but Mr. Edwards had requested that once his Alzheimer's reached an advanced stage he wanted to stay in a nursing home where he could maintain as much anonymity as possible. "He wanted his friends to remember him the way he used to be," commented Mrs. Edwards. "And he doesn't remember anything about the house or neighborhood anymore, or recognize who we are."*

*The youngest son, who had been closest to his father, asked whether some drug could be given to end his father's suffering: "I can't bear to see him this way." Dr. Wycliff and Mrs. Edwards agreed that, as a devout Baptist, Mr. Edwards probably viewed suicide as a sin. Dr. Wycliff explained that cough syrup and other medications could provide symptomatic relief and that he would give as much medicine as necessary to relieve pain, but that with advanced Alzheimer's Mr. Edwards probably felt little pain. Moreover, Mr. Edwards would most likely die very soon. Dr. Wycliff commented that the real pain was for those who had to watch him die. There was a long silence, then one by one family members held Mr. Edwards's hand, cried, and recalled the good times they had had together.*

*Two days later Mr. Edwards died in the nursing home, his youngest son holding his hand and his dog Pete at his side. The family asked Dr. Wycliff to read Mr. Edwards's eulogy at the funeral, which was attended by hundreds of Mr. Edwards's neighbors, co-workers, relatives, and friends, each of whom remembered Tom Edwards as a friendly, outgoing member of the community.*

## DEATH, DYING, AND DECISION-MAKING

One of the most difficult areas of ethical decision-making for patients, physicians, and families involves serious illness and death. Pain, suffering, loss of control, fear of the unknown, anticipation of loss, grief, guilt, and the life review process all evoke strong feelings at a time when difficult decisions must be made. To help ease the decision-making process, the following framework may be useful: prevention, clarification, and review.

### Step 1. Prevention

Ethicists, like emergency room physicians, thrive on "three alarm" situations, but most of the more dramatic ethical dilemmas, like most medical emergencies, can and should be prevented. It is the physician's responsibility to help the patient anticipate and prepare for the future. The patient's primary care physician should ask the patient about his values and preferences regarding life, death, and end-of-life choices. These conversations should be documented in the chart and, where appropriate, shared with family members and close friends. The physician should also encourage the patient to consider writing an advance directive and assigning someone as a Durable Power of Attorney for Health Care.

Advance directives, or living wills, give the patient an opportunity to express, in writing, his wishes regarding end-of-life treatment should the patient become terminally ill, incapacitated, and unable to express his preferences (see Fig. 26.1). Advance directives apply only to situations in which the patient has no reasonable hope of recovery; they do not apply to acute situations such as a car accident or bullet wound in which aggressive treatment might save the life of the patient and return him to good health. Physicians should encourage patients to indicate, verbally and in writing, any specific concerns. For example, some patients who do not want to be placed on respirators or given antibiotics may still wish, for religious or other reasons, to receive food and fluids.

Once the advance directive is signed and witnessed, it is legally binding although it can be revoked at any time. Physicians should encourage patients to submit copies for their clinic and hospital charts and to give copies to close friends, relatives, and clergy.

Sometimes family members ask physicians to continue providing curative treatments in violation of the expressed will of their loved one. Sometimes physicians feel uncomfortable complying with patients' requests for no heroic treatment. The purpose of the advance directive is to protect the patient from well-meaning but misdirected physicians and family members, such as Mr. Edwards's sons.

Like the Durable Power of Attorney, which enables a person to assign someone as proxy for legal and financial decisions should he become incapacitated, the Durable Power of Attorney for Health Care enables a patient to assign someone as a proxy for medical decisions (see Fig. 26.2). Many end-of-life decisions are difficult to anticipate, and the advance directive is so general that physicians should encourage patients to complete this document, even if they have also written an advance directive. This way the patient is assured that, if he should become incapacitated, his medical decisions will be made by someone who knows his values and preferences well. The physician should encourage the patient to discuss his values and preferences with his proxy decision-maker so that the proxy will indeed know what to do and will have the courage to make tough decisions if and when the time comes. The physician should also encourage the patient to assign a backup proxy; after all, the patient might outlive the proxy, or the proxy might be out of town or for some other reason unavailable.

Whenever a patient is hospitalized or admitted to a nursing home, the physician and patient should discuss code status. This will be a stressful time for the patient, family, and physician, but careful attention to this matter can alleviate many future difficulties. Some patients, and some physicians as well, mistakenly believe that once aggressive treatments have been initiated, they must be continued until death. In the initial stages of a crisis, if there is uncertainty as to how to treat the patient, it is best to begin with aggressive treatment and then, as soon as an assessment is possible, to consider withdrawing treatment if it does not seem to be benefiting the patient or fitting the wishes of the patient.

## Step 2. Clarification

Most ethical problems can be avoided by careful attention to preventive ethics. Sometimes, however, there will be conflicts as a result of the intense emotions surrounding the suffering and death of a loved one. Mr. and Mrs. Edwards and Dr. Wycliff did an excellent job of anticipating the debilitating effects of Alzheimer's, but they failed to communicate Mr. Edwards's preferences to his sons. Perhaps the sons were not ready to face these issues.

When the conflicts arose, they had the potential to subvert Mr. Edwards's plan of how to face death. They also had the potential to divide the family at a time when unity was most needed. Dr. Wycliff succeeded at averting these catastrophes by recognizing the misunderstandings and motives of each son, and clarifying each.

DIRECTIVE TO PHYSICIANS

Directive made this _____ day of _____ 20 _____.

I, _____ being of sound mind, willfully and voluntarily make known my desire that my life shall not be artificially prolonged under the circumstances set forth below, and do hereby declare:

1. If at any time I should have an incurable or irreversible condition caused by injury, disease, or illness certified to be a terminal condition by two physicians, and where the application of life-sustaining procedures would serve only to artificially prolong the moment of my death and where my attending physician determines that my death is imminent or will result within a relatively short time without application of life-sustaining procedures, I direct that such procedures be withheld or withdrawn, and that I be permitted to die naturally.

2. In the absence of my ability to give directions regarding the use of such life-sustaining procedures, it is my intention that this directive shall be honored by my family and physicians as the final expression of my legal right to refuse medical or surgical treatment and accept the consequences from such refusal.

3. (Optional) If I should be comatose, incompetent, or otherwise mentally or physically incapable of communication, I hereby designate the following individual to make any necessary treatment decisions for me:

   Name of Individual: _____

   Relationship to me: _____

4. If I have been diagnosed as pregnant and that diagnosis is known to my physician, this directive shall have no force or effect during the course of my pregnancy.

5. This directive shall be in effect until it is revoked.

6. I understand the full import of this directive and I am emotionally and mentally competent to make this directive.

7. I understand that I may revoke this at any time.

8. Other directions:

   _____

   _____

   _____

   _____

   Signed: _____

   City, County, and State of Residence: _____

I am not related to the declarant by blood or marriage, nor would I be entitled to any portion of the declarant's estate on his decease, nor am I the attending physician of the declarant or an employee of the attending physician, nor am I a patient in a healthcare facility in which the declarant is a patient, or any person who has a claim against any portion of the estate of the declarant upon his decease. Furthermore, if I am an employee of a health facility in which the declarant is a patient, I am not involved in providing direct patient care to the declarant nor am I directly involved in the financial affairs of the health facility.

Witness: _____     Witness: _____

**Figure 26.1.** A living will or advance directive. Requirements vary somewhat from state to state so the student is advised to check with an attorney.

DURABLE POWER OF ATTORNEY FOR HEALTH CARE

DESIGNATION OF HEALTH CARE AGENT.

I, _____, an adult being of sound mind hereby appoint:

Name: _____ Phone: _____

Address: _____

as my agent to make any and all healthcare decisions for me, except to the extent I state otherwise in this document. This power of attorney shall not terminate on my disability. This durable power of attorney for healthcare takes effect if I become unable to make my own healthcare decisions and this fact is certified in writing by my physician.

LIMITATIONS ON THE DECISION MAKING AUTHORITY OF MY AGENT ARE AS FOLLOWS:

_____

_____

_____

DESIGNATION OF ALTERNATE AGENT.

(You are not required to designate an alternate agent but you may do so. An alternate agent may make some of the same healthcare decisions as the designated agent if the designated agent is unable or unwilling to act as your agent. If the agent designated is your spouse, the designation is automatically revoked by law if your marriage is dissolved.)

If the person designated as my agent is unable or unwilling to make healthcare decisions for me, I designate the following person(s) to serve as my agent to make healthcare decisions for me as authorized by this document, who will serve in the following order:

A. First Alternate Agent

Name: _____ Phone: _____

Address: _____

B. Second Alternate Agent

Name: _____ Phone: _____

Address: _____

The original of this document is kept at:

_____

The following individuals or institutions have signed copies:

Name: _____ Phone: _____

Address: _____

DURATION

I understand that this power of attorney exists indefinitely from the date I execute this document unless I establish a shorter time or revoke the power of attorney. If I am unable to make healthcare decisions myself when this power of attorney expires, the authority I have granted my agent continues to exist until I become better able to make healthcare decisions for myself.

(IF APPLICABLE) This power of attorney ends on the following date: _____

PRIOR DESIGNATIONS REVOKED.

I revoke any prior power of attorney for healthcare.

ACKNOWLEDGMENT OF DISCLOSURE STATEMENT.

I have been provided with a disclosure statement explaining the effect of this document. I have read and understood that information contained in the disclosure statement.

(YOU MUST DATE AND SIGN THIS POWER OF ATTORNEY)

I sign my name to this durable power of attorney for healthcare on:

_____ day of _____ 20_____ at

_____ City & State

_____
Signature

_____
Print Name

STATEMENT OF WITNESS

I declare under penalty of perjury that the principal has identified himself or herself to me, that the principal signed or acknowledged this durable power of attorney in my presence, that I believe the principal to be sound of mind, that the principal has affirmed that the principal is aware of the nature of the document and is signing it voluntarily and free from duress, that the principal requested that I serve as witness to the principal's execution of this document, and that I am not the person appointed as agent by this document and that I am not a provider of health or residential care, the operator of a community care facility, or an employee of an operator of a health-care facility.

I declare that I am not related to the principal by blood, marriage, or adoption and that to the best of my knowledge I am not entitled to any part of the estate on the death of the principal under a will or by operation of law.

Date: _____

Witness Signature: _____

Print Name: _____

Address: _____

Date: _____

Witness Signature: _____

Print Name: _____

Address: _____

**Figure 26.2.** A document assigning a proxy for healthcare decisions. Legal requirements vary somewhat from state to state so the student is advised to consult with an attorney.

The first son misunderstood the terminal nature of advanced Alzheimer's disease, the second misunderstood his father's desire for privacy, and the third misunderstood the nature of his father's suffering and his religious values regarding suicide and euthanasia. Rather than engaging the sons in an argument or turning the decision-making process into a power struggle, Dr. Wycliff clarified the facts in a way that indicated respect for each son's feelings, a solid understanding of Mr. Edwards's preferences, and careful preparation by physician, patient, and spouse for this difficult moment. Dr. Wycliff refrained from personalizing the conflict; by treating it as a series of factual misunderstandings, no one felt blame, shame, or bulldozed.

In my experience most ethical conflicts involve such misunderstandings. Sometimes the family and sometimes the caregiver jump to false conclusions. For example, the physician discovers that the parents are not giving their child the antibiotics the physician prescribed 2 days ago, and now the child is seriously ill. The physician concludes that the parents are guilty of abuse by neglect and asks for an emergency meeting of the ethics committee to consider asking a judge to remove the child from her parents' custody. The ethics committee meets with the parents and discovers that they misunderstood the physician's orders: They thought she wanted them to wait until the antihistamine prescription had run out before giving the child the new medicine. This problem could have been avoided, and with it all of the shaming associated with noncompliance and abuse, had the physician spent more time clarifying the facts of the case instead of hastily jumping to negative conclusions.

The other area requiring clarification is motives. Once Mr. Edwards's sons understood their father's motives for his choices—to save money for his family, to be remembered well by friends and neighbors, and to remain faithful to his religious convictions—the sons could accept their father's decisions. And because Dr. Wycliff recognized that the sons' motives were good ones, he did not make the mistake of insulting them at this tender moment. Some physicians in this situation might have viewed the sons as obstreperous, engaged them in a power struggle or capitulated to their demands, and would not have handled their complaints so adroitly.

## Step 3. Review the Decision-Making Process

If prevention and clarification fail, then the physician should review the decision-making process to see whether some point was overlooked or misapplied. The process we have recommended here involves attention to five basic concerns: beneficence, nonmaleficence, autonomy, justice, and values.

The principles of beneficence and nonmaleficence suggest that Dr. Wycliff has an obligation to help Mr. Edwards rather than to harm him. Keeping him comfortable in a nursing home is consistent with this principle. A related issue is whether the duties of beneficence and nonmaleficence should be applied to the patient's caretakers as well. Thus, Dr. Wycliff is appropriate in working closely with Mrs. Edwards, not only to understand her husband's treatment preferences, but also to ensure that his care does not constitute an excessive burden for her.

The principle of autonomy suggests that the definitions of benefit and harm should be shaped by Mr. Edwards's preferences. Prior to becoming demented, Mr. Edwards stated these preferences through his conversations with Dr. Wycliff and Mrs. Edwards, and through his living will. Given his desire to be remembered as he was prior to becoming demented, dying at home would constitute a harm. Given his religious beliefs, assisted suicide and euthanasia would also constitute a harm. Allowing him to live his final days at a nursing home in as much comfort as possible is consistent with Dr. Wycliff's obligation to respect the autonomy of his patients. Had Mr. Edwards requested treatment outside the standard of care, or beyond his ability to pay, Dr. Wycliff would not have been obliged to honor his wishes.

The principle of justice suggests that Dr. Wycliff has an obligation to consider the physical, emotional, and financial strain on Mrs. Edwards and the family. Had Mrs. Edwards continued to care for Mr. Edwards at home, she might herself have become exhausted, sick, and she might have preceded her husband in death. Had Mr. Edwards insisted on dying at home, Dr. Wycliff would have an obligation to help Mrs. Edwards get the assistance needed to provide around-the-clock care for her husband. If such care is not available through family or visiting nurses, Dr. Wycliff should foresee this situation, discuss it with Mr. and Mrs. Edwards prior to his becoming demented, and encourage him to choose a course of treatment that is realistic for their situation and takes into consideration his wife's physical limitations.

Finally, Dr. Wycliff's fidelity to his values is an important factor in the successful outcome of this case. Dr. Wycliff is honest with each family member regarding Mr. Edwards's wishes. Dr. Wycliff apparently was very frank with Mr. Edwards in the early stages of his illness, thus enabling Mr. Edwards to prepare for his death. Yet Dr. Wycliff does not bludgeon the sons with his honesty. He maintains a tender, compassionate tone even while telling family members things they do not want to hear. Dr. Wycliff's other virtues are courage and integrity: the courage to stand up for what his patient wants and the integrity to keep his commitments. It would be so easy at this time to give in to the requests of well-meaning family members. After all, Mr.

Edwards no longer knows what is going on. But Dr. Wycliff keeps his promise to his patient, and does so in such a way that the entire family is able to recognize and appreciate the wisdom of Mr. Edwards's decision.

## The Special Case of Euthanasia and Assisted Suicide

One of Mr. Edwards's sons asks the physician to end his father's suffering by administering a lethal medication. In the case of euthanasia and assisted suicide, there is considerable debate among physicians, ethicists, and patients regarding: whether these services constitute a benefit or a harm; whether the patient has a right to expect such a presumed benefit from the medical profession; whether legalization of such services would skid us down the slippery slope of genocide of the frail elderly and disabled, or at least create unjust pressures and incentives to eliminate those who cannot care for themselves; and whether assisting in suicide or euthanasia is consistent with the meaning and mission of the medical profession.

Some jurisdictions are beginning to experiment with euthanasia and assisted suicide. In the Netherlands, euthanasia is permitted under the following conditions:

- The patient requests euthanasia voluntarily and consistently over a reasonable period of time.
- The patient is rational and fully informed.
- The patient's suffering is intolerable despite aggressive palliative care.
- The patient's probability of improvement is low.
- Two physicians agree that the above criteria are met and are willing to carry out the request (de Wachter, 1992).

In the state of Oregon, physicians are allowed to prescribe a lethal dose of barbiturates to terminally ill patients who request it. Unlike physicians in the Netherlands, physicians in Oregon do not administer the dose; they prescribe it. As with the Netherlands, a number of conditions must be met before the prescription is legal:

- Two physicians, a primary physician and a consultant, must agree that the patient is dying of a terminal condition.
- The two physicians must agree that the patient is competent to make medical decisions.
- Patients suspected of depression or other psychiatric disorder must be referred for counseling.
- Patients must be informed of all reasonable alternatives such as comfort care and hospice care.
- Patients must make three requests, one written and two oral, and at least 15 days must separate the two oral requests.
- Patients must be adults and residents of Oregon.
- Physicians may not administer the medication, and all lethal prescriptions must be reported to the Oregon Health Division (Angell, 1999; Chin *et al.*, 1999).

Critics of euthanasia and assisted suicide state that these activities are forms of murder and suicide, that patients who choose to die are committing a sin, and that physicians who assist them are violating the Hippocratic oath and committing murder. Critics fear that permitting euthanasia and assisted suicide under limited conditions will give way to a slippery slope in which the euthanasia is not voluntary or the patients are not terminal. In this era of cost containment and managed care, patients might feel pressure to die as quickly and cheaply as possible. Supporters of the experiments in the Netherlands and Oregon maintain that prolonging the lives of terminally ill patients is a form of torture and that it is wrong to keep terminally ill patients alive against their will.

In recent years hospice physicians have made considerable progress in pain and symptom management. Unfortunately, many physicians caring for seriously ill patients still do not manage pain and symptoms aggressively or have not trained extensively in this area. As attitudes change, and as physicians become better trained in the aggressive management of pain and symptoms, the need for euthanasia and assisted suicide should decrease. Until we are able to manage effectively the pain and symptoms of all seriously ill patients, euthanasia and assisted suicide will continue to be proposed as viable alternatives to prolonging the suffering of patients.

## CONCLUSION

Far from focusing on rare or hypothetical situations, and far from being an exercise in semantics, abstract reasoning, or pondering questions that only lead to more questions, medical ethics addresses everyday clinical situations and helps provide practical, workable solutions. In this chapter I have offered a four-step process for clinical ethical problem-solving: (1) What benefits can I offer this patient, and what harms are also possible? (2) What are the patient's values and preferences? (3) What is fair in this situation? (4) Am I remaining faithful to my values and ideals, and to those of my profession? Careful attention to these four questions will usually result in ethically sound clinical decision-making. Should problems arise, the physician should clarify factual misunderstandings of the patient, family, or colleagues, as well as their motives. In most cases problems can be prevented by anticipating them and preparing for them.

In this chapter I have tried to focus on the areas in which ethical and legal consensus has been reached. Just as there are standards of care, say, in the treatment of an ear infection, there are ethical and legal standards regarding confidentiality, truth telling, and informed consent. Sometimes these standards will conflict with one another or with other important ethical and legal requirements, and sometimes physicians will disagree as to the best way to reconcile these conflicts, but the physician must make a conscientious effort to be as faithful as possible to each of these important standards of care. In so doing the physician will discover that fidelity to ethical standards of care is not just good ethics, it's good medicine.

## CASES FOR DISCUSSION

### CASE 1

*Dr. Zhao calls the home of a 15-year-old patient, Mary Lou Reece, to tell her the results of her lab tests, which indicate that she has gonorrhea. Her mother, who is unaware of her daughter's problem, answers the phone and asks why the physician is calling her daughter. Dr. Zhao states that it is a confidential matter between physician and patient. The mother states that she is the legal guardian of a minor, and has the right to know what's going on. Unsure what to do, Dr. Zhao hangs up on the mother.*

1. *What ethical considerations are most important in the treatment of a 15-year-old patient?*
2. *Dr. Zhao could think of no better solution than hanging up. Can you think of a better way out of this embarrassing situation?*
3. *Now that the mother is suspicious, what should the physician do to ameliorate the situation?*
4. *How might this problem have been prevented?*

### CASE 2

*Mrs. Cruz, an 83-year-old woman, presented to a family practice clinic with a large, deep ulceration on her lower leg and foot resulting from an injury from a dog chain that had denuded the skin 4 years previously. Grafting efforts had been only marginally successful. Mrs. Cruz had not been seen in the clinic for 2 years—she reported being treated by a cardiologist in Mexico—and since that time the ulceration had been reinjured, had worsened considerably, and osteomyelitis had set in. The physician, Dr. Lumicao, admitted the patient to the hospital and requested an orthopedic consultation. The consultant felt that antibiotics were unlikely to help and recommended amputation within the next few days. Mrs. Cruz stated that she'd rather die than lose her foot.*

1. *What options are available to the primary physician?*
2. *Should either physician try to persuade the patient to change her mind?*

3. *Is this patient incompetent? Why or why not?*
4. *Imagine that the orthopedist had "stolen" the patient from the family physician and was trying to coerce her to undergo surgery. What should the family physician do in such a situation? What should the family physician have done to prevent this from happening?*

## CASE 3

*During a routine preplacement examination Sapna, a 25-year-old college graduate, volunteers that she smokes marijuana once or twice per month and asks the physician, Dr. Bloem, whether she thinks she ought to quit. She also reports smoking a pack of cigarettes per day. In filing her report with the employer, Dr. Bloem indicates that Sapna is "fit for employment" but notes that she occasionally smokes marijuana.*

*One week later Sapna returns to see Dr. Bloem, angry because she has been fired from her job. She threatens to sue Dr. Bloem for releasing confidential information to a third party.*

1. *Was Dr. Bloem correct in sharing this information with the employer? Why or why not?*
2. *Would this information be relevant if the patient were operating heavy machinery? Working as a security guard? Flying an airplane?*
3. *What are the physician's obligations to the employer? What are the physician's obligations to the patient-employee?*
4. *What should the physician say to the angry patient? What should the physician do to rectify the situation?*
5. *If Sapna had been a regular patient of Dr. Bloem, would Dr. Bloem's responsibilities be any different?*

## CASE 4

*Russell Eisen, a 51-year-old geologist, has been a patient of Dr. Davis's private practice for the past 12 years. One year ago he lost his job and with it his health insurance. He has been unsuccessful in finding other employment and recently lost his home through foreclosure. For the past few weeks he has lived on the streets and in shelters for the homeless. His only source of income is a few dollars per day from picking up aluminum cans.*

*He presents to Dr. Davis today with depression and also with inflamed feet due to walking, worn-out shoes, and standing in lines. He worries that if his feet worsen, he will no longer be able to pick up cans. Dr. Davis worries that if she refers Mr. Eisen to the local public hospital, he will have difficulty getting transportation there, will not establish a close relationship with a primary care physician, and will not get the quality of care necessary to be healed of these problems.*

1. *Is Mr. Eisen still Dr. Davis's patient?*
2. *What are Dr. Davis's ethical responsibilities to Mr. Eisen?*
3. *What are physicians' responsibilities to patients who cannot pay?*
4. *What are the public's responsibilities to patients who cannot pay?*

## CASE 5

*A 30-year-old patient, Flavio, has recently tested positive for HIV. He expresses an unwillingness to tell his past sexual partners that they may have been exposed to the AIDS virus but states that he will always use a condom in the future. In accordance with the law, his physician, Dr. Jerson, has reported the positive test result to the local health department but still feels uneasy about the situation. The health department is backlogged and unlikely to work on the case for several months. At least two of Flavio's recent partners are Dr. Jerson's long-time patients.*

1. *What are the physician's obligations to each of the affected individuals?*
2. *Would the physician be ethically justified in contacting individuals he believes to have been exposed to HIV? Are his obligations different to those individuals who are his patients?*
3. *Would the physician be justified in using persuasion to try to get the patient to change his mind? Coercion?*
4. *What responsibilities do patients have to physicians?*
5. *Under what circumstances might a physician legitimately "fire" a patient? Is this such a situation?*

# RECOMMENDED READINGS

Beauchamp TL, Childress JF: *Principles of Biomedical Ethics*. London, Oxford University Press, 2001.

> The most widely used introduction to the foundations of medical ethics. Topics covered include ethical theory, professional–patient relationships, and professional virtues.

Beauchamp TL, Walters L (eds): *Contemporary Issues in Bioethics*, ed 5. Belmont, Calif, Wadsworth Publishing Co, 1999.

> An anthology of the most influential scholarly essays and judicial decisions in modern medical ethics, on topics ranging from abortion and euthanasia to the physician–patient relationship to research, health policy, and allocation of medical resources.

Brody H: *The Healer's Power*. New Haven, Yale University Press, 1992.

> The author, an ethicist and family physician, identifies the types of power that physicians bring to the physician-patient relationship and examines negative and positive ways of utilizing that power.

# REFERENCES

American Medical Association. Principles of medical ethics, 1957, in Reiser SJ, Dyck AJ, Curran WJ (eds): *Ethics in Medicine: Historical Perspectives and Contemporary Concerns*. Cambridge, Mass, MIT Press, 1977, p 39.

Angell M: Caring for the dying—Congressional mischief. *N Engl J Med* 341:1923, 1999.

Beauchamp TL, Childress JF: *Principles of Biomedical Ethics*. London, Oxford University Press, 1989.

Brennan TA: AIDS and the limits of confidentiality: The physician's duty to warn contacts of seropositive individuals. *J Gen Intern Med* 4:242–246, 1989.

Brody H: *Placebos and the Philosophy of Medicine*. Chicago, University of Chicago Press, 1980.

Chin AE, Hedberg K, Higginson GK, Fleming DW: Legalized physician-assisted suicide in Oregon—The first year's experience. *N Engl J Med* 340:577, 1999.

Cooper AE: Duty to warn third parties. JAMA 248:431-432, 1982.

De Wachter MAM: Euthanasia in the Netherlands. *Hastings Cent Rep* 22:23, 1992.

Dickins BM: Legal limits of AIDS confidentiality. JAMA 259:3449–3451, 1988.

Edinger W, Smucker DR: Outpatients' attitudes regarding advance directives. *J Fam Pract* 35:650–653, 1992.

Faden RR, Beauchamp TL: *A History and Theory of Informed Consent*. London, Oxford University Press, 1986.

Garr DR, Marsh FJ: Medical malpractice and the primary care physician: Lowering the risks. *South Med J* 79:1280–1284, 1986.

Holleman WL, Edwards DC, Matson CC: Obligations of physicians to patients and third-party payers. *J Clin Ethics* 5:113–120, 1994.

Holleman WL, Holleman MC: School and work release evaluations. *JAMA* 260:3629–3634, 1988.

Holleman WL, Holleman MC, Moy JG: Are ethics and managed care strange bedfellows or a marriage made in heaven? *Lancet* 349:350–351, 1997.

Holleman WL, Holleman MC, Moy JG: Continuity of care, informed consent, and fiduciary responsibilities in for-profit managed care systems. *Arch Fam Med* 9:21–25, 2000.

Kubler-Ross E: *On Death and Dying*. New York, Macmillan Publishing Co, Inc, 1970.

McCullough LKB, Ashton CM: A methodology for teaching ethics in the clinical setting: A clinical handbook for medical ethics. *Theor Med* 15:39–52, 1994.

Miller TE: Managed care regulation: In the laboratory of the states. *JAMA* 278:1102–1109, 1997.

Morreim EH: *Balancing Act: The New Medical Ethics of Medicine's New Economics*. Dordrecht, Kluwer Academic Publishers, 1991.

Pellegrino ED, Thomasma DC: *The Virtues in Medical Practice*. London, Oxford University Press, 1993.

Peterson LM, Brennan T: Medical ethics and medical injuries: Taking our duties seriously. *J Clin Ethics* 1:207–211, 1990.

Reich WT: Speaking of suffering: A moral account of compassion. *Soundings: An Interdisciplinary Journal* 72:83–108, 1989.

Reiser SJ: Selections from the Hippocratic corpus: 'Oath,' 'precepts,' 'the art,' 'epidemics I,' 'the physician,' 'decorum,' and 'law,' in Reiser SJ, Dyck AJ, Curran WJ (eds): *Ethics in Medicine: Historical Perspectives and Contemporary Concerns*. Cambridge, Mass, MIT Press, 1977, pp 5–7.

*Salgo v. Leland Stanford, Jr. University Board of Trustees*, 154 C A 2d 560; 317 P 2d 170.

*Schloendorff v. Society of New York Hospital*, 211 NY, 1914 (NY Sup Ct).

Siegler M: Confidentiality in medicine—a decrepit concept. *N Engl J Med* 307:1518–1521, 1982.

*Tarasoff v. Regents of the University of California*, 551 P 2d 334 (Cal 1976) [Cal Sup Ct].

*Truman v. Thomas*, 165 Cal. Rptr. 308, 611 P. 2d 902 (1980), in Faden RR, Beauchamp TL: *A History and Theory of Informed Consent*. London, Oxford University Press, 1986.

Weisman AD: *On Dying and Denying: A Psychiatric Study of Terminality*. New York, Behavioral Publications, Inc, 1972.

## CHAPTER 27

# Health Policy and Economics

*Christopher J. Mansfield and Ann C. Jobe*

## CASE 27-1

*Mr. Olds, a patient of Dr. Wellman's with Alzheimer's disease, had a fall in the nursing home from what a nurse suggested might be a minor stroke. Dr. Wellman thought an MRI would be useful to confirm that possibility. He was advising Mr. Olds's daughter, Jane, about treatment options when she broke into tears. Jane stated that she is overwhelmed by problems in her life. Dr. Wellman had provided prenatal care and delivered her two children but had seen neither the children nor Jane in the last 4 years. In exploring the nature of her distress, he discovered that Jane divorced shortly after the birth of her last child. She has been working full time since then at the local minimart and "making do the best I can." Jane feels guilty that she can visit her father only on Sundays. She is worried about a lump on her breast and her 4-year-old who still suffers from frequent earaches. Dr. Wellman asks her to make an appointment for herself. Jane has postponed seeing a physician because she doesn't have health insurance. Jane asks Dr. Wellman how much the visit will cost.*

## EDUCATIONAL OBJECTIVES

1. Describe components and trends in the U.S. healthcare system in economic terms
2. Understand how two basic economic concepts, the production function and theories of supply and demand, are used to model, guide, and predict performance of the healthcare system
3. Understand and use basic tools of economics for selecting and optimizing resources to improve medical care and health
4. Understand the potential and limits of both free enterprise and government to deliver health
5. Understand the basic economic principles of managed care
6. Understand the interaction of agendas, alternatives, and policy windows in the development of health policy.

One cannot begin to understand health policy without considering the economics of healthcare. Economic concerns accompany virtually all health policy issues and certainly underlie two of the most intractable policy problems: providing financial access to care and controlling the cost of healthcare. Jane's situation in Case 27-1 is not unique. She is one of the 44.3 million Americans without health insurance in 1998. One out of five working age adults are uninsured.

Almost half (48%) of the poor who, like Jane, work full time have no health insurance (U.S. Census Bureau, 1999). Health insurance has been a social and political issue throughout the century but has been an increasingly acute issue during the last decade, as the percentage of uninsured has grown from 12.9% to 16.3% of the population.

Control of healthcare costs has been on the agenda of every President's agenda since 1969, when Richard Nixon called it a crisis (Starr, 1982). Healthcare financing is a constant issue in the state legislatures.

Figure 27.1 plots the increase in spending for healthcare in the United States since 1950.

The proportion of spending devoted to healthcare increased steadily through 1995 and the upward trend is likely to resume (Smith *et al.*, 1999). "So what," you might argue: "Health is important and cost should not be an issue in a nation as wealthy as the United States." The United States enjoys a high standard of living, but it is clear from Fig. 27.1 that spending for health must have some limits. Money spent for health means less to spend on other, perhaps equally beneficial, products and services. Healthcare services now account for more than we spend on either education or national defense; in fact, more than we spend on education and defense combined. And the higher the cost of healthcare, the more unaffordable it becomes and the less likely that small businesses will provide it as an employee benefit or that individuals will purchase private coverage.

Healthcare spending in the United States for 1998 was estimated to be $1.15 trillion, amounting to 13.5% of the nation's gross domestic product (GDP) (Levit *et al.*, 2000). This means that out of every $100 spent in the United States, $13.50 is for healthcare. U.S. health spending is currently divided among healthcare providers and institutions as shown in Fig. 27.2. The largest share (33%) is for hospital services, followed by physician services (20%). The share devoted to physician services has remained about the same over the years but the proportions of other key components of the health system have changed, as shown in Fig. 27.3. It is notable that the proportion of national health expenditures (NHE) ascribed to hospital care declined from 42% in 1980 to 33% in 1998, and the percentage for drugs increased from 5% to 11%. Home health is a small but new and expanding component (growing from 1% to 3% of NHE). Program administration and the net cost of

## UNINSURED PEOPLE BY RACE, POVERTY, AND WORK STATUS, PERCENTAGES—1998

|  | Uninsured | |
|---|---|---|
|  | All people | Poor people |
| All races/ethnicity | 16 | 32 |
| White | 15 | 34 |
| Black | 22 | 29 |
| Hispanic | 35 | 44 |
| Adults 18–64, in millions | 20 | 44 |
| Worked full time | 17 | 48 |
| Worked part time | 23 | 45 |

U.S. Census Bureau, October 1999, P60-208.

## PERCENTAGE OF AMERICANS WITHOUT HEALTH INSURANCE: 1987–1998

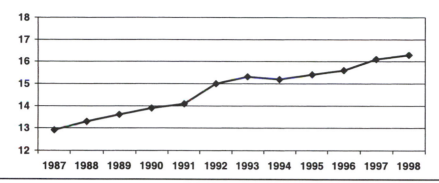

private health insurance has been relatively constant at 5% but rose to 6% for the period 1989 to 1994, a period during which utilization controls resulted in increased profits for insurance companies. The size of the spending pie, measured in constant dollars, itself is more than five times larger than it was in 1965. We can attribute the increase not only to population growth but also to greater utilization of services and intensity of care. Though only 20% of total spending goes to physicians, about 70% is for services that physicians prescribe.

You may have heard someone say, "Sure, the cost of healthcare is high in the United States, but we have the best medical care system in the world." And you may know that Americans live much longer than they

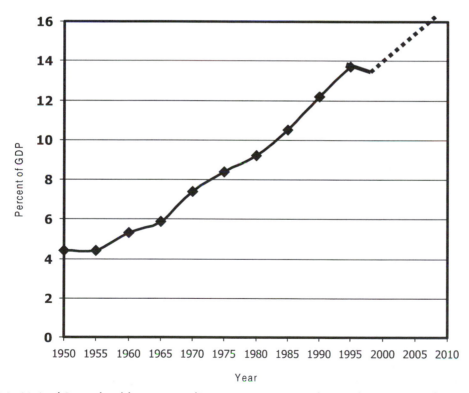

**Figure 27.1.** United States healthcare spending as a percentage of gross domestic product, 1950–1998 and projection to 2008. Sources: Health Care Financing Administration (HCFA) per Levit *et al.*, 2000. Projection to 2008 from Smith *et al.*, 1999.

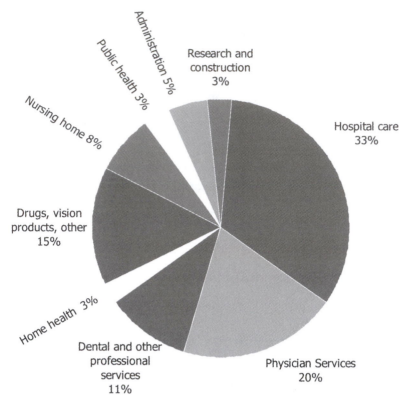

**Figure 27.2.** Components of national health expenditures in the United States, 1998 ($1.149 trillion total). Source: Levit *et al.*, 2000.

used to: Life expectancy in the United States has increased from 47 years to nearly 77 years since the turn of the century (U.S. DHHS, 2000). But are extra dollars spent today likely to increase our life expectancy? Figure 27.4 depicts U.S. spending for health as a proportion of GDP along with increasing life expectancy.

## CASE 27-2

*Dr. Wellman has been pondering an MRI scan for Mr. Olds. He typically orders one for stroke patients. He knows it is expensive but figures that insurance will usually pay. On his way to the hospital board meeting, he thinks how ironic that Mr. Olds's daughter has not sought to have her breast lump examined.*

*On the agenda for the county hospital board that evening is the question of whether the hospital should purchase an MRI unit for its next expansion and renovation. The hospital currently contracts with Dr. Ray's private radiology group, which operates its own MRI, but Dr. Ray says she would be happy to recruit another radiologist to use the hospital's unit. Bonds guaranteed by the county would pay for the MRI. One of the board members Mrs. Steward, is a member of the county board of supervisors. She questions whether the MRI is needed. She argues that one MRI ought to be sufficient and that managed care will decrease demand for the service in the future. She reminds the board that the county is ultimately liable for the bonds and says the county needs a 100% childhood immunization program more than another MRI device. Dr. Wellman interrupts. He says that the two issues are completely unrelated and have different sources of financing. The board votes to include the MRI in the expansion plans and directs the administrator to negotiate with Dr. Ray for professional services. Mrs. Steward wonders if this will improve the health of the community.*

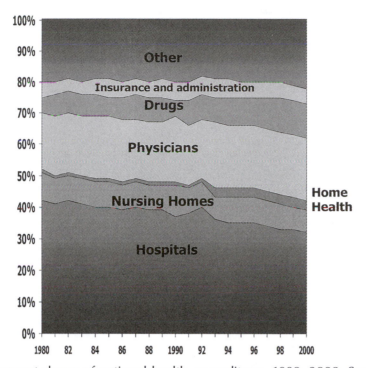

**Figure 27.3.** Component shares of national health expenditures, 1980–2000. Sources: Health Care Financing Administration, various publications.

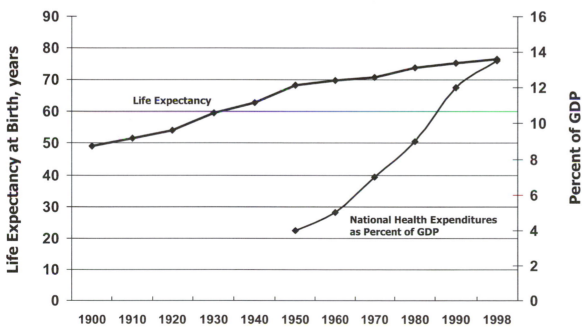

**Figure 27.4.** Trends in U.S. life expectancy and national health expenditures, 1900–1998. Sources: Statistical Bulletin, HIAA 1998; Levit, 2000.

## WHY PHYSICIANS SHOULD UNDERSTAND PUBLIC POLICY AND ECONOMICS

*1. Healthcare is a trillion dollar business and growing larger each year. Government purchases half of all medical care and the proportion is increasing, but government must balance the public's desire for healthcare with the public's reluctance to pay taxes. To contain public spending it has chosen principally to let the free market control the healthcare industry. To preserve autonomy and financial opportunity the physician must understand economic foundations of the business of health.*

*2. The practice of medicine is a privilege granted by government and government is expected to regulate the profession by public policy in the public interest. Government can regulate not only the profession of medicine but also business interests that control it. To preserve autonomy and professional opportunity the physician must understand and participate in the policymaking process.*

# ECONOMICS

Mastery of human biology and the science of medicine is an immense and worthy intellectual challenge. As Case 27-2 suggests, however, understanding the allocation of medical resources is also an important endeavor. How can we best spend scarce resources to produce health? Can we afford to provide medical care to everyone? All the care that people want? All that might be of benefit? If not, how might we choose which kinds of care? For whom? While philosophy and ethics help us understand the moral issues of rationing, economic concepts allow us to develop the specifics of health policy.

Economics is the study of how scarce resources are allocated. It offers concepts and tools to describe, predict, and optimize resource allocation.

> Economics is the study of how people and society end up *choosing*, with or without the use of money, to employ *scarce* productive resources that could have alternative uses—to *produce* various commodities and *distribute* them for consumption, now or in the future, among various persons and groups in society. Economics analyzes the costs and benefits of improving patterns of resource use. (Samuelson, 1980, p. 2)

Economic theory and empirical methods help policymakers measure how much is spent on health, understand how best to produce health services, and how they should be distributed. Economics is based on the fundamental assumption that people act rationally and make choices that maximize their self interest; i.e., in making choices they maximize the *marginal utility* (incremental value) of each investment, production, or consumption decision. This assumption allows economists to construct theoretical models of human behavior. One of the most familiar models of behavior describes the two essential features of any market for goods or services—supply and demand.

## Fundamental Economic Concepts

### Models of Supply and Demand

The less there is of a commodity, given a particular demand for it in an open market, the higher the price. Conversely, if its price is lowered, more of the commodity will be demanded (sold). If the price goes up, consumers do with less or find substitutes. This is the law of downward-sloping *demand*, which is plotted as d–d in Fig. 27.5. *Supply* in relation to price and quantity can be similarly described. Amount supplied is plotted as the upward-sloping curve, s–s. It describes the amount that producers are willing to supply at a

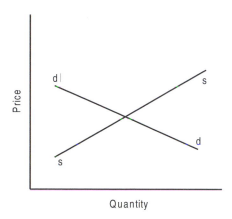

**Figure 27.5.** Supply and demand curves for land.

given price. The slopes of supply and demand curves for different goods and services vary. Land is an example of a market operating according to the curves in Fig. 27.5. It describes the market for land that might be available in a rural area where there is typically substantial choice on the part of both sellers and buyers about buying or selling a particular property at a given price. This figure could also describe the market for automobiles, personal computers, or home appliances. Variations in price would produce larger variations in demand.

In contrast, Fig. 27.6 portrays the market for medical services, where buyers (patients) have little choice of services and sellers have little competition. Much of medical care is perceived by the consumer to be a necessity and variations in price may have little effect on demand. How much the consumer has to spend does make a difference, however. Two demand curves are shown in Fig. 27.6, depicting the demand of people with different purchasing ability. The more vertical one (d–d) applies to people like Mr. Olds who have health insurance. Having insurance makes the consumer even less sensitive to price and the demand curve is steep, i.e., less price elastic. The less steep curve (d$^1$–d$^1$) applies to those in Jane's circumstance, who because they must pay out of pocket at the time of purchase are more sensitive to price. An increase or decrease in price has a larger effect on the volume of services demanded by those without health insurance than those with it. The supply–demand model is useful for understanding elementary markets where the elements of free enterprise operate with simplicity. If there is more product or service supplied, price will drop and consumers (in total) are inclined to buy more. Consider what should happen to price in Fig. 27.6 when supply is increased, say by more physicians locating in the medical service area. The supply curve would shift out to the right. A fall in

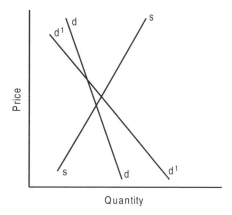

**Figure 27.6.** Supply and demand curves for medical care with and without insurance.

prices should occur in the absence of monopoly conditions. Conversely, if consumers demand more, price will rise and suppliers will be inclined to sell more. At the point where supply and demand curves cross, an "equilibrium price" is established. The market "clears" at the "going" price and is in balance. This theoretic model of behavior is supported by considerable empirical evidence in simple commodity markets. It has been argued, and many believe, that the market alone is the most efficient way of allocating resources and government intervention is not necessary. This thesis is explored below but we must ask if there are any external considerations and reasons why classic, free-market theory may not be the best description of the healthcare system or the best prescription for allocating resources. Explore first, though, how medical care became an economic issue.

## Monetarization of Medical Care

Before the turn of the century, there was not much medical care to purchase. Medicine offered the patient little hope or "marginal utility," in the economists' vernacular. This began to change with the application of science to medicine. Yet until the 1940s most people paid for medical care out of their own pockets at the time of service or incurred a personal debt for their care. Most hospitals were voluntary, not-for-profit community institutions that originated out of philanthropy and depended heavily on local charity for capital as well as operating revenue (Stevens, 1989). Physicians provided charity care or discounted their fees according to a patient's financial circumstances. Proposals for nationally sponsored or compulsory health insurance were considered in the United States after Chancellor Bismarck introduced it as a social reform in Germany in 1883. Such coverage has generally been opposed by organized medicine and others as being a form of socialism inappropriate for the United States (Starr, 1982).

As medical care became more effective and dependent on technology, hospital care became important, but widespread poverty during the Depression limited access. Thus, the need for hospital insurance increased and the Blue Cross movement began in the late 1930s. This voluntary, private insurance, which paid for hospital care, was followed by private insurance, Blue Shield, for physicians' services. A government ruling that exempted health insurance from wage and price controls during World War II set a precedent for excluding the cost of employer-provided health insurance from an employee's taxable income. Employer-paid, private health insurance is therefore subsidized by the government through these tax breaks (about $100 billion per year as of 1998). This historical artifact of tax policy is the foundation of the United States's unique employment-based, private health insurance system.

With the proliferation of private insurance after the war, hospital revenues came principally from private insurance. New capital came to the industry through the federal government's postwar Hill–Burton program for hospital construction. As a result of these developments, along with passage of Medicare insurance for the elderly and Medicaid for the poor in the mid-1960s, philanthropy is now a very small part of hospitals' budgets. Liberal reimbursement policies of public and private health insurance companies encouraged hospitals to expand services and invest in high technology with virtually no financial risk.

New money came also for the pursuit of science and its application to medicine. Billions of federal dollars were pumped into the National Institutes of Health to support the research enterprise of academic medical centers. State and federal tax dollars now fund much of medical education. Private and public insurance increased demand and payment for physicians' services, and physicians' incomes increased significantly in relation to the average worker's. These events greatly contributed to the phenomenal growth in healthcare spending, a trend characterized by Eli Ginzberg (1984) as the "monetarization of medical care."

## Insurance Principles

People are inclined to buy insurance when confronted with the possibility of expenses for which they cannot budget, or when they are averse to the risk of incurring expense. Few people can budget for major healthcare expenses. The average charge for a coronary bypass in 1995 was $51,000 (HCFA, 1997). Charges for a normal, vaginal delivery can be over $7000 (HIAA, 1998). For the poor and most of the middle class, budgeting merely for routine, primary medical care is difficult. Health insurance is a solution, made particularly attractive when offered by an employer or the government at a subsidized rate. Typical forms of health insurance provide an *indemnity benefit*, a *service benefit*, or a *prepaid benefit*. Indemnity insurance, often referred to as commercial insurance, reimburses the beneficiary for specified expenses incurred. Typically this type of insurance paid whatever the provider charged. Insurance providing a service benefit (traditional Blue Cross) pays a specified amount to the provider directly for each particular service, i.e., a *fee for service*. Sometimes the payment is a percentage of the cost involved (say 80%), with the insured person liable for the balance. Health maintenance organizations (HMOs) provide comprehensive benefits for a prepaid premium.

Indemnity and service-benefit insurance may require the insured first to spend some portion of his or her own money before any service is reimbursed. This is called a *deductible*. Typically, the deductible amount must be met each year before the insurance starts paying. When insurance plans require the insured to pay a portion of the cost of services, the self-pay fraction is called a *copayment*. Some policies may include a *stop-loss* provision that sets a limit on the amount of the copayment. HMOs typically require no deductible or copayments for most services, especially not for prevention and primary care, but premiums are usually higher. Insurance policies may have a *cap* on the amount of reimbursement for a specific service event or for lifetime benefits.

All health insurance policies specify the range of services covered in what is called a *benefit plan*. The benefit plan may exclude specific services or kinds of providers. The *premium*, i.e., price paid by the buyer, reflects the range of benefits, amount of deductible, copayment proportion, reimbursement limit, and the actuarial risk for the individual or group enrolled by the insurer, cost of marketing and administration, reimbursement rates for providers, and the profit expectation of the insurance company.

The actuarial risk can reflect either the experience of the insured group or that of the entire community. Healthy groups typically use fewer services and may be offered lower rates. An essential concept of insurance is the *pooling of risk*, i.e., spreading it over a large population. When the risk is pooled, the costs of expensive but rare events are shared among many. Age, health status, and size of the insured group determine the financial risk assumed by the insurer and the premium that will be charged. If policies are offered to small groups of older people or less healthy people, premiums will be very high.

Economic incentives motivate for-profit insurance companies to compete for the enrollment of healthy groups. The practice of selectively offering health insurance to healthier groups is referred to as *cherry picking*. Do you think a for-profit insurance company would be interested in having many enrollees like Mr. Olds or his daughter Jane?

Insurance companies may make individual business decisions that are at odds with the collective good of society; so also may the individual consumers, physicians, and other providers. The primary reason to have copayments and deductibles is to keep the individual patient involved in the economic calculus. Americans now pay for only about a fifth of their healthcare out of pocket.

Not having a substantial and immediate personal expense cost can encourage use of preventive services but may lead to overuse of unnecessary services, called *moral hazard* (Pauly, 1968). Having insurance with no copayment at the point of service, the individual is motivated to use as much service as may potentially be of benefit. Thinking of the supply and demand curves in Fig. 27.6, the slope of the demand curve for people like Mr. Olds in Case 27-1 is more vertical, *i.e., price inelastic*, than the one for those like his daughter who must pay out of pocket. As more people have such insurance, volume of services increases. If the demand curve shifts outward but the supply curve does not, the equilibrium price will go up if not regulated. The physician has little incentive to limit services. Professional culture encourages doing all that may be of benefit for the patient, what Victor Fuchs (1990) has described as the *technological imperative*.

With no monetary cost at the point of service, the rational act (maximizing utility) for the patient is to take as much medical service as is perceived to be of benefit. Advice or prescriptions of physicians may induce demand. The phenomenon of *physician-induced demand* is related to moral hazard. It happens when a physician provides or orders more services than the patient would be willing to purchase if the patient knew as much as the physician. It may also occur when the physician has income expectations and reimbursement is assured. "Wallet biopsy" is the euphemistic term for the latter phenomena. The induced demand effect (Mitchell & Sunshine, 1992; Rice & Labelle, 1988; Wilensky & Rossiter, 1983) is in contrast to the situation in which HMOs may provide financial incentives to physicians to limit services. HMOs can enhance profit by reducing use of services or limiting costs. The biggest cost is the labor of physicians, nurses, and other personnel. Profitability of HMOs has come to be characterized by the term *medical loss ratio*, i.e., the percentage of premium that goes for medical care. Investors are inclined to buy stock in HMOs with a low medical loss ratio. The conflicting roles of physician as *gatekeeper* for the investors versus purchasing agent for the patient begs a distinction between consumer demand and clinical need. The *clinical need* for medical or public health services may be more or less than expressed demand. Consider Jane's case and that of her father in Case 27-1. Medical need is a professional judgment; demand is consumer behavior. We may want to encourage the use of preventive services but our decisions should be guided by evidence, logic, and professional judgment.

---

### CASE 27-3

*Dr. Wellman was surprised recently to read in a review article that chronic obstructive pulmonary disease (COPD) is now the fourth leading cause of death in the United States and the only cause that is increasing. A number of his older patients have this problem and he has been meaning to research the new therapies available. The bronchodilators he prescribes for some patients have reduced their symptoms and improved exercise tolerance but he wonders if they actually slow the progression of the disease. He has put some of his more severely affected patients on home oxygen therapy and he has prescribed inhaled corticosteroids for many of these. He notes a claim in the article that lung-volume-reduction surgery offers some promise. He wonders if this might be appropriate for his patients with the most severe COPD and makes a note to himself to get the research articles cited and look into the effectiveness and cost of this surgery.*

## The Health Production Function

Economic theory will never replace clinical judgment of physicians but it provides a basis for logic and evidence useful not only to the health policymaker but to the physician as well. Economic theory provides the tools for selecting, organizing, and optimizing resources to produce a desired output. At the micro level, it can guide providers to assemble an effective and efficient array of inputs to produce medical care services. At the macro level, it can guide policymakers in obtaining the final product hoped for, better health of the population.

A production function describes the relationship between combinations of inputs and a resulting output (Feldstein, 1979). If the output is medical care, the most important inputs are clinical personnel ($p1$), support personnel ($p2$), facilities ($f$), supplies ($s$), and technology ($t$), i.e., *medical care* $= f(p_1, p_2, f, s, t)$.

Each resource (input) will have costs and relative contributions to the output. The output, in this case, could be measured in patient encounters, procedures, or courses of treatment for a particular condition. Within the clinical personnel component, different mixes of physicians (and specialties), nurses, nurse practitioners, and physician assistants will produce different costs, volumes, and perhaps quality of services. These empirical relationships can determine optimum staffing ratios and employment of technology and other resources, i.e., the cost accounting that measures efficiency or profitability of delivering any kind of healthcare service.

At the macro level, a production function for health (in contrast to medical care) itself can be described. In this case, medical care is an input rather than the output. Figure 27.7 describes a production function for health (Evans & Stoddart, 1990), that has been widely adopted as a model of the determinants of health (Institute of Medicine, 1997; Kindig, 1997; U.S. DHHS, 2000). In this production function, health is a product

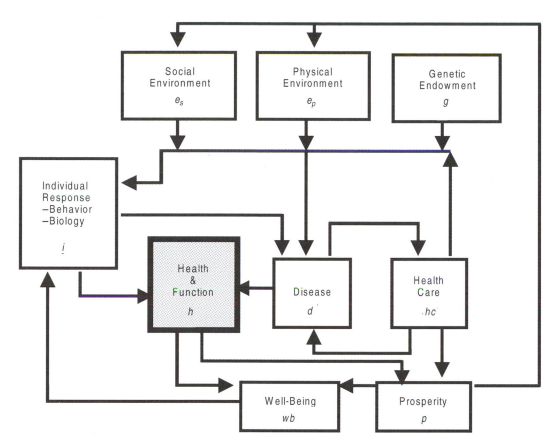

**Figure 27.7.** Health production function based on health field model of Evans and Stoddart, 1990.

not only of the indirect effect of healthcare on disease but also of disease itself and the individual's response. Individual response to disease and health depends on both behavior and biology, which are, in turn, dependent of one's genetic endowment and the physical and social environment. Each of these elements has been shown to have a strong association with health. Algebraically, this production function is specified as *health* = $f(e_s$, $e_p$, $g$, $i$, $d$, $hc$, $wb$, $p$). It is a useful tool for health policy and allows us to keep the potential contributions of medical care to health in perspective. It also allows us to consider the role of prosperity in producing health and, conversely, the role of healthcare in improving prosperity (Bloom & Canning, 2000). When crafting policy for health improvement, the contribution of each of these health fields should be considered in relation to each other and medical care in particular. Evaluating Case 27-3 in the context of the health production function (the Evans and Stoddart model), Dr. Wellman is focusing on inputs of medical care, assuming or hoping that particular therapies might cure or slow progression of COPD. Some therapies might be better than others in slowing progression but none have been shown to reverse the disease (Barnes, 2000). Health and ability to function are the actual desired outputs; medical care is only one of many inputs. The health production formula helps us to look more broadly, holistically, and more prospectively. The principal risk factors for COPD are cigarette smoking and environmental pollutants. There is likely to be greater benefit for all of his patients if he were to focus on their individual behaviors and the social and physical environments in which they live. Helping patients to avoid or quit smoking is critical but changing the social environment that promotes smoking and maintaining a healthy physical environment are important too. What skills, knowledge, abilities, and obligations does the physician have to affect these inputs? Education of all patients at an early age about the effect of smoking on pulmonary function (as well as risk of cancer and contribution to other diseases) and early pulmonary rehabilitation in the first stages of COPD can change patient behavior. At a community level, the physician can participate in local health education and smoking cessation programs, such as through the American Lung Association's Project Assist. The physician can also change the social environment that encourages smoking by bringing professional knowledge and advocacy to the policymaking

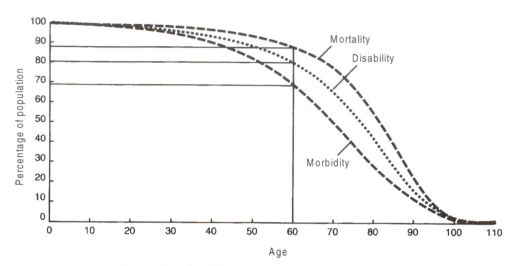

**Figure 27.8.** Percentage of mortality, disability, and morbidity in a population by age. Adapted from Verbrugge, 1989.

process. He or she may have more impact on the population's health through components in the production function other than medical care.

What are the effects and limits of medical care in improving health? How should the challenge of improving health be conceptualized and measured? Figure 27.8 represents the challenge. The percentage of the population alive, disabled, and experiencing disease morbidity is plotted at each age up to 100 years. The outer curve is the percent alive at each age (a survival curve). The lower curve is the percent experiencing morbidity. The area in between the curves measures disability. The challenge for improving population health is to push both curves outward and make them square, compressing morbidity against mortality. Medical care can contribute to squaring and compressing the curves but so can the other factors in the health production function. The effect of availability of medical care may be much less than the effect of social factors and individual behaviors. Each factor has limits. and a variable contribution that must be considered.

## Cost versus Benefit, Effectiveness, and Utility

Each successive gain from medical intervention comes at an increasing cost, particularly in treating chronic disease. We are confronted not only by the limits of affordability but also by the point of diminishing returns. Physicians are accustomed to evaluating *risks* versus *benefits* objectively, but they frequently make very subjective judgments about *cost* versus *benefit*. Economic concepts help structure the discussion of cost versus benefit and make it more systematic. Consider the theoretical plot of cost against benefit in Fig. 27.9. Dollar values of medical expense and benefit are plotted against amount of service provided. The services could be diagnostic tests, physician visits, hospital days, physical therapy sessions, and the like. Cost increases are typically linear. Benefit is typically curvilinear, initially increasing and likely to have a much higher value than cost, but increasing at a diminishing rate. At some point, the benefit curve flattens and additional services produce less incremental benefit. At some point, more medical services may even begin to do harm.

Each increment in service should be prescribed in terms of expected incremental benefit weighed against the increment in cost. Economists call incremental cost *marginal cost* and measure it against *marginal benefit*. There is a much more favorable ratio of marginal benefit to marginal cost between points A and B than between points C and D. The economist's prescription is to continue providing service until the marginal benefit is equal to the marginal cost. Most objective assessments would put the marginal benefit of Mr. Olds's MRI relatively low compared with cost, but Jane's mammogram would be high benefit versus cost.

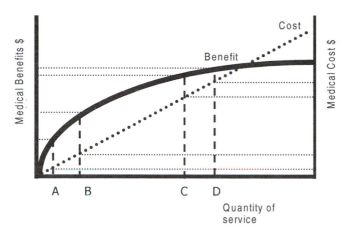

**Figure 27.9.** Medical costs versus medical benefit. Adapted from Fuchs, 1990.

The health policy analyst uses these concepts in *cost–benefit analysis* (CBA) and *cost–effectiveness analysis*, to estimate the value of a new program or compare alternative programs, services, or therapies. CBA is applied to investments of capital, applications of new technologies, or making choices between alternative services. Case 27-2 is an example of where such an analysis is helpful. Dr. Wellman was correct when he said that the MRI unit and immunization were unrelated and funded by different income streams, but only from his or the hospital's limited point of view. Mrs. Steward, taking a more global view, might well wish to compare the additional MRI unit to immunization services as alternative societal expenditures. CBA quantifies benefits and costs in dollar terms, measuring both direct and indirect costs and benefits. The result is expressed as a ratio of dollars of benefit to dollars of cost. Intangible costs and benefits accruing to the patient or society may also be identified but are often difficult to quantify. The focus of CBA is usually on long-term policies, programs, or capital commitments. Table 27.1 displays the elements of CBA for a childhood immunization program.

Though CBA is useful in policy analysis and forces the consideration of many nonclinical concerns, it is difficult to quantify all costs and benefits in monetary terms. What monetary value should be ascribed to a

**Table 27.1**
Elements of Cost–Benefit Analysis of Comprehensive Childhood Immunization Program[a]

| Costs | Benefits |
|---|---|
| Direct | Direct |
| Medical | Deaths averted, savings in life years |
| Cost of vaccine, physician fees, nursing and other personnel costs, administration | Savings in future medical costs averted, morbidity and institutionalization avoided |
| Nonmedical | |
| Parents' time | |
| Indirect | Indirect |
| Medical | Reduced loss of school days |
| Management of adverse reactions | Reduced loss of work days |
| Nonmedical | |
| Loss of work for parents from adverse reaction | |
| Intangible | Intangible |
| Incompatibility with values and religious beliefs of some citizens | Reduced suffering |
| | Level of herd immunity gained |
| Suffering and potential loss from adverse reactions | Protection afforded the nonimmunized |
| | Reduced loss of loved ones |

[a]All benefits and costs are expressed in dollar value.

human life, to the potential life of an infant versus an octogenarian? What cost for suffering, the value to individuals of herd immunity? *Cost–effectiveness analysis* (CEA) avoids some of these problems. CEA can be used for evaluating specific clinical services and choosing between specific therapies or diagnostic procedures that have similar ends or purposes. Cost–effectiveness is a ratio of cost per unit of service or desired outcome; e.g., the net cost per death averted because of one intervention compared with another, the cost per vaccination, or the cost per life year saved. CEA, applied to clinical trials or outcomes research, attaches dollar value to measures of clinical efficacy. It would be useful in examining, for instance, the efficacy of coronary artery bypass graft surgery versus lipid-lowering pharmacological therapy, or one pharmacological agent versus another. It could also be used to compare the various therapies for COPD mentioned in Case 27-3. If the outcome of interest were cost per day of remaining life without oxygen therapy, where would lung-reduction surgery be on the cost–effectiveness curve (Fig. 27.9) versus therapy to assist smoking cessation or pulmonary rehabilitation?

We could also use CEA to compare different antibiotics for treating otitis media with each other and with watchful waiting. Table 27.2 presents a hypothetical CEA of two antibiotics compared with a placebo. The comparison is limited to children aged 1 to 3 who have been diagnosed by reliable techniques as having OME for at least 6 weeks, but less than 4 months, and who are otherwise healthy. Note that two cost–effectiveness ratios are given, one for a short-term outcome and one for a long-term outcome. In the short-term, drug A appears twice as effective but less cost-effective than drug B. By 24 weeks, however, it was less effective and much less cost-effective (by a factor of 3). Contrast both, however, to a choice of watchful waiting in this hypothetical situation

With any of these techniques, it is necessary to identify the perspective of the analysis. Is it being done from the perspective of society (a population approach), the individual patient, a provider (clinical approach), or a payer (bottom-line approach)? The intervention must be carefully defined, as well as what it is being compared with. Is it to be compared with doing nothing, with a placebo, a similar intervention, different medical intervention, or with a form of primary prevention? Are all relevant costs and benefits specified and measured? What assumptions are used in measuring the costs and benefits? These techniques may be used by policymakers, payers, and physicians for different ends. For physicians, they are an aid to judgment about wise use of resources, not a substitute for clinical decision-making.

## Free Enterprise and Competition versus Government Intervention in Markets

Economic theory such as supply and demand, the production function, and techniques like those above are useful; but to see the larger picture of health policy, an understanding of economic philosophy is neces-

**Table 27.2**
Cost-Effectiveness Analysis of Two Antibiotics for Otitis Media with Effusion, Compared to Placebo
in Otherwise Healthy Children Aged 1–3 Years Having Clearly Diagnosed OME of 6 to 16 Weeks' Duration (Hypothetical)

| Group | N | OME cases Clear at 3 wks | OME cases Clear at 24 wks | Direct cost Drug cost | Indirect costs Side effects Rashes, diarrhea | Indirect costs Side effects Unit cost | Indirect costs Future drug resistance proxy cost | Total net cost | Net cost per case cleared at 3 wks | Net cost per case cleared at 24 wks |
|---|---|---|---|---|---|---|---|---|---|---|
| Drug A | 100 | 48 | 46 | $2936 | 3 | $150 | $25 | $3411 | $71.06 | $74.15 |
| Drug B | 100 | 24 | 52 | 524 | 6 | 125 | 25 | 1299 | 54.13 | 24.98 |
| Control | 100 | 18 | 42 | 0 | | 0 | 0 | 0 | 0 | 0 |

Synopsis of methods and materials
1. Measurement of clearance of fluid from ear by otoscopic judgment and tympanometry
2. Confounding variables controlled by randomization and equivalent counseling to parents regarding environmental risk reduction
3. Cost effectiveness = Net cost per cases cleared
4. Net cost = Direct cost (total drug cost per treatment group) + Indirect cost ($25 for each side effect noted in chart, representing a cost to patient's parent for consultation) and $25 proxy for cost of potential future drug resistance is assumed
5. Price of antibiotic A to pharmacist—$5.24 for 10-day treatment; price of antibiotic B to pharmacist—$29.36 for 10-day treatment

sary. The choices for constructing any nation's economic system are found within the spectrum defined by free markets on one end and authority systems on the other (Lindblom, 1977; Marx, 1888; Smith, 1776). The United States's free enterprise system is based on the philosophical principle of private property—the right to have, use, and exchange it freely. Adam Smith's economic philosophy supported both that right and claims that free markets are the most efficient way to allocate resources. The classical, free-enterprise system is one of paramount simplicity, promising self-regulating efficiency, equity, and dynamic flexibility. Efficient *allocation* of private goods occurs where the supply and demand curves cross. In situations of perfect competition for private goods, the market is the most efficient way to allocate resources. *Allocation* is not the same as *distribution,* however, and *private goods* must be distinguished from *public goods*. The market can allocate private goods efficiently, but does not necessarily distribute either private or public goods fairly.

The market is inefficient if benefits and/or costs accrue to others external to the transaction. Everyone benefits from national defense, police and fire protection, pure water sources, medical education, immunization, and construction of hospitals. In the economists' jargon, there are *externalities,* a concept that helps define what goods or services should be considered public.

*Private goods* are ones for which the benefits and costs of consumption are internalized and consumption is rival (Musgrave & Musgrave, 1984, pp. 47–69). Markets will not allocate efficiently when consumption of a good is *nonrival* or when benefits or costs are not internalized. If you buy and eat an ice cream cone, no one else can consume it (a rival good) but a street light shines on all that who walk beneath it (nonrival). For

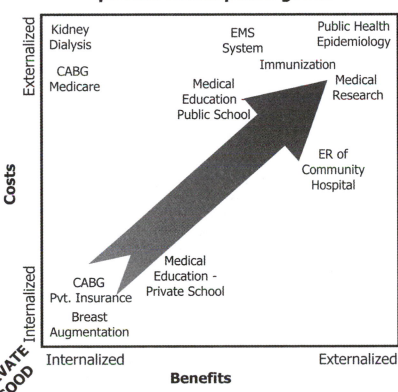

some goods and services, consumption may be rival but benefits cannot be limited to individuals. Exclusion based on payment may be neither possible nor good social policy, so for some services or goods, "free-riders" are allowed. Libraries, public education, the Internet, and treatment at the emergency room of a public hospital are public goods. Entire consumption of benefit and incidence of costs cannot be internalized or limited to individuals involved in immediate transactions so all or a portion of the costs are borne by society as a whole. Some believe that all medical care *should* be considered a public good, access to a basic minimum of which is a matter of democratic justice, and of benefit to all of society. Medical care is principally a private good in the United States, however. Those who believe that it should be a private good and base their argument on economic theory or assumptions should understand that medical services are not delivered in the perfect market of classical economic theory.

Perfect competition requires: sufficient numbers of both buyers and sellers so that decisions of an individual cannot determine market price; complete knowledge of market conditions for both buyers and sellers; substitutability of products and services; and, mobility of resources into and out of the market. Ask yourself if each of these elements is present in the healthcare system. Has the market failed?

When markets fail, government frequently intervenes. Electrical power, gas, water, sewer, taxis, cable TV, and telephone services are common examples. Government may step in to produce the good or service or to restructure the market and provide incentives for it to work more efficiently. In medical care, government has intervened in many ways. Medical education, which is heavily subsidized by government, is an example. How many students could afford or find loans for the full cost of a medical education—approximately half a million dollars? As neither the full cost nor the full benefit of training is borne by the physician, there are externalities involved. Entry into the health professions has been not only subsidized but limited as well, isolating both physician training and practice from imperatives of the market. Other examples of healthcare as a public good are the construction of hospitals with public funds and the conducting of biomedical research. On the demand side, government has selectively provided or subsidized health insurance for four-fifths (or so) of the population.

Government has certainly "messed with the market" to limit public spending on health. Public strategies to limit spending include: *certificate of need* laws to restrain investment in facilities and expensive devices; prospectively setting reimbursement rates for hospital services with *diagnosis related groups* (DRGs) and the *resource-based relative value scale* (R-BRVS) for physicians; increases in *copayments and deductibles* for Medicare and Medicaid; and subsidy of technology assessment, *outcomes research*, and *clinical practice guidelines*. Recently public strategies have promoted development of managed care.

## Basic Economic Principles of Managed Care

There are many kinds of managed care organizations and almost all insurance plans now have mechanisms to manage the cost and utilization of medical care. All managed care organizations are not HMOs, however. An HMO is an organized system of health services delivery offering a comprehensive set of benefits to a defined population for a fixed, prepaid fee. Acceptance of the fixed fee (capitation) is a strong incentive to manage services in a cost-effective manner. The HMO must limit utilization of expensive services, substitute more cost-effective alternatives, and provide preventive and primary care services that reduce the need for chronic or acute care services. By accepting financial risk for defined populations, HMOs are guided daily by the concepts of cost-effectiveness portrayed in Fig. 27.9. Depending on the corporate motives of the organization, managed care is a philosophy leading either to good medicine or to good business. Preventive services, improved continuity of care, and a focus on efficacy issues improve quality but may also improve profit margins.

Managed care organizations are distinguishable not only by profit motive but also by how much risk they assume and how they relate to their participating physicians. The distinctions are becoming increasingly blurred. At one end of the spectrum is the "managed" indemnity or service plan that only employs utilization controls like preapproval and case management for certain high-cost services. Many state Medicaid programs now selectively contract with primary care physicians to manage care of patients, paying a modest monthly per capita fee for case management while reimbursing specific services on a fee-for-service basis. Next in the spectrum would be the insurance plan that contracts with preferred provider organizations (PPOs). Physicians in a PPO agree to abide by utilization management procedures of the insurance company and accept discounted rates for services provided to their PPO patients. Patients with this type of insurance may go to any physician but are encouraged by lower premiums, copayments, or deductibles to go to the "preferred" physicians, hospitals, or other providers. The insurance company selects "preferred" providers based on documentation of costwise practices

Somewhere between the PPO and the HMO is the point of service (POS) plan. This plan offers the patient greater choice of physicians. In the POS option, the patient may be required to go through a primary care physician acting as a "gatekeeper" but is allowed to go to an out-of-network provider typically with a copayment to do so. The managed indemnity plan, PPO, and POS plan accept increasing risk for managing within a fixed budget but do not have nearly as much risk as the HMO, which is obligated to provide defined services for a capitated rate. With the HMO, there is no deductible and copayments are minimal but there is limited choice of physician and no opportunity to go to out-of-plan providers without prior authorization. HMOs may be for-profit or not-for-profit organizations. They may also be defined by how physicians share in their governance, administration, and profits. In regard to physician participation, HMOs are described as a staff model, group model, or independent practice association (IPA).

The staff model HMO employs a panel of salaried, generalist physicians from which enrollees choose their primary care physician. The staff model may employ some specialists but contract with specialists needed least frequently. The staff model HMO usually contracts for hospital care and other services. By these contracts, the staff model HMO organizes a (more or less) comprehensive and cost-effective delivery system for its enrollees and can control how its physicians use resources. In addition to salary, physicians in some staff model HMOs receive a share of profits or bonuses for achieving productivity targets.

In the IPA and group model, the HMO is a separate entity that contracts with a panel of physicians in the IPA or a medical group practice to care for its prepaid plan enrollees. Physicians are either self-employed (as in the IPA) or employed by the medical group, not by the HMO. In the IPA model, the IPA negotiates with the HMO. In either the IPA or group model, physicians may have fee-for-service patients but accept the HMO's patients at a capitated or discounted rate. The HMO may create networks of multiple groups and IPAs. In the IPA and group model, the HMO controls the system which serves its enrollees rather than controlling the behavior of individual physicians. These HMOs may also offer financial incentives to participating physicians to limit use of specialist or hospital services by holding back some percentage of reimbursement until an end-of-year review of the physicians' and plan's performance. A potential for conflict of interest exists whenever physicians have a financial stake in the utilization of health services, regardless of whether the HMO is a staff, IPA, or group model. Financial incentives put the physician on a slippery slope. "The first duty of physicians must be to the individual patient … and … financial incentives should not result in the withholding of appropriate medical services or in denial of patient access to such services" (AMA, 1999).

The shift of financial risk for care from the insurer to the provider is an important concept. Risk shifted to physicians is greatest with the fully capitated plans. Managed care has fundamentally changed the way medicine is practiced and the market for indemnity health insurance is diminishing. It is estimated that some 79 million Americans were enrolled in HMOs in 1998, an increase of 91% from 1993 (InterStudy, 1999). Another 89 million or so were estimated to be in PPOs, up from 47% in 1993 (Hoechst Marion Roussel, 1998).

Managed care has given business and government some control over spending but opinion is mixed on whether it is the best way to finance medical care. Evaluation of managed care in terms of long-term efficiency of resource use, quality, and patient satisfaction is difficult. There is no clear evidence that HMOs are better or worse than fee-for-service plans on these dimensions (Miller & Luft, 1997). There is, however, an increas-

## BASIC QUESTIONS A PHYSICIAN
## SHOULD ASK BEFORE JOINING AN HMO

1. *Will the HMO help me be a better physician?*
2. *Will the HMO be better for my patients?*
3. *Will the HMO be better for society by making the healthcare system more efficient and optimizing population health?*
4. *Will my participation in the HMO be of advantage to me financially or in regard to other personal goals?*
5. *How much do I value my autonomy and how much of it might I have to give up?*
6. *What will I lose if I don't join?*

ingly critical tone in the coverage of managed care by the media (Brodie *et al.*, 1998). Physicians are becoming disenchanted with the system and many states have now passed or are considering laws to regulate managed care. The issues to be regulated are ones such as: prohibiting financial incentives to physicians, adoption of "prudent layperson" standards regarding use of emergency room services without prior authorization, allowing women to see an obstetrician or gynecologist without referral by a gatekeeper, allowing patients to keep their physician if the physician is dropped by a plan, and allowing patients to sue their insurance company (Families USA, 1999). At the federal level, a patients' bill of rights incorporating many of these concerns has been debated in Congress at length.

There are advantages and disadvantages in managed care. The consumer in particular must evaluate options in terms of comprehensiveness of benefits, the importance of preventive services, continuity of care, cost, and how much choice of provider is desired. Physicians must decide how to negotiate with managed care organizations and the extent to which they are willing to be gatekeepers. Society must determine how much oversight is needed. Government's role is managing the competition, ensuring patients' rights, and deciding whether all, or which, citizens have financial access to care. It could also choose to control the resources that are available to the healthcare system.

A fundamental characteristic of a healthcare system is whether it is open or closed. An HMO is a closed system for its enrollees. It must operate within a fixed budget by closely estimating revenues and utilization, and carefully managing utilization and costs. The U.S. healthcare enterprise is a very open system. A major reason the cost of healthcare has been out of control is precisely that the system is so open. With so many different providers and types of insurance plans, with so many unbundled and unmanaged services, so many people (44 million) not explicitly in the system, so many disjointed attempts to fix it, and so many interest groups trying to preserve their stake in the existing system, control will remain elusive. Perhaps healthcare will remain an open, pluralistic system because that is what Americans want. However, the essential feature that distinguishes our system from that of the Canadians and the British is the notion of a fixed budget. Once a budget is fixed and a commitment made to include all citizens in the care that budget will buy, there is a stronger requirement to manage the entire system. If the hospital in Case 27-2 became an HMO and obligated to serve all people in its service area, do you think the Board would have voted to purchase the MRI unit?

## CASE 27-4

*Following the 1992 election, national health reform seemed inevitable. The President placed health reform high on the agenda. A Task Force analyzed and selected alternatives, and delivered a complex legislative draft of proposals to the Congress. By the time of the fall 1994 elections, no proposals had been approved.*

*Following the 1998 elections, Medicare reform, the uninsured, and managed care reform were the highest healthcare priorities of voters for the new Congress. Managed care reform had the greatest public consensus. In 1999 the public outcry against managed care, especially denial of services, increased. The debate on both sides of Congress was intense, with numerous bills introduced. In the summer of 2001, a patient protection bill passed the Senate (S. 1052), followed by a similar one in the House of Representatives (HR. 2563), which was then sent to the Senate for resolution of significant differences that would determine the degree to which the bill protected patients versus the interests of insurance companies.*

## HEALTH POLICY

Public policymaking, including the development of health policy, can be considered a set of processes, which include the setting of the agenda, the specification of alternatives from which a choice can be made, an authoritative choice among the specified alternatives, and the implementation of the decision (Kingdon, 1984).

At any given time, the agenda is the list of subjects, concerns, problems, or issues to which governmental officials and people outside government are devoting time and attention. The agenda-setting process narrows these to the ones that become the focus of attention. Problems or concerns can be brought to prominence by systematic indicators (e.g., percentage of GDP spent on healthcare, number of uninsured), by a focusing event such as a crisis or disaster, or by feedback from current program operation. An agenda item has a higher likelihood of rising to prominence if it is congruent with the current national mood, has interest group support or lack of organized opposition, and fits the orientation of prevailing legislative coalitions and the current administration. In Case 27-4, healthcare reform became a focus of attention as a campaign issue because of the rising cost of healthcare and the number of individuals without health insurance. Managed care reform, in Case 27-5, was congruent with the national mood, with over 78% of voters favoring patient protection legislation.

The process of specifying alternatives narrows the choices to proposals that will be most seriously considered and potentially become legislation. In Case 27-4, a number of alternatives, such as managed competition, increased regulation of insurance companies, or comprehensive national health insurance, were considered. Proposals that are technically and budgetarily feasible, consistent with dominant values and the current national mood, and that have political support or lack organized opposition, have the highest likelihood of surviving long enough for serious consideration. In Case 27-4, so many alternatives were under consideration that few had enough political support to remain under consideration. More importantly, in both Cases 27-4 and 27-5, most of the alternatives had substantial organized opposition.

Various participants, including the President, the Congress, bureaucrats, and individuals and forces outside of government (e.g., media, interest groups, political parties, and the general public), can be sources of agenda items and alternatives. The administration, including the President and his political appointees, is central to agenda setting, but has much less influence or control over the process of considering alternatives. In Case 27-4, the President was able to focus attention on health reform, but failed to bring forward a set of alternatives that survived long enough for serious consideration. Congress is central to both setting the agenda and specifying alternatives; legislators tend to have more impact on the agenda while their staffers concentrate more on the alternatives. Outside of government, interest groups affect policy agendas and most often do so by devoting their efforts to negative, blocking activities. A group that mobilizes support by motivating its

---

*"Medicine is social science, and politics is nothing more than medicine on a large scale."*
*Rudolf Virchow, 1848*

constituents to write letters and visit legislators, and stimulates its allies to do the same, can get the attention of legislators. In Case 27-4, a media campaign by the Health Insurance Association of America featured some very effective television advertisements featuring a young couple, "Harry and Louise", who communicated their fears about the government becoming the sole agent for managing the delivery of healthcare services (Blumenthal, 1995). In Case 27-5, the American Association of Health Plans, the Health Benefits Coalition, and the American Medical Association launched extensive media and grass-roots campaigns. The American Medical Association, Families USA, and the Consumers Union mobilized their members, organizing letter-writing and telephone campaigns and Washington visits. Organized interests are heard more in the political process than are unorganized interests.

Mass media clearly affect the public opinion agenda, and this affects politicians. Media's role is to report, interpret, and magnify events rather than originate them, but media can also serve as a venue for interest groups to express their support or opposition to alternatives. Public opinion through national surveys has a powerful impact on the policymaking process and can have either positive or negative effects. Some items become part of the governmental agenda because a sufficient number of voters interested in the issue make it popular for vote-seeking politicians. More often than not, public opinion constrains government action. In Case 27-4, numerous alternatives were debated in the fall of 1994. Public opinion contributed significantly to the failure to pass any legislation before the November election. In Case 27-5, public frustration with healthcare was at a peak in the summer of 1999, and in light of a pending election, both parties and both sides of Congress were motivated to finalize legislation, but no definitive action was taken by the Congress. Healthcare issues will be a significant component of the political campaigns but campaign promises don't always lead to action.

In a rational, comprehensive decision-making model, policymakers would first define their goals clearly and then set levels of achieving the goals. They would then identify and study all alternatives that might achieve these goals, compare alternatives systematically, determining costs and benefits, and after thorough analysis, choose alternatives that would meet goals at the least cost. Typically, however, instead of considering each program or issue afresh, decision makers take what they currently are doing as given and make small adjustments to what is currently being implemented. This is known as incrementalism and results in gradual policy changes. Incrementalism tends to characterize more the process of generating and selecting alternatives. In Case 27-4, the election and the abrupt change in ideas about implementing comprehensive health reform that followed are examples of nonincremental change. This abrupt change was consistent with neither other dominant public philosophy about the role of government nor the interest of major professions and the insurance business.

Incorporated within policymaking are three processes that develop and operate largely independently of one another, except at critical times: (1) the recognition of problems, (2) the formation and refining of policy proposals, and (3) the politics of enactment and implementation. When these processes or streams are linked, policy is more likely to change.

People recognize problems and generate proposals for policy change. They engage in political activities such as election campaigns and pressure-group lobbying, acting as either an impetus or a constraint. The key to understanding policy change is the coupling of these processes. A problem is recognized, a solution is available, the political climate makes the time right for change, and the constraints do not prohibit action. For any of this to occur, there must be at least one significant policy entrepreneur. Policy entrepreneurs are advocates willing to invest their time, energy, reputation, and money to promote a position or attach a problem to a solution, joining problems, policies, and politics (Kingdon, 1984). They hook solutions to problems, proposals to political momentum, and political events to policy problems.

Governmental and nongovernmental agencies routinely monitor various indicators, such as the amount of GDP spent on healthcare or the total Medicare dollars used for healthcare. Sometimes a focusing event, such as a crisis or disaster, or the personal experience of a policymaker, may call attention to a problem. Feedback is provided to governmental officials and decision makers about the operations of existing programs that may indicate a problem in a program, that goals are not being met, that costs are higher than anticipated, or that there may be unanticipated consequences of a public policy. People must be convinced that change is needed for a specific condition to be defined as a problem. In Case 27-5, many people argued that patients had been deprived of their rights of choice and access to healthcare services in the current managed care environment. Others did not believe the feedback or indicators and argued, like the CEO of Aetna Inc., that the real problem was the number of individuals without health insurance. To focus attention on a problem, participants will highlight indicators through press releases, speeches, or during hearings or committee testimony. Other strategies include associating with experiences of influential people and generating attention by letters, visits to decision makers, testimony before Congress, and protest activity. The process of fixing attention on one problem rather than another is crucial to agenda setting. In Case 27-4, many problems related to healthcare were identified and competed for attention. Without focused attention and agreement as to the problem(s), identifying and choosing alternatives became impossible.

Introducing bills and making speeches are used to test a proposal and gauge receptivity to an idea. For a proposal to survive, it must be technically feasible, compatible with the values of the policy community and powerful interest groups, have an acceptable cost, and have a high likelihood of being positively received among elected decision makers and the public. As proposals are developed, they move through a long process of consideration, discussion, debate, revision, and testing. The process emphasizes persuasion, building coalitions, striking bargains, and providing concessions. The goal is to gain enough votes to pass the proposal out of committee and through the Congress, which takes a minimum of 218 Representatives and 51 Senators.

Policy windows provide necessary opportunities for action on given initiatives to occur. They open for short periods for varying reasons. A window may open because of a change in the political stream, as in the change in administration that occurred in Case 27-4, or a redistribution of representation in Congress, as happened in the November 1994 elections. It can also occur through the efforts of individuals or policy entrepreneurs. In Case 27-5, a handful of physician members of the House of Representatives pledged support for a more extensive patient protection package and moved this idea forward in a bipartisan compromise bill. Problems may become more pressing (number of employed individuals without health insurance, potential bankruptcy of Medicare Trust Fund), creating an opportunity for advocates to attach their solutions to the problems. Policy windows present opportunities for problems, proposals, and politics to come together, and hence opportunities to move them up the decision agenda. In Case 27-4, the initial phases of the health reform debate caught the attention of the media, the public, and most legislators, creating a policy window. What did not occur during this process was the coupling of the identified problems, proposals, and political stream. In Case 27-5, there was considerable support for a bill that would guarantee patients' rights to medical care and allow them to sue insurance companies for injury in the denial of care. The American Medical Association and over forty professional associations supported such legislation but it was strongly opposed by insurance companies and employers. Representative Norwood, a Republican and dentist with an honorary MD, introduced an amendment to the house bill in 2001 that he claimed would make it acceptable to President George W. Bush. The Norwood amendment limited damaged awards in suits against HMOs and took such suits out of state courts and into federal courts, which tend to be less sympathetic to plaintiffs (patients) in such tort cases. The house bill, with the Norwood amendment, narrowly passed and was put on the calendar in the Senate by the end of August 2001. It seemed like a conference committee would easily resolve the differences and send the bill to the president. Political priorities changed dramatically with events in the fall, however. As of press time for this text, differences in the two patient protection bills had not been resolved. The September 11 terrorist attack on the New York World Trade Center, response to bioterrorism, war in Afghanistan, and economic recession displaced the issue as high priority. The policy window closed. It could be a long time before there is a critical alignment of problem, proposal, and political stream for this issue.

## CONCLUSION

This overview of the policymaking process is not designed to make you an expert but to provide a perspective of how the health policy that affects the delivery of healthcare, research, and education is determined. The process is complex, multifactorial, and dynamic. The principal issues are ones of economics, distributive justice, and control of the political decision-making process. The questions of who shall receive care, amount and kind, and how it shall be rationed, cannot be avoided. These questions will be decided by either the market or government. Government has the responsibility and authority to decide which, or what, balance between the two basic systems to employ.

Policy will be determined in a political process. The key to understanding policy changes and the policymaking process is not where the idea came from, but what made it become a focus of attention and what sustained that focus. It is critical that health professionals understand the components of this coupled process and where their involvement can help develop effective and relevant health policies for the future.

As a physician, you must continue to remember the challenges of the Hippocratic oath (Relman, 1980; Relman & Reinhardt, 1986) regarding the role of the physician as a member of a profession and not a business enterprise, and maintain your primary interest in the welfare of your patients. As you strive to improve the healthcare status of individuals by participating in the policymaking process, you must remember that "the primary concern of professionals must not be the self-interest of the professional group or the corporation. If someday physicians and their organizations do become primarily self-interest groups, society—which has given them the privilege of being called professionals—will rise up and take that privilege away. And the profession will be no more!" (Lundberg, 1995).

## CASES FOR DISCUSSION

### CASE 1

*Mr. A., a 54-year-old salesman, had a coronary artery bypass graft (CABG). Six months after the surgery he is doing well but he is sedentary, 40 pounds overweight, and continues to smoke cigarettes. His response to your concern about his lifestyle choices and the impact on his heart disease is: "Gee, Doc, I can't imagine what the quality of my life would be like without my cigarettes. I've tried to change my diet but that is really hard. If the arteries block up again you can do another surgery." The likelihood of re-occlusion in 2–4 years is very high if risk factors are not modified.*

1. *Is there a difference in the value of a CABG for one individual versus a free immunization program for children? In this situation, would a cost–effectiveness analysis (CEA) assist in determining guidelines?*
2. *In Great Britain, an individual who refused to quit smoking was refused a second CABG. Will this lead to an equitable allocation of resources?*
3. *How does the calculus or result of the economic analysis of the CABG change according to the perspective or interest of the analyst? How might the analysis be differently structured by the cardiothoracic surgeon, the cardiologist, general physician, patient, policy analyst, insurance company?*

### CASE 2

*Medicare currently provides approximately $6.1 billion for graduate medical education (GME) to academic health centers (medical schools and teaching hospitals). Each year approximately 17,000 individuals graduate from U.S. allopathic and osteopathic medical schools and begin residency training. In 1993, 106,000 residents were in postgraduate training, and of those 25,000 were in first-year positions. More than 25% of all first-year slots were occupied by international medical graduates (IMGs—individuals who have graduated from medical schools other than the United States). A large percentage of Medicare GME funds are directed to two northeastern states, each of which has 45–50% of their residency positions filled by IMGs. The cost of healthcare continues to rise each year and a significant proportion of that rise is Medicare-related expenditures, including funds for GME. The Congress is aware of the problem of escalating healthcare costs and is evaluating whether reducing the number of residency positions or the amount of GME funding through Medicare would move toward a balanced budget.*

1. *What participants and/or special interest groups would be involved in responding to a proposal for legislation to reduce the number of residency positions?*
2. *How might they position themselves, and what strategies might they utilize to support or oppose such a proposal?*
3. *Are there special interest groups that might work together in these efforts?*

## CASE 3

You are chairman of the medical society's political action committee. The two leading candidates in the gubernatorial election each promise health insurance initiatives, new social programs, and health system reforms. Leo proposes to improve financial access to health services for children by allowing parents to enroll them in the state's Medicaid program. Billy Bob's proposal is to give a credit on state income tax for purchase of private health insurance for children. Leo's Medicaid expansion plan would be offered to families earning less than 200% of zhe poverty level. Billy Bob's tax credit would be up to $500 per year for the cost of a child's health insurance premium for families making up to 250% of the poverty level. The fiscal research office of the state legislature estimates that under Leo's proposal, Medicaid would be extended to half of the 120,000 children presently uninsured at a cost of $48 million. Billy Bob's proposal is estimated to cover about 60,000 children at a cost of $30 million. Billy Bob claims his proposal will be more efficient because it will allow more choice of physician and that many parents will enroll their children in HMOs. Billy Bob supports a lottery to raise $1 billion to improve public education through decreasing class size, increasing teacher salaries, and investments in computers and the Internet. He has promised physicians that he will work for a cap on damage awards for medical malpractice. Leo hasn't staked out a position on education reform but has proposed a package of public health measures amounting to $300 million. His proposed public health initiatives include: childhood injury control, lead screening and abatement, childhood obesity interventions, drug programs, and adolescent pregnancy prevention. He has proposed a program to address medical error that would cost $25 million in new data systems and make hospital error rates public knowledge.

1. Which health insurance proposal will be the most cost-effective?
2. Which set of social programs would have the greatest long-term effect on population health, Billy Bob's education reform or Leo's public health initiatives? Would either be more effective than increasing access to care?
3. Which would have the greatest impact on healthcare costs, the malpractice damage cap or the program to address medical error?
4. Which candidate should the medical society endorse?

## CASE 4

Drs. R. and P. joined a physician organization (PO) that recently merged with a regional hospital to form a physician hospital organization (PHO). The administrator of the hospital is eager to develop shared-risk, capitated agreements with several insurance companies moving into the region who want to develop an integrated network and delivery system. In addition to being members of this network, Drs. R. and P. are being offered stock options and investment possibilities in the corporate entity of this network.

1. What are the implications of these agreements for Drs. R. and P.? For the hospital?
2. Whose interests will be represented when Drs. R. and P. provide healthcare services for patients within this network? Is there a conflict of interest?

## CASE 5

County General Hospital (CGH), a private, not-for-profit, 650-bed tertiary care center, is planning to form an integrated delivery network. It has well over half the hospital business in the service area and an entrepreneurial CEO who wants to develop managed care plans before another hospital or insurance company does. CGH's new network, called Regional Integrated Comprehensive Health System (RICHSys), would offer its own health insurance plan as an HMO. RICHSys is quietly negotiating with some of the local primary care physicians to join the HMO as salaried staff but also says it will contract with one or more IPAs for physician services. A national, for-profit insurance group, called MicroMedManagement (MMM), is also planning to enter the managed care market in the region. It will negotiate a discount on each physician's fees on a yearly basis and offer a holdback that may be paid if the MMM plan performs well.

1. Should you contract with or join one of these organizations? If so, which one?
2. What do you think is the hospital's interest in managed care?
3. Why do you think CGH is interested in bringing managed care to the region?
4. Why do you think MMM is interested in bringing managed care to the region?
5. How might cost-control strategies of RICHSys and MMM differ?

## RECOMMENDED READINGS

Himmelstein DU, Woolhandler S, *et al*: A national health program for the United States. *N Engl J Med* 1989; 320(2):102–108.

A proposal for a comprehensive, single-payer system.

Kindig DA: *Purchasing Population Health*. Ann Arbor, University of Michigan Press, 1997.

Defines outputs of the health production function and financial incentives for their achievement.

Kingdon, JW. *Agendas, Alternatives, and Public Policies*. Boston, Little Brown & Co, 1984

A very readable, concise description of how issues get on the political, policymaking agenda, who the government and non-government participants are, and what has to happen for action to occur.

Starr, P. *The Social Transformation of American Medicine*. New York: Basic Books Inc, 1982.

A description of "the rise of a sovereign profession and the making of a vast industry" which will help medical students place the career they have chosen in the context of social systems and U.S. politics.

## REFERENCES

AMA, Council on Medical Service. *Principles of Managed Care*, ed 4, 1999.

Barnes PJ: Chronic obstructive pulmonary disease. *N Engl J Med* 343(4):269–280, 2000.

Bloom DE, Canning D: The health and wealth of nations. *Science* 287:1207–1209, 2000.

Blumenthal D: Health care reform—Past and future. *N Engl J Med* 332:465–468, 1995.

Brodie M, Brady LA, Altman D: Media and managed care: Is there a negative bias? *Health Affairs* 17(1):9–25, 1998.

Evans RG, Stoddart GL: Producing health, consuming healthcare. *Soc Sci Med* 31(12):1347–1363, 1990.

Families USA: *State Managed Care Patient Protections*. October 1999. (http://FAMILIESUSA.org)

Feldstein PJ: *Health Economics*. New York, John Wiley & Sons Inc, 1979.

Fuchs V: Has cost containment gone too far? in Lee PR, Estes CL (eds). *The Nation's Health*. Boston, Jones & Bartlett, 1990.

Ginzberg E: The monetarization of medical care. *N Engl J Med* 310:1162–1165, 1984.

Health Care Financing Administration: *1997 Data Compendium*. Baltimore, U.S. Department of Health and Human Services, 1997.

Health Insurance Association of America: *Source Book of Health Insurance Data*. Washington, DC, Health Insurance Association of America, 1998.

Hoechst Marion Roussel: HMO-PPO Digest. 1998.

Institute of Medicine: *Improving Health in the Community*. Washington, DC, National Academy Press, 1997.

InterStudy: *The Competitive Edge 9.1: HMO Industry Report*. 1999.

Kindig DA: *Purchasing Population Health*. Ann Arbor, University of Michigan Press, 1997.

Kingdon JW: *Agendas, Alternatives, and Public Policies*. Boston, Little Brown & Co, 1984.

Levit KR *et al* : Health spending in 1998: Signals of change. *Health Affairs* 19(1):124–132, 2000.

Lindblom, CE: *Politics and Markets: The World's Political and Economic Systems*. New York, Basic Books, Inc, 1977.

Lundberg GD: The failure of organized health system reform—now what? *Caveat aeger*—Let the patient beware. *JAMA* 273:1539–1541, 1995.

Marx, K: *Manifesto of the Communist Party*. London, 1888.

Miller RH, Luft HS: Managed care performance: Is quality of care better or worse? *J Health Affairs* 16(5):7–25, 1997.

Mitchell JM, Sunshine JH: Consequences of physician's ownership of healthcare facilities—joint ventures in radiation therapy. *N Engl J Med* 327:1497–1501, 1992.

Musgrave RA, Musgrave PB: *Public Finance in Theory and Practice*. New York, McGraw-Hill Book Co, 1984.

Pauly M: The economics of moral hazard: Comment. *American Economic Review* June 1968.

Relman AS: The new medical industrial complex. *N Engl J Med* 303:963–970, 1980.

Relman AS, Reinhardt UE: Debating for-profit healthcare and the ethics of physicians. *Health Affairs* Summer:5–31, 1986.

Rice TH, Labelle RJ: Do physicians induce demand for medical services? *Health Policy Politics Law* 14:587–600, 1988.

Samuelson PA: *Economics*, ed 11. New York, McGraw-Hill Book Co, 1980.

Smith A: *An Inquiry into the Nature and Causes of the Wealth of Nations*. London, 1776.

Smith S, *et al* : The next decade of health spending: A new outlook. *Health Affairs* 18(4):86–95, 1999.

Starr P: *The Social Transformation of American Medicine*. New York, Basic Books, Inc, 1982.

Stevens R: *In Sickness and in Wealth: American Hospitals in the Twentieth Century*. New York, Basic Books, Inc, 1989.

U.S. Census Bureau: Health Insurance Coverage 1998. P60-208. Washington, DC, Department of Commerce, Economics and Statistics Administration, 1999.

U.S. Department of Health and Human Services. *Healthy People 2010*. Washington, DC, 2000.

Verbrugge LM: Recent, present and future health of American adults. *Annu Rev Public Health* 10:333–361, 1989.

Virchow R: The charity physician. *Medicinische Reform*, 18:33, 1848. In Rather LJ (ed): *Rudolf Virchow, Collected Essays on Public Health and Epidemiology*. Canton, Mass, Watson Publishing International, 1985.

Wilensky GR, Rossiter LF: The relative importance of physician-induced demand for medical care. *Milbank Mem Fund Q* 61:252–277, 1983.

## CHAPTER 28

# The Law and Medicine

*Cyndi Jewell Baily, J.D., M.P.H.*

CASE 28-1

*Dr. C was treating Ms. T for alcoholism. Ms. T worked as a nurse at a local psychiatric hospital. Although she had HMO coverage, Ms. T elected to pay for the treatment herself because of fears her supervisors would find out about her addiction if she submitted information to her insurance company. Dr. C admitted Ms. T for experimental inpatient treatment at Community Hospital under a study that had been approved by the Community Hospital Institutional Review Board. Dr. C verbally explained the experimental treatment procedure to Ms. T before beginning treatment. Ms. T verbally indicated to Dr. C that she understood the risks and benefits of the treatment. Complications, which Dr. C previously explained to Ms. T, arose and Ms. T had to remain hospitalized for several days. Ms. T was eventually discharged and the treatment was successful. One week later, Dr. C received a fax of a medical excuse form from the hospital where Ms. T was employed. Dr. C completed the form and provided specific information regarding Ms. T's diagnosis and treatment for alcoholism. Ms. T was then fired for misleading her employer as to the reason for hospitalization. Ms. T filed a complaint against Dr. C with the state physician licensing agency in which she claimed Dr. C violated patient confidentiality by providing information to her employer without her consent. Ms. T also hired an attorney and sued Dr. C for violating her confidentiality rights, for medical malpractice due to the complications she experienced, and for failure to fully inform her of the risks of the experimental procedure.*

*This case contains several issues that will be addressed in this chapter and represents how a variety of legal issues are implicated in the daily practice of medicine.*

## EDUCATIONAL OBJECTIVES

1. Identify specific legal issues commonly faced by physicians
2. Understand basic risk management techniques to reduce the likelihood of medical malpractice lawsuits
3. Recognize and comply with laws and regulations governing the practice of medicine
4. Give examples of how legal concerns conflict with patient care concerns
5. Understand generally the interaction between the law and the practice of medicine

# INTRODUCTION

Health law is the law related to the delivery of healthcare. It defines the rights and responsibilities of the individuals involved. As Case 28-1 illustrates, many aspects of healthcare in general, once considered solely matters of ethics, are now the subject of legislation, litigation, and regulation. For example, informed consent is now a legally recognized principle of the provision of medical care in the United States and is no longer solely an ethical obligation (Rozovsky, 1990). In Case 28-1, although Dr. C verbally explained the experimental procedure to Ms. T, his failure to do so in written form as well likely violates federal law and also likely will make the malpractice case more difficult to defend. A system of third-party private payers, as well as Medicare and Medicaid, has propagated more regulation of the delivery of medical care. Some medico-legal concepts are consistent throughout the United States. Many concepts, however, are unique to the state in which a physician practices. Whether the result of case law or statutory regulation, legal issues in medicine increasingly affect physicians and medical practice (American Society of Law and Medicine, 1985). It is imperative that medical students learn what the law requires of them and their profession. The goal of this chapter is to survey laws affecting the physician–patient relationship and the practice of medicine.

## CASE 28-2

*After completing his residency and obtaining his state medical license, Dr. R joined a large group practice in a suburban area. The group's patient population was largely managed care and Dr. R applied successfully for credentials for the provider physician panels of the managed care companies with which his practice held contracts. He also applied for, and was granted, staff privileges at the local hospital. Over the next 2 years, Dr. R focused all of his energies on building his medical practice.*

*One day, Dr. R performed a rectal examination on a 7-year-old girl who was exhibiting symptoms of severe gastrointestinal disease. Prior to the examination, Dr. R had discussed at length its necessity with the mother, and during the examination both the mother and a nurse were present. However, the mother became very upset. A few days later, she filed a complaint with the state licensing agency. The agency began an investigation.*

*Because Dr. R was under investigation by the state licensing agency, he was required, under the terms of the group's managed care contracts and of the hospital's medical staff bylaws, to notify the managed care companies and the hospital of this investigation. The hospital and the managed care companies suspended Dr. R while the investigation was pending. Although the state board dismissed the complaint for lack of merit, Dr. R and his practice suffered considerable damage.*

## REGULATION OF MEDICAL PRACTICE

Fortunately for Dr. R the complaint against him was found to be frivolous. In many other situations, however, physicians lose their license as a result of legitimate complaints made by patients, often ranging from inadequate medical care to inappropriate sexual relations with patients. As the following section demonstrates, a physician's license to practice medicine is a privilege, not a right. Violation of this privilege could end a medical career. Therefore, it is essential for physicians to understand the legal parameters of this privilege.

In the United States, there is no national or federal system for licensing physicians, and the practice of medicine is regulated on a state-by-state basis. Except in very specific instances, such as U.S. Uniformed Services or public health service personnel, physicians must hold a license in each state in which they practice. The licensing function is typically carried out by an administrative agency or board appointed by the governor of the state and comprised of medical doctors, osteopathic physicians, and public representatives. The licensing board establishes qualifications for applicants and often creates license categories, e.g., temporary license. The most common form of license is physician licensure by examination. Graduates of foreign medical schools commonly must meet additional criteria prior to licensure, including certification by the Educational Commission for Foreign Medical Graduates (ECFMG).

Physicians not otherwise licensed by the state board who are participating in graduate medical education programs usually practice under a permit that restricts their practice to their educational program.

Most states require annual renewal of licenses and a minimum number of continuing medical education hours per year. Most states include a course in medical ethics and/or professional responsibility among their annual requirements.

State licensing boards also have the authority to discipline a physician. Discipline includes reprimand (public or private), probation, suspension, or revocation of a physician's license. Grounds for discipline include: (1) submission of a false or misleading statement in an application for licensure; (2) conviction of a felony or crime of a lesser degree that involves moral turpitude; (3) intemperate use of alcohol or drugs that could, in the opinion of the licensing board, endanger the lives of patients; (4) unprofessional or dishonorable conduct that is likely to deceive, defraud, or injure the public (includes persistently or flagrantly overcharging or overtreating patients); (5) failing to supervise adequately the activities of those acting under the supervision of the physician; or (6) using any advertising statement that is false, misleading, or deceptive.

Methods of discipline vary and often depend on the seriousness of the infraction. The disciplinary process begins with the filing of a complaint against a physician. Frequently, as in Dr. R's case, complaints are initiated by patients and may be anonymous. Next, an investigation by the licensing board occurs. If, as a result of its investigation, the licensing board decides to initiate formal charges against a physician, a hearing is held. Physicians usually have the right to appeal decisions of the state licensing board to a state district court. In most cases, however, courts grant only cursory reviews and defer to the board's decision. Physicians must report any adverse action against their license to managed care companies and to hospitals where they hold staff privileges.

Licensing boards often establish mandatory reporting requirements for public welfare concerns. For example, in Texas, any physician licensed to practice medicine, any graduate medical student, or any medical student must report relevant information to the state licensing board relating to the acts of any physician if in the opinion of the physician or medical student, the physician poses a continuing threat to the public welfare through his or her practice. The most common circumstance when this reporting duty arises is when a physician has reasonable cause to believe that another physician is impaired due to alcohol or drug abuse. Other examples include impairment due to illness, injury, or old age, or making inappropriate sexual advances toward patients.

Recent advances in telecommunications technology and accessibility are fueling an expansion in "telemedicine"—the use of telecommunications technology to diagnose and treat patients at a distance from the medical provider. As mentioned earlier, each of the states regulates the practice of medicine through individual licensure laws. By definition, telemedicine involves the potential for treating patients outside the physician's state of licensure. Consequently, physicians must be aware of the additional licensure requirements created by the practice of medicine outside of state lines. A number of states have recognized the special licensing issues created by telemedicine and have begun to address them. The typical statutes and pending legislation bring telemedicine within the definition of "practice of medicine" but make exceptions for consultations, emergency diagnoses and treatments, and educational lectures and demonstration. Connecticut, for example, requires that out-of-state physicians practicing telemedicine on Connecticut patients be licensed to practice medicine in Connecticut, but makes exceptions for emergencies and consultations: "Any person who furnishes medical or surgical assistance in cases of sudden emergency ... any person residing out of state who is employed to come into this state to render temporary assistance to consult with a physician or surgeon who has been licensed in conformity [with Connecticut law] ... [or] a nonresident physician who, while located outside this state, consults ... with a medical school for educational or medical training purposes" [1996 Conn. Acts, 148 (Reg. Sess.)].

## PRESCRIBING NARCOTICS: PROCEED WITH CAUTION

*One of the easiest ways for newly practicing physicians to get into legal trouble involves the prescription of narcotics. To prevent such trouble, physicians should be familiar with the laws and regulations pertaining to the prescription of narcotics. Some common errors include:*

- *Overprescribing*
- *Unnecessary prescribing*
- *Prescribing to staff members or family members*
- *Prescribing to self*

A corollary issue to physician licensure laws is the area of drug law. Most states and the federal government have a complex system of laws governing the availability and dispensing of dangerous drugs and controlled substances. The Drug Enforcement Agency (DEA) is the federal agency and, for example, the Department of Public Safety (DPS) is the Texas agency that regulates controlled substances. The federal and Texas laws require that persons who manufacture, distribute, administer, dispense, or prescribe controlled substances must be registered with these agencies.

A controlled substance is a drug with a potential for abuse that may lead to physical or psychological dependence. Federal law creates five "schedules" of controlled substances [21 U.S.C. §812(b)]. Schedule I drugs are drugs that have no accepted medical use in treatment in the United States and include heroin, phencyclidine (PCP), and lysergic acid diethylamide (LSD). Schedules II–V contain drugs that are used in medical treatment and range from "high potential for abuse and dependence" (Schedule II) to "low potential for abuse and dependence" (Schedule V). Schedule I and II controlled substances may not be ordered or distributed by a registrant to or from another registrant except pursuant to a federal triplicate order form. Physicians do not need to use triplicate order forms for Schedules III to V. Physicians may obtain the drugs by ordering from the pharmaceutical wholesaler. A physician receiving Schedules III to V controlled substances must maintain records of the transactions by filing the supplier's invoices or maintaining a log book.

Physicians who administer or dispense drugs from their office are required to maintain a separate DEA registration for each office where drugs are administered or dispensed. Physicians who only prescribe drugs are required to maintain a single DEA registration at their principal place of business. DEA registration must be renewed every 3 years and maintained at the registered location for official inspection. Grounds for revocation or suspension of a physician's DEA registration include the following: (1) furnishing false or fraudulent material on application; (2) felony conviction; (3) suspension or revocation of physician's license; (4) failure to establish and maintain effective controls against diversion of controlled substances into other than the legitimate medical, scientific, or industrial channels; (5) willful failure to maintain required records; (6) willful or unreasonable refusal to allow inspection; (7) commission of acts that would render registration inconsistent with the public interest; or (8) exclusion from the Medicare program.

## CASE 28-3

*A 14½-year-old-girl was brought to Dr. M by her mother with complaints of abdominal pain for several weeks. Dr. M had not met the family before, but they came on the recommendation of friends whose children Dr. M has taken care of for several years. After obtaining an initial history from mother and daughter together, Dr. M prudently decides to see the girl by herself. From the girl's sulky demeanor and the mother's angry, overbearing tone, it is apparent that there are serious problems between them.*

*Dr. M assures the girl of confidentiality and learns that she has been sexually active for more than 6 months, without any contraception. For the last week she has experienced increasingly severe pelvic pain. She now has a fever, an elevated erythrocyte sedimentation rate, and bilateral adnexal tenderness on pelvic examination. Dr. M is certain the girl has pelvic inflammatory disease and wishes to admit her to the hospital for intravenous antibiotic treatment.*

*Dr. M discusses the situation with the girl herself. While accepting admission to the hospital, she begs Dr. M not to tell her mother the cause of her illness. The mother, a registered nurse, is certain to know that pelvic infection generally results from being sexually active. She and the father have, on several occasions, expressed to their daughter stern disapproval of such behavior. After talking further with the girl about family dynamics, Dr. M concludes that if the parents discover their daughter is sexually active, they are more likely to be punitive and rejecting than supportive.*

# CONSENT TO TREATMENT AND INFORMED CONSENT

## Consent to Treatment—Capacity and Competency

The doctrine of consent is founded on recognition by the courts and sometimes by legislatures of the rights of patients to make decisions regarding their medical care. The duty of a physician to obtain consent is defined primarily by the liability that has been imposed when this right is not properly honored. Issues surrounding consent to treatment have come to the forefront in recent years because of a growing emphasis on patients' autonomy, i.e., the right of patients to control the course of their medical treatment and the obligation of physicians to provide them the necessary information to enable them to do so. The duty to obtain consent was created by common law, but increasingly this duty is imposed also through the statutory/regulatory process.

Consent encompasses two separate but closely related doctrines: (1) consent to treatment and (2) informed consent.

Failure to obtain consent to treatment may result in a civil tort claim for battery. Some courts have held that a physician must obtain the patient's permission prior to treating him. Failure to do so constitutes a battery—an unlawful touching.

Adult patients have the right to consent for themselves unless they lack the mental capacity to do so. Various standards have been suggested for determining capacity to consent. In general, courts are reluctant to second-guess patient decisions and consider a patient competent to consent if he understands the consequences of his decision, even if the decision is not one that a reasonable person would make or the reasons for it are irrational. Although "competency" as a legal matter can only be determined by a court, most determinations of mental capacity to consent are made by physicians. For most patients, the determination is clear, but if it is not, the question may be referred to a court for decision, particularly if the patient is objecting to the treatment.

If the adult patient lacks the capacity to consent, consent should be obtained from a third party. Unless the patient has a legal guardian appointed or has designated a surrogate decision maker, consent laws usually mandate that consent be obtained from next of kin. Some states have statutes authorizing consent from family members in a hierarchical fashion. For example, Texas law ranks the following order of priority and availability of who should consent to treatment for an adult patient who is incapable of doing so: (1) patient's spouse; (2) an adult child of the patient who has the waiver and consent of all other qualified adult children of the patient to act as the sole decision-maker; (3) a majority of the patient's reasonably available adult children; (4) the patient's parents; or (5) the individual clearly identified to act for the patient by the patient when he became incapacitated, the patient's nearest living relative, or a member of the clergy [Tex. Health & Safety Code Ann., §313.004 (a) (Vernon 1998)]. A few states permit patients to designate someone to act on their behalf. For example, Arizona law allows persons to execute three types of healthcare directives to deal with his or her future healthcare decisions: a living will, a healthcare power of attorney, and a prehospital medical directive (Ariz. Rev. Stat. §36-3201 *et seq.*).

If a patient has no surrogate decision maker, the only absolutely safe course is to obtain judicial authorization of treatment or have a guardian appointed and empowered to make medical care treatment decisions on the patient's behalf.

When a patient is a minor, consent to medical treatment must be obtained from the parent or legal guardian. In most states, children under the age of 18 are defined as minors. An emancipated minor is a child who is no longer under the control of his parents; he is in effect acting as an adult and is permitted to consent to medical care. Although the law varies from state to state, in general children are considered emancipated if they are married, a parent, or financially self-supporting and living away from home. A physician may treat "emancipated minors" in the same manner as adults for purposes of consent to treatment and confidentiality laws. When a child is close to the age of adulthood (i.e., 18) and has the mental capacity to consent on his own behalf, courts occasionally have absolved physicians from liability for failure to obtain parental consent even if the child could not be considered emancipated. This is commonly referred to as the "mature minor" exception. A mature minor exception has been recognized in several states for treatment for venereal disease, pregnancy, and alcohol and drug abuse. A minor's right to consent to abortion was established by the United States Supreme Court in *Planned Parenthood v. Danforth* (1976), but the Supreme Court has upheld the power of states to require parental consent as well (*Planned Parenthood v. Casey*, 1991). The Court upheld Pennsylvania's requirement of parental consent but struck down the law's spousal notification requirement. In Dr. M's case, if the patient's parents demanded information about their daughter's condition, Dr. M may be legally justified in withholding the information on the basis of the mature minor exception. However, because this exception varies considerably among states, a physician faced with a situation similar to Dr. M's should seek legal advice prior to disclosing or withholding information.

Parents who consent to treatment on behalf of the child must act in the child's best interest. Many state child neglect laws include in the definition of "neglect" the failure of the parent to provide necessary medical care. The religious objections of parents may not justify a refusal to consent to treatment of minors: "Parents may be free to become martyrs themselves. But it does not follow that they are free . . . to make martyrs of their own children before they have reached the age of full and legal discretion when they can make that choice for themselves" (*Prince v. Massachusetts*, 1944). Although this principle is well established, the question of how far parents may go in refusing appropriate care is unresolved, and court decisions vary significantly. Parents have been permitted, both by court decision and by statute, to discontinue life-sustaining treatment for minor children who are in a persistent vegetative state. But, generally, parents cannot refuse lifesaving treatment for a child who is not terminally ill, and Jehovah's Witness children are often given blood transfusions over their parents' objections. Parents have been subject to criminal prosecution for failure to provide medical treatment, as in the case of *Walker v. Superior Court* (1988), in which the parents were held responsible for the death of their child who died of meningitis after being treated by prayer alone. Parents have in some cases been permitted to decline conventional treatment in favor of a more unorthodox approach, such as laetrile treatment for cancer, or when a child's prognosis is poor.

Some of the most difficult determinations in this area have involved refusal of treatment for severely damaged or premature newborns. Although the federal government's attempt to regulate this area was unsuccessful, the federal Child Abuse Amendments of 1984 require states that wish to receive federal grants for their child abuse prevention programs to include in their definition of child neglect the failure to provide certain treatment to newborns.

A very problematic issue is determining the proper legal approach when parents of minor children disagree about the proper course of treatment. In a 1991 trial court opinion from Fulton County, Georgia, a judge ruled that a hospital could not reduce the level of treatment provided to an incompetent minor patient or enforce a do-not-resuscitate order because one of the child's parents did not agree with the withdrawal of treatment (*In re Doe*, 1991).

Although liability today is more likely to arise from lack of informed consent (i.e., the physician did not fully inform the patient of the risks of the procedure before the patient consented to the procedure), cases based on failure to obtain consent (i.e., the physician touched and/or treated the patient without consent) still do occasionally arise. At least one case has held that a patient may give conditional consent, and violation of the patient's consent could lead to a civil battery action. In the case of *Ashcraft v. King* (1991), a patient's consent to treatment allegedly was conditioned on use of family blood in transfusions. The patient sued when nonfamily blood was used and the patient subsequently was infected with the human immunodeficiency virus.

## Informed Consent

"A physician violates his duty to his patient and subjects himself to liability if he withholds any facts which are necessary to form the basis of an intelligent consent by the patient to the proposed treatment" (*Salgo v. Leland Stanford, Jr. University Board of Trustees*, 1957). Beginning in the 1970s, many states adopted informed consent laws.

A major issue in informed consent litigation is the scope of the explanation the physician must give about the proposed treatment. Generally, courts have required that the patient be told: (1) the nature and purpose of the procedure, (2) the risks and consequences related to the procedure, (3) alternatives to the proposed treatment, and (4) the risks of foregoing the proposed treatment. Failure to disclose a risk is the most common source of liability.

One of the most difficult questions for courts has been how much detail the physician is required to provide. Two standards have emerged: the "professional practice standard," which requires the physician to make such disclosure as a reasonable medical practitioner in similar circumstances would make (*Retkwa v. Orentreich*, 1992) and the reasonable patient or "materiality standard," which requires the physician to disclose the information that a reasonable person in the patient's position would consider material in deciding whether to undergo the proposed therapy (*Griffith v. Jones*, 1991).

The professional practice standard looks to the medical community to set the standard for required disclosure. To add more certainty to disclosure requirements related to informed consent, some states have formed medical disclosure panels authorized to specify the list of procedures for which informed consent must be obtained and the risks that must be disclosed. For example, Texas's medical disclosure panel has determined that the following potential risks must be disclosed to a patient before an abdominal hysterectomy is performed: (1) uncontrollable leakage of urine, (2) injury to bladder, (3) sterility, (4) injury to the tube (ureter) between the kidney and bladder, and/or (5) injury to the bowel and/or intestinal obstruction.

In a lawsuit, the patient must prove the standard in the community by expert testimony including the physician alleged to have violated the standard. No expert testimony is required under the materiality standard; whether disclosure was appropriate is decided by the jury. Some courts have rejected the materiality standard because of the "potential danger that a jury, composed of laymen and gifted with the benefit of hindsight, will divine the breach of a disclosure obligation largely on the basis of the unfortunate result" (*Wooley v. Henderson*, 1980).

Several legal exceptions exist to the doctrine of informed consent. The most widely recognized exception is in emergency situations. That is, if the delay in treatment necessary to obtain the patient's consent would result in significant harm to the patient, the physician may proceed to treat the patient without express consent. The treatment at issue need not be lifesaving as long as time is critical and the possible harm to the patient is more than trivial. Another legal exception involves unanticipated conditions during surgery. If a patient is under general anesthesia and the physician discovers an unanticipated condition that requires attention, the physician may treat the condition. This exception protects the patient from the need for a second surgical procedure. The condition must be unanticipated in order for an exception to apply. Reliance by the surgeon on this exception is more risky when the unanticipated procedure involves removal of an organ, affects reproductive capacity, or significantly increases the risks of the surgery. Alternatively, the surgeon's position is enhanced if before the surgery he or she discussed with the patient the possibility that an unanticipated condition might arise or this possibility was disclosed on the consent form (*Douget v. Touro Infirmary*, 1988).

The "therapeutic" exception to the informed consent doctrine allows a physician to withhold information from the patient if he reasonably believes that the patient's mental or physical well-being would suffer as a result of learning the information. Merely being upset is not sufficient; disclosure must pose a serious threat to the patient's health [N.Y. Pub. Health Law §2805-d (McKinney Supp. 2000)].

Finally, under the "waiver" exception, a physician need not make disclosure of risks when the patient requests that he not be so informed.

Under a theory of negligence, a patient may file a lawsuit against a physician for failure to obtain informed consent. As in any negligence action, to prevail the patient must establish not only that the physician has breached the duty to obtain consent, but also that the elements of "causation" and "injury" are present. The patient must prove that he would not have consented to the procedure or treatment if the physician had properly disclosed the risks and side effects. Most courts have adopted an objective test for causation: Would a reasonable person have consented if he had known the risk? Causation requirements should prevent many informed consent lawsuits because studies have shown that for most medically indicated procedures, patients are likely to consent even if the risks are explained in great detail (Alfidi, 1971).

## Obtaining the Patient's Consent—Practical Tips

In most states, it is the treating physician's obligation to obtain the patient's consent. Ideally, the consent responsibility should not be delegated to nurses or residents. Legally, even if he delegates the responsibility, the physician remains ultimately responsible. Consent to specialty procedures should be obtained by the physician performing the specialty procedure. When one or more physicians are involved in the treatment of a patient, the failure of the patient to present evidence regarding which physician had the duty to obtain informed consent has been found to be grounds to set aside a jury verdict in favor of the patient (*Mason v. Walsh*, 1991). That is, it is the patient's obligation to prove which physician on a treatment team had the ultimate obligation to obtain consent.

The physician should talk with the patient regarding the proposed treatment. This conversation can be supplemented with videotapes and brochures. The explanation should be in a nontechnical language that the patient can understand and translation should be provided for non-English-speaking patients.

If possible, consent should be obtained sufficiently prior to the proposed treatment to provide the patient with adequate time to deliberate, but not so far in advance that the patient's physical condition may change. Consent should be documented to provide a record in the event a question is later raised. An example of a consent form is provided in Fig. 28.1. The form should never be used in place of a discussion between the physician and the patient.

There are certain consent decisions that may warrant, for either legal or special risk situations, separate consent policies or at least a form designed for the particular purpose. Examples are blood transfusion, abortion, sterilization, autopsies, and HIV testing.

## Informed Consent and Experimental Drugs or Devices

When medical treatment involves experimental drugs or devices, it is particularly important that informed consent be obtained, and that the patient be provided with adequate information on which to base consent. For example, in a recent New York case, the patient/plaintiff was permitted to submit evidence that a physician working with liquid silicone in 1982 should have informed his or her patients that liquid silicone was not approved by the Federal Food and Drug Administration (FDA).

A substantial body of federal regulations governs the protection of human subjects involved in research that is funded, conducted, or regulated by federal agencies. Some state laws also protect human research subjects. Because the federal and state requirements may differ, it is important to determine which provisions apply and to then follow the applicable procedures.

Patient _____ Date _____

Time _____ a.m./p.m.

1. I authorize the following operation(s) or procedure(s) _____
   (state nature and extent of each operation or other procedure) to be performed by Dr. _____ and
   associates and assistants of the doctor's choice upon the patient named above.

2. I consent to additional and different operations and procedures as may be necessary or advisable in the
   course of the operation or procedure described above.

3. I consent to use of anesthetics, as appropriate, except _____
   (if none, write none). I understand that anesthesia may involve serious risk to the patient even though done in
   a careful manner. I understand that a patient should not drive, operate equipment, or drink alcoholic
   beverages for at least 24 hours after general anesthesia (being put to sleep).

4. The following are true: My physician has explained to me the nature, purpose and possible consequences of
   each operation or procedure as well as significant risks involved, possible complications and possible
   alternative methods of treatment. I understand that the explanation I have received is not exhaustive and that
   there may be other, more remote risks and consequences. I have been advised that a more detailed
   explanation will be given me if I so desire. I do not want further explanation. I have received no guarantees
   from anyone of the results that may be obtained.

5. I consent to the photographing or televising of the operations or procedures showing portions of my body, for
   medical, scientific or educational purposes, providing my identity is not revealed by the pictures or by tests
   accompanying them. To advance medical education, I consent to observation of care given pursuant to this
   consent.

6. I understand that the physicians in attendance at such operation or procedure for the purpose of administering anesthesia, and the physicians performing services involving pathology and radiology, are not the
   agents, servants or employees of the hospital nor of any surgeon, but are independent contractors.

7. I consent to the hospital and the pathologist to preserve for scientific or teaching purposes, to use in the
   treatment of other living persons, to use in the treatment of other living persons, or to use their discretion in
   the disposal of any severed tissue, parts or organs resulting from the operation or procedure authorized
   above.

8. I have been advised that dental devices such as dentures, bridges, caps, crowns, fillings, etc., are more
   subject to damage than normal teeth. I have also been advised that all removable teeth should be removed
   before going to surgery and I agree that responsibility for loss or damage will be mine if I fail to remove such
   teeth.

9. Any special circumstances are hereby noted (if none, write "None")

   _____

   (Cross out and initial any paragraphs above which do not apply.)

   My signature below constitutes my acknowledgement (1) that I have read or have had read to me and
agreed to the foregoing; and (2) that the proposed operation or procedure have been satisfactorily explained to
me by my attending physician and that I have all of the information that I desire.

   All blank spaces in this document have been either completed or crossed off before my signing.

                               Patient: _____
                               Witness: _____
If patient is unable to consent, state reasons: _____

_____

                    Authorized Representative: _____
                    Relationship to patient: _____
                    Witness: _____
                    Witness: _____

**PHYSICIAN'S STATEMENT:**
I certify that I have obtained the patient's informed consent after discussing with the patient the matters
described in the paragraphs above.
Date: _____ Physician: _____

**Figure 28.1.** Consent to operation and other procedure, anesthetics, and other medical services.

On June 18, 1991, a uniform federal policy for the protection of human research subjects was adopted by 16 federal agencies. Commonly referred to as the "Common Rule," this policy applies to research conducted or funded by these agencies (45 C.F.R. Part 46—Protection of Human Subjects). The FDA regulations are similar but not identical to the Common Rule. Under the Common Rule, no individual conducting research may "involve a human being as a research subject" without first obtaining informed consent. Consent may be sought only under conditions that (1) provide a sufficient opportunity for the prospective subject or his legally authorized representative to consider whether to participate and (2) minimize the likelihood of coercion or undue influence. The regulations specify a number of basic elements of informed consent that must be provided to each prospective subject in language that is understandable. These elements include a description of any reasonably foreseeable risks of the study, a description of any benefits to the subject or to others that may reasonably be expected from the research, and a disclosure of appropriate alternative procedures or courses of treatment, if any, that may be advantageous to the subject. Like informed consent to medical treatment, informed consent for medical research must be documented.

An institutional review board (IRB) is a committee or board of an institution at which research is conducted. IRBs are charged with reviewing research proposals to ensure that federal requirements have been satisfied. Part of an IRB's function when reviewing research is to ensure that the informed consent requirements have been met. Thus, an IRB must review the consent procedure and the consent form before they may be used (45 C.F.R. 46.109).

# The Opposite of Treatment: Terminating a Physician–Patient Relationship

Finally, an ancillary issue to consent to treatment and informed consent is termination of the physician–patient relationship. Once a physician begins treating a patient, the physician has a legal and ethical duty to continue to provide services to the patient until treatment is no longer necessary, absent extenuating circumstances. Such circumstances often include discord in the relationship due to the patient's willful noncompliance with a treatment regimen or the patient's disruptive behavior (e.g., rudeness to staff or frequent cancellation of appointments).

No specific laws exist that delineate the process for terminating a physician–patient relationship. However, in September 1998, the American Medical Association issued an ethics opinion titled "Ending the Patient–Physician Relationship." This opinion provides physicians with excellent guidance. Specifically, the AMA opinion recommends the following steps: (1) give the patient written notice, preferably by certified or registered mail, return receipt requested (retain returned card for records as proof of patient's receipt); (2) provide the patient with explanation for terminating the relationship; (3) agree to continue to provide treatment and access to services for a reasonable period of time, such as 30 days, to allow a patient to secure care from another physician; (4) provide resources and/or recommendations to help the patient locate another physician; and (5) offer to transfer copies of the patient's records to a newly designated physician on receipt of an authorization signed by the patient.

How a physician handles termination of the relationship is very important. If the relationship is not properly terminated, the physician is vulnerable to legal claims of negligence and "patient abandonment." The easiest way to avoid such a claim is to follow the AMA's guidelines.

## CASE 28-4

*In January, John Fox was injured in a car accident. He was taken to a local emergency room and treated for superficial cuts and abrasions. In addition, Mr. Fox was suspected of driving while intoxicated (DWI) and a blood alcohol level was obtained. The next morning, Mr. Fox awoke with back pain and made an appointment to see his family practitioner, Dr. Day. During the appointment,*

*Mr. Fox told Dr. Day about the accident and also reluctantly revealed recent test results showing Mr. Fox to be HIV positive. Dr. Day recorded all of the information in his office records. Six months later, Mr. Fox's girlfriend, Ms. Green, comes to see Dr. Day for her annual physical and informs him of her plans to marry Mr. Fox. On the same day, Dr. Day receives a subpoena issued by the grand jury in the county in the case of State v. Fox requesting a copy of all medical records pertaining to Mr. Fox in Dr. Day's possession, even though Dr. Day knows nothing about the DWI charge. Dr. Day is faced with several dilemmas. First, can Dr. Day discuss Mr. Fox's HIV status with Ms. Green? Second, should Dr. Day release Mr. Fox's records to the grand jury without Mr. Fox's consent, including the records pertaining to his HIV test results?*

## PATIENT CONFIDENTIALITY ISSUES

This situation faced by the mythical Dr. Day is a common reality experienced by most medical practitioners at one time or another. The purpose of the following section is to identify patient confidentiality issues commonly encountered by physicians.

Historically, patient confidentiality has been an amalgam of ethical and legal concerns. The Hippocratic Oath states "whatsoever things I see or hear concerning the life of men in my attendance of the sick or even a part therefrom, which ought not to be noised abroad, I will keep silence thereon counting such things to be holy secrets." The American Medical Association's Code of Medical Ethics declares that "the physician should not reveal confidential communications or information without the express consent of the patients" [AMA Code of Medical Ethics §5.05 (1996–1997)]. The concept of "privacy" has been found by courts as arising out of the First, Fourth, Fifth, and Ninth Amendments to the U.S. Constitution.

There are no federal laws recognizing a physician's duty to protect the confidentiality of his or her patient's medical information (also known as the "physician–patient privilege"). Confidentiality laws were enacted on a state-by-state basis. The federal Health Insurance Portability and Accountability Act of 1996 (HIPAA) contains standards related to privacy and security of "electronic health information" [42 U.S.C. §1320d-6 (West 1999)]. However, the HIPAA regulations implementing these privacy standards are not effective until April 2003. Therefore, physicians still must look primarily to state law for guidance on confidentiality matters.

Laws exist that protect both patient records and communications between a physician and patient. However, despite this general rule of confidentiality, public policy requires extensive exceptions to this rule. Common exceptions are found in areas of child abuse and other criminal acts. Under both state and federal law, there is no privilege in criminal cases. For example, a judge in a criminal case may order a physician to testify about his patient's condition, with or without the patient's consent or, in Dr. Day's case, order a physician to release Mr. Fox's medical records without his consent. Further, other exceptions exist for billing requirements and communicable disease reporting.

Texas, like most states, has an extensive number of laws regarding the confidentiality of medical information. There are currently 313 Texas statutory laws and regulations that address medical information. The general rules of confidentiality in Texas provide the following protections:

1. Communications between one licensed to practice medicine, relative to or in connection with any professional services as a physician to a patient, are confidential and privileged, unless otherwise stated under law.
2. Records of the identity, diagnosis, evaluation, or treatment of a patient by a physician that are created or maintained by a physician are confidential and privileged unless otherwise provided.

The protection is very broad and, simply speaking, medical information is any information given or collected, in any form, in anticipation of receiving healthcare.

These prohibitions continue to apply to confidential communications or records concerning any patient irrespective of when the physician treated the patient. That is, the physician's duty to maintain confidentiality is not limited in time and even exists after the patient's death. A physician may not reveal any information to anyone other than the patient without written consent unless a legal exception applies. Physicians should not assume that they may always discuss medical treatment with the patients' family (or, as in Case 28-1, with a patient's employer). Rather, the physician should ask the patient for permission and document it in the patient's medical record. The privilege of confidentiality may be claimed by the patient or the physician acting on the patient's behalf and thus the physician must assert the patient's confidentiality rights when he receives a request for information about a patient.

Recognizing the sensitivity of certain types of medical information, special laws create limits on disclosure of this information. For example, a federal law protects the disclosure of mental health records containing the diagnosis or treatment of chemical dependency or substance abuse. Among other things, this law prohibits, without a patient's consent or court order, a person from acknowledging the presence of a patient in a facility publicly identified as a place that only treats substance abuse patients and contains very restrictive criteria about disclosure of any treatment information.

State laws often give physicians extensive latitude for the release of confidential information. Some common exceptions are as follows:

- Patient or legal representative who consents to the release of the information
- Lawsuit by physician against patient to collect debt for services rendered
- Court-ordered examinations involving the patient's mental or emotional condition or disorder
- Governmental agencies when disclosure is required by law
- Medical or law enforcement personnel when the physician determines that there is a probability of imminent physical injury by the patient to himself or others
- Other physicians or professionals and personnel under the direction of a physician who also are participating in the diagnosis, evaluation, and treatment of a patient
- In certain judicial or administrative proceedings such as in a will contest if the patient's physical or mental condition is relevant to the execution of the will

---

## SUBPOENAS AND THE CONFIDENTIALITY LAWS

*A subpoena is a legal document typically issued by a court at the request of a party to a civil or criminal legal proceeding directing the person named in the subpoena to appear at a specified date, place, and time in order to testify and/or produce records specified in the subpoena. There are two types of subpoenas. One requires the person to whom it is addressed to appear to give testimony, and the other type of subpoena (Latin translation, "subpoena duces tecum") requires a person to appear with documents and may also require testimony.*

*If a physician receives (is "served with") a subpoena, the following guidelines for handling are recommended:*

- *Read the subpoena thoroughly to determine precisely what is sought (testimony and/or records).*
- *Do not accept a subpoena that is not directed to you personally.*
- *Consult with legal counsel regarding whether a legal exception exists that would allow testimony and/or disclosure of records without the patient's written authorization.*
- *If required, obtain patient's written authorization before complying with subpoena.*
- *Do not ignore a subpoena. Because a subpoena is issued under court authority, it requires a response. If no response is made, a court has the power to find you in contempt of court and impose a monetary fine or imprisonment for failure to respond.*

---

In a few instances, a physician can face criminal penalties for improper disclosure, but generally, physicians may be sued by a patient in civil court for improper disclosure or breach of patient confidentiality and the patient may recover monetary damages. Recently in Missouri, a patient sued a health center that had released her medical records to her ex-husband's attorney. The attorney sought the records because the husband was trying to get custody of the couple's children. The husband's attorney wrongly told the health center that the patient's attorney consented to release. The jury awarded the patient several thousand dollars.

Records and information regarding mental healthcare and treatment are afforded heightened confidentiality protections under many states' laws. One area of particular controversy is whether a mental health professional may disclose a patient's confidential information when a patient threatens another person during the course of treatment. Under California law, a mental healthcare professional has a duty to warn the intended victim when the professional determines, in the exercise of his expert skill and knowledge, that this patient presents a serious danger of violence to another (*Tarasoff v. Regents of University of California*, 1976). In stark contrast, the Texas Supreme Court recently decided that due to a mental health professional's statutory duty of confidentiality, such professionals should not have a duty to warn third parties of their patients' threats (*Thapar v. Zezulka*, 1999). The Texas decision does represent the minority view among the states. Nevertheless, physicians should be very cautious before disclosing information in these circumstances.

In certain circumstances, lawmakers have created not only an exception to the physician's duty of confidentiality but also a duty to report information about a patient. Many states require a physician to make a report to the child welfare agency if the physician believes that a child's physical or mental health or welfare has been or may be adversely affected by abuse or neglect by any person. Usually, the law requires that the report be made within a certain time frame and imposes a penalty for failing to report. In Texas, a physician commits a criminal offense if he intentionally fails to report child abuse or neglect. Other instances of required reporting include elder abuse or abuse of disabled persons; patient abuse, neglect, and sexual exploitation, particularly in mental health and skilled nursing care facilities; and certain crime information such as gunshot wounds.

Many states have statutes that deal with compelled testing for HIV and the confidentiality of HIV records. These laws generally provide that HIV test results are confidential and may not be released or disclosed except in certain instances. These instances often include release to the state and local health department, the Centers for Disease Control, and the physician who ordered the test. Also, many state laws allow a positive HIV test result to be released to the spouse of the person tested but few, if any, state laws permit or require disclosure of results to nonspouse sex partners. In Dr. Day's case, he likely would be legally prohibited from disclosing Mr. Fox's HIV test results to Ms. Green, Mr. Fox's fiancée.

Changes in the U.S. healthcare delivery system, particularly managed care, have accelerated the movement of medical records into health information systems, thus raising the opportunity for leakage of confidential patient information to unauthorized persons. The need for rapid access to patient data in

---

## DOCTORS AS POLICE AGENTS?

*The United States Supreme Court recently reviewed a case focusing on this question. In* Ferguson v. Charleston, S.C., *the Court examined a South Carolina public hospital's former policy of conducting warrantless drug testing of certain pregnant women and turning positive cocaine results over to the police. The U.S. Supreme Court considered whether the policy fell under the "special needs" exception to the Fourth Amendment to the Constitution (which prohibits unreasonable searches and seizures). The Court's challenge was to balance the purpose of the policy—to prevent pregnant women from harming their children by using cocaine—with a patient's expectation of privacy in the physician–patient relationship. The Court ultimately ruled that hospital tests cannot legally be used to obtain evidence in law enforcement programs, unless the patient consents to the disclosure of the test result.*

utilization review and outcome studies fuels the demand for such data to be placed in electronic databases. Further, although the electronic medical record provides numerous efficiencies to the delivery of patient care, it creates a host of new challenges to patient confidentiality. The risks of breach of security of patient data are increased and the existence of patient information in an electronic form can lead to inadvertent or casual disclosure to unauthorized persons. For example, recently an Ohio hospital employee was charged with a crime after finding a friend's AIDS diagnosis in the hospital computer and sharing it with other hospital employees. With the advent of electronic technology into medical practice, and in particular into the medical records, physicians must learn new methods of safeguarding the confidentiality of these records. Security controls such as password protection and encryption may have prevented the Ohio hospital employee from gaining access to her friend's record.

## CASE 28-5

*Mr. Smith, a 67-year-old slightly overweight man, is brought to the Emergency Department of Teaching Hospital on July 1, 2000, at 2310 by his 15-year-old niece. He tells the nurse that he hasn't been able to catch his breath for the last 3 days, his heart feels like it is pounding, and he is tired due to lack of sleep. He has trouble sleeping because he can't breathe if he lies down. Mr. Smith gives the following information to Dr. ER: that he has never smoked or used recreational drugs; that he is not allergic to any foods or medications; that he never experienced these symptoms at any time in the past; and that he drank a six pack of beer every day until the age of 30, at which time he quit drinking completely. Mr. Smith states he suffered a gunshot wound to his left thigh while in the service in 1963 and underwent an appendectomy at age 40. He is an investment broker and retired Marine colonel. His blood pressure is 180/110. His other vital signs are within normal limits. He denies any chest pains and denies taking any medications, prescribed or over-the-counter, other than a daily aspirin as a blood thinner. His EKG results and blood gases are normal. Blood enzymes are ordered STAT. The nursing staff calls Dr. PCP, Mr. Smith's primary care physician, who arrives and admits Mr. Smith for observation at 2400. Dr. PCP has seen Mr. Smith in the past only for his yearly physicals, the results of which have all been normal.*

*Mrs. Smith, the patient's young wife, soon arrives and tells Dr. PCP that her husband has never been sick a day in the 10 years she has known him. In fact, he works out at a local gym four times a week to keep his strength up and weight down. Mrs. Smith is an aerobics instructor at the same gym. She insists everything must be done to make her husband well. Due to Mr. Smith's distress, the niece has read all of the hospital consent forms to Mr. Smith and signed them for him in his presence. The blood enzyme results are forwarded from the Emergency Department to the floor; all results are within the normal range. A second set of enzymes and a CBC are ordered STAT at 0030. Finally, Dr. PCP requests a pulmonary consult.*

*Mr. Smith is given the information and forms for medical power of attorney and a physician's directive. He completes both, designating his wife as the person to make healthcare decisions for him in case he cannot. Mr. Smith's three adult children arrive at the hospital and request their father's chart. Dr. PCP obliges their request. They dispute that Mrs. Smith is their father's wife, stating that she is only living with him in common law. Before they leave for the night, they insist she not be allowed into their father's room at any time in the future.*

*Dr. PCP also leaves for the night and requests the nurse call him at home if the STAT enzymes or CBC results come back abnormal. He leaves the Teaching Hospital at 0130. The nurse calls him at home at 0200 and reports all laboratory results are normal except for an elevated white count of 17,000 and a platelet count of 40,000 confirmed by differential. The differential report also notes 3+ schistocytes. Dr. PCP orders a repeat STAT CBC along with coagulation studies with results expected by 0230 and tells the nurse he is on his way back to the hospital. Before Dr. PCP returns, however, Mr. Smith suffers a pulmonary embolism followed quickly by several strokes that neurologically devastate him. He is unable to communicate or feed himself and is transferred first to a local rehabilitation hospital for therapy and then to a nursing home.*

Physicians in the United States may be sued by their patients for improper care or treatment. This type of lawsuit is generally referred to as *medical malpractice*. A medical malpractice case is a civil matter, as opposed to a criminal matter. The penalty is not prison time but monetary compensation. As shown in Fig. 28.2, the frequency with which a physician is sued is in part related to the physician's areas of specialty.

A medical malpractice case involves an allegation of "negligence" on the part of the physician and consists of four basic elements:

1. Duty—the standard of care
2. Breach of duty—a deviation from the standard of care
3. Proximate cause—a direct and generally foreseeable, causal relationship between the deviation from the standard of care and an injury-producing event
4. Damages—legally cognizable injuries that result from the event.

It is these four elements that the patient (referred to in litigation as the *plaintiff* or *complainant*) must prove to win her case against the physician. The patient has the burden to prove her case by "a preponderance of the evidence," i.e., that it was more likely than not that the physician was negligent, the patient was injured, and that the negligence caused her injuries. This is a lesser burden than the "beyond a reasonable doubt" standard used in criminal cases.

Negligence is the lack of ordinary care, which is that degree of care that a reasonably prudent physician would have exercised under the same or similar circumstances. In medical malpractice cases, a patient usually alleges several acts of negligence on the part of one or more physicians and other healthcare professionals. Figure 28.3 illustrates common allegations of negligence against physicians in medical malpractice cases filed in Texas from 1990 to 2000.

The standard of care generally must be established by expert testimony (i.e., a physician) since the subject matter of most medical malpractice cases is outside the common knowledge of lay jurors. An expert need not be of the same practice specialty as the physician being sued and need not be from the same locale. Experts are usually required to be qualified based on their training and experience to offer an expert opinion regarding the accepted standards of medical care. An exception to the expert witness rule sometimes exists when the negligence is so obvious that it would be understood by a jury of lay people: for example, when a surgeon operates on the wrong limb or other portion of the body.

The negligence of the physician must have "proximately caused" the damage to the patient. Proximate cause has two subparts: cause-in-fact and foreseeability. Cause-in-fact requires the alleged negligence to have been a cause, which in a natural and continuing sequence produces an event, and without which the event would not have occurred (the "but for" test). Foreseeability exists when a physician of ordinary skill, knowledge, care, and prudence, in the exercise of ordinary care, would have been able reasonably to anticipate and foresee that the event, or some similar event, would have occurred as a natural and probable consequence of his conduct. In most circumstances, expert medical testimony is required on proximate cause.

When a physician's negligent conduct aggravates a patient's preexisting condition, the physician is responsible to the extent that the injuries were not already manifest and would not have otherwise persisted. For most cases, the fact-finder apportions fault between the patient and the physician. If the jury finds that the patient was negligent ("contributory negligence"), and such negligence is a proximate cause of the injuries, such contributory negligence is included in the jury's apportionment of fault and ultimately the award, if any, of money damages. For example, if a patient fails to take her prescribed antibiotics and develops a postsurgical infection that causes her leg to be amputated, in any subsequent medical malpractice action the physician could claim that the patient was contributorily negligent because she failed to follow the physician's instructions and that her wrongful conduct was the cause of her injuries.

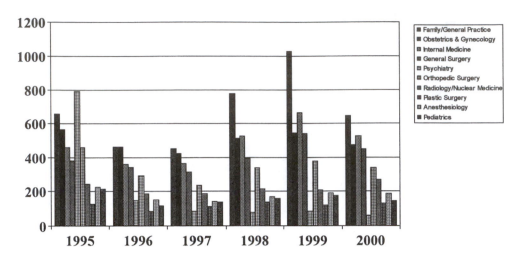

**Figure 28.2.** Total claims filed by physician's primary specialty, as of 2/28/01. Source: Texas State Board of Medical Examiners, Professional Liability Statistics for Physicians Practicing in Texas.

There are generally two types of damages in a medical malpractice case. "Actual" damages are money damages that may be awarded by the jury. These include past and future physical pain, mental anguish, disfigurement, physical disability, medical expenses, loss of wage earning capacity, death, and funeral expenses. Depending on the facts of the case and the particular state law, others (patient's spouse, parents, and children) also may be entitled to damages. In some states, the jury may award damages to punish the physician and to deter the physician from committing similar acts in the future. These damages are known as *exemplary* or *punitive damages*.

There are a variety of precipitating factors in a medical malpractice case. A major factor in medical malpractice cases is poor recordkeeping (usually omissions or imprecise entries). Physician and hospital personnel should be very careful to record complete, accurate, and detailed information. In litigation, the patient's attorney often will contend that "if it is not in the record, it did not happen." Positive signs and symptoms, as well as negative signs and symptoms, should be recorded.

A second factor is criticism of one physician by another. Criticizing a colleague often results in the physician being called to testify as an expert witness against that colleague in a medical malpractice case. A physician should always be cautious regarding any criticism of a colleague, especially if the physician was not present when the care in question was rendered. Important facts may not be reflected in the records; therefore, it would be inappropriate to criticize without knowledge of all of the facts. A physician should never criticize a colleague in a medical record.

A third factor in medical malpractice litigation is self-criticism by the physician. Being critical of a physician's own care and treatment may also be reason for a patient to consider a medical malpractice case. In a medical malpractice trial, the patient is permitted to testify about any comments the physician makes regarding the physician's care and treatment. As a result, a physician is faced with both ethical and legal dilemmas when considering whether to disclose a medical error to a patient. There may be times when a physician may believe it is morally and ethically right to disclose a mistake to a patient, even if such disclosure means a higher likelihood of being sued. Further, disclosure of mistakes is not necessarily harmful to a physician's defense but often can be helpful in defending the physician's actions. However, the manner in which disclosure of mistakes occurs can cause difficulties in the defense of a medical malpractice case. As a result, a physician should carefully choose his or her words when providing self-criticism to patients. Being honest and forthright is certainly encouraged, but thinking before speaking is always advisable.

Other factors include: poor communication, poor continuity of care, misleading the patient, and poor outcomes. Failure to establish or maintain good communications with the patient can lead to dissatisfaction

| Year | Total no. of claims filed | Not yet determined | Failure to diagnose | Failure to operate | Failure to treat | Negligent diagnosis | Negligent surgery | Negligent treatment | Failure to obtain informed consent | Breach of confidentiality | Unnecessary surgery/ treatment |
|---|---|---|---|---|---|---|---|---|---|---|---|
| 1990 | 2,987 | 439 | 553 | 3 | 15 | 65 | 638 | 1,216 | 28 | 0 | 32 |
| 1991 | 3,706 | 505 | 594 | 1 | 32 | 106 | 639 | 1,757 | 42 | 3 | 27 |
| 1992 | 5,049 | 519 | 623 | 6 | 65 | 96 | 1,162 | 2,484 | 54 | 2 | 38 |
| 1993 | 5,515 | 918 | 680 | 10 | 120 | 202 | 1,098 | 2,400 | 47 | 4 | 36 |
| 1994 | 4,494 | 642 | 721 | 8 | 95 | 167 | 751 | 1,998 | 51 | 12 | 49 |
| 1995 | 5,414 | 881 | 776 | 8 | 83 | 147 | 706 | 2,682 | 49 | 3 | 79 |
| 1996 | 3,551 | 817 | 599 | 2 | 57 | 96 | 460 | 1,469 | 29 | 1 | 21 |
| 1997 | 3,326 | 1,182 | 447 | 3 | 19 | 78 | 400 | 1,149 | 30 | 0 | 18 |
| 1998 | 4,554 | 1,984 | 500 | 7 | 90 | 140 | 525 | 1,235 | 50 | 1 | 22 |
| 1999 | 5,337 | 2,566 | 503 | 9 | 81 | 100 | 726 | 1,282 | 39 | 1 | 30 |
| 2000 | 4,502 | 2,198 | 409 | 8 | 139 | 26 | 529 | 1,163 | 7 | 2 | 21 |

**Figure 28.3.** Types of alleged negligence, 1990–2000. As of 2/28/01. Source: Texas State Board of Medical Examiners, Professional Liability Statistics for Physicians Practicing in Texas.

with treatment. Infrequent visits with the patient in the hospital or failure to follow up on the patient may also lead to patient dissatisfaction and precipitate an allegation of medical malpractice. "Ghost surgery"—having another physician do the surgery without advising the patient—is another significant precipitating factor. A devastating injury to a relatively healthy individual undergoing a minor procedure often leads to the filing of a lawsuit as does an injury that devastates a family financially or emotionally. Finally, putting a patient into collections who has had a serious complication is a near-certain invitation to litigation.

In Mr. Smith's case, numerous factors can be identified as indicators for a medical malpractice action: (1) the dissension among Mr. Smith's relatives and the claim that Mrs. Smith, as a common law wife, did not have authority to consent to the procedure; (2) Dr. PCP's failure to ensure that the pulmonary consult occurred before leaving the hospital for the night; (3) the problematic laboratory reports and potential misdiagnosis; and (4) the devastating injury.

When a patient sues a physician for medical malpractice, state law often provides a physician with various available defenses. The most common defense is the "statute of limitations," which is the time period in which a patient may file suit. Statutes of limitation are premised on the theory that a person should be given a reasonable time to discover, investigate, and file a suit but that this time should be limited to allow for preservation of key witnesses and information and to provide certainty and finality to certain relationships. In Texas, for competent adult patients, there is a 2-year statute of limitations from the date of the occurrence of the "injury" or from the date the medical treatment that is the subject of the lawsuit is completed. In most states, children and incompetent patients generally are afforded longer periods of time to file a medical malpractice action.

Another, although much less common, defense recognized in many states is the "Good Samaritan" defense: A person who in good faith administers emergency care at the scene of an emergency is not liable in civil damages for an act performed during an emergency unless the act is willfully or wantonly negligent. The Good Samaritan defense does not usually apply to emergencies occurring in a hospital or other medical facility or in a medical transport vehicle nor does it apply to care administered by someone for or in expectation of payment.

With the advent of managed care, traditional liabilities for malpractice and bad outcomes are triangulated among the patient, managed care organizations (MCOs), and physician. Because continuing developments in the healthcare marketplace create ever more complex relationships, courts are facing new theories of liability when lawsuits are filed. Because, unlike physicians, MCOs are not licensed to practice medicine, they cannot be sued under a theory of medical malpractice. Some states have enacted laws that permit a patient to sue an MCO. The validity of these laws in many circumstances, however, is being challenged on the theory that the federal Employment Retirement Income Security Act (ERISA) preempts these state laws and thus substantially limits a patient's remedies against an MCO. Nonetheless, several huge verdicts have been awarded by juries against MCOs, indicating perhaps the public's dissatisfaction with managed care. A California jury recently handed down a record-setting $120 million judgment against Aetna U.S. Healthcare of California for denying experimental cancer treatment to an HMO enrollee. In *Goodrich v. Aetna*, the attorneys for Mr. Goodrich's estate argued that Aetna had delayed and denied medical treatment for Mr. Goodrich's rare form of stomach cancer over the course of 2½ years. The jury awarded $4.45 million to Mr. Goodrich's widow for medical expenses and loss of companionship, concluding that Aetna's treatment coverage denial had shortened Mr. Goodrich's life, and $116 million in punitive damages, finding that Aetna had acted with "malice, oppression, and fraud" (*Goodrich v. Aetna*, 1999 WL 181418).

## CASE 28-6

*After completing his residency, Dr. B took over a practice in his home state. The position looked promising. The internist Dr. B. would replace was retiring from a busy practice to raise her third child, and the hospital agreed to cover Dr. B's practice overhead expenses for the first 6 months, as well as guarantee him a salary of $100,000 for the first year. Dr. B barely read the contract before* *he signed it. In his first 2 weeks of practice, Dr. B realized that he was seeing only three or four patients a day. The staff informed him that most of the patients were women who refused to see a male physician. A few months later Dr. B was surprised when his accountant informed him that his quarterly estimated taxes were due since he was self-employed. By the end of the year Dr. B realized that, under the terms of the contract, he was obligated to repay the hospital every penny it extended to Dr. B for overhead. In fact, the hospital administrator informed him that it would be illegal for the hospital not to be repaid. At that point, Dr. B began to consider filing for bankruptcy.*

## LEGAL/BUSINESS ISSUES

The current business environment of healthcare is undergoing considerable change due to the impact of managed care and other developments at both the state and national levels. Additionally, due to perceptions of fraud and abuse at both levels, the government is scrutinizing the business aspects of medicine. As demonstrated in Dr. B's case, to survive today's clinical practice environment, physicians must understand the legal aspects of the medical business practice environment.

Historically, three primary types of business organizations have been used for the practice of medicine: sole proprietorships, partnerships, and professional associations. (The exact names may vary from state to state.) In these organizations, physicians are typically owners or shareholders and not necessarily employees, as in Dr. B's case.

In recent years, alternative business structure models have developed for physician practices including staff model HMOs and physician practice management companies. A legal doctrine known as the "corporate practice of medicine prohibition" affects the business structures of medical practices. This doctrine in the strictest sense prohibits corporations, especially for-profit corporations such as hospitals and HMOs, from employing physicians. The doctrine developed primarily out of the concern that if physicians were employed by lay corporations, corporations would ultimately control all aspects of the physician's medical practice, including methods of diagnosis and treatment, their relationships with patients, and their income. Currently, at least 38 states recognize some form of this doctrine (Wiorlek, 1987). In Dr. B's case, the hospital may have been legally prevented from employing him directly.

Whether a physician is an employee or is buying a medical practice, such as Dr. B, the physician often signs a contract, which governs the terms and conditions of the business relationship. As demonstrated by Dr. B's case, careful review of a contract prior to signing it is crucial.

In today's competitive medical marketplace, physician contracts often contain provisions restricting a physician's right to practice during the term of the current contract or after the contract terminates. These restrictive provisions are known as covenants not to compete and are the subject of increasing debate in the medical business community. A covenant not to compete is a contractual agreement by a physician not to compete for business with an employer or purchaser of his practice for a certain period of time within a specified geographic area. For example, Dr. B's contract with the hospital may have stated that if the contract terminated, Dr. B was prohibited from practicing medicine for 2 years within a 50-mile radius of the hospital. To be enforceable, covenants not to compete usually must be reasonable in time and geographic scope. Although not all states recognize the validity of covenants not to compete, these restrictive prohibitions are enforced more and more frequently by courts.

A Tennessee court recently ruled that a physician's employment agreement not to compete with a state college of medicine for 5 years after resigning should be enforced because a viable academic hospital is in the public interest (*Medical Education Assistance Corp. v. Mehta*, 1999). In some states, specific statutes regulate physicians' covenants not to compete in order to balance business concerns and patient needs. Texas's law, which was enacted in 1999, requires that for a covenant to be valid it (1) must not deny the physician access to a list of patients whom he or she has seen or treated within 1 year of the termination of the contract; (2) must affirmatively state that patients have access to, and copies of, their medical records; and (3) must provide that the physician will not be prohibited from providing continuing care and treatment to a specific patient or patients during the course of an illness even after the covenant not to compete becomes effective [Tex. Bus. & Commerce Code Ann. §15.50 (Vernon Supp. 1999)].

The investigation and prosecution of healthcare fraud is the second highest priority for federal law enforcement agencies. (Drug crimes are first.) The federal government estimates that of the $100 billion annually paid by the federal Medicare program to the healthcare industry, $23 billion represents Medicare overpayments. The federal government, and many state governments, are devoting extraordinary resources of both time and money to the investigation, civil enforcement, and criminal prosecution of fraud (or perceived fraud) related to Medicare, Medicaid, and the federal healthcare programs. Several laws have been passed in recent years to provide the government with weapons to combat healthcare fraud. Existing laws, such as the 100-year-old federal False Claims Act, have been used as well. The federal Medicare and Medicaid Fraud and Abuse law, commonly known as the anti-kickback law, established criminal penalties for individuals or entities participating in the Medicare and Medicaid program that give or receive illegal remuneration. Generally, illegal remuneration includes bribes, kickbacks, or rebates given in return for patient referrals or other business generation. In Dr. B's case, he had entered into a contract with the local hospital, which had agreed to cover his practice overhead expenses for 1 year. Because of the anti-kickback law, as well as several other applicable laws, the hospital also had to require Dr. B to reimburse the hospital for these payments or these payments would likely have been viewed by the government as improper payments to induce the physician to admit or refer patients to the hospital.

For every $1 spent investigating healthcare fraud, the federal government recovers $13. In the last few years, multimillion dollar settlements have been made between the federal government and some of the nation's largest healthcare organizations. Government enforcement efforts are likely to increase in the foreseeable future. Physicians must keep abreast of these developments to ensure compliance with these complex laws.

## CONCLUSION

A basic understanding of the major areas of health law and their rationale is essential for the practice of medicine. Physicians should be familiar with the rights and restrictions of their medical license, their legal responsibilities to their patients, reports they may be obligated to file, potential lawsuits in which they might be involved, and the legal complexities of the healthcare business environment. This familiarity will enable physicians to adapt to and comply with the vast number of laws and regulations that affect the practice of medicine and a physician's relationship with his or her patients.

## CASES FOR DISCUSSION

### CASE 1

*Your patient is scheduled to undergo ERCP (endoscopic retrograde cholangiopancreatography) for evaluation of persistent increased amylase. As you, the intern, are preparing to go home at 8 PM, the upper level resident tells you to get consent for the procedure, which is scheduled for 7 AM the next day. You are unfamiliar with the procedure.*

*1. Should you or the resident obtain the patient's informed consent?*
*2. Should you ask the supervising nurse to do so?*
*3. What if you explain the ERCP procedure to the patient and the attending physician confirms that you did?*

### CASE 2

*At 7 PM, your elderly demented patient develops an acute abdomen with hypotension requiring emergent laparotomy. You call the patient's daughter but she has left for a movie and isn't expected back for 3 hours and has no cell phone. No other family members are available.*

1. *Should you proceed with the operation?*
2. *Do you need to document the patient's emergent condition?*
3. *What if the patient was a child?*

## CASE 3

*A 2-year-old visits you in your clinic with complaints of abdominal pain. Your examination reveals a well-developed child who verbalizes very little. You note two large areas of bruising on the back and consider the possibility of abuse.*

1. *Should you call the state children's protection agency immediately?*
2. *What if the parents want to take the child home against your medical advice?*
3. *Can the parents sue you for making a report?*

## CASE 4

*A patient presents to the ambulatory clinic for medication refills. This is his first visit to the clinic. He changed physicians because of a change in insurance and job status. He reports that he suffers from epilepsy and continues to have seizures on a regular basis, about once every other week. He did not report his seizures to the Department of Public Safety (DPS) and continues to drive and work in a job that is potentially hazardous to himself and others. He states that if he loses his driver's license, he would continue to drive because it is the only way he can continue to work. He also states that he always has an aura before a seizure and can therefore take appropriate action.*

1. *Should you report the patient to DPS?*
2. *What about the patient's confidentiality rights?*
3. *Are you liable if you fail to report and the patient has a seizure while driving and injures someone?*

## CASE 5

*A patient presents to you with abdominal pain. In the course of the examination she states that her previous physician fondled her in the examination room.*

1. *How should you respond to the patient?*
2. *What should you write in the chart?*
3. *Should you report this information to anyone? If so, to whom?*
4. *What are the possible repercussions for her previous physician?*

# RECOMMENDED READINGS

*American Journal of Law and Medicine.*

> This periodical, published by the American Society of Law, Medicine & Ethics, provides articles on an array of health law issues. Its articles typically combine legal and ethical viewpoints in an effective and practical manner.

Furrow BR, Johnson SH, Jost TS, Schwartz RL: *Health Law: Cases, Materials, and Problems*, ed 3. St. Paul, Minn, West Publishing Co, 1987.

> This is one of the most widely used texts and works well for students with a variety of backgrounds including medical students. The book shows how law affects the professionals and institutions that deliver healthcare in the United States. It focuses on legal and regulatory mechanisms related to health services organizations, market-driven changes in healthcare financing and delivery, and the relationship of physician and patient.

Gosfield AG (ed): *Health Law Handbook*. St. Paul, Minn, West Publishing Co, 1999.

> This annual publication is an excellent survey of health law issues in a variety of areas. It contains current analyses and information on developing legal issues affecting the healthcare professional, such as telemedicine and reimbursement.

Alfidi: Informed consent: A study of patient reaction. *JAMA* 216:1325, 1971.

AMA Code of Medical Ethics §5.50 (1996–1997)

American Society of Law and Medicine, Health Law and Professional Education: *The Report of the Task Force on Health Law Curricula of the American Society of Law & Medicine*, 1985.

Ariz. Rev. Stat. §36-3201 et seq.

*Ashcraft v. King*, 228 Cal. App. 3d 604, 278, Cal. Rptr. 900 (1991).

Code of Federal Regulations, 45 C.F.R. Part 46—Protection of Human Subjects.

Conn. Acts 148 (Reg. Sess.) 1996.

*Douget v. Touro Infirmary*, 537 So.2d 251 (La. App. 1988).

*Ferguson v. City of Charleston*, 532 U.S.67 (2001).

*Goodrich v. Aetna U.S. Healthcare of California, Inc.*, 1999 WL 181418 (Cal. Super.).

*Griffith v. Jones*, 577 N.E. 2d 250 (Ind. App. 1991).

HIPAA: Health Insurance Portability and Accountability Act; 42 U.S.C. §1320d-6 (West 1999).

*In re Doe*, No. D-93064 (Fulton Cnty, Ga. Sup. Ct. Oct 17, 1991), aff'd 262 Ga389, 418 S.E.2d (1992).

*Mason v. Walsh*, 600 A.2d 326 (Conn. App. 1991).

*Medical Education Assistance Corp. v. Metha*, Tenn. Ct. App., No. 03A01-9908-CH-00289, 12/16/99.

N.Y. Pub. Health Law §2805-d (McKinney Supp. 2000).

*Planned Parenthood v. Casey*, 112 S.Ct. 2791 (1991).

*Planned Parenthood v. Danforth*, 428 U.S. 52 (1976).

*Prince v. Massachusetts*, 321 U.S. 158 (1944).

*Retkwa v. Orentreich*, 584 N.Y.S.2d 710 (Sup. Ct. 1992).

Rozovsky FA: *Consent to Treatment: A Practical Guide*, at 1-98, ed 2, 1990.

*Salgo v. Leland Stanford, Jr. University Board of Trustees*, 317 P.2d 170, 181 (1957).

*Tarasoff v. Regents of University of California*, 551 P.2d 334 (Cal. 1976).

Tex. Bus. & Commerce Code Ann. §15.50 (Vernon Supp. 1999)

Tex. Health & Safety Code Ann. §313.004(a) (Vernon 1998).

*Thapar v. Zezulka*, 994 S.W.2d 635 (Tex. 1999).

United States Code, Schedules of Controlled Substances, 21 U.S.C. §812(b).

*Walker v. Superior Court*, 763 P.2d 852 (1988).

Wiorlek J: The corporate practice of medicine doctrine: An outmoded theory in need of modification. *J Legal Med* 8:465, 1987.

*Wooley v. Henderson*, 418 A.2d 1123 (Me. 1980).

## CHAPTER 29

# Spirituality and Medicine

*Dana E. King*

*Allison Lee, a 49-year-old housewife, underwent surgery to remove a ruptured diverticulum and had to stay in the hospital 10 days because of infection complications. She was mildly depressed when she went home to continue her recovery. Over the next few weeks her depression worsened; she would not get out of bed, she would not eat, and she would hardly speak. Her family dutifully waited on her, bringing her meals which she barely touched, spongebathing her since she would not bathe, and encouraging her to get up and be more active. They repeatedly asked why she felt so poorly, but she would not or could not explain. When 3 weeks had passed since the surgery with no improvement, her husband Charlie called her family physician.*

*The physician made a house call since the patient refused to come to the office. He found the patient in bed, unwilling to speak except for one-word answers. Her abdominal wound was healing well. She had no fever and her pulse and respiration were normal. The patient's severe depression was evident, and the physician recommended immediate psychiatric hospitalization and treatment with antidepressant medication.*

*The patient refused both antidepressant therapy and hospitalization. Her husband explained that according to the health beliefs in their native culture, it was humiliating to be dependent on others, and even more humiliating to have depression. Depression was a sign of weakness of moral character, not a medical illness. Accepting treatment would communicate to others a character weakness; she should help herself instead. The husband was torn about what to say or do, since his spiritual faith seemed to conflict with the health beliefs of his and his wife's culture. His spiritual belief was that accepting treatment from a physician was often part of God's plan. The husband then asked the doctor, "What should we do?"*

## EDUCATIONAL OBJECTIVES

1. Recognize the prevalence of religion and spirituality in patients' lives
2. Identify the health beliefs of various religious groups

3. Know how to take a spiritual history
4. Evaluate the ethics of spiritual inquiry

---

# INTRODUCTION

Patients' religious and spiritual beliefs play an important role in their views of life and medical illness. In one study hospitalized patients indicated their spiritual health to be as important as their physical health, and most wanted the physician to consider their spiritual needs (King & Bushwick, 1994). Spirituality is broadly defined as the beliefs that give transcendent meaning to one's life (Puchalski & Larson, 1998). Religion can be considered a subset of spirituality with a more formal set of beliefs, rituals, and practices. Most people express their spirituality in religious terms: over 90% of Americans identify with a particular religious denomination and 75% say that religion is an important part of their daily lives (Gallup, 1990, 1997). Many religions include specific guidelines regarding healthcare decisions, such as the Jehovah's Witness prohibition against the use of human blood products and the Roman Catholic proscription against abortion. As Case 29-1 indicates, sometimes patients' cultural beliefs conflict with their spiritual beliefs. Often such conflicts are hidden from the clinician and not openly discussed as part of medical decision-making.

Imagine counseling the family in Case 29-1 without understanding or considering the family's spiritual or religious beliefs. Many clinicians fail to consider that every patient has spiritual views that provide a context for interpreting the meaning of illness. Every patient asks these questions at one time or another: Why must I suffer? What is the value of living? Why am I here? Is there life after death? Failure to address the patients' spiritual beliefs and concerns can frustrate the medical decision-making process because of lack of communication about fundamental issues. Physicians cannot allow themselves to have undue influence over the religious views of their patients, but neither can they afford to ignore the beliefs that give the patients' lives meaning. Physicians must learn to inquire about patients' religious and spiritual lives in such a way as to communicate compassion and care for the whole person, and initiate referral to a minister or chaplain for assistance with complex issues.

Determining patients' spiritual and religious beliefs and how they affect health beliefs can be a challenge. Clinicians are often uncomfortable discussing patients' religious beliefs because of a lack of training in religion and spirituality, and because of fears about the ethics of discussing religion with their patients (Ellis *et al.*, 1999).

This chapter will present the rationale for considering patients' spiritual well-being as well as their physical well-being, review the health beliefs of certain religious groups, explore ways to obtain a spiritual history, and consider the ethics of obtaining a spiritual history.

---

# PATIENTS' RELIGIOUS AND SPIRITUAL LIVES

## General Population

The Gallup organization has tracked U.S. religious beliefs over the last 60 years (Gallup, 1997) and has documented a consistent pattern of religiousness and denomination identification. Ninety-five percent of Americans believe in God, and 92% express a particular religious denomination. Eighty-seven percent are Christian, with 53% Protestant, 26% Catholic, and 8% other Christian. Two percent are Jewish, 2% are Muslim, and 2% are other religions.

The most common formal religious activity is attendance at worship services. Over 40% of Americans attend worship services weekly. Other frequent formal religious activities include scripture study classes, baptisms, weddings, and funerals. Private religious activity is also prevalent, the most common of which is prayer (Levin & Taylor, 1997). Several sources indicate that 99% of Americans pray, and over half pray daily or more often (Gallup, 1997; Levin & Taylor, 1997). Other frequent private activities include reading devotional materials, watching religious programming on television, and listening to religious programming on the radio (Taylor & Chatters, 1991).

Many people who are not involved in formal religious activities have spiritual beliefs and activities that influence their attitudes and behaviors and serve as a guide for living (McBride *et al.*, 1998). Having an internal or intrinsic spiritual orientation has been associated with decreased stress-related medical symptoms, regardless of whether a formal religious affiliation is present (Kass *et al.*, 1991).

PATIENTS' RELIGIOUS AND SPIRITUAL LIVES

## Patients

One of the most important reasons to address patients' spiritual and religious beliefs in the healthcare setting is their impact on health-related decisions and behaviors. Sixty-one percent of Americans state that their religion is the most important influence in their daily lives (Gallup, 1990). Patients undergoing inpatient or outpatient medical treatment express strong religious and spiritual orientations (King & Bushwick, 1994; Maugans & Wadland, 1991). Maugans and Wadland's survey of 150 outpatients demonstrated that over 90% believed in God, 85% used prayer, and 74% felt close to God. King and Bushwick's survey of inpatients at two hospitals revealed that 98% believed in God and that 93% were very strong or somewhat strong in their beliefs. Seventy-three percent prayed daily or more often. Ninety-four percent agreed that spiritual health is as important as physical health. Spiritual concerns are almost universal among hospitalized patients.

The Joint Council for Accreditation of Healthcare Organizations (JCAHO) has recognized the influence of spirituality on hospitalized patients by requiring a hospital chaplain or access to pastoral services in the standards for accreditation of all hospitals (JCAHO, 1999). According to the JCAHO, a spiritual assessment should be performed on every patient, identifying, "at a minimum," the patient's denomination, beliefs, and spiritual practices. The JCAHO also recommends asking patients and family numerous other questions about spirituality and health.

---

### CASE 29-2

*A 19-year-old woman comes to the office complaining of nausea every day for the last week. The physician examines her and finds no abdominal tenderness or distension. On further questioning, the patient states she has missed her last two periods. Her pregnancy test is positive. The patient is*

---

### QUESTIONS TO ASK PATIENTS AND FAMILIES

*From where do you get your strength and hope?*
*Do you pray?*
*How do you express your spirituality?*
*How would you describe your philosophy of life?*
*What type of spiritual/religious support do you want at this time?*
*What is the name of your minister, chaplain, pastor, rabbi?*
*How do you cope with your suffering?*
*How do you interpret the meaning of your suffering?*
*Do you ever think about death?*
*What does dying mean to you?*
*What are your spiritual goals?*
*What role, if any, does church, synagogue, or some other religious community play in your
    life?*
*Has belief in God been important in your life?*
*How does your faith help you cope with illness?*
*How has this illness affected you and the others around you?*
*Adapted from the JCAHO Web site: (www.jcaho.org/standard/clarif/pe_spirtass.html)*

*unmarried and seems distraught by the news of her pregnancy. Seeing her distress, the physician suggests that she consider an abortion. The patient, who is Catholic, recoils at the suggestion and becomes more upset.*

## HEALTH BELIEFS OF RELIGIOUS GROUPS

Clinicians should be aware of the more common health beliefs of religious groups in their practice, so that they will be able to better counsel and care for their patients. Health beliefs vary according to culture, education, and experience. Religious beliefs can be very strong and can be the deciding factor in medical decisions such as abortion or withdrawal of life support.

Many factors add to the complexity of the interaction of religious and health beliefs, including differing beliefs between patients and their families, between the patient and physician, between patients and their religious traditions, and inconsistencies within patients. Case 29-2 illustrates some of these factors. The patient has not followed the guidelines of the Catholic faith by becoming pregnant out of wedlock, but she is still very interested in following the Catholic proscription against abortion. The physician likely has different views from the patient, since Catholic physicians would not readily suggest abortion as a solution. The family may have different views than either the patient or the physician. While purely medical factors may play some role in the scenario in Case 29-2, the religious factors are likely to play an equal or greater role in the upcoming medical decisions.

While individuals' beliefs do not always coincide with the principles of a specific religious code, health professionals should be aware of the major moral and religious norms that guide the medical decision-making of many patients. Physicians should be especially mindful of potentially strong religion-based health beliefs when discussing life and death issues, contraception, abortion, and euthanasia. The brief summaries below serve as an introduction and illustration of some of the key health beliefs of the major faith traditions regarding contraception and family issues, death and dying, and some special and unique beliefs. Those desiring more in-depth information should consult the bibliography for resources.

## Catholicism

Catholics are the largest single denomination in the United States, representing about 25% of the population. Their concept of God is monotheistic yet Trinitarian, with God the Father, God the Son, and God the Holy Spirit comprising a mystical unity of three in one (Fellows, 1979; Manning, 1986). The Pope has final

### RESOURCES FOR HEALTH BELIEFS OF DIFFERENT FAITHS

*The Park Ridge Center has produced a series on "Health and Medicine in the Faith Traditions" that explores the ways in which many of the major religions relate to health and medical issues. Available guides include the Reformed tradition, Catholic, Anglican, Methodist, Christian Science, Hindu, Eastern Orthodox, Latter-day Saints, and Islamic. You may find the guides in your medical library. For more information, contact the Park Ridge Center, 211 E. Ontario, Suite 800, Chicago, IL 60611-3215. Phone: (312)266-2222, or go to their Web site at www.prchfe.org <http://www.prchfe.org/>.*

*For assistance with understanding the religious basis for health and medical decisions, the Park Ridge Center also publishes a series of handbooks on "Religious Traditions and Healthcare Decisions." This series focuses on beliefs and moral traditions regarding specific clinical issues and medical procedures. Contact and ordering information are the same as above.*

authority over church matters on earth. Catholic beliefs about health are based on the dignity of human life, the Catholic tradition of holistic health, the belief that suffering can have meaning, and that death is a natural transition to life with God (Hamel, 1996). The Church's guidance in moral and health matters comes from a commitment to truth based on the accumulated experience and wisdom of the community of faith (Hamel, 1996).

## Family, Sexuality, and Procreation

Church leaders have the highest regard for marriage and family. The Catholic Church does not permit use of any medication, instrument, or procedure before, during, or after sexual intercourse to prevent conception (Hamel, 1996). Human life is regarded as sacred and the direct intent to interfere with the solemn purpose of intercourse as a sin. The Church condemns sterilization for the same reason (e.g., vasectomy or tubal ligation).

On the subject of abortion, the Guidelines for Catholic Healthcare Institutions state that "Since all human life deserves respect and protection, every reasonable effort must be made to nourish, support, and protect life in the womb. Thus, abortion has been rejected by the Church" (McCormick, 1987). The Catholic Church has maintained a consistent position on this issue despite many technological advances in our understanding of fetal development. The ovum is considered human life; any attempt to terminate that life is considered a direct abortion. The Church does allow indirect abortion, a situation that occurs when treatment for another serious pathological condition (e.g., cancer of the uterus in a pregnant woman) has an abortive effect (Hamel, 1996).

## Death and Dying

Death is viewed as part of the human condition and is a natural transition to life with God. Life is a good gift from the Creator and we are considered stewards of that precious gift. Catholics have a duty to preserve life and to do nothing intentionally to end it. The church commends the relief of pain and suffering in the dying patient. Analgesics should be used to relieve pain even though their use may shorten life (Hamel, 1996). The Vatican's "Declaration on Euthanasia" (Hamel, 1996) specifies that no one is permitted to kill an innocent human being whether it is an older person, someone who is dying, or someone suffering from an incurable disease.

# Judaism

The Jewish faith tradition extends back at least 4000 years and is based on beliefs in the oneness of God, the goodness of God's creation, and life as a gift of God. Orthodox Jews adhere more strictly to the religious and ceremonial laws, whereas Reform and Conservative Jews use the Scriptures more as a guide than as an absolute authority (Levi, 1986). In all branches of Judaism, maintaining a healthy body as well as soul is a religious imperative (Feldman, 1986).

## Family, Sexuality, and Procreation

Marriage and children are considered the epitome of blessing in the Jewish view (Dorff, 1996). Propagation of the race is a command as well as a blessing, although contraception is permitted. In managing difficult pregnancies, the mother's life is of paramount importance; thus, abortion is permissible when the mother's life is threatened. Most Jews would also allow abortion if there were substantial risk of congenital deformity (Levi, 1986). There may be a gap between the official position of the Jewish faith (abortion restricted to certain circumstances) and a more permissive tradition present among contemporary Jews (Dorff, 1996). While all Jewish sources would permit abortion to preserve the life or organs of the mother, authorities differ widely on how much of a threat justifies such an action.

## Death and Dying

Jewish law prohibits the taking of an innocent human life in all circumstances. The body belongs to God, not the individual person. There is some difference among Jewish authorities regarding when the obligation to save life and cure ends and when the permission to let nature take its course begins (Dorff, 1996). The judgment of the attending physician is accepted and used as a reasonable standard when absolutes are not known. Unlike Catholics, Jews observe no sacraments or "last rites," but do have an active and complex calendar of holy days and observances throughout the year.

### Special or Unique Views

Jewish male children must be circumcised on the eighth day unless there is danger to the child's life, in which case it may be delayed. Whereas boys of other faith traditions are often circumcised for cultural and perceived health reasons, in Judaism there is a religious obligation, as a way of setting apart Jews as God's "chosen people." The circumcision is performed by a specially trained rabbi.

## Islam

Islamic moral guidelines are based on the Holy Quran which is the supreme scripture from Allah (God) recited by Muhammad the Prophet, and the hadiths, which are the recorded actions and sayings of Muhammad (Fellows, 1979). Islam has grown quickly and now is prevalent in many parts of the world including Asia, the Middle East, North Africa, and to a lesser degree in North America. An early schism (circa 656 A.D.) led to two main sects, the Shiites (Imams provide religious leadership) and the Sunnis (leadership from religious scholars) (Waugh, 1996).

### Family, Sexuality, and Procreation

Marriage is an important part of the social order. Sexuality in marriage is proper and good as long as the reproductive dimension remains paramount (Waugh, 1996). Similar to the Jewish and Christian Bible's command to "go forth and multiply," Muslims are advised to "reproduce and increase in numbers" (Rahman, 1987). Contraception is allowed but sterilization is considered contrary to religious requirements (Waugh, 1996).

Exact guidelines regarding abortion are lacking, possibly due to a lack of a uniform definition of the fetus. Some scholars refer to a process of "ensoulment" or formation of the soul that takes place between 40 and 120 days of gestation, after which interference with life would be murder (Waugh, 1996). Abortion after the fetus is formed (note no specific time element or definition) is considered a crime among more conservative Muslims; an exception may be made if continuation of the pregnancy threatens the life of the mother (Rahman, 1987).

### Death and Dying

Allah is the creator and possessor of life, and therefore active euthanasia is not permitted (Rahman, 1987). The dying process is a community and family event and accompanied by prayers for a "good death." Unbelievers are thought to face an eternity of torture that can be foreseen at the moment of death by its bleakness (Waugh, 1996). Forgiveness is very important; if the dying person has done wrong to anyone, then he must seek forgiveness so that he will be forgiven by God. Heroic measures near death must be tempered by awareness of the religious beliefs of Muslims that they are going on to an eternal life. Intravenous feedings or mechanical ventilation for the sole purpose of maintaining mechanical bodily functions are not required and can be stopped in a dying patient, since it is Allah who determines the time of death.

## Jehovah's Witness

Jehovah's Witnesses are a fundamentalist Christian group adhering to a strict and literal interpretation of the Bible, particularly the Old Testament laws. Church policies and health beliefs are outlined in the Watch Tower Bible and Tract Society publications. Scripture is used as a guide for all aspects of life, including diet, hygiene, and health (DuBose, 1996).

## Family, Sexuality, and Procreation

Jehovah's Witnesses strongly emphasize families, children, and moral values. They agree with the traditional Christian view of restricting sexual activity to heterosexual marriage. Contraception use is determined by the conscience of the individual in light of the general principle of sanctity of life and is considered a personal matter (DuBose, 1996). Sterilization was originally discouraged due to the disruption of procreation in the family but is considered a personal matter now that reversal of sterilization is technically possible. Abortion is opposed even when the life of the mother is in danger; it is held that life begins at conception (MacLean, 1986).

## Death and Dying

Death is a transition to eternal life in a New World. Preparation for death includes prayer with a focus on repentance and forgiveness. Family, spiritual, and community support is important, but there are no formal last rites or ceremonies. Jehovah's Witnesses may decide to forego life-sustaining treatment when death is imminent or when treatment is futile. Jehovah's Witnesses oppose active euthanasia.

## Special Beliefs

Jehovah's Witnesses are best known for their prohibition of blood transfusions. Their views are based on proscriptions against ingesting blood in both the Old and New Testaments (Genesis 9:3–4, Leviticus 17: 10–14, Acts 15:28–29). As a general rule, they do not accept blood or blood products, nor will they accept re-infusion of their own blood.

With the advent of fractionated blood products, artificial plasma, and highly processed blood-based products, the policies of Jehovah's Witnesses have undergone some clarification (*The Watchtower*, 2000). Jehovah's Witnesses hold that accepting whole blood or any of the four primary components (red cells, white cells, platelets, and plasma) violates God's law. However, since blood can be processed beyond those primary components, questions arise about fractions derived from the primary blood components. Should Christians accept these fractions in medical treatment? Jehovah's Witnesses authorities cannot say for sure. The Bible does not give details, so a Jehovah's Witness must make his or her own conscientious decision before God. They will accept blood substitutes such as intravenous fluids, Ringer's solution, and others.

Since adherence to these restrictions varies according to the individual's commitment to the principles of Jehovah's Witnesses, clarification of views should be made in every case. Many hospitals have formed committees to address questions and mediate discussion between parties when opinions differ. This is particularly important when treating children who are Jehovah's Witnesses. Church policy maintains that parents have the God-given duty to make medical decisions for their offspring (DuBose, 1996). In cases where the child's life is endangered, the ethical and legal consensus in the United States is that the physician should act to save the life of the child even if the parents oppose such action. When the physician, family, hospital representatives, and church representatives sit down to understand each other's concerns, creative solutions and compromises are possible.

# Christian Science

## Death and Dying

The Christian Science denomination was formed by Mary Baker Eddy in the latter nineteenth century. Eddy taught that the spirit is real and eternal, that matter is unreal and temporal (Peel, 1988), and that death is not an end but a passage into the presence of God. According to this view, illness—being a material entity—is an illusion caused by a lack of faith.

## Special or Unique Beliefs

Many Christian Science followers eschew traditional medical care and turn to Christian Scientist practitioners for prayer and healing. When the decision to use Christian Science healing includes a rejection of modern healthcare treatment, conflicts may arise. Recent cases involving minor children have caused great distress in the medical community due to what is perceived as religiously motivated medical neglect. A recent review analyzed the documented cases of children who died between 1975 and 1995 after their parents withheld medical care for religious reasons and for which the probability of survival with medical care would have exceeded 90%. Of the 172 cases identified, 28 were Christian Scientist (Asser & Swan, 1998). Hope for better outcomes in the future is based on the emergence of leaders in the Christian Science community and other faith-healing communities who use both conventional treatment and spiritual healing. Better laws are also needed to protect children from medical neglect (Benson & Dusek, 1999).

## Protestantism

Protestant churches include a wide variety of denominations with different styles of worship, church organization, moral beliefs, and social concerns. The style of worship ranges from formal to informal, with some focusing on preaching, others on the sacraments, and others on prayer or praise or healing. Some are intellectually oriented, others are oriented toward feelings. Some Protestant churches adhere to a literal interpretation of the scriptures, while others don't. Some Protestant churches have a hierarchical form of church government much like the Catholics, while others place the decision-making in the individual congregations. On moral and social issues Protestant groups range from very liberal to ultraconservative.

### Family, Sexuality, and Procreation

Marriage and family are central to most Protestant denominations. Many groups prohibit homosexual relationships on the basis of biblical teachings, but some denominations have recently embraced homosexual participation and even marriage.

Regarding abortion, the divergence among Protestants in the interpretation of scripture is quite diverse. Liberal Protestants such as the American Baptists, the United Church of Christ, Unitarians, and Quakers tend to allow freedom of conscience with regard to such issues as abortion, assisted suicide, and means of contraception that destroy a fertilized egg (Nehring, 1996). Conservative Protestants such as the Southern Baptists, the Assembly of God, and other evangelical Protestant groups tend to express strong opposition to abortion, assisted suicide, and euthanasia. Many of the so-called mainline Protestant denominations, such as the Methodists, Episcopalians, and Presbyterians, currently find themselves split on these issues (Holifield, 1996). All Protestant denominations allow traditional forms of contraception.

### Death and Dying

Death is considered a transition to eternal life. Most conservative and moderate Protestants believe in Heaven and Hell, and one's ultimate destiny is based on decisions made while here in this life, namely, salvation through Christ. Acceptance of the gift of salvation from God can take place at any time, even on the deathbed. Dying persons receive comfort from loved ones and clergy when nearing death, using prayer as a means of coping. Forgiveness and reconciliation are often stressed. End-of-life decisions about life support and resuscitation are left to the prayerful consideration of the patient and family (Morgan *et al.*, 1986; Nehring, 1996). Except among the more liberal Protestants, active euthanasia and assisted suicide are not endorsed. Each person is valuable in the eyes of God and worthy of love and protection (Baptist Faith and Message, 2000), so actively taking a life is presuming on God's sovereignty.

## Mormon (Church of Jesus Christ of Latter-Day Saints)

The Mormon church was founded in 1830 by Joseph Smith who claimed to have received multiple revelations from God. An angel provided him with plates of gold engraved with holy scriptures called the Book of Mormon. The Mormon church (LDS) now claims 4.5 million members in the United States. They are perhaps best known for their tradition of door-to-door evangelism by young men in the church. Mormons see scientific revelation as being from God and as such see religion and science as complementary (Harris-Abbott, 1996).

## Family, Sexuality, and Procreation

Family life and marriage are a prominent part of LDS life and teaching. One unique view is that faithful couples will continue to be together in the afterlife and bonded to their children (Harris-Abbott, 1996). The church originally opposed contraception, but since 1989 it has been allowed as a personal decision of families, with an emphasis on spacing children rather than limiting procreation. Sterilization is not viewed as benignly and is strictly opposed.

The LDS church strictly opposes elective abortion on the basis of the sanctity of life. Abortion is allowed in extreme cases to protect the life of the mother, or in cases of rape or incest, but consultation with a bishop and prayer is recommended (Harris-Abbott, 1996).

## Death and Dying

Death is a transition to an eternal spiritual life. No formal declaration has been made as to determining the time of death or on the use of palliative care. LDS members should not feel obligated to extend mortal life by means that are unreasonable. They should seek guidance through fasting and prayer. The church proscribes assisted suicide and euthanasia (Harris-Abbott, 1996).

## Special Beliefs

Like many conservative traditions, Mormans eschew the use of alcohol and tobacco. In addition, most Mormans believe that the consumption of coffee and tea is proscribed by their scripture's prohibition against "hot drinks" (Doctrine and Covenants 89:9). Some LDS members view caffeinated soft drinks and cough syrup containing alcohol as also forbidden. Physicians treating LDS patients should discuss with them their beliefs before prescribing or recommending medicines, food, or beverages containing alcohol or caffeine.

# Hinduism

The vast majority of India's 900 million citizens are practicing Hindus. Approximately 1 million Hindus live in North America, and most U.S. cities have a large Hindu community. Many Americans who are not Hindus practice yoga, a form of meditation, exercise, and health maintenance rooted in Hinduism. In the Hindu world-view, life has four aims: virtue, purpose or wealth, pleasure, and release or liberation from the cycle of rebirth.

## Death, Rebirth, and Release

Hindus believe in reincarnation: that those who die will be reborn, and that our degree of virtue in this life will determine whether we are reborn to a higher or lower form of being. The ultimate goal is to be released from bondage to the physical world with its cycle of pain, suffering, old age, death, and rebirth. The goal is to liberate the atman, the spiritual or transcendental self, from its bondage to the ahankara, the physical, public, or phenomenal self.

Cremation, rather than embalming and burial, is the preferred method of disposing of the deceased body. Fire purifies that which is impure, and fire most quickly and effectively returns bodies to their original form. The family of the deceased is responsible for offering the body to the fire and the ashes to the holy waters (Desai, 1989).

## Family, Sexuality, and Procreation

In traditional Hinduism, marriage is arranged by the parents and involves payment of a dowry by the wife's family to the husband's family. Divorce is forbidden.

In traditional Hinduism, premarital sexual intercourse is strictly forbidden. To reduce temptation, individuals are encouraged to marry at an early age. Girls are considered sexually mature at the time of their first menstruation, and in the past their fathers were supposed to arrange their marriages by this time.

Hinduism strongly encourages procreation, particularly of male children. But the tradition also supports birth control and family planning. In ancient Hinduism, abortion was regarded as murder, except where necessary to save the life of the mother. Today, abortion is legal and widely practiced in Hindu cultures.

Homosexual relationships are taboo in Hindu culture. Historically, those caught engaging in homosexual acts were excluded from their caste under both religious and secular law. In recent years the Hindu religion has become more tolerant toward homosexuality than Hindu culture (Park Ridge Center, 2000).

## The Status of Women

In the past, Hindu women played very traditional roles in family and society. Some changes are taking place, as evidenced, for example, by the rise to power of Indira Ghandi. Sati (the self-immolation of widows), female infanticide, abortion of female fetuses, child marriage, and dowry-murder are now exceptions rather than the rule, and are no longer sanctioned by religious or secular law (Park Ridge Center, 2000).

# Buddhism

The global Buddhist population has been estimated at 354 million, the vast majority of whom live in southeast Asia and Japan. There are approximately 2.5 million Buddhists in North America.

Buddhism evolved out of the Hindu tradition and its teaching is rooted in the Four Noble Truths, which offer a solution to the problem of pain, suffering, and evil.

## Pain, Suffering, and Death

The first Noble Truth is that suffering exists and is universally experienced; the second truth: desire and attachment are the causes of suffering; the third and fourth truths: a person can be liberated from suffering through the cessation of desire (the desire not to suffer) and by journeying on the Eightfold Path. The Eightfold Path consists of: right understanding, right thought, right speech, right action, right livelihood, right effort, right mindfulness, and right concentration. When one develops these disciplines, one learns to stop worrying about the past or future, to live fully in the present: to be fully present wherever one is, and whatever one is doing. This, according to the Buddhists, is the secret to good mental and physical health.

## Family, Sexuality, and Procreation

The cultures that gave birth to Buddhism hold a strong reverence for marriage and family. Buddhist teaching values marriage as an important way of promising fidelity to one's spouse, but does not view marriage as the only place where sex is permitted. Buddhist moral teaching permits adult sexual relations wherever there is mutual consent, selflessness, and love. Buddhist teaching regarding adolescent sexual

---

### THE SECRET OF GOOD HEALTH

*The secret of health for both mind and body*
*is not to mourn for the past,*
*not to worry about the future,*
*or not to anticipate troubles,*
*but to live the present moment wisely and earnestly.*
*—Gautama Buddha*

activity ranges from traditional views promoting filial piety and prohibiting premarital sexual activity, to more liberal views of affirming sex when based on love. Buddhist moral teaching is ambivalent on the subject of homosexual activity (Park Ridge Center, 2000).

Birth control and family planning are permissible within the Buddhist tradition, except perhaps for those forms that are abortifacient. Some Buddhists consider abortion a violation of the Buddha's prohibition of killing, while others do not (Park Ridge Center, 2000).

## The Status of Women

Unlike Hindu tradition, Buddhist moral teaching emphasizes the equality of all beings and the Buddha opposed discrimination against women. Yet due perhaps to pre-Buddhist cultural influences, Buddhist women still do not enjoy equality in many Asian societies. Buddhist nuns today still protest their inequal status vis-à-vis Buddhist monks (Park Ridge Center, 2000).

### CASE 29-3

*Mander Wilson was a 44-year-old-man with type II diabetes who came to the hospital because of pain and swelling in his left lower extremity. He had had a below-knee amputation 3 weeks previously and had noticed pain and swelling for several days. He had not checked his sugar lately and he wasn't sure whether he had taken his insulin. His left leg stump was red, swollen, tender, and oozing and he had a temperature of 102 degrees. His blood sugar was 670 but he was not in ketoacidosis. The on-call medical team admitted him to the hospital, started him on antibiotics, and gave him insulin.*

*The next morning he was no longer running a fever but looked tired and depressed. The daytime physician took his history and examined him. In the process of inquiring about symptoms of depression, he asked the patient whether he felt like giving up. The patient looked up and made eye contact with the physician for the first time that morning. "No, I don't want to give up." Sensing a renewed spirit of determination in the patient, the physician pressed further. "But you don't take care of yourself, you skip your insulin, you miss appointments—all these point to a person who has given up and just doesn't care anymore," the physician challenged. "But I haven't given up. I want to get better. If I can just get this leg straight..." he replied. "Where will you find the strength? What is going to change?" the physician asked. "I don't know," was the reply. He sunk back into his pillow.*

*"Do you have family, friends, a minister that will come and visit you?"*

*"My wife will be in later. I don't have a minister."*

*"Do you have a faith or religion that is important to you?"*

*"I used to be a Baptist, and my sister-in-law is a minister, but she doesn't live around here."*

*"We have chaplains in the hospital who could come by and visit you. Would you like me to ask one of them to come and see you?"*

*"Yes, doc, I'd sure appreciate it."*

## TAKING A SPIRITUAL HISTORY

Patients' spirituality should be assessed for several reasons: patients have views that affect their health; many patients want their spiritual needs addressed in the medical setting; and patients often use their faith as a source for coping with an illness (Gallup, 1990; King & Bushwick, 1994; Koenig *et al.*, 1992, 1998). Clinicians need to know whether the patient's religious or spiritual views may affect medical decision-making. Hospitalized patients have expressed the desire to have their spiritual needs addressed and some would like physicians to pray with them (Yankelovich, 1996). Koenig and colleagues have documented the prevalence of religious coping in hospitalized patients, and that patients who use religious coping have less depression and better health (Koenig *et al.*, 1992, 1998). Case 29-3 illustrates that spiritual issues may be hidden from view but will surface quickly once inquiry is made. It may take little more than asking the simple question "Do you have a faith or religion that is important to you?" to open a dialogue about spiritual or religious needs or concerns the patient may have.

Taking a spiritual history is the process of gathering relevant information from a patient about spiritual values, religious beliefs, spiritual needs and concerns, and whatever gives the patient's life and illness meaning. It should also include questions about how their religious and spiritual views affect their health, whether they use religious coping, whether they have specific spiritual concerns at the time, and whether they have a minister or other spiritual counselor on whom to call. Case 29-3 illustrates taking a spiritual history in the context of a patient with depression. The physician inquired about the social and spiritual resources to help the patient deal with his acute hospitalization and his chronic illness. After finding a past religious affiliation, the physician offered spiritual support in the form of a chaplain visit. The patient readily accepted the offer, which is consistent with my experience of seeing the vast majority of patients willingly and eagerly accept an offer of chaplain support. Most patients (85%) believe in God and express a denominational affiliation, but only 40% are members of a particular congregation (Gallup, 1997). Thus, many hospitalized patients do not have their own minister or spiritual counselor; for them, chaplains are an important spiritual resource.

Taking a spiritual history should be incorporated into the workup of all hospital patients and should be a part of any complete history and physical examination. Several clinicians have developed tools for taking a spiritual history that aid in the process and make the topics to cover easier to remember, including the SPIRITual history (Table 29.1) and the FICA tool (Table 29.2).

A simple approach is to ask about "FAITH" (King, 2000) which is summarized in Table 29.3. The first question deals with whether the patient has a faith or religion that is important to him or her. Discovering

**Table 29.1**
Sample Questions for the SPIRITual History[a]

| Mnemonic | Questions |
|---|---|
| S—Spiritual belief system | What is your formal religious affiliation? |
| | Name or describe your spiritual belief system. |
| P—Personal spirituality | Describe the beliefs and practices of your religion or spiritual system that you personally accept. |
| | Describe the beliefs or practices you do not accept. |
| | Do you accept or believe … (specific tenet or practice)? |
| | What does your spirituality/religion mean to you? |
| | What is the importance of your spirituality/religion in daily life? |
| I—Integration with a spiritual community | Do you belong to any spiritual or religious group or community? |
| | What is your position or role? |
| | What importance does this group have to you? |
| | Is it a source of support? In what ways? |
| | Does or could this group provide help in dealing with health issues? |
| R—Ritualized practices and restrictions | Are there any specific practices that you carry out as part of your religion/spirituality (e.g., prayer or meditation)? |
| | Are there certain lifestyle activities or practices that your religion/spirituality encourages or forbids? Do you comply? |
| | What significance do these practices and restrictions have for you? |
| | Are there specific elements of medical care that you forbid on the basis of religious/spiritual grounds? |
| I—Implications | What aspects of your religion/spirituality would you like me to keep in mind as I care for you? |
| | Would you like to discuss religious or spiritual implications of health care? |
| | What knowledge or understanding would strengthen our relationship as physician and patient? |
| | Are there any barriers to our relationship based on religious or spiritual issues? |
| T—Terminal events planning | As we plan for your care near the end of life, how does your faith impact on your decisions? |
| | Are there particular aspects of care that you wish to forgo or have withheld because of your faith? |

[a]Adapted from Maugans TA. The SPIRITual history. *Arch Fam Med* 5:11–16, 1996.

**Table 29.2**
FICA Spiritual Assessment Tool[a]

| | |
|---|---|
| F—Faith | What is your faith tradition? |
| I—Important | How important is your faith to you? |
| C—Church | What is your church or community of faith? |
| A—Apply | How do your religious and spiritual beliefs apply to your health? |

[a]Adapted from Puchalski CM. Taking a spiritual history: FICA. *Spirituality and Medicine Connection*, 3(1):1, 1999.

whether the patient has a particular denominational affiliation can give the clinician clues to particular health beliefs (see Health Beliefs of Religious Groups above) and also offers a relatively "safe" starting point for further inquiry. In my experience, few patients object to the question about faith or religion—when they do, it is often a red flag indicating that this is not a comfortable subject for them and perhaps such inquiry should be postponed.

The next question to resolve is how the patient's beliefs apply to their health. Are there any dietary restrictions the healthcare team needs to know about? Are there any important religious holidays coming up that would affect the patient? Are fasting, set times for prayer, or other customs followed that might affect health important to holiday observance? Are there any restrictions about the use of blood or other blood products? Many religious traditions have customs or rituals about diet, prayer, religious holidays or observances, end-of-life times, and other beliefs that may affect medical decisions.

Involvement in a faith community is helpful in understanding the patient's available social and spiritual support. Is the patient's involvement regular and current? Some patients have past connections they wish to renew in times of stress and illness, as in Case 29-3. Others may wish to see their own minister, priest, or rabbi while they are in the hospital.

Treatment decisions may hinge on spiritual beliefs, especially end-of-life decisions about continuing or withholding treatment. Patients who believe in an afterlife may have an outlook different from those who do not. I have seen family and clergy praying by the bedside in gratitude to God regarding a moribund dying patient in families who have strong belief in an afterlife, communicating a sense of peace and joy at the transition to an afterlife with God. In contrast, I have also seen great emotional upheaval and decompensation in other families who believe that the earthly life is all there is even when death has been long expected. Patients with AIDS or liver failure or even prostate cancer may feel that their illness is a punishment from God—or that their suffering is redemptive—and may be reluctant to address important end-of-life issues (Kaldjian *et al.*, 1998). Inquiring about spiritual beliefs is critical when dealing with patients who are making medical decisions about life and death issues.

Asking how you as a health provider can help the patient with any spiritual concerns is an excellent way to open the dialogue about the patient's concerns. Patients may share some conflicts or questions, request to see the chaplain, ask for prayer, or ask you to pray with them. Many providers will not be comfortable praying with patients, but each provider should be prepared to respond in a constructive way and be knowledgeable

**Table 29.3**
FAITH Spiritual History[a]

| | |
|---|---|
| F—Faith | Do you have a Faith or religion that is important to you? |
| A—Apply | How do your beliefs Apply to your health? |
| I—Involved | Are you Involved in a church or faith community? |
| T—Treatment | How do your spiritual beliefs affect your views about end-of-life Treatment? |
| H—Help | How can I Help you with any spiritual concerns? |

[a]Adapted from King DE. *Faith, Spirituality and Medicine: Toward the Making of a Healing Practitioner*. New York, Haworth Press, 2000.

about available chaplains and spiritual counselors. Often the most important thing to do is listen. Patients are sometimes surprised to know that you are interested in their spiritual concerns; in my experience, most are grateful that you care about them as a "whole person." Listening to the patient's struggles with the meaning and value of life can be therapeutic for the patient and enlightening to the provider as well.

Few providers have been trained to counsel patients in religious or spiritual matters, nor would it be ethically appropriate to use the power of the physician's position. Patients in whom the physician identifies spiritual needs or concerns should be referred to a certified chaplain or qualified minister.

Care and compassion demand that we acknowledge and address the spiritual needs of our patients. Sometimes we will address these needs directly, especially when the need is simply to listen empathetically; other times through referral to clergy. Helping patients find meaning and peace in their suffering is part of what helps make medicine a profession rather than a purely technical enterprise.

## CASE 29-4

*Miss Winter came to the office complaining of headaches, backache, and abdominal pain. She had significant stress in her life, including an 8-month-old baby, a new house, and a husband who had recently lost his job. The physician examined her and found no physical pathology. He diagnosed depression and recommended medication and psychotherapy for the situational problems she was facing. He concluded his recommendation with a question regarding the person's religious background. She replied that she had no religious affiliation and did not believe in God. She believed that every person had some good in them and that each person should find meaning in helping one another. The physician replied that she would be better off seeking true meaning from a saving relationship with Jesus Christ, and gave her a pamphlet describing the steps to becoming a believer.*

## ETHICS OF SPIRITUAL INQUIRY

Some physicians have cautioned against any integration of spirituality into clinical medicine because of concerns about boundaries, power, autonomy, and nonmaleficence (Sloan *et al.*, 1999). Others have promoted more spiritual involvement as part of the ethical obligation to benefit the patient and, in the case of religious patients, to enhance their autonomy (Matthews *et al.*, 1998). Case 29-4 illustrates the scenario of evangelical proselytizing in the examination room, a situation full of ethical issues and one that is often cited as the reason to keep religion and medicine separate. Most authors would agree that proselytizing in the examination room is inappropriate. But what if the patient brings up the issue first? What if the patient asks the physician about his faith?

Further reflection and deliberation are needed on the ethical dimensions of integrating spirituality and religion into the medical realm (Ellis *et al.*, 1999). Are taking a spiritual history, being sensitive to spiritual concerns, and referring patients to chaplains appropriate clinically? Are they, or should they be, within the standard of care? If so, in what manner, and under what circumstances should physicians question patients regarding spiritual matters?

The first step in addressing the ethics of spiritual involvement is determining whether it is ethically acceptable to inquire about patients' religious and spiritual beliefs. Such a determination should be based on the importance of obtaining the information as well as the rights and responsibilities of physicians and patients. Information obtained during a medical history should respect patients' basic rights of autonomy, confidentiality, and privacy.

Obtaining important medical information is one ethical justification for spiritual inquiry (Matthews *et al.*, 1998). Because much disease, illness, and injury is the result of lifestyle choices rooted in cultural and spiritual values rather than distinct organic pathology, ignoring the cultural and spiritual dimensions is on a par with making a diagnosis without an adequate physical examination (Jamison, 1995). Just as treating patients with heart attacks without knowing the social and psychological status is incomplete care, so treating patients without knowledge of their spiritual context may be inappropriate. In Case 29-4, the physician may have been justified in finding out more about the patient's spiritual life, since he was investigating other psychosocial issues to determine the context for the depression. Including religious influences in medical assessment and decision-making produces a more complete basis for choosing treatment in the healthcare setting. Lack of spiritual inquiry may omit important information regarding patients' health, health beliefs, and personal behaviors that affect health.

A counterargument is that inquiring about patients' spiritual concerns is inherently "nonmedical" and therefore outside the realm of appropriate inquiry. Physicians could use their power to influence improperly the religious beliefs of patients, or to cause patients to suffer from guilt or depression when they do not recover after using prayer. Case 29-4 shows that physicians can easily move over the line and become religious advocates rather than listeners. Miss Winter did not ask for spiritual advice. Her world-view, while different from the physician's, is her own choice and within the realm of her autonomy as a patient and a human being. The physician is acting on the basis of his own agenda rather than that of the patient. While some critics make an allowance for "taking into account" religious factors that affect medical choices and medical care, inquiry leading to nonmedical or spiritual interventions would be considered inappropriate (Sloan et al., 1999).

The rights and responsibilities of physicians and patients should also be considered. Physicians have the right to inquire about spiritual concerns that may have an impact on health or health beliefs. Patients have the right to accept or decline such inquiry. One survey of physicians and patients in Vermont investigated the rights and responsibilities of religious inquiry and found that 89% of physicians and 52% of patients agreed with the right of the physician to inquire about religion and religious concerns (Maugans & Wadland, 1991). Fifty-two percent of physicians and 21% of patients felt it was the responsibility of the physician to inquire. This study illustrates the divided views of physicians and patients regarding religious inquiry. In my experience patients rarely decline to respond to compassionate inquiry about spiritual concerns. When patients ask for the reason behind my inquiry, an explanation about my interest in them as a whole person usually satisfies their curiosity and they proceed to answer. Patients who are concerned about sharing private information can often be reassured about the confidentiality of the medical record. In my own experience, most patients are quite willing to share their religious or spiritual views and experiences as they relate to health.

Some patients may prefer that physicians assess the relevant information for making medical decisions without inquiring about the religious or spiritual basis for a patient's views. When the patient's desire for privacy conflicts with the clinician's need to obtain important medical information, compassionate explanation of the relevance of spiritual issues and understanding of the intimacy of spiritual experience will help in negotiating a solution. If there are no medical consequences evident from omitting religious inquiry, then the patient's wishes should be followed.

Once spiritual issues are identified, the provider must decide how best to address them. Many providers feel uncomfortable inquiring about religious and spiritual concerns; few would feel qualified and prepared to counsel patients directly about such matters (Ellis et al., 1999; Sloan et al., 2000). The well-trained clinician should be able to assess patients' concerns and then refer the patient to a qualified spiritual counselor such as a certified chaplain.

Chaplains offer expertise and experience in spiritual counseling that physicians do not possess; using better trained professionals should improve the quality of care. If one agrees that it is an obligation of physicians to inquire about spiritual concerns that relate to health, and such concerns are identified, then it seems the ethics and professionalism of the physician should compel him or her to seek assistance from a chaplain.

## QUALIFICATIONS AND TRAINING OF CHAPLAINS

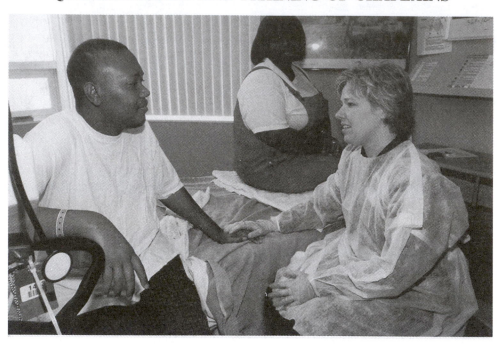

*Chaplains must hold an undergraduate degree from an accredited college or university. Board certification requires theological education at the graduate professional level, usually at least 3 years at an accredited seminary or graduate school earning the master of theology or master of divinity degree. Hospital chaplains then undergo an additional 1–2 years of training in a clinical pastoral care residency at an acute care hospital. Certification as a hospital chaplain also requires being ordained or commissioned by a religious organization. Ordination is recognition of commitment to ministry after recommendation from peers. An additional requirement for certification is ecclesiastical endorsement by a faith group for ministry in a specialized setting. Board certification is granted by the Association of Professional Chaplains (APC) after receipt of required letters of recommendation and documentation of completion of clinical pastoral education. The APC offers associate chaplain status to ordained ministers with 2 years of graduate training. (Information from the Association of Professional Chaplains, Schaumberg, IL 60173; more information can be obtained by email to info@professionalchaplains.org <mailto: info@professionalchaplains.org>). Photo courtesy of the Department of Pastoral Care, Emory University Hospital.*

## CONCLUSION

Physicians who are sensitive to the biopsychosocial needs of patients should also consider patients' spiritual needs. The prominent role of religious commitment and spirituality in medical decision-making and their use as a source of coping provide further rationale for physicians to address spirituality in the clinical setting. Taking a spiritual history and referring patients with spiritual concerns to chaplains or ministers are basic clinical skills. Spiritual inquiry is justified by the need to obtain important medical information and explore the patient's point of view, but must be done in such a way that respects the patient's privacy, confidentiality, and autonomy. Effectively integrating spiritual sensitivity into clinical practice is a challenge that should be addressed by all physicians.

# THE COLLABORATIVE MODEL

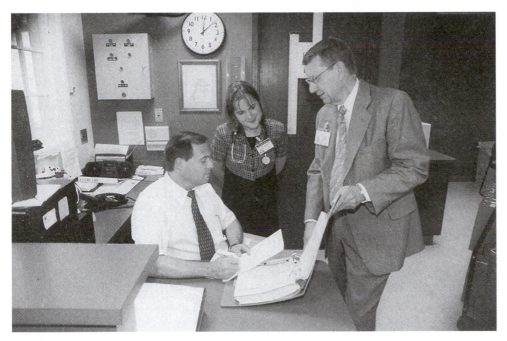

*Patients in hospitals and nursing homes often have spiritual needs that exceed the expertise, professional boundaries, and time boundaries of the physician. Consultation and collaboration with chaplains, ministers, priests, and rabbis is essential to effective care. Photo courtesy of the Department of Pastoral Care, Emory University Hospital.*

## CASES FOR DISCUSSION

### CASE 1

Mrs. Badger is a 72-year-old widow who came into the emergency room after a fall that broke her right arm. Her arm was put in a cast, but she had to be admitted to the hospital because of an exacerbation of her diabetes and a possible stroke. After admission, she began feeling much better. Her stroke symptoms resolved and were judged to be a consequence of her altered glucose metabolism. Mrs. Badger was not anxious to go home, however. After talking with her further, the treating physician discovered that the patient had recently moved to an "eldercare" apartment. She felt she was being "kicked out" of her daughter's house and was very anxious about living alone. She had no help to get settled in the new apartment, she had boxes to unpack, and she had a broken arm with which to deal. Social services did not include helpers for moving and unpacking. The patient was distraught despite her physical improvement.

1. What would be your reaction to the woman's predicament?
2. Would you discharge her knowing that her home care situation was unresolved? Why or why not?
3. Would you take a spiritual history on this patient? What resources might that illuminate?

### CASE 2

Brad Gaston is a 36-year-old sociology professor at the local college. You know from a previous encounter that he is a nature lover and environmentalist. You are seeing him for a scrape on his knee and thigh he sustained while riding his bike to the school. You note an infection developing and recommend antibiotic treatment and a tetanus shot. The patient balks *and says he only wants "natural" therapy, no "artificial" remedies. He believes in natural healing. He believes in a God-like force in nature but has no formal religious affiliation. You do not share his views, but feel he has a right to his opinions. You feel he is risking more serious infection and consequences by refusing antibiotics.*

1. *What would be your advice to the patient?*
2. *What would you do to address his beliefs?*
3. *Would you try to convince him to take the medication? If so, why?*
4. *How would you do it?*

## CASE 3

*Lisa Nowell is a 23-year-old woman being treated by a cardiologist for postpartum cardiomyopathy, a condition that causes heart failure. She was initially improving at home on multiple medications. However, despite medical advice to the contrary, she has become pregnant again. Her cardiologist has explained to her the high risk of worsening heart failure and even death should she continue the pregnancy and has recommended abortion. She has come to you because you are her obstetrician.*

1. *What would be your advice to the patient in this situation?*
2. *What would you like to know about her spiritual and religious beliefs before giving her advice?*
3. *On which values would you base your advice?*
4. *In what way might your own beliefs and values affect the way you counsel Ms. Nowell?*

## CASE 4

*An 82-year-old man with a history of multiple medical problems comes into the emergency room with severe shortness of breath. You admit him with a diagnosis of severe exacerbation of COPD. His condition worsens and you speak with his family about resuscitation status, since he is unable to speak because of hypoxia and dyspnea. You suggest that resuscitation would be fruitless and recommend he be moved to Do Not Resuscitate status. His family seems very upset at this suggestion. You try to explain the medical situation further, but this seems to upset them even more.*

1. *What other strategies could you use to clarify the family's wishes?*
2. *How might taking a spiritual history assist in this situation?*
3. *What is the physician's agenda and what is the patient's family's agenda in the above situation?*

## CASE 5

*A 45-year-old man comes to your office for a physical. In the course of taking a history, you ask him whether he has a faith or religion that is important to him. He asks why you want to know. You respond by saying it will help you to know him better and may provide some information about health beliefs and behavior. He says he has no religion, no beliefs, and appears irritated.*

1. *What would be your next step?*
2. *Should you pursue the issue by asking why the question upsets him? Why or why not?*
3. *Would you ask your next patient about his or her religious/spiritual beliefs?*

## RECOMMENDED READINGS

King DE: *Faith, Spirituality, and Medicine: Toward the Making of a Healing Practitioner.* New York, Haworth Press, 2000.

This textbook reviews how to take a spiritual history, reviews the rationale for exploring patients' spirituality, and explores the ethics of spiritual inquiry. The book gives practical guidance to physicians and other health professionals. Dr. King provides a biopsychosocial-spiritual model that stresses the importance of viewing the patient as a physical, psychological, social, and spiritual being. Timely use of chaplain services and the special role of religion and spirituality in the care of dying patients are also addressed. The book also examines the impact that spirituality plays in the lives of health professionals, with an exploration of how this may affect the quality of care that they provide and the fulfillment and satisfaction they experience in their vocation.

Koenig HG: *Is Religion Good for Your Health? The Effects of Religion on Physical and Mental Health*. New York, Haworth Press, 1997.

This book examines the findings of research on the relationships between religion and mental health and between religion and physical health. It explores possible psychological, social, and physiological pathways on which these relationships might be based. Dr. Koenig also reviews the implications of these findings for physicians, researchers, and laypersons.

Koenig HG: *The Healing Power of Faith: Science Explores Medicine's Last Great Frontier*. New York, Simon & Schuster, 1999.

Dr. Koenig expands his discussion of new breakthroughs in medical research about health, including findings involving healthier immune systems, lower blood pressure, and prolonged survival of people with strong religious commitment. The book is filled with heartwarming stories of people of many faiths including Protestants, Catholics, Orthodox Jews, and others who have found faith beneficial for health, marriage difficulties, and addictions.

Matthews DA: *The Faith Factor: Proof of the Healing Power of Prayer*. New York, Viking, 1998.

Dr. Matthews is an advocate of taking a spiritual history in all patients. He uses the information to encourage patients in whatever faith motivates them to better themselves. His book is filled with case histories of people who believe in the power of prayer for healing. He uses recent research findings to bolster his advocacy of incorporating religion and spiritual health into everyday practice.

Pargament KI: *The Psychology of Religion and Coping: Theory, Research, and Practice*. New York, Guilford Press, 1997.

This book brings religion and psychology together onto common ground using research, personal experience, and clinical insight. The author provides a rationale for being more sensitive to religion and spirituality in the context of psychological counseling and suggests several ways to address these issues in therapy.

## REFERENCES

Asser SM, Swan R: Child fatalities from religion-motivated medical neglect. *Pediatrics* 101(4): 625–629, 1998.

Baptist Faith and Message 2000 (Statement of faith by the Southern Baptist Convention): www. <http://www.sbc.net/> sbc.netBM _Hlt486303938

Benson H, Dusek JA: Self-reported health, and illness and the use of conventional and unconventional medicine and mind/body healing by Christian Scientists and others. *J Nerv Ment Dis* 187(9): 539–548, 1999.

Desai PN: *Health and Medicine in the Hindu Tradition*. New York, Crossroad, 1989.

Dorff EN: The Jewish tradition: Religious beliefs and healthcare decisions. In "Religious Beliefs and Healthcare Decisions," 1996, Park Ridge Center, Chicago.

DuBose ER: The Jehovah's Witness tradition: In "Religious Beliefs and Healthcare Decisions," 1996, Park Ridge Center, Chicago.

Ellis MR, Vinson DC, Ewigman B: Addressing spiritual concern of patients: Family physicians' attitudes and practices. *J Fam Pract* 48(2): 105–109, 1999.

Ewers GA: Four viewpoints: Churches of Christ. *Aust Fam Physician* 15(8):1024, 1986.

Feldman DM: *Health and Medicine in the Jewish Tradition*. New York, Crossroad, 1986.

Fellows, WJ: *Religious East and West*. New York, Holt, Rinehart & Winston, 1979.

Gallup G: Religion in America 1990. Princeton, NJ, The Princeton Religion Research Center, 1990.

Gallup G: The Gallup Poll. Public Opinion 1997. Wilmington, Del, Scholarly Resources, Inc, 1998.

Hamel RP: The Roman Catholic tradition: Religious beliefs and healthcare decisions. In "Religious Traditions and Healthcare Decisions," 1996, Park Ridge Center, Chicago.

Harris-Abbott D: The Latter-Day Saints: Religious beliefs and healthcare decisions. In "Religious Traditions and Healthcare Decisions," 1996, Park Ridge Center, Chicago.

Holifield EB: Health & medicine in the Methodist tradition. In "Religious Traditions and Healthcare Decisions," 1996, Park Ridge Center, Chicago.

Jamison JE: Spirituality and medical ethics. *Am J Hospice Palliative Care*, May/June 1995, pp 41–45.

Joint Council for Accreditation of Healthcare Organizations, Standards Manual 1999.

Kaldjian LC, Jekel JF, Friedland G: End-of-life decisions in HIV-positive patients: The role of spiritual beliefs. *AIDS* 12:103–107, 1998.

Kass JD: Contributions of religious experience to psychological and physical well-being: Research evidence and explanatory model. *Care Giver J* 8:4–11, 1991.

Kass JD, Friedman R, Leserman J, Zuttermeister PC, Benson H: Health outcomes and a new index of spiritual experience. *J Sci Study Religion* 30:203–211, 1991.

Khan SN: The Islamic viewpoint. *Aust Fam Physician* 15(2):179–180, 1986.

King DE: *Faith, Spirituality, and Medicine: Toward the Making of a Healing Practitioner*. New York, Haworth Press, 2000.

King DE, Bushwick B: Beliefs and attitudes of hospital inpatients about faith healing and prayer. *J Fam Pract* 39(4):349–352, 1994.

Koenig HG, Cohen HJ, Blazer DG, et al: Religious coping and depression among elderly, hospitalized, medically ill men. *Am J Psychiatry* 149 (12):1693–1700, 1992.

Koenig HG, George LK, Peterson BL: Religiosity and remission from depression in medically ill older patients. *Am J Psychiatry* 155:536–542, 1998.

Levi JS: Jewish medical ethics. *Aust Fam Physician* 15(1):17–19, 1986.

Levin JS, Taylor RJ: Age differences in patterns and correlates of the frequency of prayer. *Gerontologist* 37(1):75–88, 1997.

MacLean D: Jehovah's Witnesses. *Aust Fam Physician* 15(6):772–774, 1986.

Manning KM: A Catholic viewpoint. *Aust Fam Physician* 15(4):493–497, 1986.

Marty ME: *Health and Medicine in the Lutheran Tradition.* New York, Crossroad, 1986.

Matthews DA, McCullough ME, Larson DB, Koenig HG, Swyers JP, Milano MG: Religious commitment and health status. *Arch Fam Med* 7:118–124, 1998.

Maugans TA, Wadland WC: Religion and family medicine: A survey of physicians and patients. *J Fam Pract* 32:210–213, 1991.

McBride JL, Arthur G, Brooks R, Pilkington L: The relationship between patients' spirituality and health experiences. *Fam Med* 30(2): 122–126, 1998.

McCormick RA: *Health and Medicine in the Catholic Tradition.* New York, Crossroad, 1987.

Morgan JL, Henley J, McCaughey D: The Anglican and Uniting Church viewpoints. *Aust Fam Physician* 15(3): 264–265, 1986.

Nehring AK: United Church of Christ: Religious beliefs and health care decisions. In "Religious Traditions and Healthcare Decisions," 1996, Park Ridge Center, Chicago.

Oats WN: Four viewpoints: The Religious Society of Friends (Quakers). *Aust Fam Physician* 15(8):1025, 1986.

Park Ridge Center: Religion, Sexuality, and Public Policy: Overview of World Religions, 2000. www.prchfe.org <http://www.prchfe.org/>.

Peel R: *Health and Medicine in the Christian Science Tradition.* New York, Crossroad, 1988.

Puchalski CM, Larson DB: Developing curricula in spirituality and medicine. *Acad Med* 73 (9):970–974, 1998.

Rahman F: *Health and Medicine in the Islamic Tradition.* New York, Crossroad, 1987.

Sloan RP, Bagiella E, Powell T: Religion, spirituality, and medicine. *Lancet* 353:664–667, 1999.

Sloan RP, Bagiella E, VandeCreek L, Hasan Y, Puolos P: Should physicians prescribe religious activities? *N Engl J Med* 342(25), 2000.

Taylor RJ, Chatters LM: Nonorganizational religious participation among elderly black adults. *J Gerontol* 46(2): S103–S111, 1991.

Watch Tower Bible and Tract Society. Questions from Readers. *The Watchtower*, June 15:29–31, 2000.

Waugh EH. The Islamic tradition: Religious beliefs and healthcare decisions. In "Religious Traditions and Healthcare Decisions," 1996, Park Ridge Center, Chicago.

Yankelovich Partners, Inc, in Kaplan M: Ambushed by spirituality. *TIME*, June 24: 62, 1996.

## CHAPTER 30

C. Special Problems

# The Tobacco Pandemic

*Alan M. Blum and Eric J. Solberg*

*Jane L., a 28-year-old graduate student, is waiting to see her family physician for her annual well-woman examination. She is concerned about an article that she recently read in* **Mademoiselle.** *The author warned of dangers associated with the use of oral contraceptives by women who smoke. Jane L. smokes one pack a day of Marlboro Lights 100s. Accordingly, she has decided she would like to stop taking the pill and get fitted for a diaphragm. Rather than simply acquiescing to the patient's request, the physician seized the opportunity to help the patient make the connection between health improvement and cessation of smoking, and to explain the relative risk of smoking compared with oral contraceptives. The patient expressed a desire to stop smoking and asked for help in doing so.*

## EDUCATIONAL OBJECTIVES

1. Identify obstacles to tackling tobacco problems, from challenges in working with individuals who smoke to barriers in curbing tobacco industry marketing practices
2. Better understand common myths surrounding tobacco use and its promotion, and be able to identify the origins of those myths
3. Develop positive, office-based strategies in dealing with tobacco use, including strategies for the overall office environment and clinical strategies for assisting individuals who smoke
4. Distinguish the differences between the traditional medical/pharmacological model of smoking cessation and consumerist/behavioral approaches to smoking cessation
5. Understand the forces that shape individual and public attitudes regarding tobacco use and its promotion.

## INTRODUCTION

As Case 30-1 illustrates, in only a few minutes there is much a physician can do to motivate patients to stop smoking. Such active interventions are more effective than relegating this task to ancillary personnel, a smoking cessation clinic, or a pamphlet off the shelf.

The biggest obstacle to tackling the tobacco problem is complacency—on the part of the public and health professionals alike—stemming from the belief that the war on smoking has been won (Blum, 1992). Although there is hardly a child or adult who has not heard that smoking is dangerous to health, the fact remains that the incidence of smoking has declined by less than 1% per year in the United States over the past decade. Moreover, women, teenagers, blue-collar workers, and minority groups in general are not appreciably reducing their cigarette consumption (Blum, 1993; Department of Health and Human Services, 1998).

Cigarette smoking is the chief avoidable cause of death and disease in our society. Each year smoking is responsible for 18% of all deaths in the United States (Pollin & Ravenholt, 1984). Approximately 40% of all deaths from cancer and 21% of deaths from cardiovascular disease are caused by smoking (DHHS, 1989). Tobacco use contributes to more than 400,000 deaths annually in the United States, and more than 3 million annually worldwide (Centers for Disease Control, 1994). Although cigarette smoking among adults declined from 42% to 27% in the United States during the 23 years following publication of the first Surgeon General's report on smoking and health in 1964, 26.4% of men and 22% of women continue to use tobacco regularly (Centers for Disease Control, 2000; McGinnis & Foege, 1993; Pierce et al., 1989).

Ending the tobacco pandemic is not a *static* effort whereby health professionals educate the public about the adverse health effects of smoking in the hope that individuals will change their behavior, but rather a *dynamic* one whereby the tobacco industry changes its tactics to anticipate all efforts to discourage tobacco use (Blum & Solberg, 1992). As physicians and other health professionals work with their patients to end their smoking, cigarette companies continue to advertise their products, spending more than $6.7 billion on advertising each year, touting low-tar, implicitly "safer" cigarettes, with reduced prices and coupons for increased savings (Federal Trade Commission, 2000). Physicians should point out to patients who smoke that buying a $3 pack of cigarettes is a real "rip-off," especially considering that a pack costs less than 25 cents to manufacture. One patient, after smoking more than two packs a day for 20 years, realized he had "smoked a Porsche."

Concerns about smoking have long been raised in the scientific community. In 1928 Lombard and Doering reported a higher incidence of smoking among patients with cancer than among controls (Lombard & Doering, 1928). Ten years later, Pearl reported that persons who smoked heavily had a shorter life expectancy than those who did not smoke (Pearl, 1938). In 1939 Ochsner and DeBakey began reporting their observations on the relationship between smoking and lung cancer (Ochsner & DeBakey, 1939). They and other outspoken opponents of smoking, such as Dwight Harkin and William Overholt, were met with derision by the medical profession, more than two-thirds of whom smoked.

Not until the epidemiological work in the 1950s of Doll and Hill (1956) in the United Kingdom and Hammond and Horn (1958) in the United States did the medical profession begin to take the problem seriously. Since that time, information about the health risks associated with smoking has been well publicized in the medical literature. The first U.S. Surgeon General's Report on Smoking and Health in 1964 concluded that cigarette smoking was the major cause of lung cancer in men. Besides lung cancer, smoking is a major cause of cancers of the larynx, oral cavity, and esophagus. It is a contributory factor in cancers of the pancreas, bladder, kidney, stomach, and cervix. Recent studies implicate smoking in leukemia, colon cancer, Graves' disease, depression, and renal disease in persons with diabetes mellitus (Blum, 1993). A dose–response relationship exists between smoking and all of these diseases.

Cigarette smoking is a primary risk factor for coronary heart disease (CHD). Overall, those who smoke have a 70% greater CHD death rate, a two- to fourfold greater incidence of CHD, and a two- to fourfold greater risk for sudden death than nonsmokers (DHHS, 1982). The risk of stroke increases with the number of cigarettes smoked. The incidence of stroke among persons who smoke is 50% higher than among persons who do not smoke (Wolf et al., 1988). Cigarette smoking is also the main cause of chronic obstructive pulmonary disease (COPD), which is the leading cause of disability in the United States.

More than 44 million Americans have stopped smoking cigarettes. Unfortunately, some 47 million Americans continue to smoke cigarettes (which represents only a slight decline in actual numbers since 1964), despite the consequences of smoking to their health (CDC, 2000). Moreover, the cohort of smokers is younger than ever. Smoking cessation has major and immediate health benefits for men and women of all ages. The 1990 Report of the Surgeon General outlines the benefits of smoking cessation. The report concludes that smoking cessation decreases the risk of lung cancer, other cancers, heart attack, stroke, and chronic lung disease. For example, after 10 years of abstinence, the risk of lung cancer is about 30 to 50% of the risk in people who continue to smoke, and after 15 years of abstinence, the risk of CHD is similar to that of persons who have never smoked (DHHS, 1990a).

## CASE 30-2

*Dr. Susan Murphy was invited to speak to a health class of junior high school students. She began by asking the students to recall advertising images from the most familiar cigarette and spitting tobacco brands. The students reported that Latino- and African-American men often smoked menthol brands, such as Newport, Salem, and Kool; several members of a low-riders club used Skoal; and most of the teenage girls who smoked bought Marlboro Lights. The students began to discover the effectiveness of the advertising and marketing efforts of the tobacco companies. Several students mentioned that their parents bought Basic, Doral, or GPC because these were cheaper.*

## WOMEN AND MINORITIES

In 1964, at the time of the first Surgeon General's Report discussing the smoking epidemic, lung cancer was the leading cause of death due to cancer in men and the fifth leading cause of cancer mortality among women (Blum, 1993). This difference in lung cancer mortality between the genders can be explained by the fact that until the 1920s, it was socially unacceptable—and in some states illegal—for women to smoke. Men had taken up cigarette smoking in large numbers toward the end of the nineteenth century—in part because antispitting ordinances to curtail the spread of tuberculosis had led the tobacco companies to switch from the promotion of chewing tobacco and cigars to the inhalation of tobacco smoke by means of the cigarette (Blum, 1993). Smoking did not take hold among women until the American Tobacco Company began a mass media advertising campaign for its Lucky Strike brand with the enticement, "To keep a slender figure, reach for a Lucky instead of a sweet." Cigarette smoking among women rose steadily. In the 1960s the women's liberation movement led cigarette companies to introduce brands such as Virginia Slims, with the slogan, "You've come a long way, baby."

By 1985 more women than men smoked, and lung cancer had surpassed breast cancer as the leading cause of cancer deaths among women. Cigarette smoking leads to other problems for women, especially during pregnancy. There is a confirmed association between maternal smoking and low-birth-weight infants, and there is an increased incidence of premature birth, spontaneous abortion, stillbirth, and neonatal death (Centers for Disease Control and Prevention, 1988; Rakel & Blum, 1995).

African-Americans and Latino-Americans have the highest rates of lung cancer and cardiovascular disease in the United States (DHHS, 1985). The disproportionately high rates of smoking-related diseases among ethnic minorities can be attributed to the successful marketing of tobacco products to minority communities (Blum, 1989). Until their removal in 1998, billboards advertising cigarettes appeared four to five times more often in inner-city neighborhoods than in middle-class suburbs (Scenic America, 1990). Cigarette advertising in black and Hispanic magazines and newspapers continues to represent a major source of revenue for these publications. In more than 40 years of publication, the leading black-oriented magazine, *Ebony*, has carried almost no articles on smoking; not surprisingly, cigarette companies are leading advertisers (Blum, 1989).

The tobacco industry has been especially adept at exploiting racial identity in defining a profitable market among ethnic minorities. R.J. Reynolds Tobacco Company, maker of Salem, More, Camel, and

## WOMEN AND SMOKING

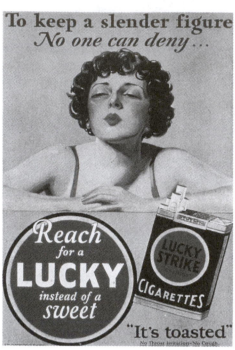

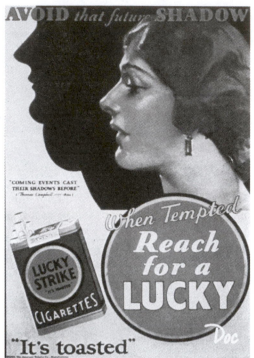

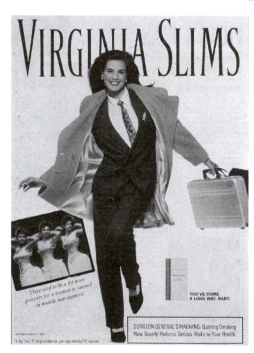

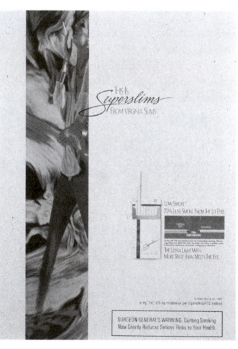

At the turn of the twentieth century, cigarette smoking was socially unacceptable for women. In fact, smoking by women in public places met considerable opposition. In 1904, a policeman in New York City arrested a woman for smoking a cigarette in an automobile, with the admonition, "You can't do that on Fifth Avenue" (Sullivan, 1932). Smoking by female schoolteachers was considered grounds for dismissal (Sobel, 1978). In 1910, Alice

*Longworth, President Roosevelt's daughter, was scolded for smoking in the White House and retorted she would smoke on the roof (Sullivan, 1932). (She later appeared in an advertisement for Lucky Strikes cigarettes).*

*In 1923, only 5% of all cigarettes were consumed by women, increasing to 12% by 1929. The increase in smoking rates among women coincides with the direct appeal to women in cigarette advertising beginning in the mid-1920s. Marlboro cigarettes were first designed as a brand only for women, and were promoted with slogans such as "Mild as May" and "Red Tips for your Pretty Lips."*

*The most renowned advertising campaign of the period directed at women was the association of cigarette smoking with staying slim, launched in 1928 with advertisements carrying the slogan "Reach for a Lucky Instead of a Sweet." To this day, the Lucky Strike campaign is considered one of the greatest successes in advertising history.*

*By the mid-1960s and the launch of Virginia Slims cigarettes, 33% of women in the United States smoked cigarettes. Because of Virginia Slims's perceived popularity (attained through intense advertising and promotion through women's professional tennis tournaments), it is often believed that Virginia Slims is the leading women's cigarette. In fact, women who smoke today buy Marlboro Lights more than any other brand.*

Winston, has sponsored street fairs and fashion shows in Latino- and African-American neighborhoods. Throughout the 1980s Brown and Williamson Tobacco Company, manufacturer of Kool, presented annual Kool Achiever awards to people who improved the "quality of life in inner-city communities." For decades, major African-American and Latino civic organizations, such as the NAACP, the Urban League, the United Negro College Fund, and La Raza, have received funding from tobacco companies.

The result of such successful marketing targeted to ethnic minorities is a higher rate of smoking among African-Americans and an increase in smoking among Hispanic women. Data from the 1998 Surgeon General's Report reveal that 26.5% of African-Americans smoke compared with 25% of the white, non-Hispanic population (CDC, 2000; DHHS, 1998).

## CASE 30-3

*Billy J. is an 8-year-old who presents with a persistent cough. This is his third visit over the past 3 months, during which time he has missed several days of school. The principal has requested a physician's note to explain Billy's absences. Billy's parents are frustrated and believe that Billy is faking or exaggerating his symptoms to avoid school. Neither Billy nor his parents smoke, but the woman who takes care of him after school smokes in her house.*

## INVOLUNTARY OR PASSIVE SMOKING

Billy's parents should be made aware that two-thirds of the smoke from a burning cigarette never reaches the lungs of the person who smokes, but instead goes directly into the air (DHHS, 1986). The 1986 Report of the Surgeon General, dedicated to a discussion of involuntary or passive smoking, defined environmental tobacco smoke (ETS)—also called secondhand smoke—as the combination of sidestream smoke that is emitted into the air from a burning cigarette between puffs and the fraction of mainstream smoke that is exhaled by one who smokes.

The effects of tobacco smoke on nonsmokers can be significant. An estimated 3000 nonsmokers die each year from secondhand smoke (National Institutes of Health, 1993). Fifteen percent of the U.S. public is allergic to cigarette smoke. Numerous studies have explored the health risks of the nonsmoker who is exposed to ETS. The toxic and carcinogenic effects of ETS are similar to those of tobacco smoke inhaled by active smokers. At least 14 studies have demonstrated a risk of lung cancer in nonsmoking wives exposed to the secondhand smoke of their husbands (Rakel & Blum, 1995). Some studies have found that passive smoking increases the risk of leukemia, lymphoma, and cancer of the breast and uterine cervix.

The risks of passive smoking extend beyond cancer. It is estimated that tobacco smoke in the home and workplace could be responsible for the deaths of 46,000 nonsmokers annually in the United States (NIH, 1993). Most of these, 32,000, are the result of heart disease, making passive smoking the third leading preventable cause of death after smoking and the consumption of alcohol.

Parents who smoke are more likely to have children who will smoke. The risk of a child taking up smoking increases with each additional adult family member who smokes (Rakel & Blum, 1995). Over 50% of children under 5 years of age live in homes with at least one adult who smokes. Children of smoking parents are more likely to suffer from otitis media, bronchitis, and pneumonia. Numerous studies have shown that the increased incidence of cough, bronchitis, and pneumonia in children of smoking parents is proportional to the number of cigarettes smoked by the parents, particularly the mother (Rantakallio, 1978). Asthma is also more prevalent, and passive smoking has been linked to some instances of sudden infant death syndrome (Rantakallio, 1978).

## CASE 30-4

*Tim S. is a fourth-year medical student completing a dermatology elective. A patient he has seen for dry skin returned for a follow-up visit to get a renewal on a prescription for a moisturizing lotion. While she is waiting to speak with her physician, Tim recognizes her and asks if she has stopped smoking yet. She replies by saying she really did try, but that the stress at work and home have been unbearable, and she does not want to gain back the weight that she just lost. "I'm not ready to quit," she explains. However, she adds that she switched to a lower-tar brand and now actually smokes more cigarettes per day than ever before. Tim tells her that her smoking may contribute to her skin problem, and that if she doesn't stop she may not see much improvement. Tim tells her that her stress is just an excuse for not quitting, and warns her of the serious danger smoking is to her health.*

## SMOKING CESSATION

Rather than scold his patient for not listening to him previously about the adverse health effects of smoking and the importance of stopping in Case 30-4, Tim should have used this opportunity to serve as a consumer advocate as much as a health nanny. Tim could have helped this patient not by remonstrating, but rather by suggesting that the stress she feels impelling her to light up a cigarette may in large measure reflect her dependence on nicotine and by correcting the myth that smoking low-tar cigarettes is safer.

### Low Tar Means Low Poison

In the 1950s, confronted with declining cigarette sales after the publication of studies linking smoking to lung cancer, tobacco companies began producing filter-tipped brands and claimed that these filters removed certain components of smoke (which manufacturers have never acknowledged to be harmful) (Miller, 1985). Brown and Williamson Tobacco Company purchased advertising space in the Medicine section of Time to claim that Viceroy cigarettes offered "double-barrel health protection," and advertisements for Liggett and Myers's filter L & Ms claimed they were "just what the doctor ordered." Until the 1960s (and until the 1980s in Kentucky) tobacco companies promoted cigarettes at meetings of the American Medical Association and state medical associations by means of scientific exhibits that sought to demonstrate the alleged benefits of one brand over another (Blum, 1992). Consumer demand soared. Currently, 97% of those who smoke buy filtered brands.

In the late 1960s, to allay public anxiety about cancer, tobacco companies began marketing brands with purportedly lower levels of "tar" and nicotine. Throughout the 1970s the American Cancer Society, the National Cancer Institute, and most major health organizations promoted the concept of a safer cigarette in the belief that most people who smoke cannot stop. Persons who switch to allegedly low-tar cigarettes have been found to employ compensatory smoking, whereby they inhale more frequently and more deeply to maintain a satisfying level of nicotine (Miller, 1985; Rickert, 1983). More simply, for the purpose of educating the patient who smokes, "low tar" can be translated as "low poison." Tar is a composite of more than 4000 separate solid poisons, including at least 43 known carcinogens. Cigarettes with reduced yields of tar, nicotine, and carbon monoxide are not safer. A recommendation to switch to such brands is misguided.

## Debunking Common Myths

An important myth surrounding smoking is that it relieves stress. This idea can be debunked by pointing out that the stress that is relieved is that which resulted from being dependent on nicotine—this is the essence of addiction. At the same time, deep breathing has a relaxing effect. The physician can suggest that the patient try to postpone for 5 minutes every time she intends to light up, then breathe slowly and deeply for 5 minutes, then reconsider whether the cigarette is important.

Another myth reinforced in advertisements for Virginia Slims and other cigarettes aimed at women and girls is that smoking keeps weight off. The woman who stops smoking need not gain weight if she relearns the joy of walking and other activities as much as she relearns the taste of food. By no means will all persons who stop smoking gain weight. Even among those who do, the average weight gain is less than 5 pounds (DHHS, 1990a).

Perhaps the biggest myth that has been encouraged in the medical literature is that the patient must be "ready to quit." Although common sense dictates that those who express a greater interest in smoking cessation will have a greater success rate, those patients who do not express an interest in smoking cessation symbolize the overall challenge to be faced in ending the pandemic. Setting a quit date, the essential element of the smoking cessation literature, may rationalize the continuation of an adverse health practice and may strengthen denial. It is helpful to remind patients that they can stop now.

## Consumer Advocacy Role

Traditional office-based approaches begin by asking, "Do you smoke?" "How much do you smoke?" and "When did you start smoking?" Although this may provide the physician with relevant data for charting purposes, this approach is too often a signal for the patient to become defensive and resistant to further discussion, especially if the patient had no intention to stop smoking. There are alternative ways of obtaining information and at the same time piquing the patient's interest in the subject. By using and identifying with the vocabulary used by the consumer of cigarettes, the physician can adopt and be perceived in the role of consumer advocate as opposed to medical finger-wagger. The most important and nonthreatening questions to ask are, "What brand do you buy?" and "How much do you spend on cigarettes?" The patient is likely to be surprised and intrigued by these questions, which can be asked at any time in the course of the interview, because they appear to be nonjudgmental. They suggest that the physician is not a know-it-all and a polemicist. A question about the cost of cigarettes shows concern for the patient's financial well-being.

Promotions for various pharmacologic agents, mail-order gadgets, and clinics in smoking cessation reinforce the notion that cigarette smoking is primarily a medical problem with a simple, easy-to-prescribe, nonindividualized solution. When a patient requests a "drug that will help me stop smoking," the physician must confront the dilemma of not wanting to dash the patient's expectation while emphasizing that a drug or device is, at best, an adjunct and not a means of smoking cessation.

Ironically, as pharmacies in the United States in recent years have become sites for screening of blood pressure, reading of Hemoccult tests, and monitoring of diabetes, cigarettes have become a staple of chain drug stores. Is there any doubt that some patients who smoke rationalize their adverse health behavior by pointing to the sale of cigarettes at the very place where they are directed by physicians to obtain medications (Richards & Blum, 1985)? Although independently owned pharmacies by and large began discontinuing the sale of tobacco products in the late 1970s, more and more of these pharmacies have been acquired by the major chain drug stores, including Eckerd, Walgreens, Rite-Aid, and CVS, all of which prominently display cigarettes at the checkout counter. (Moreover, major supermarkets and discount stores such as Walmart also maintain both pharmacies and tobacco products sections). Thus, incredible as it may seem, the number of pharmacies in the United States that sell cigarettes has actually risen as a result of the concentration of ownership by large chains. In contrast, then, to their staunch support of health fairs and programs to detect and treat hypertension, diabetes, and colon cancer, no retail pharmacy chain has either stopped selling cigarettes or supported paid mass media campaigns to reduce demand for tobacco products. The problem is compounded by the fact that health insurance companies continue to award major employee prescription drug plan contracts to the large chain pharmacies. As a consequence, independent pharmacies cannot compete on price, and many small communities have seen the last local corner pharmacies absorbed by conglomerates.

## Personalize and Individualize

In addition to debunking common myths surrounding smoking, the physician can learn to personalize approaches to smoking cessation by carefully screening the pamphlets and other audiovisual aids available in the office. It is essential to scrutinize all such material, as one would with a new drug or medical device. Personally handing a brochure to a patient while pointing out and underlining certain passages or illustrations will provide an important reinforcing message. Individualizing the message to the patient is the cornerstone of success in patient education. The same cigarette counseling method cannot be used for a high school girl, a construction worker, and an executive already showing signs of heart disease. In the case of a high school girl, the physician should not focus on such abstract concepts as emphysema and lung cancer, but rather emphasize the cosmetic unattractiveness of yellow teeth, bad breath, the loss of athletic ability, and the financial drain that results from buying cigarettes. As for the construction worker, the physician might suggest the likelihood of fewer lost paydays, greater physical strength, and even a lengthier sex life were he to stop smoking cigarettes.

In any event, such dialogue must be practiced over and over again like any medical procedure, and individualized to the patient. The counseling should be designed to call attention not only to the inevitable risks of smoking cigarettes but also to the chemically adulterated tobacco product itself, its inflated price, and the ubiquitous and ludicrous way in which the person's brand is promoted. In effect, the physician can shift the focus away from a resistant or guilt-ridden smoker and onto the product.

### CASE 30-5

*Dan Glatt, a fourth-year medical student and delegate to the American Medical Association's (AMA) Student Section, worked collaboratively with peers and colleagues to submit a resolution in 1992 for the AMA to adopt a policy stating that the AMA would no longer accept financial support from tobacco companies. A separate resolution submitted by another section of the AMA called for the AMA to "discourage all medical schools and their parent universities from accepting research funding from the tobacco industry."*

## TOBACCO USE AND SOCIETY

In 1964, the AMA refused to join other health organizations in immediately endorsing the Surgeon's General's Report on Smoking and Health. Between 1964 and 1978 the AMA accepted upwards of $18 million from the tobacco industry, purportedly to conduct additional research to verify the findings of the Surgeon General's Report.

The ethical issues described in Case 30-5 arose primarily from a $250,000 grant that Fleischmann's Margarine gave the AMA for an anticholesterol campaign. Fleischmann's, at that time, was owned by tobacco giant R.J. Reynolds. Similarly, the AMA received advertising revenue from tobacco company-owned products, such as Philip Morris-owned Kraft and R.J. Reynolds-owned Nabisco, for their cable television ventures. The AMA's Board of Trustees defended their acceptance of money from tobacco company "subsidiaries" by saying that they funded important public health programs.

The proposals by Dan Glatt and his colleagues were referred to the Board of Trustees, as the AMA House of Delegates directed the Board to report back in 6 months with a "definition" of a tobacco company (Wolinsky & Brune, 1995). The resulting definition would thus apply to any AMA policy on nonacceptance of funds from tobacco companies and the AMA's encouragement of medical schools to end their acceptance of research support from the tobacco industry.

These proposals did not represent the first time that the AMA's ties with the tobacco industry were called into question. Nor was it the first time that medical students and residents were the originators of the debate. In 1979 a few resident physicians learned that the AMA's Members Retirement Fund owned $1.4 million in tobacco securities (Blum, 1983b). In 1980, a handful of residents persuaded the AMA Resident Physicians Section to present a resolution to the House of Delegates declaring "the AMA fiduciary responsibility to the public is greater than its fiduciary responsibility to its investment portfolio," and asked for the divestment of the tobacco stock (Wolinsky & Brune, 1995). The AMA Board's finance committee chairman argued that the purpose of the pension fund was to make the biggest buck, not to make social statements. Other AMA officials attempted to minimize the issue by noting that tobacco companies were highly diversified and were involved in nontobacco industries.

The residents' resolution was defeated by the AMA, but after the resulting bad publicity the AMA received in national media for defeating the proposal, the portfolio managers sold the tobacco stock. In 1985, the AMA officially informed its investment brokers that tobacco securities could not be purchased without prior approval by the AMA Board or its finance committee (Wolinsky & Brune, 1995).

Dan Glatt in Case 30-5 and his colleagues in the Medical Student and Resident Physicians Sections of the AMA knew that their resolutions to end financial support of the AMA and medical schools by tobacco companies would not be well received by executives at the AMA, nor by the deans of medical schools and their parent universities. In June 1993, the AMA Board unveiled its definition of the tobacco industry. The AMA defined the tobacco industry as "companies or corporate divisions that directly produce or market tobacco products along with their research and lobbying groups including the Council for Tobacco Research and the Tobacco Institute" (American Medical Association, 1993). The definition continued that "a company or corporate division that does not produce or market tobacco products, but that has a tobacco producing company as or among its owners should not be considered a prohibited part of the tobacco industry." In other words, under the definition the AMA could not deal directly with tobacco companies, but could continue to trade with the companies' subsidiaries so long as they were not involved in the promotion of tobacco products, leaving the ethical question open for further debate.

By the late 1990s, without ever having either acknowledged or apologized for its own role in aiding and abetting the tobacco industry during the crucial years following publication of the Surgeon General's Report, the AMA had positioned itself as a visible player in the public relations campaign against smoking. Its flagship journal published a considerable number of antitobacco articles, and in 2000 the AMA served as a co-host of the 11th World Conference on Tobacco OR Health. Yet in spite of increased awareness on the part of both the medical community and the general public of the devastating health and economic toll taken by the use of tobacco, concerted efforts to curtail demand for these products have been undermined by both direct and covert financial ties between the tobacco industry and respected sectors of society.

In 2000, in the face of a jury's decision that tobacco companies must pay $144.8 billion to Floridians

# WHEN DOCTORS SMOKED

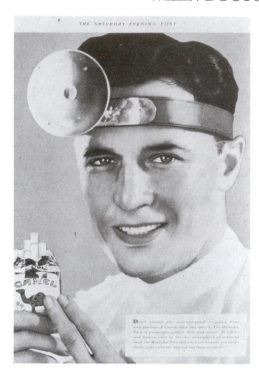

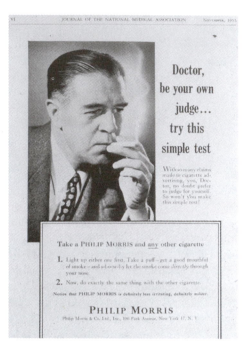

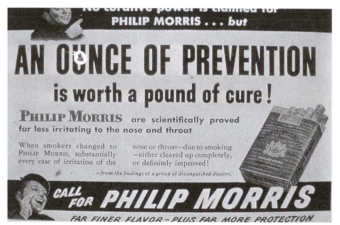

*Even before the first widely publicized scientific reports were published linking smoking to a host of diseases, tobacco companies were using health claims in cigarette advertisements. Lucky Strikes, the top-selling and most advertised brand in the 1930s, used health-oriented slogans like "No throat irritation, No cough," while Old Gold's claimed "Not a Cough in a Carload." A number of such health claims originated in cigarette advertisements in medical journals. Between 1933 and 1954, cigarette advertisements appeared regularly in peer-reviewed medical journals such as JAMA, state medical society journals, and even The Laryngoscope and the Women's Medical Journal. A number of tobacco companies used physicians in their advertisements, such as Philip Morris's "Doctor, be your own judge," which encouraged physicians to try Philip Morris cigarettes and advise their patients to switch to the "less irritating, definitely milder" Philip Morris brand. "More Doctors smoke Camels" was a popular theme for R.J. Reynolds in the 1940s that made its way to the popular press and prime-time radio and television. Beginning in 1942, R.J. Reynolds invited physicians to visit the Camel cigarette exhibit at the convention of the*

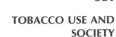

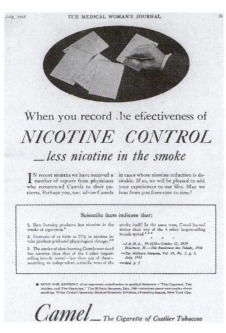
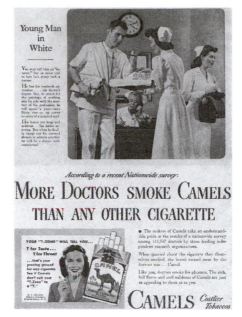

*American Medical Association. More than 40 years after cigarette advertisements disappeared from peer-reviewed medical journals, it seems inconceivable that they ever could have been accepted in the first place. Yet many of the throw-away medical magazines continued to accept cigarette advertising throughout the 1960s and 1970s. At least one magazine,* Physician East, *published in Boston, accepted cigarette advertising as late as 1983 (Blum, 1983a).*

made ill by smoking (the largest punitive damages award in legal history), investment firms attempted to bolster public confidence in the tobacco industry. After predicting solid returns for investors in tobacco, Credit Suisse First Boston underwrote $3 billion in bonds for Philip Morris. *The New York Times*, which proudly proclaimed in 1999 that it would decline cigarette advertisements, joined the television networks and most major newspaper and magazine publishers in continuing to accept advertisements from cigarette manufacturers touting their charitable endeavors. Philip Morris, renamed in the advertisements "the Philip Morris Family of Companies," spent four times the amount of its charitable contributions on promoting its good deeds.

Most glaringly, most pension funds and university endowments continue to invest in tobacco stocks. In 2000, while administering the $22 million Tobacco-Related Diseases Research Program funded by taxes, the Board of Regents of the University of California also oversaw an investment of $55 million in tobacco companies from the university's endowment and pension funds. Ironically, the University has been sued twice by the tobacco industry aimed at derailing academic research into industry activities.

Although in 1999 Yale University joined a handful of other educational institutions in banning the sale of tobacco products on campus, Yale's president stated he did not feel that the University's ongoing investments in tobacco stocks are unethical. Similarly, in the mid-1990s Rice University, among the leaders in academia in tobacco investments, rebuffed a call by 80 alumni to divest its $33 million in tobacco holdings, reasoning that the high stock dividends helped hold down tuition. In 1998 and 1999, Rice earned several hundred thousand dollars for hosting the George Strait Country Music Festival on its campus, two of the most prominent sponsors of which were GPC cigarettes, manufactured by Brown & Williamson Tobacco Company, and Skoal, made by the United States Smokeless Tobacco Company (UST). Free samples of cigarettes and spitting tobacco were distributed at the events, and UST passed out fliers urging voters to turn down all tobacco tax increases. When a lecturer in a premedical course on cancer posed questions about the University's role in aiding the tobacco companies, the president of Rice refused to respond.

One of the most open relationships between an educational institution and the tobacco industry (apart from agricultural colleges working to improve the crop) can be found at Syracuse University, which participates in Philip Morris's Student Ambassador Program. Undergraduates hired by the company for summer internships are paid to promote the image of the company to faculty, administrators, and fellow students. While highlighting the company's charitable endeavors and food product divisions, Philip Morris recruits students at campus job fairs for positions as "Territory Sales Managers," which in reality involve promoting Marlboro at retail outlets. Also at Syracuse, the Louis Bantle Institute, named for a past chairman of UST, has invited leaders of the tobacco industry to speak on campus. It was endowed by an alumnus and trustee who is credited with having popularized smokeless tobacco use throughout the United States by means of clever marketing and having propelled sales into the billions of dollars (personal communication, Leon Blum, 2001).

## CASE 30-6

*Susan Evans, a first-year resident in family medicine, worked as a volunteer of the community-based health charity as part of the requirements for a preventive medicine and health promotion curriculum of her residency program. The organization asked her to help them develop a curriculum for tobacco prevention to be implemented in area schools.*

*Susan began her work by researching resources and other agencies that work on the tobacco issue. In addition to the information she received from traditional voluntary health agencies, primarily restricted to pamphlets about the dangers of smoking, one organization called DOC (Doctors Ought to Care) provided her with materials developed for health professionals to present in the school classroom. To Susan's credit, she did her homework. Rather than try to reinvent the wheel, Susan discovered that much of the initial work and research had already been done, and she simply needed to focus on implementation.*

## MEDICAL ACTIVISM: BEYOND THE EXAMINING ROOM

DOC, the example provided in Case 30-6, was founded in 1977 to educate the public, especially young people, about the major causes of poor health and high medical costs. One of DOC's primary objectives has been to tap the highest possible level of commitment from every health professional to combat the promotion of lethal lifestyles in the mass media. Unfortunately, public health issues and health promotion do not receive the attention they should in medical schools and residency programs. Indeed, within the medical profession, incentives for health promotion have never been strong. Put in these challenging terms, there is understandable discomfort, skepticism, and even resistance by many physicians to health promotion efforts. Many physicians question why the responsibility, or onus, of health promotion should fall to the physician. To the busy practitioner, health promotion does not appear to be time-effective or cost-effective. For these reasons, a more concerted effort is needed to involve medical students, residents, and physicians in health promotion efforts.

To confront the tobacco pandemic, numerous strategies can be implemented in the clinic, classroom, and community (Blum, 1992). Some of the clinical approaches have been described earlier in this chapter. But the messages imparted in the clinic must be reinforced outside the office. To this end, school-based programs must be made more engaging, placing an equal emphasis on what could be called the "three Ps": peer pressure, parental modeling, and propaganda. Too few educational programs in or out of the classroom, especially in primary schools, go beyond scare tactics and cognitive objectives about the dangers of smoking.

## MEDICAL ACTIVISM

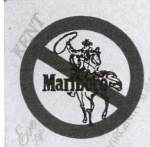

Many of the ads in this magazine are misleading, deceptive and/or a rip off.

For example, smoking does not make one glamorous, macho, successful, or athletic. It does make one sick, poor and dead.

We care about you and your health.

Love,

*Doc*
Doctors Ought to Care

BEND & PEEL THIS STRIP FIRST

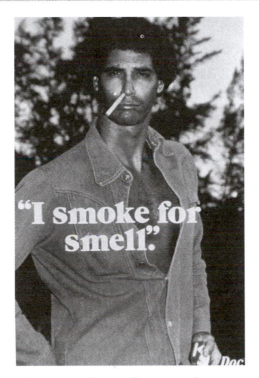

*In any clinical setting, the entire office staff must work to create an environment that encourages nonsmoking behavior. Even before a physician's individual encounter with a patient, steps can be taken to provide positive health messages. As part of the professional office, the reception area automatically grants credibility and implies endorsement to whatever editorial or commercial material it may contain. Indeed,* Time, Newsweek, Sports Illustrated, Better Homes and Garden, Ladies Home Journal, *and* People—*the most frequently purchased magazines for doctors' offices (National Cancer Institute, 1994)— have many advertisements encouraging and glamorizing tobacco use. Healthcare professionals can send a message to patients and publishers alike by canceling subscriptions to these publications and subscribing to publications that do not promote tobacco (NCI, 1994). An alternative technique is to call attention to the harmful and untruthful nature of these advertisements by pasting stickers on them such as the one developed by DOC (Doctors Ought to Care) in the illustration on the left. Other areas of the office, such as restrooms and even the ceilings of examination rooms, can be provided with eye-catching posters that poke fun at tobacco use and its promotion.*

By analyzing and satirizing the promotional techniques of tobacco companies and their media allies, students can delight in turning the tables on the firms that create cigarette advertisements. In studying the long arm of the tobacco industry around the world and making the connection between tobacco advertising and the deaths of family members and friends from tobacco-related diseases, students may learn to redirect their anger from teachers, parents, and health professionals to the authority figures in society who attempt to promote unhealthy products to children.

Physicians and other healthcare professionals can begin their own secondary education in this effort by learning more about the tobacco industry, its products, and the way tobacco is promoted in society. The three essential tools for such research are a map, a calendar, and a camera. With these tools, one can monitor the promotional strategies of the tobacco industry in one's own community and utilize the results as part of a larger school-based or community-based educational effort.

Legislation and policy initiatives, such as a ban on tobacco advertising and promotion, would also be helpful but lack sufficient support from Congress. On the other hand, enforcement by the U.S. attorney general of existing laws that regulate tobacco advertising could be a major step forward. For example, the Public Health Cigarette Smoking Act of 1969, which prohibits the promotion of cigarette brands on television, calls for a $10,000 fine for each violation of the law. If this law could be applied to national telecasts of tobacco-sponsored sporting events, levying fines of up to tens of millions of dollars per event—based on the hundreds of tobacco brand names shown on television during an auto race—neither media corporations nor tobacco companies could afford to continue televising tobacco-sponsored sporting events (Blum, 1991).

Until such action is taken by federal agencies, it is important to counteract such promotions at the community level. By lampooning brand names as part of paid counteradvertising and sponsoring antismoking events, DOC has been instrumental in pointing out the vulnerability of the tobacco industry. From 1978 throughout the 1990s, DOC used its version of the Virginia Slims Tennis Tournament—the Emphysema Slims, with the slogan "You've coughed up long enough, baby"—to counter tobacco sponsorship of sports.

The passage of smoke-free indoor legislation has been the single major advance in the United States in terms of reducing cigarette consumption, thanks to the efforts of nonsmokers' rights groups. In simple terms, when adults learn of policies prohibiting smoking in public places and at work, they don't light up. Among teenagers, preventive measures should focus on demand reduction, encouraging young people not to *buy* these products and to save their money.

There is great need for a no-holds-barred revocabularization, i.e., a new set of terms, images, and other symbols with which to communicate to the public about tobacco products and manufacturers (Blum, 1980). A crucial phase in U.S. public health will be reached when the six major tobacco companies in the United States are recognized as cancer's leading warning signs: Philip Morris (makers of Marlboro and Virginia Slims), RJR/Nabisco (R.J. Reynolds Tobacco Company: Winston, Salem, and Camel), Loews (Newport and Kent), Brown and Williamson (Kool and Carlton), Liggett (generics), and UST (United States Smokeless Tobacco: Skoal and Copenhagen spitting tobaccos). Similarly, the leading preventable cause of death and disease in our society is not lung cancer, heart disease, or emphysema, but rather Marlboro, which is the leading brand among adults and adolescents.

To the physician, hard-hitting satirical counteradvertising that shifts the public focus away from the substance (tobacco, nicotine), the user (smoker), and the effects of the substance (lung cancer) to the manufactured product, the way in which it is promoted, and the promoters may seem overly political and at risk of invoking the wrath of the tobacco industry and its allies. This effect is precisely the intention. Cigarette sales have not been seriously damaged by warnings of the dangers of smoking, because danger has become part of the formula for selling cigarettes, especially to the fearless adolescent. Tobacco companies have blithely responded to thousands of research reports describing the dangers of smoking by funding hundreds more to seek further proof.

A concerted effort that includes physicians, researchers, nurses, dentists, pharmacists, and other health professionals is essential for ending the tobacco pandemic. By better understanding the opposition to this public health tragedy, with the knowledge that complacency plays a major role as a barrier to a well-coordinated effort, health professionals will gain the skills needed to become more effective in their efforts.

By studying and counteracting the tobacco industry like a parasitic disease, health professionals can begin to immunize children and change societal attitudes about smoking through humorous, positive health strategies implemented in the clinic, classroom, and community.

## CASES FOR DISCUSSION

### CASE 1

*A medical student, on completion of an oncology elective, learns that one of the trustees on the board of the major New York City cancer center also serves on the board of Philip Morris, which is also headquartered in New York. The medical student, who has just seen firsthand the toll that tobacco use takes on patients and their families, feels compelled to present this issue to the board of trustees by encouraging a colleague to introduce the problem through a faculty committee.*

1. *Is it a conflict of interest for a trustee of the cancer center to also serve on the board of a tobacco company?*
2. *Is the medical student acting appropriately by calling attention to this issue, or should this be left to those who set policy for the cancer center?*
3. *Should the medical student alert others inside and outside the cancer center to this issue (i.e., the local news media)?*

### CASE 2

*A family physician is approached by one of his patients to speak on her behalf to her employer who permits smoking throughout her worksite. The patient is allergic to tobacco smoke and, when exposed to it for long periods, experiences headaches, sneezing, and itchy, watery eyes.*

1. *Does the physician's obligation for his patient's health and well-being extend to such interventions at the worksite?*
2. *Should the physician risk the alienation of his patient by her employer?*
3. *What information can the physician share with the employer without breaching the trust and confidentiality of his patient?*
4. *How could/should the physician approach his patient's employer?*

### CASE 3

*An otolaryngologist specializing in voice problems is invited to serve as the physician for the Houston Grand Opera. As one who enjoys the performing arts, he feels this is a good opportunity to participate in civic activities and help promote his clinic. The next morning, he reads in a newspaper report that the opera has just received a large grant from the nation's largest tobacco company, Philip Morris, which gives millions each year to support arts groups.*

1. *Should the physician question the support of the opera by the tobacco company?*
2. *Can the physician accept this position and then utilize the position to draw attention to the tobacco company's contribution?*
3. *Should the physician turn down the position?*
4. *Should the American Medical Association urge its members not to serve on the boards of opera companies, museums, and other institutions that accept money from tobacco manufacturers?*

| CASE 4 |
| --- |

*A physician and faculty member at a leading medical school has accepted the position of editor of a peer-reviewed medical journal. In considering manuscripts for an upcoming issue devoted to lung disorders, he is informed by a reviewer that one manuscript was submitted by researchers who formerly received funding from the tobacco industry-supported Council for Tobacco Research.*

1. *Is it appropriate for the editor to question the researchers about their former ties to tobacco money?*
2. *Should the editor reject the manuscript solely based on the source of funding provided for the study?*
3. *Should a pharmaceutical company that manufactures a nicotine replacement product be permitted to underwrite the cost of a special issue of the journal on smoking cessation?*
4. *Should researchers who have accepted funding from the tobacco industry be eligible to receive research grants from the American Legacy Foundation, which was established in 1998 with funds from the national tobacco settlement?*

## RECOMMENDED READINGS

Blum A (ed): *The Cigarette Underworld.* Secaucus, NJ, Lyle Stuart, 1985.

> This book was published as a second printing of the December 1983 issue of the *New York State Journal of Medicine* (Vol. 83, No. 13), the first medical journal ever to devote an entire issue to a consideration of the world tobacco pandemic. Rather than a discussion of the adverse health effects associated with smoking, this book focuses on the social and political history of the leading cause of death in the twentieth century, namely, the tobacco industry.

Smith S, Smith J (eds): *Medical Activism: DOC's Approach to Countering the Tobacco Pandemic.* Houston, Tex, DOC (Doctors Ought to Care), 1992.

> Outlined in this guide is a blueprint for health professionals to become more active in counteracting tobacco use and promotion. Strategies designed for the clinic, classroom, and community are highlighted, and successful examples are shared.

Wolinsky H, Brune T: *The Serpent on the Staff: The Unhealthy Politics of the American Medical Association.* New York, Tarcher/Purman, 1995.

> This book provides an inside look at some of the policies developed within the American Medical Association, whose political intentions often conflict with the organization's stated public health mission.

## REFERENCES

American Medical Association: Report of the Board of Trustees (SS, A-93), presented by Scalettar R. Chicago, American Medical Association, 1993.

Blum A: Medicine vs. Madison Avenue: Fighting smoke with smoke. *JAMA* 243:739–740, 1980.

Blum A: When 'More doctors smoked Camels': Cigarette advertising in the Journal. *NY State J Med,* 83(13):1347–1352, 1983a.

Blum A: The AMA tackles smoking: "A strong stand." *NY State J Med* 83:1363–1365, 1983b.

Blum A: Targeting of minority groups by the tobacco industry, in Jones L (ed): *Minorities and Cancer.* Berlin, Springer-Verlag, 1989, pp 153–162.

Blum A: The Marlboro Grand Prix: Circumvention of the television ad ban on tobacco advertising. *N Engl J Med* 324:913–916, 1991.

Blum A: Role of the health professional in ending the tobacco pandemic: Clinic, classroom, and community. *JNCI* 12:37–43, 1992.

Blum A: Curtailing the tobacco pandemic, in DeVita VT, Hellman S, Rosenberg SA (eds): *Cancer: Principles and Practice of Oncology,* ed 4. Philadelphia, JB Lippincott Co, 1993, pp 480–491.

Blum A, Solberg E: The role of the family physician in ending the tobacco pandemic. *J Fam Pract* 43(6):697–700, 1992.

Centers for Disease Control: Cigarette smoking among adults—United States, 1993. *MMWR* 43(50):925–930, 1994.

Centers for Disease Control: Cigarette smoking among adults—United States, 1998. *MMWR* 49(39):881–884, 2000.

Centers for Disease Control and Prevention (CDC): State-specific estimates of smoking-attributable mortality and years of potential life lost—United States, 1985. *MMWR* 37, 1988.

Department of Health and Human Services, Public Health Service, Centers for Disease Control, Office on Smoking and Health: *The Health Consequences of Smoking: Cardiovascular Disease.* A Report of the Surgeon General. DHHS Publication No. (PHS) 82-50179, 1982.

Department of Health and Human Services. *Report of the Task Force on Black and Minority Health.* Washington, DC, DHHS, 1985.

Department of Health and Human Services, Public Health Service, Centers for Disease Control, Office on Smoking and Health. *The Health Consequences of Involuntary Smoking.* A Report of the Surgeon General. DHHS Publication No. (CDC) 87-8398, 1986.

Department of Health and Human Services, Public Health Service, Centers for Disease Control, Office on Smoking and Health. *Reducing the Health Consequences of Smoking: 25 Years of Progress.* A Report of the Surgeon General. DHHS Publication No. (CDC) 89-8411, 1989.

Department of Health and Human Services, Public Health Service, Centers for Disease Control, Office on Smoking and Health. *The Health Benefits of Smoking Cessation.* A Report of the Surgeon General. DHHS Publication No. (CDC) 90-8416, 1990a.

Department of Health and Human Services, Public Health Service, National Institutes of Health, National Cancer Institute. *Smoking Tobacco and Cancer Programs: 1985–1989 Status Report.* NIH Publication No. 90-3107, 1990b.

Department of Health and Human Services. *Tobacco Use Among U.S. Racial/Ethnic Minority Groups—African Americans, American Indians and Alaska Natives, Asian Americans and Pacific Islanders, and Hispanics.* A Report of the Surgeon General. Department of Health and Human Services, Centers for Disease Control and Prevention, National Center for Chronic Disease Prevention and Health Promotion, Office on Smoking and Health, 1998.

Department of Health and Human Services: *Reducing Tobacco Use.* A Report of the Surgeon General. Department of Health and Human Services, Centers for Disease Control and Prevention, National Center for Chronic Disease Prevention and Health Promotion, Office on Smoking and Health, 2000.

Doll R, Hill AB: Lung cancer and other causes of death in relation to smoking: Second report on mortality of British doctors. *Br Med J* 2:1071–1081, 1956.

Federal Trade Commission: *Federal Trade Commission Report to Congress for 1998 Pursuant to the Federal Cigarette Labeling and Advertising Act,* 2000.

Hammond EL, Horn D: Smoking and death rates—Report on forty-four months of follow-up of 187,783 men. *JAMA* 166:1294–1308, 1958.

Lombard HL, Doering CR: Cancer studies in Massachusetts: Habits, characteristics, and environment of individuals with and without cancer. *N Engl J Med* 198:481–487, 1928.

McGinnis JM, Foege WH: Actual causes of death in the United States. *JAMA* 270:2207, 1993.

Miller GH: The "less hazardous" cigarette: A deadly delusion. *NY State J Med* 85:313–317, 1985.

National Cancer Institute: Tobacco and the Clinician: Interventions for Medical and Dental Practice. Smoking and Tobacco Control Monograph No. 5. Bethesda, Md, U.S. Department of Health and Human Services, National Institutes of Health, National Cancer Institute, 1994; pp 38–39.

National Institutes of Health: *Respiratory Health Effects of Passive Smoking: Lung Cancer and Other Disorders.* The Report of the U.S. Environmental Protection Agency. Department of Health and Human Services, Public Health Service, National Institutes of Health, Environmental Protection Agency. HIN Publication No. 93-3605, 1993.

Ochsner A, DeBakey ME: Primary pulmonary malignancy: Treatment by total pneumonectomy. Analysis of 79 collected cases and presentation of 7 personal cases. *Surg Gynecol Obstet* 68:435–441, 1939.

Pearl R: Tobacco smoking and longevity. *Science* 87:216–217, 1938.

Pierce P, Fiore MC, Novotny TE, *et al*: Trends in cigarette smoking in the United States. *JAMA* 261:61, 1989.

Pollin W, Ravenholt RT: Tobacco addiction and tobacco mortality. *JAMA* 252:2849, 1984.

Rakel RE, Blum A: Nicotine addiction, in Rakel RE (ed): *Textbook of Family Practice,* ed 5. Philadelphia, WB Saunders Co, 1995, pp 1549–1564.

Rantakallio P: Relationship of maternal smoking to morbidity and mortality of the child up to age five. *Acta Paediatr Scand* 67:621–629, 1978.

Richards JW, Blum A: Pharmacists who disperse cigarettes. *NY State J Med* 85:350–353, 1985.

Rickert WS: "Less hazardous" cigarettes: Fact or fiction? *NY State J Med* 83:1269–1272, 1983.

Scenic America: *Citizens Action Handbook on Tobacco and Alcohol Billboard Advertising.* Washington, DC, Scenic America, 1990.

Sobel R: *They Satisfy: The Cigarette in American Life,* New York, Anchor Press/Doubleday, 1978.

Sullivan M: *Our Times: The United States 1900–1925,* vol 4. New York, Charles Scribner's Sons, 1932.

Wolf PA, D'Agostino RB, Sannel WB, *et al*: Cigarette smoking as a risk factor for stroke: The Framingham Study. *JAMA* 259:1025–1029, 1988.

Wolinsky H, Brune T: *The Serpent on the Staff: The Unhealthy Politics of the American Medical Association.* New York, Tarcher/Purman, 1995.

## CHAPTER 31

# Alcohol and Drug Abuse

*Kristen Lawton Barry*

## CASE 31-1

*Frank Jones is a 38-year-old married auto mechanic who came to see Dr. Smith today for a follow-up visit to assess his hypertension. Dr. Smith has been working with Mr. Jones for 1 year and his hypertension has remained labile despite varying medication regimes. At this visit, Mr. Jones mentioned that he has also had pains in his stomach for the last month and attributed it to arguments with his wife. When asked, he said that he doesn't drink much—just a few beers a day.*

## EDUCATIONAL OBJECTIVES

1. Feel more comfortable treating patients with alcohol and drug problems
2. Understand techniques for prevention, intervention, and referral
3. Recognize low-risk use, at-risk use, problem use, and alcohol/drug dependence, and the interventions appropriate to each
4. Understand variables in treating special populations such as adolescents and elderly
5. Understand the importance of physician attitudes in working with patients regarding alcohol and drug problems
6. Know specific strategies that can be used in a busy practice to screen, assess, intervene, and refer patients with problems related to alcohol/drug use

## INTRODUCTION

Alcohol and drug disorders are among the most common medical problems primary care physicians encounter in their practices (Brown, 1992). Like Mr. Jones in Case 31-1, many other patients present us with opportunities to intervene before alcohol and drug problems have advanced to the most serious consequences. Consensus statements recommend that primary care physicians routinely screen all patients for substance use disorders, including adolescents and older patients (American Society of Addiction Medicine, 1997; Institute of Medicine, 1997; US Preventive Services Task Force, 1996).

Unfortunately, working with patients around issues of alcohol and drug abuse is commonly perceived as a "can of worms" best left unopened. The fear is that once the worms are wriggling all over the office, it's difficult to get them back in the can, especially during a standard 15- to 30-minute office visit. The purpose of this chapter is to help students overcome these fears by providing them with time-efficient techniques for screening, assessing, intervening, and referring patients with alcohol and drug problems.

---

# PREVALENCE

## Definitions and Terms

The terms presented in this chapter are derived from both the clinical and research expertise of professionals in the field of addiction medicine (Fleming & Barry, 1992). The term *addictive disorders* includes the clinical problems of alcohol and drug dependence as well as other disorders that have often been classified as addictions, such as eating and gambling disorders. *Alcohol or drug disorder* is often used to describe the spectrum of problems associated with the negative consequences of mood-altering drugs. *Substance abuse* and *substance dependence* (alcohol or drug dependence) are terms based on standardized alcohol and drug criteria such as those from the fourth edition of the *Diagnostic and Statistical Manual of Mental Disorders* (DSM-IV) (American Psychiatric Association, 1994). These terms are often used for insurance reimbursement and are generally accepted by the medical community.

To diagnose alcohol and drug disorders, clinicians look for behavioral factors such as the inability to cut down or stop, social and emotional consequences such as family problems or work and school problems, and physiological symptoms such as insomnia, gastrointestinal pain, liver toxicity, tolerance (over time it takes more of the substance to feel an effect), and withdrawal. One of the limitations in the alcohol and drug field is that, unlike many other medical problems, there are no laboratory tests to make a definitive diagnosis of alcohol or drug abuse or dependence. Liver function and other laboratory tests detect end organ damage but do not detect the primary disorder. Although a number of alcohol marker indicators are potential diagnostic tools for detection of alcohol abuse or dependence, the performance of all tests is too low to be useful for screening procedures in a general population (Meerkerk *et al.*, 1999; Sillanaukee *et al.*, 1998; for further discussion see below). Numerous studies indicate that increased alcohol consumption is related to increased health risk for mortality as well as a host of serious illnesses, including various cancers, cardiovascular disease, and cirrhosis.

Psychoactive drugs may be sanctioned medically to modify or control moods. However, any use of a psychoactive substance to change the state of mind that is harmful to oneself or others is considered abuse. *Abuse* and *dependence* pertain to both alcohol and drugs. Definitions regarding low-risk, at-risk, and problem use focus primarily, but not exclusively, on alcohol.

---

## CASE 31-2

*Josh Sanderson is a 28-year-old married car salesman with two small children and no family history of alcohol-related problems. He got drunk a few times in college but did not like the aftereffect. Since he married and had children, most of his activities have centered around his family and other friends with small children. Alcohol is not often a part of family activities. Mr. Jones generally drinks one or two beers twice a week.*

## Low-Risk Use

Psychoactive substance use as in Case 31-2 that does not lead to problems is called low-risk use. Persons in this category can set reasonable limits on alcohol consumption and do not drink when pregnant or trying to conceive, driving a car or boat, operating heavy machinery, or using contraindicated medications. They do not engage in binge drinking—more than 2 or 4 drinks per occasion for women and men, respectively—or in excessive regular drinking—more than 7 drinks a week for women or 14 drinks a week for men (NIAAA Guide, 1995). An example of low-risk use of medications/drugs would be taking a prescribed antianxiety drug for an acute anxiety state following the physician's prescription (Trachtenberg & Fleming, 1994).

---

### CASE 31-3

*Maria Adelman is a 26-year-old single graduate student who drinks three or four beers two or three times a week, mostly on the weekends. She smokes marijuana about once a month when she gets together with an old friend from college. She has no family history of alcoholism. She usually drives home after drinking with friends but has had no accidents. She reports that she does not always practice safe sex when she has been drinking but has no other consequences of alcohol or drug use.*

## At-Risk Use

*At-risk use* is use that increases the chances that a person will develop problems and complications related to the use of alcohol as in Case 31-3. These individuals will consume more than 7 or 14 drinks per week for women and men, respectively, or they will drink in risky situations. They do not currently have a health problem caused by alcohol, but if this drinking pattern continues over time problems might result.

---

### CASE 31-4

*Mark Lorenzo is a 51-year-old executive with a large marketing firm. He has had an alcohol and tobacco problem for many years resulting in abdominal pain, hypertension, and one auto accident while driving under the influence. He stopped using both substances 3 years ago after much discussion with his physician, family, and employer who explained the risks to his health, family life, and career. He reported that the major problems associated with his alcohol use were continuing. Once he made up his mind to stop, he did so without withdrawal symptoms and has remained abstinent for 3 years.*

## Problem Use

*Problem use* refers to a level of use that has already resulted in adverse medical, psychological, or social consequences as in Case 31-4. Potential consequences include accidents and injuries, legal problems, and sexual behavior that increases the risk of HIV infection. Although most problem drinkers consume more than the low-risk limits, some people who drink smaller amounts may experience alcohol-related problems, such as the elderly and persons with severe medical or psychiatric problems.

---

### CASE 31-5

*Karen Crawford is a 36-year-old single physician who was discovered using intravenous fentanyl while on call in the second year of her residency. She said she was only experimenting. Although she used alcohol and marijuana in college, she reported no blackouts and said she was always able to control her use. Both her family and the residency director intervened with her and she entered an intensive inpatient treatment program. The urine drug screen taken when she entered treatment revealed she had also been using cocaine and marijuana. After she completed the treatment program, her urine drug screens were negative and she remained abstinent at 6-year follow-up.*

## CASE 31-6

*Samuel Jackson is a 52-year-old construction worker. He has had chronic abdominal pain and unresolved hypertension for the past 8 years. Two years ago, after experiencing withdrawal symptoms during a hospital admission for a work-related injury, he entered an alcohol treatment program. After 1 year of abstinence, Mr. Jackson began drinking again. He now drinks approximately eight beers a day plus some additional liquor once a week. His physician is aware that this is a chronic relapsing disorder and continues to work with Mr. Jackson to help him stabilize his medical conditions and find longer-term help for his primary alcohol dependence.*

## Drug and Alcohol Dependence

As Cases 31-5 and 31-6 indicate, those patients who use at the level of *alcohol or drug dependence* have a medical disorder characterized by loss of control and preoccupation with alcohol or drugs. They continue to use despite adverse consequences and suffer physiological symptoms such as tolerance and withdrawal (American Psychiatric Association, 1994). A wide range of legal and illegal substances can be addictive.

## CASE 31-7

*Kathryn Sampson is a 65-year-old widow living alone in an apartment in a housing project. She broke her ankle a month ago and has been cared for since then by a visiting nurse. She came to the clinic for routine follow-up for her ankle. When asked by the physician to talk about how the accident happened, she was evasive. The physician then asked some questions about her general health and Mrs. Sampson reported, "I'm so tired all the time and I don't sleep well. I must need stronger sleeping pills. I've been taking the kind I can buy myself in the drugstore. I've been taking that medicine [Zantac] for my stomach, but things don't seem much better." Because the effect of alcohol is exacerbated by age, Zantac, and over-the-counter sleeping pills, her physician discussed with her these risks and her desire to remain as independent as possible. She reported drinking one glass of wine a day before dinner just as she and her husband did when they were younger. The physician encouraged her to work with the community services available to find outside activities and to stop the use of alcohol. She felt that she would be able to follow her physician's recommendations.*

## Special Population: Older Adults

The elderly pose special concerns when setting drinking and medication use criteria. Compared with younger people, older adults have an increased sensitivity to alcohol and over-the-counter and prescription medications. There is an age-related decrease in lean body mass versus total volume of fat, and the resultant decrease in total body volume increases the total distribution of alcohol and other mood-altering chemicals in the body. Liver enzymes that metabolize alcohol and certain other drugs are less efficient with age and central nervous system sensitivity increases with age. Of particular concern in this age group is the potential interaction of medication and alcohol. For some patients, any alcohol use, coupled with the use of specific over-the-counter or prescription medications, can be problematic as in Case 31-7.

Primary care physicians often may "underdetect" alcohol use disorders among older patients (Reid *et al.*, 1998). In contrast to most studies of the general population, surveys conducted in healthcare settings have found increasing prevalence of alcoholism among the older population (Adams, 1997). A recent study found that the incidence of current alcohol abuse or dependence in patients aged 60 or older treated in primary care settings was 2.3% (Lyness *et al.*, 1999). Intervention with this population has promising potential, as elderly persons with alcohol problems are at least as likely as younger persons to benefit from alcoholism treatment (National Institute on Alcohol Abuse and Alcoholism, 1998). Because of age-related body changes in both men and women, the National Institute on Alcohol Abuse and Alcoholism recommends that persons older than 65 consume no more than one drink per day (Dufour *et al.*, 1992). With some patients, such as Mrs. Sampson, even this may be too much.

---

### CASE 31-8

*Gregg Herberger is a 16-year-old high school student who lives with his father, mother, and older sister in a midsized city in the Midwest. He is on the basketball and baseball teams at his school and has been a B student. In the past 6 months, his grades have deteriorated and his principal has called about his belligerent behavior toward a teacher. He spends most evenings home alone in his room, seldom eats dinner with the family anymore, and his mother found a half-empty bottle of alcohol and some marijuana in his room. He recently broke up with his girlfriend and hangs out with new friends unknown to his family. His parents tried grounding him but he threatened to move out. As part of a sports physical for basketball season, his physician asked him how things were going at school and at home. Gregg said that everyone was hassling him, that he had some bad teachers, and that his folks were really difficult, "par for the course." The physician provider empathized with Gregg and asked him about health behaviors such as nutrition, exercise, seat belts, safe sex, smoking, and alcohol use. Gregg said that he mostly drank on weekends, "like everyone else," and that his parents were "on my back about it." He denied drug use. The physician discussed with Gregg the possible relationship between the alcohol use and problems at home and school. She made a follow-up appointment to review test results and explained that they would talk more about alcohol use at that time. She made an agreement with Gregg not to drink and drive before the next office visit. At the follow-up visit the physician referred Gregg for an alcohol and drug assessment, as well as an assessment of his potential depression. Gregg met for four sessions with a psychotherapist, cut back to two beers on the weekend, did not drink and drive, and stopped the use of any illicit drugs.*

## Special Population: Adolescents

As Case 31-8 illustrates, children and teens are especially susceptible to influences that encourage risk-taking and experimentation with substances. The age at which adolescents begin to use alcohol and illicit drugs, particularly if it is before the age of 15, is a strong predictor of later problems with substances (Institute for Health Policy, 1993). The incidence of binge drinking five or more drinks in a row for teens was at an all-time high of 41% in the early 1980s and decreased to 29.8% in 1995. Thirteen- to fifteen-year-olds are at high risk to begin drinking (Johnston *et al.*, 1995). According to results of an annual survey of students in grades, 8, 10, and 12, 26% of 8th graders, 40% of 10th graders, and 51% of 12th graders reported drinking alcohol within the past month (University of Michigan, 1996).

Risk factors for adolescent alcohol use, abuse, and dependence include genetic risk factors (parental alcoholism), biological markers (a low P300 amplitude), childhood aggressiveness or antisocial behavior, psychiatric disorders (such as conduct disorder, attention deficit hyperactivity disorder, anxiety disorder, major depressive disorder), suicidal behavior, and a host of psychosocial risk factors, including parenting, family environment, peer influences, positive expectancies regarding drinking, child abuse, and other traumas, and alcohol advertising. Health consequences of adolescent alcohol use include increased automobile crash risk due to drinking and driving, risky sexual behavior and increased vulnerability to coercive sexual activity, risky behavior and victimization, possible risk of delayed puberty and slowed bone growth, and risk of the development of alcohol abuse and alcohol dependence (National Institute on Alcohol Abuse and Alcoholism, 1997).

Alcohol and tobacco are often referred to as "gateway" drugs because teens who progress to substance abuse often start with these two drugs. Statistics indicate that those who use tobacco are at risk for other substance use: most teenagers who smoke cigarettes have also used an illegal drug. Two-thirds of tobacco smokers aged 12 to 17 have also used an illegal drug (Morrison, 1990). Although there was a downward trend in the use of illicit drugs by teens in the late 1980s and early 1990s, use increased significantly between 1992 and 1993, and the trend continued through 1995 (Brasseux *et al.*, 1998). At that time the lifetime incidence of any illicit drug use was 42.9% while the incidence in the year before sampling was 31% (*HHS News*, January 31, 1994). A community sample of adolescents (mean age 15.7 years) in Quebec, Canada, reported almost one-third had used illegal drugs more than five times. Of this group, more than 70% reported going to school high on drugs, and the majority reported playing sports while high and using drugs (Zoccolillo *et al.*, 1999).

From a clinical perspective, it is important to ask all adolescents about tobacco, alcohol, and other drug use. An effective technique is to begin by asking about use at their school and friends' use as lead-ins to questions about their own behavior. Sports physicals are also a good time to address these issues.

## National Prevalence Data

Alcohol dependence and abuse are current problems for nearly 10% of the U.S. population (Kessler *et al.*, 1994). Recent research reports 14 million Americans are dependent on alcohol; another 14 million Americans use illicit drugs (McGinnis & Foege, 1999). More than 20% of adults in primary care settings have a past or current substance use disorder, and many physicians are unaware of their patients' substance use histories (Buchsbaum *et al.*, 1995; Robins *et al.*, 1984).

Prevalence in the United States is often measured through national telephone surveys, face-to-face large-scale clinical surveys, and tax receipts. Figure 31.1 plots data collected from 1979 to 1998 on trends in alcohol, tobacco, cocaine, amphetamine, and marijuana use in a series of annual telephone surveys based on national probability samples. The data presented only include subjects between 18 and 25 years old, but changes in other age groups reflect similar trends.

The Epidemiological Catchment Area (ECA) Study (Regier & Robins, 1991) is a landmark study conducted in five sites in the 1980s. It used face-to-face interviews based on DSM-III criteria for substance abuse or dependence. In this community-based sample of 20,291 adults, approximately 16.7% of the persons sampled had a lifetime substance abuse disorder, 6.1% had problems in the previous 6 months, and 3.8% reported problems in the last month. More recently, in a large multistage study with a sample size of 42,861 U.S. respondents aged 18 or older, Grant and colleagues reported a combined incidence of alcohol abuse or alcohol dependence (DSM-IV definitions) of 7.4% (Grant *et al.*, 1994).

National data on alcohol use are based on tax receipt reports to calculate per capita consumption. "Apparent per capita consumption" is determined by dividing alcohol sales data (or shipment data) from every state and the District of Columbia by the U.S. population aged 14 and older (Williams *et al.*, 1994). These estimates attribute average consumption to all members of the population; they do not consider actual individual consumption. Per capita consumption is measured in gallons of pure alcohol. Historically, following a period of stable alcohol use from 1947 to 1961, alcohol use steadily increased from the early 1960s,

*One out of every five adult patients in a primary care clinic has or has had a substance abuse problem. Oftentimes, their physician doesn't have a clue. (Sources: Buchsbaum et al., 1995; Robins et al., 1984)*

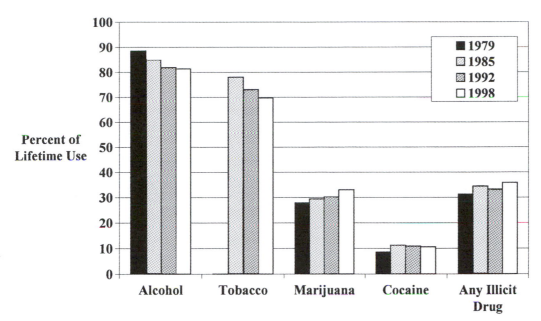

**FIGURE 31-1.** Percentages reporting lifetime use of alcohol, tobacco, and illicit drugs in the U.S. population aged 12 and older, 1979–1998.

reached a peak in 1980 and 1981, and subsequently began to decline. The 1993 per capita alcohol consumption level was down to its lowest level since 1964, at 2.25 gallons of pure alcohol per person (Williams *et al.*, 1995). This translates to approximately 541 twelve-ounce cans of beer per adult American per year or 1.48 cans/day (a standard 12-ounce light beer has approximately 96 calories, a standard regular beer approximately 156 calories). The number of abstainers has increased slightly. The Behavioral Risk Factors Study (BRFS), which is conducted in most states in coordination with the Centers for Disease Control, is used to obtain data on abstinence by state. In this survey, people aged 18 and over are asked to report alcohol consumption in the last month. The District of Columbia, Alaska, and Wisconsin have the highest rates of per capita consumption (3.28, 4.23, and 2.97 gallons, respectively), while Wisconsin has the lowest percentage of abstainers (30.1%).

## Primary Care Incidence Data

Studies that address the prevalence of alcohol and drug problems in primary care practices are important because they provide an estimate of the extent of these problems. Incidence estimates in primary care range from 4 to 29% for hazardous or at-risk drinking and from less than 1 to 10% for harmful or problem drinking (Reid *et al.*, 1999). Further, patients with alcohol involvement are typically overrepresented in primary care settings (Searight, 1992).

Using methods similar to those used in the ECA Study, Fleming and Barry (1991) estimated lifetime and 12-month incidence of alcohol and drug disorders in five family medicine clinics in three counties in Wisconsin in 1988. Lifetime incidence ranged from 16 to 28% in the five clinics. The 12-month incidence ranged from 9 to 15%. The lifetime incidence of drug disorders was 7 to 9%. Three percent of the sample had drug problems in the previous year. Although the 12-month incidence of alcohol disorders is high, there is an even larger group of patients in primary care practices who are problem drinkers. As part of a large clinical

*The average adult American consumes each year the amount of alcohol found in 541 cans of beer. (Source: Williams et al., 1995)*

trial testing the effectiveness of brief physician advice with problem drinkers, Fleming *et al.* (1997) screened approximately 20,000 adults in primary care practices in Wisconsin. Findings from the survey indicated that the incidence of problem drinking is age dependent and ranges from 15 to 20% for men and from 8 to 10% for women. Approximately one-fifth of the men had more than 15 drinks a week and one in eight had 3 or more drinks a day. Women engaged in problem drinking less often than men.

Clinicians who are finding fewer cases of problem drinking and alcohol or drug disorders in their own practices may want to begin screening programs. Because patients with a previous history of problems with alcohol or other drugs are at risk for relapse, establishing a history of use can provide important clues for future problems. A majority of patients with a history of alcohol abuse or other drug problems seen in the primary care setting are in recovery (O'Connor & Samet, 1996; Samet *et al.*, 1995). Working within a supportive patient–physician relationship, the primary care physician can help recovering patients decrease their susceptibility to relapse, recognize and manage high-risk situations, and find and utilize available resources (Friedmann *et al.*, 1998).

## CASE 31-9

*Carlotta Brown is a 26-year-old woman who grew up in the inner city of a large metropolitan area. She has a 2-year-old son and is living with her mother. She has been unable to work and is insured by Medicaid. Ms. Brown was in the emergency department last night reporting chronic headaches and fatigue and asking for some pain medication for her headaches. She was given a prescription for one night and told to visit her regular physician, Dr. Jones, today. He knows that she is under a lot of stress but is unsure if she is drug seeking and suggests some alternatives to medications. Further probing about her current use of drugs and alcohol angers her. As she leaves she states that Dr. Jones is "just like those other doctors who think I'm an addict and don't care if I hurt."*

## CASE 31-10

*Jane Morrow is a 46-year-old housewife married to an insurance executive in the community. She has two children, both boys, who are 20 and 18. She has been a patient in this particular practice for 10 years. She comes to the clinic today with abdominal pain and headaches. She has been taking Fiorinal for headaches during the last year. When asked about any stress or changes in her life she mentioned that her sons were both off at school and her husband was so busy that she felt very lonely. Mrs. Morrow said, however, that her bridge club and other groups help her to forget some of her loneliness and that they all take turns finding exotic food and drinks to serve. She is a well-known hostess and active volunteer in civic causes.*

## Physician Attitudes

Ramsey *et al.* (1998) found that physicians asked 60% of their patients about alcohol use (range 6% to 94%) and screened 41% of patients about noninjection recreational drugs (range 0% to 100%). Implementing practice procedures to detect alcohol and drug disorders can be hampered not only by a variety of institutional factors, such as including screening administration and lack of standardized follow-up procedures, but also by the attitudes of physicians and staff.

Societal stereotypes about people who have alcohol and drug problems can be misleading since alcohol and drug problems are shared by every class, race, and religion. For example, a study in primary care practices found that male patients were 1.5 times as likely to have been warned about alcohol and three times as likely to have been told to stop or modify their consumption compared with female patients. Patients with lower educational attainment were more likely to have been warned, while the likelihood of ever being told to stop or modify consumption increased with age (Volk *et al.*, 1996). A number of factors in addition to basic societal stereotypes affect clinician attitudes about substance abuse. All of these factors can, in turn, affect the quality of care provided to patients with alcohol and drug disorders. The failure to diagnose and treat alcohol and drug disorders may result from inadequate training, a sense of futility about the effectiveness of treatment, and denial stemming from the physician's own family history (Waller & Casey, 1990).

Until the last decade medical schools and residencies devoted little curriculum time to issues of substance abuse. In a review of changes in medical education about substance abuse in six clinical departments (psychiatry, family medicine, internal medicine, pediatrics, emergency medicine, and obstetrics-gynecology) in the 126 U.S. medical schools from 1976 to 1992, Fleming *et al.* (1994) found significant increases in the numbers of required and elective curriculum units for medical students between 1986–1987 and 1991–1992. The number of medical schools requiring courses in substance abuse treatment increased from 5 to 8. The number of curriculum units for residents in family medicine and pediatrics increased significantly. Almost every medical school (116) reported curricular units on substance abuse for medical students or residents, and for these schools the average number of faculty specializing in addictions was 4.1. There were 45 fellowships in addiction medicine identified in 1991–1992, with a total of 61 fellows in training. While these findings confirm positive changes, 118 of 126 programs still do not require such courses for medical students. Curriculum time and number of faculty with expertise in this field does not compare well with other areas with similar prevalence, such as cancer and heart disease. Training for primary care physicians in the recognition, diagnosis, treatment, and referral of alcohol and other drug problems still remains a concern.

The sense of futility physicians sometimes feel in the treatment of alcohol and drug problems often begins early in medical school. Rotations on medical services and in the emergency department often expose students to patients suffering from severe complications of alcohol and drug disorders. Students seldom work with patients at earlier stages of the problem when brief interventions are most effective and the results of the professional's efforts are more readily apparent. Medical students are more likely to see drug-seeking patients such as Carlotta Brown (Case 31-9) on rotations in the emergency department than they are to see patients like Jane Morrow (Case 31-10) whose symptoms are less apparent in part because we are less likely to look for symptoms in patients who have better coping skills and support systems in the community.

In addition, in inpatient and emergency situations, students seldom have the opportunity for longer-term follow-up that would allow them to see the positive results of their efforts. Classes and clinical rotations with primary care physicians who understand addictions are beginning to provide learners with a more balanced picture of these disorders and will hopefully change attitudes and behaviors in the process. Recent research indicates that physicians who have a special interest and some experience with addictions regard patients with a substance abuse diagnosis as much less difficult to manage than do their colleagues with less interest and training (Farrell & Lewis, 1990). Training in a brief intervention protocol, cues to counsel high-risk drinking patients, and support by a primary care office system have also been shown to help physicians and other healthcare providers address alcohol use with their patients (Adams *et al.*, 1998).

Many of the newer innovative programs designed to teach medical students, residents, and practicing physicians about alcohol and other drug disorders work not only to change attitudes but also to change behaviors. Research has indicated that a change in attitude toward the treatment of alcohol and drug disorders does *not* necessarily lead to a change in actual practice behavior. Useful practice experiences seem to have the greatest impact on future behavior. Practice experience can come through working with primary physicians with alcohol and other drug abuse expertise, attending open Alcoholics Anonymous meetings and talking to members, spending time at a treatment center, and role-playing situations with patients when alcohol and drug questions need to be addressed. Finally, a personal or family history of alcohol or drug problems can affect a physician's ability to adequately treat patients with symptoms of these disorders. With the increasing national awareness of the effects of alcohol and drug problems, medical schools are beginning to institute student assistance programs to help medical students deal with personal concerns that have an impact on their education and future careers. An awareness of the impact that alcohol and drugs have had in any of our lives is the first step toward confronting the issues from both a personal and a professional perspective.

*Larry Simmons is a 45-year-old marketing analyst who lost his job 5 months ago during corporate layoffs. He has been treated by Dr. Adams for the last 8 years. Dr. Adams has worked with him in the past to cut back or stop his use of alcohol but he continues to have six or seven mixed drinks a day during the week with more on weekends. He has a history of chronic hypertension and has been unable to stop smoking. Mr. Simmons was recently hospitalized for acute pancreatitis related to his alcohol use. While in the hospital he was referred to an alcohol and drug program for evaluation. Dr. Adams is continuing to help him stabilize his medical conditions and is working with the alcohol and drug program to help him obtain longer-term help for his primary alcohol and nicotine dependence.*

# MORBIDITY AND MORTALITY

Excessive alcohol consumption and drug use can affect every organ system in the body depending on the individual's genetic predisposition and the amount, length, and pattern of use. Alcohol and drug use are a significant cause of mortality and morbidity in the United States (McGinnis & Foege, 1999). The presence of other diseases is also a cofactor that can increase risk. Alcohol is a risk factor for coronary heart disease, cancers, and overall mortality. Prolonged consumption of large amounts of alcohol is known to lead to addiction, fatal and nonfatal injuries, and several chronic diseases (Haapanen-Niemi *et al.*, 1999). Abstainers have modestly higher mortality than moderate drinkers but considerably lower mortality than heavy drinkers. The lowest risk of death seems to be at the average intake level of one drink per day (Poikolainen, 1995). Causes of death associated with drinking are cirrhosis and alcoholism; cancers of the mouth, esophagus, pharynx, larynx, and liver combined; breast cancer in women; and injuries and other external causes in men (Thun *et al.*, 1997). Alcohol is involved in an estimated 44% of the 45,000 annual traffic fatalities in the United States (National Highway Traffic Safety Administration, 1994).

In 1992, HIV infection became the number one cause of death among men aged 25–44 years (Centers for Disease Control, 1993). Morbidity and mortality reports regarding illicit drugs often do not include HIV/AIDS statistics for intravenous drug users. Death rates almost double when this group is included in the analysis.

This section will briefly review the most salient findings regarding alcohol and drugs and health risk. For more complete reviews, see Anderson *et al.* (1993) and the Ninth Special Report to the U.S. Congress on Alcohol and Health (NIAAA, 1997).

## Alcohol-Induced Liver Disease

Alcohol-induced liver disease is a major cause of illness and death in the United States. Approximately 10 to 35% of heavy drinkers develop alcoholic hepatitis and 10 to 20% develop cirrhosis, with limited treatment options and often fatal outcomes (NIAAA, 1993). Between 10,000 and 24,000 deaths from cirrhosis are attributable to alcohol consumption each year (DeBakey *et al.*, 1996). Past and current alcohol drinking are strongly related to cirrhosis risk (Klatsky & Armstrong, 1992). In the past alcohol-induced liver cirrhosis was thought to come from nutritional deficiencies common in heavy drinkers, but now the evidence suggests that the products generated during alcohol metabolism (e.g., acetaldehyde) are toxic (NIAAA, 1993). Further, alcohol consumption limits the body's natural defenses against free radicals (which damage liver cells and promote inflammation) and increases cytokine levels (implicated in the scar formation and oxygen depletion associated with cirrhosis) (McClain *et al.*, 1997).

Susceptibility to alcohol-induced liver disease varies substantially among individuals. Possible factors contributing to risk include genetic factors, dietary factors, gender, and hepatitis C (Dannenberg & Nanji, 1998; Maher, 1997). Prospective studies indicate that the risk of cirrhosis becomes significant when intake is, on average, above 80 g/day (6.2 ounces) for men or 20 g/day (1.55 ounces) for women (Grant *et al.*, 1988). Women develop liver disease after consuming lower levels of alcohol over a shorter period of time than men

(Gavaler & Arria, 1995), and have a higher incidence of alcoholic hepatitis and a higher mortality rate from cirrhosis than men (Hall, 1995). The higher risk for women may occur because they have higher peak blood alcohol levels and a slightly higher rate of hepatic metabolism of alcohol resulting in a higher production of acetaldehyde, which may play a part in alcohol-induced liver injury. Another possible link is found in the hypoxia hypothesis (Saltatos & Soranno, 1991), which predicts that women are more susceptible to alcoholic liver damage because they have lower hematocrits, lower hemoglobin levels, and a higher prevalence of anemia. The average duration of heavy drinking for cirrhotic patients is between 10 and 20 years. The regular consumption of alcohol accelerates the disease progression of hepatitis C virus to cirrhosis, HCC, and end-stage liver disease (Imperial, 1999).

## Pancreatitis

The effects of alcohol on the pancreas are well established. Alcohol abuse can lead to chronic pancreatic inflammation, atrophy, and fibrosis. Approximately 65% of all cases of pancreatitis are alcohol related (Balart & Ferrante, 1982). Alcoholic pancreatitis may be one of the most serious adverse consequences of alcohol abuse, although the mechanisms leading to alcoholic pancreatitis are poorly understood (NIAAA, 1997). Mild pancreatitis usually resolves acutely with alcohol abstention and supportive therapy. Severe pancreatitis has a significant morbidity and mortality, mainly related to the degree of pancreatic necrosis and infection (Schenker & Montalvo, 1998). Women are also more likely to have pancreatitis with a shorter duration of heavy alcohol use than men. Both acute and chronic pancreatitis can result in diabetes mellitus (Greenhouse & Lardinois, 1996). Although some research has causally associated pancreatitis with a long-term risk of pancreatic cancer, this relationship has not been definitively substantiated (Karlson et al., 1997).

## Cardiovascular Disease

Cardiovascular disorders continue to be the leading cause of death in the United States (NIAAA, 1993). Alcohol-related cardiovascular disease includes hypertension, cerebrovascular hemorrhage (stroke), arrhythmias (disturbances in heart rhythm), cardiomyopathy (heart muscle disease), and coronary heart disease, including sudden coronary death. Disparities in the relationships between alcohol consumption and various cardiovascular conditions are now evident, with complex interrelationships between conditions. An inverse relationship of alcohol use to coronary heart disease is supported by many population studies. Interpretation of these data as a protective effect of alcohol against coronary disease is strengthened by plausible mechanisms. Epidemiological and intervention studies have now firmly established an association between heavy drinking and hypertension, but a mechanism remains elusive (Klatsky, 1998). While there is increasing evidence that light to moderate alcohol consumption decreases the risk of death from coronary heart disease (CHD), chronic heavy drinking is associated with many of the other cardiovascular diseases (Lands & Zakhari, 1990; NIAAA, 1997).

Numerous studies have shown a lower risk for CHD for light to moderate drinkers, generally one to two drinks a day, compared with abstainers (Anderson et al., 1993; NIAAA, 1999). There is a "J"-shaped curve wherein nondrinkers have a slightly higher rate of CHD than light drinkers, with risk increasing as consumption increases (Klatsky, 1996; Rosenberg et al., 1981; Stampfer et al., 1988). Substantial evidence has discounted speculation that abstainers include a large proportion of former heavy drinkers with preexisting health problems (i.e., "sick quitters") (Hennekens, 1996). Health-related lifestyle factors that correlate consistently with drinking level might account for some of the association between alcohol and lower risk for CHD, including such factors as exercise and diet (Ashley, 1984; Barrett et al., 1995; Berlin & Colditz, 1990; Klatsky, 1994; Rimm et al., 1991). The findings regarding moderate alcohol consumption and lowered CHD risk need to be weighed against the risk of other diseases associated with alcohol use for both men and women, such as hypertension, cardiomyopathy, stroke, and some cancers. Women and younger persons appear more susceptible to the increased mortality risk of heavy drinking. The reduced cardiovascular risk of lighter drinkers is more pronounced in older persons. Lower coronary disease prevalence may reduce the noncardiovascular mortality risk of lighter drinkers (Klatsky et al., 1992). The National Institute on Alcohol Abuse and Alcoholism reviewed epidemiologic evidence regarding this issue in its October 1999 Alcohol Alert (NIAAA, 1999).

Alcohol can act as an antioxidant and an oxidant, and its intake seems to exert both beneficial and untoward effects on stroke, depending on drinking habits. Light or moderate regular alcohol intake has been suggested to protect against internal carotid artery atherosclerosis, a major cause of ischemic stroke. On the other hand, recent heavy drinking has been observed to worsen vasospastic ischemia caused by subarachnoid bleeding (Hillbom, 1999). Potentially protective against heart attack, the anticlotting ability of alcohol may increase the risk of hemorrhagic stroke, or bleeding within the brain (Stampfer et al., 1988).

Cocaine abuse can lead to serious cardiac complications (Bunn & Giannini, 1993), including myocardial ischemia and infarction, myocarditis, cardiomyopathy, and arrhythmias. Hepatic transformation from the use of alcohol and cocaine together can produce cocaethylene, now thought to be primarily responsible for many cocaine abuser deaths. Treatment of cardiovascular complications has focused on cocaine-induced ischemia, hypertension, and arrhythmias. Thrombolytic agents have been used in the treatment of myocardial infarction but their use with this population remains controversial.

# Cancers

Alcohol and the risk of cancer has been comprehensively reviewed (Anderson et al., 1993; Eighth Special Report, 1993). The International Agency for Research on Cancer's monograph reviewed cancers and alcohol risk and concluded that alcohol is causally related to cancers of the oral cavity, pharynx, larynx, esophagus, and liver (Thomas, 1995). Holman et al. (1996) found increased risk of cancers of the pharynx, esophagus, liver, larynx and female breast with increasing alcohol intake level. Alcohol consumption is strongly related to the risk of colon cancer in both men and women (Meyer & White, 1993). The joint effects of alcohol and smoking are greater than additive, and are probably multiplicative, suggesting biological synergism (Thomas, 1995).

The role of alcohol in cancers of the gastrointestinal tract is still controversial. Risks of cancers of the distal stomach, pancreas, and rectum have not been consistently related to alcohol (Bouchardy et al., 1990; Ferraroni et al., 1989; Nomura et al., 1990), although possible relationships between alcohol and rectal carcinoma (Stemmerman et al., 1990) and between heavy use of alcohol and pancreatic cancer (as mentioned above) warrant further study (Thomas, 1995).

As expected, alcohol abuse plays an important role in the development of primary liver cancer. Some research has indicated that hepatitis B viral infection is an important risk factor in the development of primary liver cancer, while other research shows that heavy alcohol use, even without hepatitis B, is causally linked to liver cancer (Ohnishi et al., 1987). Hepatocellular carcinoma develops frequently in patients with hepatitis C viral infection, a disease that progresses more rapidly with regular alcohol use (Imperial, 1999).

Alcohol consumption is associated with a linear increase in breast cancer incidence in women over the range of consumption reported by most women. Among women who consume alcohol regularly, reducing alcohol consumption is a potential means to reduce breast cancer risk (Smith-Warner et al., 1998). Of the 17 studies of breast cancer in women reviewed by Anderson et al. (1993), 11 showed a significant positive association with alcohol consumption, including all 5 of the cohort studies in their sample. The consistency of the 5 large cohort studies is compelling evidence to counsel women to limit their use of alcohol. Several of the studies indicate that risk increases slightly with an intake above one drink a day. Zhang et al. (1999) found that the light consumption of alcohol or any type of alcoholic beverage, however, is not associated with increased breast cancer risk. Alcohol has not been implicated in other female cancers such as endometrial or cervical cancer.

# HIV/AIDS

There are two major areas of concern regarding alcohol and drug use in relationship to HIV/AIDS. The first is the public health concern related to the relationship between alcohol and drug use and unsafe sex, which has the potential to lead to HIV transmission. This concern has been the focus of many prevention messages, both in the media and in clinical settings. The second major concern is the sharing of contaminated injection equipment which is the primary means of HIV transmission among intravenous drug users. Recent reports indicate that the drug use in this population has changed to include widespread use of cocaine. In the United States, approximately 34% of all cases of AIDS in adults have occurred either in injection drug users or in their sexual partners (O'Connor *et al.*, 1994). When HIV/AIDS is included in the statistics for illicit drug mortality, the numbers double. In 1990, roughly 20,000 deaths were attributed to the use of illicit drugs, with 9000 HIV related (DesJarlais *et al.*, 1992).

Of particular importance to the medical community is the documented observation that HIV-related complications among injection drug users differ somewhat from those of other HIV-infected population groups. Physicians treating these individuals need to address clinical and psychosocial issues related to both drug dependence and HIV infection. These patients are more likely than other HIV patients to have frequent occurrences of pyogenic bacterial infections, particularly pneumonia, endocarditis, and septis, HIV-related tuberculosis, and sexually transmitted diseases such as syphilis and human papilloma virus. They are also more likely to have hepatitis, other retroviral infections, and cancer, such as lung and cervix. The 1992 revised AIDS case definition of the Centers for Disease Control and Prevention includes recurrent bacterial pneumonia, pulmonary tuberculosis, and cervical carcinoma as AIDS-defining illnesses in patients with HIV infection (1993 Revised Classification, *Morbidity and Mortality Weekly Report*, 1992; 41) (No. RR0-17). This change should provide better epidemiological data on HIV by more accurately reflecting the illnesses seen in drug users and women.

# Other

## Gender Differences

Women develop many alcohol-related medical problems at lower levels of consumption than men, likely reflecting women's lower total body water, gender differences in alcohol metabolism, and effects of alcohol on postmenopausal estrogen levels. Women who report drinking more than two drinks daily have increased rates of mortality and breast cancer. Women are more likely to die from all causes and alcohol-related liver disease than are men who report drinking the same amount of alcohol. High levels of alcohol consumption increase women's risk for infertility, spontaneous abortion, and menstrual symptoms, while variable amounts of alcohol use in women increase the risk for fetal alcohol syndrome. Women and men who drink alcohol have similar risks for hypertension, stroke, injury, and cardiovascular mortality (Bradley *et al.*, 1998).

## Fetal Problems

Fetal alcohol syndrome (FAS) is estimated to occur at a rate of 9.7 per 10,000 live births in the general obstetric population (Abel, 1995). Among heavy drinkers, 4.3% of children born annually have FAS, more than 2000 cases per year in the United States. Mental handicaps and hyperactivity are probably the most debilitating aspects of FAS (Streissguth *et al.*, 1989), and prenatal alcohol exposure is one of the leading known causes of mental retardation (Abel & Sokol, 1986). Problems with learning, attention, memory, and problem solving are common, along with incoordination, impulsiveness, and speech and hearing impairment (NIAAA, 1997; Streissguth & LaDue, 1985).

Cocaine use during pregnancy has been associated with such maternal complications as hypertension, cardiac arrhythmias, decreased uterine blood flow, abruptio placentae, precipitous labor, seizures, and even death and such fetal complications as cerebral hemorrhages, fetal distress, edema, meconium staining, low birth weight, premature birth, hypoxia, and stillbirth (Brown *et al.*, 1992; Church *et al.*, 1991; Slutsker, 1992). The interpretation of data from epidemiologic studies to assess the association between adverse pregnancy outcomes and cocaine use is limited by misclassification of users, reporting bias confounded by socioeconomic factors, and inaccurate measurement of cocaine use. Some evidence shows that increased sensitivity to cocaine may be mediated by estrogen or progesterone, suggesting that the cocaine-abusing woman is at increased risk for cocaine-induced morbidities whenever levels of these hormones are elevated, such as during the final stages of pregnancy or possibly when taking oral contraceptives (Church & Subramanian, 1997).

Although chronic alcohol dependence is associated with reduced cerebral blood flow (CBF), changes in CBF after marijuana smoking are variable: increases and decreases having been reported (Mathew & Wilson, 1991). Chronic use of marijuana, however, seems to reduce CBF. Most inhalants and solvents are vasodilators, with chronic abuse also showing a decrease in CBF. These decreases are at least partially reversible with abstinence.

## Injury and Violence

Substance abuse plays a significant role in many injuries, particularly those related to motor vehicle crashes, falls, fires, and drownings (NIAAA, 1997). Injuries resulting from motor vehicle crashes are the leading cause of death in the United States among people aged 1 to 34 (National Center for Health Statistics, 1994); approximately 41% of the 40,676 traffic fatalities in 1994 were related to alcohol (National Highway Traffic Safety Administration, 1995). Two of five people in the United States will be involved in an alcohol-related motor vehicle crash at some time during their lives (Fell & Nash, 1989). Problem drinkers utilize injury-related medical care at higher rates than nonproblem drinkers and experience injury-related medical care costs three times as high (Blose & Holder, 1991). Alcohol consumption is also linked to family and marital violence (Martin, 1992). For example, a recent study conducted among 375 men in family medicine clinics found that men with increased alcohol consumption were more likely to report violent behavior (Oriel & Fleming, 1998). High rates of alcohol and other drug use have also been associated with suicide (Goodman *et al.*, 1991), increased risk of violent death (Rivara *et al.*, 1997), high-risk sexual behavior (Strunin & Hingson, 1992, 1993), homicide, physical assault, and involvement in other criminal activities (Martin, 1992).

### CASE 31-12

*Jeanine Jefferson is an eighth-grade student in a suburban middle school. She is an athlete on the soccer and basketball teams. She and her friends enjoy sports in general and meet to watch sporting events on television. While watching the women's soccer playoffs they noticed a really great ad featuring a new type of beer. The music and slogans were very attractive and appealed to young women in particular. One of the girls mentioned that her older sister in college had some of the beer at home and maybe they could try it.*

## SOCIETY'S ROLE IN SUBSTANCE ABUSE

Because the use of addictive substances typically begins at an early age, and because early onset of use is one of the predictors of later health problems, it is important to consider society's role in the problem. Despite all of the evidence to the contrary, and despite the huge economic, social, and emotional costs of alcohol problems, the alcohol industry insists that its marketing techniques do not influence those under the legal drinking limit. Studies in the United States and other countries indicate the powerful potential of alcohol advertising. Grube and Wallack (1994) tested fifth and sixth graders' awareness of beer advertising and their retention of information contained in the advertisements. They found that awareness and retention of the information influenced the children's beliefs, knowledge, and intentions regarding the use of alcohol. The children who were more familiar with specific advertisements were more likely to have positive attitudes about alcohol. In a second study, Madden and Grube (1994) analyzed the number of alcohol and tobacco advertisements included in a random sample of televised sports events. They included the appearance of stadium billboards, on-site promotions, and product sponsorship announcements and advertisements. These programs primarily aired beer commercials with a number of the advertisements portraying activities with high trauma risk such as water sports while drinking. Studies commissioned by the Surgeon General in 1991 revealed that young people were inaccurately informed about alcohol, found the packaging of alcohol confusing, and were attracted to wine coolers and beer, which are packaged and advertised to be attractive to this age group.

The main conclusion of these and other studies is that the most important effect of alcohol advertisement is not on immediate use but in its pervasive influence on society's view of alcohol. Alcohol is associated with some of our most important life events, yet the negative potential of the drug is not discussed. The only programs that have been found to be successful in working with societal impressions of alcohol have been social influence programs that include information, decision-making, and resistance skills training. These techniques are used in programs with children and adolescents and have also been successfully used in brief advice protocols in primary care settings. Prevention and brief intervention strategies in primary care settings can play a crucial part in a public health effort to address these problems throughout the life span.

---

### CASE 31-13

*Judy Field is a 35-year-old patient of Dr. Martin. She is married and has two daughters, aged 9 and 7. Ms. Field has been Dr. Martin's patient for 10 years since moving to this community. During an annual physical examination Dr. Martin asked her to complete a short questionnaire about her health habits regarding nutrition, exercise, smoking, alcohol, and other drug/medication use. Ms. Field reported that she drank two glasses of wine every day of the week and two additional cocktails on the weekend. Because she met the criteria for at-risk drinking, Dr. Martin asked further questions to assess use and discovered that Ms. Field had been under more stress at work, was experiencing some new gastric distress, and was not sleeping well. Her alcohol use had increased as the work problems increased in the last year. Dr. Martin and her nurse, Melissa Enders, worked with Ms. Field to cut back on her drinking using a brief intervention model. Her gastric distress improved. At the end of 1 year, she was consuming approximately one drink 3 days a week, was sleeping better, and was better able to handle the changes on her job.*

## THE PHYSICIAN'S ROLE IN TREATMENT AND PREVENTION ———

The link between substance use and health risk naturally leads to an examination of the role of primary care practitioners in the detection and treatment of people with these disorders. As the statistics in the prevalence section of this chapter suggest, detecting at-risk and problem drinkers is as important as recognizing patients who are alcohol dependent. In fact, the majority of people experiencing health problems secondary to their alcohol or other drug use are at-risk users rather than alcohol or drug dependent. Intervention at this stage has the potential to prevent longer-term medical, social, and psychological consequences. *This means that primary care physicians have a crucial role in the prevention and early intervention of alcohol and drug problems in their patients* (Saunders *et al.*, 1993).

## Screening/Asking the First Questions

To be able to practice prevention and early intervention with patients, clinicians need to screen for alcohol and drug problems. Screening can be done as part of a routine health examination and updated annually, before prescribing medications, or in response to problems that may be alcohol or drug related.

The common signs and symptoms of alcohol problems seen in primary care settings are listed in Table 31.1.

As mentioned earlier, *any current use of tobacco or illicit drugs is considered at-risk behavior*. The initial screening questions listed in Table 31.2 for alcohol can be used for other drugs with any positive responses indicating risk (see also Table 31.3).

**TABLE 31-1**
Signs and Symptoms of Alcohol Problems

| Medical signs | Family patterns |
|---|---|
| ☐ Stomach/abdominal pain | ☐ Frequent visits by other family members |
| ☐ Elevated blood pressure | ☐ Unexplained symptoms, such as headaches or |
| ☐ Chronic tension headaches |    abdominal pain in a child |
| ☐ Insomnia (accompanied by a medication request) | ☐ Trauma secondary to physical abuse |
| ☐ Sexually transmitted diseases | ☐ School problems in a child |
| ☐ Frequent accidents and trauma | ☐ Depression or anxiety disorders in a family member |
| ☐ Fatigue | |
| ☐ Chronic depression | |
| ☐ Chronic diarrhea | |
| ☐ Memory loss | |

However, because of the relationship between alcohol consumption and health problems, questions about consumption (quantity and frequency of use) provide a method to categorize patients into levels of risk for alcohol use. The traditional assumption that all patients who drink have a tendency to underreport their alcohol use is not supported by research (Babor *et al.*, 1989). People who are not alcohol dependent often give accurate information.

Physicians can get more accurate histories by asking questions about the recent past; embedding the alcohol use questions in the context of other health behaviors (e.g., exercise, weight, smoking); and paying attention to nonverbal cues that suggest the patient is minimizing use (e.g., blushing, turning away, fidgeting, looking at the floor, change in breathing pattern). Screening questions can be asked by verbal interview, by paper-and-pencil questionnaire, or by computerized questionnaire. All three methods have equivalent reliability and validity (Greist *et al.*, 1987; Barry & Fleming, 1990). Any positive responses can lead to further questions about consequences. *To successfully incorporate alcohol (and other drug) screening into your practice, it should be simple and consistent with other screening procedures already in place.*

## Assessing/What to Ask Next?

Assessment helps the clinician to determine the severity of the alcohol problem—whether or not the patient is an at-risk drinker, a problem drinker, or alcohol dependent. The following are some general guidelines for clinicians to adapt to each particular patient and situation. Physicians can follow questions about consumption with the CAGE questions (Ewing, 1984) adapted to include drugs of abuse (Brown, 1992) plus a question on the consequences of alcohol use (Table 31.4). The Alcohol Use Disorders Identification Test (AUDIT), an instrument specifically designed to identify at-risk and problem drinking, is recommended as an additional assessment tool (Reid *et al.*, 1999).

*Screening and assessment can be completed during a standard 15-minute office visit.*

It is appropriate to conduct laboratory tests such as liver function tests on patients who are heavy drinkers. A number of alcohol marker indicators are potential diagnostic tools for detection of early phase

**TABLE 31-2**
Specific Recommended Questions for Alcohol Screening (Often Asked in the Context of a Series of Health Behaviors)

☐ Do you drink alcohol? (If no, is that a change?) If *yes*:
   ☐ About how many days a week do you drink alcohol?
   ☐ On a day when you drink, how much do you drink?
   ☐ How many days a month do you drink four or more drinks?

Screening *positive* for men is drinking more than 14 drinks/week, for women is drinking more than 7 drinks/week, and for men or women is a report of ANY single occasion when they have consumed more than 4 drinks in the past month.

**TABLE 31-3**
Specific Recommended Questions for Drug Screening

☐ Do you:
    a. use prescribed or over-the-counter drugs in excess of the directions,
    b. use any nonmedical drugs?
If no, is that a change?)
If yes:
    ☐ What medications/drugs are you using?

Screening is *positive* if any use of prescription or over-the-counter drugs in excess of the directions is present, and if there is any use of nonmedical drugs.

heavy drinkers for brief intervention treatment, including carbohydrate-deficient transferrin (CDT), mean corpuscular volume (MCV), aspartate aminotransferase (AST), alanine aminotransferase (ALT), and gamma-glutamyltransferase (GGT). Some research has shown that marker combinations, especially those including CDT, are more sensitive in detecting heavy alcohol use (Sillanaukee *et al.*, 1998). In these patients, physical findings such as elevated laboratory values can be a powerful motivator to change behavior. Test results can also be used to monitor compliance with a treatment program.

To assess *dependence* in patients who report alcohol-related problems, have a history of failed attempts to stop or cut back, or report withdrawal symptoms such as tremors, the questions in Table 31.5 may be helpful. *These questions can also be adapted to other drugs*. Physicians should refer any patient thought to be alcohol or drug dependent for a diagnostic evaluation and possible specialized alcohol and other drug treatment.

Assessing the use of other drugs includes asking the patient about prescriptions, particularly antidepressants, benzodiazepines, and codeine; over-the-counter drugs; and illicit drugs (particularly marijuana, cocaine, and heroin). If there is evidence for either prescription drug abuse or illicit drug use, the patient should be referred to a specialist for a diagnostic assessment and possible specialized treatment. For a more comprehensive discussion of the diagnosis and treatment specifically of *drug abuse* in primary care, see Trachtenberg and Fleming (1994).

## Brief Intervention

Although traditional approaches to alcohol and other drug problems have focused on long-term counseling, there is increasing evidence that brief intervention, delivered by a physician, can effectively reduce drinking in at-risk and problem drinkers, persons who are not alcohol dependent. The clinical trials of brief advice with at-risk drinkers have been based, in part, on the original "stop smoking" trials. Studies in the United States and Europe have demonstrated a significant (10 to 20%) reduction in drinking by persons in the experimental groups when compared with control groups that did not receive the advice (Fleming & Barry, 1995; Fleming *et al.*, 1997, 1999; Kristenson *et al.*, 1983; Saunders *et al.*, 1993). These findings are consistent

**TABLE 31-4**
The CAGE Questions

☐ "Have you ever felt you should CUT down or stop drinking/drug use?"
☐ "Have people ANNOYED you by criticizing your drinking/drug use?"
☐ "Have you ever felt bad or GUILTY about your drinking/drug use?"
☐ "Have you ever had a drink /drug first thing in the morning or after rising to steady your nerves or get over a hangover (EYE opener)?"

Additional question
☐ "Has your drinking/drug use ever caused you problems (for example, problems with family, work, school, sleep, accidents, or injuries)?"

Adapted from the CAGE/AID, R. Brown, 1992.

**TABLE 31-5**

Dependence Questions

☐ Are you ever unable to stop drinking once you start?
☐ How many drinks does it take to get high? Does it take more drinks than it used to get high?
☐ Do you drink in the morning to get over a hangover or stop the shakes?
☐ Do you have strong urges to drink? Do many of your everyday activities revolve around drinking?

across more than ten trials. The effectiveness rates are similar to those found with at-risk and problem drinkers in traditional alcohol treatment.

A brief alcohol intervention (see TIP) consists of the following steps. These steps can be used with or without an accompanying workbook or pamphlet covering the action steps for the patient.

1. *Summary of health habits.* Customized feedback on screening questions relating to drinking patterns and other health habits (may also include smoking, nutrition, tobacco use, seat belt use, safe sex, and so on). This information can be derived from screening and preassessment questionnaires or from the patient during this session.

2. *Discuss the types of drinkers in the population, and where the patient's drinking patterns fit into the population norms for their age group.* The purpose of this step is to introduce drinking guidelines (women under 65: no more than one drink/day; men under 65: no more than two drinks/day; women and men 65 and over: no more than one drink/day or seven drinks/week), the idea that patients' alcohol use can be related to their physical and emotional health, and that their level of drinking can put them at risk for more health-related problems. This brief discussion may evoke a number of strong reactions from patients (e.g., argumentation, minimizing, acceptance, concern, tearfulness, embarrassment, hostility). Avoid creating additional resistance by "rolling with the patient's resistance" and being empathic.

3. *Consequences of at-risk and problem drinking.* Relate this to any potential or ongoing health problem that is currently important in the care of this patient (e.g., hypertension, gastrointestinal problems). It should be noted that some patients might also begin to recognize that their drinking is problematic. This may facilitate a change in drinking behavior.

4. *Reasons to quit or cut down on drinking.* This is a very brief discussion of how changing drinking levels could have important benefits for the individual.

5. *Introduce the concept of standard drinks* (see sidebar). This discussion focuses on the equivalence of alcohol content across various beverage types. This concept provides the context for a discussion of sensible drinking limits.

6. *Drinking agreement* (see sidebar). Agreed-on drinking limits in the form of an agreement or "prescription" can be negotiated and signed by the patient and the clinician. *Patients take this "prescription" with them when they leave the office.* This "formal" agreement is a particularly effective tool in changing

---

## STANDARD DRINKS: KEY POINTS

- *One standard drink = 12 oz beer or ale; 1.5-oz. shot of distilled spirits; 4–5 oz wine; 4 oz sherry; 4 oz liqueur).*
- *When pouring wine, sherry, or distilled spirits, measuring is important to ensure that the patient is consuming standard drinks.*
- *Alcohol is alcohol. Some patients may think that they do not use alcohol because they "only drink beer or wine." Some view "hard" and "soft" alcoholic beverages as different in their effects.*
- *Review standard drinks briefly. Avoid disputes about details regarding the alcohol content of specific beverages.*

---

## KEY POINTS

- *Give guidance on abstinence versus cutting down. Patients who have a serious health problem or take medications that interact with alcohol should be advised to abstain. Others may be appropriate candidates to cut down on drinking to below recommended limits.*
- *Complete the* negotiated *agreement/prescription.*
- *Provide guidance by recommending a low level of alcohol use or abstinence. Remember, you may have to negotiate "up" so start low.*
- *The prescription-type form contains a space to write what you have negotiated with the patient: (1) stop or cut down on drinking; (2) when to begin; (3) how frequently to drink.*
- *If the patient is reluctant to sign a contract, try to determine the reason for his or her reluctance and address his or her concerns if possible.*

  *Be sensitive to the patient's reactions including concern, embarrassment, defensiveness, minimization of drinking problems, or hostility and "roll with the patient's resistance." Avoid disputes over these guidelines and ask the patient's patience in considering how alcohol could affect his life.*

drinking patterns. A follow-up visit or phone call can help the patient stay on track with any changes in drinking patterns.

It helps have the patient record any alcohol use on a calendar to keep track of it for discussion at a follow-up visit.

7. *Coping with risky situations.* Social isolation, boredom, and negative family interactions can present special problems. The patient will need to identify situations and moods that are related to drinking too much alcohol, and to identify some individualized cognitive and behavioral coping alternatives.

8. *Summary of the session.* The summary should include a review of the agreed-on drinking goals and a discussion of the drinking diary calendar to be completed.

## Specialized Treatment

Brief advice is not appropriate for all patients with alcohol problems. People with more severe alcohol dependence or with serious psychiatric or other drug use disorders are likely to participate in specialized alcoholism treatment programs. For example, in 1993 an estimated 708,255 clients were treated for alcoholism across the United States, 13.5% as inpatients and 86.5% as outpatients (NIAAA, 1997).

Successful treatment of alcohol and drug dependence began in 1935 with the development of Alcoholics Anonymous (AA), the first of the 12-step self-help groups. Programs like the Minnesota model of alcoholism

---

## DRINKING AGREEMENT

*Date* _____

*Start date:* _____

*Agreement:* _____

_____

*Patient signature* _____

*Clinician signature* _____

## SUMMARY OF BRIEF INTERVENTION PROCESS AND DIALOG EXAMPLES

- *The physician offers clear advice to cut down or stop drinking, often in the context of a health, social, or family problem. For example:*

  I'm concerned about your [particular symptom(s), e.g., high blood pressure, sleep problem, abdominal pain] and I think your alcohol use may be a part of the problem.

  *Based on clinical judgment regarding the seriousness of the alcohol problem, the clinician will decide if the patient should cut down or abstain. For example:* I want you to stop drinking any alcohol for the next month so we can see if your abdominal pain decreases,

  or

  I want you to cut back your drinking to no more than one drink every other day. How do you feel about that?
- *This last statement provides the opportunity to negotiate and empowers the patient to be a part of the decision-making process.*
- *These approaches can also be tests to determine the seriousness of the patient's alcohol problem. If the patient cannot abstain or cut down, it suggests a more serious problem that requires referral and follow-up.*
- *Brief interventions often include the use of a behavior modification pamphlet or self-help book that includes levels of drinking in the general population, a discussion of consequences, an agreement to cut back, a discussion of risky situations, ways to cope with setbacks, and ways for the patient to reward herself for success.*
- *A follow-up phone call 2 weeks after the office visit to determine if the patient is able to keep the agreement and follow-up office visits (at 1-month intervals) are often beneficial.*
- *Brief interventions can be completed during a standard 15-minute office visit.*

treatment, which includes an abstinence-oriented treatment program with education, individual and group therapy, and participation in AA, have been the mainstay of alcoholism treatment in the United States (Cook, 1988) but have only been tested in controlled clinical trials recently (Keso & Salaspuro, 1991). In a comparison between the Minnesota model and a traditional model based on individual, group, family, and work therapy without AA or a goal of abstinence, 26% of the patients in the Minnesota model were abstinent at the end of 1 year compared with 10% in the traditional model.

In the last decade, the alcohol and other drug abuse (AODA) field has moved away from 28-day inpatient programs to outpatient programs and several other models of treatment. These treatment models include cognitive–behavioral therapy, cue therapy, and motivational enhancement techniques. Trends in AODA treatment reflect more freedom to choose programs that will best meet the needs of individual patients. The choice of treatment depends on motivation to change, co-occurring medical and psychiatric problems, and family issues to be resolved, as well as what treatment options are available in the community. Studies of treatment matching are underway to determine characteristics of patients who benefit from each of the types of treatment modalities.

## Use of Alcohol-Sensitizing and Anticraving Agents

Medications with alcohol-sensitizing effects, like disulfiram (Antabuse), have been used to stop patients' alcohol use during treatment. The disulfiram–alcohol reaction includes flushing, nausea, vomiting, and cardiovascular changes (Christensen *et al.*, 1991). Treatment programs and practitioners show great variability in prescribing disulfiram. This variability often depends on philosophy and administrative approaches (Eighth Special Report, 1993, p. 333) rather than on patient characteristics or treatment setting. Fuller *et al.* (1986), in a controlled clinical trial, found that disulfiram had no long-term effect on abstinence but that patients who received 250 mg/day had fewer drinking days than those on smaller doses or on placebo. In a comprehensive review of techniques to improve patient compliance, Allen and Litten (1992) concluded that, in general, patient incentives, treatment contracts, and medication instructions have improved the consistency of disulfiram use and reduced alcohol consumption, at least during the medication period.

There is continued concern about the side effects and toxicity of disulfiram (Christensen *et al.*, 1991). Because of this concern, other aversive agents, such as calcium carbamide, which does not have the drowsiness and lethargy associated with disulfiram (Peachey *et al.*, 1989), are being tested. Calcium carbamide, however, is not approved for use in the United States and is contraindicated for patients with thyroid disease. Disulfiram should not be used in the absence of an ongoing treatment and monitoring program, and may not benefit patients who have difficulty following medication regimens.

Naltrexone (ReVia®) was approved in December 1994 by the U.S. Food and Drug Administration for the treatment of alcoholism. Clinical trials have shown naltrexone to decrease alcohol craving and drinking days among patients participating in psychosocial treatment, with risk of relapse less than half that of placebo-treated patients (O'Malley *et al.*, 1992; Volpicelli *et al.*, 1992). Further, naltrexone also prevented relapse to heavy drinking (five or more drinks consumed per occasion) among those patients who resumed drinking alcohol. In one study, naltrexone has been found to work best with patients who received supportive psychotherapy in addition to the medication (Jaffe *et al.*, 1996). A randomized controlled trial study of cognitive–behavioral therapy (CBT) and naltrexone found that patients with moderate alcohol dependence were treated with greater effectiveness when naltrexone was used in conjunction with CBT (Anton *et al.*, 1999). Naltrexone increased control over alcohol urges and improved cognitive resistance to thoughts about drinking.

## Referral

Identifying the particular expertise of specialists in the community is important if treatment matching (matching the needs of the patient with the available programs) is to occur. Physicians may use the following steps to determine their community resources (Barry & Fleming, 1994): (1) Ask colleagues for names of treatment programs or individual providers; (2) contact an AODA treatment program or specialist, mental health center, or hospital for consultation about a specific patient problem; (3) call the state alcohol and drug abuse agency for the names of publicly and privately funded treatment programs; (4) call employee assistance programs in the area; and (5) complete the Community Alcohol and Drug Treatment Resource Guide (see Table 31.6) including telephone numbers of key professionals in the community, and post the guide in the nursing station, reception area, or examination room.

When referring patients to a specialist, it helps to tell the patient that a second opinion from a specialist is needed, to make telephone calls to the AODA specialist to set up the assessment while the patient is in the office, and to ask the specialist to call once she has completed the evaluation. This allows the physician to participate in long-term follow-up and provides continuity of care to patients who are in need of ongoing support.

Sometimes patients refuse to see specialists or do not have the financial or family resources to go into treatment, e.g., childcare is unavailable, older adults are afraid to leave home for treatment because they might not be able to return home again. When this happens, physicians can take two steps to help these patients. First, they can identify recovering alcoholics in their own practices who are willing to meet with persons with AODA problems to discuss ways to change drinking behavior. Second, they can ask the patient to attend self-help groups such as AA. The patient may need to attend more than one group to find one that is comfortable, e.g., smoking versus nonsmoking groups. Two types of group meetings that do not follow a 12-step model are Rational Recovery and Women for Sobriety. These groups are most often found in midsized and larger cities.

**TABLE 31-6**
Community Alcohol/Drug Treatment resources

1. **Alcohol and Drug Specialist:**

Name _____ Ph. Number _____

Name _____ Ph. Number _____

2. **Physician** with expertise in alcohol and drug disorders

Name _____ Ph. Number _____

3. AA phone numbers _____

_____

4. Community substance abuse services (publicly funded)

Name _____ Phone _____

Contact Person _____

Type of facility (circle)        residential        outpatient        evening        adolescent/adult

Specialized program _____

5. **Other treatment programs**

Name _____ Phone _____

Hours _____ Contact Person _____

Type of facility (circle):        residential        outpatient        evening        adolescent        adult

Specialized program _____

Name _____ Phone _____

Type of facility (circle):        residential        outpatient        evening        adolescent        adult

Specialized program _____

# Prevention and Motivation

As mentioned earlier, the majority of persons who drink suffer no adverse consequences. For those patients who do not drink above the at-risk cutoffs, do not abuse prescription drugs, and do not use illicit drugs, a clear positive message reinforcing that behavior is appropriate:

*Our goal is to prevent future health problems. Your exercise program looks good and your weight has remained stable. Since you have no family history of alcohol or drug problems and are taking no medication to interfere with alcohol, not exceeding a glass of wine once or twice a week should not cause any additional medical problems for you.*

It is often easier to remember to intervene with problems than to provide verbal support for healthful behaviors. There are few opportunities in clinical medicine to make significant long-lasting changes in the lives of patients, and helping a patient to avoid the consequences of an alcohol or drug disorder is one such opportunity.

For the patient struggling with an alcohol or drug disorder, hope is a powerful motivator. Treatment programs that focus on recovering professionals report 5-year success rates of over 80%. No other chronic condition has such a high potential cure rate. Proven models for screening, assessment, brief advice, and referral are now available (NIAAA, *Physician's Guide to Helping Patients with Alcohol Problems*, 1995).

## RECOVERY HAPPENS!

*The 5-year success rate of some recovery programs is 80%. (Source NIAAA, Physician's* Guide to Helping Patients with Alcohol Problems, *1995)*

# CONCLUSION

This chapter provides background data concerning the importance of prevention and early intervention in the area of alcohol and other drug problems, effective screening procedures for at-risk drinkers and drug users, a brief intervention protocol to be used with patients who are not alcohol or drug dependent, and steps to establish a referral network for patients who need specialized treatment. As healthcare in the United States changes, the role of primary care physicians in the prevention and treatment of alcohol and other drug problems will broaden.

# CASES FOR DISCUSSION

## CASE 1

*George Williams is a 63-year-old white school custodian whom you have seen a few times in the last 3 years after his previous physician, Dr. James, retired. You admitted him to the hospital for pneumonia last year and found that he had mild emphysema from a long history of smoking. He had been treated for hypertension for 5 years. His blood pressure was stable in the hospital, so you discontinued the medication and advised him to avoid salt in his diet. He came to the office last week for a yearly physical, the results of which were within normal limits except for the mild emphysema and an elevated blood pressure of 160/105 mm Hg. At his insistence you continued Dr. James's prescription for triazolam 0.125 hs, prn (at bedtime as needed) for insomnia. You asked him to return in 1 week (today) for a blood pressure recheck and planned to spend more time discussing his smoking. His laboratory tests came back today and you discovered that he has an elevated GGT and an MCV of 98 (normal = 80 to 96). During the physical examination he stated that he drinks a few days a week with his friends at the corner bar. You are also concerned that he has been calling for prescription renewals increasingly early in the last 3 months.*

1. *What additional screening questions will you ask him?*
2. *What areas should be assessed for more severe alcohol or other drug problems?*
3. *Do you think he will be a candidate for brief advice?*
4. *If you think Mr. Williams needs an assessment by an AODA specialist, how will you approach the subject with him?*

## CASE 2

*Dr. Pendleton is a 48-year-old primary care physician who has been the medical director of a clinic in a small rural community in the Midwest for the last 3 years. He grew up in a large city and moved to a smaller community for his residency program. He engaged in binge drinking in college with his fraternity brothers, used marijuana regularly, and experimented with cocaine a few times. During his residency program he and the other residents had in-home parties every few weeks. He noticed that he was able to drink more than anyone else and was a little irritated that none of them seemed to want to go out drinking as often as he did. His use of marijuana and cocaine stopped during his years in the residency program. After completing his residency, his drinking also tapered off because he was so busy with his new practice and young family. During the last 3 years Dr. Pendleton's binge drinking has increased but has generally been confined to evenings although his nurse has noticed changes in his personality and has smelled alcohol on his breath during working hours on one occasion. His wife recently filed for divorce. He had three instances of being intoxicated while on call in the last few months, one of which you and another junior colleague witnessed. You were uncertain if you should report this or talk to him yourselves. After checking into what help was available, you decided to get some help from the impaired physicians program of the state medical society. The physician intervenors assured you that the information you both provided would be kept confidential and that they would work with Dr. Pendleton. They met with Dr. Pendleton and explained that there were reports of alcohol-related problems in his job performance. Although he initially denied problems related to his drinking, the committee arranged for an alcohol and drug assessment as well as a urine drug screen. In addition to binge drinking, Dr. Pendleton was using benzodiazepines on a regular basis. He entered a treatment program for professionals and was clean and sober at 1 year posttreatment.*

1. *Would you have confronted Dr. Pendleton yourself first? If yes, what would you say? If no, why not?*
2. *Would you have confronted someone who was a colleague without seniority or a subordinate? If yes, what would you say? If no, why not?*
3. *How could an impaired physicians program help a physician such as Dr. Pendleton?*
4. *How can you find out about an impaired physicians program in your area?*

## CASE 3

*Sal Franco is a 74-year-old man living alone in an apartment in a complex for older adults. He owned a grocery store with his wife Mary for 44 years. He and Mary sold the business to their son Dominique when Sal was 70 with plans to travel and enjoy their remaining years together. Shortly after their retirement, Mary was diagnosed with bone cancer and died within 6 months of the diagnosis. Mr. Franco has been alone for the last 3 years. Although he was a "hard drinker" as he described it in his 20s and 30s, because of gastritis and high blood pressure, his use of alcohol was limited to his weekly poker games and Sunday family meals for many years. Because Sal and Mary spent most of their time working at the grocery store and involved in family activities, there was little time left for friends. Now he has time on his hands and uses alcohol to alleviate some of the pain and stress of his loneliness, generally having three drinks a day. He has developed few outside interests and doesn't know where to start. He came to the clinic for follow-up of his labile hypertension and gastritis. You asked Mr. Franco how he was feeling and received this response, "Oh, Doctor, I guess I'm OK for an old widower. I sometimes think it really doesn't matter how I feel at this age." You followed up with some questions about what Sal does with his time and discovered that he uses alcohol to excess along with taking over-the-counter medication to sleep.*

1. *What assessment questions would you ask to determine the extent of the problem?*
2. *How would you work with Mr. Franco to cut back or stop his use of alcohol?*
3. *What outside agencies and activities might be useful to Mr. Franco, who is spending most of his time alone? What would you suggest to him?*
4. *How would you help him get connected with programs or agencies in the community that could provide some interests in life for him? Are there other professionals in your clinic who could be of assistance with this issue?*

## CASE 4

*Josh Kendrick is an 18-year-old high school senior who is graduating this year. He came to the office for his physical examination before he leaves to be a camp counselor for the summer and attends a local university in the fall. He was on the wrestling and baseball teams all 4 years of high school and has been active in extracurricular activities sponsored by the school. His grades have been good, mostly Bs and a few As. As part of your routine physical examination you ask questions about alcohol and drug use. Josh reports that he drinks about once a month at parties and uses marijuana at least once a week with friends.*

1. *What other questions would you ask about his use of alcohol and drugs?*
2. *If he was not so forthcoming about his use, what types of questions would be a good lead-in to questions about his use?*
3. *Is Josh's use problematic at this time? If yes, what would you do next? If no, what will you say next?*
4. *What prevention messages would you give him as he goes off to college?*

## CASE 5

*Mandy Quist is a 25-year old married computer programmer who has been in your practice for three years. At her last physical she indicated that she drank a glass of wine three times a week. She experimented with marijuana in college but has not used any illicit drugs in the last 2 years. She exercises three times a week in an aerobics class at the YWCA, does not smoke, and her weight has remained stable since she entered your practice. Mrs. Quist has been trying to conceive and is here for a pregnancy test.*

1. *What advice will you give her regarding the use of alcohol, medications, and drugs?*
2. *What prevention messages will you give her about her other health behaviors?*
3. *What advice would you give her regarding her health behaviors during pregnancy?*

## RECOMMENDED READINGS

Barry KL (Chair): Brief Interventions and Brief Therapies for Substance Abuse. Rockville, Md, U.S. Department of Health and Human Services, Public Health Service, Substance Abuse and Mental Health Services Administration, Center for Substance Abuse Treatment, 1999. Treatment Improvement Protocol (TIP) Series #36.

> This TIP was developed by a national expert panel of clinicians and researchers and provides state-of-the-art best practice guidelines for the use of brief interventions with persons who have problems related to alcohol use. This and the other manuals in the TIP series are available free of charge from the Center for Substance Abuse Treatment @ http://www.samhsa.gov/csat/

National Institute of Alcohol Abuse and Alcoholism: NIAAA Physician Intervention Guide, 1995. For development information contact Francis Cotter, MPH, NIAAA, Willco Building, 600 Executive Blvd, Rockville, Md 20892-7003.

> The NIAAA with the cooperation and help of experts in the alcohol field from around the United States have developed a physician intervention guide to aid the identification, assessment, and treatment of persons with alcohol-related problems in the office setting.

Ninth Special Report to the U.S. Congress on Alcohol and Health: U.S. Department of Health and Human Services, Public Health Service, National Institutes of Health, National Institute of Alcohol Abuse and Alcoholism, NIH Publication No. 97-4017, 1997.

> This state-of-the-art publication is a very useful reference covering the effects of alcohol on health in a variety of areas. It includes sections on the nature and extent of alcohol use and alcohol-related problems, causes of alcohol abuse and alcohol dependence, consequences of use, abuse, and dependence, prevention and early intervention, treatment approaches, and alcohol health services research.

## REFERENCES

Abel EL: An update on incidence of FAS: FAS is not an equal opportunity birth defect. *Neurotoxicol Teratol* 17(4):437–443, 1995.

Abel EL, Sokol RJ: Fetal alcohol syndrome is now leading cause of mental retardation. *Lancet* 2:1222, 1986.

Adams A, Ockene JK, Wheller EV, Hurley TG: Alcohol counseling: Physicians will do it. *J Gen Intern Med* 13(10):692–698, 1998.

Adams W: Interactions between alcohol and other drugs, in Gurnack AM (ed): *Older Adults' Misuse of Alcohol, Medicines, and Other Drugs: Research and Practice Issues.* Berlin, Springer, 1997, pp 185–205.

Allen JP, Litten RZ: Techniques to enhance compliance with disulfiram. *Alcohol Clin Exp Res* 16(6):1035–1041, 1992.

American Psychiatric Association. *Diagnostic and Statistical Manual of Mental Disorders*, ed 4. Washington, DC, American Psychiatric Association, 1994.

American Society of Addiction Medicine: Public policy statement on screening for addiction in primary care settings. *ASAM News* 17:17–18, 1997.

Anderson P, Cremona A, Paton A, Turner C, Wallace P: Alcohol and risk. *Addiction* 88:1493–1508, 1993.

Anton RF, Moak DH, Waid R, Latham PK, Malcolm RJ, Dias JK: Naltrexone and cognitive behavioral therapy for the treatment of outpatient alcoholics: Results of a placebo-controlled trial. *Am J Psychiatry* 156(1):1758–1764, 1999.

Ashley MJ: Alcohol consumption and ischemic heart disease: The epidemiologic evidence, in Smart RG, Cappell HD, Glaser FB, *et al* (eds): *Research Advances in Alcohol and Drug Problems.* New York, Plenum Press, 1984, vol 1, pp 99–147.

Babor TF, Kranzler HR, Laverman RJ: Early detection of harmful alcohol consumption: Comparison of clinical, laboratory, and self-report screening procedures. *Addict Behav* 14(2):139–157, 1989.

Balart LA, Ferrante WA: Pathophysiology of acute and chronic pancreatitis. *Arch Intern Med* 142:113–177, 1982.

Barrett, DH, Anda RF, Croft JB, *et al*: The association between alcohol use and health behaviors related to the risk of cardiovascular disease: The South Carolina Cardiovascular Disease Prevention Project. *J Stud Alcohol* 56(1):9–15, 1995.

Barry KL, Fleming MF: The family physician. *Alcohol Health Res World* 18(1):105–109, 1994.

Berlin JA, Colditz GA: A meta-analysis of physical activity in the prevention of coronary heart disease. *Am J Epidemiol* 132(4):612–628, 1990.

Blose JO, Holder HD: Injury-related medical care utilization in a problem drinking population. *Am J Public Health* 81(12):1571–1575, 1991.

Bouchardy, C, Clavel F, LaVecchia C, Raymond L, Boyle P: Alcohol, beer, and cancer of the pancreas. *Int J Cancer* 45(5):842–846, 1990.

Bradley KA, Badrinath S, Bush K, Boyd-Wickizer J, Anawalt B: Medical risks for women who drink alcohol. *J Gen Intern Med* 13(9):627–639, 1998.

Brasseux C, D'Angelo LJ, Guagliardo M, Hicks J: The changing pattern of substance abuse in urban adolescents [see comments]. *Arch Pediatr Adolesc Med* 152(3):234–237, 1998.

Brown E, Prager J, Lee HY, Ramsey RG: CNS complications of cocaine abuse: Prevalence, pathophysiology, and neuroradiology. *Am J Roentgenol* 159(1):137–147, 1992.

Brown R: Identification and office management of alcohol and drug disorders, in Fleming MF, Barry KL (eds): *Addictive Disorders*. St. Louis, Mosby Year Book Medical Publishers, 1992, pp 25–43.

Buchsbaum DG, Welsh J, Buchanan RG, Elswick RK: Screening for drinking problems by patients' self-report. *Arch Intern Med* 155:104–108, 1995.

Bunn WH, Giannini AJ: Cardiovascular complications of cocaine abuse. *Am Fam Physician* 47(5): 1072, 1993.

Centers for Disease Control: Leads from the Morbidity and Mortality Weekly Report, Atlanta, Ga: Update: Mortality Attributable to HIV Infection Among Persons Aged 25-44 Years —United States, 1991 and 1992. 270(22):2672, 1993.

Church MW, Subramanian GG: Cocaine's lethality increases during late gestation in the rat: A study of "critical periods" of exposure. *Am J Obstet Gynecol* 176:901–906, 1997.

Church MW, Kaufmann RA, Keenan JA, Martier SS, Savoy-Moore RT, Ostrea EM, *et al*: Effects of prenatal cocaine, in Watson RR (ed). *Biochemistry and Physiology of Substance Abuse*, Boca Raton, Fla, CRC Press, 1991, vol 3, pp 179–204.

Christensen JK, Moller IW, Ronsted P, Angelo HR, Johansson B: Dose–effect relationship of disulfiram in human volunteers: 1. Clinical studies. *Pharmacol Toxicol* 68(3):163–165, 1991.

Cook CCH: The Minnesota Model in the management of drug and alcohol dependency: Miracle, method or myth? Part I. The philosophy and the programme. *Br J Addict* 83(6):625–634, 1988.

Dannenberg AJ, Nanji AA: Dietary saturated fatty acids: A novel treatment for alcoholic liver disease. *Alcoholism Clin Exp Res* 22(3):750–752, 1998.

DeBakey SF, Stinson FS, Grant BF, Dufour MC: Surveillance Report #41. *Liver Cirrhosis Mortality in the United States, 1970–93.* Bethesda, Md, National Institute on Alcohol Abuse and Alcoholism, 1996.

DesJarlais DC, Friedman SR, Choopanya K, Vanichseni S, Ward TP: International epidemiology of HIV and AIDS among injecting drug users. *AIDS* 6:1053–1068, 1992.

Dufour MC, Archer L, Gordis E: Alcohol and the elderly. *Clin Geriatr Med* 8(1):127–141, 1992.

Eighth Special Report to the U.S. Congress on Alcohol and Health. Department of Health and Human Services, Public Health Service, National Institutes of Health, National Institute of Alcohol Abuse and Alcoholism. Publication No. ADM-281-91-0003, 1993.

Ewing JA: Detecting alcoholism: The CAGE questionnaire. *JAMA* 252:1905–1907, 1984.

Farrell M, Lewis G: Discrimination on the grounds of diagnosis. *Br J Addict* 85(7):883–890, 1990.

Fell JC, Nash CE: The nature of the alcohol problem in US fatal crashes. *Health Educ Q* 16:335–343, 1989.

Ferraroni M, Negri E, LaVecchia C, DaVanzo B, Franceshi S: Socioeconomic indicators, tobacco and alcohol in the etiology of digestive tract neoplasms. *Int J Epidemiol* 18(3):556–562, 1989.

Fleming MF, Barry KL: The effectiveness of alcoholism screening in an ambulatory care setting. *J Stud Alcohol* 52(1):33–36, 1991.

Fleming MF, Barry KL (eds): *Addictive Disorders*. St. Louis, Mosby Year Book Medical Publishers, 1992.

Fleming MF, Barry KL: The effectiveness of brief physician advice with at-risk drinkers. Results of a clinical trial. Unpublished, 1995.

Fleming MF, Barry KL, Davis A, Kropp S, Kahn R, Riva M: Medical education about substance abuse: Changes in curriculum and faculty between 1976 and 1992. *Acad Med* 69(5): 362–369, 1994.

Fleming MF, Barry KL, Manwell LB, Johnson K, London R: Brief physician advice for problem alcohol drinkers: A randomized controlled trial in community-based primary care practices. *JAMA* 277:1039–1045, 1997.

Fleming M, Manwell LB, Barry KL, Adams W, Johnson K: Guiding older adult lifestyles (Project GOAL): The effectiveness of brief physician advice for alcohol problems in older adults, *J Fam Pract* 48(5):378–384, 1999.

Friedmann PD, Saitz R, Samet JH: Management of adults recovering from alcohol or other drug problems: relapse prevention in primary care. *JAMA* 279(15):1227–1231, 1998.

Fuller RK, Branchey L, Brightwell DR, *et al*: Disulfiram treatment of alcoholism. A Veteran's Administration cooperative study. *JAMA* 256:1449–1455, 1986.

Gavaler JS, Arria AM: Increased susceptibility of women to alcoholic liver disease: Artifactual or real? in Hall P (ed): *Alcoholic Liver Disease: Pathology and Pathogenesis*, ed 2. London, Edward Arnold, 1995, pp 123–133.

Goodman RA, Istre GR, Jordan FB, Herndon JL, Kelaghan J: Alcohol and fatal injuries in Oklahoma. *J Stud Alcohol* 52:156–161, 1991.

Grant BF, Dufour M, Harford TC: Epidemiology of alcoholic liver disease. *Semin Liver Dis* 8(1):12–25, 1988.

Grant BF, Harford TC, Dawson DA, Chou P, Dufour M, Pickering R: Prevalence of DSM-IV alcohol abuse and dependence: United States, 1992. *Alcohol Health Res World* 18(3):243–248, 1994.

Greenhouse L, Lardinois CK: Alcohol-associated diabetes mellitus: A review of the impact of alcohol consumption on carbohydrate metabolism [Clinical Review]. *Arch Fam Med* 5(4):229–233, 1996.

Greist J, Klein M, Erdman H, Bires J, *et al*: Comparison of computer- and interviewer-administered versions of the Diagnostic Interview Schedule. *Hosp Community Psychiatry* 38(12):1304–1311, 1987.

Grube JW, Wallack L: Television beer advertising and drinking knowledge, beliefs, and intentions among school children. *Am J Public Health* 84:254–259, 1994.

Haapanen-Niemi N, Miilunpalo S, Vuori I, Pasanen M, Oja P: The impact of smoking, alcohol consumption, and physical activity on use of hospital services. *Am J Public Health* 89(5):691–698, 1999.

Hall P: Factors influencing individual susceptibility to alcoholic liver disease, in Hall P (ed): *Alcoholic Liver Disease: Pathology and Pathogenesis*, ed 2. London, Edward Arnold, 1995, pp 299–316.

Hennekens CH: Alcohol and risk of coronary events, in Zakhari S, Wassef M (eds): *Alcohol and the Cardiovascular System*. NIAAA Research Monograph No. 31. NIH Publication No. 96-4133. Washington, DC, US Government Printing Office 1996, pp 15–24.

*HHS News*. Rockville, Md, U.S. Department of Health and Human Services, January 31, 1994.

Hillbom M: Oxidants, antioxidants, alcohol and stroke [Review]. *Front Biosci* 4:67–71, 1999.

Holman CD, English DR, Milne E, Winter MG: Meta-analysis of alcohol and all-cause mortality: A validation of NHMRC recommendations [see comments]. *Med J Aust.* 164(3):141–145, 1996.

Imperial JC: Natural history of chronic hepatitis B and C. *J Gastroenterol Hepatol* 14(suppl):S1–S5, 1999.

Institute for Health Policy, Brandeis University. *Substance Abuse: The Nation's Number One Health Problem; Key Indicators for Policy.* Princeton, NJ, Robert Wood Johnson Foundation, 1993.

Institute of Medicine Committee to Study Fetal Alcohol Syndrome. Washington, DC, National Academy Press, 1996.

Institute of Medicine: *Dispelling the Myths About Addiction.* Washington, DC, National Academy Press, 1997.

Jaffe AJ, Rounsaville B, Chang G, Schottenfeld RS, Meyer RE, O'Malley SS: Naltrexone, relapse prevention, and supportive therapy with alcoholics: An analysis of patient treatment matching. *J Consult Clin Psychol* 64:1044–1053, 1996.

Johnston LD, *et al*: *National Survey Results on Drug Use from the Monitoring the Future Study, 1975–1994: Volume 1. Secondary School Students.* Rockville, Md, National Institute on Drug Abuse, 1995.

Karlson BM, Ekbom A, Josefsson S, McLaughlin JK, Fraumeni JF Jr, Nyren O: The risk of pancreatic cancer following pancreatitis: An association due to confounding?. *Gastroenterology* 113(2):587–592, 1997.

Keso L, Salaspuro M: Inpatient treatment of employed alcoholics: A randomized clinical trial on Hazelden-type and traditional treatment. *Alcoholism Clin Exp Res* 14(4):584–589, 1991.

Kessler RC, McGonagle KA, Zhao S, Nelson CH, Hughes M, Eshleman S, Wittchen HU, Kendler K: Lifetime and 12-month prevalence of DSM-III-R psychiatric disorders in the United States. *Arch Gen Psychiatry* 51(1):8–19, 1994.

Klatsky AL: Epidemiology of coronary heart disease—Influence of alcohol. *Alcohol Clin Exp Res* 18(1):88–96, 1994.

Klatsky AL: Alcohol, coronary disease, and hypertension [Review]. *Annu Rev Med* 47:149–160, 1996.

Klatsky AL: Alcohol and cardiovascular diseases: A historical overview. *Novartis Foundation Symposium* 216:2–12, discussion 12–18, 152–158, 1998.

Klatsky AL, Armstrong MA: Alcohol, smoking, coffee, and cirrhosis. *Am J Epidemiol* 136(10):1248–1257, 1992.

Klatsky AL, Armstrong MA, Friedman GD: Alcohol and mortality. *Ann Intern Med* 117(8):646–654, 1992.

Kristenson H, Ohlin H, Hulten-Nosslin MB, Trell E, Hood B: Identification and intervention of heavy drinking in middle-aged men: Results and follow-up of 24–60 months of long-term study with randomized controls. *Alcoholism Clin Res Exp* 7(2):203–209, 1983.

Lands WEM, Zakhari, S: Alcohol and cardiovascular disease. *Alcohol Health Res World* 14:304–312, 1990.

Lyness JM, Caine ED, King DA, Cox C, Yoediono Z: Psychiatric disorders in older primary care patients. *J Gen Intern Med* 14(4): 249–254, 1999.

Madden PA, Grube JW: The frequency and nature of alcohol and tobacco advertising in televised sports. *Am J Public Health* 84:297–299, 1994.

Maher JJ: Exploring alcohol's effects on liver function. *Alcohol Health Res World* 21(1):5–12, 1997.

Martin SE: The epidemiology of alcohol-related interpersonal violence. *Alcohol Health Res World* 16(3):230–237, 1992.

Mathew RJ, Wilson WH: Substance abuse and cerebral blood flow. *Am J Psychiatry* 148(3):292–305, 1991

McClain CJ, Shedlofsky S, Barve S, Hill DB: Cytokines and alcoholic liver disease. *Alcohol Health Res World* 21(4):317–320, 1997.

McGinnis JM, Foege WH: Mortality and morbidity attributable to use of addictive substances in the United States. *Proc Assoc Am Physicians* 111(2):109–118, 1999.

Meerkerk GJ, Njoo KH, Bongers IM, Trienekens P, van Oers JA: Comparing the diagnostic accuracy of carbohydrate-deficient transferrin, gamma-glutamyltransferase, and mean cell volume in a general practice population. *Alcoholism: Clin Exp Res* 23(6):1052–1059, 1999.

Meyer F, White E: Alcohol and nutrients in relation to colon cancer in middle-aged adults. *Am J Epidemiol* 138(4):225–236, 1993.

Morrison MA: Addiction in adolescents. *West J Med* 152:543–546, 1990.

National Center for Health Statistics: Health, United States, 1993. US Department of Health and Human Services Publication PHS 94-1232. Hyattsville, Md, Public Health Service, 1994.

National Highway Traffic Safety Administration: Traffic Safety Facts 1993: A Compilation of Motor Vehicle Crash Data from the Fatal Accident Reporting System and the General Estimates System. DOT HS 808 169. Washington, DC, US Department of Transportation, National Center for Statistics and Analysis, 1994.

National Highway Traffic Safety Administration: Traffic Safety Facts, 1994: Alcohol. Washington, DC, US Department of Transportation, National Highway Traffic Safety Administration, 1995.

National Institute on Alcohol Abuse and Alcoholism: *Alcohol Alert No. 19: Alcohol and the Liver.* PH 329. 1993.

National Institute on Alcohol Abuse and Alcoholism: NIAAA Physician Intervention Guide 1995. For development information, contact Francis Cotter, MPH, NIAAA, Willco Building, 600 Executive Blvd, Rockville, Md 20892-7003.

National Institute on Alcohol Abuse and Alcoholism: *Ninth Special Report to the U.S. Congress on Alcohol and Health.* NIH Publication No. 97-4017. Rockville, Md, National Institutes of Health. 1997.

National Institute on Alcohol Abuse and Alcoholism: *Alcohol Alert No. 40: Alcohol and Aging.* 1998.

National Institute on Alcohol Abuse and Alcoholism: *Alcohol Alert No. 45: Alcohol and Coronary Heart Disease.* 1999.

Nomura A, Grove JS, Stemmerman GN, Severson RK: A prospective study of stomach cancer and its relation to diet, cigarettes, and alcohol consumption. *Cancer Res* 50(3):627–631, 1990.

O'Connor PG, Samet JH: Prevalence and assessment of readiness for behavioral change of illicit drug use among primary care patients [abstract]. *J Gen Intern Med* 11(suppl):53, 1996.

O'Connor PO, Selwyn PA, Schottenfeld RS: Medical care for injection drug users with human immunodeficiency virus infection. *N Engl J Med* 331:450–459, 1994.

Ohnishi K, Terabayashi H, Unuma T, Takahashi A, Okuda K: Effects of habitual alcohol intake and cigarette smoking on the development of hepatocellular carcinoma. *Alcoholism Clin Exp Res* 11(1):45–48, 1987.

O'Malley SS, Jaffe AJ, Chang G, Schottenfeld RS, Meyer RE, Rounsaville B: Naltrexone and coping skills therapy for alcohol dependence: A controlled study. *Arch Gen Psychiatry* 49(11):881–887, 1992.

Oriel KA, Fleming MF: Screening men for partner violence in a primary care setting. A new strategy for detecting domestic violence. *J Fam Pract* 46(6):493–498, 1998.

Peachey JE, Annis HM, Bornstein ER, Sykora K, Maylana SM, Shamai S: Calcium carbamide in alcoholism treatment. Part 1. A placebo-controlled, double-blind clinical trial of short-term efficacy. *Br J Addict* 84(8):877–887, 1989.

Poikolainen K: Alcohol and mortality: A review [published erratum appears in *J Clin Epidemiol* 48(9):I, 1995] *J Clin Epidemiol* 48(4):455–465, 1995.

Ramsey PG, Curtis JR, Paauw DS, Carline JD, Wenrich MD: History-taking and preventive medicine skills among primary care physicians: An assessment using standardized patients. *Am J Med* 104(2):152–158, 1998.

Regier DA, Robins LN (eds): *Psychiatric Disorders in America: The Epidemiological Catchment Area Study*. New York, The Free Press, 1991.

Reid MC, Tinetti ME, Brown CJ, Concato J: Physician awareness of alcohol use disorders among older patients. *J Gen Intern Med* 13(11):729–734, 1998.

Reid MC, Fiellin DA, O'Connor PG: Hazardous and harmful alcohol consumption in primary care. *Arch Intern Med* 159(15):1681–1689, 1999.

Rimm EB, Giovannucci EL, Willett WC, *et al*: Prospective study of alcohol consumption and risk of coronary disease in men. *Lancet* 338:464–468, 1991.

Rivara FP, Mueller BA, Somes G, Mendoza CT, Rushforth NB, Kellermann AL: Alcohol and illicit drug abuse and the risk of violent death in the home. *JAMA* 278:569–575, 1997.

Robins LN, Helzer JE, Weissman MM, *et al*: Lifetime prevalence of specific psychiatric disorders in three sites. *Arch Gen Psychiatry* 41:949–958, 1984.

Rosenberg L, Slone D, Shapiro S, Kaufman DW, Miettinen OS, Stolley PD: Alcoholic beverages and myocardial infarction in young women. *Am J Public Health* 71(1):82–85, 1981.

Saltatos LG, Soranno TM: Alcohol-induced liver disease, in Watson RR (ed): *Biochemistry and Physiology of Substance Abuse*, vol 3. Boca Raton, Fla, CRC Press, 1991, pp 73–92.

Samet JH, Vega M, Nuciforo S, Williams C: Assessment of readiness for behavioral change of substance abusers in primary care [abstract]. *J Gen Intern Med* 10(suppl):48, 1995.

Saunders J, Aasland O, Amundsen, Grant M: Alcohol consumption and related problems among primary health care patients: WHO collaborative project on early detection of persons with harmful alcohol-consumption-1. *Addiction* 88:349–362, 1993.

Schenker S, Montalvo R: Alcohol and the pancreas. *Recent Dev Alcoholism* 14:41–65, 1998.

Searight HR: Screening for alcohol abuse in primary care: Current status and research needs. *Fam Pract Res J* 12(2):193–204, 1992.

Sillanaukee P, Aalto M, Seppa K: Carbohydrate-deficient transferrin and conventional alcohol markers as indicators for brief intervention among heavy drinkers in primary health care. *Alcoholism Clin Exp Res* 22(4):892–896, 1998.

Slutsker L: Risks associated with cocaine during pregnancy. *Obstet Gynecol* 79(5):778–789, 1992.

Smith-Warner SA, Spiegelman D, Yaun SS, van den Brandt PA, Folsom AR, Goldbohm RA, Graham S, Holmberg L, Howe GR, Marshall JR, Miller AB, Potter JD, Speizer FE, Willett WC, Wolk A, Hunter DJ: Alcohol and breast cancer in women: A pooled analysis of cohort studies. *JAMA* 279(7):535–540, 1998.

Stampfer MJ, Colditz GA, Willett WC, Speizer FE, Hennekens CH: A prospective study of moderate alcohol consumption and the risk of coronary disease and stroke in women. *N Engl J Med* 319:267–273, 1988.

Stemmerman GN, Nomura AMY, Chyou P, Yoshizawa C: Prospective study of alcohol intake and large bowel cancer. *Dig Dis Sci* 35(11):1414–1420, 1990.

Streissguth AP, LaDue RA: Psychological and behavioral effects in children prenatally exposed to alcohol. *Alcohol Health Res World* 10(1):6–12, 1985.

Streissguth AP, Sampson PD, Barr HM: Neurobehavioral dose–response effects of prenatal alcohol exposure in humans from infancy to adulthood. *Ann NY Acad Sci* 562:145–158, 1989.

Strunin L, Hingson R: Alcohol, drugs and adolescent sexual behavior. *Int J Addict* 27(2):129–146, 1992.

Strunin L, Hingson R: Alcohol use and risk for HIV infection. *Alcohol Health Res World* 17(1):35–38, 1993.

Trachtenberg AI, Fleming MF: Diagnosis and Treatment of Drug Abuse in Family Practice. Am Fam Phy, Kansas City, MO, Summer 1994.

Thomas DB: Alcohol as a cause of cancer. *Environ Health Persp* 103(suppl 8):153–160, 1995.

Thun MJ, Peto R, Lopez AD, Monaco JH, Henley SJ, Heath CW Jr, Doll R: Alcohol consumption and mortality among middle-aged and elderly U.S. adults. *N Engl J Med* 337(24):1705–1714, 1997.

University of Michigan: The rise of drug use among American teens continues in 1996. News and Information Services press release [early results of annual Monitoring the Future Study] 1996.

US Preventive Services Task Force: *Guide to Clinical Preventive Services*, ed 2. Alexandria, Va, International Medical Publishing, 1996.

Volk RJ, Steinbauer JR, Cantor SB: Patient factors influencing variation in the use of preventive interventions for alcohol abuse by primary care physicians. *J Stud Alcohol* 57(2):203–209, 1996.

Volpicelli JR, Alterman AI, Hayashida M, O'Brien CP: Naltrexone in the treatment of alcohol dependence. *Arch Gen Psychiatry* 49(11): 876–880, 1992.

Waller JA, Casey R: Teaching about substance abuse in medical school. *Br J Addict* 85(11):1451–1455, 1990.

Williams GD, Clem DA, Dufour MC: Apparent per Capita Alcohol Consumption: National, State and Regional Trends, 1977–92. Surveillance Report No. 31. Rockville, Md, National Institute on Alcohol Abuse and Alcoholism, Division of Biometry and Epidemiology, Alcohol Epidemiologic Data System, 1994.

Williams GD, Clem DA, Dufour MC: Apparent per Capita Alcohol Consumption: National, State and Regional Trends, 1977–92. Surveillance Report No. 35. Rockville, Md, National Institute on Alcohol Abuse and Alcoholism, Division of Biometry and Epidemiology, Alcohol Epidemiologic Data System, 1995.

Zhang Y, Kreger BE, Dorgan JF, Splansky GL, Cupples LA, Ellison RC: Alcohol consumption and risk of breast cancer: The Framingham Study revisited. *Am J Epidemiol* 149(2):93–101, 1999.

Zoccolillo M, Vitaro F, Tremblay RE: Problem drug and alcohol use in a community sample of adolescents. *J Am Acad Child Adolesc Psychiatry* 38(7):900–907, 1999.

## CHAPTER 32

# Violence

*L. Kevin Hamberger and Bruce Ambuel*

## CASE 32-1

*Betty, 23 years old, brings her newborn son to the office for a well-baby check and postpartum examination. She has a large hickey on her neck. The baby is healthy and Betty says that both she and Joe (the father) are very happy with the baby. The baby sleeps well, has a good appetite, and mostly has a good disposition.*

*Betty is somewhat concerned that the baby has "spells" when he just seems to cry and cry. During these "spells" Betty reports feeling somewhat tense and uncertain about what to do. Putting him in his crib and shutting his door helps somewhat. She states that Joe sometimes wonders why the child "won't mind" and "just be a good boy, like he's supposed to." She accepts information on child development and assures the physician that the baby is in no danger of being abused. She states that both she and Joe "went through that as kids" and have no intention of putting their kids through it. She does express openness, however, to being contacted by someone from the county Home Aid office for a little extra help and learning some parenting tips. Betty is not sure, however, whether Joe will go along with the idea.*

*With this last comment, the physician, referring to Betty's hickey, noted half-jokingly, "I thought I instructed 'no sex' for at least a month after the birth." Betty, looking to the floor, quietly replied, "I guess Joe couldn't wait." Betty's examination was essentially negative, she was healing as expected, and she was scheduled for another well-baby check in 6 months.*

*The physician had an uneasy feeling about Betty and Joe, but was uncertain about the precise nature of those concerns and how to go about evaluating them. The following history was collected during Betty's prenatal course. Betty completed the 11th grade and then left school because of pregnancy, though she later miscarried. Throughout her most recent obstetrical course, Betty was reasonably compliant with her diet and nutrition and showed adequate weight gain and appropriate interest in her pregnancy. She reported her relationship with Joe was stable and that he was looking forward to the baby's arrival. She has lived with Joe for 3 years.*

*Joe is 24 years old and completed the 11th grade. For the past 3 years, he has been self-employed in a tree removal business. Betty moved in with Joe 3 years ago because she "couldn't take" living with her previous partner. She reported that Joe works hard trying to make his business succeed. Joe came to a couple of the OB visits but was very quiet and did not disclose much about himself. He participated in the prenatal classes and the birth of their son.*

---

## EDUCATIONAL OBJECTIVES

1. Understand key definitions of intentional injury, violence, partner violence, child abuse, and elder abuse
2. Understand the natural history of violence in interpersonal relationships, including the use of violence to dominate, control, or punish
3. Know incidence and prevalence of major types of intentional injury
4. Know the acute and long-term impact of violence on health
5. Understand the important role of the healthcare system and the physician in identifying, treating, and preventing violence

---

## PATTERNS OF VIOLENCE

The physician's uneasy but unarticulated feelings about Betty and Joe in Case 32-1 are justified by their history, if it were known.

*Betty.* As a child, Betty was sexually abused by her grandfather. He would fondle her vaginal area and have her perform oral sex, beginning when Betty was 5 years old. When Betty was 12, her grandfather had intercourse with her for the first time. She was threatened with harm if she ever told anyone of the abuse. Betty tried to tell her mother, who spanked and slapped her, and warned her to "never say such things again."

At age 15, Betty moved in with her 17-year-old boyfriend. He rarely worked and, although Betty continued to go to school, both "partied" a great deal with alcohol and drugs. He was very violent with Betty, beating her with his fists, throwing dishes at her, and, on one occasion, trying to drown her in the bathtub. She tried to return home once, but her parents told her, "You made your bed, now lie in it." She became pregnant and decided to drop out of school and prepare to give birth. At 26 weeks she miscarried but did not return to school because "I just didn't feel like going back." Her boyfriend blamed her for losing the baby and beat her as punishment. She escaped to a battered women's shelter and ended the relationship.

Betty met Joe. He treated her well and worked hard. Betty told Joe about her prior abusive relationship, and he promised never to hurt her or do anything to make her afraid. He was going to "take care of her." Six months into their relationship, however, they had a big fight over Joe's drinking and he slapped her. Following the fight, Joe felt remorse and expressed fear that Betty would leave him. He mentioned that he ought to just kill himself now and get it over with, if he couldn't have her. Betty feared being responsible for Joe's death if she left and he killed himself. She stayed. Three months later Joe wanted to have sex, and Betty refused. He grabbed her breasts and pushed against her with his body, telling her "You're mine and I'll have you if I want." At other times, Joe would "remind" Betty that he "could" do to her what her ex-boyfriend did. This type of statement gained her compliance without having to resort to physical violence.

*Joe.* Joe grew up the oldest of three children, with a younger brother and sister. Joe's father physically beat his mother, or "tore up the house" after nights of heavy drinking. Joe recalled staying awake nights, fearful that his father would come home and hurt someone and fearful that he wouldn't come home at all. At times his father would round all the children up in the middle of the night to make them watch and "learn a lesson" as he beat one of them with an extension cord for some rule infraction. Once when Joe was 11 years old, his father took him hunting in the woods. Joe's father made him kneel down and placed the shotgun to his mouth, asking Joe if he "trusted" his father. Joe never told anyone of the incident. At age 15, Joe ran away from home, living in the streets and surviving on odd jobs. Prior to meeting Betty, Joe socialized mostly in bars, fighting several times a week. On one occasion he was shot, sustaining a flesh wound, while trying to help a friend in a fight.

*Typical pattern.* The story of Betty and Joe is fairly typical. Many men who batter their partners were themselves victims of child abuse and witnessed abuse in the family of origin (Hamberger *et al.*, 1996). Children who are abused are at risk for becoming violent offenders as adults. Further, many men who abuse their partners are also violent outside of their immediate relationship (Hamberger *et al.*, 1996; Saunders, 1992). Hence, it is not surprising that Joe often fought in bars and was himself the victim of violence in such settings.

In Betty's case, child sexual abuse is not viewed as a "cause" of her victimization as an adult. However, the degradation and hopelessness she experienced in a nonsupportive family limited her choices and led directly to her decision to leave home early. Her lack of preparation for independent living and the effect of the sexual abuse on her self-image left her vulnerable to involvement in relationships with men who abused her.

This case also illustrates that, even though an individual or couple may present with one particular "type" of violence issue at any given time, both victims and perpetrators often exhibit complex histories. If these histories are not known or well understood, our patients may do things that seem pathological, inexplicable, or "proof" of noncompliance. Such misunderstanding can lead to victim-blaming and assignment of pejorative diagnostic labels, such as "hysterical" or "borderline personality."

Another problem that can arise from such misunderstanding is the application of inappropriate or inadequate interventions. For example, a friendly pat on the back may seem innocuous to the healthcare provider, but if your patient is a survivor of childhood sexual abuse, that pat on the back may be emotionally overwhelming. A doctorly scolding may be therapeutic to some individuals to enhance compliance, but a man who learned to distrust authority through beatings and abuse may react by leaving the practice and rejecting all encouragement to seek help.

# THE NATURE AND PREVALENCE OF VIOLENCE

## What Is Violence?

Violence is "the threatened or actual use of physical force or power against oneself or against a group or community which either results in, or has a high likelihood of resulting in injury, death or deprivation" (Rosenberg, 1994). Violence is functional, intended to dominate, punish, or control another individual, group, or community. The concept of violence brings to mind images of extreme destructive acts such as a recent case in which a man bludgeoned his wife with a sledgehammer and watched her die over a 6-hour period, or the serial killer who cut up and cannibalized his victims. However, violence actually is multidimensional, consisting of acts that vary according to type, severity, frequency, and impact. Violence can be considered legitimate, as when a law enforcement officer subdues and neutralizes a dangerous criminal with a nightstick. Violence can also be considered illegitimate, as when an angry husband kicks down a door that his wife is hiding behind for safety or when a police officer uses excessive force.

Within the field of spouse abuse, Anne Ganley (1989) has identified and defined four basic types of violence. Although developed primarily for understanding partner violence, this typology can serve as a heuristic for understanding virtually any type of interpersonal violence.

## Dimensions of Violence

### Physical Violence

The first type of violence is actual physical violence, involving direct physical attacks on the victim's body. Physical violence includes a wide range of actions from grabbing and restraining to pushing and shoving to slapping, punching, kicking, clubbing, choking, drowning, burning, stabbing, and shooting. Note that physical violence constitutes a continuum of actions ranging from apparently less severe behaviors such as pushing and shoving to more severe and even life-threatening behaviors, such as using a knife or a gun.

## QUICK FACTS: HOW COMMON IS FAMILY VIOLENCE?

- *Women experience physical and sexual violence in relationships*
  - *16% have been physically assaulted by their partner in the past year*
  - *25% have been physically assaulted during their marriage*

  *(Gelles & Straus, 1988)*

  - *22% report being forced, by a man, to do something sexual they did not want to do*
  - *14 to 25% of adult women have been raped*

  *(Koss, 1993; Michael et al., 1994)*

- *Children (aged 3–17) physically abused by parents:*
  - *8.6% experience* physical assault *each year (kicks, bites, hitting, and more severe violence)*
  - *3.8% experience* severe physical assault *each year (beating up, striking with an object, threatening or assaulting with a weapon)*

  *(Gelles & Straus, 1988)*

- *Children sexually abused*
  - *Girls before age 18: 10–50% are* sexually abused by physical contact *(e.g., forced touching of the victim or perpetrator, intercourse, oral and anal intercourse). Our analysis of the literature leads us to conclude that 1 in 3 girls are sexually abused by physical contact before age 18.*
  - *Boys before age 18: 10–30% are* sexually abused *(contact and noncontact abuse). Our analysis of research leads us to conclude that 1 in 6 boys are sexually abused by physical contact before age 18.*

  *(Haugaard & Reppucci, 1988)*

Even perceived less severe violent behaviors, however, can have great injury potential. One of us (L.K.H.) has conducted over 1000 assessments of domestically violent offenders, many of whom insisted that they "only" pushed their partners. In-depth assessment of these "pushing" incidents has frequently indicated that the impact has been severe. For example, one offender who reported he had "only pushed" his partner later admitted that he tried to push her out of a closed second-floor window. Another reported succeeding in pushing his partner off a second-floor balcony, resulting in multiple fractures. Still another reported shoving his partner down a flight of concrete steps, causing her serious head injuries. Hence, although an offender may report using seemingly less severe violence in an assaultive act, it is important to assess carefully the context and consequences of the violence.

### Sexual Violence

A second form of violence is sexual. Sexual violence involves any actual or threatened assault of a sexual nature against a victim's body. This can range from unwanted fondling or touching to forced sexual acts. Sexual violence also includes coercive, threatening statements, exposure, and other actions that induce fear in the victim for purposes of sexual gratification and control in the perpetrator. This could include threatening to carry out sexual acts against the victim's wishes or threatening violence if sex is not provided. With children in particular, sexual violence can include exposure to pornography, taking pictures for adult gratification, exposure to genitals, or adult sexual contact.

As with physical violence, sexual violence usually involves direct action against a victim's body and constitutes a continuum of acts. As with physical violence, however, it is important not to assume that so-called minor acts of sexual violence are not serious. For example, many battered women report feeling degraded and humiliated after being coercively touched and fondled by their partners. Likewise, victims of sexual harassment are not always directly physically assaulted. Nevertheless, such victims often report experiencing intense emotional distress.

## Property and Pet Destruction

A third form of violence is property and animal destruction. This type of violence typically does not involve direct physical attacks against a victim's body but is nevertheless directed toward a victim. Examples include breaking down doors or windows or destroying cars, household items, and favorite personal possessions. Violence toward animals includes injuring and killing of pets, which may be displayed prominently in the victim's view. These actions communicate the perpetrator's destructive power and willingness to use violence to accomplish some goal, while terrorizing the victim.

## Psychological Violence and Terror

The fourth type of violence is psychological violence. Psychological violence includes a wide range of behaviors, such as name-calling and insults, following and stalking, forcing someone to do degrading things, and controlling the victim's movements and relationships within the community. In domestic violence situations, controlling economic resources and manipulating children is also part of psychological violence.

# The Function of Violence

People use violence intentionally to achieve certain outcomes that have value to the perpetrator. The outcomes are reinforcing and thus increase the probability that violence will be used again in subsequent similar situations. One key to preventing violence is to determine how it functions to reinforce, then change the value of the reinforcers. For example, in the field of partner violence, Ganley (1989) suggests that violence functions to dominate, control, or punish one's partner. Research by Hamberger *et al.* (1997) appears to confirm Ganley's assertion. The researchers found that the most common reason for abuse given by men participating in a domestic violence abatement program was to control or dominate their partner. The second most typical reason given was to reduce aversive tension built up during conflict. In Case 32-1, Joe indicated he battered Betty in an effort to get her to "quit bugging him" when he came home from work tired. On other occasions he threatened to hit her (psychological battery) to keep her from associating with her friend in the neighborhood. Although Joe never actually said the words "dominate and control" in describing how violence worked for him, the themes in his explanations clearly indicated these functions of violence for him.

From a societal level, violence may function to dominate or oppress an entire class or group of people. Violence toward women, for example, can be analyzed as part of a larger, historical pattern of male domination of women, through the development, by males, of social systems that favor men and oppress women (Yllo, 1993). In the home, women perform a disproportionate amount of childcare and "domestic" duties, and our society provides few resources for childcare (Mederos, 1987). In the workplace, women occupy a disproportionate number of lower-paying, lower-status jobs, and experience greater difficulty being promoted to higher-level management jobs than men. In divorce cases, women typically experience a greater drop in standard of living than do men. This creates societally sanctioned economic disincentives for women to leave abusive partners, thus maintaining the cycle of violence. Physical and sexual violence, or the threat of such violence, also reinforces the broader social-level inequities (Barnett *et al.*, 1997). Thus, domestic violence, together with societal maintaining factors, disenfranchises and devalues women, not only affecting battered women, but also functioning to oppress the entire group.

Sometimes violence has a protective function. In our work with battered women, we have learned that many women use physical force to resist the violence and coercion of their abusive partners. As noted above, a recent study comparing male and female perpetrators' reasons for using violence showed that over two-thirds of male perpetrators reported using violence to dominate, control, or punish. In contrast, two-thirds of the women reported using violence to defend against an attack or retaliate for a previous attack against them (Hamberger *et al.*, 1997). Hence, it is important to assess carefully the function of violence for a particular patient prior to developing conclusions about its meaning.

## CASE 32-2

*D. J., a healthy, active 9-year-old, was spending the beautiful Saturday afternoon at his neighborhood park, hanging out with his friends and watching some older men play basketball. A heated argument broke out on the court, and one of the men involved in the game pulled out a gun. He repeatedly fired the gun, clearing the area around the basketball court. When the violence had subsided, D. J. was found lying in a pool of blood. He was dead, killed by a bullet wound to the head. That evening, some neighborhood leaders called for the closing of that park. The next day, a team of counselors was dispatched to D. J.'s school to talk with his friends and classmates. Many spoke of their fears of being harmed and of not feeling safe anywhere, including their own homes.*

## Family versus Stranger Violence

Although the specific forms of violent behaviors may appear similar when directed toward strangers or family members, there are significant differences between violent crimes involving strangers and violent crimes within the family. These differences may affect how individuals may react and how the system, including healthcare providers, may react.

Contrary to popular belief, most violence occurs between people who know each other, not between strangers. For example, a woman is more likely to be raped by an acquaintance, friend, or partner than by a stranger (American Medical Association, 1992). Child abuse is primarily a problem of parents or caretakers hurting the children under their care. Contrary to the idea that child sexual abuse is perpetrated by strangers, most is perpetrated by family or caretaking adults and older children (Haugaard & Reppucci, 1988). Elder abuse is also more likely to be committed by an adult child than by a stranger (Costa & Anetzberger, 1997).

Whereas stranger violence may damage the notion that the world is basically a safe place, family violence destroys or undermines any sense of safety and trust within life's most intimate relationships. Survivors of stranger violence may be able to avoid the scene of their victimization. They may also be willing to cooperate in criminal justice and prosecution efforts to bring the offender to justice. For victims of family violence, however, leaving the offender or the household may not be an option, at least immediately.

A child victim may tell another parent or adult, only to be met with disbelief or, worse, punishment for "causing trouble." Child victims may be told that if they report the violence, it will be their fault if the offensive family member is incarcerated or put out of the family. Child victims are often threatened with more violence if they disclose the abuse. In addition to being dependent on and frightened of their abuser, child victims may also love the abuser, creating tremendous conflict about disclosing abuse. They may also have been blamed for the abuse, which was characterized by the abuser as "discipline" and "for your own good."

Similarly, victims of elder abuse and partner violence face many obstacles to reporting the violence or leaving the violent offender. These obstacles include financial and emotional dependency, acceptance of blame for the abuse, fear of retribution for efforts to end the abuse, and fear of death at the hands of the offender. Many family violence victims have been threatened with death if the abuse is reported or if they try to leave the perpetrator. Because past threats have been backed up by the offender, the victim may legitimately fear for her life when contemplating leaving. As with child victims, victims of elder and partner violence may love the offender and be hopeful that the violence will end. Sometimes, particularly with elders, physical infirmities preclude the option of leaving an abuser.

Because of the complexities of family violence, it is important to withhold judgment and prescriptive advice prior to conducting a thorough assessment of dangerousness and resources. Providing advice to victims of family violence on the basis of principles appropriate to stranger violence could further victimize the patient, particularly in the area of leaving the offender. Research has shown that the most dangerous time in a victim's life is when she attempts to end the relationship with her abuser (Rasche, 1988). Methods for asking about child maltreatment and partner violence are summarized in Tables 32.1 to 32.3.

**Table 32.1**

Identifying Child Abuse or Neglect: General Signs and Symptoms

1. General signs of distress in a child that warrant further assessment
   - Symptoms of anxiety or depression
   - Social withdrawal
   - Aggressive, mean, or violent behavior toward others
   - Low self-esteem
   - Attention problems, failure to learn, or developmental delay
   - Extreme perfectionism, fearfulness, or intolerance of own mistakes
   - Extreme need for attention
   - Regressive or childlike behavior
   - Inappropriate hygiene
   - Parental child: child takes parental role with siblings or has excessive domestic responsibilities
   - Sudden change in behavior or school performance
   - In late childhood and adolescence: eating disorders; sexually active before age 15, or multiple partners; pregnancy; self-mutilation; attempted suicide; running away
2. Action (when you observe general signs and distress)
   - Interview the parent(s) and child
   - Document in the chart
     S: What the child and parent(s) said. Use quotation marks to document exact words
     O: What behavior, signs, and symptoms you observed
     A: Your assessment of stress-related problems
     P: Describe follow-up plans
   - Schedule follow-up appointments to assess changes over time
   - Refer to a mental health professional with training in child development and request a report
   - Consult schoolteacher or counselor

©B. Ambuel, Family Peace Project, Family & Community Medicine, Medical College of Wisconsin, 210 NW Barstow, #201, Waukesha, Wisc 53188, (414) 548-6903. Reprinted with permission of the author.

**Table 32.2**

Identifying Child Abuse or Neglect: Specific Signs and Symptoms

1. Specific signs and symptoms of child abuse and neglect that warrant action
   - Unusual or suspicious bruises, burns, rectal or genital pain or bleeding, or injury inconsistent with reported event
   - Sexually explicit play with dolls or other children, including play with dolls or other children that illustrates intercourse, oral intercourse, or anal intercouse (distinguish from normal self-exploration and masturbation)
   - Inappropriate touching of other children's private areas (buttocks, genital area)
   - Specific comments or complaints about being maltreated, neglected, or sexually touched
   - Lack of basic needs (e.g., food, clothing, medical and dental care)
   - Grossly inappropriate hygiene
   - A child left unsupervised for long periods of time
   - In your professional opinion, you suspect the child is being abused or neglected
2. Action (when you observe specific signs or abuse or neglect)
   - *Immediately* file a report with child protective service (CPS) and engage your clinic's protocol. Involve parents in filing the report when this does not place the child at risk
   - Hospitalize the child when necessary to treat injuries or place the child in a safe environment
   - Document the nature of injury and observations carefully in the child's chart
     S: What the child and parent(s) said. Use quotation marks to document exact words
     O: What behavior and injuries you observed. Drawings and photographs describe location and quality of injuries. Include a ruler in photos for scale, and victim's face for identity
     A: Your assessment of potential child abuse
     P: Describe and safety and follow-up plans
   - If you are unsure about reporting, consult a trusted colleague, a local expert, or a child abuse caseworker at child protective services. Discuss a hypothetical situation to maintain confidentiality. Trust your own professional judgment
   - Develop a treatment plan for the child and family that engages clinic and community resources

©B. Ambuel, Family Peace Project, Family & Community Medicine, Medical College of Wisconsin, 210 NW Barstow, #201, Waukesha, Wisc 53188, (414) 548-6903. Reprinted with permission of the author.

**Table 32.3**

Screening and Case Finding for Relationship Violence: Summary of Interview Strategies

A. Screening for current partner violence
  - "Are you in any relationships where you are afraid for your personal safety, or where someone is hurting you, threatening you, forcing sexual contact, or trying to control your life?"
B. Screening for past violence
  - "As an adult, have you even been a victim of violence, such as assault or sexual assault?"
  - "Have you ever been in a relationship where your partner hurt you, threatened you, forced sexual contact, or tried to control your life?"
  - "When you were a child or adolescent, did anyone ever physically hurt you, force sexual contact, or hurt you psychologically (for example, by telling you that you were worthless or unwanted)?"
C. Case finding with general signs of distress
  - "In my experience, these types of symptoms are sometimes caused or made worse by stress. Are there any sources of stress in your personal life, family life, or at work?"
  - Screen for current violence (A) and past violence (B)
  - Screen for other causes of distress (e.g., positive and negative life events; family problems; depression or anxiety)
D. Case finding with specific signs of violence
  - "In my experience, this type of injury is sometimes caused by other people's actions. Are you safe? Is anyone hurting or threatening you?"
  - Screen for current violence (A)
E. When you suspect abuse but the patient denies abuse
  - "I'm concerned about your safety and would like to tell you about several community resources you can use if you ever need them."
  - Describe resources, offer follow-up, and document as in protocol
  - Do not confront or challenge the patient

©B. Ambuel and L.K Hamberger, Family Peace Project, Family & Community Medicine, Medical College of Wisconsin, 210 NW Barstow, #201, Waukesha, Wisc 53188, (414) 548-6903. Reprinted with permission of the authors.

# Prevalence of Violence in Society

Violence is difficult to measure. Official statistics gathered through government agencies often use narrow definitions of violence and provide information only on cases brought to the attention of authorities (Gaquin, 1977–78). Thus, such studies underestimate true incidence and prevalence rates. Others utilizing random samples recruited from the community studies (e.g., Straus & Gelles, 1986) may be more representative but may also suffer from underreporting as survey participants may not want to report that they have been victimized or have perpetrated violence. Violence is also difficult to define, adding to reporting difficulties. In the field of child sexual abuse, for example, there is wide agreement that forced intercourse constitutes abuse. On the other hand, there may be less agreement about whether a parent taking nude photographs of his children constitutes abuse.

## Child Physical and Sexual Abuse

Based on national surveys, 11% of children are physically assaulted by a parent each year. Such assaults include kicking, biting, hitting, or more severe physical violence (Gelles & Straus, 1988). Further, 2% of children are estimated to experience severe physical assault by a parent—beating, striking with an object, threatening, or assaulting with a weapon (Gelles & Straus, 1988). Based on retrospective studies with adults, it is estimated that at least 20% of girls and 5 to 10% of boys experience sexual abuse before age 18 (Finkelhor, 1994).

## Adolescent Violence

Adolescents are exposed to more violence in the home, in the neighborhood, and at school than any other age group in our society. Exposure to violence is high for girls and boys from all income and racial/ethnic groups. Singer *et al.* (1994) found that between 27 and 56% of high school students reported being slapped, hit, or punched at home in the past year, 14 to 44% reported being slapped, punched, or hit at school, and 3 to 10% beaten or mugged at school. Boys reported higher rates of physical assault in their neighborhood and at school, while girls reported higher rates of sexual assault and higher rates of physical assault at home. In a nationwide survey of high school youth, 37% reported being involved in a physical fight in the past 12 months, and 3.5% reported being injured.

## Partner Violence

Each year about 16% of married women are assaulted by their husbands (Straus & Gelles, 1986; Straus *et al.*, 1980). Higher rates have been found among nonmarried, dating couples (Hamberger & Ambuel, 1998). Although gay and lesbian couples have been more difficult to study, available data suggest rates of violence among gay and lesbian couples are about the same as those for heterosexuals (Island & Letellier, 1991).

## Elder Abuse

Sparse data suggest that each year between 300,000 and 1.5 million elders are abused. The most common form of elder abuse is failure of the family or significant support group to provide needed support to elders who stop caring for themselves (Tatara, 1993).

## Sexual Assault

Sexual assault of women is believed to be a highly underreported form of violence. Official FBI statistics show that, in 1988, over 92,000 rapes were reported to police, but experts estimate that 90% of sexual assaults go unreported (Bryant, 1990). Epidemiological studies indicate that about 20% of adult women and 15% of college women report being sexually assaulted during their lifetime (Koss, 1993). Rates of sexual assault are believed to be higher among women of color (Koss, 1993).

## Firearm Violence

Violence involving firearms deserves special attention because firearms are such a lethal mechanism of injury. Callahan and Rivara (1992) found that 33% of high school handgun owners reported having shot at someone. Over 9% of female students reported involvement of firearms in the suicide or homicide of family members. Six percent of male high school students reported carrying a gun to school at some time. Among urban youth, the firearm-related homicide rate was 13.7 per 100,000. Among rural youth, the firearm homicide rate was 2.9 per 100,000 (Fingerhut *et al.*, 1992). Black youths had the highest rates of death from firearms. Further, Fingerhut *et al.* found that between 1979 and 1987 rates of firearm homicides increased dramatically. In contrast, during the same time period non-firearm-related homicides decreased or remained stable. Most intentional firearm violence occurs between people who know each other (Kellerman *et al.*, 1993) or is self-inflicted (Goldberg, 1997). In addition, for every firearm homicide, there are approximately 7.5 nonfatal firearm-related injuries (Rice & McKenzie, 1989).

## Witnessing Violence

Although physical violence directly claims many victims, there are also many indirect victims. Indirect victims are those who have witnessed violence or who are somehow associated with victims of violence. Such individuals include child observers of parental violence, relatives of violence and homicide victims, or victims of other forms of violence. According to the American Psychological Association (1993), for example, 73% of eighth-graders surveyed in Chicago had seen someone shot, stabbed, robbed, or killed. Untold thousands of children observe parental violence. Such witnessing of violence can have profound effects on the mental well-being of the observer, including posttraumatic stress (Rossman *et al.*, 1997).

# Prevalence of Patients Who Have Experienced Violence in Medical Settings

Rates of victimization among patients attending hospital emergency rooms and outpatient primary care and specialty clinics vary. Koss *et al.* (1991) found that 57% of women attending a health maintenance organization had been victims of crime, including rape, physical assault, and noncontact crimes. Greenwood *et al.* (1990) found that 5% of male and female patients at a multispecialty clinic reported having been physically abused as children. Among female patients, 16.9% reported child sexual abuse. No men reported childhood sexual abuse. Drossman *et al.* (1990) studied violence in the backgrounds of women attending a gastrointestinal disorders clinic. The authors found that 44% of the women reported physical or sexual abuse in either childhood or adulthood. Women are frequently victims of partner violence during pregnancy. One study (Hillard, 1985) found that 10.9% of women in an obstetrical clinic reported being battered. Helton *et al.* (1987) observed violence occurring in the lives of 8% of women during their pregnancy. In a family practice setting, it was found that about 23% of women reported being assaulted by a partner in the past year. Nearly 40% reported assault at some time in a relationship during their adult life (Hamberger *et al.*, 1992; Johnson & Elliott, 1997).

There is little question that violence is a prevalent reality in the United States. Victims and perpetrators of violence are all around us, both in our communities and in our healthcare settings. In addition to routine health concerns, they seek medical treatment for injuries sustained from violence and for stress-related health concerns that follow victimization. Further, victims also often carry the emotional scars of violence, both directly experienced and observed, in other areas of their lives. Hence, physicians can expect to encounter numerous victims and perpetrators of violence in their practice.

Patients are not the only victims or survivors of violence. Physicians themselves may suffer the burdens of violence in their own lives. These personal experiences and knowledge can affect the attitudes and practices of physicians in treating victims and perpetrators. Case 32-3 illustrates physician attitudes toward a pregnant woman with signs of abuse.

## CASE 32-3

*Judy, 23 years old, came to the clinic for her first OB visit. She has two other children with Bill, her partner for 5 years. While taking her vital signs, the nurse noticed a handprint bruise on her right bicep. She subsequently notified the physician of her concern that Judy might have been "roughed up" by someone. After the examination, the following exchange took place:*

DOCTOR: *How are things going with Bill?*
JUDY: *Good.*
DOCTOR: *How does he feel about the pregnancy?*
JUDY: *He's not real excited.*
DOCTOR: *Oh, why is that?*
JUDY: *He blames me for getting pregnant.*
DOCTOR: *Well, just tell him it takes two to tango!*
JUDY: *I'll say!*
DOCTOR: *How did you get that bruise on your right arm?*
JUDY: *We tangoed the other night.*
DOCTOR: *Well, you've got to be careful now. After all, you're going to have a baby. We'll see you next month.*

## PHYSICIANS' ATTITUDES TOWARD VICTIMS AND PERPETRATORS OF VIOLENCE

In Case 32-3, Judy provided two very powerful signs that she might be battered—the bruise and the "tango" quip—yet the physician never responded directly to these signs. When the opportunity presented itself, Judy instead got a patronizing lecture. Why didn't the physician delve more deeply into the violence in Judy's life?

First, it is important to know that Judy is not alone in not being asked about violence by her physician. Hamberger *et al.* (1992) found that only 1.7% of women in a family practice center were asked by their physician about violence. Other studies have found similar low physician inquiry rates in ambulatory settings (Rath *et al.*, 1989) and emergency settings (Stark *et al.*, 1979).

Common reasons for not asking about violence even when clear indications of violence are evident include fear of being overwhelmed with what they may be told. In addition, not having enough time to deal with a victim in crisis is another reason frequently given for not asking about violence. Some physicians do not believe that domestic violence is a true "medical" issue. Other physicians express some desire to ask about violence but do not do so because of lack of knowledge of subsequent steps to take if battering is disclosed. Still others believe that there are no victims or perpetrators of partner violence in their practices. Finally, in our experience, many physicians and other healthcare professionals do not know how to ask about violence, or else fear angering their patients for being "too intrusive." (Sugg & Innui, 1992).

## CASE 32-4

*Jill came to her physician's office because of right rib pain. She told the physician that her husband had punched her several times three nights ago and might have cracked her ribs. The physician offhandedly mentioned that she "should either take up boxing or else learn to be a better wife." Jill felt humiliated and decided it was simply not safe to talk about violence with a physician.*

## CASE 32-5

*Sue had a slightly different experience. After telling her physician about being battered, she initially felt supported by his empathy. Some time after Sue left the office, the physician called Sue's husband and "counseled" him to stop hurting her. Three days later, she came into the emergency room with a broken nose. Sue's husband punished her for telling the physician.*

## Countertherapeutic Reactions to Victimization

In Case 32-3, the physician felt uncomfortable and chose to avoid the issue by making an inappropriate comment rather than asking direct questions to gather more information. Cases 32-4 and 32-5 illustrate inappropriate and detrimental actions. Other inappropriate actions include medically treating symptoms without working to end the violence. Examples include medicating anxiety or depression symptoms or suturing a wound, but failing to provide resource information or to conduct safety planning.

## CASE 32-6

*Jackson is a 25-year-old steelworker who came to the clinic for evaluation of a back injury. The physician noticed alcohol on his breath, so as part of the evaluation, alcohol abuse was also assessed. Because the physician had read that alcohol abuse is often associated with domestic violence, the following exchange took place:*

DOCTOR: *How does your drinking affect your relationship with Barb [his wife]?*
JACKSON: *Well, she gets on my case when I've had a few, sometimes.*
DOCTOR: *When she gets on your case, how do you react?*
JACKSON: *It depends. If I get tired of it and don't want to hear any more of her lip, I might let her know.*

DOCTOR: *Do you ever let her know by, say, yelling at her?*

JACKSON: *Sometimes. After all, if she yells at me, I can yell at her, can't I?*

DOCTOR: *I suppose we all need a good scolding now and then. Tell me, do you ever lay a hand on her when you two are arguing?*

JACKSON: *Sometimes she gets right up in my face or stands in my way when I want to leave, so I have to move her out of the way.*

DOCTOR: *Well, it's easy to see why you'd get upset with someone getting in your space during a dispute.*

## Perpetrators

As with victims of violence, perpetrators often remain invisible in medical settings. Sometimes physicians collude with perpetrators by providing tacit support for the violence, as in Case 32-6. Although reports of violence were elicited, the physician failed to respond appropriately to the findings. Twice the physician responded to reports of abusive behavior with "understanding" and supportive comments, rather than therapeutically confronting the violence. To Jackson's report of yelling at his partner, the physician acknowledged the occasional need for a "scolding." Later, in response to Jackson's report of using physical force, the physician excused Jackson for being upset, did not mention his use of force, and placed responsibility for Jackson's behavior on his partner for "getting in [his] space." Rather than therapeutically confronting Jackson's aggressive and controlling behavior, the physician's actions actually provided Jackson emotional support and justification. Hence, the violence was minimized as the primary problem, and his partner's "negative" behavior became the focus and reason for Jackson's aggression.

Sometimes failure to confront violence results from fear that such confrontation might result in aggression from the patient. Violence evokes painful and fearful images, even among healthcare providers. The thought of confronting someone who batters his partner or is violent on the street may be accompanied by fears that the healthcare provider will also be assaulted. A natural defense against such fear is to avoid asking about or confronting a patient with the wrongfulness of violent behavior. However, in the authors' experience in a typical outpatient setting with nondelusional or nonpsychotic patients, the risk of assault is low.

Still other inappropriate physician responses include becoming overly moralistic or righteously indignant with a perpetrator. Violence as a social problem is rightly viewed as an evil that destroys families and individual lives. Further, all concerned citizens should be angry about it and work to end violence. However, angry or moralistic pronouncements to an offending patient will usually bring denial, loss from the practice, and possible renewed violence toward the partner. A more appropriate and effective approach is to deal with violence issues in a matter-of-fact, collaborative, and concerned manner. The concern is for all involved,

---

### COMMUNITY-BASED ACTIVITY

*You can learn a great deal about violence and community efforts to prevent and end it by visiting agencies that work in the field, as well as those affected by the violence.*

*Arrange to visit a shelter for battered women or a rape crisis center.*

*Interview agency staff, asking about the scope of their work. Ask how clients access their services. Inquire about their relationship with other agencies charged with ending violence. What are their ideas about the physician's role in ending violence?*

*If possible, ask permission to interview clients of the agency. Listen to their stories of how violence has affected their lives, including health. Determine what struggles and barriers they faced obtaining help. How did they overcome the barriers?*

*Identify the types of physician behaviors that facilitate effective interventions with patients affected by violence. Identify negative and ineffective physician behaviors and attitudes.*

---

including the perpetrator, his partner, and his children. By getting a perpetrator to realize the damage he does to his entire family, he is more likely to consider the need to change. By helping a perpetrator focus on his need to change, the physician can motivate him and provide appropriate referral information for abuse abatement counseling (Chelmowski & Hamberger, 1994).

## CASE 32-7

*Jimmy is 19 years old. He has been a member of the Scorpions, a street gang, for as long as he can remember. His parents were never married, and Jimmy can't remember the last time he saw his father, who is in prison for armed robbery. Jimmy had three older brothers, but the next oldest was killed in a gang-related shooting 3 years ago. Jimmy never completed the eighth grade because of fighting and truancy. Since that time he has survived on the streets, hustling odd jobs, selling drugs, and assaulting people for pay.*

*Tonight, Jimmy comes to the emergency room with a gunshot wound that shattered his lower spine, and a bullet that penetrated his left brain. He was shot when he and his friends encountered a rival gang in an area on the border of their turf. Three years ago, Jimmy sustained a flesh wound in another fight. He bragged that he was invincible. Tonight's wound will leave him paralyzed. In addition to being confined to a wheelchair, he will experience chronic pain and require the use of a colostomy bag. His head wound will result in loss of use of his right arm and compromise visual–spatial abilities. He will require about a year to rehabilitate, and another 6 months for assisted independent living.*

## WHY IS VIOLENCE A HEALTH PROBLEM?

It is clear that violence is pervasive and epidemic. Moreover, no group is immune from violence. Research indicates that violence is responsible for both medical and emotional injuries (Saltzman *et al.*, 1992) and death (Fingerhut *et al.*, 1992). Therefore, physicians and other healthcare providers have begun to consider violence to be a health problem that is a significant cause of morbidity and mortality among their patients, as illustrated in Case 32-7.

Throughout this ordeal, Jimmy in Case 32-7 will require the services of a neurosurgeon, neurologist, internist, specialized nursing staff, medical assistants and home health aides, rehabilitation psychologists, transportation aids, and vocational rehabilitation specialists. Following rehabilitation, Jimmy will require lifetime care of his colostomy, medication and rehabilitation for chronic pain, and disability support because of his limited prospects for vocational rehabilitation. He is at risk of infections, decubitus ulcers, drug addiction (to pain medications), depression, and numerous other complications secondary to the paralysis and brain injury. Violence, in all its forms, affects both the medical and emotional status of those who are victimized. Violence also affects medical system utilization. Koss *et al.* (1990) also found that female violence victims sought healthcare services about twice as frequently as nonvictimized women. In addition, Bergman and Brismar (1991) found that, compared with a matched group of nonbattered women, battered women were admitted to the hospital significantly more often for both trauma and nontrauma-related surgery, medical problems, miscarriage and elective abortion, alcohol and drug abuse, and psychiatric problems. In the outpatient setting, Johnson and Elliott (1997) found that battered women were significantly less likely than nonbattered women to attend the clinic for routine health maintenance, but did attend significantly more often for episodic care. In addition, Wisner *et al.* (1999) studied the differential annual healthcare costs for battered versus nonbattered women in a managed healthcare plan. The research showed that, compared with nonbattered women, healthcare costs for battered women totaled $1,775 more per year. Hence, violence has a significant effect on medical care costs as well as health and quality of life.

These effects of violence accrue not only to those directly victimized, but also to the patient's family. For example, Jimmy's baby daughter will miss out on many activities that she might otherwise have experienced with her father. Although he receives disability checks, Jimmy has limited earning potential. Society loses out because of Jimmy's injury, as a result of his loss of productivity, and the demands his disabilities place on the healthcare and social welfare systems.

---

## CASE 32-8

*Bill and Joy were high school sweethearts. They have been married for 8 years and have three children, aged 2, 3, and 7. Bill works as a sales representative for a sporting goods wholesaler. Joy is a homemaker. After they married, Bill insisted that Joy stay home and "keep the home fires burning." He frequently stated proudly that Joy would "never have to work as long as he was the man of the house." She has no marketable job skills.*

*Shortly after marriage, Bill punched Joy in the nose and ribs during an argument. She called the police, but they did not arrest Bill, stating that if Joy wanted to press charges, she would have to go down to the courthouse the next day to press charges herself. She decided against pressing charges this time but brought the matter to the attention of her mother during a get-together a week later. Her mother instructed Joy not to bother her with such complaints, since Joy "made her bed and now she has to lie in it."*

*Three months later, Bill pulled Joy's hair, kicked her in the leg, and threw her onto the floor. This time, Joy went to the DA's office to press charges, just as the police instructed her. The assistant DA who took her complaint told Joy that she had better not "crap out" on him by dropping charges, like so many battered women do.*

*One year later, following another beating in which Bill broke Joy's nose, she went to the emergency room for medical attention. The ER physician expressed indignation that "couples these days can't seem to solve their problems without violence." He further advised her to get away from Bill, if she knew what was good for her.*

*Five months later, Bill blackened both of Joy's eyes. She went to speak with her pastor about the abuse. The pastor encouraged her to keep the faith, pray for the strength to forgive her husband, and try to be the best wife and mother she could.*

*One year later, Joy did attempt to leave Bill. Because all of the assets were in his name, however, she was unable to take more than the weekly $75 grocery money with her. She applied for food stamps and welfare benefits but because she was still married and the family income was too high, she didn't qualify for assistance. She did not have a work history or job skills to qualify for any but the most basic employment—insufficient to support her and her children.*

*Joy returned home and 2 months later suffered a back injury after Bill threw her to the floor. The examining physician was familiar with her case and that she had left Bill before, only to return. The physician concluded that she had a masochistic personality and recorded this in her chart. There was no discussion about safety planning or provision of information about battered women's advocacy services. Joy returned home once again.*

---

# WHY DOES THE PROBLEM EXIST?

The problem of violence is deep and multifaceted, supported by social structures, practices, and beliefs that value violence or promote the oppression of certain groups. Beliefs devaluing people of a given age, sex, race, economic class, or sexual orientation are used to justify or tolerate violence toward individual members of those groups. Violence is learned at home, in the neighborhood, and through the media. It seems that many of us view violence as "normal" even as we speak against it. Solving—or even mitigating—the problem calls for complex and pervasive changes.

In Case 32-8, Bill used violence with impunity because no one held him responsible for the violence or for stopping it. Conversely, Joy received the message that the violence was her responsibility wherever she sought help: from her family, the criminal justice system, the medical establishment, her church, and the social welfare system.

Other factors contributing to the pervasiveness of violence in U.S. society are television, readily available handguns, high unemployment of young minority men, economically depressed and physically deteriorating cities, and decreased resources for coping and conflict resolution.

## Societal Interventions

In-depth discussion of social interventions needed to stop violence is outside the scope of this chapter. However, physicians and other healthcare providers have a vested interest in community responses to the problems of violence. The medical system is one of the front lines of violence intervention, in the form of

---

### INTERNET RESOURCES ON VIOLENCE PREVENTION

*The Family Peace Project, http://www.family.mcw.edu/FamilyPeaceProject.htm*
*Family violence prevention resources for healthcare professionals including clinical protocols, a fact sheet, and a discussion forum.*

*A Systematic Approach to Partner Violence in Health Care Lecture, http://www.medinfo. ufl.edu/cme/grounds/violence/*
*A 1-hour CME lecture by Bruce Ambuel, PhD, offered via the University of Florida Medical School CME Web site.*

*Kathy's page, http://www.mcs.net/%7Ekathyw/abuse.html*

*Minnesota Center Against Violence and Abuse, http://www.mincava.umn.edu/*
*This site offers extensive resources for the prevention of violence and abuse, and the promotion of peace.*

*The Child Abuse Prevention Network, Cornell University, http://child-abuse.com*
*An initiative of Family Life Development Center at Cornell University and sponsored by LifeNET, Inc. The Child Abuse Prevention Network is dedicated to enhancing Internet resources for the prevention of child abuse and neglect, and reducing the negative conditions in the family and the community that lead to child maltreatment.*

*The Family Violence Prevention Fund, http://www.fvpf.org/*
*The FVPF is a national nonprofit organization that focuses on domestic violence education, prevention, and public policy reform. This Web organization offers excellent resources for healthcare professionals and the general public.*

*The US Department of Justice, Bureau of Justice Statistics, http://www.ojp.usdoj.gov/bjs/ welcome.html*
*This Bureau of Justice Statistics offers many government reports on the incidence and prevalence of various types of violence. Many reports are available online.*

*The US Violence Against Women Office, http://www.ojp.usdoj.gov/vawgo/*
*Offers many resources on violence against women, including facts and figures, grant information, and other government resources.*

*The US Centers for Disease Control and Prevention, http://www.cdc.gov/*
*Offers information on family violence prevention programs, research grants, and other resources.*

*The American Medical Association, http://www.ama-assn.org/*
*Offers a variety of resources on violence prevention for physicians.*

*The American Medical Women's Association, http://www.amwa-doc.org/*
*Provides a variety of resources for health professionals including an online course on partner violence.*

*The American Psychological Association, http://www.apa.org/*
*Information and resources for violence prevention within families and communities.*

*Physicians for a Violence Free Society, http://www.pvs.org/*
*Many resources on violence prevention, including a course on how physicians should document intentional injury.*

---

trauma and emergency medicine. Thus, healthcare providers often begin the process of providing preventive care or connecting patients to other support services. Screening for potential victims, educating all patients about ways to avoid violence, providing safe places for people fleeing or fearing violence, and supporting perpetrators to find nonviolent ways of behaving are all areas in which physicians can exert far more impact than they may be having currently.

But the medical system is only one point in a web of services and interventions. Also essential are strengthening:

- Criminal justice system policies that hold offenders responsible, including arrest, prosecution, and appropriate penalties
- Social service systems that effectively advocate for victims and provide necessary services and benefits
- Community programs such as caregiver respite services, recreational programs, job and skills training, mentoring, and conflict resolution
- Religious/spiritual support through integration with churches to provide healing, intervention with at-risk individuals, and guidance along constructive paths
- School and other educational programming around prevention and intervention, including respectful conflict containment, peer mediation, and identification of abused or neglected children.

## CASE 32-9

*Sue is a 16-year-old high school sophomore who comes to the clinic for her basketball athletic physical. Her family is well known to clinic physicians. Her father is an alcoholic and her mother has struggled with depression for several years. There has been some concern that Sue's father abused her mother, but nothing was ever confirmed. Last year, Sue came to the emergency room for acute alcohol intoxication and was encouraged to see a counselor. She comments to the physician that, for the past 6 months, she has been dating Chuck. She likes him, but feels that he is too possessive and won't give her any space. She denies that she is sexually active but reports that Chuck has been putting heavy pressure on her lately.*

## CASE 32-10

*Bill is a 76-year-old widower who lives with his 52-year-old unmarried son, Jake. Bill has been coming to the clinic for several years for monitoring of his heart medication and arthritis. Jake, an unemployed factory worker, usually brings Bill and accompanies him to the examination. Today, Bill has several bruises on his right arm and shoulder. When asked how it happened, Jake answered that he fell in the garage. The physician believes that the explanation for the injury is not consistent with the pattern of bruising. Furthermore, there were several other bruises in various stages of healing on other parts of Bill's body.*

## CASE 32-11

*Dr. Smith presented a comprehensive training program to third-year medical students on identification, dynamics, and help for victims of family violence. In addition to lecture, Dr. Smith showed slides depicting graphic photographs of abuse injuries for children, adults, and elders. The session was further punctuated by the stories of violence, oppression, and terror, as well as escape from violence provided by a panel of survivors. Finally, the professor completed the session by having the students role-play identifying and helping family violence victims in healthcare settings. Students took turns playing the roles of victims and physicians. Immediately after the session, Susan, a student in the class, met with Dr. Smith. She was angry with him and challenged "You had no right to make me do this!" Susan went on to explain that, as a child, she was abused and battered. She worked hard to put it all behind her, and did not want to ever have to think of abuse issues again. Susan stated she felt blindsided by the program presentation, did not feel she had the option to not participate, and was especially distressed by the graphic pictures of abuse-related injuries. Another student, Jill, came into the professor's office a day later. Jill stated "I'm living in an abusive relationship. That program opened my eyes. But, I don't know what to do, and since the program, I've been having trouble concentrating and sleeping, and I'm afraid my grades will suffer." That same day, John, who also had participated in the domestic violence training, called the professor and reported "I really think the program was helpful and important. But, my problem is that I have a good friend here at the medical school who is involved with a guy who I think is hurting her. I'm not sure what to do." Later that day, Bill made an appointment with Dr. Smith to offer that, as a child, he had witnessed his father beat his mother severely and regularly. Though Bill had never assaulted an intimate partner, he frequently wondered, as a physician, if he would be able to effectively help other victims.*

# WHAT PHYSICIANS CAN DO: PREVENTION AND INTERVENTION

Sue's case, 32-9, presents many opportunities for preventive action. First, since athletic physicals are the primary types of visits for healthy adolescents, the setting alone provides an opportunity to ask about Sue's concerns for her safety, at home, in her relationship with Chuck, and at school. Although Sue might deny any concerns at present, she will appreciate being asked and will identify the physician's office as a resource for safety information if she ever needs it. Her decision-making about sex with Chuck can be validated and reinforced. She can be asked about her drinking as it relates to other high-risk activities (violence, sexual activity), and reinforced for making healthy choices in that part of her life as well. Finally, the physician may consider talking with Sue's mother during her next appointment about safety in the home.

In Case 32-10, the physician's role is intervention rather than prevention. Intervention first involves separating Bill and Jake and talking to Bill alone with reassurances that his disclosures are confidential. If there are mandatory reporting laws for elder abuse, these must be acknowledged and complied with. In every case, such disclosure should be done in collaboration with the elder, particularly if he is competent. Social service resources for assisting elder victims and families or caregiver perpetrators should be accessed. Once the abuse is acknowledged and out in the open, family-level interventions may be feasible, if all members are amenable and the perpetrator acknowledges the abuse. Part of the intervention might be to help Jake find respite care for Bill to reduce the pressure and isolation Jake feels in caring full-time for his father with no outside help. If Jake has a drinking problem, alcohol abuse counseling can also be offered. If Bill is competent to handle his own finances, he can be given anticipatory guidance about selecting an appropriate guardian and durable power of attorney, if Jake is not appropriate for the task. The physician can also advocate for Bill with social agencies to ensure that he receives adequate services to enable independent living for as long as he is able and willing. Such resources include visiting nurses, home health aides, senior center accessibility, mobile meals, and so on. Speaking out on behalf of elderly citizens to community groups, legislators, and policy-makers is another way physicians can intervene on a social level.

Case 32-11 illustrates that teaching medical students about partner and other forms of family violence is not always a straightforward, intellectual process. Dr. Smith was at first confused by his students' reactions. Other students gave him very enthusiastic reactions to his training program. On further reflection, Dr. Smith realized that he had an obligation as an educator to listen carefully and validate Susan's experiences. He also went to the literature and found additional evidence for the lessons he had already learned from his students. Physicians and medical students themselves may suffer the burdens of violence in their lives. Three studies (Ambuel *et al.*, 1997a; Cullinane *et al.*, 1997; deLahunta & Tulsky, 1996) of medical students show that

# SAFETY PLAN TIPS

*Healthcare providers should be prepared to help patients who are victims of violence develop a safety plan. A safety plan is a plan of action, thought out in advance, to help the victim avoid or escape future violence. Eight areas of safety should be considered when beginning to develop a safety plan. Patients can be referred to domestic violence programs for complete, in-depth safety planning.*

1. *Open the discussion.*
   - *Express concern for your patient's safety and a desire to help them develop options for safety planning.*
     - *"I'm concerned for your future safety. If you find yourself in a situation in the near future where you could be harmed, what would you do? Where would you go? How would you get there? Let's talk about that."*
2. *Safety in explosive situations.*
   - *Help the patient identify danger signals*
     - *Situational cues such as specific rooms or known dangerous places*
     - *The offender's body language, words, and mood states associated with violence*
     - *The patient's own internal cues of danger: feelings of tension or fear, tightening of neck muscles, reddening or warming of face*
     - *Interpersonal danger cues such as arguments about specific issues*
   - *Help the patient develop strategies for managing explosive situations*
   - *Develop alternative, immediate escape routes*
   - *Have the patient develop a mental map of her residence and memorize alternative escape routes*
   - *Discuss strategies for contacting help.*
   - *Discuss 911*
   - *Discuss enlisting the aid of children or signaling neighbors to call 911 in the event of new violence.*
3. *General safety in the home.*
   - *Have patient rehearse multiple escape routes from different areas or rooms of the residence*
   - *Encourage patients to position themselves, during threatening interactions, as close to doors or phones as possible.*
   - *Remind patients that bathrooms and bedrooms are dangerous because they have only one exit. Kitchens are dangerous because they contain knives and other dangerous objects*
4. *Timing of escape*
   - *Discourage the patient from telling the abusive partner of her intention to leave; this increases her danger*
   - *Discuss timing of escape so that it can occur in the abuser's absence*
5. *Identify possible and feasible shelter resources*
   - *Family and friends*
   - *Community-based shelter services*
   - *Community-based nonshelter services*
6. *Safety in public and at work*
   - *Help patient identify alternate routes to and from work*
   - *Develop work-based safety plans, including the management of harassing phone calls and managing safety in the actual workplace from unwanted intrusions*
   - *Safety in the parking lot*
   - *Develop strategies for managing "chance" encounters with the abuser in public places such as restaurants or shopping areas*
7. *Safety with temporary restraining orders*
   - *Encourage patient to call police whenever the restraining order is violated*
   - *Encourage patient to maintain possession of the restraining order at all times*
   - *Encourage patient to give trusted friends or family members copies of the order*
8. *Develop an "escape bag"*

## ITEMS TO PLACE IN AN "ESCAPE BAG"

*Sometimes battered victims must leave home with little more than the clothes on their backs. Victims of violence should keep ready a bag or small suitcase of important items to take when escaping an abusive environment. The following items should be in the bag.*

*Legal Papers*
   *Restraining order*
   *Divorce papers*
   *Lease, rental agreement and/or house deed*
   *Insurance and automobile registration papers*
   *Children's birth certificates and school records*
   *Custody papers*
   *Work permits, green card, visa, passport*
*Financial Records*
   *Bank account numbers and/or books*
   *Telephone calling card*
   *Credit cards and/or cash*

*Identification*
   *Social Security card*
   *Personal and children's birth certificates*
   *Baptismal record*
   *Driver's license*
*Miscellaneous*
   *Jewelry*
   *Address book*
   *Clothes for self and the children*
   *Children's favorite toys, blankets, pillows*
   *Medications*
   *Important keys*
   *Pictures*
   *Toiletries/diapers*

---

between 13 and 30% have experienced child physical or sexual abuse, 13 to 23% have experienced partner violence, and 7 to 10% have been sexually assaulted as an adult. Medical students' lifetime prevalence for any type of severe interpersonal violence ranged from 24 to 53%. Personal experience and knowledge can affect a physician's work with victims and perpetrators. In some cases, personal experience may be a valuable resource that enhances a medical student's or physician's understanding. However, some medical students and physicians experience difficulty working with patients who are victims of violence. Ambuel *et al.* (1997) found that students who have experienced more types of severe violence have more symptoms of depression and anticipate more difficulty working effectively with patients who are victims of violence.

Instructors must be mindful of the fact that violence affects the lives of persons across all educational and socioeconomic strata. Moreover, any given learner's response to violence education is variable and highly personal. One way to guard against surprises is to acknowledge at the outset of training sessions, the potentially upsetting nature of the issues to be discussed and practiced. The instructor can also inform students of available support services for those who experience upset, including personal discussion and debriefing with the instructor, and giving students the option to fulfill course requirements through alternative means.

## CONCLUSION

Violence is a complex phenomenon that includes psychosocial, political, and medical issues. Traditionally, medical practitioners have treated primarily the biomedical sequelae of violence. The reluctance to intervene at psychosocial and political levels has been rooted in traditions that emphasize pathophysiology and biophysical mechanics of injury and rehabilitation. Etiology of violence-produced injuries has often been ignored or dismissed as outside the domain of "true" medical practice (Warshaw & Poirier, 1991). As a result, injuries have been examined outside the context of their cause. Further, medical treatments have been administered and documented in ways that dissociate the injuries from the violence that caused them.

More recently, epidemiological surveys have begun to illuminate the high incidence and prevalence of many forms of violence. These studies demonstrate that violence is not rare or aberrant in our society but is a major epidemic with profound implications for the well-being of our society. Medical implications include

## POPULAR FILMS

*A number of popular films explore the dynamics and consequences of family violence. After reading this chapter, you may be interested in viewing some of them.*

*Donner, Richard (Director). (1992).* Radio Flyer. *Running time: 114 minutes.*
*Figgis, Mike (Director). (1986).* Leaving Las Vegas. *Running time: 111 minutes.*
*Gibson, Brian (Director). (1993).* What's Love Got To Do With It? *Running time: 118 minutes.*
*Greenwald, Robert (Director).(1984).* The Burning Bed. *Running time: 95 minutes.*
*Hackford, Taylor (Director). (1995)* Dolores Claiborne. *Running time: 131 minutes.*
*Kaplin, Jonathon (Director). (1988).* The Accused. *Running time: 110 minutes*
*Reiner, Rob (Director). (1990).* Misery. *Running time: 107 minutes.*
*Rubin, Joseph (Director). (1991).* Sleeping with the Enemy. *Running time: 99 minutes.*
*Scorcese, Martin (Director). (1986).* Casino. *Running time: 179 minutes.*
*Spielberg, Steven (Director). (1985).* The Color Purple. *Running time: 154 minutes.*
*Streisand, Barbra (Director). (1991).* Prince of Tides. *Running time: 132 minutes.*
*Young, Robert M. (Director). (1986).* Extremities. *Running time: 89 minutes.*
*Zemeckis, Robert (Director). (1994).* Forrest Gump. *Running time: 142 minutes.*

morbidity and mortality, which have personal, familial, and communitywide implications. These include decreased quality of life, increased stress, and economic factors such as loss of productivity, costs of medical treatment, and costs for law enforcement and justice-making.

Increased attention to violence as a social problem allows the development of a public health perspective and thus a role for the practicing physician (Ambuel *et al.*, 1997b). On the level of the patient and family, physicians can make violence screening a routine practice. Given the prevalence of violence in our society, there is little doubt that such screening will prove beneficial. Interventions include empathic and supportive listening and providing information about violence risks and resources for help. Intervention also includes appropriate follow-up with patients around violence issues and documentation.

Physicians can and should become involved in community and societal-level violence prevention initiatives. Such initiatives include community task forces on violence prevention and setting policy to prevent violence. One model of such an initiative is the Family Peace Project (Ambuel *et al.*, 1997b). The Family Peace Project is an interdisciplinary initiative to provide healthcare professionals with the knowledge, skills, and attitudes to work with patients who are struggling with violence issues. The Project provides intensive didactic training, which includes direct contact with victim survivors and various agencies that deliver services to victims and perpetrators of violence. Physicians bring to such projects expertise and credibility as community leaders. These contributions facilitate violence prevention efforts to enhance safety for vulnerable societal members.

## CASES FOR DISCUSSION

## CASE 1

*John is a 22-year-old drywall contractor who is coming to the office for referral for an alcohol assessment. He has a number of tattoos, including the letters L-O-V-E on his right fingers and H-A-T-E on his left fingers. He wears a large knife on his belt. His attire is consistent with someone who belongs to a motorcycle club. While giving him a "once over" the physician notices that the knuckles of both hands are scraped and scabbed. He makes numerous references to "partying" and "rock 'n rolling" in bars and with his "old lady."*

1. Has John given any hints that he may be involved in violent behavior? Explain.
2. How would you ask about John's use of violence?
3. How would John's cultural context support his use of violence?
4. What community resources might be helpful to John?

## CASE 2

Jenny is a 24-year-old single mother who is bringing her 13-month-old son, Jason, for a well-child check. Jenny lives with her mother and works as a waitress at the local truck stop. Jason's father is out of the picture, providing no support or visitation. During the exam, Jenny begins to talk about how Jason frequently "drives me nuts" with his "bad behavior." She reports feeling extremely tense during those episodes and copes by screaming at him and locking him in his room. Her mother, who is divorced, works and is reluctant to use her spare time watching Jason since she feels she is helpful enough by giving Jenny and Jason a place to live. As Jenny talks about her stress she begins to cry and states "I hope I don't end up doing to Jason what my mother did to me."

1. Should this mother be reported to Child Protective Services? Why or why not?
2. What community supports are needed to help Jenny cope with her situation?
3. What family interventions would facilitate Jenny's efforts to cope?
4. How would you ask Jenny about possible abuse of Jason?

## CASE 3

Marie is 40 years old and is seeking medicine for "stress." She describes symptoms of anxiety that she relates to problems at work and at home. She relates that she and her husband argue a lot about sex and that he frequently calls her "frigid." These arguments last into the night, resulting in fatigue and reduced job performance the next day. In describing the problem briefly, Marie notes that sex is painful and that her husband criticizes her for not wanting sex. She adds that he states, "I don't care if you want it or not, I'm just gonna take it!"

1. Does this couple need sexual dysfunction counseling?
2. Would you prescribe antianxiety medications to Marie?
3. Would it be proper to assess Marie for a history of child sexual abuse?
4. To which community resources would you direct Marie?

## CASE 4

Josh is a 29-year-old engineer coming to the clinic for help with depression and sleep disturbances. He relates that he hasn't eaten well for 2 weeks and has lost about 10 pounds. Josh further states that 2 weeks ago, his wife, Melinda, to whom he has been married for 10 years, filed for divorce. They have three children, aged 8, 6, and 3. During the discussion, Josh mentions that "I've given her everything, and now she is taking it all away." Later on he states, "I don't think I can live with this. I'm gonna have to do something to make it right."

1. Is Josh suicidal? Is it appropriate to assess suicide in this case?
2. Is Josh homicidal? If so, who could be a foreseeable target?
3. Should Josh be hospitalized?
4. Should the police be contacted?
5. Is antidepressant medication indicated?
6. Should Josh's estranged wife be warned about risks to her safety?

## CASE 5

Ben is 14 years old and lives with his mother and two older sisters in an economically depressed part of town. His mother works two jobs to support the family. Ben is going to school and wants to go to college some day. The area around school *and the school itself is divided by two gangs that frequently fight. Ben does not belong to any gang, but lately has been receiving a lot of pressure to join one. He is hassled on the way to school, pushed around at school, and 2 weeks ago someone threw a rock through a window of his house while his mother was at work. He is coming to the office today for an athletic physical.*

    *1. What community resources can help support Ben's efforts to avoid gang involvement?*
    *2. Does Ben's mother need to spend more time with him?*
    *3. How should Ben be counseled to cope with being assaulted?*

## RECOMMENDED READINGS

American Medical Association: *JAMA* 267(22):2985–3108, 1992.

    This special issue of *JAMA* provides several empirical studies and essays on societal violence. A major focus is on firearms as a primary cause of violence.

American Medical Association: *JAMA* 267(23):3109–3240, 1992.

    This issue of *JAMA* is largely devoted to violence against women and children. Ethical and value considerations for physician involvement in violence prevention are also discussed.

American Psychological Association: *Violence and Youth: Psychology's Response*. Washington, DC, American Psychological Association, 1993.

    This report provides a comprehensive overview of the causes of violence and experiences of victims of violence. Recommendations for research and public policy are presented.

Hamberger LK, Burge SK, Graham AV, Costa AJ (eds): *Violence Issues for Healthcare Educators and Providers*. Binghamton, NY, The Haworth Maltreatment and Trauma Press, 1997.

    This edited work provides state-of-the-art information for both medical educators and healthcare providers on developing and implementing training and clinical programs to prevent and intervene into violence in the lives of their patients, both in the clinic and in the community.

Hendricks-Matthews M, Costa AJ (eds): *Family Violence. Report of the First Ross Roundtable on Critical Issues in Family Medicine*. Columbus, Ohio, Ross Laboratories, 1993.

    This work provides an in-depth overview on the different types of family violence. The physician's role in violence prevention is also described.

## REFERENCES

Ambuel B, Butler D, Hamberger LK, Lawrence S, Guse C: Medical students' personal exposure to violence. Paper presented at the 5th International Family Violence Research Conference, Durham, NH, 1997a.

Ambuel B, Hamberger LK, Lahti J: The Family Peace Project: A model for training for health care professionals to identify, treat, and prevent partner violence, in Hamberger LK, Burge S, Graham A, Costa A (eds): *Violence Issues for Health Care Educators and Providers*. Binghampton, NY, The Haworth Press, 1997b, pp 55–81.

American Medical Association, Council on Scientific Affairs. Violence against women. *JAMA* 267: 3184–3189, 1992.

American Psychological Association Commission on Youth and Violence: *Violence and Youth: Psychology's Response*. Washington, DC, American Psychological Association, 1993.

Barnett OW, Miller-Perrin CL, Perrin R: *Family Violence Across the Lifespan*. Newbury Park, Calif, Sage Publications, Inc, 1997.

Bergman B, Brismar B: A 5-year follow-up study of 117 battered women. *Am J Public Health* 81:1486–1488, 1991.

Bryant BE: *Statistics Abstract of the United States, 110th edition*. Washington, DC, US Bureau of the Census, 1990, p 173.

Callahan CM, Rivara FP: Urban high school youth and handguns: A school-based survey. *JAMA* 267: 3038–3042, 1992.

Chelmowski M, Hamberger LK: Screening men for domestic violence in your medical practice. *Wis Med J* December: 623–626, 1994.

Costa AJ, Anetzberger GJ: Elder abuse, in Hamberger LK, Burge S, Graham A, Costa A (eds): *Violence Issues for Health Care Educators and Providers*. Binghamton, NY, The Haworth Press, 1997, pp 243–260.

Cullinane PM, Alpert EJ, Freund KM: First year medical students' knowledge of, attitudes toward, and personal histories of family violence. *Acad Med* 72(1):48–50, 1997.

deLahunta EA, Tulsky AA: Personal exposure of faculty and medical students to family violence. *JAMA* 275(24):1903–1906, 1996.

Drossman DA, Leserman J, Nachman G, Li Z, Gluck H, Toomey TC, Mitchell M: Sexual and physical abuse in women with functional or organic gastrointestinal disorders. *Ann Intern Med* 113: 828–833, 1990.

Fingerhut LA, Ingram DD, Feldman JJ: Firearm and non-firearm homicide among persons 15 through 19 years of age: Differences by level of urbanization, United States, 1979 through 1989. *JAMA* 267: 3048–3053, 1992.

Finkelhor D: Current information on the scope and nature of child sexual abuse. *The Future of Children* 4:31–53, 1994.

Ganley A: Integrating feminist and social learning analyses or aggression: Creating multiple models for intervention with men who batter, in Caesar PL, Hamberger LK (eds): *Treating Men Who Batter: Theory, Practice and Programs*. Berlin, Springer, 1989, pp 196–235.

Gaquin DA: Spouse abuse. Data from the National Crime Survey. *Victimology* 2:632–642, 1977–78.

Gelles RJ, Straus MA: *Intimate Violence*. New York, Simon & Schuster, Inc, 1988.

Goldberg BW: Preventing firearm violence, in Hamberger LK, Burge S, Graham A, Costa A (eds): *Violence Issues for Health Care Educators and Providers*. Binghamton, NY, The Haworth Press, 1997, pp 99–111.

Greenwood CL, Tangalos EG, Maruta T: Prevalence of sexual abuse, physical abuse, and concurrent traumatic life events in a general medical population. *Mayo Clin Proc* 65:1067–1071, 1990.

Hamberger LK, Ambuel B: Dating violence. *Pediatr Clin North Am* 45: 381–390, 1998.

Hamberger LK, Saunders DG, Hovey M: The prevalence of domestic violence in community family practice and rate of physician inquiry. *Fam Med* 24:283–287, 1992.

Hamberger LK, Lohr JM, Bonge D, Tolin D: A large sample empirical typology of male spouse abusers and its relationship to dimensions of abuse. *Violence and Victims* 11:277–292, 1996.

Hamberger LK, Lohr JM, Bonge D, Tolin D: An empirical classification of motivations for domestic violence. *Violence Against Women* 3:401–423, 1997.

Haugaard JJ, Reppucci ND: *The Sexual Abuse of Children*. San Francisco, Calif, Jossey–Bass Publishers Inc, 1988.

Helton AS, McFarlane J, Anderson ET: Battered and pregnant: A prevalence study. *Am J Public Health* 77:1337–1339, 1987.

Hillard PH: Physical violence in pregnancy. *Obstet Gynecol* 66:185–190, 1985.

Island D, Letellier P: *Men Who Beat the Men Who Love Them*. New York, Harrington Park Press, 1991.

Johnson M, Elliott BA: Domestic violence among family practice patients in midsized and rural communities. *J Fam Pract* 44: 391–399, 1997.

Kellerman AL, Rivara FP, Rushforth NB, *et al*: Gun ownership as a risk factor for homicide in the home. *N Engl J Med* 329:1084–1088, 1993.

Koss MP: Rape: Scope, impact, interventions and public policy responses. *Am Psychol* 48:1062–1069, 1993.

Koss MP, Woodruff WJ, Koss PG: Relation of criminal victimization to health perceptions among women medical patients. *J Consult Clin Psychol* 58:147–152, 1990.

Koss MP, Koss PG, Woodruff WJ: Deleterious effects of criminal victimization on women's health and medical utilization. *Arch Intern Med* 151:342–347, 1991.

Mederos FR: Men who abuse women and "normal" men: Theorizing continuities and discontinuities. Paper presented at the Third National Family Violence Research Conference. Durham, NH, 1987.

Michael RT, Gagnon JH, Lauman EO, Kolata G: *Sex in America*. Boston, Little Brown & Co, 1994.

Rasche C: Domestic murder-suicides: Characteristics and comparisons to non-suicidal mate killing. Paper presented at the meeting of the American Society of Criminology, Chicago, 1988.

Rath GD, Jarratt LG, Leonardson G: Rates of domestic violence against adult women by men partners. *J Am Bd Fam Prac* 2:227–233, 1989.

Rice DP, McKenzie EJ: Cost of injury in the United States: A report to Congress. San Francisco. Institute for Health and Aging, University of California and Injury Prevention Center, The Johns Hopkins University, 1989.

Rosenberg ML: Violence prevention. Paper presented at the United States Attorneys Conference, Washington, DC, January 20, 1994.

Rossman BB, Bingham RD, Emde RN: Symptomatology and adaptive functioning for children exposed to normative stressors, dog attack, and parental violence. *J Am Acad Child Adolesc Psychiatry* 36: 1089–1097, 1997.

Saltzman LE, Mercy JA, O'Carroll PW, Rosenberg ML, Rhodes PH: Weapon involvement and injury outcomes in family and intimate assaults. *JAMA* 267:3043–3047, 1992.

Saunders DG: A typology of men who batter women: Three types derived from cluster analysis. *Am J Orthopsychiatry* 62:264–275, 1992.

Singer MI, Anglin TM, Song L, Lunghofer L: Adolescents' exposure to violence and associated symptoms of psychological trauma. *JAMA* 273(6):477–482, 1994.

Stark E, Flitcraft A, Frazier W: Medicine and patriarchal violence: The social construction of a "private" event. *Int J Health Serv* 9: 461–493, 1979.

Straus MA, Gelles RJ: Societal change and change in family violence from 1975 to 1985 as revealed by two national surveys. *J Marriage Fam* 4:161–180, 1986.

Straus MA, Gelles RJ, Steinmetz SK: *Behind Closed Doors: Violence in the American Family*. Garden City, NY, Anchor Press, 1980.

Sugg NK, Inui T: Primary care physicians' response to domestic violence: Opening Pandora's box. *JAMA* 267:3157–3160, 1992.

Tatara T: Understanding the nature and scope of domestic elder abuse with the use of state aggregate data: Summaries of the key findings of a national survey of state APS and aging agencies. *J Elder Abuse Neglect* 5:35–57, 1993.

Warshaw C, Poirier S: Hidden stories of women. *Second Opinion*, p 61, October 1991.

Wisner CL, Gilmer TP, Saltzman LE, Zink TM: Intimate partner violence against women: Do victims cost health plans more? *J Fam Pract* 48: 439–443, 1999.

Yllo KA: Through a feminist lens: Gender, power, and violence, in Gelles RJ, Loseke DR (eds): *Current Controversies on Family Violence*. Newbury Park, Calif, Sage Publications, Inc, 1993, pp 47–62.

# Mental Illness

*Frank Verloin deGruy III*

*Louise Davis is a 35-year-old bank teller who is in Dr. Abel's office, sobbing uncontrollably. Her troubles started about 3 months ago, when she began having problems with sleep. She falls asleep at about 11 o'clock at night, but awakens at 3 or 4 am unable to return to sleep. Now she always feels exhausted and has begun having difficulty concentrating at work. She notices that she frequently forgets to follow through on tasks, and has made calculation errors, something she never did previously. She has lost interest in all of her hobbies, has stopped going to church, and has stopped visiting her friends. She wonders if she should be replaced at work by someone more valuable to the company.*

## EDUCATIONAL OBJECTIVES

1. Identify the most common types of mental illness
2. Describe the impact of these disorders on patients, physicians, and society
3. Understand the most effective ways for physicians to respond to mentally ill patients.

## INTRODUCTION

Mental illness is now recognized as an important health problem in this country. In 2000, the Surgeon General issued a Report on Mental Health pointing out that 4 of the 10 leading causes of disability worldwide are mental disorders and calling for action to deal with this problem (Satcher, 2000). Mental disorders are common, they cause significant distress and impairment, and they are frequently overlooked and undertreated (Higgins, 1994). This chapter will describe the extent of diagnosable mental illness in the United States, list the most common mental disorders and the health consequences of each, describe the sources of care for people with mental illness, and describe the adequacy of care for patients with mental illness.

## FACTS ABOUT MENTAL ILLNESS

- *Mental illnesses are more common than cancer, diabetes, or heart disease.*
- *In any given year, more than 5 million Americans suffer from an acute episode of mental illness.*
- *The treatment success rate for schizophrenia is 60%, 65% for major depression, and 80% for bipolar disorder. Comparatively, the success rate for treatments of heart disease ranges from 41 to 52%.*
- *The No. 1 reason for hospital admissions in the United States is a biological psychiatric condition. At any moment, 20% of all hospital beds are filled by people with a mental illness.*
- *The price tag of mental illnesses in the United States is $81 billion, including direct costs (hospitalizations, medications) and indirect costs (lost wages, family caregiving, losses due to suicide).*
- *On any given day, 150,000 people with severe mental illness are homeless, living on the streets or in public shelters.*

*Source: National Alliance for the Mentally Ill: http://www.nami.org/fact.htm*

## Definition of Mental Illness

Every proposed definition of mental illness and mental disorder has limitations. Moreover, there are fundamental disagreements over whether certain conditions should be regarded as mental illness and whether the basic problem is best understood as within the individual or within the system of relationships in which the individual is located. This disagreement has very important implications. For example, a woman who is experiencing severe abuse from her husband may well exhibit criterion symptoms for major depression. While one may define the problem as depression, an assessment at the level of the family system might yield a diagnosis such as Severe Interpersonal Conflict with Physical Abuse of an Adult; in this instance the depressive symptoms might be viewed as a normal response to an abnormal situation. These two formulations have drastically different management implications.

With these caveats in mind, I will offer the definition of mental illness given in the American Psychiatric Association's *Diagnostic and Statistical Manual of Mental Disorders*, fourth edition—DSM-IV (American Psychiatric Association, 1994). This definition is widely accepted, and quite useful. A mental disorder is a distinct psychological or behavioral syndrome or pattern that is associated with *distress* or *impaired function*, or the *risk* of pain, disability, loss of freedom, or death. The syndrome must not be an expectable response to a traumatic event. Deviant behavior per se, and conflicts between an individual and society, are not considered mental disorders unless the deviance or conflict is a symptom of a dysfunction within the individual.

## Mind–Body Dualism and the Biopsychosocial Model

While it is convenient and useful to think of mental disorders as "real" entities, this convention can mislead the clinician into fundamentally misunderstanding the patient's predicament and thereby making serious management mistakes. In 1641, Rene Descartes published *Meditations on First Philosophy*, in which he postulated a dualistic reality: the external physical world and the internal mental world. Much of what we know as science rests on this formulation, and much of what we know in medicine rests on science. Nevertheless, this separation of mind from body seduces us into overlooking the deep, extensive, and inherent connections between these two domains. (Connections, incidentally, that were not lost on Descartes himself.) Mental disorders always feature physical symptoms, and physical disorders always feature mental symptoms. The two simply cannot be separated, and we do so here for heuristic purposes only. Thus, it must be kept in mind that mental illness is an inherently incomplete construct—a mental diagnosis can only partly describe the condition of a person so afflicted. The clinician who desires a more comprehensive perspective will be

**MISCONCEPTIONS ABOUT MENTAL ILLNESS**

*In a recent survey regarding the causes of mental illness*

- *71% believed that mental illness is caused by emotional weakness*
- *65% believed that mental illness is caused by bad parenting*
- *35% believed that mental illness is caused by sinful or immoral behavior*
- *43% believed that mental illness is brought on in some way by the individual*

*Source: National Mental Health Association: http://www.nmha.org/infoctr/didyou.cfm*

better served by a biopsychosocial formulation, in which physical, psychological, and social domains are systemically assessed and integrated (Engel, 1977). Some would add a fourth dimension, the spiritual, to this model.

## Diagnostic Variability and Cultural Considerations

In the United States most of the mental health community has agreed to codify mental illnesses by the conventions established in the DSM-IV. In fact, the DSM-IV diagnostic conventions have enjoyed worldwide acceptance. However, a number of authors have voiced reservations about the assumptions and implications of the DSM diagnostic system (Denton, 1996; Klerman *et al.*, 1984; Ritchie, 1989); I would encourage the reader to review one or more of these critiques for a broader perspective on our practice of making mental diagnoses. A DSM-IV diagnostic entity generally consists of a list of criterion symptoms; the patient must exhibit or report a specified number of them. One might infer from this that mental illness manifests identically, or at least similarly, in all people, from all cultures. While certain core symptoms of a given disorder do seem to occur across cultures, there is much transcultural variation in the manifestations of mental illness (Kleinman, 1980). For example, certain Chinese and Latina groups tend to "somatize" their distress, such that the presenting complaints of mental disorders are more likely physical symptoms (Escobar, 1987; Lin *et al.*, 1985). Moreover, some syndromes are limited to one or a few cultural settings. An example of this might be *susto*, an illness that occurs in Latina peoples. It is said to be an illness caused by intense fright, which dislodges the soul from the body. Symptoms include insomnia, irritability, fatigue, anorexia, weight loss, restlessness, and outbursts of hysteria and fainting (Trotter, 1985).

---

### CASE 33-2

*Dr. James Ray is a family physician in a small town in the Midwest. The first six patients on his visit list this morning were:*

*Terry Lopez, a 4-year-old boy returning for an ear check after 10 days of antibiotics for otitis media.*

*Marvin Simon, a 37-year-old plumber with shoulder pain, probably the result of a rotator cuff injury.*

*Tonya Tolliver, a 49-year-old secretary who returns with abdominal pain. She feels overwhelmed at work and has an adolescent son who was arrested last week.*

*Jerry Davis, a 50-year-old salesman who came in to get a prescription for insomnia. He drinks about 12 beers a night while he is on the road, which is four or five nights a week.*

*Angela Barnes, an 80-year-old woman who complains of constipation. Her son, with whom she lives, reports that she has worsening forgetfulness, disorientation, and crying spells.*

*Chelsea McGovern, a 25-year-old physical therapist who came in for a Pap smear and oral contraceptives.*

## FAMOUS PEOPLE WHO ARE BELIEVED
## TO HAVE SUFFERED WITH A MENTAL ILLNESS

*Depression*
   *Charles Dickens*
   *Thomas Eagleton*
   *Betty Ford*
   *Tipper Gore*
   *Ernest Hemingway*
   *John Lennon*
   *Abraham Lincoln*
   *Carmen Miranda*
   *Marilyn Monroe*
   *Eugene O'Neill*
   *Sylvia Plath*
   *Rembrandt*
   *Mike Wallace*
   *Tennessee Williams*

*Bipolar disorder*
   *Alvin Ailey*
   *Ludwig van Beethoven*
   *Winston Churchill*
   *Patty Duke*
   *Goya*
   *Graham Greene*
   *Vivien Leigh*
   *Edgar Allan Poe*
   *Robert Schumann*
   *Virginia Woolf*

*Schizophrenia*
   *Lionel Aldridge*
   *Syd Barrett*
   *Vincent van Gogh*
   *Mary Todd Lincoln*
   *John Forbes Nash, Jr.*
   *Vaslav Nijinsky*
   *Ezra Pound*
*Obsessive–compulsive disorder*
   *Howard Hughes*
*Panic disorder*
   *Charles Darwin*
*Social anxiety disorder*
   *Donny Osmond*
*Eating disorder*
   *Princess Diana*
   *Karen Carpenter*

*Note: In the case of persons who lived more than 50 years ago, a definitive diagnosis is not possible, but their symptoms suggest the above diagnoses. Many others had definite symptoms of mental illness, although there is not enough information to identify the particular diagnosis. These include John Keats, Leo Tolstoy, Sir Isaac Newton, and Michelangelo.*

# PREVALENCE AND INCIDENCE OF MENTAL DISORDERS IN THE UNITED STATES

Of the six patients in Case 33-2, two (Jerry Davis and Angela Barnes) have strong evidence for a mental diagnosis, and another (Tonya Tolliver) has a physical symptom that seems related to her mental distress. This would be a fairly typical clinical experience for a primary care physician, and reflects the frequency with which mental illness and symptoms appear in the population that primary physicians serve.

## The Epidemiologic Studies
### The ECA Study

The edifice of knowledge in medicine is uneven, and in some places entirely absent. Happily, this situation does not apply to our knowledge of the nature and extent of mental disorders in the United States. Thanks to an extraordinary study—the Epidemiological Catchment Area (ECA) Study—we know a great deal about the mental illnesses that affect our citizenry, which subgroups are particularly affected, who receives services for these disorders, and where these services are rendered (Robins & Regier, 1991). This study was conducted in the 1980s, and consisted of careful diagnostic interviews with over 20,000 subjects randomly selected from five sites. One of the most important general findings from this study was that 32% of Americans had experienced a mental disorder at some time in their lives, and 20% had an active disorder. Thus, this is a problem of enormous magnitude—which is why mental healthcare education, research, and provision of services have become national priorities.

In the ECA Study there were important differences in prevalence by site, from a high of 41% lifetime and 27% current diagnosis rate in Baltimore, to a low of 28% lifetime and 18% current in New Haven. From this and other epidemiologic studies we also learned that most people seeking care for mental disorders do so in a primary care, rather than a mental healthcare, setting.

**745**

PREVALENCE AND
INCIDENCE OF
MENTAL DISORDERS
IN THE UNITED
STATES

There are quite a lot of population-based data on specific mental disorders, or particular aspects of specific disorders, that augment and corroborate the ECA data set and that sometimes address important issues not dealt with in the ECA Study. I have largely ignored this literature, electing instead the path of parsimony and simplicity: The reader can find most of the salient findings of the ECA Study collected under one volume, to which I have made extensive reference (Robins & Regier, 1991).

## The MOS Study

The ECA Study was population-based and selected subjects at their homes. An equally ambitious study (or set of studies) has been conducted with *patients*—people who were selected from the waiting rooms of physicians' offices in three cities—to learn about their illnesses and symptoms. This study, the Medical Outcomes Study (MOS), was not concerned specifically with mental disorders, but assessed patients with certain tracer conditions: hypertension, coronary artery disease, diabetes, chronic lung disease, and depression (Wells *et al.*, 1988). The MOS contains much detail about the functional consequences of these conditions and the adequacy of care rendered for patients with these conditions. This was the first study to show, for example, that depression was a serious medical illness, with impairment equal to or exceeding other chronic medical conditions (Wells *et al.*, 1989). Depression was the only mental disorder selected as a tracer condition in this study.

## The PRIME-MD 1000 Study

This study, which was undertaken in four U.S. primary care practices, aimed to develop and validate an instrument for making rapid and accurate mental diagnoses in primary care settings (Spitzer *et al.*, 1994). The PRIME-MD study documented the incidence and profiled the characteristics of patients in this setting with any of 24 mental diagnoses. This study measured the extent of comorbidity between diagnoses, and compared the impairment associated with these disorders with that of common physical disorders. One of the principal findings of this study was that 26% of primary care patients currently suffer from a mental disorder, and another 13% qualify for a "subthreshold" diagnosis, not sufficient to meet DSM criteria, but sufficient to show significant functional impairment. It is noteworthy that there was considerable variation across sites—the site range for any PRIME-MD diagnosis was 30–52%. Another important finding from this study was the demonstration that functional impairments and disability in primary care patients were much more strongly related to mental disorders than physical diagnoses (Spitzer *et al.*, 1995).

## International Perspective

Much work from the international perspective has been directed by the World Health Organization. For example, their recently completed Collaborative Study on Psychological Problems in General Health Care detailed the relative prevalence and functional consequences of mental illnesses in primary healthcare facilities in 14 cities around the world (Ormel *et al.*, 1994). This study, which included over 5000 patients, showed an overall prevalence of current mental disorder of 21%, with a dramatic range across sites, from a high of 53% for patients in Santiago, to a low of 8% for patients in Shanghai.

---

## CASE 33-3

*Peter Bosarge is a 41-year-old evangelical preacher who came to the emergency room because of chest pain. For the last month, every time he begins to preach, he develops a sharp left-sided chest pain, a feeling of breathlessness, diaphoresis, and an overwhelming fear that he is going to die. Immediately thereafter he develops diarrhea, and then the episode passes. Early this morning he was awakened from a sound sleep with another attack. His father, also a preacher, died in the pulpit of a*

## THE PREVALENCE OF MENTAL ILLNESS

- *One in five adults has a diagnosable mental disorder.*
- *One in four families will have a member with a mental illness.*
- *Mental health problems affect one in every five young people at any given time.*
- *Fewer than one-third of the children under age 18 with a serious mental disorder receive any mental health services.*
- *Suicide is the third leading cause of death for 15- to 24-year-olds and the sixth leading cause of death for 5- to 15-year-olds.*

*Source: National Mental Health Association: http://www.nmha.org/infoctr/didyou.cfm*

*heart attack at age 41. Mr. Bosarge has undergone exhaustive cardiac evaluation, including two catheterizations, and no heart disease is present. He has become so fearful of another attack that he has stopped preaching.*

# THE DIAGNOSTIC ENTITIES

## The Disorders

There are over 250 mental disorders listed in the DSM-IV manual. Most of these diagnoses have a relatively large medical literature associated with them. It is far beyond the scope of this chapter to even mention all of these illnesses, let alone describe them. Our purposes will be better served by simply grouping mental illnesses into general categories and describing a few selected disorders within these categories. I will therefore attempt to describe only those mental diagnoses that, because of their frequency, seriousness, or impact on medical or mental health practice, are of the most consequence to the health of our nation.

## CASE 33-4

*Jerry Baker was 39 years old when he finally made an appointment to see his wife's family physician. He had been extremely successful in his business career, having acquired and successfully run almost a dozen companies. He had always been an exceptionally hardworking man—his wife described him as obsessed with work—but for the past 6 months he had experienced progressively more difficulty doing his work. He described two problems: loss of motivation and difficulty actually attending to the details. His mind would drift, and he began forgetting to do things. His motivation became so impaired that he refused to go to work for an entire week, a behavior that cost one of his companies several hundred thousand dollars. This precipitated his visit to the physician. He described himself as a "shell" of his former self: He didn't enjoy work any more. He didn't enjoy anything any more; even his passion for good food had disappeared. He had begun sleeping up to 14 hours a day, and still was fatigued. He had actually begun thinking that he and his family would be better off if he were dead.*

*His physician conducted a thorough physical evaluation, and discovered no abnormalities, other than profound sadness and slowing of thought and movement in this previously energetic, optimistic man.*

## Depression and Other Mood Disorders

More people are afflicted by mood disorders than any other category of mental illness. We will concern ourselves here with three diagnoses within this general category: major depression, dysthymia, and bipolar

---

## SYMPTOMS OF A MAJOR DEPRESSIVE EPISODE

*At least five symptoms, present for most of the time, which cause significant distress or impairment for at least 2 weeks, and are not due to medications, a medical condition, or another mental condition. At least one of the symptoms must be either:*

  *Depressed mood, or*
  *Loss of interest or pleasure in previously enjoyable activities.*

*Other symptoms include:*

  *Significant weight loss or weight gain;*
  *Insomnia or hypersomnia;*
  *Psychomotor retardation or agitation;*
  *Fatigue;*
  *Feelings of worthlessness or guilt;*
  *Difficulty concentrating or deciding; and*
  *Recurrent thoughts of death or suicide.*

*Source: American Psychiatric Association,* Diagnostic and Statistical Manual of Mental Disorders, *ed 4, Washington, DC, American Psychiatric Press, 1994.*

---

disorder. What are these disorders? What do people who have them look like? Case 33-1, which opened this chapter, and Case 33-4, just above, describe people who are suffering from a major depressive episode. The salient symptoms are sadness, a loss of interest in previously enjoyable activities, insomnia or hypersomnia, fatigue, psychomotor retardation (or agitation), diminished ability to concentrate, and feelings of worthlessness, including suicidal thoughts. In the general medical setting, about 25% of adults are suffering from a mood disorder (Spitzer *et al.*, 1994). The distribution of diagnoses within this category and the general demographic breakdown parallel those of the general population.

While symptoms must have been present for only 2 weeks for a major depressive episode, the diagnostic criteria for dysthymic disorder require the presence of symptoms most of the time for at least 2 years. During this time, the person must have had a depressed mood and at least two other symptoms such as poor appetite (or overeating), insomnia (or hypersomnia), fatigue, difficulty concentrating, poor self-esteem, or feelings of hopelessness.

Dysthymia is a chronic, mild to moderate depression that often goes undiagnosed. Persons with dysthymia can often mask their symptoms and appear to function normally. A person with major depression, on the other hand, cycles from a normal mood down to a severe expression of symptoms, during which time it would be extremely difficult to function at work or home.

Bipolar disorder is characterized by episodes of mania or hypomania, usually also interspersed with depressive episodes. A manic episode is dramatic to behold and terrible to experience. It consists of at least 1 week of elevated, expansive, or irritable mood, in conjunction with grandiosity, decreased need for sleep, pressure of speech, racing thoughts and flight of ideas, easy distractibility, and excessive pursuit of pleasurable, often risky, behavior. People experiencing a manic episode often feel invulnerable and cannot be persuaded that their behavior is inappropriate; therefore, treatment is difficult to initiate.

In the U.S. population, about 8% of adults have met criteria for one of the mood diagnoses in their lifetimes: 5% have suffered a major depressive episode, 3% meet criteria for dysthymia, and less than 1% have experienced a manic episode. In the general population, women are affected by mood disorders at about twice the rate as men; diagnostic rates tend to decrease with age, and are roughly comparable across racial and ethnic categories (Robins & Regier, 1991). There is some evidence for a genetic predisposition, particularly for the bipolar disorders; divorce and unemployment seem to be risk factors for depression (American

## SIGECAPS

*Many medical students find the SIGECAPS acronym helpful for remembering the symptoms of depression that generally accompany depressed mood:*

S  *Sleep*
I  *Interest, pleasure*
G  *Guilt, worthlessness*
E  *Energy*
C  *Concentration*
A  *Appetite*
P  *Psychomotor*
S  *Suicidal*

Psychiatric Association, 1994). People with bipolar and major depressive disorders use far more health services, both psychiatric and medical, than their unaffected counterparts (Leaf, 1994).

## CASE 33-5

*Miriam Welch had shredded three tissues in the first 3 minutes of her office visit. She was so fidgety that her physician was beginning to feel nervous just being in the room with her. Miriam was 29 years old and on the verge of remarrying. She came in for a contraception examination, but it was clear she had something else on her mind: "I have always been a worrier, but this has gotten ridiculous. For the last year or two, I have stayed on edge about everything. Everything worries me now. My new marriage might not work out. I probably will get laid off when our company reorganizes, then I won't make my rent and will get evicted, and on and on. I get headaches all the time, and I've gotten to where I can't keep my mind on anything more than a minute. I can't even read the newspaper any more, for being so distracted. I just feel so tired and irritable and on edge!"*

## Anxiety Disorders

The anxiety disorders include panic disorder, phobias, obsessive–compulsive disorder, posttraumatic stress disorder, acute stress disorder, and generalized anxiety disorder. As a group, these disorders are almost as common as the mood disorders. Each condition has its own characteristic clinical presentation; the most common ones will be summarized briefly here.

Peter Bosarge, described in Case 33-3, is suffering from panic disorder and is developing secondary phobias. Note the sudden appearance of intense fear and discomfort. This patient's panic attacks are associated with cardiac symptoms, but the symptoms can also be gastrointestinal (diarrhea, nausea), neurological (numbness, dizziness), or psychological (fear of dying or going crazy). The person must have either recurrent attacks or a persistent fear of recurrence. One of the most problematic complications of panic attacks is the development of avoidance behaviors, or phobias. This is a fear of being in a place or situation in which help might not be available or escape might be difficult in case of a panic attack. Such phobias can severely limit a person's ability to carry on a normal life—people with severe phobias may become completely homebound. About 2–3% of people have at some time qualified for panic disorder, and about half of them have an associated agoraphobia (Robins & Regier, 1991). Like depression, the disorder is found in about twice as many women as men.

People with obsessive–compulsive disorder are burdened with either recurrent obsessions or compulsions that are time-consuming or cause significant distress or impairment. The affected person can see that this

## SYMPTOMS OF A PANIC ATTACK

*A sudden attack of intense fear, in which at least four of the following symptoms occur:*

- *Pounding or racing heart*
- *Sweating*
- *Trembling or shaking*
- *Shortness of breath or smothering*
- *Choking sensation*
- *Chest pain*
- *Nausea or abdominal distress*

- *Dizziness or lightheadedness*
- *Feelings of unreality or of being outside oneself*
- *Fear of going crazy or losing control*
- *Fear of dying*
- *Numbness or tingling*
- *Chills or hot flushes*

*Source: American Psychiatric Association,* Diagnostic and Statistical Manual of Mental Disorders, *ed 4, Washington, DC, American Psychiatric Press, 1994.*

is unreasonable, but is unable to prevent the intrusive thoughts or behaviors. Obsessions are persistent thoughts or impulses, usually unrelated to a real-life problem, such as concern over contamination from shaking hands, fear that one has left the door unlocked or the stove on, intrusive sexual imagery or aggressive impulses. These thoughts or impulses cause distress. Compulsions are repetitive behaviors (e.g., repetitive hand washing) or mental acts (e.g., counting, repeating words) employed to reduce the distress. The ECA data suggest a lifetime incidence of 2.6% for obsessive–compulsive disorder, which is surprisingly high in light of the much lower incidence measured in mental health and general medical settings. This suggests that many people with obsessive–compulsive disorder do not seek help for their condition, at least from a medical or mental health professional. This condition is equally common in males and females, and usually begins in adolescence or early adulthood.

Acute stress disorder and posttraumatic stress disorder (PTSD) can be thought of as essentially two versions of the same disorder separated by time. After an extremely traumatic stressor, such as witnessing a murder, being raped or tortured, or learning of the unexpected or violent death of a family member, a person may develop a characteristic set of symptoms. These symptoms involve flashbacks or dreams about the event; avoidance behavior or numbing of feelings associated with the trauma; and symptoms of agitation, insomnia, irritability, or hypervigilance. If these symptoms have persisted less than 1 month, the person may qualify for the diagnosis of acute stress disorder. If the symptoms have persisted for more than 1 month, PTSD would be the more appropriate diagnosis. Estimates vary, but probably 25% of the population have suffered from one of these conditions at some time. Certain forms of severe, prolonged sexual and physical abuse, particularly within families, lead to a variant of PTSD characterized by certain personality deformations, severe depression, somatizing behavior, and a tendency toward panic and other anxiety symptoms. These patients are surprisingly common in the primary care setting—the prevalence is probably 2–3%, based on a sample of 300 patients in three family practices (Dickinson *et al.*, 1999).

## OCD

*2.3% of the U.S. population has OCD in a given year.*
*OCD affects men and women equally.*
*OCD typically begins during adolescence or childhood.*
*OCD costs the United States $8.4 billion in 1990 in social and economic losses, nearly 6% of the total mental health bill of $148 billion.*

*Source: National Mental Health Association: http://www.nmha.org/pbedu/anxiety/ocd.cfm*

## SYMPTOMS OF PTSD

- *Exposure to a severely traumatic event that evoked intense fear, helplessness, or horror*
- *The event is persistently reexperienced as intrusive memories, recurrent dreams, flashbacks, or strong reactions to reminders of the event*
- *Avoidance or numbing, which includes efforts to avoid thoughts, events associated with the trauma, the inability to remember, a feeling of detachment from others, or restrictions on certain feelings*
- *Hypervigilance, including difficulty falling asleep, irritability, difficulty concentrating, and an exaggerated startle response*
- *Symptoms have been present for at least a month, and impair normal functioning*

*American Psychiatric Association,* Diagnostic and Statistical Manual of Mental Disorders, *ed 4, Washington, DC, American Psychiatric Press, 1994.*

Generalized anxiety disorder is characterized by excessive, uncontrollable, free-floating worry and anxiety. Miriam Welch, described in Case 33-5, exemplifies this condition. In order to meet DSM-IV criteria, this anxiety must have been present for at least 6 months, and must be accompanied by three of the following: muscle tension, fatigue or irritability, difficulty concentrating, insomnia, restlessness. About 5% of adults have met criteria for this disorder at some time, and about twice as many women as men are affected. Unfortunately, the symptoms of anxiety tend to be chronic, and often persist, with variable intensity, over the course of a lifetime. Symptoms of generalized anxiety, whether or not they reach the diagnostic threshold, accompany most medical illnesses, and so anxiety symptoms are extremely common in the medical setting. About 7% of adults in the PRIME-MD Study met criteria for current generalized anxiety disorder, with a site range of 2–13%.

## CASE 33-6

*Dr. Fletcher looked with dismay over his morning clinic schedule. There, third from the top, was Daria Ruhle. This would be a long morning. Ms. Ruhle faithfully appeared on the schedule at least twice a month; she usually came in with a list of physical complaints at least two pages long, and two or three of these were sure to be severe. She had the thickest chart in the practice, having had innumerable diagnostic workups over the years. All of these workups had been negative, but this did little to remove the symptoms themselves, or her concern that there was a physical explanation for these symptoms. In the past year she had been evaluated for recurrent headaches, abdominal pain, leg numbness, blurry vision, nausea, passing out, wrist pain, knee pain, chest pain, weakness, and difficulty urinating.*

### Somatoform Disorders

The somatoform disorders are characterized by the presence of physical symptoms that cannot be explained by a general medical condition. These symptoms are not intentional and not under voluntary control, and are thereby distinct from Factitious Disorders and Malingering. The symptoms must cause significant functional impairment or result in medical treatment. Only the most severe of the somatoform disorders will be discussed here, namely, somatization disorder.

Somatization disorder is characterized by multiple unexplained physical complaints, as exemplified by Ms. Ruhle in Case 33-6. There is some controversy about the proper diagnostic disposition of patients with multiple somatic complaints, and a number of alternative classifications exist. The DSM-IV diagnosis requires at least four different pain symptoms, two gastrointestinal symptoms, one sexual symptom, and one pseudoneurological symptom. Somatization disorder is rare in the population: The pooled incidence in the ECA Study was 0.13%. Such a rare condition would not ordinarily merit consideration in this overview, but patients affected with this condition are far more common in the general medical setting, and their medical care is extremely expensive. The prevalence is about 5–15% in primary care practices, where these patients appear frequently for care. By one estimate, physicians expend nine times as much money on their healthcare than the population average (Smith *et al.*, 1986a). This is generally thought to be related in part to unnecessary diagnostic evaluation by physicians. Somatization disorder has a much higher prevalence among women than men, generally by a ratio of about ten to one (Smith *et al.*, 1985). There are interesting familial patterns associated with this disorder, including somatization and depression in female family members and antisocial characteristics and substance abuse in male family members (Cloninger *et al.*, 1986; Guze, 1993; Guze *et al.*, 1986). There is a strong association between a history of sexual or physical abuse and subsequent somatizing behavior (deGruy *et al.*, 1994).

## CASE 33-7

*Eric Nelson was a loner. He had grown up as the only child of a drill press operator and a textile mill worker in the Deep South. He had done well through high school, but his classmates hardly knew the sound of his voice. He seemed nice enough, but he certainly kept to himself. In fact, he had never had a friend. During his first semester away from home at college, he began receiving messages through the fillings in his teeth. At first he thought these messages were from his father, but as they became more clear and understandable, he realized that they were from angels warning him about various dangers. He would receive information about which routes to walk on his way to class, and even what to avoid eating and drinking. Soon he began having conversations, aloud, with his guardian angels, and began wearing a ski mask over his face at all times to protect himself from poisonous gases on the campus.*

## Schizophrenia

Schizophrenia is perhaps the most devastating of the mental illnesses. While there are a number of subtypes of schizophrenia, all are characterized by two or more of the following symptoms:

- Delusions, usually bizarre and often persecutory
- Hallucinations, usually auditory
- Disorganized, loose, tangential speech
- Disorganized, inappropriate behavior
- Negative symptoms such as loss of normal emotional expressiveness, poverty of speech, inability to begin and maintain goal-directed activities

## WHAT'S THE DIFFERENCE BETWEEN A DELUSION AND A HALLUCINATION?

*A delusion is an erroneous belief that cannot be dislodged despite strong contradictory evidence. Schizophrenic delusions are typically bizarre, meaning they are clearly implausible, not understandable, and do not derive from ordinary life experiences. A hallucination is the perception with one of the senses of an experience that "is not out there," such as hearing voices or seeing things that no one else can hear or see. The hallucinations most characteristic of schizophrenia involve hearing voices.*

## SYMPTOMS OF SCHIZOPHRENIA

*The presence for at least a month of two or more of the following:*

- *Delusions*
- *Hallucinations*
- *Disorganized speech*
- *Grossly disorganized behavior*
- *Negative symptoms, such as loss of emotional expressiveness, loss of volition, and lack of speech volition*

*These symptoms must cause major social or occupational impairment.*

*American Psychiatric Association,* Diagnostic and Statistical Manual of Mental Disorders, ed 4, Washington, DC, American Psychiatric Press, 1994.

Although schizophrenia is relatively rare, occurring in 1.3% of the population, it tends to appear during late adolescence or early adulthood, completely removes people from their normal spheres of activity, and most of the time causes at least some lifelong impairment. Most people with schizophrenia do not marry, are unemployed or employed at low-level jobs, and have limited social contacts, although there are exceptions to this pattern. Men and women are equally affected. Schizophrenia has a strong familial predilection, although environmental factors also contribute to the appearance of this illness.

Most of the conditions described in this chapter have been characterized as frequent in general medical practice. Schizophrenia is an exception to this rule. While patients with schizophrenia definitely have pronounced physical symptomatology, the mental symptoms are usually so severe and so clearly mental that most of these patients get their care in mental health settings. In fact, the NAMCS data suggest that about one-third of the content of ambulatory psychiatry consists of management of patients with schizophrenia.

## PEDIATRIC MENTAL HEALTH

Less information is available about mental diagnoses among children, particularly information describing the associated impairment and costs of treatment, than about adults. This is not because mental disorders are less common in children, but simply because they are less well studied.

The Great Smoky Mountain Study examined a representative sample of 1000 children aged 9, 11, and 13 years drawn from 11 counties in the southeastern United States (Costello *et al.*, 1996). Twenty percent of these children met criteria for a DSM-III-R axis I mental disorder. The most common diagnoses were anxiety disorders (6%), enuresis (5%), tic disorders (4%), conduct disorder (3%), oppositional defiant disorder (3%), and hyperactivity (2%). Depression was relatively uncommon, with an incidence of about 1.5% for any depressive disorder.

The prevalences in primary care are slightly different, as evidenced by the Psychosocial Problems in Children in Primary Care study, conducted by Kelleher and colleagues (Kelleher *et al.*, 1997). Approximately 18% of children in pediatric practice show evidence of a psychosocial problem of some type, and 10% of children show evidence of behavioral problems severe enough to cause functional impairment. Half of these children have a "disruptive" behavioral disorder. By far the most common of these is attention deficit hyperactivity disorder, which is present in 8% of children visiting primary care clinicians (Wasserman *et al.*, 1999). This condition is diagnosed more frequently in boys than in girls, and has been the subject of controversy, accounting as it does for 80% of psychotropic prescriptions written in the primary care setting (Hoagwood, 1996; Kelleher *et al.*, 1989). Symptoms of ADHD include severe hyperactivity, impulsivity, and an inability to maintain attention. To be diagnosed as ADHD the child's symptoms should be so severe as to impair functioning at school and home.

While few dispute the fact that stimulant medications produce an improvement in disruptive, hyperactive behavior, these medications have a host of side effects, some of which can be serious. This has prompted a debate about whether we are inappropriately drugging our nation's children in order to enforce "good" behavior. It has also provoked an evaluation of alternative treatment strategies, such as biofeedback, behavior modification, and environmental adjustments. These recent events will undoubtedly bring changes in the way we regard and approach mental disorders in children in the next few years.

## SUBTHRESHOLD CONDITIONS

As a general rule, a condition is called a mental illness if two criteria are met: A specified set of symptoms must be present, and these symptoms must collectively cause some sort of impairment. In recent years the assessment of functional health has enjoyed considerable development, so that the measurement of impairment has become much more specific and refined. This development has created an interesting situation in the field of mental health. It turns out that significant functional impairment frequently occurs before the requisite symptom count threshold has been exceeded. Thus arises the concept of *subthreshold conditions*—symptoms too few or too mild to meet diagnostic criteria, but sufficient to cause significant impairment. This creates quite a sharp dilemma: On the one hand we do not wish to "pathologize" or "medicalize" every twitch and tic, every stress and complaint that occurs in life; on the other hand we do not wish to overlook the plight of people who are suffering significant impairment in their functional health. So there is some instability in the field with respect to the concept of diagnostic threshold, and we can expect that diagnostic criteria will most likely undergo adjustments as clinicians and researchers come to grips with the functional impairment associated with various symptom constellations.

This issue is most salient with respect to depression, somatization, and perhaps panic and other anxiety disorders.

With respect to depression, severe and persistent symptoms have occurred in up to one-third of the population; minor depression (consisting of at least two of the criterion symptoms for at least 2 weeks) is more common than major depression, and almost as disabling. This is true of the population in general (Robins & Regier, 1991) and of medical patients in particular (Broadhead *et al.*, 1990; Spitzer *et al.*, 1994; Wells *et al.*, 1989).

With respect to somatization, almost 12% of the population meet criteria for lifetime abridged somatization, consisting of four or more symptoms for men, and six or more for women (Escobar *et al.*, 1989). This is 100 times the incidence of somatization disorder. These patients having abridged somatization are more likely to be unemployed and to be on welfare than their unaffected counterparts; those who are employed received significantly less pay than employed nonsomatizing people. This pattern repeats in the clinical realm. Subthreshold or abridged somatization is far more common than somatization disorder, and the patients so affected exhibit significantly higher utilization of medical resources and lower levels of functional health than matched nonsomatizing patients.

## CASE 33-8

*Sandra Fulcher is a 34-year-old woman with a long history of physical complaints that her physician has been unable to explain: On separate occasions in the past 5 years she has been evaluated for shortness of breath, chest pain, back pain, joint pain, headaches, fatigue, dizziness, blurry vision, nausea, abdominal bloating, burning with urination, pain with intercourse, and painful menstrua-*

*tion. At the last visit her physician completed a thorough mental evaluation, and discovered that she met criteria for major depression, panic disorder, and PTSD. The implicated stressor in her diagnosis of PTSD was prolonged, severe sexual abuse by her father when she was a child.*

## THE PROBLEM OF COMORBIDITY

### The Extent and Nature of Comorbidity

Case 33-8 illustrates that people with one mental disorder frequently have at least one other. The ECA Study made the surprising discovery that all subjects meeting criteria for somatization disorder met criteria for at least one other DSM diagnosis (Robins & Regier, 1991). Those most commonly implicated were phobias, major depression, and panic disorder. This pattern is also found in the medical setting, wherein patients with both somatization disorder and intermediate somatization exhibit an extraordinarily high likelihood of having other mental diagnoses (Brown *et al.*, 1990). Moreover, the mere presence of unexplained physical symptoms increases the likelihood that a primary care patient meets criteria for a mental diagnosis, and this likelihood rises with the number of unexplained symptoms (Kroenke *et al.*, 1994).

We have identified a subset of female patients who meet diagnostic criteria for somatization disorder, who came out of dangerous, abusive families, and who themselves have been abused; these women have an average of over four additional DSM-III-R diagnoses (usually depression, panic, PTSD, other anxiety diagnoses, and substance abuse) and are suffering profound functional impairment (deGruy *et al.*, 1994). This comorbidity is so extensive as to call into question the appropriateness of the diagnosis of somatization disorder. When comorbidity is extensive, one must question whether a more fundamental, comprehensive diagnostic formulation might be more fitting. In this case, some variation of extreme PTSD might more accurately (and more sympathetically) portray this condition.

Somatization is not the only condition implicated in this web of comorbidity. For example, the WHO Study cited earlier demonstrated that all specific psychiatric disorders had comorbidity rates above 50% except alcohol dependence, which had a comorbidity rate of 43% (Ormel *et al.*, 1994). Seventy-one percent of patients with panic disorder had another ICD-10 psychiatric diagnosis, and 62% of patients with a major depressive episode had a comorbid diagnosis.

---

### CASE 33-9

*Thomas Layton is a 58-year-old man who suffered a myocardial infarction 3 months ago. His hospital course was uncomplicated, although he was pessimistic about his prospects of returning to a normal life, and he was discharged home to a cardiac rehabilitation program consisting of dietary instruction and a graded exercise regimen. His physician advised him that he should be able to return to normal work activities as a draftsman in about a month. On returning home, however, he expressed increasing pessimism about his future, refused participation in the cardiac rehabilitation program, and showed no interest in returning to work. He became increasingly irritable and agitated and refused visitors. He repeatedly told his wife that "his life was over." Indeed, 4 months after discharge, he died in his sleep.*

---

## THE HEALTH CONSEQUENCES OF MENTAL ILLNESS

### Mortality

Numerous studies have convincingly and repeatedly demonstrated a strong association between mental illness and mortality. The ECA Study documented that people over 55 years of age were four times more likely to die in the ensuing 15 months if they were suffering from major depression than if they were not (Robins & Regier, 1991). In a well-done study of 500 psychiatric outpatients with a wide range of diagnoses followed for an average of 7 years, this cohort had nearly twice the mortality rate of the age-, sex-, and race-adjusted reference population (Martin *et al.*, 1985).

As Mr. Layton's story in Case 33-9 suggests, patients who sustain a myocardial infarction are at increased risk. One study documented a fourfold increased likelihood of death in the following 6 months for those who are depressed at the time of discharge compared with those who are not (Smith *et al.*, 1993). Of course, some of the mortality associated with mental illness is direct: Approximately 15% of patients with severe depression will commit suicide (Fawcett, 1988), and patients with severe panic disorder may be even more likely to kill themselves (Weissman *et al.*, 1989). It is interesting to note that patients with somatization disorder do not appear to be at increased risk of death because of this disorder (Coryell & Norten, 1981).

## Morbidity

Patients with mental disorders suffer poor health. There are at least two aspects to this relationship. First, mental disorders themselves are associated with significant functional impairment. For example, the MOS Study demonstrated that patients suffering from depression are equally or more impaired than comparable patients suffering from medical problems such as hypertension, arthritis, or chronic lung disease (Wells *et al.*, 1989). Even more startling is the finding reported from the PRIME-MD 1000 Study that, among primary care patients, the proportion of functional impairment attributable to mental disorders far outweighs the proportion attributable to physical disorders (Spitzer *et al.*, 1995). In other words, mental disorders themselves seem to cause profound impairment.

The second aspect of this association between mental illness and poor health is related to the comorbidity between mental and medical disorders, such that about two-thirds of patients with a mental diagnosis will have a significant medical problem, with its attendant morbidity (Bridges & Goldberg, 1985; Kroenke *et al.*, 1994). Conversely, patients with medical disorders have a two- to threefold increased likelihood of having a mental diagnosis (Weyerer, 1990). A special case of this mental–medical comorbidity is the peculiar relationship between certain medical disorders, such as stroke or cancer, and mental diagnoses (Wells *et al.*, 1988). It appears that when one has a stroke, for example, one is particularly vulnerable to depression, and when both appear together, the patient is likely to be severely impaired.

## USE OF HEALTHCARE RESOURCES

Patients with mental disorders use more healthcare resources than their unaffected counterparts. Much of this evidence is indirect and in need of confirmation, but several interesting patterns have emerged.

- A study of distressed high utilizers (top 10% healthcare expenditures) in a primary care setting found that over half qualified for a mental diagnosis (Katon *et al.*, 1990). A study of primary care patients with DSM diagnoses showed about a twofold increase in their healthcare utilization compared with patients without mental diagnoses (Shapiro *et al.*, 1984).
- A study of patients diagnosed with a depressive episode showed a rise in visit frequency during the 6 months prior to a diagnosis of depression being made, with a tapering off of visit frequency after the diagnosis has been made and treatment instituted (Widmer & Cadoret, 1978).
- A study of family practice patients with somatization disorder found that their charts were twice as thick, and visit frequencies to the primary care physician nearly twice as great, as matched controls (deGruy *et al.*, 1987).
- Another study of primary care patients with conspicuous somatizing behavior documented a *ninefold* increased rate of overall expenditure for healthcare, relative to the general population (Smith *et al.*, 1986a).

*Nadine Carney recognized what was happening to her: She had been down this road before. She and her husband had retired last July, but since moving to her new home on the Gulf Coast, she had not enjoyed the sense of freedom and leisure she had anticipated. In fact, she felt terrible, even though part of her felt "great." She was becoming more agitated, irritable, and talkative. She was beginning to stay awake at night, and felt the pressure of thoughts crowding into her head, demanding action. She was beginning to feel as though she was having the most profound, important ideas a human had ever had, and this spelled trouble—her mania was returning. She had been admitted to a private psychiatric hospital 14 years ago, after her symptoms had gotten completely out of control, but had returned to her normal mental state after beginning lithium. She took this medication for 10 years, initially under the direction of her admitting psychiatrist, but eventually her family physician assumed responsibility for monitoring her mental status and her lithium levels; when he retired 3 years ago she simply stopped refilling her prescriptions. Now she was getting in trouble again. She knew she needed to begin treatment quickly, before she was "over the edge" again, but didn't know whether to seek psychiatric admission, see a private psychiatrist, visit her family physician, or simply start taking lithium.*

## RESPONSES TO THE PROBLEM

### Society's Response to Mental Illness

One might organize a brief outline of how we as a nation have responded to the problem of mental illness among our citizenry by using as a point of departure the President's Commission on Mental Health, spearheaded by Rosalynn Carter in 1978 (President's Commission on Mental Health, 1978). Prior to this time, several events had occurred that laid the groundwork for the questions raised and programs begun by that commission. In 1961, the Joint Commission on Mental Illness and Health, drawing on census data from mental institutions and early, rough epidemiological data, recommended the Community Mental Health Centers Program as a means of dealing with the mental health needs of the poor and of avoiding unnecessary hospitalization for the mentally ill. Subsequently, many patients with mental illnesses were deinstitutionalized. Concurrently, diagnostic nomenclature and criteria became more valid and reliable, and by the time DSM-III was developed, it was possible to diagnose the "same" mental disorders across settings. Nevertheless, at the time of the President's Commission, there were still few answers to a number of critically important questions: we knew something about the range of disorders affecting patients currently or formerly in mental institutions, but what proportion of the total national burden of mental illness did this represent? How many of our citizens suffer from mental disorders? In what populations do these disorders occur? What are the health consequences of these disorders? Do these people seek care for their problems? Where? How adequate is the care that is rendered in various settings, and how effective are the treatments even when adequately rendered? A number of ambitious programs were instituted to address these questions, including programs of research and training in the mental health specialty and primary care medical sectors and the extraordinary ECA program, which mapped the mental health of the United States.

While we can be encouraged by the enormous progress in our knowledge about and treatment of mental illness, this progress is seriously deficient in certain areas. At this time only about 20% of patients with mental diagnoses seek help for their condition (Robins & Regier, 1991, p. 341). Moreover, the structure of our healthcare system and our funding priorities practically guarantee that important problems with the care of the mentally ill will persist. The mental healthcare of children and the elderly is seriously deficient, and we still have a need for improved care of ambulatory patients with serious mental illnesses. Perhaps two of the most important problems are the generally inadequate—and deteriorating—health insurance benefit for mental healthcare, and the difficulty incorporating mental healthcare into the incentives and practice structure of the primary healthcare system. The Surgeon General has recently issued a Report on Mental Health that gives an excellent overview of the problem, and proposes a set of actions to address these problems, including:

- Building the science base
- Overcoming stigma
- Improving public awareness of effective treatment
- Ensuring an adequate supply of services and providers
- Ensuring delivery of treatments
- Tailoring treatments to age, race, gender, and culture
- Facilitating entry into treatment
- Reducing financial barriers to treatment (Satcher, 2000)

## The Clinician's Response to Mental Illness

It is generally conceded that, while most mental health care transpires in the primary care medical setting, the quality and extent of this care are less than optimal. This problem has received extensive discussion recently, and is the subject of considerable research. At the risk of oversimplifying the present state of affairs, I would venture the following summary:

People who present to primary care physicians with mental symptoms and disorders are different from those who appear for care in a mental health care setting. They often present with physical rather than psychological complaints (Bridges & Goldberg, 1985); when this happens, the clinician is less likely to diagnose a mental disorder (Kirmayer *et al.*, 1993). Comorbidity is extensive, and patients tend to have confusing constellations of symptoms that do not fit very well into the existing classifications.

While primary care physicians tend to have incomplete knowledge of the diagnostic criteria for mental diagnoses (Badger *et al.*, 1994), simple education has little effect on diagnostic accuracy. In fact, provision of diagnostic information or even clinical diagnoses appears to have little effect on management of mental disorders in primary care (Magruder-Habib *et al.*, 1989).

While protocol-type interventions for specific mental disorders, such as depression (Schulberg *et al.*, 1995) or somatization (Smith *et al.*, 1986b, 1995), have been shown to result in improved outcomes, these have proven difficult to implement or maintain in the primary care setting. Even though patients may be extremely resistant to accepting a referral to a mental health professional (Olfson, 1991), they are also resistant to accepting and staying in treatment by their primary care physician (Schulberg *et al.*, 1995). Moreover, even

---

### MISSING MENTAL DISORDERS

*About half of the patients who come to the office of a primary care physician and who are depressed are not diagnosed with depression. About half of those who are diagnosed are either not treated or are treated inadequately. Why? There are good reasons for this apparent deficiency.*

- *The average visit lasts less than 15 minutes, yet most patients have up to six problems on their problem list, and they are there for a reason other than depression. Moreover, the primary care clinician may wish to spend some time on prevention, health maintenance, and other health issues. In other words, depression gets crowded out by other competing demands.*
- *Many patients with depression do not wish to have this diagnosis on their chart. It can interfere with a patient's insurability, and it can be a source of embarrassment for and discrimination against the patient.*
- *Certain insurance companies will not pay for a primary care clinician to take care of this problem.*
- *Many patients with depression get better without treatment, and many physicians are waiting until we have a better way of recognizing just those patients who will benefit from treatment.*

---

the primary care physician who likes to deal with psychosocial issues faces a number of disincentives, such as a long list of competing demands for the 10–15 minutes allotted for the patient's visit (including dealing with the presenting complaint and with health maintenance issues), the stigma to the patient of a mental diagnosis, and the unwillingness of third parties to pay for mental health services rendered in this setting. Some managed care plans insist that all patients with mental diagnoses be referred to mental health specialists for care, even though the patients refuse to accept the referral.

Nevertheless, there is progress. For example, the PRIME-MD and the SDDS-PC are two of a new generation of instruments that can quickly and accurately make multiple mental diagnoses in the primary care setting. These are powerful case-finding tools that lend a new impetus to the search for effective management strategies within the primary care setting. In fact, several interesting management strategies are currently under investigation, and some have been shown to be effective and cost-effective in the primary care setting, notwithstanding the difficulty of their implementation. For example, Schulberg and colleagues have demonstrated that primary care patients who are randomized into a protocol involving careful administration either of an antidepressant or of psychotherapy, both administered in the primary care setting, fare substantially better than similar patients exposed to usual care (Schulberg *et al.*, 1995). It is beginning to look like a combination of pharmacotherapy and psychotherapy (specifically, cognitive–behavioral therapy) might be particularly effective against depression in the primary care setting (Keller *et al.*, 2000). Katon and colleagues demonstrated that primary care patients who receive a consultation visit with a psychiatrist have significantly better outcomes than those receiving usual care (Katon *et al.*, 1995). Smith and colleagues have demonstrated that primary care patients with somatization disorder and with abridged somatization (6–12 unexplained symptoms) benefit if their primary care physician receives a consultation letter from a psychiatrist; group therapy also helps these patients (Smith *et al.*, 1986b, 1995). At this time there are a score of clinical trials underway testing a variety of interventions against mental disorders in the primary care setting; many of these trials are collaborative efforts taking place within the primary care setting.

## CONCLUSION

Recently we have learned about the startling degree to which mental disorders affect our nation's health. These disorders are surprisingly common, both in the general population and in various medical settings. They are also surprisingly debilitating. We are accustomed to regarding chronic medical illnesses as causing functional impairment, but mental illnesses have been shown to be as much or more injurious to a person's ability to function normally. Add to this two important barriers: (1) that people do not wish to be known as mentally ill, and will resist seeking care for these problems, and (2) when they do seek care, it is most often in a medical setting, with their mental distress disguised by physical complaints or confounded with physical illness. The training of medical practitioners and the structure of their practices work against the successful management of mental disorders, and the management of these disorders in segregated mental health specialty settings is fraught with problems—the inherent inseparability of the mental and the physical, the resistance of many patients to accepting care in a mental health specialty setting, and the tendency of care to become fragmented and redundant.

Despite these important obstacles, much progress has been made. We have evolved a reliable and exceptionally powerful diagnostic system for mental disorders. We now have an accurate profile of these disorders and their constituent symptoms as they occur in the population and in various medical and mental health care settings. We have begun to learn about the functional consequences of these disorders, and we have begun to learn a great deal about the care people with mental illness need and receive. We continue to discover more efficacious treatments for the various mental disorders, and are likewise learning how to apply these treatments more effectively. Despite the enormous islands of ignorance remaining in our knowledge of mental illness, and the equally enormous discrepancy between the knowledge we have and the service we actually render, we can take hope that sufficient infrastructure, investigators, and providers are in place to feed the stream of progress in the field. We have good reason to be optimistic about the future of this long-neglected domain, even though we have far to go before we can rest assured that the mental health care needs of our citizens and our patients are adequately addressed.

## BIOGRAPHIES AND AUTOBIOGRAPHIES
## OF PERSONS WITH MENTAL ILLNESS

Darkness Visible, *by William Styron. Major depression*
Mrs. Dalloway, *by Virginia Woolf. PTSD, suicide*
Ladder of Years, *by Anne Tyler. Depression*
An Unquiet Mind, *by Kay Redfield Jamison. Bipolar Disorder*
The Outsider: A Journey into my Father's Struggle with Madness, *by Nathaniel Lachen-meyer. Paranoid schizophrenia*
The Tennis Partner, *by Abraham Verghese. Depression, substance abuse, suicide*

# CASES FOR DISCUSSION

## CASE 1

*Eddie Nelson was having trouble with his bowels. Since childhood he had suffered from trouble with constipation, and now he knew why. His food was being poisoned by the FBI, who wanted to keep him quiet about their secret operations in the West. For years he had harbored a suspicion that our government was intruding illegally into his life. Two years ago he had joined the CFF, a well-funded and well-organized group dedicated to eliminating these illegal violations of privacy. Lately, however, he had stopped going to meetings and stopped talking to CFF members. The FBI had begun planting distracting thoughts in his head, buzzing about the weather conspiracy and their agents who worked for the television and newspaper companies. He had taken to humming loudly as a way of keeping the buzzing from driving him crazy. He knew*

## FILMS ABOUT PERSONS WITH MENTAL ILLNESS

Captain Neuman, MD *(1963), with Gregory Peck, Tony Curtis, and Angie Dickinson. PTSD*
Sling Blade *(1996), with Billy Bob Thornton. Mental Retardation*
Shine *(1996), with Geoffrey Rush and Armin Mueller-Stahl. Schizophrenia*
Ordinary People *(1980), with Donald Sutherland, Mary Tyler Moore, and Timothy Hutton. Abnormal Grief Reaction*
Girl, Interrupted *(2000), with Winona Ryder and Angelina Jolie. Depression*
Primal Fear *(1998), with Richard Gere and Edward Norton. Sociopathic Personality Disorder and feigned Dissociative Identity Disorder*
As Good as It Gets *(1997), with Jack Nicholson and Helen Hunt. OCD*
What About Bob? *(1991), with Bill Murray and Richard Dreyfuss. Anxiety (agoraphobia, hypochondriasis), Dependent Personality Disorder*
Don Juan De Marco *(1995), with Marlon Brando and Johnny Depp. Delusional Disorder*
Mr. Jones *(1993), with Richard Gere and Lena Olin. Bipolar Disorder*
The Three Faces of Eve *(1958), with Joann Woodward. Dissociative Identity Disorder*
Hannah and Her Sisters *(1986), with Mia Farrow. Hypochondriasis, substance abuse.*
Fatal Attraction *(1987), with Glenn Close and Michael Douglas. Borderline Personality Disorder*
Jacknife *(1989), with Robert DeNiro and Ed Harris. PTSD.*
A Beautiful Mind *(2001), with Russell Crowe, Ed Harris, and Jennifer Connelly. Schizophrenia*

*that the woman posing as his physician was also trying to poison him with the medication she was giving him, and he avoided taking it whenever possible.*

*His parents first got worried about a year ago, when he became much more reclusive and suspicious than usual. For almost 6 months prior to his hospitalization, he had refused to leave his room; his mother had sought help for her son when he began defecating in his room to avoid the bathroom, which he believed to be bugged. Initially he had responded dramatically to medication, but lately his old symptoms were returning.*

1. *Does Eddie Nelson have a mental disorder? If so, what are the symptoms that suggest mental illness?*
2. *Did he have a mental illness 5 years ago? If not, at what point would you say his mental illness began?*
3. *Eddie does not wish to take medication, which he believes steals his awareness of what the FBI is trying to do to him. His parents wanted him to take medication. Is it ethical to force him to take medication over his objections? If his parents wished him left unmedicated, what would be the proper thing to do?*

## CASE 2

*"Twelve more years before retirement. I don't think I can make it. I don't think I can make it for another month. I used to love my work, but now I just don't care. All I want to do is stay in my recliner and watch the tube. Not that I enjoy that either, but I don't feel like doing anything else. I don't have the energy to do anything. I don't eat, I can't sleep, I can't think clearly. I dunno, I give up. I just can't go on living like this." Two months ago Regina Jacobi had been promoted to floor supervisor, a position she'd had her eye on for 4 years. While this promotion brought new stresses, these were neither unmanageable nor entirely unwelcome. Then her mother died unexpectedly. Shortly thereafter "the color began to go out" of her life, and the symptoms described above began.*

1. *Does Ms. Jacobi have a mental disorder? If so, what would you call it? If you can't decide or don't know, what additional information would you like to have?*
2. *What role does stress and loss play in her symptoms? Would the presence of these factors change the way the physician manages this situation?*
3. *What are the management options here? Is this something that should be handled in the primary care medical setting? In the mental health setting? In the hospital?*

## CASE 3

*Nicole Dunnagan told a horrible story. Her life had been normal—boring, even—until last New Year's Eve, when she went to a party at a friend's house. Shortly after midnight she left for home, but was assaulted in the parking lot as she got into her car. Her assailant abducted her at knifepoint, drove her deep into the woods, and brutally raped and beat her. She suffered facial fractures, laryngeal edema from strangulation, a laceration of her right breast, and severe genital trauma. It took her body 6 months to recover, but even after her physical injuries healed, she continued to have nightmares about her ordeal. She awakened almost nightly in a panic, with her heart racing, unable to catch her breath, her stomach in knots. It was hours before she could calm down enough to go back to sleep. She had become so fearful that she couldn't drive any more and refused to go out with her friends. Sounds would startle her, and the very thought of having sex caused her to become physically ill.*

1. *What is going on here? Is Ms. Dunnagan having a normal reaction? Does she have a mental illness? If so, what?*
2. *What can be done to help her? Who should do it?*
3. *What is her prognosis? Does she have a chance to return to her normal, old self?*

## CASE 4

*Veronica Thomas was worried. Her chest pain was more frequent and severe, and she wanted some answers. Her cardiologist argued that her age (25 years), her previous normal catheterization, her low risk factor profile, and her atypical symptoms meant her heart was almost surely normal. He refused any further cardiac workup, and suggested she see a gastroenterologist about a GI workup. She did—last week she had an endoscopy, which was normal. Today she is in your office, saying: "I know this pain is not in my head. This pain is real! Something is wrong, and I want you to find out what it is!" You perform a physical examination, which is entirely within normal limits.*

1. *What further tests do you want at this point?*
2. *Assume any further tests are also normal. What do you think accounts for Ms. Thomas's pain? How do you explain this to her?*
3. *In 3 weeks Ms. Thomas returns with steady, severe midabdominal pain. Your initial examination is normal. What tests would you order at this point? If these tests are normal, does this suggest a diagnosis?*

## CASE 5

*Arthur Campbell has returned for his annual visit to get his medication refilled. He takes an ACE inhibitor for hypertension, which has completely controlled his blood pressure for the past 4 years. Today his pressure is 156/96. He states that he never missed a dose until last month, when he forgot his pill twice. He says that he has been forgetful lately. This prompts you to ask a series of questions that yield the following facts: Mr. Campbell's forgetfulness seems to be related to a difficulty in concentrating; he has been very restless and fidgety, and has begun worrying about things that didn't previously bother him, such as his marriage, his kids, his job, and his waning physical capacities. These worries have been present for about 4 months, but more worrisome to him is his loss of interest in his hobbies. He is a gun collector and a hunter, and has not hunted once this season. His sleep, appetite, sex drive, and job performance are unimpaired. On some days he feels fine, but on most days he does not.*

1. *Mr. Campbell did not come in complaining of these psychological symptoms, but only wanted his blood pressure medication refilled. Do you regard his symptoms as a problem? Does he have a mental disorder? How will you discuss this with him?*
2. *After a careful diagnostic assessment, you learn that Mr. Campbell has symptoms of depression and anxiety, but meets diagnostic criteria for neither. Does he have a mental illness? How would you chart his problem, and how would you follow it?*
3. *Is treatment indicated for Mr. Campbell's mental symptoms? If so, what treatment?*

## RECOMMENDED READINGS

American Psychiatric Association: *Diagnostic and Statistical Manual of Mental Disorders*, ed 4 (DSM-IV). Washington, DC, American Psychiatric Association, 1994.

> This is the current version of the standard psychiatric diagnostic nomenclature and criteria. This volume is dry and somewhat difficult to navigate, but is packed with useful diagnostic clinical material.

American *Psychiatric Association: Diagnostic and Statistical Manual of Mental Disorders*, ed 4: *Primary Care Version* (DSM-IV-PC). Washington, DC, American Psychiatric Association, 1995.

> This is a psychiatric diagnostic manual written for primary care clinicians. It is much simpler and briefer than the full DSM-IV manual, and is organized into diagnostic algorithms that lead the clinician to a diagnosis from presenting symptoms.

Miranda J, Hohmann AA, Attkisson CC, Larson DB (eds): *Mental Disorders in Primary Care*. San Francisco, Jossey–Bass Inc, Publishers, 1994.

> As the title implies, this interesting volume summarizes what we know, and what we need to know and do, about mental disorders as they occur in the primary care setting.

Robins LN, Regier DA: *Psychiatric Disorders in America: The Epidemiologic Catchment Area Study*. New York, The Free Press, 1991.

> This is a one-volume summary of many of the findings from one of the most ambitious mental health studies ever undertaken, the ECA Study.

## REFERENCES

American Psychiatric Association: *Diagnostic and Statistical Manual of Mental Disorders*, ed 4, Washington, DC, American Psychiatric Press, 1994a.

American Psychiatric Association. *Diagnostic and Statistical Manual of Mental Disorders*, ed 4, primary care version (DSM-IV-PC). Washington, DC, American Psychiatric Press, 1994b.

Badger LW, deGruy FV, Hartman J, Plant MA, Leeper J, Ficken R, Maxwell A, Rand E, Anderson R, Templeton B: Psychosocial interest, medical interviews, and the recognition of depression. *Arch Fam Med* 3:899–907, 1994.

Bridges KW, Goldberg DP: Somatic presentation of DSM III psychiatric disorders in primary care. *J Psychosom Res* 29:563–569, 1985.

Broadhead WE, Blazer DG, George LK, Tse CK: Depression, disability days, and days lost from work in a prospective epidemiologic survey. *JAMA* 264:2524–2528, 1990.

Brown FW, Golding JM, Smith GR: Psychiatric comorbidity in primary care somatization disorder. *Psychosom Med* 52:445–451, 1990.

Cloninger CR, Martin RL, Guze SB, Clayton PJ: A prospective follow-up and family study of somatization in men and women. *Am J Psychiatry* 143:873–878, 1986.

Coryell W, Norten SG: Briquet's syndrome (somatization disorder) and primary depression: Comparison of background and outcome. *Compr Psychiatry* 22:249–256, 1981.

Costello EJ, Angold A, Burns BJ, Stangl DK, Tweed DL, Erkanli A, Worthman CM. The Great Smoky Mountains study of youth: Goals, design, methods, and the prevalence of DSM-III-R disorders. *Arch Gen Psychiatry* 53:1129–1136, 1996.

deGruy FV, Columbia L, Dickinson WP: Somatization disorder in a family practice. *J Fam Pract* 25:45–51, 1987.

deGruy FV, Dickinson I, Dickinson P: Patterns of somatization in primary care. Paper presented at the Eighth Annual NIMH International Research Conference on Mental Health Problems in the General Health Care Sector, McLean, VA, 1994.

Denton WH: Problems encountered in reconciling individual and relational diagnoses, in Kaslow FW (ed): *Handbook of Relational Diagnoses*. New York, John Wiley & Sons, Inc, 1996, p 450.

Dickinson LM, deGruy FV, Dickinson WP, Candib LM: Health-related quality of life and symptom profiles of female sexual abuse survivors. *Arch Fam Med* 8:35–43, 1999.

Engel GL: The need for a new medical model: A challenge for biomedicine. *Science* 196:129–136, 1977.

Escobar JI: Cross-cultural aspects of the somatization trait. *Hosp Community Psychiatry* 38:174–180, 1987.

Escobar JI, Rubio-Stipec M, Canino G, Karno M: Somatic symptom index (SSI): A new and abridged somatization construct: Prevalence and epidemiological correlates in two large community samples. *J Nerv Ment Dis* 177:140–146, 1989.

Fawcett J: Predictors of early suicide: Identification and appropriate intervention. *J Clin Psychiatry* 49:7–8, 1988.

Guze SB: Genetics of Briquet's syndrome and somatization disorder. *Ann Clin Psychiatry* 5:225–230, 1993.

Guze SB, Cloninger CR, Martin RI, Clayton PJ: A follow-up and family study of Briquet's syndrome. *Br J Psychiatry* 149:17–23, 1986.

Higgins ES: A review of unrecognized mental illness in primary care: Prevalence, natural history, and efforts to change the course. *Arch Fam Med* 3:908–917, 1994.

Hoagwood K: Outcomes of mental health care for children and adolescents: I. Comprehensive conceptual model. *J Am Acad Child Adolesc Psychiatry* 35:1055–1063, 1996.

Katon W, Von Korff M, Lin E, Lipscomb P, Russo J, Wagner E, Polk E: Distressed high utilizers of medical care: DSM-III-R diagnoses and treatment needs. *Gen Hosp Psychiatry* 12:355–362, 1990.

Katon W, Von Korff M, Lin E, Walker E, Simon GE, Bush T, Robinson P, Russo J: Collaborative management to achieve treatment guidelines: Impact on depression in primary care. *JAMA* 273:1026–1031, 1995.

Kelleher KJ, Hohmann A, Larson D: Prescription of psychotropic drugs in office-based practices. *Am J Dis Child* 143:855–859, 1989.

Kelleher K, Childs G, Wasserman R, McInerny T, Nutting P, Gardner W: Insurance status and recognition of psychosocial problems: A report from PROS and ASPN. *Arch Pediatr Adolesc Med* 151:1109–1115, 1997.

Keller MB, McCullough JP, Klein D: A comparison of nefazodone, the cognitive behavioral-analysis system of psychotherapy, and their combination for the treatment of chronic depression. *N Engl J Med* 342:1462–1470, 2000.

Kirmayer LJ, Robbins JM, Dworkind M, Yaffe MJ: Somatization and the recognition of depression and anxiety in primary care. *Am J Psychiatry* 150:734–741, 1993.

Kleinman AM: *Patients and Healers in the Context of Culture: An Exploration of the Borderland between Anthropology, Medicine, and Psychiatry*. Los Angeles, University of California Press, 1980.

Klerman GL, Vaillant GE, Spitzer RL, Michels R: A debate on DSM-III. *Am J Psychiatry* 141:539–553, 1984.

Kroenke K, Spitzer RI, Williams JB, Linzer M, Hahn S, deGruy F, Brody D: Physical symptoms in primary care: Predictors of psychiatric disorders and functional impairment. *Arch Fam Med* 3:774–779, 1994.

Leaf PJ: Psychiatric disorders and the use of health services, in Miranda J, Hohmann AA, Attkisson CC, Larson DB (eds): *Mental Disorders in Primary Care*. San Francisco, Jossey–Bass Inc, Publishers, 1994, pp 377–401.

Lin EH, Carter WB, Kleinman AM: An exploration of somatization among Asian refugees and immigrants in primary care. *Am J Public Health* 75:1080–1084, 1985.

Magruder-Habib K, Zung W, Feussner J, Alling W, Saunders W, Stevens H: Management of general medical patients with symptoms of depression. *Gen Hosp Psychiatry* 11:201–206, 1989.

Martin RI, Cloninger CR, Guze SB, Clayton PH: Mortality in a followup of 500 psychiatric outpatients: I. Total mortality. *Arch Gen Psychiatry* 42:47–54, 1985.

Olfson M: Primary care patients who refuse specialized mental health services. *Arch Intern Med* 151:129–132, 1991.

Ormel J, Von Korff M, Ustun B, Pini S, Korten A, Oldehinkel T: Common mental disorders and disability across cultures: Results from the WHO collaborative study on psychological problems in general healthcare. *JAMA* 272:1741–1748, 1994.

President's Commission on Mental Health: *Report to the President from the President's Commission on Mental Health* (040-000-00390-8, vol 1). Washington, DC, Government Printing Office, 1978.

Ritchie K: The little woman meets son of DSM-III. *J Med Philos* 14:695–708, 1989.

Robins LN, Regier DA: *Psychiatric Disorders in America: The Epidemiologic Catchment Area Study*. New York, The Free Press, 1991.

Satcher D: *Mental Health: A Report from the Surgeon General*. 2000. http://www.surgeongeneral.gov/library/mentalhealth/home.html

Schulberg HC, Block MR, Madonia JJ, Rodriguez E, Scott CP, Lave J: Applicability of clinical pharmacotherapy guidelines for major depression in primary care settings. *Arch Fam Med* 4:106–112, 1995.

Shapiro S, Skinner EA, Kessler LG, Von Korff M, German PS, Tischler GL, Leaf P, Benham L, Cottler L, Regier DA: Utilization of health and mental health services: Three epidemiologic catchment area sites. *Arch Gen Psychiatry* 41:971–978, 1984.

Smith GR, Monson RA, Livingston RL: Somatization disorder in men. *Gen Hosp Psychiatry* 7:4–8, 1985.

Smith GR, Monson RA, Ray DC: Patients with multiple unexplained symptoms: Their characteristics, functional health, and health care utilization. *Arch Intern Med* 149:69–72, 1986a.

Smith GR, Monson RA, Ray DC: Psychiatric consultation in somatizations disorder: A randomized controlled study. *N Engl J Med* 314:1407–1413, 1986b.

Smith GR, Rost K, Kashner TM: A trial of the effect of a standardized psychiatric consultation on health outcomes and costs in somatizing patients. *Arch Gen Psychiatry* 52:238–243, 1995.

Smith NF, Lesperance F, Talajic M: Depression following myocardial infarction: Impact on 6-month survival. *JAMA* 270:1819–1861, 1993.

Spitzer RL, Williams JB, Kroenke K, Linzer M, deGruy FV, Hahn SR, Brody D, Johnson JG: Utility of a new procedure for diagnosing mental disorders in primary care: The PRIME-MD 1000 Study. *JAMA* 272:1749–1756, 1994.

Spitzer RL, Kroenke K, Linzer M, Hahn SR, Williams JBW, deGruy FV, Brody D, Davies M: Health-related quality of life in primary care patients with mental disorders: Results from the PRIME-MD 1000 Study. *JAMA* 274:1511–1517, 1995.

Trotter RT: Folk medicine in the Southwest. *Postgrad Med* 78:167–179, 1985.

Wasserman R, Kelleher K, Bocian A, Baker A, Chids GE, Indacochea F, Stulp C, Gardner WP: Identification of attentional and hyperactivity problems in primary care: A report from PROS and ASPN. *Pediatrics* 103:E38, 1999.

Weissman WM, Klerman GL, Markowitz JS, Ouellette R: Suicidal ideation and suicide attempts in panic disorder and attacks. *N Engl J Med* 321:1209–1214, 1989.

Wells KB, Golding JM, Burnam MA: Psychiatric disorder in a sample of the general population with and without chronic medical condition. *Am J Psychiatry* 145:976–981, 1988.

Wells KB, Stewart A, Hays RD, Burnam A, Rogers W, Daniels M, Berry S, Greenfield S, Ware J: The functioning and well-being of depressed patients. *JAMA* 626:914–919, 1989.

Weyerer S: Relationships between physical and psychological disorders, in Sartorius N, Goldberg D, de Girolamo G, Cost e Silva J, Lecrubier Y, Wittchen U (eds): *Psychological Disorders in General Medical Settings.* Toronto, Hogrefe & Huber, 1990, pp 34–46.

Widmer RB, Cadoret RJ: Depression in primary care changes in pattern of patient visits and complaints during a developing depression. *J Fam Pract* 7:293–302, 1978.

# Sexually Transmitted Diseases

*Peggy B. Smith*

*Sarah, an 18-year-old African-American woman, came to the clinic for a pregnancy test. Her test was positive. She was also tested for gonorrhea, chlamydia, and syphilis, and was reactive for syphilis. This was her third pregnancy. She had one living child, a previous abortion, and planned to terminate this pregnancy. All three pregnancies resulted from unprotected intercourse with her 22-year-old boyfriend of 3½ years. This was her second case of syphilis from this partner. She was in denial regarding her partner's infidelity and her risk of pregnancy. She also doubted the diagnosis of syphilis.*

## EDUCATIONAL OBJECTIVES

1. Differentiate the consequences to the patient of various sexually transmitted diseases (STDs)
2. Evaluate life circumstances that place patients at risk for infection or reinfection with an STD
3. Identify social values that might act as barriers to effective treatment

## INTRODUCTION

As Case 34-1 indicates, physicians must deal with a number of sensitive and troubling issues when treating patients with STDs. Changing lifestyles, serial monogamy, partner age, and early initiation of sexual activity have increased the prevalence of STDs. No age group is spared, although 65% of infections are found among individuals 16 to 24 years of age. Although viewed by many as an affliction of minorities and the poor, STDs are prevalent among all social, economic, and racial groups.

Social issues and partner selection factors as well as epidemiological trends affect the prevalence of STDs and therefore need to be addressed proactively. It is only when these illnesses are evaluated systematically, holistically, and contextually that the patient can be treated effectively.

As Case 34-1 suggests, a large number of STDs are asymptomatic or have such mild symptoms that the patient ignores them. For a subset of individuals, discharges from genital organs, even when odoriferous, are seen as normal. Another important point is that some STDs covary; this is often the case with gonorrhea and chlamydia and with syphilis and HIV. Because of this covariance, diagnostic procedures have been developed that are sensitive to both infections and should be the screening method of choice.

Another point concerns the way that pregnancy testing and other service options can function as gateways to preventive primary healthcare. Pregnancy testing for women of reproductive age provides a flexible access point to diagnose and treat STDs and other illnesses. A complete physical examination along with appropriate screening for STDs should be routine. Even if the pregnancy test is negative, public health interventions can be initiated. If syphilis is detected, for example, treatment and cure can be initiated so that if a future pregnancy is conceived, the fetus will be protected. The trends toward use of urine-based detection methods may affect the clinical screening of high-risk groups for other reproductive health concerns.

Classically, STDs have included syphilis, herpes, chlamydia, and gonorrhea as major entities. HIV/ AIDS, by virtue of its form of transmission, has also been added by some to the major category. Since many other diseases are now known to be capable of passage by sexual activity, such as hepatitis B, the list of sexually transmitted diseases has grown (see Table 34.1). Most of these infections involve the genital area, but rectal, pharyngeal, and other areas of infection are increasingly common.

**Table 34.1**
Sexually Transmitted Diseases[a]

| Disease | Organism |
|---|---|
| | Bacteria |
| Gonorrhea | *Neisseria gonorrhoeae* |
| Vulvovaginitis, urethritis | *Haemophilus vaginalis* and other anaerobic bacteria, chlamydia also |
| Chancroid | *Haemophilus ducreyi* |
| Granuloma | *Calymmatobacterium granulomatis* |
| Syphilis | *Treponema pallidum* |
| Dysentery | *Shigella* |
| Gasterenteritis, enteric fever | *Salmonella* |
| Neonatal and infant infections | Group B *Streptococcus* |
| Lymphogranuloma venereum | *Chlamydia trachomatis* |
| Inclusion cervicitis, vaginitis, and urethritis | Trachoma inclusion conjunctivitis agent |
| | Fungus |
| Vulvovaginitis | *Candida albicans* |
| Tinea cruris | *Epidermophyton inguinale* |
| | Metazoa |
| Pediculosis pubis | *Phthirus pubis* |
| Scabies | *Acarus* |
| | Mycoplasma |
| Cervicitis, vaginitis, urethritis | *Mycoplasma hominis* or *T. mycoplasma* |
| | Protozoa |
| Vulvovaginitis | *Trichomonas vaginalis* |
| | Viruses |
| Vulvovaginalis | Herpes simplex virus type 2 |
| Conduloma acuminatum | Papilloma virus |
| Genital dermatitis | Molluscum contagiosum virus |
| Cervicitis, urethritis | Cytomegalovirus |
| Hepatitis | Hepatitis B or C |
| AIDS | Human immunodeficiency virus (HIV) |

[a]Adapted from Smith PB, Mumford DM (eds): *Adolescent Pregnancy Perspectives for the Health Professional.* Boston, GK Hall & Co, 1986.

*As oral sex rates have increased so have the rates of pharyngeal infections of gonorrhea.*
*This is an important new infection location.*

With increasing sexual activity, especially among the young, venereal disease incidence continues to rise. For example, the incidence of gonorrhea has increased rapidly over the past 10 years (Hatcher *et al.*, 1998). The increase in gonorrhea incidence in the teenage group continues to be much faster than in the general population. Moreover, changing legislation on serological screening for marriage licenses in many states, the covariance of sexual intercourse with IV drug use, and the emergence of large homeless populations have changed the typical patient profile of many STDs. Social trends, such as delay of first marriage, also contribute to the influence of multiple sexual partners on STD acquisition. Additionally, it is not unusual for some patients to contract more than one infection, remain with symptoms over an extended period of time, and if treatment is obtained, either refuse to complete the prescription regimen or become reinfected quickly after cure.

In the following pages we will review the major and minor types of STDs: their incidence, their etiology, their symptoms, and the best means of treatment. We then consider how the physician's attitudes, experience, and training can adversely affect the quality of care for patients with STDs. Next we examine the impact of STDs on patients' lives, focusing particularly on the changes brought about in the relationships of patients, their partners, and their physicians. In the fourth section we ask why STDs are so prevalent and consider such factors as survival sex, family dysfunction, sexual abuse, incest, ignorance, taboos, social stigmas, multiple sexual partners, changing sexual practices, becoming sexually active at a young age, partner selection issues, and the asymptomatic nature of many STDs. In the fifth section we focus on a problem long overlooked by physicians, public health officials, and law enforcement officers: the impact of possible infection on victims of sexual assault. Finally, we consider the physician's role in the community and the need for leadership in educating the public about the risks of acquiring STDs and the most realistic means of prevention.

## CASE 34-2

*A 29-year-old white woman presented for her annual examination at a clinic where she had been a patient for 6 years. She reported being sexually active since age 15, being pregnant twice, and having had only one sex partner. No previous STDs had been diagnosed. The patient reported no vaginal discharge but had experienced itching and an odor for 2 weeks. Her cultures for gonorrhea and chlamydia returned with a positive diagnosis. Her partner reported no symptoms.*

# MAJOR TYPES OF STDs

## Gonorrhea

Gonorrhea is one of the most common STDs. The estimated incidence of gonorrhea in the United States is over 800,000 annually (Institute of Medicine, 1996). Although gonorrhea declined in the United States nearly 60% from 1980 to 1996, the 1996 rate of 124/100,000 was 26 times greater than the rate for Germany (*MMWR*, July 31, 1998). In the United States, reinfection and intercourse with multiple partners continue to fuel the disease. Sixty percent of those afflicted with gonorrhea are said to be males, but some authorities place the estimate closer to 50%. Rates for adolescents are 30% greater than established year 2000 U.S. health goals. Acute gonococcal infection is on the rise among children and adolescents under the age of 15 years. Sexual assault, sexual abuse, and incest contribute significantly to this trend.

Asymptomatic infection of the cervix is the most common form of gonorrhea in women. The symptoms are mild and include vaginal discharge, dysuria, pelvic pain, and uterine bleeding. Uncomplicated gonorrhea is usually limited to the cervix, but disseminated gonorrhea infections may occur. Complicated gonorrhea may involve acute gonococcal salpingitis with fever, chills, abdominal pain during premenstrual intervals, and eventually pelvic inflammatory disease.

Infertility, pain, and ectopic pregnancies often result from this infection. Untreated gonorrhea can scar a woman's tubes and block the transport of a fertilized egg into the uterus. Joint and orthopedic problems can be attributed to gonorrhea. The most common form of disseminated gonococcal infection is the arthritis–dermatitis syndrome.

In men, gonorrhea may cause a discharge, urinary symptoms, and pain in the perineal, suprapubic, or inguinal areas. Fever may also be present, along with pain and swelling of the scrotum. Anorectal gonorrhea can result from anal intercourse. This infection is usually asymptomatic but may cause rectal burning, discharge, or bleeding. Another prevalent form of this infection is oropharyngeal gonorrhea. Estimates suggest that 20% of individuals with genital gonorrhea also have an infection in the pharyngeal area. As the practice of oral sex increases in various populations, so has this infection location.

Women are much more vulnerable to this disease then men. Several authors state that the risk of a woman acquiring gonorrhea from an infected man is 80 to 90%, whereas the man has an estimated 22% risk of being infected by a woman with gonorrhea (Smith & Mumford, 1980). There is much discussion concerning the difference in symptomatology. Age may also play a factor in contagion, as the vaginal tissue of adolescents may be more susceptible to infection than that of adult women. Some believe asymptomatic gonorrhea to be present in 80 to 90% of women, but a more likely figure is 50 to 60%. As seen in Case 34-2, men are more likely to be asymptomatic.

Treatment regimens for this entity have gradually shifted for several reasons. Relative resistance of gonorrhea to penicillin varies and gonorrhea can be resistant to other antibiotics, such as tetracycline, as well. Thus, penicillin or ampicillin treatment failure patients should be monitored after initial treatment and treated with a more powerful antibiotic. The initial emergence in this country of *Neisseria gonorrhoeae* resistant (QRNG) to fluoroquinolones from Asia is now detected with less than 1% reported from designated cities (*MMWR*, 1998), so that current regimens can be automatically used as first-line treatment. However, culture for this entity should be recommended for patients with apparent treatment failure. To facilitate compliance, especially for high-risk populations, single doses of cefixime (400 mg orally), ceftriaxone (125 mg i.m.), ciprofloxacin (500 mg orally), or azithromycin (1 g orally) are the recommended regimens (Centers for Disease Control and Prevention [CDC], 1998). However, cost considerations may force public clinics to utilize doxycycline (100 mg orally/day/7 days) as the treatment of choice. Because doxycycline is also effective against chlamydia, such a treatment may be warranted as estimates suggest that one-fourth of men and two-fifths of women have coexisting infections (Hatcher *et al.*, 1998).

# Syphilis

In 1997, the incidence for all ages of primary and secondary syphilis was 3.2 per 100,000, reflecting a decline of 84% from 1990 to 1997. Numerous have been cited for this steep decline. Since the mid-1980s, increased state and federal public health funding has targeted syphilis. Second, the use of crack cocaine and the exchanging of sex for drugs has declined. Third, the adoption of nontraditional modes of outreach was utilized, and finally the halo effect of HIV education has extended to other STDs. Some researchers have also suggested that some populations are developing a natural immunity (Garnett *et al.*, 1997). In addition to being transferred sexually, syphilis can be transferred vertically from mother to fetus after the third or fourth month of pregnancy. This form of the disease, called congenital syphilis (CS), had, in 1998, a reported rate of 20.6 per 100,000 live births (*MMWR*, September 3, 1999).

The syphilis spirochetes, found only in humans, are slender corkscrew organisms with 6 to 14 regular spirals. Syphilis is traditionally diagnosed through serological testing, the most common tests being the Venereal Disease Research Laboratory (VDRL) and the RPR Card. A variety of conditions such as mononucleosis, collagen diseases, malaria, drug addiction, and in some cases pregnancy can cause false positives.

*Major risk factors for congenital syphilis include no penicillin treatment and/or no prenatal care.*

In addition, syphilis is usually described as having three stages: primary, secondary, and tertiary syphilis. A latent phase occurs between the secondary and tertiary stages. In its early stages syphilis may be unrecognized. It usually takes 3 to 4 weeks of incubation before a chancre or painless sore erupts. The lesion is an ulcer with a clear base and a raised, firm ridge and is found in the genitalia, pharynx, or perianal areas. The VDRL test usually becomes positive 1 or 2 weeks after the chancre is noticed. The spirochete can be found in most lesions, thus making it possible to distinguish the infection from other genital ulcers such as genital herpes, lymphogranuloma venereum, or chancroid.

Parenteral penicillin G has been used effectively for 4 decades to treat syphilis. Nonpregnant or pregnant allergic patients with primary or secondary syphilis can be treated with doxycycline 100 mg orally two times a day for 2 weeks or tetracycline 500 mg orally four times a day for 2 weeks. Penicillin allergic patients need to be desensitized.

If primary syphilis is not treated, secondary syphilis may follow after a period of a few weeks to 6 months. *Treponema pallidum* may produce systemic signs and symptoms such as fever, myalgia, headaches, loss of appetite, a generalized skin rash, mucous membrane lesions including patches and ulcers, condylomata lata from weeping papules in moist skin areas, sore throat, patchy hair loss, and generalized nontender lymphadenopathy. Because of the long incubation period and the variety of manifestations, patients with secondary syphilis may not remember the primary lesion.

Latent or hidden syphilis is the "sleeping" phase, which occurs after the subsidence of secondary symptoms but before the appearance of tertiary ones. If symptoms recur in the first 3 to 5 years after primary infection (so-called "relapsing" syphilis), the stage is defined as early latency; if after 5 years, the latent phase. During the latent phase, positive serology persists.

Tertiary syphilis can be benign when it responds to rapid therapy or it can be more damaging especially where there is central nervous system involvement. Symptoms of neurosyphilis, which is found in 20% of tertiary syphilis cases, are progressive and can be lethal, and include dementia, neurologic deficits, and pain. The cardiovascular system may also be involved, with dissection of the ascending aortic arch, universally fatal, being characteristic.

Undetected, syphilis can also cause serious damage to the fetus, midtrimester abortion, or death. As a preventive measure it is recommended that all women be screened in the first and third trimester for this infection. For populations at risk, screening at delivery is also recommended. Because of the action of the placenta, the fetus is usually protected from transplacental passage of the infection during the first 4 months of pregnancy. Major risk factors for CS include no penicillin treatment during pregnancy (81%) or lack of prenatal care (35.8%) (*MMWR*, June 26, 1998).

The fetus infected with CS may have a variety of symptoms. Syphilitic pemphigus is usually found on the bottoms of the feet and the palms of the hands. These lesions usually contain the spirochete. Mucous membrane involvement with classic sniffle and enlargement of the spleen and lymph nodes accompanied by anemia are also common. Because the onsets of symptoms vary, the neonate may not develop signs of CS before 2 years of age. Continued evaluation of the newborn born during the first year of life is recommended.

*Half of all syphilis cases occur in only 1% of U.S. counties.*

Following increased incidence of primary and secondary syphilis, epidemics of CS are observed. The most recent case was in Baltimore in 1996, which experienced a subsequent increase of CS from 62 to 282 per 100,000 live-born infants (*MMWR*, October 30, 1998).

While the prevalence of primary, secondary, and congenital syphilis has declined since 1991, it demonstrates certain regional and ethnic distributions. Most cases are concentrated in the southern United States (Risser *et al.*, 1999). Although rates have declined 80% since 1990 (*MMWR*, June 26, 1998), the Institute of Medicine (1996) suggests that half of reported cases are found in only 1% of U.S. counties. In addition, rates of primary and secondary syphilis for blacks remained substantially higher than for non-Hispanic whites and Hispanics. In 1997, the rate of primary and secondary syphilis for blacks was 220 per 100,000, compared with 1.6 Hispanic and 0.5 for non-Hispanic whites. Similarly, while CS declined 78.2% from 1992 to 1998, rates were also disproportionately high in the South and among certain ethnic populations, which may reflect other factors such as poverty and nonaccess to healthcare.

# Herpes Simplex Viruses

The herpes simplex viruses (HSV) consist of a group of at least 25 viruses, 5 of which are known to infect humans. These infections include herpes simplex virus types 1 and 2, cytomegalovirus, varicella-zoster, and Epstein–Barr viruses. The last two types usually are not associated with venereal infections.

HSV type 1 causes fever blisters and cold sores, whereas HSV type 2 causes genital lesions and neonatal herpes. Definitive diagnosis of HSV is made through tissue culture, although clinical diagnosis can be made by noting the characteristics of the lesions. Classified into two stages, primary HSV and recurrent or secondary HSV, genital herpes infections are characterized by latency periods and asymptomatic viral shedding stages. In addition, when a person is infected, recurrent lesions often reappear in the same place. Physical and emotional triggers, the presence of an immunosuppressant disease, intense sunlight, or increased stress can reactivate the infection. Based on serologic studies, 45 million people in the United States have been diagnosed HSV-2.

There is no cure for HSV and its treatment is uncertain, often unsatisfactory, and usually directed toward symptomatic relief. The antiviral drugs acyclovir, famciclovir, and valacyclovir have offered some comfort in reducing initial symptoms and suppressing recurring outbreaks. Daily dosage of acyclovir (400 mg × 2) helps control outbreaks in 75% of cases but does not eliminate viral shedding and the possibility of infectivity. The time-honored remedies of sitz baths and astringent solutions give some comfort. Local analgesic ointments, such as 2% lidocaine, may limit intense pain, but should be used sparingly and for short periods (i.e., less than 2 weeks) to prevent sensitization. Topical acyclovir may be necessary during the ulceration stages but is not as successful as the oral form and is useful only for the first clinical episode. Local antibiotic application to prevent secondary infections is often ineffective. Since *Candida albicans* is a common secondary invader, some authorities recommend azoles or nystatin vaginal suppositories.

HSV, if active, can also attack the central nervous system of the neonate during delivery. Neonatal herpes is severe and often fatal. Transmission occurs as the child passes through the birth canal. If a patient with an active case of genital herpes is pregnant, a cesarean section should be performed within 4 hours of the rupture of the membranes to reduce the risk of transmission. The risk of transmission from an infected mother is highest among women with a primary herpes infection but low among women with recurrent herpes. Infants delivered through an infected birth canal should be cultured, followed carefully, and treated with systemic acyclovir. As some women shed virus while asymptomic, a more conservative course may recommend cesarean sections for all infected mothers.

# Chlamydia

The chlamydiae are a group of large, intracellular parasites closely related to gram-negative bacteria. Two species exist, *Chlamydia psittaci*, responsible for the disease in birds (which may be transferred to humans) and *Chlamydia trachomatis*, which has been implicated in a variety of infections including pelvic inflammatory disease, nongonococcal urethritis, and epididymitis.

An estimated 4 million new cases of chlamydiae occur annually. The majority of infected women have few or no symptoms, and asymptomatic infection in women can persist for up to 15 months (Hatcher *et al.*, 1998). Infection can progress in women to involve the upper reproductive tract and may result in serious complications. To identify patients who may have chlamydial infections, the CDC has recommended routine testing based on age, risk behavior, and clinical findings, especially in clinics and group practices that provide reproductive health care to adolescents. The CDC reports that the incidence of chlamydiae continues to increase and is now the most prevalent STD. Adolescents are seen as especially prone to this infection; at-risk teens should be screened twice a year.

Diagnosis of chlamydiae has been enhanced through the development of DNA amplification techniques using urine samples. However, such diagnostic tests are more expensive and are not a substitute for clinical examinations that may detect other STDs or reproductive health conditions.

## HIV/AIDS

HIV type 1 (HIV-1) was identified in 1984 and is found in blood, semen, and vaginal secretions. The virus causes a defect in the body's immune system by invading and then multiplying within certain white blood cells. Once released from the infected cells, the virus attacks more cells and multiplies with time. Other infections that activate the immune system, including other STDs, may act as cofactors that speed further multiplication of the virus. Casual contact or insect bites do not pass the infection. In 1986 a second type of HIV called HIV-2 was isolated from AIDS patients in West Africa. While similarities exist, individuals infected with HIV-2 are less infectious early in the course of infection. With advancing disease, the infectiousness of HIV-2 increases. As less than 100 cases have been diagnosed in the United States, the CDC does not recommend screening for this infection unless a person has a link to an infected partner in West Africa.

The longer a person is infected with HIV, the more likely the immune system will be impaired, thus leaving the infected person vulnerable to many opportunistic diseases, including cancers and pneumonias. In the absence of effective inhibition of HIV replication by antiviral therapy, nearly all people will suffer progressive deterioration of immune function. HIV infections persist for the life of the infected individual, as there is no cure. For adults, in developed countries, the average progression of HIV to AIDS in the absence of a drug regimen is 10–11 years.

In the initial stages of the outbreak, gay men were considered at greater risk for the infection. Vigorous educational and behavioral interventions have had some success in leveling the increasing prevalence of this infection among this cohort. Younger gay men appear to be less worried about being infected and have been less consistent in their sexual practices. As a result, reemergence of the infection has been seen in some homosexual areas. The heterosexual population is also experiencing a growing infection rate. A combination of factors is often cited, including IV drug use among men and sporadic use of condoms by men. A factor that may contribute to marginal condom usage is the attitudes and practices of the female partners. Women, while knowledgeable on the need for condom use, may not apply the information to their behavior. Valdiserre *et al.* (1989) found that among women who acknowledged the importance of such practices, only 14% currently used condoms. As a result, marginal condom use, especially by older men, has been a significant factor in the spread of HIV, especially among adolescent girls.

*There is more than 1 type of HIV! HIV-1 is still the most prevalent, however, and fewer than 100 cases of HIV-2 have been seen in the US.*

As of June 1999, the U.S. Department of Health and Human Services reported 592,552 male and 118,789 female AIDS cases. Data from prevalence surveys and from HIV and AIDS case surveillance continue to reflect the disproportionate impact of the epidemic on racial/ethnic minority populations, especially women, youth, and children. At the same time, prevalence surveys suggest that young men who have sex with men remain a population at high risk for HIV infection. Declines in AIDS incidence and deaths, first reported in 1996, continued through 1997 and provide evidence of the widespread beneficial effects of new treatment regimens. The data highlight the importance of HIV prevention strategies such as promoting knowledge of HIV risk behaviors and ways to reduce the risk of infection, increasing the number of HIV-infected people who are aware of their status, and improving access to effective care and treatment programs to improve health and survival among persons who are already infected.

The CD4+ T-lymphocyte count is the best laboratory indicator of clinical progression, and comprehensive management strategies for HIV infection are typically stratified by CD4 count. Patients with CD4+ counts > 500 usually do not demonstrate evidence of clinical immunosuppression. Patients with 200–500 CD4+ cells are more likely to develop HIV-related symptoms and to require medical intervention. Patients with CD4+ counts < 200 cells, and those with higher CD4+ counts who develop thrush or unexplained fever are at increased risk for developing complicated HIV disease.

Over the last 10 years the profile of HIV in the United States has transitioned from a short-term to a long-term disease. HIV infection in young men and women continues to increase while the rate of AIDS death has slowed. Age-adjusted death rates from HIV infection in the United States declined 47% from 1996 to 1997, and HIV infection fell from 8th to 14th among leading causes of death in the United States over the same time. For those aged 25–44, HIV dropped from the leading cause of death in 1995 to 3rd leading in 1996, and 5th leading in 1997. The age-adjusted HIV death rate of 5.9 per 100,000 is the lowest rate since 1987, the first year mortality data were available for the disease. The 1997 rate is less than one-half the 1992 rate (12.6) and almost one-third the 1995 rate (15.6). The decline in AIDS deaths is primarily due to the continuing impact of highly active antiretroviral therapy in helping people with HIV live longer and healthier lives. At the same time, success in treating those with HIV does not mean the issue has gone away. Prior to the introduction of antiviral therapies the AIDS incidence increased 5% per year.

A closer look at the trends for AIDS in the United States reveals a shift in the epidemic's profile. While there appears to be a declining trend in AIDS diagnosis, HIV diagnosis reveals a higher proportion of HIV cases among women and minorities. Between 1995 and 1996 HIV diagnosis declined slightly among men (−3% from 10,762 to 10,395) but increased among women (+3% from 4126 to 4253). Racial shifts have also occurred during this time frame with HIV diagnosis declining slightly among African-Americans (−3% from 8569 to 8300) and among whites (−2% from 5093 to 4966) but increased among Hispanics (+10% from 971 to 1,070).

AIDS continues to be an affliction of the young. The greatest proportion of cases has always been among Americans aged 25–44. In 1996, 75% of Americans diagnosed with AIDS were in this age range, 21% were among those over 44, and less than 4% were among those aged 13–24. It should be noted, however, that 11% of all cases occur among Americans 50 and older (*MMWR*, January 23, 1998).

Global statistics are not encouraging. As of December 1998 over 33.4 million persons were living with AIDS worldwide. Half of all new infections are found in persons 15 to 24 years old. The global epicenter of the infection continues to be sub-Saharan Africa. Political and social factors help shape the epidemic. Wars and armed conflicts create the social instability as rural inhabitants are herded into the city or to refugee camps. The impact of HIV is also observed perinatally and during childhood in infected populations. Worldwide approximately 500,000 infants are perinatally infected with HIV each year (*MMWR*, March 6, 1998). In one study drug regimens of zidovudine orally administered to HIV-pregnant women in the second trimester, intravenously during labor, and orally to newborns for 6 weeks reduced risk for perinatal transmission by two-thirds (Sperling *et al.*, 1996). The impact of this therapy is significant; from 1996 to 1997 the number of children (under 13 years of age) who were diagnosed with AIDS declined 40% principally reflecting the continued success of promoting voluntary HIV testing and zidovudine therapy for pregnant HIV-infected women.

## CASE 34-3

*Suzie, a 15-year-old Hispanic patient, presented to the Family Planning Clinic 1 month prior to her 6-month visit, complaining of a discharge with an odor and itching for 2–3 days. She reported no "bumps or blisters" on her labia or introitus and she stated that she used condoms occasionally. Her physical examination revealed lesions at the introitus consistent with genital warts. At her previous visit she had reported a discharge but her serology and cultures were negative, and she had never tested positive for gonorrhea or chlamydia. Suzie reported being sexually active since age 13, a lifetime total of two sexual partners, and having currently had the same partner for 18 months. She also reported one induced abortion. She was treated with trichloroacetic acid one time and was instructed to return to the clinic for additional treatment if needed.*

## MINOR TYPES OF STDs

### Cytomegalovirus (CMV)

CMV, a member of the herpes family, is transmitted sexually as well as other ways. Over 80% of adults over 35 years of age in this country have antibodies against CMV. Six to eight percent of sexually active young women are estimated to have CMV in their cervix. CMV has been implicated in some cases of endometritis, cervicitis, pelvic inflammatory disease, and in men, nonspecific urethritis.

Symptomatic contacts of definitively diagnosed CMV patients may be presumed to have CMV infection as well. Otherwise, definitive diagnosis is difficult to establish because CMV is associated with nonspecific clinical syndromes, and the diagnostic tests are complex and expensive. Definitive diagnosis of CMV infection requires a rise in antibody titer, a positive immunofluorescent test, or identification of the virus in tissues or secretions known to be previously negative in a symptomatic patient. Many healthy individuals shed CMV in their saliva, cervical secretions, urine, semen, breast milk, feces, or blood. Thus, isolating those with known CMV has little value for public health.

CMV is also responsible for cytomegalic inclusion disease, a severe, and often fatal, disease of the fetus and newborn. This disease afflicts approximately 10,000 infants in the United States each year. Infants may also develop conjunctivitis or pneumonia from a mother infected with chlamydia.

Treatment is supportive, nonspecific, and symptomatic. No accepted routine therapy exists for either maternal or neonatal infection. The acquired illness is usually self-limiting among immunocompetent individuals.

### Group B Streptococcus

Group B streptococcus, transmitted both sexually and nonsexually, causes life-threatening infections in the newborn. In this country, 7500 babies each year develop Group B streptococcus infections. The infection in babies often takes severe, life-threatening forms: septicemia, pneumonia, and meningitis. Approximately 6% of these babies die. Of those who survive, as many as 20% may have brain damage, hearing loss, or blindness. Adults can carry the bacteria in the gastrointestinal tract, genital tract, or urinary tract. Of pregnant women 10 to 30% have a Group B streptococcus infection in the genital tract but have no symptoms. Since 1970, Group B streptococcus has become the leading bacterial infection causing illness and death in

*7500 babies get group B strep infections each year. 450 of them will die due to this infection.*

newborns. Adult cases are on the rise. Risk of infection is greatest among babies born 18 hours after the amniotic fluid breaks or whose mothers are teens, have a history of Group B streptococcus, or have a history of infection in a previous baby. The CDC recommends that all pregnant moms be screened between 35 and 37 weeks and be provided with antibiotics if the screen is positive.

## Condyloma Acuminatum

Condyloma acuminatum (venereal or genital warts) is caused by several types of the human papilloma-virus (HPV). Types 6 and 11 cause the visual warts; types 16, 18, 31, 33, and 35 are associated with vaginal, anal, and cervical cancer. Transmission is primarily sexual. Genital warts account for more than one million physician visits annually in the United States (Hatcher *et al.*, 1998). The exact incubation period is unknown, but the lesions are slow growing and may take up to 2 to 3 months to develop after exposure.

The lesions are usually found in the vaginal, anal, or cervical area. Condyloma is commonly associated with other infections such as moniliasis and trichomoniasis. The individual lesions are fleshy, pointed, wartlike, soft, and moist, and seem to become less infectious with time. In moist areas the growth may readily spread to adjacent regions. As Case 34-3 suggests, small lesions may not itch, but large ones do. Spontaneous remission of lesions is possible but so too are recurrences. Pregnancy often encourages exuberant growth. Rectal intercourse may result in perianal or rectal warts.

Treatment results for condyloma acuminatum vary and depend somewhat on the size of the lesions, the patient's immune competence, pregnancy status, and perhaps whether other vaginal infections coexist. Podofilax, in a 0.05% solution or gel, or trichloroacetic acid, as in Case 34-3, may be used on small lesions, but not during pregnancy because of potential toxicity to the fetus. Larger lesions are often treated with cryotherapy, surgery, podophyllin resin (10–25%) or trichloroacetic acid (80–90%).

## Molluscum Contagiosum

The virus causing molluscum contagiosum is a member of the DNA pox family. It is particularly prevalent in underdeveloped countries, and afflicts over 20% of the population in some South Pacific regions. Children are its prime target, but adults can be affected as well. Viral spread is presumably both direct and through the common use of such items as bedding and towels. However, the sexual mode of transmission seems to be increasing in adults and adolescents.

Lesions are 1 to 5 mm, smooth, rounded, firm, shiny flesh-colored to pearly white papules with character-istically umbilicated centers. They are most commonly seen on the trunk and anogenital region and are generally asymptomatic.

Infection is usually diagnosed on the basis of the typical clinical presentation. Microscopic examination of lesions or lesion material reveals the pathognomonic molluscum inclusion bodies. Lesions may resolve spontaneously without scarring. However, they may be removed by curettage after anesthesia. Caustic chemical therapy (podophyllin, trichloroacetic acid, silver nitrate) and cryotherapy (liquid nitrogen) have also been used successfully.

## Bacterial Vaginosis

Bacterial vaginosis, a significant vaginal infection in women, is a clinical syndrome caused by a mixture of anaerobic organisms, *Gardnerella vaginalis* and *Mycoplasma hominis*. These entities replace the normal water-producing vaginal lactobacillus. Considered a sexually associated condition, some women are often asymptomatic. Others have mild vulvovaginal irritation with scanty to moderate, gray, slightly malodorous discharge. Anaerobic bacteria often coexist with other virulent organisms in the vagina and hence are often overlooked as a causative agent.

Diagnosis is usually made by wet mount techniques. A pH greater than 4.7, a fishy smell, referred to as the whiff test, prior or subsequent to the addition of KOH to the wet mount, and a homogeneous white discharge that smoothly coats the vaginal walls are also used by some practitioners to confirm diagnosis. Vaginal cells seen under the microscope on a wet mount may have small dark particles adherent to them, called *clue cells*, that also identify the syndrome. Cultures for *G. vaginalis* are not recommended because they are not specific.

Systemic and topical modes of treatment are available. Clindamycin cream (2%) can be used topically. Treatment with oral metronidazole is greater than 80% effective. Treatment of the male sexual partner is still controversial, although it is useful in women with recurrent infections. Controversy exists as to whether or not to treat women in their first trimester with metronidazole. Some research suggests that bacterial vaginosis, left untreated, can be the causative agent in preterm delivery. The potential for this infection influences some practitioners to treat prophylactically for bacterial vaginosis. The patient should be counseled to avoid alcohol while using metronidazole.

## Pediculosis Pubis (Crab Lice)

Crab lice (*Phthirus pubis*) are bloodsucking parasites, which are more apt to be transmitted sexually than from shared contact with clothes or linen. Adult lice lay eggs (nits) at the base of the pubic skin hair shafts. These eggs hatch in 7 to 9 days and the new lice attach themselves to the skin of the host. Their bites may cause an erythematous papule within a matter of hours. Secondary infection is common.

The usual clinical presenting picture is that of pubic itching or the patient's simply observing lice moving on the skin surface. The lice can be positively identified when seen on a slide under a microscope or with a magnifying glass to view the lice or eggs on the pubic hair.

Treatment is with 1% gamma benzene hexachloride (Kwell) cream, lotion, or shampoo for 12 to 24 hours. Treatment should be repeated in 4 to 7 days to catch any eggs missed on the first application. Sexual partners should also be treated.

## *Candida albicans*

*Candida albicans* is a common saprophyte living in the mouth, vagina, respiratory tract, and intestines. Its presence may be detected from these sites in cultures in 25 to 50% of women. However, mere presence does not necessarily indicate infection.

Predisposing factors to *C. albicans* infections include the use of broad-spectrum antibiotics, oral contraceptives, pregnancy, diabetes mellitus, steroids or other immunosuppressive agents or events, narcotic abuse, perhaps increased carbohydrates in the diet, heat, and moisture. Pantyhose has been identified as a contributing agent because it retains heat and is not moisture absorbent.

The organism is an oval, budding, gram-positive yeast. Although *C. albicans* is, in one sense, not communicable since most individuals harbor the organism, it is now being considered a minor STD. Symptoms of candida vulvovaginitis include a discharge, vulvar itching, pain, or burning often beginning before menstruation. Painful urination and intercourse are other possible complaints. The vulva is usually red, edematous, and excoriated. The vaginal discharge characteristically is white, thick, and resembles curds of cottage cheese, usually moderate in quantity, but adherent to the vaginal wall.

Diagnosis is based on smears and cultures. *C. albicans* is associated with a vaginal pH of < 4.5. Wet mounts may demonstrate yeasts or pseudohyphae and may give a rough quantitative estimate of the number of organisms. The presence of these organisms without symptoms should be an indicator for treatment as 10–20% of women harbor candida in the vagina. Treatment of *C. albicans* is often problematic and requires careful attention to predisposing factors. Nystatin has been replaced by topically applied azoles as the drugs of choice. Oral azoles should not be used by pregnant patients. Treatment of male sexual partners is controversial, but useful in women with recurrences, as is the use of condoms. Patients should be advised that topical treatments may weaken latex condoms. Self-treatment without professional diagnosis is often incorrect. *C. albicans* is often confused with bacterial vaginosis.

## Trichomoniasis

This flagellated protozoal infection is a common cause of vaginitis in women and is transmitted through sexual intercourse. While most men are asymptomatic, most women have a malodorous, yellow-green discharge with vulvar irritation. Sharing of towels, bedding, and bathing and douche equipment may also cause transmission. Infection rates may be as high as 40% in some populations where hygiene is poor.

Diagnosis is made from wet mounts with the treatment of choice being oral metronidazole, 2 g orally in a single dose. This drug should not be used if there is a suspicion of pregnancy or if the patient is breast-feeding. Patients should abstain from drinking alcohol when taking this drug. To avoid "ping-ponging" the infection, the male partner should be treated simultaneously.

## Chancroid

Chancroid is endemic in many areas of the United States and also occurs in discrete outbreaks. Chancroid, a bacterial STD characterized by genital ulceration, has reemerged in the United States during the last decade. Chancroid has been well established as a cofactor for HIV transmission. As many as 10% of patients with chancroid may be coinfected with *T. pallidum* or HSV.

Definitive diagnosis of chancroid requires identification of *Haemophilus ducreyi* on special culture media that are not commercially available; even using these media, sensitivity is 80% at best. A probable diagnosis may be made if the person has one or more painful genital ulcers and no evidence of *T. pallidum* infection. Patients should be tested for HIV infection at the time of diagnosis. Patients also should be tested 3 months later for both syphilis and HIV, if initial results are negative.

Treatment involves the use of erythromycin 500 mg taken orally, four times a day for 7 days, or ceftriaxone 250 mg, i.m. in a single dose. An alternative is trimethoprim/sulfamethoxazole, double-strength tablet (160/800 mg) taken orally, twice a day for 7 days. The susceptibility of *H. ducreyi* to this combination of antimicrobial agents varies throughout the world. The practitioner should evaluate the results of therapy after a maximum of 7 days, and continue therapy until ulcers or lymph nodes have healed. Fluctuant lymph nodes should be aspirated through healthy, adjacent, normal skin. Incision and drainage or excision of nodes will delay healing and are contraindicated. All sexual partners should be simultaneously treated.

## Hepatitis B

Hepatitis B virus (HBV) infection is a common STD. Sexual transmission accounts for one-third to two-thirds of the 200,000 to 300,000 new HBV infections that occurred annually in the United States during the past 10 years. Of persons infected as adults, 6–10% become chronic HBV carriers. The risk for perinatal HBV transmission among infants of infected mothers is 10–85% depending on the mother's hepatitis B antigen.

*Hepatitis B leads to over 6000 deaths annually, even though there is a vaccine that can prevent HBV infection.*

Chronic HBV carriers are capable of transmitting HBV to others and are at risk for developing fatal complications. HBV leads to an estimated 6000 deaths annually in the United States from cirrhosis of the liver and hepatocellular carcinoma. Hepatitis B vaccine is the most effective way to prevent this infection.

Persons known to be at high risk for acquiring HBV should be advised of their risk for HBV infection (as well as HIV infection) and the means to reduce their risk. Persons at specific risk include sexually active homosexual and bisexual men, individuals who have recently acquired another STD, and persons in nonmonogamous relationships. Such individuals should be vaccinated unless they are immune to HBV as a result of past infection or vaccination. There is currently no treatment or cure for either acute infections or the carrier state.

## CASE 34-4

*A 37-year-old white middle-class woman presents to her private practice gynecologist for her annual examination and to assess the cause of chronic pelvic pain. During the medical history she reveals that she and her husband have been living apart. CBC, Pap smear, and blood pressure are assessed, but no serology or cultures are taken by the physician. Undiagnosed, the woman has contracted asymptomatic chlamydia and anal gonorrhea.*

## CASE 34-5

*A 25-year-old African-American woman was seen at her HMO clinic requesting HIV testing. She reported a total of four heterosexual partners in the past 3 years and frequent unprotected vaginal intercourse. She recently began a new sexual relationship and both partners have agreed to HIV screening. Her partner's HIV test was negative. Her HIV test was positive. She did not plan to tell her family, and her partner was sworn to secrecy. She was referred to an early intervention program.*

*Two weeks later, the clinic staff received a long-distance collect phone call from her partner. While the woman was visiting her grandmother 200 miles away, she became ill, unconscious, and was on a respirator in a small rural community hospital. He reported that the physicians had treated her pneumonia and were surprised that none of the medications were working. The staff told him the pneumonia might be related to her positive HIV status, and that this matter should be discussed with her physicians. The partner stated he had sworn not to tell anyone and therefore could not tell the physicians.*

## CASE 34-6

*A 50-year-old white ob-gyn private practitioner was informed of the presence of trichomoniasis in an African-American patient. He refused to treat the patient, stating that the disease was "endemic in this population" and "treatment would not be effective."*

*Cultural sensitivity can be the most important factor in ensuring good patient–physician rapport.*

Physicians often harbor unspoken value judgments and personal expectations concerning how to treat and communicate information about STDs. One perception concerning STDs involves the role of ethnic or social class. In Cases 34-4 and 34-6 the decision to screen and treat was based on stereotypes that a middle-class white patient would not need screening and that an African-American patient would not benefit from treatment. While certain risk factors may exist, attending physicians should consider every sexually active individual at risk for contracting an STD. Some physicians hesitate to offer STD screening for married women for fear that the husband may ask why and may, in fact, refuse payment. Nevertheless, STD screening is essential to good primary and reproductive care, especially since a large number of women who have contracted an STD are asymptomatic.

Case 34-5 involves a value judgment about confidentiality and the exceptions about guarding such confidences. While in most cases it is imperative to protect the patient's confidentiality regarding HIV status, physician and patient should discuss at the outset circumstances that might require the waiving of such confidential agreements. In particular, the physician should gain permission to discuss the patient's HIV status with other health professionals involved in her care. Such discussions should be noted in the patient's chart.

## Physician Training

Physician experiences, beliefs, and exposure to STDs can affect knowledge and attitudes which in turn can affect one's ability to diagnose these infections. First, the skills necessary to diagnose new strains of STDs are constantly changing. Improved diagnostic tests and assays developed in the last 10 years require continuing medical education to enhance the ability of practitioners to diagnose and treat such infections. For example, chlamydia, a major disease entity, cannot be diagnosed without current new technology. Urine-based assays offer diagnostic tests appropriate for hard-to-reach populations. While the merits of such advances may be familiar to young physicians with recent training, these scientific breakthroughs may not reach those physicians with earlier training experiences. In addition, newer and more complicated expressions of STDs may go unnoticed by older practitioners.

Second, many physicians have had limited exposure to human sexuality in their medical training. Many medical schools do not require such courses and their elective status and emphasis on psychosocial issues hinders their attractiveness to budding clinical scientists. Residency requirements in pediatrics, internal medicine, and family medicine now mandate a structured experience including didactic and clinical programs that cover family planning, STDs, and gynecology.

A recent study of residency education suggests additional reforms are needed. Fifty percent of graduates had performed fewer than 20 pelvic examinations, 30% had never prescribed oral contraceptive pills, and 14% lacked a single experience in diagnosing or treating gonorrhea (Braverman & Strasburger, 1994). Only 68% of graduates reported adequate training in sexuality counseling and knowledge, with 64% reporting adequate training in pregnancy and only 46% expressing comfort with abortion counseling.

## Physician Comfort Level

Physician discomfort with STDs often relates to personal beliefs and experience in the area of sexuality. Success in medical and premedical education requires dedication to studies rather than social life and focus on the sciences rather than the humanities. This lack of interpersonal experiences may retard both the development of empathic skills necessary for patient rapport and limit the medical student's understanding of the complexities of sexual decision-making and several practices. For those medical students with little or no sexual experience, treating patients for STDs can create considerable discomfort. In addition, limited sexual exposure can reduce the student's knowledge and raise the student's inhibitions regarding fellatio, anal intercourse, and other alternate forms of sexual expression.

*Lack of condom use with HIV+ patients may be due to fears that requests for condom use will "reveal their secret."*

## Physician Social Attitudes

Healthcare professionals hold widely divergent views regarding the social and moral aspects of treating patients with STDs. One survey showed that one-third of physicians believed reproductive services such as screening for STDs should be provided without parental or spousal consent. Another third, however, would require parental and spousal notification and participation.

At the heart of this disagreement are cultural and religiously influenced definitions of the purpose of sexuality. Influenced by their backgrounds and beliefs, many medical students fail to appreciate the erotic, as opposed to the reproductive dimension of sexuality. Unfortunately, medical education has focused almost exclusively on reproductive sexuality, while the erotic function has been either ignored or limited to pathology. Erotic pleasures are an integral part of sexual experience and are independent of the consequences of STDs.

Some healthcare professionals interpret the contraction of an STD as a judgment on the behavior of the infected patient. Such a belief is particularly prevalent when the diagnosis of HIV seropositivity occurs. Other physicians choose to empathize with and advocate for their patients, but feel in conflict with their religious backgrounds and traditions. This conflict is particularly difficult for religiously conservative medical students and residents who must deal with abortion in their training.

### CASE 34-7

*A 26-year-old Hispanic woman had attended a clinic for general family planning for 4 years. Her sister, a single 17-year-old and also a clinic patient, had a chronically ill 1½-year-old. The baby was tested and found to be HIV positive. Both sisters were tested and found to be HIV positive. The only risk factor was multiple heterosexual partners.*

*Following family planning and lifestyle counseling, a pregnancy test was performed on the older sister, and the result was positive. Not interested in a pregnancy termination, she subsequently delivered an HIV-positive baby. Despite counseling, 9 months later she conceived again and delivered another HIV-positive infant.*

## IMPACT OF STDs ON PATIENTS' LIVES

Case 34-7 suggests the consequences of HIV seropositivity often conflict directly with life goals and desires. For such women, especially those who are poorly educated, the decision to avoid childbearing violates cultural norms. The emotional need to be a mother and to acquire the associated social status outweighs the public health or long-term negative consequences of an HIV-positive baby for many women. Educational and counseling efforts must take such issues into account.

*Chancroids are an important co-factor. As many as 1 in 10 of patients with chancroids also have HIV or* T. pallidum.

Treatment of patients with STDs often requires attention to serious ethical and legal issues. Physicians should discuss the risk of transmission to others and ways of reducing these risks. STD-infected individuals should be counseled to use condoms, preferably in combination with foam. Patients who refuse to protect or notify their partners present an ethical quandary for their physicians. For infections such as HSV and HIV, case laws permit charges and convictions against individuals who knowingly infect others. Regardless of the type of STD, sexual responsibility should be encouraged, but physicians will vary as to the means of doing so.

A patient infected with HSV with primary or recurrent blisters will infect a partner if unprotected intercourse or other forms of sexual activity occur. While abstinence is urged, condom use is mandated if the first alternative is not adopted. Even if an active case is not present, studies suggest that viral shedding of covert lesions occurs among some women. Thus, the infection can be contracted even if no external lesions are present. Caution dictates continual condom use for such individuals.

Because HIV infections are asymptomatic by definition, at-risk individuals often choose not to be tested to determine their status. Such behavior, though understandable, represents not only psychological avoidance and denial but also, if the patient continues to be sexually active, a shirking of ethical responsibility. Epidemiological projections suggest that as many as 1 million people in the United States are HIV positive with the largest increases occurring among women and heterosexual populations. The iceberg effect increases the pool of risk to the heterosexual population (Hatcher et al., 1998).

Even more problematic are those heterosexual and homosexual individuals who have tested positive for HIV yet continue to practice unprotected sex. While sexual acting out and irresponsibility are implicit in such behaviors, dislike of condoms is often a contributing factor. Some individuals lie about their status and fear that condom use will reveal their secret. Adolescents who partner with older men also have trouble convincing their partners to use this method. As Case 34-7 indicates, some women choose not to use condoms because they desire to become pregnant. Since transplacental transmission of HIV approximates 30%, the soundness of such decisions is highly questionable.

Most physicians and ethicists agree that HIV infections and other STDs require specific changes in sexual behaviors. Abstinence and safe-sex practices, including the use of condoms, dental dams, and the refraining from rectal intercourse, are recommended. Data indicate that these safe-sex practices can reduce the infection risk (Ku et al., 1992).

Because of the chronicity of both HSV and HIV, many believe that life changes may prevent recurrent outbreaks of HSV and lower an HIV-infected individual's T-cell count. The most commonly recommended interventions include stress reduction, nutritional counseling, and visualization and meditation, as well as acupuncture, massage, and therapeutic touch. Complementary to these methods are support groups, "worried well," and "next step" groups for HIV-positive individuals. In various combinations such behavioral interventions allow individuals to take control of their lives and reduce stress.

Other STDs, while less acute, can still devastate the mental health and personal outlook of the infected individual. In addition to the discomfort, the presence of an STD can negatively affect an individual's sexual self-esteem and self-image. For the conscientious, the possibility of infecting another individual or guilt regarding past behavior can effectively eliminate any interest in sexual activity.

## CASE 34-8

*A single white woman in her early 20s was hospitalized for the second time with pelvic inflammatory disease (PID). She stated that she was in a monogamous relationship with a man. The continuing etiology of her PID was chlamydia, and her partner had never been treated. The physician informed the partner that the condition would recur if he didn't receive treatment, and he agreed to be treated by his partner's physician. Although the male partner received treatment for his infection, subsequent attempts on the part of the couple to conceive were unsuccessful.*

## Partner Treatment

When asymptomatic venereal diseases are diagnosed from complications resulting from non- or inadequate treatment, the physician must ascertain whether the patient is still sexually active and whether her partner has been screened and treated concomitantly. In some communities protocols support the treatment of partners without testing if the woman is symptomatic. Without simultaneous treatment for such conditions, reinfection is almost guaranteed as illustrated in Case 34-8.

A secondary issue is whether the woman was adequately informed of the need for partner treatment. A good STD treatment protocol is enhanced by a strong educational component. A final consideration is whether access to treatment was convenient for the infected partner. Otherwise, he is unlikely to be cured and he will continue to infect his partner. Typically STD clinics and family planning clinics do not attract asymptomatic partners. Practitioners should actively encourage their infected patients to return with their partners for treatment. Special arrangements could be made through the woman's private physician so that services can be accessed in an easy and unobtrusive way.

## Association with Cervical Cancer

Women who have a history of STDs, especially HPV, are at increased risk for cervical cancer, and women attending STD clinics may have additional characteristics that place them at even higher risk. Prevalence studies have found that precursor lesions for cervical cancer occur approximately five times more often among women attending STD clinics than among women attending family planning clinics. The Pap smear is an effective and relatively low-cost screening test for invasive cervical cancer and squamous intraepithelial lesions, the precursors of cervical cancer. An annual Pap is recommended for all sexually active women, especially those who have a history of STDs.

---

### CASE 34-9

*A 20-year-old Anglo white woman is living in an abandoned car with her 26-year-old boyfriend. The patient had been unable to bathe for over a month. She was only able to "wash up" in the sink of a gas station. She presented to the clinic with complaints of a foul vaginal odor. The patient was found to have trichomoniasis and was treated with metronidazole. The patient was instructed to bring her partner in for treatment. When she told him about the infection, she reported that he beat her. He came the next day for treatment and expressed severe anger about her "infidelity." The staff provided educational information. She denied any partner other than him. He abandoned her due to the infection.*

---

### CASE 34-10

*Jane, a 13-year-old white girl, was living with her mom, stepfather, and 3½ year-old stepsister when her father came to the home and murdered her mother. Jane witnessed the crime. Her father was convicted and incarcerated. Jane's stepfather began to sexually abuse her stepsister. Jane called Children's Protective Services who prosecuted the stepfather and he also was imprisoned. Jane, now 14, was "given" to an aunt. Unhappy with the living arrangements, Jane ran away. During this time she became pregnant and put the baby up for adoption. Jane then met Lazaro, the boyfriend of her aunt. Jane was rejected by her aunt, and Lazaro, a 27-year-old undocumented worker, went to court and was appointed Jane's legal guardian. They started having sex and he fathered two children. By age 16, she had three babies. Periodic STD screening diagnosed recurrent trichomoniasis and gonorrhea.*

*One day Jane came to the clinic with bruises on her body reportedly from fighting with Lazaro. She also stated that he was beating the children. She moved out with a friend but left the three children and said she would come back in a few days. Social welfare was called and took custody of the children.*

*Jane then became involved with another illegal alien. She had one abortion and two more children by age 19. She again tested positive for gonorrhea. The clinic staff encouraged Jane to have a bilateral tubal ligation, since she was a poor contraceptor. As she could not qualify for subsidized medical services, permanent sterilization services were donated. She became pregnant again and was scheduled to have a bilateral tubal ligation after delivery. However, she changed her mind after counseling.*

## WHY DOES THIS PROBLEM EXIST?

One of the first steps in providing intervention and treatment for a public health concern, whether it be tuberculosis or STDs, is to evaluate the level of personal control that patients can exercise over their lives. If the basics of survival, food, shelter, and clothing are inadequate, curing a communicable disease will be difficult and the compliance necessary for the completion of a drug regimen will be compromised. In Case 34-9 the lack of running water and facilities for personal hygiene compromised basic public health compliance. If medical intervention is to be successful, social services must often complement the work of the physician. In Cases 34-9 and 34-10 it is not surprising that STDs continued to recur.

With regard to STD, homeless individuals and runaway youth are especially vulnerable. New technologies of diagnosis through the utilization of oral swabs for HIV detection or urine assessment for chlamydia are appropriate for this group. In Cases 34-9 and 34-10 the women involved made sexual choices in response to personal needs and to procure the basic commodities of life. This is known as survival sex: sexual intercourse performed in exchange for goods or money.

Another factor that plays a role in the spread of STD is dysfunctional family behavior and the correlates of domestic violence, sexual abuse, and incest. A healthy family unit, however it is defined, can provide some prophylaxis for such culturally abnormal behavior. When family units are compromised, some of the taboos associated with interfamilial sexual behavior evaporate. Family secrets can enhance and perpetuate inappropriate sexual behavior that promotes the contraction of an STD. Approximately 20% of all women experience domestic violence which may include sexual abuse.

In addition to inappropriate sexual behavior, decision-making skills associated with those behaviors are also compromised. In addition to the history of sexual abuse, domestic violence and emotional abuse can also covary with these behaviors. For a variety of reasons, individuals often appear to be paralyzed by their circumstances and cannot mobilize the psychological energy necessary to extract themselves from their surroundings. To be effective in such cases, physicians should be familiar with victim service agencies, which can provide emergency care or legal counsel.

Dealing with the chronic nature of STDs requires an appreciation of the various forces that impede treatment. First, many individuals, including those who are highly educated, lack basic understanding of the different types of infections and common means of transmission. Sexual behavior, by its very nature, is shrouded in taboos and values that discourage frank discussion, thus limiting the knowledge and vocabulary necessary to explain the associated aspects of these diseases. Religiosity, personal myths, and ignorance combine to inhibit the development of sound cognitive skills in human sexuality that are the prerequisite for decision-making regarding risky sexual behaviors.

Second, becoming sexually active at an early age and having multiple sexual partners over time enhances the risk of contracting an STD. Surveys conducted over the last 30 years indicate that the age at onset of

*Some young adults feel that they will probably not live past 30 years old, so sexual risk taking is common with perceived minor consequences.*

sexual activity among teens has decreased significantly (Youth Risk Behavior Surveillance, 1998). In addition, the number of sexual partners has increased during that time among adolescents.

A third factor in the increase of certain types of STDs is related to their asymptomatic nature in both the carrier and the individual who becomes infected. Among women, gonorrhea and chlamydia can cause significant damage to the reproductive system without prior signs of the infection. Unfortunately, physicians in private practice may not perform routine screening for these infections, allowing these diseases to go unchecked.

The social stigma attached to being infected with an STD can be a powerful deterrent to seeking treatment. When treatment centers are difficult to access or are lacking in privacy, treatment is likely to be avoided. Inadequate access may justify sending medications home for treatment of the sexual partner.

## CASE 34-11

*A 20-year-old nulliparous woman presented to a general health clinic reporting an aggravated sexual assault. The patient reported that the attack was her second sexual experience. A 25-year-old African-American male was identified as the perpetrator. She said that she had dated him twice before and on this latest occasion he stated that they were going "party hopping." After attending two separate events, he told her that the third party was at a hotel and that it would be the "best ever." After entering the hotel room, which turned out to be vacant, she attempted to leave. She was forcibly assaulted at gun point and was raped orally, vaginally, and anally four times.*

*He threatened that if she told anyone he would kill her. He also stated that no one would believe her because they had been dating. She did not seek medical treatment for 3 weeks. She subsequently presented herself to the emergency room and was cultured for gonorrhea, the result of which was positive. She was then referred to a clinic for a general work up where she was diagnosed with trichomoniasis. After signing a separate consent form she was also tested for HIV. The results came back positive. The patient was visibly upset and because a family member had died of the disease she became very fatalistic about her own demise. Subsequent to counseling, her mother became involved and provided family support so that the woman would attend an HIV-positive support group. The possibility of pressing charges against the man was explored with clinic staff but the family refused because they did not want to undergo the headache of subjecting themselves to the legal process.*

## SEXUAL ASSAULT

Little attention has been given to the impact of possible infection with an STD or HIV in survivors of sexual assault. This may be due in part to society's conflicting attitudes and beliefs concerning STDs, AIDS, and rape. This problem is compounded in that rape is a crime that is often hidden and underdocumented. The National Women's Study (1988) reported that 22% of female victims were under age 12, 32.4% were aged 12–17, and 29.4% were 18–24 years old. Significant numbers of adolescents and children are victims of sexual assaults often involving multiple encounters. More than half of all rapes (61%) involved victims under the age of 18. The risk of contracting an STD or HIV often depends on the health status of the assailant, the type of sexual assault, and the frequency of assaults. The type of sexual exposure (vaginal, anal, or oral), the associated trauma, the presence of other STDs, and the exposure to bodily fluids affect the risk of infection.

Gonorrhea, syphilis, or hepatitis B may have per-contact infectivity rates as high as 20%. Bacterial vaginosis, trichomoniasis, and chlamydia have also been frequently diagnosed among assaulted victims. Compared with these diseases the estimate of per-contact HIV infectivity rate from male to female via penile–vaginal intercourse is less than two per 1000 contacts.

The presence of lesions or blood from violent assaults may increase the chance of transmission of HIV and other STDs. Genital ulcerative STDs also have been associated with increased infectiousness, as well as susceptibility to HIV. Another factor is the strength of the viral strain. Violence, trauma, and blood exposure or the presence of inflammatory or ulcerative STDs increases the risk. Women are of special concern because of ascending chlamydial and gonococcal infections.

Physicians counseling rape victims need to educate their patients, help survivors regain a sense of control over their lives, and allow survivors to make decisions regarding STD screening and HIV testing. Information and counseling should be provided in a nondirective manner, offering survivors the opportunity for open-ended discussions of their questions in a nonjudgmental manner. As some of the acquired infections may not have produced sufficient concentrations of organisms to cause positive results at the medical examination, STD examinations should be repeated 2 weeks after the assault.

Some professionals may question whether survivors of sexual assaults should be offered AZT as a prophylactic for HIV infection. Antiretroviral therapy has proven efficacious in inhibiting HIV replication. Many major healthcare facilities offer postexposure zidovudine treatment for workers who sustain injuries with contaminated needles, even though the efficacy of zidovudine in preventing HIV infection after initial exposure remains unproved. Similarly, postexposure hepatitis B vaccine should be administered to assault victims at the time of the exposure. Follow-up dosage at 1–2 months and 4–6 weeks should also be followed.

## CASE 34-12

*A large metropolitan school board in the southern United States, after analyzing the prevalence of STDs and pregnancy in a predominantly Hispanic public high school, passed a resolution for the establishment of a school-based health clinic. The goal was to provide primary health and screening services to the student body and their siblings. Subsequent to board approval, local community groups demanded a public meeting. At this forum, various parents and community members expressed concern that providing information and services for the treatment of STDs encouraged irresponsible sexual behavior. Furthermore, in spite of the morbidity statistics, the parents insisted that the students were not sexually active and were not at risk for STDs. A great fear was expressed that as part of any prevention strategy condoms would become available on campus. The presence of these items was perceived by a group of parents as sending the wrong message to the community and the students who attended the high school.*

*Based on the expressed concerns, a multidisciplinary team comprised of a pediatrician, psychologist, nurse, health educator, and social worker initiated a series of parent focus groups. At these meetings the various constituencies were given the opportunity to express their concerns. Their input was solicited as to the scope of services to provide and the type of consent procedures required for participation in the medical services.*

## THE PHYSICIAN'S ROLE IN THE COMMUNITY

Dealing successfully with STDs will require leadership from the medical community to assuage the public's fears and prejudices. Oftentimes attempts to deal directly with issues associated with sexuality are misconstrued as attempts to provide liberal interpretations of sex education or encouragement to initiate early sexual activity. These fears are exacerbated when one deals with certain cultures. The Hispanic and Asian communities, for example, have historically maintained a conservative posture on issues relating to human sexuality and STDs. In spite of the increasing prevalence of HIV and STD among these populations, there is reticence to deal proactively with these delicate subjects. The physician in Case 34-12, in order to provide these proposed services, had to gain the confidence and support of this conservative group.

STD education in the community and in schools, while attempting to reach many individuals, tends to be brief and nonspecific. Information is often provided after adolescents are sexually active. Community attitudes toward STD and HIV are also problematic. Many communities believe that public education on sexual issues may be a subtle reinforcer of sexual behavior. As a result misinformation and ignorance abound. Heterosexual populations, for example, find it difficult to concretize their risk because they do not understand transmission issues. In the case of HIV, teens especially may not view AIDS as a "real disease." They have difficulty grasping the notion that a healthy, robust person could transmit a deadly, fatal disease. Many adults still identify AIDS as a "gay disease" that does not affect a healthy heterosexual. Risk behaviors such as school drop-out, drug and alcohol use, and sexual misconduct are predictive of nonuse of condoms, STDs, and denial of risk. Persons who engage in these behaviors are difficult to reach and may not appear at healthcare facilities until they are symptomatic.

Scare tactics and calls for abstinence seldom work. While federal initiatives have invested $50 million in abstinence-only programs as of 1999, no substantive evaluation documents significant effects for this curriculum. Innovative educational programs are needed to motivate the public to practice safer sex. Educational methods appropriate for some populations may be insufficient or even inappropriate for other groups. For example, the gay community is probably more aware that negotiation skills must be learned in making sexual choices, especially as it relates to safe sex. Moreover, certain terms may be interpreted differently. Physicians need to know, for example, that a teen's definition of monogamy may mean being with a person for a week or a month or a year.

Education about STDs must take a positive approach to teaching about all types of sexuality in a manner that is frank and gender appropriate. Use of condoms requires the cooperation of the man, and many men resist using them, leaving their partners vulnerable. Ethnic concepts of sexuality must also be considered when attempting to teach good decision-making skills to high-risk young women. Discussing sex is considered inappropriate in many Latin American and Asian communities, making it difficult to educate patients concerning the use of condoms, previous sexual partners, and sexual practices between men and women. This is an example of why cross-cultural training should be an essential part of medical school and residency.

The needs of community populations at risk for HIV infection will increase. Knowledge and preparation for decision-making skills are not sufficient without access to medical, social, and even legal services. Community-minded physicians should also be aware that women face a difficult set of negotiation challenges regarding abstinence or safer sex behaviors. Asking for assistance with condom purchases in stores or pharmacies may not always be an easy request.

Because of the consequences of STDs discussed previously, various efforts have been undertaken to encourage abstinence, postpone sexual involvement, or promote safe-sex practices. Such efforts have met with varying levels of success. First, for certain populations, such as adolescents, the ability to ascertain the risk of acquiring an infection is perceived to be low. It is not surprising that the rates of many STDs are the highest among adolescents (*MMWR*, 1998). Second, some population cohorts lack adequate knowledge about diseases and their contagion. Third, there are groups of young adults who express the feelings that they will not live past their 30s, so sexual risk-taking has relatively minor consequences.

Programs developed to enhance life skills associated with sexual decision-making are varied and have

---

*To be effective, STD education must be both frank, gender appropriate, and culturally appropriate.*

different degrees of success. Most programs designed to prevent STDs focus on high-risk individuals who are already sexually active. While some forms of sex education have succeeded at postponing sexual involvement among youth (Ku et al., 1992), training in condom utilization skills is probably a more realistic approach to the problem. Such classes focus on either skills associated with mechanical use or social factors associated with using condoms with a partner, or both. While some change was found in students who participated in these classes (Cohen et al., 1992), large numbers continued with unsafe sexual practices. Some programs have emphasized increasing availability of condoms as perhaps a way of encouraging use (Calsyn et al. 1992). However, even among educated groups such as college students, condoms were not used consistently and those with greatest risk were least likely to practice safe sex (Oswalt & Matsen, 1993).

## CONCLUSION

The risks associated with sexual activity are serious and complicated. Past stereotypes are misleading and may inhibit treatment options. Changes in the age of fertility, in the nuclear family, and in the educational and economic opportunities for women have all played a role in increasing exposure of individuals to a variety of STDs. Data indicating that 53% of all infants in the United States in 1998 were born out of wedlock reflect the magnitude of the shift in sexual mores in our culture.

Epidemiological trends indicate ways STDs are expressed in contemporary populations and suggest strategies physicians should adopt to address them. First, physicians must communicate that all individuals who are sexually active and do not practice safe sex are at risk for STD and HIV/AIDS. Opportunities to stress the risk to patients should be acknowledged and utilized. Testing for such infections, while requiring a separate consent form for HIV/AIDS, should be routine in all primary care settings. In addition to testing, physicians should discuss frankly the availability and use of condoms and the sexual practices of their patients as a routine part of the standard clinical visit. Desensitizing patients and perhaps providing the opportunity to role-play can facilitate safe-sex practices. Partners of infected patients should also be encouraged to receive treatment.

A second trend is the growing tendency to contract multiple diseases and infections. A patient may have several infections in addition to the one for which treatment is sought. In addition, physicians should consider the throat and rectal areas as sites for infection.

A final consideration involves the role that changing lifestyles and economics are playing in the transmission of various diseases. Homelessness, drug and alcohol use, and gay lifestyles all influence how individuals express their sexuality. Traditional models defining sexual behavior are no longer appropriate or broad enough to adequately assess, treat, and prevent STDs.

## CASES FOR DISCUSSION

### CASE 1

In October, a 20-year-old African-American man came to the clinic concerned with a small sore on his penis and lip. He also reported "flulike" symptoms and a possible weight loss. He was tested for GC, chlamydia, herpes, chancroid, and syphilis. Staff also provided pretest counseling for HIV and he agreed to testing due to unprotected heterosexual contact with 18 partners in the preceding 5 years. He denied or was unaware of his partners' possible risks. He also denied any history of i.v. drug use or a blood transfusion. Lab results were negative for GC, chlamydia, herpes, chancroid, and syphilis. The test for HIV was positive. The young man returned in 2 weeks for posttest counseling and had lost 16 pounds. Posttest counseling was provided and the man agreed to meet an HIV case manager at the county AIDS clinic the next morning. He did not show up and future contacts were unsuccessful. In February, a female patient came to the family planning clinic and showed the newspaper obituary of his death from AIDS complications.

1. Should pre- and posttest counseling be offered to the friends of the HIV-positive adolescent?
2. Are there any cultural issues that should be addressed with this population?
3. If HIV testing is performed, what consent procedures are required?

## CASE 2

In 1984, Linda, a 13-year-old African-American adolescent, was brought in by her mom for a rape evaluation regarding an encounter that had occurred 3–4 days earlier. Although she was referred elsewhere, she continued to come for primary care to the clinic. At the next visit, Linda came to the clinic with a gash in her foot requiring stitches. A member of the clinic staff walked to the adjoining housing project where Linda lived to obtain parental consent for treatment. The staff member found the mother in bed with a man. The mom said she would attend to the problem but did not.

At age 16, Linda married an African man and desperately desired to become pregnant. She frequently came in for pregnancy testing. When she was 18, her husband was killed by a car while standing at a bus stop. His survivors received an insurance settlement, which was held in trust for her by the executor of the estate, a professor at a nearby university. After the death of her husband Linda went out of control, congregated with drug users, and became a user herself. The next time Linda came in, she had what appeared to be shingles. After a medical history, an HIV-ELISA test was performed and results were positive. The Western blot results were also positive. The staff tried to explain the consequences of being sero-positive. However, Linda continued to express her desire to become pregnant. She even reported chewing food and feeding it to an infant in the family.

Linda later brought family members to the clinic and asked the staff to explain HIV. She had a bad cough and purple spots all over her body. She failed to keep her next clinic appointment. The clinic staff tried to locate her because a Pap smear showed severe dysplasia. Linda refused to come in and did not answer any of her correspondence.

1. Should other tests be performed if the HIV test is positive?
2. What other service options should be offered to this client?
3. Are there issues associated with informed consent?
4. Are there any reporting requirements that must be addressed?
5. If the results are HIV positive, what are the physician's obligations to the sexual partner?

## CASE 3

A 30-year-old homeless African-American woman was sexually active with two adult homeless men. She behaved in a manner that suggested schizophrenia and drank on a daily basis. She has been diagnosed with trichomoniasis repeatedly. The indication is that the three of them continue to reinfect each other.

1. How does the practitioner manage an STD-infected patient who has multiple partners?
2. What role does alcohol abuse play in this behavior?
3. What sort of social service interventions would be appropriate?

## CASE 4

A 25-year-old Caucasian white woman with mental health problems had been diagnosed with chlamydia four times. She was sent home with doxycycline and instructions. She returned for test of cure, but was still positive. The patient reported that she could only take doxycycline with ice cream, which reduces the drug's absorption. Arrangements to provide liquid erythromycin were made due to her refusal to comply with the medical instructions.

1. What are physicians' responsibilities to spouses or partners when STD results continue to be positive? How do practitioners address frequent reinfections among their patients?
2. Are there any other ways to encourage difficult patients to cooperate with treatment regimens?

## CASE 5

*In November 1994, a divorced 37-year-old white businessman developed a sexual relationship with a single woman in Europe. The relationship continued until 1997 when the man subsequently met and married a woman in the United States. In 1998 when his wife was 20 weeks pregnant he received a call from his former lover who revealed that she had tested positive for HIV and suggested that he be tested. His HIV test was positive although he was still asymptomatic. Tests for other STDs were negative. His wife tested negative for HIV infection.*

1. *Should the wife be retested for HIV?*
2. *What are some perinatal considerations for the couple?*
3. *What are the issues associated with the sexual relationship of the couple?*

## RECOMMENDED READINGS

The Boston Women's Health Book Collective (eds): *The New Our Bodies, Ourselves.* New York, Simon & Schuster, Inc, 1981.

This work approaches sexuality from a woman's perspective and empowers women to take control of their sexual decisions.

Carrera M (ed): *Sex: The Facts, The Acts & Your Feelings.* New York, Crown Publishers, Inc, 1993.

This is a comprehensive work generated from experience with college students. It covers a wide array of sexual issues in a direct but tasteful way.

Hatcher RA, Stewart F, Trussell J, Kowal D, Guest F, Stewart GK, Cates W (eds): *Contraceptive Technology 1990–1992—15th Revised Edition.* New York, Irvington Publishers, Inc, 1992.

This text provides a comprehensive integration of reproductive health, contraception, and prevention of STDs. Practitioners should consider this a thorough reference on how human reproduction in the life cycle is affected by a variety of infections, practices, and changing mores.

Morbidity and Mortality Weekly Report: *1998 Sexually Transmitted Diseases Treatment Guidelines.* 42, No. RR-14, 1993.

This short text describes all current treatment regimens for STDs. In addition, it provides up-to-date epidemiological trends and changes in contagion and disease expression among various populations.

## REFERENCES

Braverman PK, Strasburger VC: The practitioner's role. *Clin Pediatr* 33(2):100–109, 1994.

Calsyn DA, Meinecke C, Saxon AJ, Stanton V: Risk reduction in sexual behaviors: A condom giveaway program in a drug abuse treatment clinic. *Am J Public Health* 82(11):1536–1538, 1992.

Centers for Disease Control and Prevention: Trends in the HIV and AIDS Epidemic—1998, pp 1–13.

Cohen CA, Dent C, MacKinnon D, Hahn G: Condoms for men, not women: Results of brief promotion and programs. *Sex Transm Dis* 19(5):245–251, 1992.

Garnett GP, Aral SO, Hoyle DV, Cates W, Anderson RM: The natural history of syphilis: Implications for the transmission dynamics and control of infection. *Sex Transm Dis* 24:185–200, 1997.

Hatcher RA, Stewart F, Trussell J, *et al* (eds): *Contraceptive Technology 1996–1997 17th Revised Edition.* New York, Irvington Publishers Inc, 1998.

Institute of Medicine: *The Hidden Epidemic: Confronting Sexually Transmitted Diseases*, Eng TR (ed), Butler WT (preface), Washington, National Academy Press, 1997.

Ku LC, Sonenstein FL, Pleck JH: The association of AIDS education and sex education with sexual behavior and condom use among teenage men. *Fam Plann Persp* 24(3):100–106, 1992.

Morbidity and Mortality Weekly Report. *Ectopic pregnancy—United States, 1988–1989.* 41(32):591–594, 1992.

Morbidity and Mortality Weekly Report. *AIDS among persons aged ≥ 50 years—United States 1991—January 23, 1998.* 47(2):825–829, 1996.

Morbidity and Mortality Weekly Report. *Administration of zidovudine during late pregnancy and delivery to prevent perinatal HIV transmission—Thailand 1996.* 47(8):151–154, 1998.

Morbidity and Mortality Weekly Report. Primary and secondary syphilis—United States, 1997. 47(24):493–497, June 26, 1998.

Morbidity and Mortality Weekly Report. *HIV prevention through early detection and treatment of other sexually transmitted diseases—United States.* 47(RR-12):1–24, July 31, 1998.

Morbidity and Mortality Weekly Report Update: *Adoption of hospital policies for prevention of perinatal group B streptococcal disease—United States 1997.* 47(32):665–670, August 21, 1998.

Morbidity and Mortality Weekly Report. *Epidemic of congenital syphilis—Baltimore, 1996–1997.* 47(42):904–907, October 30, 1998.

Morbidity and Mortality Weekly Report. *HIV testing among populations at risk for HIV infection—nine states.* 47(50):1091–1093, December 1998.

Morbidity and Mortality Weekly Report. *1998 Guidelines for the treatment of sexually transmitted diseases—1998*. 47(RR-1), 1998

*National Women's Study*. Charleston, Crime Victims Research and Treatment Center, Medical University of South Carolina, 1988.

Oswalt R, Matsen K: Sex, AIDS, and the use of condoms: A survey of compliance in college students. *Psychol Rep* 72(1):764–766, 1993.

Risser JMH, Hwony L, Risser WL, Hollins L, Paffe J: The epidemiology of syphilis in the waning years of an epidemic: Houston, Texas, 1991–1997. *Sex Transm Dis* 26(3):121–126, 1999.

Smith PB, Mumford DM (eds): *Adolescent Pregnancy—Perspectives for the Health Professional*. Boston, GK Hall & Co, 1980.

Snabes MC, Weinman ML, Smith PB: Prevalence of HIV seropositivity among inner-city adolescents in 1988 and 1992. *Tex Med* 90(12): 48–51, 1994.

Sperling RS, Shapiro DE, Coombs RW, *et al*: Maternal viral load, zidovudine treatment and the risk of transmission of human immunodeficiency virus type 1 from mother to infant. *N Engl J Med* 335: 1621–1629, 1996.

Valdiserre RO, Arena VC, Proctor D, Bonati FA: The relationship between women's attitudes about condoms and their use: Implications for condom promotion programs. *Am J Public Health* 79(4):499–501, 1989.

Wyatt GE, Newcomb MD, Riederle MH (eds): *Sexual Abuse and Consensual Sex*. Newbury Park, Calif, Sage Publications, 1990.

Youth Risk Behavior Surveillance—United States, 1997. US Department of Health and Human Services, August 14, 1998, 47(SS-3).

## CHAPTER 35

# Maternal and Child Health

*Larry Culpepper, Sara G. Shields, and Mark Loafman*

## CASE 35-1

*Sandy Kopenski is an unscheduled walk-in who appears depressed and upset as Dr. Fields enters the examining room. Six months ago she had come in with her boyfriend Tom to see Dr. Fields for her first prenatal visit. She is 19 and worked in a nearby factory to pay for tuition at the community college she attended part-time. Dr. Fields has cared for Sandy and her family for years. He knew this unplanned pregnancy had caused considerable tension in the Kopenski family, who always have been outspoken about their strong religious beliefs.*

*Since Sandy was unsure of her last menstrual period, Dr. Fields performed an ultrasound to help establish the baby's gestational age. The ultrasound showed a 20-week fetus that appeared to have an abnormality in the continuity of its vertebrae. He referred Sandy to the regional medical center where a targeted ultrasound examination confirmed the presence of a meningomyelocele. She returned to Dr. Fields who explained that the infant might be neurologically impaired and unable to walk or attain bowel and bladder control. They discussed options, including termination, and how best to involve her family for support.*

*The pregnancy continued until 37 weeks of gestation when Sandy went into labor. As planned, she was transferred by ambulance from their community hospital to the medical center in anticipation of the need for neonatal intensive care. The baby was delivered by elective cesarean section and was found to have significant neurologic involvement. The NICU staff was supportive but Sandy felt overwhelmed by the technology, numerous physicians, and the many decisions that had to be made regarding surgery and related care of her infant. Dr. Fields discussed the case with the neurosurgeon and neonatologist, then held a family meeting with the Kopenskis to discuss their options and begin discharge planning. The infant subsequently underwent surgery and was eventually discharged to the care of Sandy, her family, and Dr. Fields. They worked closely with the staff at the regional neurodevelopmental unit and used the visiting nurse service. A referral to an early intervention program also was arranged.*

*Although Sandy appreciates her family's support, she has not resolved her feelings of guilt surrounding the unplanned and out-of-wedlock birth. Her boyfriend Tom is afraid of the baby and is becoming detached. Sandy is becoming more isolated and depressed, and fears that Dr. Fields will be unable to help.*

1. Discuss the main components of maternity care
2. Understand how preconception care can improve pregnancy outcomes
3. Understand the relationship between psychosocial and obstetric problems and the rationale for comprehensive care for pregnant women and their families
4. Identify the special challenges and benefits of care management of women at high risk for poor pregnancy outcomes
5. Discuss community-based approaches using multidisciplinary team resources for pregnant adolescents and other high-risk women

## INTRODUCTION

Physicians who provide obstetric services consider the care of women and their families during pregnancy and early childhood one of the most essential and rewarding aspects of practice. The family physician is perhaps the best positioned of all physicians to fulfill the goals of care during this time in a family's life, as defined by the federal Expert Panel on the Content of Prenatal Care (Rosen *et al.*, 1989). These goals of care include goals for the pregnant woman, the fetus and infant, and the family (see Table 35.1). Success requires that the physician identify and respond in an organized manner to the broad variety of problems that might arise during this time in a family's life. These problems might be of an urgent obstetric or medical nature, of a psychiatric nature, or relate to a family's behaviors and social circumstances.

The preconception and prenatal interval are critical to the health of the fetus and future child, and the care provided during this interval might dramatically alter the entire life of the child and family. Effective preventive interventions can alter conditions that otherwise might lead to permanent disability. In addition, the birth of the first child involves fundamental changes in the relationship between husband and wife; subsequent children further redefine this relationship and the parent–child dynamics of the family.

While this can be a time of growth and joy for the family, it is also a time of risk. Extramarital relationships involving the husband are most likely to start during the first pregnancy. Pregnancy is also a time of heightened risk for physical and emotional abuse (Helton *et al.*, 1987; Newberger *et al.*, 1992), with 2.6 to 5.4% of women in each state reporting physical abuse during pregnancy (Colley Gilbert *et al.*, 1999). Indeed, abuse paradoxically also may lead women and adolescents to become pregnant or to rapidly have repeat pregnancies (Jacoby *et al.*, 1999). Many women and families are not prepared for the birth of a child and need assistance in fundamental ways. The family physician is often the person to whom a family turns to for help with these issues. Often, effective care of medical and obstetric problems is not possible until psychosocial

---

**Table 35.1**
The Goals of Prenatal Care Defined by the Expert Panel on the Content of Prenatal Care

Objectives for the pregnant woman
- Increase her well-being before, during, and after pregnancy and improve her self-image and self-care
- Reduce maternal mortality and morbidity, fetal loss, and unnecessary pregnancy interventions
- Reduce risks to health prior to future pregnancies and beyond childbearing years
- Promote development of parenting skills

Objectives for the infant
- Increase well-being
- Reduce preterm birth, intrauterine growth retardation, congenital anomalies, and failure to thrive
- Promote healthy growth and development, immunization, and health supervision
- Reduce neurologic, developmental, and other morbidities
- Reduce child abuse and neglect, injuries, preventable acute and chronic illness, and need for extended hospitalization after birth

Objectives for the family
- Promote family development and positive parent–infant interaction
- Reduce unintended pregnancies
- Identify for treatment behavior disorders leading to child neglect and family violence

## BABIES DELIVERED BY FAMILY PHYSICIANS

| Practice location | % delivering one or more babies in past year | Mean number of babies delivered annually |
|---|---|---|
| South Atlantic | 13.9 | 26.3 |
| New England | 31.1 | 18.6 |
| East South Central | 16.4 | 42.7 |
| Middle Atlantic | 17.1 | 28.2 |
| West South Central | 26.4 | 40.2 |
| East North Central | 37.3 | 23.9 |
| Mountain | 38.0 | 32.1 |
| West North Central | 52.6 | 28.5 |
| Pacific | 33.2 | 27.3 |
| National average | 29.3 | 28.6 |

*Includes only active member respondents of the American Academy of Family Physicians.*
*Source: American Academy of Family Physicians, Practice Profile I Survey, May 1998.*

problems are addressed. For example, the woman who does not have transportation or childcare for her other children, possibly because of a dysfunctional relationship with the father of her children, is not likely to seek early or adequate care for preeclampsia, an often asymptomatic condition involving increased blood pressure and decreased uterine perfusion that can lead to prematurity and low birth weight.

As in Case 35-1, for families with infants born prematurely or with a chronic problem, and for women with chronic medical problems, the coordination of care from prior to conception through pregnancy, and from delivery through ongoing care after discharge is important. A young woman with a child who has a congenital defect might find herself cared for initially during pregnancy in her local community and its hospital facilities, then in a tertiary care center by maternal–fetal medicine specialists, delivering at the tertiary care center with subsequent involvement of a neonatologist and neonatal intensive care unit team, and then discharged back to her community with intended follow-up with a variety of pediatric specialists and a community-based team of services for children with special needs. The decisions she must make for her infant, the variety of information she will receive, the feelings of self-blame and guilt for her infant's condition, and the alterations expected for her own life all might be overwhelming.

In these circumstances, the steady presence of a physician who knows the woman and her family, who has developed an understanding of her strengths and ability to cope, as well as her weaknesses, and who is trusted to help with the adjustments and decisions to be made can dramatically alter the outcome for all involved. Thus, core principles of primary care—comprehensiveness, coordination, and continuity—are critical to the provision of high-quality care to women, their families, and children during the childbearing years.

## CASE 35-2

*Catherine Jones related to Dr. Fields the mixed emotions she felt last week as she watched her home pregnancy test turn positive. Although she has wanted a baby for several years, her two previous miscarriages had been devastating. In each case, she developed pain and bleeding late in the first trimester. A thorough evaluation had failed to detect any abnormalities or risk factors for miscarriage. Dr. Fields discussed the various screening tests that were available and set up a schedule of frequent visits to monitor Catherine and her pregnancy. They had already discussed the role of nutrition, lifestyle modifications, and emotional preparation for pregnancy.*

*As the pregnancy approached the 10th week, Catherine experienced some painless vaginal bleeding. An ultrasound was reassuring and she was asked to restrict her physical activity. Her employer requested that she either perform her usual duties or take a full medical leave. She asked Dr. Fields to intervene on her behalf.*

*The bleeding resolved and the pregnancy continued without complication until 32 weeks of gestation when Catherine noticed several episodes of premature contractions. Again, frequent visits and patient education were undertaken along with a series of outpatient visits to the hospital for monitoring.*

## COMPONENTS OF PRENATAL CARE

As Case 35-2 illustrates, prenatal care involves three basic activities: early and continuing risk assessment, health promotion, and medical and psychosocial interventions in response to risks and problems identified. A comprehensive risk assessment done at initial contact and then regularly updated provides the information around which all other prenatal care is organized. While pregnancy should be viewed as a normal (rather than illness) event, only about 40% of women will be found to have no risk requiring professional intervention (Alexander & Keirse, 1989; Selwyn, 1990). For most mothers, the family physician might need to pursue further investigations and intervene accordingly.

Risk assessment includes history taking, physical examination, and diagnostic tests. Table 35.2 lists the risks that have been documented as influencing birth outcomes (Fry, 2000; Rosen *et al.*, 1989). As can be seen, a great variety of medical, obstetric, nutritional, psychological, health behavior, and social risks can adversely affect pregnancy outcomes. Risks, especially those of a psychosocial nature, are simply characteristics that have been associated with adverse birth outcomes. While they are all markers of poor outcomes, they might not be the direct cause. Instead, as illustrated in Fig. 35.1, such factors might play a role in a complex set of processes leading to poor outcome. The content, timing, and number of prenatal visits will vary depending on the woman's risks.

While risks can be separated into medical (organic) and psychosocial groups, the physician must respond to all risks in an integrated manner. Medical risks can lead to psychosocial risks and vice versa. For example, a woman placed at bed rest early in pregnancy because of a medical complication might lose income and thus require additional support from other family members, leading to other stresses. High levels of stress might in turn lead to blood pressure alterations, increased uterine irritability, and premature labor. For this reason, the biopsychosocial model of care is particularly appropriate for reproductive age families (Culpepper & Jack, 1993; Jack *et al.*, 1998).

For all women, including those at low risk, a series of health promotion activities is required (Rosen *et al.*, 1989). These activities are listed in Table 35.3 and can be provided one on one or in group settings. Their purpose is to help the woman and her family adjust to the changes that occur during pregnancy and to prepare for the coming of the newborn. They include counseling to promote and support healthy behaviors, education regarding pregnancy and parenting, and provision of information about proposed care. While some activities are likely to be most effective if done early in pregnancy, others become more relevant to the family later in

---

## PRECONCEPTION AND PRENATAL CARE INCLUDES:

- *Early and continuing risk assessment*
- *Health promotion*
- *Medical and psychosocial interventions in response to risks and problems identified*

**Table 35.2**
Conditions to Be Targeted during Prenatal Risk Assessment[a]

History
  Sociodemographic
    Age*
    Income and educational level*
    Household size, geographic location
    Level of financial resources for pregnancy*
    Nature of support network for pregnant woman and
      family*
    Adequacy of housing
    Availability of transportation*
    Availability of childcare
    Fluency and literacy in English language*
    Mental or physical disabilities*
  Psychological
    Major life events and stressors
    Family function*
    Extremes of maternal stress and anxiety*
    Abuse or family violence*
    Mental status and illness*
    Readiness for pregnancy*
    Readiness for parenting (attitudes, knowledge, skills)*
    Adjustment problems*
    Suicide risk*
  Menstrual/gynecologic
    Onset, duration, frequency, and character of menses
    Last menstrual period (LMP) and last normal menstrual
      period (LNMP)*
    Infections such as pelvic inflammatory disease (PID)*
    Gynecologic surgery
  Contraceptive and sexual
    Whether pregnancy is planned or wanted*
    Contraceptive methods used*
    Current sexual relationship, partners
  Past obstetric
    Prior pregnancies, length and timing
    Previous intrauterine growth retardation (IUGR) infant or
      preterm birth
    High parity, short birth intervals*
    Previous hemorrhage
    Stillborn or neonatal death
    Sudden infant death syndrome (SIDS) infant
  Medical and surgical
    Chronic diseases, e.g., diabetes mellitus, hypertension,
      anemias*
    Prescription medications*
    Infections, e.g., HIV, hepatitis, toxoplasmosis*
    Allergies
    Trauma
    Surgical procedures
    Blood transfusions
  Genetic—individual, spouse, and family
    Repeated spontaneous abortions*
    Chromosomal and other congenital abnormalities*
    Hemoglobinopathies, e.g., sickle-cell anemia*
    Radiation and other toxic substance exposure*
    Multiple births

History (cont.)
  Genetic (cont.)
    Family history of chronic diseases
  Nutrition
    Prepregnancy weight (height-to-weight profile)*
    Diet history with evaluation of adequacy*
    Barrier to adequate nutrition intake, e.g., financial,
      cultural, food fads, pica*
    Special dietary patterns, e.g., vegetarian, lactose
      intolerance, caffeine*
  Behavioral
    Smoking, alcohol, illicit drug use*
    Over-the-counter medications, prescription drugs*
    Rest and sleep patterns*
    Extremes of exercise or physical exertion*
    Dental care*
    History of antisocial behavior*
    Care seeking and compliance*
    Pregnancy wantedness*
  Environmental hazards, work hazards, or both
    Exposure to toxins, teratogens*
    Work—occupation, type, and level of activity
  Current pregnancy to date (first visit)
    Normal signs and symptoms
    LMP and LNMP
    Estimated date of conception, weeks gestation and present
      time
    Abnormal signs and symptoms, concerns
General physical examination
  Blood pressure
  Breast exam
  Pelvic exam
  Fetal size
  Fetal heart tones
Laboratory tests
  Hemoglobin or hematocrit*
  Blood Rh, Rh negative titer, antibody screen
  Rubella titer (if immunity not previously documented)*
  Syphilis test*
  Pap smear*
  Urine protein and glucose*
  Urine screen for urinary tract infection (UTI), kidney disease
  Gonorrheal culture*
  Hepatitis B titer*
  Screening tests offered to all women*
    HIV titer
    Drug toxicology
  Screening test in endemic areas or for women with risk
    factors*
    Toxoplasmosis, tuberculosis
    Herpes simplex, varicella
    Chlamydia
    Hemoglobinopathies
    Tay–Sachs
Fetal evaluation
  Confirm gestational age (LMP, uterine size)

[a]Asterisks identify conditions that are appropriate for preconception identification and screening.

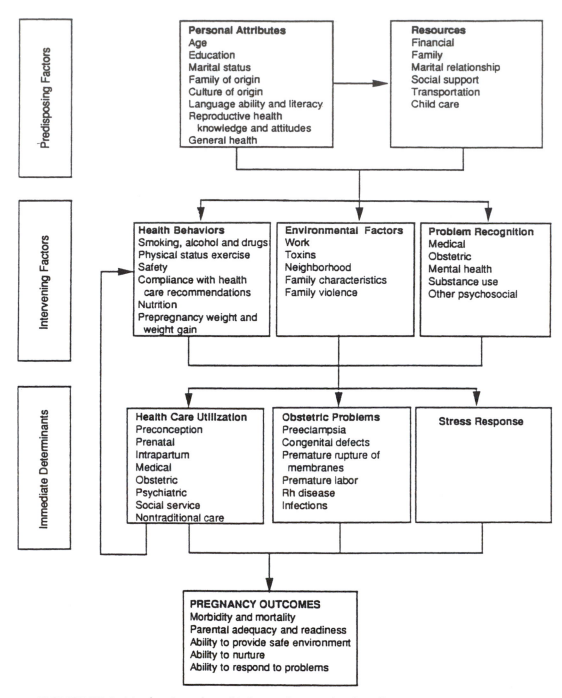

**FIGURE 35.1.** Mechanisms by which psychosocial risks affect pregnancy outcomes.

pregnancy. Consequently, some medical and midwifery practices offer both early and late prenatal classes, which may be followed by parenting classes after the birth.

In addition to risk assessment and health promotion, prenatal care includes specific interventions to alter the risks for poor pregnancy outcome, including treating existing medical and obstetric problems, and initiating psychosocial interventions.

**Table 35.3**
Health Promotion for Pregnant Women[a]

| | |
|---|---|
| Counseling to promote support healthful behaviors | General knowledge of pregnancy and parenting (*cont.*) |
|   Nutrition* |   Nutrition |
|   Smoking cessation* |   Physiologic changes |
|   Avoidance of alcohol* |   Psychological adaptation |
|   Avoidance of illicit drugs* |   Exercise for fitness |
|   Avoidance of teratogens* |   Rest and sleep patterns |
|   Safer sex* |   Infant car seat and safety |
|   Maternal seat belt use |   Preparation for childbirth |
|   Work counseling* |   Preparation for parenting |
|   Stress reduction (avoidance of heavy lifting and | Information on proposed care |
|     long standing)* |   Need for early entry into prenatal care* |
| General knowledge of pregnancy and parenting |   Preparation for screening and diagnostic tests |
|   Physiologic and emotional changes of pregnancy |   Content and timing for prenatal visits needed* |
|   Sexual counseling |   Need to report danger signs immediately |
|   Fetal growth and development |   Birth plan, expectations, and goals |
|   Self-help strategies for common discomforts |   Labor onset plans |
|   Early pregnancy classes | |

[a] Asterisks identify conditions that are appropriate for preconception study.

## CASE 35-3

*A 33-year-old woman and her husband, married 3 years, have come to Dr. Fields's office seeking advice and to interview him about being their physician. She has recently attained the seniority at her work that she wanted prior to starting a family. The couple feel they have worked through several difficult relationship issues and are emotionally and financially ready to start a family; they have bought a house and are saving for private schools. They both want advice and counseling to improve the health of their future child.*

## PRECONCEPTION CARE

Preconception care is care received by women before they become pregnant to reduce the risk of poor pregnancy outcome. Its components are the same as prenatal care: risk assessment, health promotion, and interventions to reduce risks (Culpepper & Jack, 1991). For an activity to be recommended as a part of preconception care, it must have enhanced value if it is done before conception as opposed to waiting until after conception. Conditions for which preconception identification and intervention are appropriate are identified in Tables 35.2 and 35.3.

For some risks, intervention is available only if initiated before pregnancy. For others, interventions during pregnancy are available but must be initiated early in the pregnancy. To prevent congenital defects, exposure to teratogens during the first 57 days of pregnancy, when most organogenesis occurs, must be eliminated. Unfortunately, the very nature of some risks also results in some women not seeking prenatal care until late in pregnancy, if at all. Table 35.4 lists factors associated with women obtaining prenatal care (Perez-Woods, 1990). To reach women who otherwise would not seek prenatal care promptly, physicians can use two strategies: preconception care and working with others to conduct community outreach.

A large portion of neural tube defects are prevented by folate supplementation beginning 1 to 3 months prior to conception (Thompson *et al.*, 2000), supplementation that did not occur in Case 35-1. Rubella syndrome can be prevented by vaccination of susceptible women prior to pregnancy, but because it involves a live vaccine, vaccination during pregnancy is contraindicated (Fineman & Walton, 2000; Lee *et al.*, 1992). Alcohol consumption during pregnancy is the number one cause of mental retardation. Avoidance of

**Table 35.4**
Factors Associated with Beginning and Remaining in Prenatal Care (Perez-Woods, 1990)

Characteristics of prenatal care
  Individualized psychosocial services available, including
    feedback and advice
  Communication patterns
  Affordable at a reasonable cost or covered by insurance
    other than Medicaid
  Geographic accessibility (distance < 1 mile, safe public
    transportation available)
  Conservative (traditional birthing arrangements unless
    previous experience, or social norms associated with
    innovation)
  Education and information available
  Care provided by a multidisciplinary team
  Care provided by nurse midwives and nurses
  Availability publicized in news media
The pregnant woman's social network
  Availability of psychosocial support
  Social norms support need for care
  Family supports use of service
Characteristics of the pregnant woman—psychological
  Satisfied with current health services
  Feeling of self-competence
  Positive attitude about care
  Sense of power
  Hopeful about the future

Characteristics of the pregnant woman—psychological (*cont.*)
  Absence of depression, denial of pregnancy, fear about the
    future
  Low stress level
  Early developmental and physical stage of pregnancy
  Expectations about outcome
  Early acknowledgment of pregnancy
  Attitude about pregnancy
  Somatization
  Accepts innovation only after experience or confirmation by
    social network
Characteristics of the pregnant woman—social
  Previous satisfactory experience with high-risk pregnancy or
    healthcare services
  Culture
  Higher social class
  Length of time since immigration to the United States
  Higher level of education
  Being married
  Informs others about the pregnancy early
  Availability of social networks
  Age (>19 years and <35 years)
Characteristics of the pregnant woman—Cognitive
  Higher level of cognitive development

unwanted pregnancy among heavy drinkers, or interventions (which may take time) to reduce drinking before pregnancy can eliminate this risk (Herron *et al.*, 1982). For women who smoke, nicotine-containing gum might be a helpful smoking-cessation aid before pregnancy, but is not recommended for use during pregnancy. For women with epilepsy, medications can be altered to remove those with major teratogenic potential. For those who are anorexic or bulimic, interventions that improve nutritional status before conception are important, since underweight women who do not gain adequate weight during pregnancy are at increased risk for fetal death and preterm delivery (Schieve *et al.*, 2000). Genetic counseling before conception allows a couple additional options, e.g., adoption, *in vitro* fertilization, and if needed, can promote early chorionic villous sampling or amniocentesis during pregnancy. Preconception care is appropriate for both men and women, or for couples to consider together.

# NEURAL TUBE DEFECTS

*The* neural tube *is the embryonic structure that develops into the brain and spinal cord. It starts out as a flat pancake of cells, folding into a tube by the 29th day of conception. When the tube does not close completely, the fetus has a neural tube defect (NTD). In the United States about 2500 babies are born each year with NTDs.*

*The most common NTDs are spina bifida and anencephaly; meningomyelocele (Case 35-1) is a less common form.*

- *Spina bifida—defect resulting from the failure of one or more vertebral arches to fuse; subtypes are based on the degree and pattern of deformity*
- *Anencephaly—absence of the bones of the cranial vault and absent or only rudimentary formation of the cerebral hemispheres, brain stem, and basal ganglia*
- *Meningomyelocele—protrusion of the spinal cord and its membranes through a defect in the vertebral column*

## DO YOU DRINK ALCOHOL?

*Alcohol consumption during pregnancy is the number one cause of mental retardation; a large portion of women at risk are unaware of this. A single question, asked by the family physician before pregnancy starts, can lead to effective preventive education:*

*"Do you drink alcohol?"*

Perhaps one of the most important preconception risks is the risk of unplanned or unwanted pregnancy (Fischer *et al.*, 1999). Among married women, 10% of births are unwanted, and an additional 25% are unintended and mistimed: wanted, but not just now. Among unmarried women these percentages are 25 and 40%, respectively (Williams & Pratt, 1989). In some age and socioeconomic subgroups, such as among teenagers, the vast majority of pregnancies are unwanted. Many women, including teenagers, who become pregnant by "leaving it to fate" are not aware of the contraceptive options available to them. The concept of poor investment in pregnancy has been developed to describe the woman with an unwanted pregnancy (DeMuylder *et al.*, 1992; Marsiglio & Mott, 1988; Weller *et al.*, 1987). Such a woman is likely to delay the start of prenatal care, continue the use of alcohol and cigarettes, and engage in behaviors that place her pregnancy at risk. She might delay recognition and care of problems affecting her pregnancy (Joyce & Grossman, 1990). These behaviors are related to adverse outcomes such as low birth weight at delivery and child abuse after delivery. A child in a family with two unplanned pregnancies is 2.8 times more likely to be abused, and with three unplanned pregnancies the risk increases to 4.6 times, compared with a child in a family with no unplanned births (Zuravin, 1991).

Physicians have numerous opportunities to incorporate preconception care into their practices: during routine periodic health assessments, school, work, and premarital examinations, family planning visits, negative pregnancy test visits, and well-child care for another family member. Unfortunately, many of the women most likely to benefit from preconception care are least likely to have access to it because of the social, financial, health behavior, or psychological risks involved. To reach such women, physicians must work in their communities to make preconception care available in settings where such high-risk women can be reached before becoming pregnant, such as STD clinics, substance abuse treatment centers, women's shelters, halfway houses, and detention centers (Jack & Culpepper, 1990).

## CASE 35-4

*Shana is 22 years old and Dr. Fields is seeing her for the second time. She was late in her pregnancy and had come to his office for her first visit the previous week. At that time, the office nurse performed a rapid review of relevant risks, which Dr. Fields subsequently confirmed, and sent blood samples for basic screening lab tests based on her risk status. Shana has had five previous pregnancies including two that aborted. One of her three children had been born premature and subsequently died at home in unclear circumstances at 3 months of age. Her other children were placed in foster care by Child Protective Services. Shana currently smokes two packs a day, drinks regularly, and until midpregnancy supported herself in part through prostitution. She first came to Dr. Fields because she was destitute; her boyfriend had kicked her out of his apartment. She is underweight and had not eaten well in weeks. She complained of burning on urination, and a urinalysis revealed numerous white cells, highly suggestive of a urinary tract infection, which he treated with amoxicillin. An ultrasound and pelvic examination on the first visit indicated a pregnancy of 35 (± 3 weeks) week's gestation, assuming that the fetus was of normal size for gestational age.*

*Today she returns unhappy with the shelter to which Dr. Fields referred her, in part because of its curfew, and because the shelter's social worker insisted that Shana meet with her regularly. Her laboratory results suggest that she is a hepatitis B carrier. She confides that she has mainlined a variety of substances in the past and uses crack when her boyfriend makes it available. When asked to consent to HIV testing, she declines. Since the weather has improved, she is thinking of leaving the shelter. She also confides her belief that she can get control of her problems, if only she can keep this baby.*

## CARE OF WOMEN AT HIGH RISK

Low birth weight, congenital birth defects, and problems arising during labor and delivery are the major immediate causes of the delivery of newborns who have serious problems with long-term consequences. However, underlying problems that are responsive to prenatal care interventions often precede these immediate causes. These include acute problems, especially infections, and chronic medical conditions, particularly hypertensive disorders and diabetes mellitus, which affect the adequacy of the fetal–placental unit and its ability to maintain a supportive intrauterine environment, and conditions, such as epilepsy, that require chronic medications of a potentially teratogenic nature. In addition, women often have psychosocial risks, including psychological difficulties, social problems, and adverse health behaviors, which can contribute to poor pregnancy outcomes. These latter risks also can lead to problems arising after pregnancy, such as failure to thrive, accidents, and developmental delay.

## Congenital Defects

Approximately 3% of newborns are affected by genetic defects. Mendelian (single gene), chromosomal, multifactorial (both high and low heritability conditions), infectious, and environmental etiologies (e.g., radiation, toxin, and drug exposures) contribute to the spectrum of congenital defects (Yang *et al.*, 1997). The number of chromosomal abnormalities that can be detected in prospective parents is increasing rapidly, as a result of the current emphasis on genome research and advances in DNA probe techniques. Ultrasound, MRI, chorionic villous sampling techniques, and early amniocentesis all provide additional diagnostic and therapeutic options once conception has occurred. Early experience with *in utero* therapy for conditions such as fetal urinary tract obstruction, hydrocephalus, or diaphragmatic hernia are promising.

However, the development of genetic screening tests and interventions with potential clinical application result in a variety of considerations for families and their physicians. For many conditions, the undertaking of preconception or prenatal testing for congenital defects currently is limited to those couples known to be at high risk, such as screening for Tay–Sachs disease among Ashkenazi Jews, and hemoglobinopathies among those of Greek and Italian descent. For a number of conditions, screening could be of some benefit if routinely performed; this results in a number of controversial issues.

Cystic fibrosis, one of the most common congenital defects, illustrates the complexity of the issues involved in deciding who should be screened. Preconception screening for cystic fibrosis provides a couple with increased options including not bearing children, artificial insemination, *in vitro* fertilization, surrogate pregnancy, adoption, as well as conception with early pregnancy testing and selective abortion. Diagnosis during pregnancy does not appear to improve outcomes for infants subsequently born with cystic fibrosis. At least through age 4, there is no evidence that presymptomatic diagnosis of cystic fibrosis is of therapeutic benefit to the child (Lemna *et al.*, 1990).

In a general population, a sequential strategy of testing one member of the couple initially, and the second only if the first is positive, can identify 75% of anticipated cystic fibrosis births at a cost of $367,000 each. This figure does not include the lifetime medical costs of caring for a patient with cystic fibrosis (which would largely offset this cost over time), and assumes that couples who identify a pregnancy at risk will choose to have prenatal diagnosis and termination of affected pregnancies (Asch *et al.*, 1998). The cost per cystic fibrosis birth identified is about half this figure when couples plan two children. Thus, the cost-effectiveness of CF carrier screening depends greatly on couples' reproductive plans. At a population level, out of 11,000 couples screened, 10 would be identified who are at risk (both parents heterozygotes); of these, 8 would choose prenatal diagnosis resulting in 2 fetuses identified as having cystic fibrosis.

## CYSTIC FIBROSIS IN THE UNITED STATES

*A three-base-pair deletion in a gene on the long arm of chromosome 7 has been found responsible for*

- *75.8% of cystic fibrosis of the white population, but only*
- *49% in Hispanic,*
- *43% in Italian, and*
- *30% in Ashkenazi Jewish populations.*

The potential stigmatization and altered public perceptions of cystic fibrosis possibly resulting from dissemination of cystic fibrosis screening have been identified as areas needing further understanding to enlighten development of public policy. If cystic fibrosis is potentially preventable through screening with subsequent avoidance of pregnancy or abortion, then the public perception might shift toward subtly blaming the parents of children with cystic fibrosis, and decreased support and acceptance of them, including through publicly funded programs. As a consequence of all of these considerations, currently most physicians limit screening for cystic fibrosis and many other conditions to those couples known to be at increased risk because either they or a close relative suffer from it.

In addition to interventions related to genetic screening, physicians can prevent congenital defects through counseling regarding teratogenic exposures at work or around the home, abstinence from alcohol intake during pregnancy, maintenance of adequate folate intake (to prevent neurotubular defects), and tailoring of chronic medications.

# Low Birth Weight

Low-birth-weight infants either are born prematurely (before 37 weeks' gestation), have suffered from intrauterine growth retardation (IUGR) and consequently are born small for gestational age (SGA), or both. For all specific birth weight cohorts, the United States has the best rate of infant survival worldwide. However, relative to other developed countries, the United States has had a higher rate of low-birth-weight infants, and has seen virtually no decrease in this rate (about 7%) over the past four decades. As a result, its ranking has dropped from the 6th lowest total infant mortality rate in 1950–1955, to the mid-20s in recent decades. However, countries with the lowest infant mortality rates tended to have the lowest incidence of births less than 500 g ($r = 0.73$) and of births 500–999 g ($r = 0.81$). Furthermore, the countries with the lowest infant mortality rates report the fewest number of deaths in the first 24 hours after birth. Consequently, differences in birth registration practices for infants weighing less than 1500 g are primarily responsible for the poor, deteriorating performance by the United States in the international rankings of neonatal mortality rates (Sepkowitz, 1995).

## PRETERM DELIVERY

- *10% of all births*
    *Twice as frequent among African-American women*
- *Accounts for 70% of perinatal mortality and half of long-term neurologic morbidity*
    *Most concentrated in the 1–2% born at less than 32 weeks of gestation weighing less than 1500 g*
- *May be causally associated with chronic intrauterine infections, including ones preceding conception.*

*Source: Goldenberg et al. (2000)*

Immediate causes of preterm delivery include lethal congenital defects (10–20%); multiple pregnancy, e.g., twins (10%); elective delivery due to an obstetric problem [25–30%, including hypertension/preeclampsia (10–15%), hemorrhage (4–6%), diabetes mellitus (2–3%), IUGR (3–9%), Rh disease (1–2%) and other medical problems (5–10%)]; spontaneous rupture of membranes (SROM) (15–25%); and spontaneous preterm labor (25–35%), including about half complicated by obstetric problems similar to those leading to elective early delivery (Culpepper, 1991). Each of these immediate causes has been linked to risk factors present earlier in pregnancy or before pregnancy. Individual risk factors usually predict multiple immediate causes of low birth weight. Large portions of these are of a psychosocial nature (Institute of Medicine, 1985).

Preterm labor occurs with membranes intact, or labor onset and ROM occur together. In addition, once twin pregnancies, fetal deaths, and induced preterm deliveries are excluded, about half of the remaining cases of prematurity start with ROM prior to labor, with labor developing spontaneously or being induced. Preterm labor risk factors include psychosocial ones related to low income, inadequate prenatal care, stress, low social support, and behaviors such as smoking and substance use; acute and chronic medical conditions, including infections; and obstetric problems such as multiple gestation, abruption, and preeclampsia (Challis, 2000; Von Der Pool, 1998; Weismiller, 1999). Of note, studies in other countries have shown that poverty need not be associated with an increased risk of prematurity, as occurs in the United States (Piekkala et al., 1986).

IUGR leads to a 5- to 8-fold increase in rate of fetal death, a 2- to 5-fold increase in neonatal mortality, and a 5- to 10-fold increase in neurologic deficits in surviving offspring. Causes of IUGR are diverse, and include factors that affect the integrity of the placental transfer of nutrition such as maternal hypertension, smoking, drug use, diabetes mellitus, Rh disease, lupus, and other conditions (Prada & Tsang, 1998). Maternal behaviors such as smoking account for over 50% of IUGR. While a theoretical incidence of IUGR of under 1% might be attainable, in high-risk populations incidences of over 10% and even 20% have been found (Goldenberg et al., 1990; Kramer, 1998)

Little national consensus has emerged regarding the diverse approaches to screening, confirmation, monitoring, therapy, and timing of delivery for IUGR. Diagnostic strategies include screening techniques using umbilical height and third trimester ultrasound screening of patients with risk factors and subsequent confirmatory ultrasound investigation. Nonstress test monitoring and fetal growth ultrasound monitoring both have been used to follow fetal well-being. Measurement of fetal and umbilical blood flow by ultrasound Doppler studies holds promise for identifying fetal status including the need for urgent delivery. The value of bed rest and home versus hospital care as interventions are all unclear (Crowther & Chalmers, 1989; Ural & Nagey, 1998).

Considering all of the causes of low birth weight together, the Institute of Medicine (Institute of Medicine, 1985) concluded that the lack of prenatal care that starts early and is continuous is the most

---

## POSTDATE PREGNANCIES

*Gestations lasting beyond 42 weeks (294 days) are considered postdate*

- *Infant mortality doubles by 43 weeks and increases fivefold by 45 weeks*

*Determination of due dates is best done early in pregnancy using:*

- *Known date of conception (± 3 days)*
- *Accurate LMP (± 7 days)*
- *Early uterine size assessment (± 7 days)*
- *Ultrasound exam before 20 weeks (± 7 days)*
- *Ultrasound exam after 28 weeks (± 3 weeks)*
- *First fetal heart tones usually heard with a nonelectronic fetal stethoscope at 18 weeks (± 3 weeks)*
- *Quickening (felt fetal movements) at 18 weeks (± 4 weeks)*

---

important risk factor. It identified six major reasons for women obtaining inadequate prenatal care: financial constraints (no or inadequate health insurance); inadequate availability of healthcare service providers, especially ones willing to serve socially disadvantaged or high-risk women; insufficient prenatal services and facilities routinely used by high-risk populations, such as community health centers; the experiences, attitudes, and beliefs of pregnant women; poor or absent childcare and transportation services; and inadequate systems to recruit hard-to-reach women into care (Institute of Medicine, 1988).

## CASE 35-5

*Dr. Fields's next case is Marie Howbarth, a 39-year-old Jehovah's Witness who is returning at 24 weeks gestation. Dr. Fields has been seeing Mrs. Howbarth weekly to monitor her medical status and fetal development. Mrs. Howbarth has had three previous pregnancies, including a relatively normal first pregnancy, a second pregnancy complicated by deep vein thrombosis, preeclampsia, and gestational diabetes mellitus, and a third pregnancy resulting in a repetition of the same complications and resulting in a stillbirth at 24 weeks' gestation. Her second child was born premature, and requires developmental services for cerebral palsy and borderline mental retardation.*

*Dr. Fields had counseled the Howbarths on the importance of avoiding further pregnancies because of the likely recurrence of the same problems. This pregnancy was unwanted, and considerable tension continues between the Howbarths. Mr. Howbarth is deeply religious and determined that the pregnancy continue with minimal medical intervention; also, he blames his wife for not noticing that her IUD had been spontaneously expelled. Mrs. Howbarth is not as religious, but acquiesces to her husband's wishes. Dr. Fields suspects she would have opted for an abortion if her husband were not involved.*

*Dr. Fields has monitored fetal growth with monthly sonograms beginning at 12 weeks. In addition, he has maintained Mrs. Hobarth on home injections of heparin, with weekly partial thromboplastin time monitoring, and had planned to begin insulin with home monitoring of blood glucose levels at this visit. Mrs. Howbarth's blood pressure has risen by 15 mm Hg diastolic beginning 2 weeks ago, and she will need an antihypertensive agent. Her weight has dropped 2 pounds since last week as well.*

*However, today Dr. Fields notes that on her heparin diary, this past week Mrs. Howbarth has missed 40% of her doses. When asked about this, Mrs. Howbarth begins crying uncontrollably and notes that she has been unable to sleep or eat, feels terribly guilty about bringing another baby with problems into the world, and has lost all interest in living. When asked about suicidal thoughts, she reveals that she has had almost uncontrollable urges to run her car into the interstate bypass on her way home from picking up her child from the developmental center each afternoon.*

## RESOURCES REQUIRED TO SERVE HIGH-RISK POPULATIONS

Physicians caring for high-risk women can be most effective in improving pregnancy outcomes, and improving the health of their offspring during childhood, if they have a number of resources available to them. These include the use of a practice record system and information system, which promote the comprehensive recognition of women at increased risk and their tracking. The capacity to conduct home visiting, either in person, through the visiting nurse service, or other community program, is helpful for further assessing risks identified in the office, and for intervening to reduce a number of risks. In long-term studies among low-income unmarried women, home visiting—especially if it continues postpartum—helps reduce rates of childhood injuries and ingestions that may be associated with child abuse and neglect, and helps mothers defer subsequent pregnancies. Having fewer children enabled women to become employed, become economically self-sufficient, and eventually avoid substance abuse and criminal behavior. Their children benefited too. By the time the children were 15 years old, they had had fewer arrests and convictions, smoked and drank less, and had had fewer sexual partners (Olds *et al.*, 1999). Collaboration with community programs that offer special services is crucial to working effectively with certain pregnant women. These include smoking cessation and substance abuse programs, programs for victims of family violence, services for mentally retarded women and those with chronic mental illness, and programs for pregnant teenagers.

For a number of women, especially single parents and women living in poverty, programs to provide social support are important. Social support is postulated as having both direct effects and ones due to its mediation of the effects of stress (Culpepper & Jack, 1993). Stress might result in altered pregnancy outcomes either at birth or later in infancy through several mechanisms (Koeske & Koeske, 1990; Sheehan, 1998). Stress can divert a woman's or couple's attention from pregnancy and decrease the priority of pregnancy-related issues. This diversion can result in decreased recognition of risks, symptoms, or problems, and decrease the adequacy of response either through delaying or decreasing compliance with care. Stress can have an impact through increasing unhealthy coping behaviors including smoking, substance use, inadequate rest, and excessive work. It might alter interpersonal relations and decrease the resources available to women. The problems causing stress might concomitantly result in diversion of financial assets. Psychological mediation of effects through increased anxiety, decreased self-esteem, and related alterations have been proposed. The effects of stress have been postulated to be catecholamine, immune system, or hormonally mediated.

Social support might work to mediate the effects of stress or have unrelated direct effects. This effect can occur through increasing tangible resources such as safe shelter, food, and financial assets, improving the recognition of risks and problems, and improving responses through self-care, care seeking, and compliance with medical recommendations. Social support also might alter psychological mechanisms or be mediated by biochemical changes. The effects of stress and social support on adverse pregnancy outcomes might occur through their contributing to prenatal problems such as preeclampsia, abruption, preterm labor, or they might have influence on the adequacy of parenting and related infant outcomes (Dejin-Karlsson et al., 2000; Wilkinson et al., 1998).

While the physician treating a small number of women requiring such community services might provide or arrange for them personally, the physician working with high-risk populations can be most effective if attached to a team that also includes nursing, social service, and nutritional expertise, as well as the ability to conduct outreach. Such a team might make interventions at the community level as well as work with individual families. This is important, since communities and neighborhoods themselves may contribute to infant mortality through aspects of social impoverishment (Garbarino, 1990; Turnock & McGill, 1983). For example, infant mortality rates in the poorest third of Chicago neighborhoods are 5 to 10 times the rate of the most affluent third (Kostelny & Garbarino, 1987). Even when the effect of socioeconomic status has been adjusted for, some neighborhoods stand out as contributing to infant mortality (Garbarino & Sherman, 1980). Neighborhoods also have been demonstrated to affect entry to and value derived from prenatal care (Dejin-Karlsson et al., 2000; Wilkinson et al., 1998).

The ability of the practice to provide care coordination and case management support is critical to working successfully with high-risk women and their families. Different high-risk families require different types of support (Culpepper, 1995). Some require assistance in the recognition of problems and help in basic decision-making about their care; examples include mentally retarded parents, overwhelmed single parents, and some recent immigrants. A woman who has been subject to spousal abuse may require a provider who identifies not only her risk, but also that to her children. In some cases, the provider needs to make basic decisions for an immobilized woman. Other women might be able to identify problems but have a poor understanding of the consequences likely to be involved, and are unable to set priorities or appropriately follow through with action. A third high-risk group is able to identify the problems and understand the consequences, but is not aware of the resources available or how to use them effectively. Some families simply require information about available resources and encouragement in using them. Finally, some families can manage virtually all of their needs with only occasional support and assistance during particularly difficult times. These families occasionally need the encouragement and advocacy of the helping professionals involved with them.

While in some families the level of function is static and unlikely to change, with others there is potential for growth as the woman or couple involved learns requisite life skills and begins to deal with problems independently. Ideally, the primary care system involved will be responsive to the circumstances of these

## DEPRESSIVE SYMPTOMS FOLLOWING PREGNANCY ARE VERY COMMON, WITH SPECIFIC DIAGNOSIS REQUIRED FOR APPROPRIATE TREATMENT

*Postpartum blues*
- *Mildest postpartum mood disturbance*
- *Affects up to 85% of women following pregnancy*
- *Begins in first postpartum days*
- *Peaks at 3–7 days*
- *Resolves within 2–12 weeks*
- *Coincides with major changes in endocrine balance*
- *Requires education, reassurance, and support*

*Postpartum depression*
- *Incidence: 10–20%*
- *Up to one-fourth of adolescent mothers*
- *Develops in the first few weeks after pregnancy*
- *Majority resolve within 3–6 months*
- *Risk factors*
    - *Personal or family history of depression*
      *Prior postpartum depression: a 50% risk of recurrence*
      *Prior depression before conception: 30% risk of recurrence*
    - *Lack of social or spousal support*
    - *Poor communication with significant other*
    - *Marital difficulties*
    - *Stressful life events*
    - *Infant with health problem*
    - *Infant with disagreeable temperament*
    - *Unwanted pregnancy*
- *Treatment*
    - *Requires specific pharmacologic or psychotherapeutic treatment*

*Postpartum psychosis*
- *1–2 per 1000 births*
- *Onset within first few days to 4 weeks postpartum*
- *Hospitalization required for most, often urgently*
- *Suicide and infanticide risk is high*
- *95% improve within 3 months*

different types of families and not only ensure appropriate care, but also concomitantly foster improvement of the functioning of the family unit.

With regard to high-need families, the scope of the primary care system's responsibilities and the adequacy of the medical model are interrelated issues. Not only will the level of involvement in outreach, prioritizing, and decision-making by a case manager vary depending on the family, but their clinical needs will be diverse over time, and might include traditional primary medical care, dental care, developmental disability services, mental health services such as for substance abuse and behavioral disorders, and preventive services. In addition, the primary care system might need to respond to family dysfunction as a problem in its own right to be able to effectively care for other problems.

In contrast to the diversity of professional services a high-need family might require, primary care clinicians generally follow a medical or biopsychosocial approach. This usually is problem oriented, involving an elucidation of the history and objective findings, collection of additional information through testing,

## NEED HELP?

*Health professionals find it beneficial to develop strong referral and comanagement relationships, including agreement around communication and care management with a variety of agencies, including ones that provide the following services:*
- *Prenatal classes, including "early" classes*
- *Breast-feeding classes and support*
- *WIC (Women, Infants, and Children) Program (a federal program providing food supplements)*
- *Shelters, including for abused women and their children*
- *Mental health services*
- *Transportation*
- *Financial counseling*
- *Housing*
- *Abortion and abortion counseling*
- *Adolescent pregnancy*
- *Parenting classes*
- *Genetic counseling*
- *Social services*
- *Dental care*
- *Disability services*

obtaining consultation, or information from others including by home visit, and then development of a therapeutic plan that integrates medical, psychological, and social responses. Within a continuity setting, this then leads to ongoing monitoring of the plan with changes in therapy as needed. The physician generally relates to families in a collaborative–contractual relationship, wherein the physician provides recommendations within a framework in which the woman or family is free to follow or ignore the recommendations, including return for follow-up. The clinician generally views his or her role as being supportive to the patient, possibly including advocacy in obtaining care from other community agencies. Should a patient not return for follow-up appointments, the clinician might feel little responsibility for aggressive outreach, and indeed might dismiss families who repeatedly miss appointments.

Such a range of physician–patient relationships frequently is too limited for high-need families. Instead, at times adopting the professional relationship modes used by other disciplines is required to work effectively with some families. For example, both mental health and substance abuse treatment providers often must use confrontational tactics with which most primary care clinicians are uncomfortable. Developmental specialists often relate to parents using a developmental model rather than a problem-oriented medical model and engage parents as teachers of their children. A variety of professionals, such as those dealing with abusive or neglectful families, use a monitoring and limit-setting style that includes a variety of adverse consequences for noncompliant families. While it is not necessary for primary care clinicians to be highly skilled in all of these modes of relating to patients, nevertheless, they do need to be able to use them on occasion, and to be supportive of their use by other members of the health team.

## CASE 35-6

*Katie is a 15-year-old whose parents and younger sisters are also Dr. Fields's patients. Dr. Fields saw Katie's mother recently for worsening migraine headaches and suggested stress reduction classes as well as medication for migraine prophylaxis. Katie has not been to the physician for a couple of years.*

*Today Katie has come alone for her appointment, the last one on a busy Thursday afternoon. Dr. Fields greets her and then listens as Katie begins slowly to discuss her main concern: her period is several weeks overdue. With gentle questioning, she acknowledges having intercourse without using contraception. She has many symptoms of pregnancy, and a brief examination of her abdomen yields an enlarged uterus (halfway to her umbilicus) and audible fetal heart tones. She begins to cry and wonders aloud how she will tell her parents. Dr. Fields offers support and suggests a joint meeting with her parents, stressing the need for the prompt initiation of prenatal care.*

## ADOLESCENT PREGNANCY

Adolescents are one group of women at increased risk for poor perinatal outcomes. The care of pregnant teens demonstrates the principles applicable to many groups of high-risk women. Adolescents' increased risk is due to multiple biopsychosocial factors. By understanding and identifying these risk factors prenatally or even preconceptionally, as described earlier, physicians can play an important role in improving adolescent health outcomes in their communities. The rest of this section will focus on issues pertinent to teen pregnancy, but applicable to women with other risk factors.

In spite of recent declines in birth rates for teenagers, adolescent pregnancy remains a common public health problem in the United States (Fraser *et al.*, 1995; Goldenberg & Klerman, 1995; Ventura & Curtin, 1999). Over the last decade, the teen birth rate dropped 15% but still remains higher than in the 1980s (AAP, 1999). The most recent estimates suggest that total teen pregnancy rates (which include an estimate of abortions) have declined steadily in the 1990s. However, compared with Canada, England, or France, the United States still has twice the rate of teen pregnancy. In addition, teen pregnancy rates vary with race in the United States, with blacks and Hispanics having almost triple the rate of non-Hispanic whites (9 versus 3.6 versus 10%, respectively). Relative to women 20 to 40 years of age, teens have increased rates of premature delivery, low birth weight, and perinatal complications such as substance use and poor nutrition; they also breast-feed less often and are less likely to use contraception after pregnancy. Teen mothers are less likely to complete high school and more likely to live in poverty.

Primary care physicians are well positioned to respond to the individual and public health impact of teen pregnancy. First, physicians can promote teen pregnancy prevention programs through participation in school health programs and advocacy for education and employment for teens. Second, since they may be the first contact with the health system for teen members of families in their practice, these primary care providers can screen for and help modify many of the risks associated with teen pregnancy. They also might be a key source of contraception. Adolescents may be particularly needy regarding access to emergency contraception, a method with which all primary care clinicians should be familiar (Gold, 1997, 1999). The multifactorial risks associated with teen pregnancy lend themselves to care by clinicians such as family physicians, who are trained to address biomedical and psychosocial issues jointly and to use multidisciplinary resources in addressing these risks.

Working with any high-risk group requires outreach into the community to identify at-risk individuals, preferably prior to development of the undesired outcome for which their risk is increased, in this case

## TEENAGE PREGNANCY

*Each year in the United States, 800,000 to 900,000 adolescents under 19 years old become pregnant (rates vary more than twofold between states):*

- *6–8/1000 of those < 15 years old*
- *55–60/1000 of those 15–17 years old*
- *140–150/1000 of those 18–20 years old*

pregnancy. For pregnant teens, such outreach includes the physician's contact with school- and church-based health programs, whether that is as simple as knowing the school nurse and being available for questions or referrals, to assisting in the development or staffing of a school clinic. Physicians can advocate for school-based sex education that includes access to contraception, since there is some evidence from nonrandomized trials that such programs may decrease teen pregnancy rates. During the care of pregnant teens, one of the key issues is promoting their education, so that outreach includes working with at-risk schools to develop teen-parenting programs, including childcare for teen parents, GED programs, and classes in parenting skills.

To address effectively the multiple biopsychosocial risks associated with adolescent pregnancy, some form of case management is often necessary (Heins *et al.*, 1987). An identified case manager, perhaps a social worker affiliated with a teen parenting program or a public health nurse, can help the physician coordinate the often multiple referrals needed to provide true comprehensive care to the at-risk pregnant teen; for example, the case manager can assist with transportation to prenatal appointments, encourage adequate nutrition and healthy behaviors, and help plan for postpartum needs such as infant supplies (Buescher *et al.*, 1991; Olds *et al.*, 1986). The case manager might become involved in home visitation during prenatal care to help assess risks and plan interventions. While trials of such case management have not shown a significant difference in preterm delivery rates, women who receive home visits have demonstrated increased satisfaction with care, more medical knowledge, more access to social support, and healthier habits than women not receiving such visits (Blondel & Breart, 1995; Marcenko & Spense, 1994). Ideally the case manager acting in concordance with the physician can link the disparate prenatal, intrapartum, and postpartum resources in a community to best serve the pregnant teen and her newborn family.

Part of caring for pregnant teens by necessity involves other members of their families, whether these be biologically or geographically defined; thus, experience in multigenerational care is important (Miller, 1995). The family life-cycle changes that occur with any birth have even more impact when parents are confronting adolescent development simultaneously with becoming grandparents—the effects of "children having children" ripple beyond the teen and the new baby as all family members adjust to their new roles. The new grandparents, especially the new grandmother, might indeed be doing double-parenting once the teen mother returns to school and the newborn needs childcare. The family physician can support the entire family in its adjustments around these issues in ways that promote healthy parenting across generations. This support may include, for example, special support for the teen mother to breast-feed in spite of pressure from her mother who used formula and lacks understanding of basic lactation.

## CASE 35-7

*Joan is a 29-year-old well known to Dr. Fields primarily through the well-child care of her only child, 5-year-old Drew, who recently has been diagnosed with attention-deficit hyperactivity disorder (ADHD). Although his parents work hard learning appropriate parenting skills for their active son, Joan as the primary caregiver is often overwhelmed by his behavior and frequently has sought help from Dr. Fields. Today her appointment is for a first prenatal visit; Joan had been ambivalent about having another child after the struggle to cope with Drew's behavior, but she and her husband always have wanted a large family.*

*Dr. Fields and Joan have a half-hour appointment to review her history, discuss the nausea and fatigue that are currently bothering her at 9 weeks' gestation, and do a focused physical examination to confirm her uterine size. Because she recently has had a complete physical for work, Dr. Fields has current health maintenance records including breast examination and Pap smear, so they can spend most of the visit discussing her history and symptoms and developing a plan for her prenatal care. Dr. Fields notes that Joan looks quite fatigued, and with further questioning she reveals that between her pregnancy symptoms, her husband's recent work-related travels, and Drew's behavior, she has been especially overwhelmed and sleeping poorly. She and Dr. Fields decide that she needs to get more help from both her husband and her mother-in-law who lives*

# DISTRIBUTION OF LABOR

*How interesting that patients pay me*
*for time when I make them work.*
*Still, there are precedents:*
*teachers, coaches, midwives—*
*we are all there to aid the process.*
*I elicit details,*
*exhort insights, urge them to*
*better define the problem, issue, worry.*
*And, when at last it emerges,*
*crowning from their mouths,*
*my place is to catch and witness.*
*Only then, in this birth with two mothers,*
*can some solution or suggestion*
*resembling an answer*
*separate from within me.*
*Tugged by its conjoined question*
*it pulls away from inside my skull,*
*a placenta whose job is done.*
*We've labored together*
*yet I receive congratulations*
*for the child they carried all along.*

*Andrea Gordon, M.D.*

*nearby and who often takes Drew for afternoon visits. Joan feels her mother-in-law is better than she is at coping with Drew's behavior.*

*A month later at her next prenatal visit Joan's mother-in-law and Drew also come along. Joan's fatigue has improved slightly although she is still nauseated frequently. Drew explores the examination room in great detail while awaiting Dr. Fields, but quiets when the doctor finds the fetal heart rate. Joan's mother-in-law is teary-eyed with hearing the heartbeat. She ends up attending the rest of Joan's prenatal visits with her, helping settle Drew down in the waiting and examination rooms.*

*By her third prenatal visit, Joan has begun feeling fetal movement and although this is exciting, she also dreads having to care for a newborn when Drew continues to be so demanding. She and Dr. Fields locate a local support group for parents of kids with ADHD, which meets without the kids one evening a month and with the kids one Saturday afternoon a month.*

*The next time Dr. Fields sees Joan is just 3 weeks later at an appointment with Drew. She has been to the group and wants a referral to the local university ADHD clinic for Drew to be evaluated for a trial of medication; several of the parents in the group have suggested this clinic. Dr. Fields makes the referral while suggesting that Joan and her husband review the local library's collection of information about ADHD for parents to learn more about the disorder and the potential risks and benefits of the medication. Joan reports continued fatigue but less nausea, and has been trying to take daily walks with Drew.*

*By her third trimester, Joan and her family have decided to try a placebo-controlled trial of medication for Drew, hoping to have some idea of his response by the time his new sibling arrives. Drew's grandmother, who cares for him after school several times a week to give Joan a break, is opposed to medication and has insisted that his parents work hard around specific behavioral techniques. Dr. Fields has seen the whole family to discuss the clinical trial and offered to follow up on their observations of its success. Drew's behavior has improved somewhat with his grandmother's care, and she agrees to continue providing this after the baby's birth. The family together attends a sibling class that the local childbirth education group sponsors.*

Normal pregnancy care involves helping women cope with many of the common symptoms of pregnancy, using lay information as needed, working with community resources around childbirth education and parenting skills, and helping women juggle the demands of working during pregnancy, either in the home or at outside employment. While prenatal care must address biomedical risk factors throughout pregnancy, for most healthy women these risks are minimal, and the majority of prenatal visit time can focus on guiding families through the transitions that come with a new baby.

Encouraging the participation of the rest of the family in the pregnancy and delivery processes is an important role for the clinician as well. The increasing heterogeneity of family constellations means that providers must personalize each pregnant woman's definition of family. Frequently, one challenge is getting the fathers to participate in prenatal care. Although societal trends have encouraged fathers to be present in the delivery room, this has not extended into the primary care office as much, sometimes for logistical reasons such as work schedules, and sometimes for family reasons such as estranged or unmarried fathers. The clinician can work around this by offering evening or weekend hours for appointments, by calling the father (with the mother's permission) to ask if he has any concerns or questions, or simply by routinely asking at each prenatal visit about the father's involvement or concerns. Clinicians should also inquire about family habits and histories, since partners of pregnant women affect their smoking behavior (McBride *et al.*, 1998) and their breast-feeding choices (Humphreys *et al.*, 1998). In addition, during the 9 months of the mother's prenatal care, the clinician can encourage the father to come in for a general checkup as well, to allow him time to discuss his own health issues (McDaniel *et al.*, 1990).

Another important part of family-oriented pregnancy care is addressing the changes that a new younger sibling will bring into a family. Depending on the age difference among siblings, the parents may need help with issues such as when to have an older child wean, toilet-train, or move out of a crib, what childcare plans will work for all of the children, how to cope with sibling rivalry, what to expect with infectious diseases in a larger family, how to plan for care of the older sibling(s) during the childbirth and postpartum times, or whether or not to involve the older child in the birth of his or her new sibling. The family physician can often use local childbirth education resources for sibling preparation classes and literature to help families with some of these decisions (Fortier *et al.*, 1991; Spero, 1993). Other ways to make older children part of the prenatal visits include providing toys or books in the waiting or examination rooms, asking for their help with checking the fetal heartbeat, or asking about their opinions of the new baby's looks or name choices.

When a family is coping during pregnancy with stressful life issues, such as behavior problems with an older child, the family physician can assist by helping them locate resources within or outside their family. This especially might be important in considering postpartum support needs. A physician who has cared for the woman and her other children throughout pregnancy and will continue to follow them all, including the newborn, has particularly important insight into such needs. A physician who understands cross-generational

## DOMESTIC VIOLENCE

*Domestic violence occurs in 1 to 20% of pregnancies, depending on how and how often women are asked about violence. Risk factors for becoming a victim include:*

- *History of abuse as a child*
- *History of mental illness*
- *History of witnessing abuse as a child*
- *Immigration status*
- *Isolation of victim*
- *Power imbalance (income, employment, or education)*
- *Pregnancy*

issues can help families find support beyond the immediate nuclear family to face complicated behavioral issues. This might include involving not only the grandparents or other extended family but also community resources such as parent-support groups. Sometimes if the mother is a single parent or the father is unable to be an active participant in the prenatal care, the mother's or father's mother can fill an important support role for the pregnant woman and might provide much lay education about her own childbirth experiences. Routine prenatal care should include questions about such grandparent participation, particularly since the extended family might be involved at delivery or in the postpartum period.

## CASE 35-8

*While Dr. Fields is finishing up paperwork one afternoon, his nurse interrupts to say that the translator for Mai, one of their Vietnamese patients, is on the phone reporting that her waters have broken. Mai is a 22-year-old primiparous woman who speaks minimal English and lives with her parents and younger siblings. The father of the baby has returned to Vietnam indefinitely. Through the translator, who works as a patient advocate and labor support person for a community-based organization aiding Southeast Asian refugees, Dr. Fields arranges for Mai to be seen and evaluated.*

*The translator helps Mai arrange transportation to the office, where Dr. Fields examines Mai and notes that she is in active labor at about 3 cm dilated with ruptured membranes. They walk from Dr. Fields's office across the street to the hospital-affiliated birthing center, where Mai has chosen to give birth in its homelike setting. The translator remains with her, helping her get comfortable in the hospital room and rubbing her back during contractions. Mai's mother comes along but speaks even less English and feels uncomfortable being "in the way" until Dr. Fields through the translator reassures her that her presence is welcome. With support from the advocate, Mai's mother, Dr. Fields, and the nurse, Mai's labor progresses normally and within 4 hours she gives birth to a healthy 6-pound girl. The translator works with Mai and the nurse to help the baby breast-feed right away and to plan for teaching during Mai's short postpartum stay at the center and during her home-based postpartum care.*

*The birth center works with the local visiting nurse organization, which has a special program for new mothers to help them through the transitions of the first 2 weeks with the newborn. Dr. Fields stays in touch with the visiting nurse and with Mai through the translator in these first weeks to provide breast-feeding support in particular, so that by the time Mai brings the baby back to Dr. Fields's office for her second checkup at 1 month, the baby is thriving.*

## COMMUNITY AND CULTURAL ISSUES

Physicians providing perinatal care need to understand community resources for pregnant women and children. This is especially true for communities of potentially higher risk such as adolescents, as described earlier, or communities of diversity where multicultural issues might impact perinatal health.

Physicians also need to understand the potential "low-tech" resources available to them in working with women in labor (Brody & Thompson, 1981; Rosenblatt, 1989; Strobino *et al.*, 1988). Several studies have suggested that the simple presence of a supportive companion in labor can shorten labor and lead to fewer cesarean sections for delivery (see Table 35.5) (Hodnett, 1999; Keirse *et al.*, 1989; Kennell *et al.*, 1991). This might be particularly true for primiparous women or women who do not speak the same language as their birth attendants (Kennell *et al.*, 1991; Klaus *et al.*, 1986; Sosa *et al.*, 1980; Zhang *et al.*, 1996). Thus, a physician working in a culturally diverse community might improve her population's perinatal health by working with cross-cultural organizations to train labor advocates. Such advocates can both translate and provide labor support. Modeling the family physician's longitudinal role in providing care for a new family, advocates also can work with postpartum women and families in the crucial first weeks after a birth.

**Table 35.5**
Benefits of Doulas (Labor Support Companions)[a]

Shorter labor
More spontaneous vaginal births
   Fewer operative vaginal deliveries
   Fewer cesareans in young, disadvantaged women
Less use of pain relief medication
Less need for labor augmentation
More immediate maternal–infant bonding
More positive experiences of labor for mothers
More positive maternal views of infants in first 6 weeks
More exclusive breast-feeding at 6 weeks postpartum

[a]See Hodnett (1999), Challis (2000), Zhang et al. (1996).

Family physicians can also support institutional options in labor and delivery care such as the birth center described above. Low-risk women might have more natural childbirth experiences and improved perinatal outcomes if they can labor without continuous electronic monitoring and with freedom to choose different positions.

Another important aspect of immediate postpartum care involves successful initiation and continuation of breast-feeding (see Table 35.6). Currently about 64% of women giving birth in the United States initiate breast-feeding, and by 6 months only 24% are continuing to breast-feed (Hill, 2000). While many factors contribute to determining these rates, physicians involved in perinatal care need to emphasize the health benefits for both baby and mother of breast-feeding and need to be well versed in counseling families in common concerns and problems with breast-feeding, especially in the first few weeks postpartum. Physicians need to take charge of their own education in these issues (Freed et al., 1995) and can help in developing antenatal as well as intrapartum and postpartum processes and programs that encourage breast-feeding (Shaw & Kaczorowski, 1999; Zimmerman, 1999).

As many insurance companies and hospitals move toward early discharge of healthy mothers and babies, physicians need to work with local community resources such as visiting nurse organizations to make sure that these families receive appropriate guidance and timely medical follow-up. Sometimes such follow-up

## DOULAS

*Three meta-analyses using different approaches have been performed on the results of 12 clinical trials. Findings:*

- *Emotional and physical support significantly shortens labor and decreases the need for cesarean deliveries, forceps and vacuum extraction, oxytocin augmentation, and analgesia.*
- *Doula-supported mothers rate childbirth as less difficult and painful than do women not supported by a doula. Labor support by fathers does not appear to produce similar obstetrical benefits.*
- *Early psychosocial benefits include reductions in anxiety, positive feelings about the birth experience, and increased rates of breast-feeding initiation.*
- *Later postpartum benefits include decreased depression, improved self-esteem, exclusive breast-feeding, and increased sensitivity of the mother to her child's needs.*

*A thorough reorganization of current birth practices is recommended to ensure that every woman has access to continuous emotional and physical support during labor.*
*Source: Scott et al. (1999).*

**Table 35.6**
Increasing Breast-Feeding Rates[a]

| |
| --- |
| Inquire about breast-feeding plans at every first prenatal visit (include this in baseline breast exam) |
|   Ask "Do you have any questions about breast-feeding?" rather than "How will you feed baby?" |
| Include breast-feeding information in routine nutrition consultation during pregnancy |
| Show videotapes on breast-feeding topics in the waiting room |
| Remove all formula-company literature and advertisements from prenatal literature in waiting room |
| Provide space for monthly breast-feeding support group in your office/hospital |
|   Encourage antenatal childbirth education classes to include breast-feeding information and support |
| Work with hospital labor and delivery and nursery staff around delivery room and nursery policies that encourage breast-feeding |
|   Baby to breast within an hour of delivery |
|   Rooming-in for all breast-feeding mothers unless requested or medically indicated for infant |
|   No pacifiers or bottles or supplements for breast-feeding infants |
| Breast-feeding discharge packets in place of formula-company packets |
| Routine telephone consultation for lactation support within 1 week of discharge |
| Routine mother–baby postpartum visits in office within 1 week of discharge |

[a]Adapted from Zimmerman (1999).

may include both early phone contact with the family and/or visiting nurse, and early postpartum visits for baby and mother, sooner than the traditional 2 and 6 weeks respectively, or even postpartum home visits by the physician or other clinician. This is especially true for first-time mothers who are breast-feeding, a process that often takes longer than 24 hours to establish successfully.

## CONCLUSION

Provision of care to families during their reproductive years is a challenging, rewarding, and at times stressful endeavor. Often the interventions with the greatest impact on a family and its offspring are those low-key efforts designed to lower risks and respond to psychosocial as well as medical and obstetric concerns before crises arise. The drama of labor and delivery requires special skills that are often critical to the health of the mother and infant. They are, however, an extremely limited aspect of the care a family needs in bringing forth new life.

The continuing relationship of a family with a physician who provides comprehensive care from before conception and continuing through childhood offers opportunity for early recognition of risks that otherwise might lead to major problems. Particularly for high-risk families, the physician needs to work closely with other professionals and services in the community. For physicians in high-risk communities, the challenge involves developing and working within a healthcare team, and providing leadership to or assisting in the development of a network of services for young families. However, the results can be highly rewarding, particularly for physicians who remain in practice in the same community, caring for families as children grow, and in whose lives they were able to make a difference.

## CASES FOR DISCUSSION

All of the cases in this chapter are located in the village of Middletown. It has evolved significantly over the past 20 years from a working- and middle-class, white ethnic suburb of Providence to the ethnically diverse and socioeconomically disadvantaged community it is today. Many of the industries that employed Middletown's citizens have relocated. One large manufacturing plant and two smaller service-oriented firms remain. One of Middletown's two hospitals closed about 5 years ago, leaving Middletown Memorial as the sole healthcare institution servicing the community.

Memorial is a 250-bed, not-for-profit and nonsectarian community hospital that provides full-service primary and secondary care and has an academic affiliation with Bradford Medical School in the Tri-Cities.

Memorial Hospital struggles to maintain a "market share" among those with commercial insurance in the surrounding neighborhoods, yet the proportion of patients who are underinsured or uninsured continues to rise.

The businesses in town have enrolled most of their employees in Tri-City HMO, a local branch of a nationwide managed care organization. They have offices in Memorial's professional building. There are also several private practitioners remaining in Middletown who continue to see those patients with commercial insurance and who serve as consultants for the HMO. A community health center was developed 5 years ago in the ambulatory care center of the hospital that closed. This health center has federal and state grants that support its mission of caring for the underserved.

## CASE 1

*The triage nurse met the paramedics at the ER door. A message from the paramedics had warned that they were en route with a 22-year-old in premature labor. The paramedics gave report as they wheeled the stretcher down the corridor toward the OB unit. Tonya, the patient, thinks her due date is next month. Her contractions started 2 hours ago and she has not received prenatal care and does not have a regular physician. Tonya is crying and writhing in pain.*

*Debbie, an experienced and reassuring labor nurse, helps to get Tonya admitted. Dr. Smith, the resident on duty, examines Tonya and confirms that she is in active premature labor. Tonya is alone. Her mother wanted to come but could not find anyone to watch Tonya's little brother who is 11 months old. It was 6:00 P.M. and Dr. Smith explained that she was going off duty and Dr. Alexander was taking over.*

*Tonya labored through the evening alone except for Debbie. Dr. Alexander introduced himself and apologetically explained that there were many other patients to attend. Tonya's boyfriend, Johnny, stopped by with one of his friends. The visit felt awkward to him and Tonya was relieved to see him go. They had argued frequently the past few months and Johnny's temper outbursts had turned to violence on more than one occasion. She hoped the baby would make him calm down.*

*Feeling frightened and alone, Tonya had her baby. The 5-pound girl was a few weeks premature and appeared healthy but was taken to the nursery for observation. A drug screen, taken because of the premature labor and lack of prenatal care, is positive for cocaine. Dr. Alexander informed Tonya that if cocaine were found in the baby's system, it would be reported as child abuse. Tonya is discharged the following day while her baby awaited social service evaluation for possible placement. On discharge, Tonya is given Dr. Fields's name and office number for postpartum care.*

1. *How could prenatal care affect Tonya's case? Should prenatal care be available to everyone? Is routine prenatal care adequate for Tonya?*
2. *List and determine the appropriate further evaluation of potential risk factors, both medical and psychosocial.*
3. *What is the role of Child Protective Services in this and similar cases? Is there evidence for child abuse? What supports are needed?*
4. *How should the health care team encourage the involvement of the baby's father?*

## CASE 2

*Rosa is a 16-year-old who is in labor. Her baby is also coming a few weeks early, but unlike Tonya, Rosa is not alone. Hector, the baby's father, and Rosa's mother are at her bedside as she labors. Hector attended childbirth classes with Rosa and went to many of her prenatal visits at the community health center. Hector and Rosa's mother take turns rubbing her back and coaching Rosa through pains. Dr. Thomas, who works at the health center, is also there. He reassures Rosa and her family that the labor is progressing normally and encourages Rosa to focus on the precious little life she is miraculously and courageously bringing into this world.*

*Feeling frightened but safe and supported, Rosa has her baby. With tears of joy, Hector ceremoniously cuts the cord. Dr. Thomas places the slippery, vigorous 5-pound boy on Rosa's chest. Though 4 weeks premature, the little boy appears healthy and stays in the room with his family. Rosa begins breast-feeding as she had been encouraged to do by the staff at the health center.*

*The following day, Dr. Thomas discharged Rosa and her baby home. She is seen 3 days later at home by a home care nurse. The baby is thriving on the breast milk but Rosa is frustrated with the breast-feeding and wants to start bottle feedings. Rosa's mother is concerned that the baby is not getting enough milk because Rosa is impatient with the feedings.*

Rosa had planned to return to school after a few weeks at home, and has chosen a birth control method. However, the school nurse tells Rosa that she will be tutored at home, and may have to repeat the year. Rosa begins to have conflicts with her mother over the care and discipline of her newborn; Rosa wants to set strict limits, so the baby does not grow up to be spoiled. Hector visits after school but is uncomfortable with the baby and openly annoyed at the conflict between Rosa and her mother.

1. Review the comprehensive care system that Rosa and her family have access to, including: (a) how is it more than routine and (b) how does it extend the physician's role?
2. What are critical issues requiring continuity between the prepregnancy, prenatal, and postpartum intervals in this family's care? How is such continuity care best organized?
3. Describe the family dynamics. How can Hector be involved? What should Dr. Thomas advise, and how should he approach family members to bring about change?
4. How can Dr. Thomas intervene to help Rosa acquire parenting skills? Consider practical experience, familial modeling, and school- and community-based programs.

## CASE 3

Recall Tonya, who delivered a premature baby who was cocaine exposed. There had been little or no prenatal care and Tonya was alone with minimal family support. There was a concern about Johnny, the baby's father, who had become increasingly violent with Tonya. The case had been reported to the Department of Child Protective Services because of the drug abuse. They found no other evidence of abuse and discharged the baby home in the custody of Tonya's grandmother. A caseworker was assigned. Tonya had not seen Dr. Fields, and again was encouraged to do so.

One month later, the baby is seen in the local emergency room for a cold and diarrhea. The baby weighs 6 pounds and appears relatively healthy. The baby has not been seen for routine childcare as yet. Tonya and Johnny brought the baby to the ER. The examining physician notices some large bruises on the baby's arms and questions the young parents. They are unsure as to the cause of the bruises and had not noticed them. The cold and diarrhea symptoms are not significant.

1. Consider the alternative societal responses to suspected parenting inadequacies. Which would be appropriate for this family?
2. What obligations and options are there for the ER physician?
3. How could a comprehensive care system influence this family?
4. How should Dr. Fields become involved?

## CASE 4

A 21-year-old African American woman with two previous miscarriages makes an appointment with Dr. Fields to discuss trying to get pregnant again. She is a smoker, and on looking through her chart you see that she is rubella nonimmune. (Dr. Fields tested her at her last contraceptive appointment.)

1. What are some modifiable perinatal risk factors? Discuss smoking and immunizations prior to and during pregnancy.
2. What are other risk factors, less modifiable but still important to identify? Discuss genetic counseling around sickle cell disease, and race/ethnicity as a risk factor in pregnancy outcomes.
3. When should you do preconception care?
4. How can primary care practice be organized to support preconception and other preventive and health promotion practices? How can it best work with community-level interventions, including smoking cessation, immunization tracking, sickle cell screening and genetic counseling in the community, psychological concerns, and supporting families around perinatal loss.

## CASE 5

Recall from Case 35-6 the story of Katie, a 15-year-old girl whose family are Dr. Fields's patients. Dr. Fields last saw her 2 years ago. She came to the office by herself with a positive pregnancy test. On further questioning, she had been taking oral contraceptives intermittently and has been feeling fetal movement. She hasn't told her parents yet about the preg-

*nancy. Dr. Fields finds out that she is a smoker. The initial prenatal examination indicates that she is about 18 weeks pregnant; the Pap smear comes back abnormal.*

1. *What are some of the public health issues around teenage pregnancy?*
2. *What community resources are needed for school-aged mothers?*
3. *How can primary care offices interact with other agencies in caring for pregnant teenagers?*
4. *What are the cross-generational issues for the family's physician?*
5. *What are some of the biomedical issues regarding late prenatal care?*
6. *Discuss the biomedical and practice organizational issues involved in the management of abnormal Pap smears.*

## RECOMMENDED READINGS

Brody H, Thompson JR: The maximum strategy in modern obstetrics. *J Fam Pract* 12:977–1986, 1981.

Rosenblatt RA: The perinatal paradox: Doing more and accomplishing less. *Health Affairs* 1989, pp 158–168.

> The Brody and Rosenblatt articles describe from different perspectives the dilemmas in applying high-tech approaches to reproductive health at both the individual patient and national policy level. Together they provide considerable insight into the controversies facing both clinicians and policymakers as they choose strategies to improve birth outcomes.

Buescher PA, Roth MS, Williams D, Goforth CM: An evaluation of the impact of maternity care coordination on Medicaid birth outcomes in North Carolina. *Am J Public Health* 81(12):1625–1635, 1991.

Olds DL, Henderson CR Jr *et al*: Prenatal and infancy home visitation by nurses: Recent findings. *Future Child* 9(1):44–65, 190–191, 1999.

> These articles provide convincing evidence of the value of community-based integration of medical and psychosocial care approaches. They provide insight into how services can be organized to respond effectively to the needs of high-risk communities.

Enkin M, Keirse MJNC, Renfrew M, Neilsen J (eds): *A Guide to Effective Care in Pregnancy and Childbirth.* New York, Oxford University Press, 1995.

> This masterful work is the definitive collection of evidence related to the effectiveness of reproductive healthcare. The work of the Cochrane Center, it has led to an international initiative to promote evidence-based medicine, The Cochrane Collaboration.

Institute of Medicine Committee to Study the Prevention of Low Birthweight: *Preventing Low Birthweight.* Washington, DC, National Academy Press, 1985.

Institute of Medicine Committee to Study Outreach for Prenatal Care: *Prenatal Care: Reaching Mothers, Reaching Infants.* Washington, DC, National Academy Press, 1988.

Institute of Medicine Panel on Adolescent Pregnancy and Childbearing: *Risking the Future: Adolescent Sexuality, Pregnancy, and Childbearing.* Washington, DC, National Academy Press, 1987.

Institute of Medicine Committee on Unintended Pregnancy: *The Best Intentions. Unintended Pregnancy and the Well-Being of Children and Families.* Washington, DC, National Academy Press, 1995.

> These Institute of Medicine reports, all of which have executive summaries, are the definitive works related to MCH care of socially high risk populations in the United States.

Jack BW, Culpepper L: Preconception care: Risk reduction and health promotion in preparation for pregnancy. *JAMA* 264:1147–1149, 1990.

> This reference identifies the potential of preconception care to improve birth outcomes and discusses opportunities and impediments to implementing preconception care.

## REFERENCES

Alexander S, Keirse MJNC: Formal risk scoring during pregnancy, in Chalmers I, Enkin M, Keirse MJNC (eds): *Effective Care in Pregnancy and Childbirth.* New York, Oxford University Press, 1989, pp 345–365.

American Academy of Pediatrics, Committee on Adolescence: Adolescent pregnancy—Current trends and issues: 1998. *Pediatrics* 103(2):516–520, 1999.

Asch DA, Hershey JC, Dekay ML, Pauly MV, Patton JP, Jedrziewski MK, Frei F, Giardine R, Kant JA, Mennuti MT: Carrier screening for cystic fibrosis: Costs and clinical outcomes. *Med Decis Making* 18(2):202–212, 1998.

Blondel B, Breart G: Home visits during pregnancy: Consequences on pregnancy outcome, use of health services, and women's situations. *Semin Perinatol* 19(4):263–271, 1995.

Brody H, Thompson JR: The maximum strategy in modern obstetrics. *J Fam Pract* 12:977–986, 1981.

Buescher PA, Roth MS, Williams D, Goforth CM: An evaluation of the impact of maternity care coordination on Medicaid birth outcomes in North Carolina. *Am J Public Health* 81(12):1625–1635, 1991.

Challis JRG: Mechanism of parturition and preterm labor. *Obstet Gynecol Surv* 55(10):650–660, 2000.

Colley Gilbert BJ, Johnson CH, Morrow B, Gaffield ME, Ahluwalia I: Prevalence of selected maternal and infant characteristics, Pregnancy Risk Assessment Monitoring System (PRAMS), 1997. *Morbidity Mortality Weekly Rep CDC Surveill Summ* 48(5):1–37, 1999.

Crowther C, Chalmers I: Bed rest and hospitalization during pregnancy, in Chalmers I, Enkin M, Keirse MJNC (eds): *Effective Care in Pregnancy and Childbirth*. London, Oxford University Press, 1989, pp 624–632.

Culpepper L: Reducing infant mortality: The research gaps. Background report for the HRSA Interagency Committee on Infant Mortality, 1991.

Culpepper L: Primary care provider and system challenges in caring for high-risk children and families, in Grason HA, Guyer B (eds): *Assessing & Developing Primary Care for Children*. Arlington, VA, National Center for Education in Maternal and Child Health, 1995, pp 136–150.

Culpepper L, Jack BW: Preconception care, in Cherry SH, Merkatz IR (eds): *Complications of Pregnancy: Medical, Surgical, Gynecologic, Psychosocial and Perinatal*. Baltimore, Williams & Wilkins Co, 1991, pp 2–15.

Culpepper L, Jack B: Psychosocial issues in pregnancy. *Primary Care* 20(3):599–619, 1993.

Dejin-Karlsson E, Hanson BS, Ostergren PO, Lindgren A, Sjoberg NO, Marsal K: Association of a lack of psychosocial resources and the risk of giving birth to small for gestational age infants: A stress hypothesis. *BJOG* 107(1):89–100, 2000.

DeMuylder X, Wesel S, Dramaix M, *et al*: A woman's attitude toward pregnancy—Can it predispose her to preterm labor? *J Reprod Med* 37(4):339–342, 1992.

Fineman RM, Walton MT: Should genetic health care providers attempt to influence reproductive outcome using directive counseling techniques? A public health prospective. *Women Health* 30(3):39–47, 2000.

Fischer RC, Stanford JB, Jameson P, DeWitt MJ: Exploring the concepts of intended, planned, and wanted pregnancy. *J Fam Pract* 48(2):117–122, 1999.

Fortier JC, Carson VB, Will S, Shubkagel BL: Adjustment to a newborn: Sibling preparation makes a difference. *JOGNN* 20(1):73–79, 1991.

Fraser AM, Brockert JE, Ward RH: Association of young maternal age with adverse reproductive outcomes. *N Engl J Med* 332:113–117, 1995.

Freed GL *et al*: National assessment of physicians' breast-feeding knowledge, attitudes, training, and experience. *JAMA* 273(6):472–476, 1995.

Fry LR: Prenatal screening. *Prim Care* 27(1):55–69, 2000.

Garbarino J: The human ecology of early risk, in Meisels SJ, Shonkoff JP (eds): *Handbook of Early Childhood Interventions*. New York, Cambridge University Press, 1990, pp 78–96.

Garbarino J, Sherman D: High-risk neighborhoods and high-risk families: The human ecology of child maltreatment. *Child Dev* 51: 188–198, 1980.

Gold M: Emergency contraception: A second chance at preventing adolescent unintended pregnancy. *Curr Opin Pediatr* 9:300–309, 1997.

Gold M: Adolescent gynecology, Part II: The sexually active adolescent—Prescribing and managing oral contraceptive pills and emergency contraception for adolescents. *Pediatr Clin North Am* 46(4):695–718, 1999.

Goldenberg RL, Klerman LV: Adolescent pregnancy—another look. *N Engl J Med* 332:1161–1162, 1995.

Goldenberg RL, Davis RO, Nelson KG: Intrauterine growth retardation, in Merkatz IR, Thompson JE, Mullen PD, Goldenberg R (eds): *New Perspectives on Prenatal Care*. New York, Elsevier Science Publishing Co, Inc, 1990, pp 461–478.

Goldenberg RL, Hauth JC, Andrews WW: Intrauterine infection and preterm delivery. *N Engl J Med* 342;1500–1507, 2000.

Heins HC Jr, Nancy NW, Ferguson JE: Social support in improving perinatal outcome: The Resource Mothers Program. *Obstet Gynecol* 70(2):263–266, 1987.

Helton AS, McFarlane J, Anderson ET: Battered and pregnant: A prevalence study. *Am J Public Health* 77:1337–1339, 1987.

Herron MA, Katz M, Creasy RK: Evaluation of a preterm birth prevention program: Preliminary report. *Obstet Gynecol* 59:452–456, 1982.

Hill PD: Update on breast-feeding: Healthy People 2010 objectives. *MCN Am J Matern Child Nurs* 25(5):248–251, 2000.

Hodnett ED: Caregivers support for women during childbirth, in Neilson JP, *et al* (eds): *Pregnancy and Childbirth Module of the Cochrane Database of Systematic Reviews, Cochrane Collaboration. Issue 2*. Oxford, Update Software, 1999.

Humphreys AS *et al*: Intention to breastfeed in low-income pregnant women: The role of social support and previous experience. *Birth* 25(3):169–174, 1998.

Institute of Medicine Committee to Study Outreach for Prenatal Care: *Prenatal Care: Reaching Mothers, Reaching Infants*, Brown SS (ed). Washington, DC, National Academy Press, 1988.

Institute of Medicine Committee to Study the Prevention of Low Birthweight: *Preventing Low Birthweight*. Washington, DC, National Academy Press, 1985.

Jack BW, Culpepper L: Preconception care: Risk reduction and health promotion in preparation for pregnancy. *JAMA* 264(9):1147–1149, 1990.

Jack BW, Culpepper L, Babcock J, Kogan MD, Weismiller D: Addressing preconception risks identified at the time of a negative pregnancy test. A randomized trial. *J Fam Pract* 47(1):33–38, 1998.

Jacoby M, Gorenflo D, Black E, Wunderlich C, Eyler AE: Rapid repeat pregnancy and experiences of interpersonal violence among low-income adolescents. *Am J Prev Med* 16(4):318–321, 1999.

Joyce TJ, Grossman M: Pregnancy wantedness and the early initiation of prenatal care. *Demography* 27(1):1–17, 1990.

Keirse MJNC, Enkin M, Lumley J: Social and professional support during labor, in Chalmers I, Enkin M, Keirse MJNC (eds): *Effective Care in Pregnancy and Childbirth*. New York, Oxford University Press, 1989, pp 805–814.

Kennell JH, Klaus MH, McGrath S, Robertson SS, Hinkley C: Continuous emotional support during labor in a US hospital. *JAMA* 265(17):2197–2201, 1991.

Klaus MH, Kennell JH, Robertson SS, Sosa R: Effects of social support during parturition on maternal and infant morbidity. *Br Med J* 293:585–587, 1986.

Koeske GF, Koeske RD: The buffering effect of social support on parental stress. *Am J Orthopsychiatry* 60:440–451, 1990.

Kostelny K, Garbarino J: *The Human Ecology of Infant Mortality: An Analysis of Risk in 76 Urban Communities.* Chicago, Erikson Institute, 1987.

Kramer MS: Socioeconomic determinants of intrauterine growth retardation. *Eur J Clin Nutr* 52(suppl 1):S29–S32; discussion S32–S33, 1998.

Lee SH, Ewert DP, Frederick PD, Mascola L: Resurgence of congenital rubella syndrome in the 1990s. Report on missed opportunities and failed prevention policies among women of childbearing age. *JAMA* 267(19):2616–2620, 1992.

Lemna WK, Feldman GL, Kerem B-S, *et al*: Mutation analysis for heterozygote detection and the prenatal diagnosis of cystic fibrosis. *N Engl J Med* 322:291–296, 1990.

Marcenko MO, Spence M: Home visitation services for at-risk pregnant and postpartum women: A randomized trial. *Am J Orthopsychiatry* 64(3):468–478, 1994.

Marsiglio W, Mott FL: Does wanting to become pregnant with a first child affect subsequent maternal behaviors and infant birth weight? *J Marriage Fam* 50:1023–1036, 1988.

McBride CM, Curry SJ, Grothaus LC, Nelson JC, Lando H, Pirie PL: Partner smoking status and pregnant smoker's perceptions of support for and likelihood of smoking cessation. *Health Psychol* 17(1):63–69, 1998.

McDaniel S, Campbell T, Seaburn DB: The birth of a family: A family oriented approach to pregnancy care, in *Family Oriented Primary Care. A Manual for Medical Providers.* New York, Springer-Verlag, 1990, pp 105–122.

Miller R: Preventing adolescent pregnancy and associated risks. *Can Fam Physician* 41:1525–1531, 1995.

Newberger EH, Barkan SE, Lieberman ES: Abuse of pregnant women and adverse birth outcome: Current knowledge and implications for practice. *JAMA* 267:2370–2372, 1992.

Olds DL, Henderson CR, Tatelbaum R: Improving the delivery of prenatal care and outcome of pregnancy: A randomized trial of nurse home visitation. *Pediatrics* 77:16–28, 1986.

Olds DL, Henderson CR Jr, Kitzman HJ, Eckenrode JJ, Cole RE, Tatelbaum RC: Prenatal and infancy home visitation by nurses: Recent findings. *Future Child* 9(1):44–65, 190–191, 1999.

Perez-Woods RC: Barriers to the use of prenatal care: Critical analysis of the literature 1966–87. *J Perinat Med* 10:420–434, 1990.

Piekkala P, Kero P, Erkkola R: Perinatal events and neonatal morbidity: An analysis of 5380 cases. *Early Hum Dev* 13:249–268, 1986.

Prada JA, R. Tsang C: Biological mechanisms of environmentally induced causes of IUGR. *Eur J Clin Nutr* 52(suppl 1):S21–S27; discussion S27–S28, 1998.

Rosen MG, Culpepper L, Goldenberg RL, Gordis L, Henderson OA, Klein L, Klerman LV: *Caring for Our Future: The Content of Prenatal Care. A Report of the Public Health Service Expert Panel on the Content of Prenatal Care.* Washington, DC, Public Health Service, Department of Health and Human Services, 1989.

Rosenblatt RA: The perinatal paradox: Doing more and accomplishing less. *Health Affairs* 8(3):158–168, 1989.

Schieve LA, Cogswell ME, Scanlon KS, Perry G, Ferre C, Blackmore-Prince C, Yu SM, Rosenberg D: Prepregnancy body mass index and pregnancy weight gain: Associations with preterm delivery. The NMIHS Collaborative Study Group. *Obstet Gynecol* 96(2):194–200, 2000.

Scott KD, Klaus PH, Klaus MH: The obstetrical and postpartum benefits of continuous support during childbirth. *J Womens Health Gend Based Med* 10:1257–1264, 1999.

Selwyn BJ: The accuracy of obstetric risk assessment instruments for predicting mortality, low birth weight, and preterm birth, in Merkatz IR, Thompson JE, Mullen PD, Goldenberg R (eds): *New Perspectives on Prenatal Care.* New York, Elsevier Science Publishing Co, Inc, 1990, pp 39–65.

Sepkowitz S: International rankings of infant mortality and the United States' vital statistics natality data collecting system—failure and success. *Int J Epidemiol* 24(3):583–588, 1995.

Shaw E, Kaczorowski J: The effect of a peer counseling program on breastfeeding initiation and longevity in a low-income rural population. *J Hum Lact* 15(1):19–25, 1999.

Sheehan TJ: Stress and low birth weight: A structural modeling approach using real life stressors. *Soc Sci Med* 47(10):1503–1512, 1998.

Sosa R, Kennell JH, Klaus MH, Robertson SS, Urrutia J: The effect of a supportive companion on perinatal problems, length of labor, and mother–infant interaction. *N Engl J Med* 303:597–600, 1980.

Spero D: Sibling preparation classes. *AWOHNN Clin Issues* 4(1):122–131, 1993.

Strobino DM, Baruffi G, Dellinger WS, *et al*: Variations in pregnancy outcomes and use of obstetric procedures in two institutions with divergent philosophies of maternity care. *Med Care* 26:333–347, 1988.

Thompson S, Torres M, Stevenson R, Dean J, Best R: Periconceptional vitamin use, dietary folate and occurrent neural tube defected pregnancies in a high risk population. *Ann Epidemiol* 10(7):476, 2000.

Turnock BJ, McGill L: Approaches to reducing infant mortality in Illinois. Part II: Targeting approaches. *Ill Med J* 164:29–32, 1983.

Ural S, Nagey DA: Preventing intrauterine growth retardation with aspirin: Does it work? *Birth* 25(1):54–55, 1998.

Ventura SJ, Curtin SC: Recent trends in teen births in the United States. *Statistical Bulletin* 2–12, Jan–Mar 1999.

Von Der Pool BA: Preterm labor: Diagnosis and treatment. *Am Fam Physician* 57(10):2457–2464, 1998 [published erratum appears in *Am Fam Physician* 58(4):866, 1998].

Weismiller DG: Preterm labor. *Am Fam Physician* 59(3):593–602, 1999.

Weller RH, Eberstein JW, Bailey M: Pregnancy wantedness and maternal behavior during pregnancy. *Demography* 24:407–412, 1987.

Wilkinson DS, Korenbrot CC, Greene J: A performance indicator of psychosocial services in enhanced prenatal care of Medicaid-eligible women. *Matern Child Health J* 2(3):131–143, 1998.

Williams LB, Pratt WF: *Wanted and unwanted childbearing in the United States: 1973–88, National Survey of Family Growth.* Washington, DC, Department of Health and Human Services, Public Health Service, 1989.

Yang Q, Khoury MJ, Mannino D: Trends and patterns of mortality associated with birth defects and genetic diseases in the United States, 1979–1992: An analysis of multiple-cause mortality data. *Genet Epidemiol* 14(5):493–505, 1997.

Zhang J, Bernasko JW, Leybovich E, Fahs M, Hatch MC: Continuous labor support from labor attendant for primiparous women: A meta-analysis. *Obstet Gynecol* 88(4 pt 2):739–744, 1996.

Zimmerman DR: You can make a difference: Increasing breast-feeding rates in an inner-city clinic. *J Hum Lact* 15(3):217–220. 1999.

Zuravin SJ: Unplanned childbearing and family size: Their relationship to child neglect and abuse. *Fam Plann Perspect* 23(4):155–161, 1991.

# Index

**821**